Dedication

The eleventh edition of Healthy Healing is dedicated to the profound wonders of healing herbs.
I believe that herbs are an eye of the needle through which we can look to glimpse
the miracle of creation...because herbs help us care for each other.
They grow eyes on our hearts.

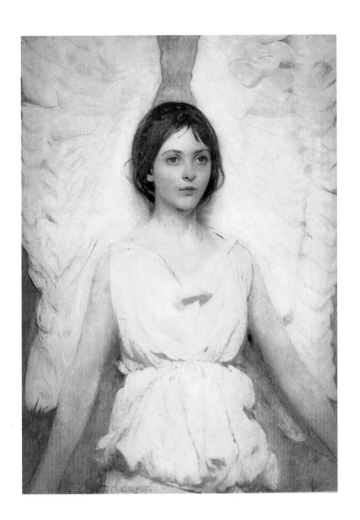

Even one miracle cure can show the value of a therapy
with the body's own healing powers.
When the evidence is good enough to affect the behavior of researchers,
why pretend it is too preliminary for consumers?
If a therapy is natural, non-invasive and does no harm,
consumers should be able to act upon it as a valid choice.

Herbs are without a doubt...UNIVERSAL.
They do not discriminate,
but embrace humans of all sorts and animals of all kinds with their benefits.
While it seems, on a day-to-day basis, that we are hopelessly divided,
in the end we are all one.
Our hopes and dreams are the same.

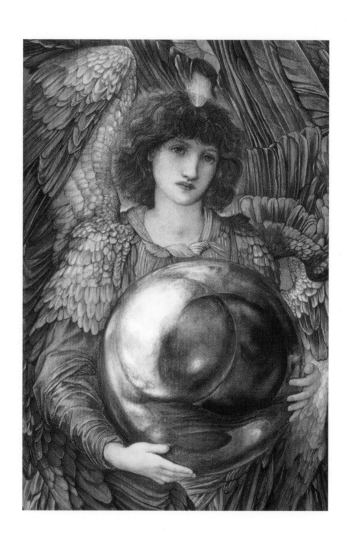

The highest calling of the healer
is to rally the mind and body against the disease.

The Earth does not belong to man.
Man belongs to the Earth.
All things are connected like the blood
which unites a family.
Man does not weave the web of life,
he is only a strand in it.
Whatever happens to the Earth
happens to all of us.
Whatever man does
to the web of life on Earth,
he does
to himself.

Native American Belief

Traditional
Inc.
Wisdom

Linda Page, N.D., Ph.D.

Long before natural foods and herbal formulas became a "chic," widely accepted method for healing, Dr. Linda Page was sharing her extensive knowledge with those who dared to listen.

Through what some would call an accident of fate but she calls a blessing, she was compelled to research alternative avenues of healing. Sequestered in a hospital with a life-threatening illness, watching her 5-foot frame wither to 69 pounds, her hair drop out, and her skin peel off, doctors told her they had no cure. With only a cursory knowledge of herbs, she began a frantic research process of testing herbal formulas and healing food combinations on herself. She read voraciously about herbal healing. Good friends shopped for herbs and she began to formulate the many compounds which would eventually save her life, revitalize her health and restore beautiful new hair and skin. It was that incident that led her to seek her degrees in Naturopathy and Nutrition.

A prolific author and educator, Dr. Page has sold over a million books including **Healthy Healing, Cooking For Healthy Healing, How To Be Your Own Herbal Pharmacist, Party Lights, Detoxification** and a popular series of 20 library books which address specific healing therapies for topics like menopause, male and female energy, colds and flu and cancer. **Healthy Healing** is a textbook for courses at UCLA, The Institute of Educational Therapy, and Clayton College of Natural Health. Dr. Page also formulates over 250 herbal formulas for Crystal Star Herbal Nutrition of Earth City, Missouri. She received one of the first herbal patents in the United States for her formulas that help balance hormones to ease menopausal symptoms.

Dr. Page is an Adjunct Professor at Clayton College of Natural Health. Dr. Page has appeared weekly on a CBS television station with a report on natural healing; she has been featured with CBS fitness reporter Bonnie Kaye on national CBS television; she is a principle speaker at national health symposiums and conventions; she is featured regularly in national magazines; she appears on hundreds of radio and television programs. Currently, Dr. Page is featured on the television program, "The World of Healthy Healing" airing on PBS television. She is also leading herbal tours to China in 2000.

Today, Dr. Page delights in having come full circle. "I feel I am living my dream. I am so grateful that knowledge of healing through herbal formulas and good foods is becoming so widespread. I see it as an opportunity for people to seize the power to heal themselves. Knowledge is power. Whether one chooses conventional medicine, alternative healing avenues, or combines them both in a complementary process, the real prescription for healing is knowledge."

Dr. Page is a member of The American Naturopathic Medical Association, The California Naturopathic Association, The American Herbalist Guild, The American Botanical Council and The Herb Research Foundation.

We need to expand our horizons about health care. There is far more to healing than a lab test or a doctor's diagnosis, or the newest drug, which may be very limited. Even today we are watching supergerms overcome the latest antibiotics.

If you think about it for a moment,
nutrition isn't the alternative healing system.
Drugs are the alternative system — far from natural.

Drugs are really a patching up system of medicine. There is no such thing as an essential drug. A drug doesn't combine with your body to restore and revitalize. At worst, especially long term, drugs hit your body with a powerful hammer that overwhelms body systems never allowing your own immune response to do its job, and in the end, so imbalances body processes that you never really normalize.

I believe drugs are at best a short term method that can arrest a harmful organism and stabilize body systems to the point where your own individual immune system can take over and reestablish health.

I believe we should have access to all types of healing.
We should honor drugs for all of the lives they've saved. I never say to throw away your doctor's phone number.

But, I also believe that today's medicine has nothing to do with the quality of life. By contrast, natural healing gives people the chance to live well — better than they could without it. Natural healers never give up. They know you can improve your life no matter what state your health is in. With natural healing, days turn into months, and then into years after a "death sentence" from modern medicine.

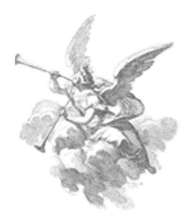

You are really your own best healer.
I believe that there is a powerful, spiritual aspect of healing that is available to each of us. It is unique to each of us because it accesses our own divine healing energy.
I have seen this phenomenon too many times to doubt it.

Never forget - there is always something more.

About 70 years ago, Albert Schweitzer said,
"The doctor of the future will be oneself."

I see that coming true almost every day as people become more
knowledgeable and take more responsibility for themselves.

If we are the doctor, what is our medicine?

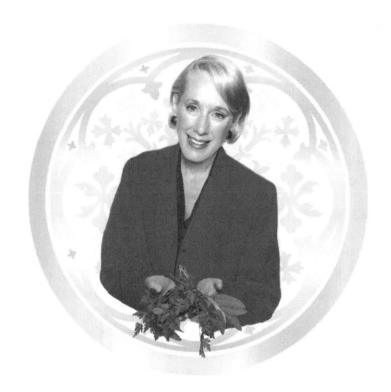

Our medicine is all around us. Our food is our pharmacy.

Herbs are our medicine. The oceans are our healers.

Our very breathing can bring us real health.

These things are truly healthy healing.
They don't need pages of warnings and lists of dangers.

Everyone can use them.

About the Cover

The "Healing of the World" cover for the new eleventh edition reminds us
that natural healing is eternal and universal.

Natural healing helps us grow in maturity because to use it
we must take a measure of responsibility for our health.
It increases our wisdom because it shows us
how to work with great diversity.
It brings us together because it helps us care for each other.

Natural healing represents timeless knowledge.
It is for everyone.

Neither drugs nor herbs nor vitamins are a cure for anything.
The body heals itself. The human body is incredibly intelligent.
It usually responds to intelligent therapies.
The healing professional can help this process
by offering intelligent therapies.

Cover Design by Barbara Howard

Thanks to hard working research associates: Sarah Abernathy, Kim Tunella and Sylvia Zamora.

This reference is to be used for educational information.
It is not a claim for cure or mitigation of disease, but rather an adjunctive approach,
supplying individual nutritional needs
that otherwise might be lacking
in today's lifestyle.

First Edition, June 1985. Copyright req. Nov. 1985.
Second Edition, January 1986.
Third Edition, Revised, September 1986.
Fourth Edition, Revised/Updated, May 1987.
Fifth Edition, November 1987.
Sixth Edition, Revised/Updated, June 1988.
Seventh Edition, Revised/Update, Jan. 1989, Sept. 1989, March 1990.
Eighth Edition, Revised/Updated/Expanded, July, 1990.
Ninth Edition, Revised/Updated/Expanded, Sept., 1992 and 1994.
Tenth Edition, Revised/Updated/Expanded, 1997 and 1998.
Eleventh Edition, Revised/Updated, March 2000.

Publisher's Cataloging-in-Publication
(Provided by Quality Books, Inc.)

Rector-Page, Linda G.
    Healthy healing : a guide to self healing for
everyone / by Linda Page. ~ 11th ed.
    p. cm.
    Includes bibliographic references and index.
    ISBN: 1-884334-89-X

    1. Holistic medicine. 2. Alternative medicine.
I. Title

R733.R43 2000   615.5
                          QB199-1886

For a free Healthy House product catalog,
call 1-888-447-2939

Visit
HEALTHY HEALING PUBLICATIONS
on the web for the latest, updated information
on natural healing techniques,
herbal remedies, the appearance and seminar
schedule for Dr. Linda Page,
and more.

www.healthyhealing.com

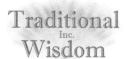

Traditional
Inc.
Wisdom

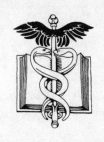

OTHER BOOKS BY

Linda Page, N.D., Ph.D.

Cooking For Healthy Healing

How To Be Your Own Herbal Pharmacist

Detoxification
All you need to know to recharge, renew and rejuvenate
your body, mind and spirit!

Party Lights

(with restaurateur Doug Vanderberg)

and

The Healthy Healing Library
Book and Guide Series

For more information about Dr. Page's books, see the last page of this book.

Table of Contents

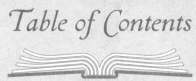

Look it up! An encyclopedia-style reference of effective alternative remedies and healing techniques that consumers can access for themselves. Over 350 entries are in this exhaustive survey.

How to Use this Book....

This book is a reference for people who are interested in a more personal kind of health care. I call it "Lifestyle Therapy." For long-lasting health, your body must do its own work. The natural healing recommendations described here help rebalance specific areas of your body so that it can function normally. They work *with* body functions, not outside them. They are free of harmful side effects and do not traumatize your body.

There are three remedy categories:
—Diet and Superfood Therapy
—Herb and Supplement Therapy
—Lifestyle Support Therapy (including Bodywork and Relaxation Techniques)

There are many effective recommendations to choose from. You can easily put together the best healing program for yourself. **Choosing one recommendation from each healing target under the interceptive therapy plan, for example, then using your choices together, may be considered a complete healing program**. All given doses are daily amounts unless otherwise specified. The rule of thumb for natural healing is one month for every year you have had the problem.

Where a remedy is especially effective for women, a female symbol ♀ appears by the recommendation.
Where a remedy is especially effective for men, a male symbol ♂ appears by the recommendation.
Where a remedy is proven effective for children, a small child's face ☺ appears by the recommendation.

No matter what your health problem is, consider your diet as your primary healing tool. The diets I recommend are "real people" diets. People with specific health conditions have used them and have related their experiences to me. Over the years, diseases change - and a person's immune response to them changes. Healthy Healing's diet programs are continually modified to meet new, changing health needs.

The "foot" and "hand" diagrams in the ailment programs show the reflexology pressure points for each body area. You can use reflexology therapy when it is indicated. In some cases, the points are very tiny, particularly for the glands. They take practice to pinpoint. The best sign that you have reached the right spot is that it will be very tender, denoting crystalline deposits or congestion in the corresponding body part. There is often a feeling of immediate relief in the area as the waste deposit breaks up for removal by your body.

You can have every confidence that the recommended remedies have been used and found to be effective, by thousands of people in some cases. I develop and work with the healing programs over the years; they are constantly updated with new information.

Every edition of Healthy Healing offers you the latest knowledge from a wide network of natural healing professionals - nutritional consultants, holistic practitioners, naturopaths, nurses, world health studies and traditional physicians in America and around the world.

The most significant information is the evidence of people who have tried the natural healing methods for themselves, experienced real improvement in their health, and wish to share their success with others.

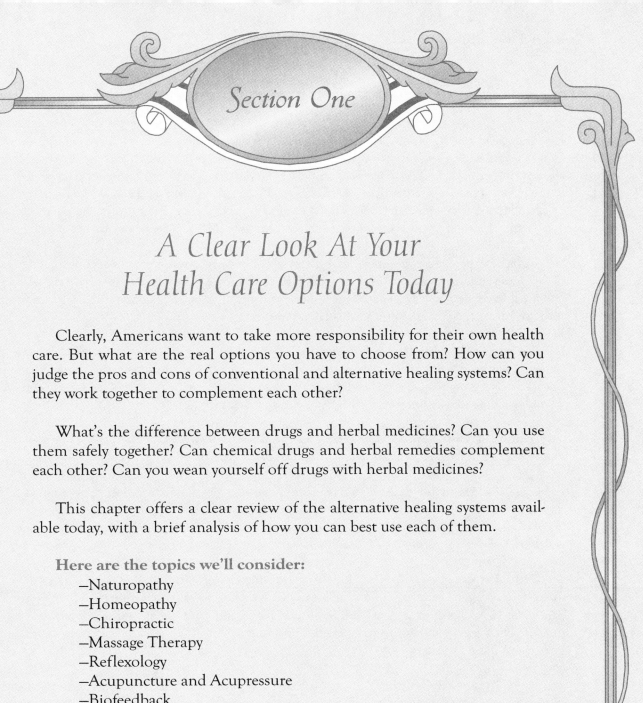

A Clear Look At Your
Health Care Options Today

Clearly, Americans want to take more responsibility for their own health care. But what are the real options you have to choose from? How can you judge the pros and cons of conventional and alternative healing systems? Can they work together to complement each other?

What's the difference between drugs and herbal medicines? Can you use them safely together? Can chemical drugs and herbal remedies complement each other? Can you wean yourself off drugs with herbal medicines?

This chapter offers a clear review of the alternative healing systems available today, with a brief analysis of how you can best use each of them.

Here are the topics we'll consider:
   —Naturopathy
   —Homeopathy
   —Chiropractic
   —Massage Therapy
   —Reflexology
   —Acupuncture and Acupressure
   —Biofeedback
   —Guided Imagery and Hypnotherapy
   —Enzyme Therapy
   —Overheating Therapy
   —Aromatherapy

and also...

   —Natural techniques for healing after surgery or serious illness.

Your Health Care Choices Today

Personal health empowerment and traditional healing knowledge in modern western populations has dropped away as medical advances and "letting the doctor do it" have become a way of life in our society. Our culture has allowed the entire health care industry to become so powerful and so disproportionately lucrative that it is now in the business of illness rather than health. In one disconcerting example, a cancer physician, returning from an extended vacation, found an empty waiting room. His colleague had been treating his patients nutritionally. The physician wailed, "This is terrible. It took me years to build a long-term, regular patient clientele!"

Thoughtful people everywhere are realizing that our doctors receive no reward for health, only for treating illness. Conventional medicine can only go so far before expense outweighs the value of the treatment. Drug and medical costs, even basic medical insurance payments, have escalated beyond the reach of most families. And, we are realizing that the doctor can't always "do it."

The turn of the twenty-first century finds many people using more natural, less drug-oriented therapies, sometimes as an alternative to conventional medicine, sometimes in a team approach along with it. As orthodox medicine becomes more invasive, and less in touch with the person who is ill, informed people are becoming more willing to take a measure of responsibility for their own health.

Health is a lifestyle process. It is based in wellness care, instead of just illness treatment. The best news is that natural remedies clearly work — often far better than prescription drugs for many health conditions.

Orthodox medicine focuses on crisis intervention. Many modern medical techniques were developed during war time, for emergency care, to do battle with an imminent threat to life. They are at their best in a "heroic mode," bringing up the big guns of surgery and drugs to search out and destroy dangerous organisms. It is the kind of treatment necessary for acute disease, accidents, emergencies and wartime life-saving.

Orthodox medicine is less successful in treating chronic illness. Respected studies show that most illnesses don't just drop out of the sky and hit us over the head. Diseases like arthritis, osteoporosis, lower back pain, high blood pressure, coronary-artery disease, ulcers and hormone imbalances are related to aging and lifestyle. The big guns and emergency measures often don't apply. They tend to overkill, and even suppress the body's own immune response.

Most illness is self-limiting. The human body is a beautifully designed healing system that can meet most of its problems without outside intervention. Even when outside help is needed, healing is enhanced if the patient can be kept free of emotional devastation, depression and panic. Emotional trauma impairs immune function by decreasing the body's interleukins, vital immune defense substances. Panic constricts blood vessels, putting additional burden on the heart. Depression intensifies existing diseases, and opens the door to others. There is a direct connection between our mental state and the ability of our immune system to do its job.

Many medical schools still don't teach disease prevention, proper diet or exercise as a part of health. Although many alternative techniques are widely accepted in Europe, American physicians downplay the interaction of mind and body, saying that a patient's state of mind does not matter to bacteria or a virus. Objective measures are emphasized - white blood cell counts, blood pressure readings, etc., instead of how the patient feels.

For all its brilliant achievements, modern medicine is still only pathology oriented. Doctors see the disease, not the person, and are only trained to use drugs, surgery, and the latest laboratory technologies. To paraphrase Abraham Maslow: "If all you're trained to use is a hammer, the whole world looks like a nail."

This approach does not sit well with the informed public today, who want more control over their health problems, and intend to be a part of the decision making process for their health needs.

Conventional medicine teaches that pain means sickness. Pain is treated as a powerful enemy, its symptoms are assaulted with prescription drugs that either mask it or drive it underground — a practice that usually means it will resurface later with increased intensity.

Alternative healers recognize that pain is also the body's way of informing us that we are doing something wrong, not necessarily that something is wrong. Pain can tell us that we are smoking too much, eating too much, or eating the wrong things. It can notify us when there is too much emotional congestion in our lives, or too much daily stress. Pain can be a friend with useful information about our health, so that we can effectively address the cause of a problem.

We are constantly pressured by the medical community to have exhaustive tests, to be screened for cholesterol, high blood pressure, breast lumps, and cancer cells. If there is acute pain or other symptoms that indicate the need for a doctor, obvious common sense dictates that a doctor should be called, or emergency medical steps taken. But mammography, pap smears, and many other tests are not prevention, simply early detection.

Many physicians have a financial interest in ordering an array of tests, in performing surgeries, and in prescribing certain medications. Many times, the pressure for testing is driven by these issues rather than for information. The fear of malpractice lawsuits also causes doctors to be overly zealous in ordering tests. Yet medical tests can be hazardous to your health. Faulty diagnoses and inaccurate readings are common in poorly trained, rushed labs. The more tests a person undergoes, the greater the odds of being told, often incorrectly, that something is wrong. Mental anxiety is brought on by needless testing, medication, or treatment, and a brusque or rushed doctor. You can literally worry yourself sick when there is nothing seriously wrong.

Not every problem requires costly, major medical attention. A sensible lifestyle, with good healthy food, regular moderate exercise and restful sleep is still the best medicine for many health conditions. The principles of nature governing health and illness are ageless; they apply equally everywhere at all times. There is no down time with the laws of nature, and they do not play favorites.

We need to be re-educated about our health — to be less intimidated by doctors and disease. I believe that the greatest ally of alternative medicine will be science itself — not the restricted view of science that assumes its basic concepts are complete, but the open-ended science that sets preconceived notions aside. Today's consumers are not only more aware of alternative health care choices, and more confident in their own healing strength, but also want to do something for themselves to get better. The time has clearly come for a partnership between health care professionals and patients, so that the healing resources from both sides can be optimally employed.

No prescription is more valuable than knowledge. This book is a ready reference for the alternative health care choices open to those wishing to take more responsibility for their own well-being. The recommended suggestions are backed up by extensive research into therapies for each ailment, and by contributing health care professionals and nutritional consultants from around the country, with many years of eyewitness and hands-on experience in natural healing results.

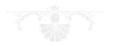

The Pros & Cons of Orthodox & Alternative Medicine
How Do They Compare?

The paradigm shift in medicine at the beginning of this century constituted vast reform for health care and medical education. The ability to isolate microbes that cause infectious disease, and to create treatments that would kill those microbes without killing the patient, meant tremendous acceptance for the practice of allopathic medicine, characterizing it as heroic and scientific. But the pendulum swung too far as the sledge hammers of drugs and surgery began to be driven by profit rather than by healing.

Today, there's another paradigm shift in health care — one that emphasizes disease prevention instead of disease treatment.

Health care had to change its focus because of the enormous rise in chronic diseases. Disorders like cancer and arthritis are the scourge of modern times. Drug and laboratory advances, the cornerstones of allopathic medicine, are less effective in treating chronic diseases. Health care systems must provide better, more protective, less invasive treatments for chronic disorders.

Conventional medicine has so far been devoted to justifying the validity, effectiveness and safety of its science and techniques, an emphasis that has resulted in an authoritarian, heavily regulated approach to its action and thinking. Many defend these rigid values and regulations because they have brought about a health care system that is arguably the most technologically advanced in the world. Yet, even with the broad medical arsenal available to doctors, they can only cure about one-fourth of the illnesses presented to them.

A recent report by the U.S. Office of Technology Assessment shows only 10 to 20% of standard medical procedures are effective!

As disease prevention becomes the watchword of wellness, medical strategies must change to avoid expensive, invasive modalities. Today's medicine depends on high-tech intervention equipment, surgical procedures, lab tests, a warehouse of antibiotics and powerful biochemicals. We know that many are hit-or-miss more often than we are willing to admit. They are frequently ineffective, and generally ignore the person in favor of the illness and its symptoms. Many have serious side effects and sometimes make the patient worse. Alternative medicine methods are less expensive, effective and much safer.

Yet, some aspects of orthodox medicine are very valuable. Most naturopathic physicians believe that building bridges with conventional medicine has tangible benefits. Medical diagnostic tools can monitor a disorder; some drugs can reduce crippling symptoms, often dramatically at first; some of the new drugs can retard progression of a disease. A broad range of healing methods makes sense.

I feel we need both types of medicine. Clearly, orthodox medicine has saved many lives. Just as clearly, alternative medicine has prevented much illness.

Our bodies are so complicated......our immune systems are almost unimaginably complex. Immune response has to take thousands of enzymes, delicate fluid balance, interlocking circulatory pathways, as well as our lifestyle, our emotions, and an unhealthy environment into account. Multiply all of this by our personal uniqueness and you can see why we need a wealth of choices for our health.

If there is no one "right" path, then multi-disciplinary health care is a better way. A team approach can take the best tools from each. A study by the New England Journal of Medicine shows American health care consumers doing just that. **One in three are using some form of complementary or alternative medicine today.**

Popular support has changed the way we look at medicine. There is clear evidence that drugs and surgery are often overused, and that human touch is vital to healing. In the field of mental health for instance, traditional doctors admit that spiritual factors influence disease. An increasing number of MD's even include holistic treatments as they see alternative approaches that are more effective, less expensive and safer than drugs.

Alternative medicine is really all about choices, something Americans consider a fundamental right. The realm of alternative medical practice is huge, because there isn't a "one-size-fits-all" for health care. Every person is an individual, and different therapies work for different people.

Here are the core principles that distinguish alternative medicine from orthodox medicine.

—Preventive medicine is the best medicine. Alternative health care emphasizes prevention over crisis intervention, seeking to improve health rather than simply to extend life by heroic means. Holistic practitioners believe healing originates within the human body, not from medicines or machines. In general, they believe that toxins in the body cause disease; using natural remedies to remove toxins helps the body regain health.

—The cure and the preventive are often the same. Most alternative healers teach that just as avoiding the causative agents will *prevent* an illness, removing them will *cure* the illness. For instance, if obesity is the condition, then the cure, a restricted diet, is the same as the preventive.

—It is important to know the cause of the disease, not just recognize the symptoms. When people seek alternative care, they're asking, "Why do I have this problem? I'm tired of having the doctor just treat the symptoms." Alternative caregivers teach that daily habits create the conditions for health or disease. Alternative practitioners believe that removing disease-causing conditions will prevent disease.

—The person is more important than the disease. Alternative treatments are highly individual. Ten people going to an alternative doctor for a headache may leave with ten different remedies. Practitioners of conventional medicine often see only the similarities and treat everyone the same.

—The body can heal itself. Alternative medicine practitioners view symptoms such as fever or inflammation, as signs that the body is mounting an immune response to heal itself. Instead of trying to eliminate symptoms, lifestyle therapy treatments work to enhance natural defenses and healing vitality.

—Alternative practitioners are also teachers who can empower you to help yourself. Many adopt the position of coach rather than doctor to give patients the power of their own healing systems.

—Lifestyle is significant. Alternative practitioners look beyond the physical symptoms and take into account a patient's mental, emotional, and even spiritual life as inseparable from physical health. Lifestyle therapy is more subtle than drugs or surgery. You should expect the healing effects of natural medicines to be slower but more permanent — a normal result of the body taking the time to do it right.
The natural healing rule of thumb is one month of healing for every year you've had the problem.

"HEALTHY HEALING" takes empowerment into account by offering a wealth of lifestyle choices for health problems...things you can do for yourself to improve almost every health condition. Even if the condition is serious, and even if you are under traditional medical care, there are always significant things you can do to help your body's healing process. Healing is both a physical process and an accomplishment of the spirit. It takes place in the physical world, and also in the universe of the soul. I have seen this to be undeniably true over the last 20 years, in case after case, regardless of the problem or its duration.

"HEALTHY HEALING" details both empirical evidence and clinical studies to offer you more choices that are non-invasive, health supporting, body balancing and disease preventing, as well as healing.
Good information is the key. Most people have a wealth of common sense and intuitive knowledge about themselves and their health problems. With access to solid information, people invariably make good choices for their health.

Naturopathy

Naturopathy, the fastest growing of all the alternative healing disciplines, represents the enormous change Americans are experiencing in their health care. Naturopathic doctors are once again becoming licensed, accredited and recognized as valuable contributors to modern healing. A leading force until the middle of this century, naturopaths have been either denied a clinical practice under American conventional medicine laws, or forced into a strictly educating posture as a way of discrediting naturopathic techniques.

As more people have become disillusioned with conventional health care, naturopathy is seen as having respect for other ways of healing.

Today, naturopaths fall into two groups. Those who are trained medically (NMD's) have extensive hands-on coursework in anatomy, physiology, biochemistry, pathology, neurosciences, histology, immunology, pharmacology, epidemiology, public health and other conventional disciplines as well as various natural therapies.

Traditionally trained naturopaths (ND's) use the naturopathy degree to consult with clients, and as an accreditation to teach, to write and to access research. One of the core beliefs of naturopathy is education – the passing on of knowledge to empower the patient.

Naturopaths are, for the most part, primary care, general practice family physicians with enormous scope. Since they specialize in non-invasive, lifestyle therapy, they can offer almost unlimited recommendations. Instead of prescribing standard treatment for a health complaint, naturopaths can offer an individual approach.

In contrast, conventional doctors have fewer choices. Since drug and surgical treatments can be so dangerous or full of side effects, they must be bound by what has been officially approved or authorized.

The strongest successes of naturopathic medicine are in the treatment of chronic and degenerative disease. Naturopathic medicine is not recommended for severe, acute trauma, such as a serious automobile accident, a childbirth emergency, or orthopedic problems that need corrective surgery, although it can contribute to faster recovery in these cases.

Although all naturopaths emphasize therapeutic choices based on individual interest and experience, they maintain a consistent philosophy. All are trained in the basic tools of natural therapeutics, and all work with diet and nutrition while specializing in one or more other therapeutic methods.

Many naturopathic physicians today have an educational background similar to that of a conventional M.D. while incorporating extensive training in other disciplines. The current scope of clinical Naturopathy covers the full practice of medicine excluding major surgery, and the prescribing of most drugs. Minor surgery, such as the removal of a mole or wart, is allowed. The orthodox medical establishment is more willing to accept clinical naturopaths than other alternative practitioners because of their rigorous schooling. They may even work in conventional hospitals.

Clinical naturopathic students are trained in therapeutic nutrition, and psychological counseling, subjects not required in traditional medical schools. They learn about herbal therapy, homeopathy, hydrotherapy, massage therapy, chiropractic, behavioral, and Oriental and Ayurvedic medicine. As NMD's, they can provide diagnostic and therapeutic services, including physical exams, lab testing and X-rays. Many can deliver babies, usually in a home setting. Others specialize in pediatrics, gynecology or geriatrics.

Naturopathic medicine sees disease as a manifestation of the natural causes by which your body heals itself, so it seeks to stimulate your body's vital healing forces. If the cause of the imbalance is not removed, the disease responses will continue either at a lower level of intensity or intermittently, to become chronic disease. Fever and inflammation are good examples of the way your body deals with an imbalance that is hindering its normal function.

Naturopathy is founded on five therapeutic principles.

A typical visit to a Naturopath generally incorporates these beliefs.

1: **Nature is a powerful healing force.** The belief that the body has considerable power to heal itself, and that the role of the physician or healer is to facilitate and enhance this process, preferably with the aid of natural, non-toxic, non-invasive therapies. Above all, the physician or healer must do no harm.

2: **The person is viewed and diagnosed as a whole.** The Naturopath must work to understand the patient's complex interaction of physical, mental, emotional, spiritual and social factors. Understanding the patient as an individual is essential when searching for factors that cause a disease.

3: **The goal is to identify and treat the cause of the problem.** Naturopathic medicine does not simply suppress symptoms, but seeks the underlying causes of a disease, especially as manifested in the four major elimination systems: the lungs, kidneys, bowels, and skin. A naturopath views symptoms as expressions of the body's attempt to heal. The causes of a disease spring from the physical, mental, emotional and spiritual levels. Healing a chronic disease requires the removal of the underlying cause.

Some illnesses are the result of spiritual disharmony, experienced as a feeling of deep unease or inadequate strength of will necessary to support the healing process. This disharmony must be overcome. Naturopathic physicians can play an important role in guiding patients to discover the appropriate action in these cases.

In acute cases such as ear infections, inflammation or fever, the naturopath addresses pain, infection and inflammation as well as the relationship of the condition to underlying causes, like diet or stress.

—Homeopathy and acupuncture are frequently used to stimulate recovery.
—Herbal medicines are frequently used as tonics and nutritive agents to strengthen weak systems.
—Dietary supplements and glandular extracts may be used to overcome nutritional deficiencies.
—Hydrotherapy and various types of physical therapy may be required.
—Relaxation techniques help alleviate emotional stress and allow the digestive system to function normally.

4: **The physician is a healing teacher.** A naturopath is foremost a teacher, educating, empowering and motivating the patient to assume more personal responsibility for their own wellness by adopting a healthy attitude, lifestyle and diet. After identifying the conditions that cause the illness, a naturopath discusses with the patient the most appropriate methods for creating a return to health.

5: **Prevention is the best cure.** Prevention is best accomplished by lifestyle habits which support health.

Care more than others think is wise.

Risk more than others think is safe.

Dream more than others think is practical.

Expect more than others think is possible.

Need to find a good naturopath? Call the California Naturopathic Assn. (530) 676-4842.

17

Homeopathy

Homeopathy is a kinder, gentler medical philosophy that sees disease as an energy imbalance, a disturbance of the body's "vital force." Its techniques are based on the premise that the body is a self healing entity, and that symptoms are the expression of the body attempting to restore its balance. Homeopathic remedies are formulated to stimulate and increase this curative ability. Each remedy has a number of symptoms that make it unique, just as each person has traits that make him or her unique. Homeopathic physicians are trained to match the patient's symptoms with the precise remedy. Even the highest potencies are non-toxic and do not create the side effects of allopathic drugs. The remedies themselves neither cover up nor destroy disease, but stimulate the body's own healing action to rid itself of the problem.

Homeopathic medicine is based on three prescription principles:

1: **The Law Of Similars:** expressed as "like curing like." From the tiny amount of the active principle in the remedy, the body learns to recognize the hostile microbe in a process similar to DNA recognition. The Law Of Similars is the reason that a little is better than a lot, and why such great precision is needed.

2: **The Minimum Dose Principle:** means diluting the "like" substance to a correct strength for the individual (strong enough to stimulate the body's vital force without overpowering it). Dilutions, usually in alcohol, are shaken or succussed, a certain number of times (3, 6, or 12 times in commercial use) to potentiate therapeutic power through a vibratory effect. Each successive dilution decreases the actual amount of the substance in the remedy. In the strongest dilutions, there is virtually none of the substance remaining, yet potentiation is the highest for healing.

3: **The Single Remedy Principle:** only one remedy is administered at a time.

Although homeopathic treatments are specific to the individual patient in private practice, I have found two things to be true about the remedies available in most stores today:

—**They work on the antidote principle.** More is not better for a homeopathic remedy. Small amounts over a period of time are more effective. Frequency of dosage is determined by individual reaction time, increasing as the first improvements are noted. When substantial improvement is evident, indicating that the body's own healing forces are stimulated and have come into play, the remedy should be discontinued.

—**They work on the trigger principle.** A good way to start a healing program is with a homeopathic medicine. The body's electrical activity, stimulated by the remedy, can mean faster response from other, succeeding therapies.

Homeopathic medicine differs from conventional medicine in two significant ways:

1: Conventional medicines usually mask or reduce the symptoms of a disease without addressing the underlying problem. Homeopathic remedies act as catalysts for the immune system to wipe out the root cause.

2: Although both medicinal systems use weak doses of a disease-causing agent to stimulate the body's defenses against that illness, homeopathy uses plants, herbs and earth minerals for this stimulation; conventional medicine uses viruses or chemicals.

The recent worldwide rise in popularity for homeopathy is due to its effectiveness in treating epidemic diseases, such as HIV-positive and other life-threatening viral conditions. Studies show that homeopathy not only treats the acute infective stages, but also reduces the need for antibiotics and other drugs that cause side effects, which further weakens an already low immune response.

In significant 1991 tests, Internal Medicine World Magazine reported six HIV-infected patients who became HIV-negative after homeopathic treatment. Following this and other reports, success with AIDS has been widely experienced by homeopaths as follows:

—**Prevention - generating resistance to the virus and subsequent infection.**
—**Support during acute illnesses - reducing the length and severity of the infection.**
—**Restoration of health - revitalizing the body so that overall health does not deteriorate.**

Here's how to take homeopathic remedies:

1: For maximum effectiveness, take $\frac{1}{2}$ dropperful under the tongue at a time, and hold for 30 seconds before swallowing; or dissolve the tiny homeopathic lactose tablets under the tongue.

2: Homeopathic remedies are designed to enter the bloodstream directly through your mouth's mucous membranes. For best absorption, do not eat, drink or smoke for 10 minutes before or after taking. Do not use with chemical medicines, caffeine, cayenne, mint or alcohol; they overpower the remedy's subtle stimulus.

3: The basic rule for dosage is to repeat the medicine as needed. You may notice aggravation of symptoms at first as your body restructures and begins to rebuild its defenses, in much the same way as a healing crisis occurs with other natural cleansing therapies. This effect usually passes in a short period of time.

4: Store homeopathic remedies at room temperature out of heat and sunlight, and away from perfumes, camphor, liniments and paints.

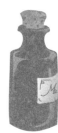

Healing can be quite long lasting.
The right homeopathic remedy can restore health on all levels.

Here are the most popular Homeopathic Remedies and how to use them:
—**APIS:** macerated bee tincture. Relieves stinging, burning and rapid swelling after bee sting or insect bites. Recommended for sunburn and other minor burns, skin irritations, hives, early stages of boils, and frostbite. Helps relieve joint pain, eye inflammation and fevers. Apis is effective against pain that is improved by cold and made worse by pressure.
—**ARNICA:** often the first medicine to take after an injury or a fall, to counter bruising, swelling, and local tenderness. Excellent for pain relief and rapid healing, particular from sports injuries like sprains, strains, stiffness or bruises. Unlike herbal preparations of Arnica, homeopathically diluted Arnica tablets are safe for internal consumption to relieve contusions, calm someone who has had a great shock, and dispel the distress that accompanies accidents and injuries. Use before and after surgery and childbirth to prevent bruising and speed recovery. Apply externally only to unbroken skin.
—**ACONITE:** for children's earaches. Helps the body deal with the trauma of sudden fright or shock.
—**ARSENICUM ALBUM:** for food poisoning accompanied by diarrhea. For allergic symptoms such as a runny nose; for asthma and colds.
—**BELLADONNA:** for fast relief of sudden fever, sunstroke or swelling. Used to treat sudden onset conditions characterized by redness, throbbing pain, and heat, including certain types of cold, high fever, earache and sore throat. Recommended for a person who has a flushed face, hot and dry skin, and dilated pupils. A remedy for teething, colds and flu, earache, fever, headache, menstrual problems, sinusitis, and sore throat.
—**BRYONIA:** for flu, fevers, coughs and colds that come on slowly. For some headaches, indigestion, muscle aches and pains. Helpful for irritability aggravated by motion. For swelling, inflammation and redness of arthritis when symptoms are worse with movement and better with cold applications.

—**CALENDULA:** promotes healing of minor cuts and scrapes; cools sunburn; relieves skin irritations.

—**CANTHARIS:** treats bladder infections and genito-urinary tract problems, especially where there is burning and urgency to urinate. Good for skin burns.

—**CAPSICUM:** a stimulating digestive aid. Apply topically to stop minor bleeding, joint pain and bruises.

—**CHAMOMILLA:** to calm fussy children during teething pain, colic and fever. Good for childhood cold symptoms of runny nose, tight cough, stringy diarrhea and earache. Treats childhood and adult restlessness, insomnia, toothache and joint pains. Recommended for those who are irascible, stubborn or inconsolable.

—**EUPHRASIA:** used as both an external and internal treatment for eye injuries, especially when there is profuse watering, burning pain, and swelling. Also used for abrasions, stuffy headache, and mucus in the throat.

—**GELSEMIUM:** to energize people with chronic lethargy. To overcome dizziness from colds or flu.

—**HYPERICUM:** used topically and internally to relieve pain and trauma related to nerves and the central nervous system. For an injury that causes shooting pain that ascends the length of a nerve, and for wounds to an area with many nerve endings, like the ends of the fingers and toes. Accelerates healing of jagged cuts and relieves the pain from dental surgery, toothaches, and tailbone injuries. Effective for depression and insomnia, A powerful anti-inflammatory for ulcers and nerve damage; also for cuts, scrapes, mild burns and sunburn.

—**IGNATIA:** a female remedy to relax emotional tension. Effective during times of great grief or loss.

—**LACHESIS:** for PMS symptoms that improve once menstrual flow begins. For menopausal hot flashes, irritability and bloating.

—**LEDUM:** for bruises. Use after Arnica treatment to fade a bruise after it becomes black and blue.

—**LYCOPODIUM:** a mood booster that often increases personal confidence. Favored by estheticians to soothe irritated complexions and as an antiseptic.

—**MAGNESIUM PHOS:** for abdominal cramping, spasmodic back pain and menstrual cramps.

—**NATRUM MURIATICUM:** for water retention and bloating during PMS.

—**NUX VOMICA:** used principally to treat headache, nausea and vomiting due to overeating or drinking. A prime remedy for hangover, recovering alcoholics and drug addiction. Beneficial for gastrointestinal tract problems, such as abdominal bloating, peptic ulcer, heartburn, flatulence, constipation and motion sickness.

—**OSCILLOCOCCINUM:** a premiere combination remedy for flu.

—**PASSIFLORA:** a prime remedy for insomnia and nervousness.

—**PODOPHYLLUM:** helps diarrhea, especially for children.

—**PULSATILLA:** for childhood asthma, allergies and earaches, when the child is tearful and passive. For colds characterized by a profusely running nose and coughing. For certain eye and ear ailments, skin eruptions, allergies, fainting, and gastric upsets, particularly when the patient is sensitive and prone to crying. Effective in homeopathic combination remedies for colds and flu, sinusitis, indigestion and insomnia.

—**RHUS TOX:** a poison ivy derivative, dilutions are taken to alleviate poison ivy and other red, swollen skin rashes, hives, and burns, as well as joint stiffness. A sports medicine for pain and swelling that affects muscles, ligaments, and tendons from sprains and overexertion. A "rusty gate" remedy, for the person who feels stiff and sore at first but better after movement. For stiffness in the joints when the pain is worse with cold, damp weather. Effective in homeopathic combination remedies for back pain, sprains and skin rashes.

—**SEPIA:** effective for treating herpes, eczema, hair loss and PMS.

—**SULPHUR:** commonly taken for certain chronic (rather than acute) conditions, skin problems, and the early stages of the flu. Treats sore throats, allergies, and earaches.

—**THUJA:** effective for treating warts and moles, and for sinusitis.

—**VALERIAN:** soothes nerves and eases muscle tension. A good sedative for insomnia.

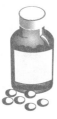

Homeopathic Cell Salts

Mineral, or tissue salts in the body can be used as healing agents for specific health problems. Homeopathic doctor, William Schuessler, discoverer of the twelve cell salts, and the Biochemic System of Medicine, felt that all forms of illness were associated with imbalances of one or more of the indispensable mineral salts. In addition, his research indicates that homeopathically prepared minerals help maintain mineral balance in our bodies, and, in fact, are used as core nutrients at the cellular level.

Cell salts are based on homeopathic remedies and may be used in healing programs that incorporate homeopathic treatment. As with other homeopathic remedies, mineral salts are used to stimulate corresponding body cell salts toward normal metabolic activity and health restoration. They re-tune the body to return it to a healthy balance. Only very small amounts are needed to properly nourish the cells.

The Twelve Cell Salts

Many of today's cell salts are extracted from organic plant sources. These medicines are available both in tinctures and as tiny lactose-based tablets that are easily dissolved under the tongue.

—**CALCAREA FLUOR:** *calcium fluoride* - contained in the elastic fibers of the skin, blood vessels, connective tissue, bones and teeth. Used in the treatment of dilated or weakened blood vessels, such as those found in hemorrhoids, varicose veins, hardened arteries and glands.

—**CALCAREA PHOS:** *calcium phosphate* - abundant in all tissues. Strengthens bones, and helps build new blood cells. Deficiency results in anemia, emaciation and weakness, slow growth and poor digestion.

—**CALCAREA SULPH:** *calcium sulphate* - found in bile; promotes continual blood cleansing. When deficient, toxic build-up occurs as skin disorders, respiratory clog, boils and ulcerations, and slow healing.

—**FERRUM PHOS:** *iron phosphate* - helps form red corpuscles to oxygenate the blood. Treats congestive colds and flu, and skin inflammation. A biochemic remedy for the first stages of inflammation or infections.

—**KALI MUR:** *potassium chloride* - deficiency results in coating of the tongue, gland swelling, scaling of the skin, and excess mucous discharge. Used after FERRUM PHOS for inflammatory arthritis and rheumatism.

—**KALI PHOS:** *potassium phosphate* - found in body fluids and tissues. Deficiency is characterized by intense body odor. Used for mental problems like depression, irritability, dizziness, headaches, nervous stomach.

—**KALI SULPH:** *potassium sulphate* - an oxygen-carrier for the skin. Deficiency causes a deposit on the tongue, and slimy nasal, eye, ear and mouth secretions.

—**MAGNESIA PHOS:** *magnesium phosphate* - an infrastructure constituent. Deficiency impairs muscle and nerve fibers, causing cramps, spasms and neuralgia pain, usually with prostration and profuse sweating.

—**NATRUM MUR:** *sodium chloride* - found throughout the body. Regulates moisture within the cells. Deficiency causes fatigue, chills, craving for salt, bloating, profuse secretions from the skin, eyes and mucous membranes, excessive salivation, and watery stools.

—**NATRUM PHOS:** *sodium phosphate* - regulates the body's acid/alkaline balance. Catalyzes lactic acid and fat emulsion. Imbalance shows a coated tongue, itchy skin, sour stomach, poor appetite, diarrhea and gas.

—**NATRUM SULPH:** *sodium sulfate* - an imbalance produces edema in the tissues, dry skin with watery eruptions, poor bile and pancreas activity, headaches, and gouty symptoms.

—**SILICEA:** *silica* - essential to healthy bones, joints, skin and glands. Deficiency produces catarrh in the respiratory system, pus discharges from the skin, slow wound healing and offensive body odor. Successful in the treatment of boils, pimples, for hair and nail health, blood cleansing, and rebuilding after illness or injury.

Need to find a good homeopath? Call the National Center for Homeopathy. (703) 548-7790.

21

Chiropractic

Overwhelming evidence has changed the medical community's attitude toward chiropractic as a method for both healing and normalizing the nervous system. With almost 15 million patients annually, and 35,000 licensed practitioners, chiropractic therapy is now America's second largest health-care system.

Meaning "done with the hands," chiropractic therapy uses physical manipulation of the spine to relieve pain and return energy to the body. The central belief of chiropractic is that proper alignment of the spinal column is essential for health, because the spinal column acts as a switchboard for the nervous system. Its practitioners feel that the nervous system holds the key to the body's healing potential because it coordinates and controls the functions of all other body systems.

Today's chiropractors incorporate physical therapy techniques, nutritional counseling and muscle rehabilitation into their practice. Since nerve obstruction is involved with a wide range of health problems, many have also branched out into treating menstrual difficulties like PMS, candida albicans yeast overgrowth, and fatigue syndromes like CFS, fibromyalgia and lupus. Respiratory conditions like asthma, digestive troubles, insomnia and circulatory problems respond well to chiropractic care.

While the most common complaint for chiropractic treatment is still lower back pain, chiropractic adjustment also helps prevent wear and tear on joints and ligaments by maintaining their proper positioning. It helps decrease scar tissue formation after injury. Evidence shows that chiropractic adjustment combined with proper nutrition can improve and help prevent joint stiffness, and, in some cases, reverse arthritis and osteoarthritis.

Most chiropractors today are no longer "back crackers." Many use a hand-held activator that delivers a controlled, light, fast thrust to the problem area. The thrust is so quick that it accelerates ahead of the body's tightening-up resistance to the adjustment. A chiropractor locates the fixated area of the spine, makes the quick adjustment, and corrects the subluxation. Other problems aggravated by the fixation usually begin to heal immediately. The gentleness of this method makes adjustments far safer and more comfortable for the patient.

The spinal column and the nervous system work together for your health:

—The spinal column is made up of twenty-four bones called vertebrae that surround and protect the spinal cord. Between each vertebra, pairs of spinal nerves reach to every part of the body, including muscles, bones, organs and glands. Each vertebra affects its neighbor and one portion of the spine may affect or damage other areas of the body.

—The nervous system is comprised of three overlapping systems: the central nervous system, the autonomic nervous system and the peripheral nervous system. Health relies upon the balance and equilibrium of all three interrelated nerve systems, which can be disrupted by misalignment, stress or illness. Almost every nerve in the body runs through the spine, and stress-caused constriction tends to accumulate in the lower back, neck and shoulders. Chiropractic adjustments therefore, can address many seemingly unrelated dysfunctions, both physical and subconscious.

Misalignments in the spine, known as *subluxations*, interrupt the electrical impulse flow from the brain to the nerve structures, resulting in both pain and lower immune response. A subluxation may also have a direct effect on organ function. A chiropractor adjusts spinal joints to remove subluxations in order to restore normal nerve function. Subluxations may not be the sole cause of a given disease, but they are a major predisposing factor to it because they prevent the nervous system from working normally.

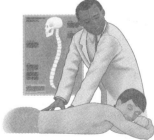

Biofeedback

Biofeedback uses high-tech electronic equipment readings to give auditory, verbal, and visual information back to the body about how it is working. Before the advent of the biofeedback machine, conventional medicine held that an individual had no control over heart rate, body temperature, brain activity, or blood pressure. When biofeedback experiments proved, in the 1960's, that people could voluntarily affect these functions, research tests began into how it might be employed for human health.

Here's how biofeedback works: The patient is wired with sensors, and by giving auditory and/or visual signals to his body, learns to control what are usually subconscious responses — like circulation to the hands and feet, tension in the jaw, or heartbeat rate. Biofeedback computers then provide a rapid, detailed analysis of the target activities within the body. Biofeedback practitioners interpret changes in the computer readings which help the patient learn to stabilize erratic and unhealthy biological functions. A normal, healthy reading includes fairly warm skin, low sweat gland activity, and a slow, even heart rate.

Today, biofeedback is being used by all kinds of health professionals — physicians, psychologists, social workers and nurses. It is seen as a useful medical tool for controlling health problems like asthma, chronic fatigue, epilepsy, drug addiction and chronic pain. It is a successful specific in the treatment of migraines, cold extremities, and psoriasis, a skin disease that has a psychological foundation.

Biofeedback is used in relaxation therapy to help overcome insomnia and anxiety. Sleep disorders, hyperactivity and other behavior problems in children, dysfunctions stemming from inadequate control over muscles, bladder incontinence, back pain, temporo-mandibular joint syndrome (TMJ), and even loss of control due to brain or nerve damage, all show improvement under biofeedback training.

Biofeedback also helps problems like heart malfunction, stress-related intestinal disorders like ulcers and irritable bowel syndrome, hiatal hernia, ringing in the ears (Meniere's syndrome), facial tics, and cerebral palsy.

The effects of biofeedback can be measured by:
1: Monitoring skin temperature influenced by blood flow beneath the skin;
2: Monitoring galvanic skin response, the electrical conductivity of the skin;
3: Observing muscle tension with an electro-myogram;
4: Tracking heart rate with an electro-cardiogram;
5: Using an electroencephalogram to monitor brain wave activity.

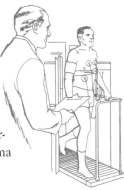

One of the most common vital signs monitored by biofeedback is muscle tension, because this can be used to treat tension headaches, muscle pain, incontinence, even partial paralysis. Another is skin temperature, which can be used to treat Reynaud's syndrome, migraines, hypertension and anxiety. Other signs are perspiration, which is used to treat anxiety and body odor; pulse, which is used to treat hypertension, stress and heart arrhythmia; and breathing rate, which is used to treat asthma and anxiety reactions.

Biofeedback is seldom used by itself, but is instead combined with other relaxation techniques and lifestyle changes. Biofeedback doesn't work for everyone. Its success stories come from people who are willing to make lifestyle improvements.

Massage Therapy

Massage therapy has been a recognized healing method for thousands of years. The ancient Romans and Greeks used massage regularly as a healing treatment. In the past decade, overwhelming scientific evidence has accumulated in support of massage therapy. Today massage therapy has joined the alternative medicine techniques of chiropractic and reflexology as a viable health discipline.

Here are some of the research findings:

—Massage therapy is helpful for pain control, stimulating the production of endorphins, the body's natural pain relievers. Special effectiveness is reported for back and shoulder pain, and spinal/nerve problems.

—Massage therapy is an effective treatment for cardiovascular disorders, actually helping to prevent future heart disease. It is often more helpful than drugs for neurological and gynecological problems like PMS.

—Massage therapy helps chronic fatigue syndromes, candida albicans infections, and gastrointestinal disorders.

—Massage therapy helps correct poor posture from spinal curvatures and whiplash.

—Massage therapy helps headaches and temporo-mandibular joint syndrome (TMJ).

—Massage therapy helps respiratory disorders like bronchial asthma and emphysema.

—Massage therapy promotes recovery from fatigue, muscle spasms and pain after exercise.

—Massage therapy helps break up scar tissue and adhesions, and remove toxins causing eczema or psoriasis.

—Massage therapy effectively treats chronic inflammatory conditions by increasing limbic circulation, especially swelling from fractures or injuries.

—Massage therapy improves blood circulation throughout the entire circulatory system.

—Massage therapy is a wonderful detox technique, promoting mucous and fluid drainage from the lungs and increasing peristaltic action in the intestines to promote fecal elimination. I recommend at least one massage treatment during a 3 to 7 day cleanse to stimulate the body's immune response and natural restorative powers.

Two types of massage therapy specifically help the detoxification-body cleansing process:

1: **Deep tissue massage** removes waste in the muscles. Deep tissue therapy uses more direct deep finger pressure across the grain of the muscles to release chronic patterns of tension, and stress accumulation. It also increases circulation to facilitate the movement of waste products out of the muscle tissue. Recent evidence shows that deep tissue massage can break up scar tissue and eliminate it.

2: **Lymphatic drainage** is a large surface, highly specialized kneading technique, a unique method that uses precise, complex hand movements to encourage the draining of lymph fluids. In comparison, normal massage techniques are much too forceful to allow drainage in the tissues and may hinder transport.

I call the lymphatic system the body's natural antibiotic. When it is flushed and clean, lymph removes body toxins as part of the auto-immune response to disease. Using slow, gentle strokes with a rhythmic pumping action, the massage technician follows the lymph pathways throughout the body to move the flow of lymph and accelerate detoxification.

Lymphatic massage has four primary effects on your body:

1: It balances the sympathetic and parasympathetic nervous systems.

2: It activates inhibitory reflex cells which decrease or even eliminate pain sensations.

3: It increases lymph flow for a decongestant effect on connective tissue, stimulates blood capillary flow and increases resorptive capacity of the blood capillaries.

4: It boosts immune response by increasing lymph flow and stimulating antibodies.

There are several popular techniques of therapeutic massage today. The choice is limited only by personal preference and desired results. For lasting benefits, use massage therapy as part of a program that includes diet improvement and exercise.

Here are the most popular massage therapy methods:

—Alexander technique - This system strives to improve posture by properly positioning the head and neck. A favorite of actors and singers, the Alexander technique works to expand the chest cavity, improve breathing and body movement. The sessions involve guided body movement as well as table-work massage procedures. To find a practitioner, call (800) 473-0620.

—Feldenkrais - This system believes that to change the way we act, we must change the way we move. Through simple body manipulations and exercises, Feldenkrais practitioners help patients change unbalanced muscle patterns and the thought patterns associated with them. To find a practitioner, call (800) 775-2118.

—Polarity therapy - Besides the muscles, glands and nerves, the human body has a magnetic field that directs these systems and maintains energy balance. A polarity practitioner works to access the magnetic current and its movement patterns to release energy blocks. (See POLARITY THERAPY, page 26.)

—Reflexology - In this system, the feet and hands are seen as end points of energy zones and associated organs and glands throughout the body. The points are manipulated to open blocked energy pathways. Since the feet serve as reflexes for the entire body, foot reflexology is most often used. Reflexology is best used in conjunction with other massage techniques. (See REFLEXOLOGY, page 35.) For a practitioner, call (727) 343-4811.

—Rolfing - Rolfers attempt to realign the body with gravity by deeply manipulating the connective tissue that contains the muscles and links them to the bones. To find a practitioner, call (303) 449-5903.

—Swedish massage uses kneading, stroking, friction, tapping and sometimes body shaking to stimulate, cleanse or relax. The techniques help muscles, joints, nerves and the endocrine system. When used before an athletic workout, they can prevent soreness, relieve swelling and tension and improve muscular performance. By stimulating the body's circulation, a Swedish massage speeds rehabilitation from injury.

Note: As wonderful as massage therapy is, there are some health conditions where massage is not a good idea.
- Don't massage a person with high fever, cancer, tuberculosis or other infections or malignant conditions which might be further spread through the body.
- Don't massage the abdomen of a person with high blood pressure or ulcers.
- Don't massage legs with varicose veins, diabetes, phlebitis or blood vessel problems.
- Massage no closer than six inches near bruises, cysts, skin breaks or broken bones.
- Massage people with swollen limbs gently, only above the swelling, towards the heart.

> When health is absent,
> Wisdom cannot reveal itself,
> Art cannot become manifest,
> Strength cannot be exerted.
> Wealth is useless,
> Reason is powerless.
> -Herophiles, 300B.C.

Polarity Therapy

Polarity therapy is a blend of art and science. Today's technology graphically shows that the human body consists of many electromagnetic patterns. We can see that energy both surrounds the body and courses through it in a continual flow of positive and negative charges. Expressed in ancient times as an aura, this magnetic field makes up our physical, mental, and emotional characteristics, directs body systems and maintains energy balance. Popular in holistic spas and detox centers today, a polarity practitioner accesses the magnetic current to release energy blocks.

Many respected researchers believe today that aberrated electromagnetic fields or wavelengths (such as EMFs) introduce an antagonistic response to man's otherwise harmonious energies frequencies. Robert Becker, M.D. author of *The Body Electric* says, "We now live in a sea of electromagnetic radiation that we cannot sense and that never before existed on this earth. New evidence suggests that this massive amount of radiation is producing stress, disease and other harmful effects by interfering with the most basic levels of brain function."

Our society is so dependent on electronics that abolishing electromagnetic radiation is out of the question. But we may be able to protect the body's life force energies with things like Polarity devices which act as "antennas" or "waveguides" to attract and reinforce healthful wave-lengths to the body. Beneficial wave-lengths, first identified by Bell Science Labs have been known since the 1950's.

Biological healing energies appear to be composed of a combination of subtle energy fields — electromagnetic

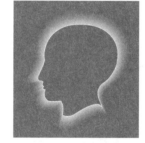

fields and quantum fields. Quantum like electromagnetic waves. They also have which helps explain how subtle energy defects. The combination of the fields apdiators. In fact, researchers say healing can to the underlying energetic fields that may

Polarizers reset vortex spins so they the Earth's equator, a toxic vortex spins clockwise. South of the equator the re- the negative vortex action, to either neu-

fields propagate without loss of energy, un- a unique ability to converge their energy, vices can focus energy to create healing effpears to boost stress-reducing biochemical me- never be explained without paying attention be primary to initiating the healing response. are consistent with positive forces. North of counter-clockwise; a healthy vortex spins verse is true. Polarizers repolarize or respin tralize it or carry it into a beneficial spin.

Is polarity therapy a new technique to reduce stress?

Polarity therapists believe that balancing the flow of energy in the body is the underlying foundation of health. Rooted in Ayurveda, polarity therapy uses diet and exercise for cleansing tissues, balancing energy, improving breath and circulation, and preventing illness.

There is clinical evidence for the effectiveness of this blend of quantum physics applied to biology and medicine. When polarity devices are brought in close contact to areas of pain or muscle tension many people report pain relief and a greater sense of well-being. In geriatrics treatment and home health nursing, numerous case studies show that polarizers make significant health improvement in many patients. Relaxation, reduced fatigue and mental confusion, improved sleep, pain relief, and allergy symptom improvement are just a few of the benefits. Polarity therapy is also helpful in treating migraines, low back pain and other stress disorders.

Gentle touch induces a relaxed, meditative state to accelerate energy flow through the body. Therapists use three types of touch: *rajasic* is gentle and stimulating, *sattvic* is a light, balancing touch, *tamasic* touch goes deeper into the muscles and tissues. Frequently, the touch is so light that one doesn't feel anything at all.

If you're interested.... SPRINGLIFE POLARIZERS, Springlife Inc., 4630 N. Paseo De Los Cerritos, Tucson, AZ 85745, 888-633-9233.

Magnet Therapy

Magnet therapy balances negative-positive energy. Science has known since the 1950's that a magnetic field is critical to normal body function and coordination. In fact, immune deficiency syndromes like chronic fatigue and fibromyalgia were first identified as magnetic field deficiency syndromes.

A positive, acid-producing field may create health conditions like arthritis, mental confusion, fatigue, pain and insomnia — and encourage fat storage. Culprits producing this field are refined foods, caffeine, nicotine, toxic chemicals in cosmetics and agriculture, auto exhaust, and many prescription drugs.

A negative, alkaline-producing field increases oxygen, encourages deep sleep, reduces swelling and fluid retention, relieves pain, and promotes mental acuity. A negative field acts like an antibiotic, helping destroy bacterial, fungal and viral infections because it lowers body acidity.

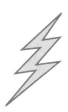

Does magnet therapy actually work? There seems to be no question that magnets can dramatically influence our health and well being. Russians used magnet therapy during World War II to ease pain, specifically from amputation. At least 50 countries including Germany, Japan and Russia have approved therapeutic magnets for healing. Magnet therapy is being enthusiastically rediscovered in the U.S. by health professionals and health conscious consumers looking for non-invasive, non-toxic solutions to chronic pain. Americans spent $500 million on therapeutic magnets in 1997 alone!

Science is still probing magnet therapy. Here is what we know so far:

1: Our blood is composed of positively and negatively charged particles. Magnets increase blood flow and therefore provide more oxygen to body areas that need healing.

2: Magnet therapy balances pH, establishing an environment unfavorable for disease, favorable for healing.

3: Magnet therapy helps breakdown scar tissue and release toxins, accelerating recovery from injury.

4: Magnet therapy speeds up the migration of calcium to help heal nerve tissue and bones, and helps eliminate excess calcium in the joints related to arthritis pain.

5: Magnet therapy stimulates enzyme activity, vital to healing.

6: Magnet therapy enlarges blood vessel diameters and reduces inflammation.

7: Magnet therapy may offset the effects of free radicals that contribute to degenerative disease by restoring the body's electrical balance.

8: Magnet therapy appears to reduce pain by modulating pain receptors or reducing neuron activity that causes pain. Magnets may stimulate the production of endorphins, our natural pain killers and mood elevators.

Here are a few examples of health benefits from magnet therapy:

—A study in November 1997 Archives of Physical Medicine and Rehabilitation reveals that patients suffering from post-polio pain experience significant, rapid relief when exposing pressure points to magnets.

—Studies conducted at the John Hopkins, Yale and NYU confirm that magnet therapy reduces pain from tendonitis, arthritis and venous ulcers. Other research finds magnet therapy relieves pain from whiplash, head and knee injuries, and menstrual cramps.

—Magnet therapy is considered a potential treatment for severe depression. An electromagnet is strapped to the left front part of the brain, underactive in depressed people, which induces an electric current in the brain causing brain cells to produce more mood elevating neurotransmitters. The treatment lasts about 5 minutes.

Magnetic sleeping pads, cushions, shoe insoles, wraps, adhesives, bracelets and necklaces and massagers are widely available. Use quality magnets with a gauss strength greater than 400 for best results. If you suffer from chronic pain from arthritis, backaches, migraines or sports injuries, magnet therapy may be a safe, effective alternative to drugs or invasive treatments. Consider Encore Technology MAGNELYFE flexible contour magnets.

Guided Imagery

Guided imagery uses the mind/body connection to help give people more control over their health. It is a communication technique for accessing the network between mind and body as a source of power in the healing process. It has its roots in the ancient Greek understanding of how the mind influences the subconscious, and has been employed under many different names throughout the history of medicine, to speed healing by reducing stress and calming the mind.

Imagery is simply a flow of thoughts that you can see, hear, feel, smell, or taste in your imagination. It's the way your nervous system processes information, so it's especially effective for the dialogue between mind and body in the healing process.

Scientifically, imagery works like a computer to program directions into the hypothalamus that a patient wants for his body. This happens almost instantaneously, traveling from the brain through the nervous system, to the endocrine system through the hypothalamus-pituitary-adrenal axis, and then through the vagus nerve for both psychological and physical accord.

Everything that is registered in our minds is registered in our bodies. Deepak Chopra M.D., a well-known expert on the mind-body connection, explains that "the mind is in every cell of the body. Every thought we think causes a release of neuropeptides that are transmitted to all the cells in the body."

Messages you send your body through imagery, for example, are immediately translated through the parasympathetic nervous system into neurotransmitters, that direct the immune system to work better against abnormal cells, or the hormone system to rebalance and stop creating abnormal cells.

Thoughts of love, for example interferon, substances that help heal. body to release cortisone and adrena- response. Peaceful thoughts release which help your body relax, adjust

The school of imagery believes cope with disease-causing factors if it high, immune response is reduced, healing. Today, guided imagery in every relaxation and stress-reduction an easy way to learn to relax, and its than other methods.

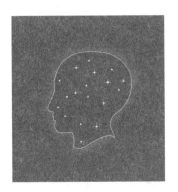

cause your body to release interleukin and Conversely, anxious thoughts cause your line, substances that suppress immune chemicals in your body similar to valium, and "take a new look" at its health state. that the body is in a better position to isn't under stress. When stress levels are so learning to relax is fundamental to self- one form or another is a part of almost technique. For many people, imagery is active nature makes it more comfortable

Guided imagery is a proven method for pain relief, for helping people tolerate medical procedures, for reducing side effects, and for stimulating healing response. It can help people find meaning in their illness, offer a way to cope, and accelerate recovery. Imagery is used to encourage athletes and performers to better performance, minimizing discomfort from all kinds of injuries, including sprains, strains, and broken bones. In healing, it is successful in overcoming chronic pain and persistent infections, and in shrinking tumor growths. Even serious, degenerative illness such as cancer has responded to guided imagery, with patients showing heightened immune activity as they imagine cancer cells being gobbled up by immune antibodies.

How does guided imagery work for stress and depression? Stress reduction techniques, like meditation and guided imagery, powerfully affect both the onset and progression of disease. Studies show that both meditation and imagery help people eliminate or reduce the severity and frequency of headaches, dramatically slow down the aging process, and manage the discomfort of lower back pain, heart disease, hypertension, irritable bowel syndrome, even cancer and AIDS.

Guided imagery is a proven method for helping people tolerate medical procedures and treatments, for reducing side effects, and for supporting a less painful, faster recuperation. Experts claim that imagery can help both physical and psychological disorders, from high blood pressure and acne, to diabetes, cancer and addictions.

Stress reactions are an excellent example of an emotional response that manifests itself in the body — often as illness. Imagery can help clarify and put in a broader perspective what's really going on in a person's life. If someone under severe stress is able to integrate his or her situation into a broader meaning of life, the feelings of loss, grief or depression will be relatively temporary.

Here's an example: a man might respond to the loss of his wife with a prolonged state of depression. His body, too, will be in a state of depression, making him susceptible to serious health problems. But if he is able to intergrate his loss into his whole life picture, by directly accessing emotions through guided imagery, his loss won't totally overwhelm him, and his grief will lessen over time. Gradually, he can develop a more wholesome view of his life, to again become a participant, rather than a victim of its circumstances.

There are two types of guided imagery techniques — receptive imagery and active imagery:

—**Receptive imagery** involves entering a relaxed state, then focusing on the area of the body with the ailment. You envision an embodiment of the illness — perhaps a mischievous demon — and ask it why it is causing the trouble. Your unconscious can provide a great deal of information about what your body needs.

—**Active imagery** involves envisioning an illness being cured. This may mean anything from imagining your immune system attacking a tumor, to picturing arm pain as a ball that rolls down your arm and out of your body.

Guided imagery therapists use a near-trance condition, induced through spoken suggestion to affect healing. Patients are asked to envision themselves in a tranquil place like a quiet woods or a mountain lake, then directed to describe what they see, hear, smell, or feel, in order to reach a deeper state of relaxation. This technique is called *sensory recruitment* because it calls on areas of the brain that control each different sense.

When relaxation has been reached, patients are asked to visualize their immune system as an energy force battling for their health. Their immune responses are analyzed in great detail. They are then asked to join forces with the immune system, by mentally envisioning the illness and then imagining their antibodies and white cells overcoming it.

Not everyone is capable of working with guided imagery treatment. An active imagination is a must, because the vividness of the image plays a role in the treatment's effectiveness. Successful subjects are those who can understand its value in relation to their problems, and who do not mentally fight it.

> *You're never given a battle you can't fight.*
>
> *You'll only know how strong you really are when you have to face adversity.*

Hypnotherapy

The power of suggestion has always played a major role in healing. Hypnosis is an artificially induced mental state that heightens receptivity to suggestion. Hypnotherapy uses both suggestion and trance to access the deepest levels of the mind in order to effect positive changes in a person's behavior. It maximizes the mind's contribution to healing by producing a multilevel relaxation state — a state which allows enhanced focus to increase tolerance to adverse stimuli, ease anxiety, or enhance affirmative imagery.

Physiologically, hypnosis stimulates the limbic system, the region of your brain linked to emotion and involuntary responses, like adrenal spurts and blood pressure. Habitual patterns of thought and reaction are temporarily suspended during hypnosis, rendering the brain capable of responding to healthy suggestions. The physiological shift can actually be observed during a hypnotic state, as can greater control of autonomic nervous system functions that are normally beyond one's ability to control. Stress and blood pressure reduction are common occurrences.

Research demonstrates that body chemistry actually changes during a hypnotic trance. In one experiment, a young girl was unable to hold her hand in a bucket of ice water for more than thirty seconds. Blood levels of cortisol in her body were high, indicating she was in severe stress. Under hypnosis, she was able to keep the same hand in ice water for thirty minutes. There was no rise in blood cortisol levels.

Hypnotherapy has healing applications for both psychological and physical disorders.

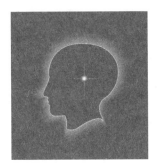

A skilled hypnotherapist can effect pro-found changes in respiration and relax-ation to create enhanced well-being. Today, hypnotherapy techniques are widely used to help you quit smoking, lose weight, or get a good night's sleep. Profes-sional sports trainers use hypnotherapy to boost athletic performance. New appli-cations with hypnotherapy help people tolerate pain during medical procedures. Some patients have even undergone surgery without anesthesia using hypnosis. It is also a method for treating medical conditions like facial neuralgia, sciatica, ar-thritis, whiplash, menstrual pain and tennis elbow. Migraines, ulcers, respiratory conditions, tension headaches, and even warts respond to hypnotherapy. Den-tists regularly use hypnosis for root ca-nal patients who can't tolerate anesthesia.

Hypnotherapy is also useful in surgical operations where regular anesthesia isn't a good option, in cases like hysterectomies, hernias, breast biopsies, hemorrhoidectomies and cesarian sections. A recent study shows that burn victims heal considerably faster with less pain and fewer complications if they are hypnotized shortly after they are injured.

Scientists are now examining a new aspect of hypnotherapy: its effect on the immune system. Recent research shows that hypnotherapy can be used to train your immune system to fight disease.

Hypnotherapy works best as a partnership between doctor and patient. Surprisingly, while most people do not think that they can be hypnotized, 90% of the population *can* achieve a trance state, (I have been one of those surprised people myself) and another 30% have a high enough susceptibility to enter a receptive state.

Three conditions are essential for successful hypnotherapy:
—A comfortable environment, free of distraction, so the patient can reach the deepest possible level.
—A trusting rapport between the hypnotist and the patient.
—A willingness and desire by the subject to be hypnotized. People who benefit most from hypnotherapy understand that hypnosis is not a surrender of personal control, but instead, an advanced form of relaxation.

Need to find a good practitioner? Call the American Board of Hypnotherapy. (800) 872-9996

Acupuncture & Acupressure

Acupuncture and acupressure are ancient systems of natural healing from the Orient. They're gaining new respect in the western world. The central belief of Traditional Chinese Medicine is that the body must be in balance to function at its peak. Acupuncture is based on this belief.

Traditional Oriental medicine believes that all emotional and physical energy, known as qi or chi, flows through the body along specific bio-electric, bio-chemical pathways called meridians, or energy pathways. The pathways regulate and coordinate the body's well-being by distributing chi energy throughout it. The meridian points are connected to specific organs and body functions. When chi energy is flowing smoothly, the body is in perfect balance. When chi energy flow is slowed down or blocked, by factors like injury, poor diet, stress or climate, then physical or emotional illness often results.

Acupuncture and acupressure are a painless, non-toxic therapy for redirecting and restoring the energy flow of chi. Most patients feel relaxed during acupuncture treatment, but response is highly individualized, relaxing some, energizing others.

Acupuncture uses hair thin needles and/or electrodes to direct and rechannel body energy. Western science believes that acupuncture needling stimulates certain nerve cells to release chemicals in the spine, muscles and brain. These biochemicals allay pain by releasing endorphins, the body's pain-relieving substances. They also stimulate the release of other chemicals and hormones that help normalize body processes. Acupuncture is used in the U.S. mainly for pain relief, but is valuable in the treatment of environmentally-induced illnesses caused by radiation poisoning or air pollution, and useful in carpal tunnel syndrome, as well as withdrawal complications from smoking, alcoholism, or drug addictions. Acupuncture is also extremely effective in treating rheumatoid conditions, bringing relief to 80% of those who suffer from arthritis.

Chinese medicine sees acupuncture as stimulating the release of blocked energy, which then flows throughout the body allowing it to begin healing itself. Because the body meridians are interconnected with the internal organs, Chinese practitioners use acupuncture to treat everything from immune disorders, like chronic fatigue syndrome, to allergies and asthma.

The World Health Organization cites 104 different conditions that acupuncture can treat including: migraines, sinusitis, the common cold, tonsillitis, eye inflammation, myopia, duodenal ulcer and other gastrointestinal disorders, neuralgia, Meniere's disease, tennis elbow, paralysis from stroke, speech aphasia and sciatica.

Acupuncturists specialize in treating people, not symptoms. They look for lifestyle patterns that affect health, and place great emphasis on balance and harmony with the patient's environment for the best results. They look first for reduced immune response caused by excesses in the patient's life, daily stress, emotional upsets, even the weather. Then they try to correct these underlying imbalances to re-establish foundation wellness, not just reduction of symptoms. Depending on the patient's needs, herbs, vitamins, exercises and changes in diet and lifestyle are part of the complete healing process. The nature of the problem determines the number of acupuncture treatments a patient will require. Someone suffering acute pain in a specific area may need only a few months of treatments; someone with a chronic disease usually requires a long-term treatment program.

Modern acupuncture also uses several adjunct treatments: **moxibustion**, a form of heat therapy in which certain herbs, like Chinese wormwood are burned near acupuncture points to radiate through the skin and influence the meridian below; **cupping**, a circulation stimulating technique, in which heated glass cups are placed over acupuncture points to draw blood to the area; and **massage therapy** to enhance circulation throughout the body.

Acupressure uses the same principles and meridian points as acupuncture, but works through finger pressure, massage and stroking rather than needles to effect stimulation. Acupressure and massage therapy are frequently combined in a healing stimulation session.

Fourteen primary meridians or channels of energy run through your body. (See diagram.) Each meridian is named for the organ or function connected to its energy flow. Stimulating these points manually releases blocked energy.

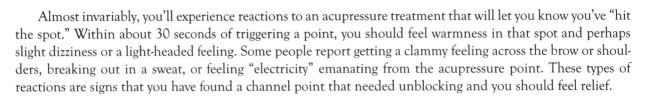

You can use some of the most effective acupressure points yourself:

The primary advantage of acupressure is that it is a self-access therapy. In fact, the Chinese consider acupressure a personal first aid method. Almost every technique can easily be done at home as needed, to relieve pain, and open up body cleansing and healing channels.

Acupressure is a two-step process. **Step one** is finding the right pressure point. They are tiny — only about the size of a pin-head — so this may be more difficult than it seems. If you can't find the exact spot on your body at first, poke around a bit — acupressure points are generally more tender than the surrounding area. **Step two** is massaging the point properly. Use the tip of your index finger, your middle finger, or both side by side. In some spots, it may be easier to use your thumb. The point should be stimulated as deeply as can be managed — in a digging kind of massage. A few seconds of pressure, repeated several times, will often be enough. You should push until you feel some discomfort.

For optimum benefits, two acupressure points may be simultaneously stimulated at the same time, one with each hand, while the part of the body in between is stretched to effect maximum energy flow between the points. Or, one can duplicate the pressure on both sides of the body. Immediately after finding and massaging the point on one side, repeat the technique on the opposite side. In most cases, points only need to be triggered about 15 seconds each to get prompt relief.

Almost invariably, you'll experience reactions to an acupressure treatment that will let you know you've "hit the spot." Within about 30 seconds of triggering a point, you should feel warmness in that spot and perhaps slight dizziness or a light-headed feeling. Some people report getting a clammy feeling across the brow or shoulders, breaking out in a sweat, or feeling "electricity" emanating from the acupressure point. These types of reactions are signs that you have found a channel point that needed unblocking and you should feel relief.

Successful acupressure can be tricky. If you don't experience relief, it may mean one of two things:
1: You did not pinpoint the correct spot. Try another one or try again. Make sure you feel the twinge when you probe and press.
2: You didn't perform the procedure correctly. Remember to use the tip of your thumb or finger, and to apply enough pressure for enough time.

Here are acupressure techniques for common health problems:
—For a sore back, press on the points on either side of the lower spine. (Look for the spot just around the corner from your bottom rib.) Press both sides simultaneously.
—For a backache, apply pressure just below the tailbone.
—For low back pain, apply strong pressure in the middle of the dip on the sides of your buttocks. For the best results, apply pressure to each side simultaneously.
—For a headache, press the point between your eyes.
—For insomnia, press two points, right at the natural hairline on either side of the spine.

—For a sore throat, press the center of your forehead about midway between the eyebrows and the natural hairline. Massage the point until the acupressure reaction occurs.

—For lower abdomen discomfort, such as bowel disorders or indigestion, run your thumb up the inner, rear edge of the shin bone directly in line with your ankle bone toward the knee. At about 3" up, you'll feel the unmistakable tingling that announces the point.

—For weight loss, locate the cleft between the bottom of the nose and top of the upper lip. Pinch it when you're hungry, and within moments your hunger will be gone.

Acupressure is an individualized approach to healing.

A skilled acupressurist works with you as an individual to treat body deficiencies and excesses. The trust of the client is integral to the success of a professional acupressure treatment. An acupressurist must ask the body's permission to his job. He then is able to relax and release blocked body meridians and correctly redistribute body chi. Both acute and chronic blockages are treated. Acute blockages are sensitive and may be hot or inflamed. Chronic blockages are more difficult to find, are cool to the touch, and the body may have adapted new habits (like limping or slouching) to keep from feeling them.

More acupressure benefits: Acupressure can improve cardiovascular disease and reduce depression. It corrects debilitating back pain, organ congestion, and, in some cases, even reverses serious problems like scoliosis. It is especially helpful when used as part of a detoxification program. Acupressure specifically cleanses the lymphatic system of toxins and fluids related to cellulite formation and immune system malfunction. (Have at least 3 acupressure treatments before an acupressure lymphatic release to strengthen elimination organs like the liver, kidneys, bladder, lungs and large intestines.)

By rebalancing body chi, acupressure can slow down aging and enhance beauty. Poor chi affects circulation, elimination, muscular tone and stresses the nervous system, all factors which affect the aging process. An acupressure facial treatment delivers oxygen to skin cells, and increases blood and lymph circulation. Improvements in skin tone, fine lines, sagging tissue or dark circles under the eyes are often reported after one month of acupressure facial treatments.

Because both acupuncture and acupressure are free of toxins and additive side effects, they have become valuable alternatives for people who used to live on Motrin, Advil and other pain pills that harm the liver. Western medicine is just beginning to realize the valuable role of acupressure and acupuncture in disease prevention care. Both methods are also effective for animals, and are often recommended for hip dysplasia and arthritis in large animals.

Acupressure is effective for general preventive care. As with other natural therapies, the aim is to regulate, balance and normalize so the body can function normally. Both acupuncture and acupressure can positively influence the course of a therapy program, and should be considered as a means of mobilizing a person's own healing energy and balance. Organ massage, reflexology and deep breathing techniques are frequently used in conjunction with acupressure. Surgery and drugs can often be avoided, and there are sometimes spectacular results. In addition, conventional doctors find that acupuncture and acupressure work well *in conjunction with* conventional medicine, an unusual benefit for western medicine.

Need to find a good acupressurist? Call the Acupressure Institute, (510) 845-1059.

33

Applied Kinesiology

Applied kinesiology is a Traditional Chinese Medicine technique now being enthusiastically rediscovered in America. The word kinesiology means the study of motion, especially the way muscles actually move our bodies. In the natural health field, kinesiology uses principles from Chinese medicine, acupressure and massage to bring the body into balance and release pain and tension.

Muscle testing is the way most Americans are familiar with applied kinesiology today. Applied kinesiology is based on the premise that muscles, glands, and organs are linked by meridians, or energy pathways throughout the body. Muscle testing is an effective method for detecting and correcting energy movements and imbalances in the body.

Muscle testing detects energy blocks.

Weak muscles indicate an energy flow blockage in one of the body's meridians. Muscle testing reliably identifies weak muscles. A kinesiologist uses stress release techniques to unblock the meridians. The muscles are then retested after visualization, massage techniques and movement exercises; if the muscles have regained strength, the restoration of the energy flow of the meridians is confirmed. Kinesiology does not heal, but rather restores balanced energy flow.

You can use personal muscle testing to determine your own individual response to a food or substance. It's a good technique to use before buying a healing remedy, because it lets you estimate the product's effectiveness for your own body before you buy. You will need a partner for the procedure.

Here's how to use muscle testing:

1: Hold your arm out straight from your side, parallel to the ground. Have a partner place one hand just below your shoulder and one hand on your forearm. Your partner then tries to force your arm down towards your side, while you exert all your strength to hold it level. Unless you are in ill health, you should easily be able to withstand this pressure and keep your arm level.

2: Then, simply hold the item that you desire to test against your diaphragm (under the breastbone) or thyroid (the point where the collarbone comes together below the neck). The item may be in or out of normal packaging, or in its raw state, like a fresh food.

3: Holding the item as above, put your arm out straight from your side as before and have your partner try to press it down again. If the test item is beneficial for you, your arm will retain its strength, and your partner will be unable to force it down. If the item is not beneficial, or would worsen your condition, your arm can be easily pushed down by your partner.

You can't save life.
You can't store it up, or hoard it,
or put it in a vault.
You've got to dive in and taste it.
The more you use it,
the more you'll have.
It's a miracle.

Hand and Foot Reflexology

Reflexology is an ancient massage therapy science that works with the body's energy zones through the hands and feet. It's based on the belief that each part of the body is interconnected through the nerve system to specific points on the feet and hands. A history of foot massage spans time and place from the Physician's Tomb in Egypt of 2300 B.C. to the Physicians Temple in Nara, Japan of 700 A.D. The ancient Egyptians are believed to have actually developed hand and foot reflexology.

The science of reflexology believes that all body parts have energy and share information. Pressure to a particular meridian point brings about better function in all parts of that meridian zone, no matter how remote the point is from the body part in need of healing. Thus, reflexology can also be used for a measure of self-diagnosis and treatment.

Reflexology is often known as zone therapy. Reflexologists look at the feet as a mini-map of the entire body, with the big toes serving as the head, the balls of the feet representing the shoulders, and the narrowing of the foot as the waist area. Ten reflexology zone meridians have been extensively mapped connecting all organs and glands, and culminating in points in the hands and feet. The nervous system is considered an electrical system. Contact can be made through the feet and hands with the electro-mechanical zones in the body to the nerve endings. The nerve endings are called reflex points. The points on the feet are reflexive, like a knee-jerk reaction. They serve as reflexes for the entire body. Any illness, injury or tension in the body produces tenderness in the corresponding foot zone. The points are manipulated to open blocked energy pathways.

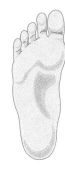

Stress is involved in over 80% of all illness. Reflexology helps the body heal itself by relaxing stress. Its goal is to clear the pathways of energy flow throughout the body, to return body balance, and increase immune response. It does this by stimulating the lymphatic system to eliminate wastes, and the blood to circulate easily to poorly functioning areas. Today, reflexology treatments are used for pain relief, and for faster recovery from injuries or illness without surgery or heavy medication.

Reflexologists rely on an inchworm-like massage motion of the thumb to produce light or deep pressure on each zone, concentrating on the tender spots, which often feel like little grains of salt under the skin.

For your own use, picture your hands and feet as your body's control panels. Get a good reflexology chart — available in health food stores. Then use your fingers or a rounded-end tool to locate the reflex points. Some points take practice to pinpoint. The best rule for knowing when you have reached the right spot is that it is usually very tender, denoting crystalline deposits brought about by poor capillary circulation of fluids, or congestion in the corresponding organ. The amount of soreness on the foot point normally indicates the size of the crystalline deposit, and the amount of time it has been accumulating. For most people, the tenderness is usually accompanied by an immediate feeling of relief in the body organ area as waste deposits break up for removal.

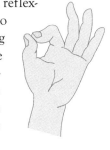

For effective reflexology, press on a reflex point 3 times for 10 seconds each time. Fifteen pounds of applied force on a reflex point is enough to send a surge of energy to remove the obstructive crystals, restore circulation and clear congestion. Use the pressure treatment for twenty to thirty minute sessions at a time, about twice a week. Sessions more often than this will not give nature the chance to use the stimulation or do its necessary repair work. Most people notice frequent and easy bowel movements in the first twenty-four hours after reflexology as the body throws off released wastes.

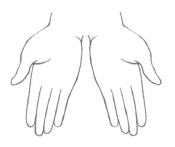

One of the best ways to become familiar with reflexology is to picture your hands and feet as your body's control panels, then locate the match on your hands and feet with the "foot" and "hand" diagrams on the ailment pages in HEALTHY HEALING. The drawings are designed to show the pressure points for each area, so that you can use reflexology to release energy blocks in your body. In some cases, the points are very tiny, particularly for the glands. They will take practice to pinpoint.

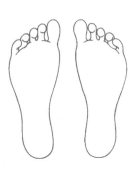

Reflexology can also be part of a good health maintenance program. You don't have to be sick to appreciate the benefits. Many people simply enjoy the tension release a session gives.

Here are some of the documented health benefits of reflexology therapy:
— **Reduces PMS.** A study published in 1993 in the journal *Obstetrics and Gynecology* finds women suffering from premenstrual syndrome experience a 40% reduction in symptoms after using reflexology treatments.
— **Improves asthma.** One case study reports a significant improvement in well being and reduction in asthma symptoms after three months of reflexology therapy.
— **Helps balance blood sugar in cases of type 2 diabetes.** Two different studies (one from China; the other from America) reveal reflexology effectively lowers high blood sugar levels in diabetics.
— **Helps restore some movement and sensation for people paralyzed from spinal cord injuries.** Case studies published in the journal *Reflexions* find some quadriplegic and paraplegic patients respond to reflexology sessions with movement. Other effects noted: some return of bowel and bladder control; induced sweating below the level of the injury; the sensation of bowel rumbling, improved muscle tone; and a decrease in bladder infections.

More:
— Medical doctor Julian Whitaker reports in his book, *199 Health Secrets*, that just two weeks of reflexology treatment helped remove a ganglion cyst on his hand.
— May help dissolve ovarian cysts. Professional reflexologist Christopher Shirley recounts the story of two women scheduled for surgery to remove ovarian cysts who experienced a mysterious disappearance of the cysts (documented by sonograms) after reflexology treatments.

> *You always have your whole life ahead of you.*
>
> —Bill Bryson

Aromatherapy

Did you know that plants have an electrical frequency? Essential plant oils carry a bio-electrical frequency expressed as hertz. Many of us today understand megahertz rates from our computers and electronic equipment. Plants have a frequency from 0 to 15Hz.; dry herbs have a frequency from 15 to 22Hz.; fresh herbs have a frequency 20 to 27Hz.; essential plant oils start at 52Hz and go to 320Hz.

Your body has an electrical hertz frequency, too. A healthy body has a frequency between 62 to 78Hz. Disease frequency rates begin at 58Hz. A higher frequency rate destroys an entity of lower frequency. Based on this knowledge, it's easy to see that certain high frequency essential oils can create an environment in which disease, bacteria, viruses and fungus cannot live.

Aromatherapy actually heals through bioelectrical frequency. In fact, a majority of essential oils can affect pathogenic organisms that are resistant to chemical antibiotics. They may turn out to be a good choice for overcoming today's virulent super germs.

Volatile liquids distilled from plants are the heart of aromatherapy. They are the plant's essential oils, the regenerating, oxygenating immune defense of the plant, and they act in plants much like hormones do in humans. Seventy-five to 100 times more concentrated than dried herbs and flowers, aromatherapy oils are some of the most potent herbal medicines. The molecules of essential aromatherapy oils carry healing nutrients to your body's cells.

Essential oils are not oily. They are non-oily, highly active fluids. They may be taken in by inhalation, steams and infusers, or applied topically to the skin. The therapeutic effects of essential oils are due both to their pharmacological properties and to their small molecule size, which allows easy penetration through the skin, the walls of the blood vessels, the lymph system and body tissues — pathways that impact the body's organ, hormonal, nervous and immune systems.

Essential oils affect people first through the **sense of smell.** Smell is the most rapid of all your senses because its information is directly re-layed to the hypothalamus. Motivation, moods, emotions and creativity all begin in the hypothala-mus, so odors affect them immediately. Some scents enhance your emotional equilibrium merely by inhaling them. Essential oil molecules work through hormone-like chemicals to produce their sensations. So odors influence the glands responsible for hormone levels, metabolism, insulin and stress levels, sex drive, body temperature and appetite.

Scents are also intimately intertwined with thought and memory. Studies on brain-waves show that scents like lavender increase alpha brain waves associated with relaxation; scents like jasmine boost beta waves linked to alertness.

Essential oils have many healing applications. For example, their value for detoxification is quite powerful. When an oil with detoxification properties is applied, certain toxins appear to be cleared from the body. Toxins such as free radicals, heavy metals, fungi, bacteria, viruses and cell wastes actually attach to the essential oil and are then excreted from the body via the skin, kidneys, urine, lungs and bowels.

Here are some other ways essential oils assist healing:

—They stimulate immune response, invigorating the production of white blood cells, and increasing the activity of T-cells, NK-cells, alveolar macrophages and serum antibodies. A new study shows all essential oils stimulate phagocytosis, the ability of white blood cells to devour harmful invading microbes.

—The molecules of essential oils have an electromagnetic charge that influences, and balances the charge on our cell magnetic fields, effective for healing.

—They are natural antioxidants which destroy free radicals and boost the body's resistance to harmful pathogens of all kinds.

—Essential oils have antibiotic properties, but each oil is effective against different pathogens. For example, tests show thyme oil, with the component thymol, is a powerful antibiotic agent against micro-organisms in candida and thrush infections. Oregano oil helps against seasonal allergies and respiratory infections.

—They cleanse the body by stimulating sluggish circulation to bring oxygen and nutrients to the tissues, and by accelerating disposal of carbon dioxide and other waste products.

—They act as blood purifiers and normalizers, generally decreasing blood stickiness. For example, rose oil helps counteract the toxic blood effects of alcohol. A rose oil and yarrow combination helps normalize a system invaded by pollen and spore allergens.

—They improve the efficiency of the lymph system, especially the body's drainage ducts, for better elimination of metabolic residues and toxins. For example, juniper oil enhances the filtration action of the kidneys.

—Eucalyptus, fennel, frankincense, ginger, peppermint and pine, are expectorants that stimulate the removal of heavy mucous from the lungs and bronchial tubes.

—Citrus oils like lemon, orange or grapefruit help fluid retention. Juniper, sandalwood and cypress release fluid wastes and cellulite. Rose oil and rosemary help normalize body chemistry, particularly against allergens. Thyme oil is an anti-fungal; marjoram promotes blood flow; cedarwood promotes lymph activity. Vetiver and cypress stimulate circulation.

—Lemon, peppermint, rosemary and thyme enhance immunity.

—Orange, juniper berry, basil and cinnamon leaf boost energy.

—Grapefruit, lavender, cypress, basil and juniper berry improve skin tone.

Most essential oils offer the best results delivered through the skin in a massage or bath oil. For best results, mix about 15 drops to 4-oz. of a carrier oil like sweet almond, sunflower, jojoba or a favorite massage oil.

Aromatherapy & Stress

Essential oils are best known for counteracting stress, with properties which can affect the mind and emotions to calm, sedate or uplift.

The immediate and profound effect of essential oils on the central nervous system makes aromatherapy an excellent method for stress management. Aromatherapy also makes us feel good in part by releasing certain mood-inducing neurochemicals in our brains. Aromatherapy relieves stress by promoting mental relaxation and alertness, quality sleep, physical relaxation, and by increasing overall energy.

How does Aromatherapy work?

How many times have you smelled something like a perfume or a food and had the taste of it instantly in your mouth? The volatile molecules of the perfume or food enter your nose and can be tasted in your mouth. Aromatherapy's oils effect different people in different ways, on different levels. Aroma itself is only one of the active healing qualities.

When inhaled, the odors stimulate a release of neurotransmitters, chemicals responsible for pleasant feelings and pain reduction. The aromas of apples and cinnamon, for example, have a powerful stabilizing effect on some people, especially those suffering from nervous anxiety. These aromas are even capable of lowering blood pressure, even preventing panic attacks.

Here's how to use aromatherapy:

Add a few drops of essential oil into a carrier oil such as almond, jojoba or a favorite massage oil. Use a diffuser or lamp, or a steam inhaler to ease respiratory distress. When inhaled into the lungs, molecules of essential oils attach to oxygen molecules, enter the bloodstream and journey throughout the body with therapeutic activity. Oils evaporate easily and completely. They don't leave marks on your clothing or towels.

1: Always dilute essential oils in a carrier oil, such as almond, apricot, canola or jojoba oil, before applying them. Essential oils are highly concentrated. Even one drop of pure essential oil applied directly to your skin may cause irritation.

2: Uncap oil bottles for a few seconds only or they'll escape. Drop oils into the palm of your hand for blending. Keep bottles tightly capped, away from sunlight and heat when not in use.

3: Follow the directions for aromatherapy blends carefully. Never add more than the recommended number of drops. When using essential oils on infants or children, dilute them.

4: Use glass containers for all blends of essential oils. Oils can damage plastic containers.

5: Don't shake essential oils. Just gently roll the bottle between your hands.

6: Inhale essential oils for short periods only; run a diffuser for only 5 to 10 minutes at a time.

7: If you experience any irritation, sensitivity, or reaction, discontinue use of the suspect oil.

8: Don't take essential oils internally, except as directed by a professional.

Note: As always, people with certain medical conditions should be cautious. Some essential oils can trigger asthma attacks or epileptic seizures in susceptible people. Some can elevate or depress blood pressure. Consult a health care professional if you have any of these conditions. Essential oils may also diminish the effectiveness of homeopathic remedies. Check with a homeopathic physician.

Reducing stress is an aromatherapy specialty

I've included some of the most popular essential aromatherapy oils you can use for stress relief and for energizing. Certain essential oils have a normalizing effect on the nervous system. For example, bergamot (geranium oil) either stimulates or sedates according to the needs of the individual.

Calming, relaxing essential oils to reduce stress:

—**Lavender:** induces sleep, exerts a calming and relaxing effect, alleviates stress, reduces depression, tension and hyperactivity. Can also be used to calm animals. Balances nerves and emotions. Pain relief for headaches. Calms the heart and lowers high blood pressure. Rub on stomach for painful menstrual periods. A tonic for the hair.

—**Marjoram:** calms anxiety. A warming analgesic for pain, stiff joints, colds, asthma, painful periods. A tonic for the heart, lowers high blood pressure. Promotes blood flow in skin. *Note:* Take a break after one month of usage.

—**Sandalwood:** relaxes; it's good for meditation and sleep. Stimulates immune response. Massage oil over the kidney area for cystitis and kidney problems. Healing and moisturizing for cracked and dry skin; relieves itching and inflammation. Many call sandalwood an aphrodisiac.

—**Clary sage:** calms edgy nerves, brings feelings of well-being, lifts the mind and reduces stress. A hormone balancer, sage is helpful for PMS cramps and muscle spasms. Useful for all types of skin inflammations and for aging skin and wrinkles.

Stress reduction and relaxation recipes:

• **Soothing Massage Oil:** to 2 ounces sweet almond oil, add 4 drops bergamot oil, 4 drops chamomile oil, 4 drops lavender oil, 4 drops sandalwood oil, 2 drops coriander oil and 2 drops frankincense oil.

• **Anti-Stress Diffuser Oil:** combine 15 drops lavender oil, 10 drops sage oil, 10 drops elemi oil, 10 drops geranium oil, 8 drops bergamot oil, 8 drops orange oil, 8 drops jasmine oil, 6 drops ylang ylang oil and 5 drops coriander oil. Add a few drops to your diffuser or lamp bowl.

Essential oils for Depression:

—**Bergamot:** an uplifting anti-depressant; relaxes nervous system; good for anxiety. Eases digestion. Helps with eczema, psoriasis and acne. An antiseptic for wounds and urinary tract infections. *Precautions:* may cause photosensitivity. Avoid hot sun right after use on skin.

—**Geranium:** both a stimulant and calmer, depending on the body's need. Acts as an antidepressant and tonic to the nervous system to reduce stress. Helpful in overcoming addictions. Helps the pituitary gland to regulate endocrine and hormone balance. Helps menopause, PMS and through its astringent action, stems heavy periods. Enhances circulation to the skin, eczema, burns and shingles. *Precautions:* Avoid during pregnancy. It's a good skin cleanser, but test first for skin sensitivity.

—**Lemon:** uplifting to the psyche. Cleanses and refreshes the skin (good for oily skin conditions).

—**Neroli:** relieves stress, depression, anxiety, nervous tension and insomnia. Helps headaches. A heart tonic, improves circulation and helps nerve pain. Useful for dry, sensitive skin.

—**Jasmine:** uplifting, soothing, very good for depression; a hormone balancer, known for its erogenous quality. Helpful for menstrual pain and uterine disorders. Helpful for respiratory difficulties, bronchial spasms, catarrh, cough and hoarseness. Especially good for dry and sensitive skin.

—**Ylang Ylang:** uplifts the mood, eases anxiety, diminishes depression, eases feelings of anger, shock, panic and fear. Balances women's hormones. Helps high blood pressure and insomnia. Balances sebum flow to stimulate the scalp for hair growth.

Essential oils for energizing and motivating:

Peppermint energizes while easing headaches. Ginger and fennel stimulate circulation from your heart to your fingertips. Rose influences hormonal activity and glandular function.

—**Lavender:** can either stimulate or sedate, according to one's physiological needs. (see previous page).

—**Cypress:** calms irritability, and stress reactions like sweating. Balances body fluids, and helps release cellulite. Helps nose bleeds, heavy periods and incontinence. Soothes sore throats. An astringent for oily skin, hemorrhoids and varicose veins. *Precautions:* Avoid in pregnancy.

—**Ginger:** sharpens senses and aids memory. Helps settle the digestive system, colds, flu and reduces fever. Helps motion sickness, nausea, gas and pain. Add to massage rubs for rheumatic pains and bone injuries, sores and bruises. *Precautions:* May irritate skin.

—**Rosemary:** encourages intuition, enlivens the brain, clears the head and enhances memory. For exhaustion, weakness and lethargy. A sinus decongestant. Pain relieving properties for arthritis or gout. A heart tonic, normalizes low blood pressure. Avoid during pregnancy, with high blood pressure or epilepsy.

Energy stimulation recipes:

•**Revitalizing Body Oil:** mix, then massage into skin in the morning, 2 ounces sweet almond oil, 6 drops lavender oil, 4 drops rosemary oil, 3 drops geranium oil, 3 drops orange oil, 2 drops coriander oil, 2 drops patchouli oil.

•**Invigorating Inhalant Oil:** in a small glass bottle, combine 8 drops rosemary oil, 6 drops cinnamon oil, 4 drops peppermint oil, 3 drops basil oil, 1 drop ginger oil. Inhale directly from the bottle.

•**Fatigue-Busting Diffuser Oil:** in a glass bottle, combine 15 drops rosemary oil, 12 drops cedar oil, 10 drops <u>each</u> lavender and lemon oil, 2 drops peppermint oil. Add a few drops to your diffuser.

•**Rejuvenating Bath:** to your bath add 4 drops rosemary oil, 2 drops each orange and thyme oil.

Note: The essential oils and blends in the aromatherapy section can be obtained from your health food store or Wyndmere Naturals 153 Ashley Road, Hopkins, MN 55343, 800-207-8538.

Flower Essence Therapy

Flower essences are part of an emerging field of life-enhancing subtle therapies, that work through human energy fields to address issues of emotional health and mind-body well-being. Even though it's new in America, the healing art of flower essences has struck a responsive chord in almost every healing discipline — medical and health practitioners, homeopaths, massage therapists, chiropractors, psychotherapists, counsellors, dentists and veterinarians.

Like homeopathy and acupuncture, flower essences are exceptions to western type science. Also like homeopathic remedies, flower essences are highly diluted from a physical point of view. Yet they are powerful healers, *potentiated* vibrational tinctures from the patterns of biomagnetic energies discharged by flowers.

Flowers are the highest concentration of the life force in a plant, the crowning experience of its growth. Flower essences are captured at the highest moment of the plant unfolding in blossom. The essence is generally prepared from a sun infusion of blossoms in a bowl of water, which is potentiated, then preserved with brandy.

The application of flower essences for specific emotions and attitudes was developed by Dr. Edward Bach, an English physician and homeopath in the 1930's. Bach's research showed that flowers discharge identifiable patterns of biomagnetic energies that can be harnessed for healing power through emotional balance. Bach's work on the relationship of stress to disease showed that the link between the mind and body is most evident during stressful times. He also showed the significance of destructive emotions like depression, hate and fear.

Bach was one of the first modern healers to realize that true healing means the manifestation of one's higher spiritual force. He saw that emotional balance strengthened the body's ability to resist disease and he used flower essences as a healing tool to assist in that balance. In the last decade, modern medicine is also beginning to see the connection between negative emotions and lower disease resistance. *"What Bach was doing with his vibrational essences was working to increase his patients' resistance by creating internal harmony and an amplification of the higher energetic systems that connect human beings to their higher selves." Richard Gerber, M.D. Vibrational Medicine.*

Bach was able to document scientifically the clinical criteria that is still used today in flower essence research. His compound, **Rescue Remedy**, is the most widely used flower essence — a gentle, effective remedy which restores emotional balance during stress or anxiety. It can also be used in emergency situations or at any time of upset, shock or trauma, like impending events which produce anxiety. RESCUE REMEDY contains essence of cherry plum for fear of losing control, clematis for resignation and fatalism, impatiens for anxiousness, rock rose for panic, and star of Bethlehem for fright. *(Nelson Bach, Wilmington Technology Park, 100 Research Drive, Wilmington MA 01887-4406, 800-319-9151.)*

Holistic Recovery From Surgery

When your body is in crisis, orthodox medicine is at its best in a heroic role. It is emergency intervention technology that can stabilize a crisis condition, or arrest a life-threatening disease long enough to give your body an opportunity to fight, a chance to heal itself. But surgery and major medical treatments are always traumatic on the body. Take healing steps **before and after** your surgery to strengthen your system, alleviate body stress, and increase your chances of rapid recovery and healing.

Pre-op techniques strengthen your body for surgery
Starting 2 to 3 weeks before your scheduled surgery:

Strengthen your immune system and supply your body with healing nutrients. Include daily:
—Extra vegetable protein. You must have protein to heal. Eat brown rice, other whole grains and sea greens.
—Vitamin C 3000mg with bioflavonoids and rutin for tissue integrity.
—B Complex 100mg with pantothenic acid 500mg for adrenal strength.
—A multivitamin/mineral with anti-oxidants, beta-carotene, zinc, calcium and magnesium for tissue repair.
—Take a full spectrum, pre-digested amino acid compound drink, about 1000mg daily.
—OPC's, pycnogenol or grape seed, 50mg 2x daily, as powerful antioxidants.
—Garlic capsules, 4-6 daily, a natural antibiotic that enhances immune function.

Strengthen your ability to heal. Include daily:
—Bromelain 750mg twice daily (with Quercetin 250mg if you expect inflammation).
—CoQ-10, 60mg 2x daily and/or germanium 150mg capsules, 2x daily - as free radical destroyers.
—CHLORELLA 15 tablets, 1 packet of powder, or Crystal Star ENERGY GREEN™ drink for chlorophyll.
—Centella asiatica (gotu kola) capsules, 2 caps 2x daily for nerve tissue strength.
—Crystal Star GINSENG SIX SUPER™ tea, 2x daily for recuperation strength.
—Vitamin K for blood clotting. Food sources: leafy greens, blackstrap molasses, alfalfa sprouts.
—Take a potassium juice (page 215), a potassium supplement liquid, or a protein-mineral drink daily.

Note 1: The medical community uses information and testing results from synthetic, rather than naturally-occurring vitamin E sources, like wheat germ and soy. Thus, many doctors insist that no vitamin E be taken four weeks prior to surgery in an effort to curb post-operative bleeding. I have not found this to be a problem with natural vitamin E, but suggest that you consult your physician if you are in doubt.

Note 2: Immediately prior to surgery, take a pinch of ginger powder (or 8 - 10 drops ginger extract) in water to relieve nausea after surgery. Don't take garlic 2 to 3 days before surgery (it's a slight blood thinner.)

Post-Op techniques for recovery when you come home.

Eat a very nutritious diet. Include frequently:
—AloeLife ALOE GOLD drink, one 8-oz. glass daily.
—A potassium broth (page 215), or a vegetable drink (page 218).
—A protein drink such as Nature's Life SUPERGREEN PRO 96, or Nutri-Tech ALL ONE multi drink.
—Plenty of fresh fruits and vegetables. **Have a green salad every day.**
—Daily sushi (at least 6 pieces), or sea greens for vitamin B_{12} and new cell growth.
—Brown rice and other whole grains with tofu for protein complementarity and more B vitamins.
—Yogurt and other cultured foods for friendly intestinal flora.

Accelerate Healing After Surgery

Herbal combinations can contribute a great deal to the success of surgery – nurturing, normalizing, and supporting healing.

Here are specific systems that herbs can help in healing:
- **Cardiovascular System and Blood Vessels** - *hawthorn, garlic and ginkgo*
- **Respiratory System** - *mullein and coltsfoot*
- **Digestive System** - *chamomile and lemon balm*
- **Glandular System** - *panax ginseng*
- **Bowel/Urinary System** - *corn silk* for the bladder; *yellow dock* for the bowel
- **Reproductive System** - women: *black cohosh, false unicorn root.* men: *saw palmetto and damiana*
- **Nervous System** - *oats and St. John's wort*
- **Musculo-Skeletal System** - *aloe vera, oatstraw, sarsaparilla*
- **Skin** - *sea vegetables, nettles, red clover, and calendula, St. John's wort* oil or cream for scarring
- **Immune System** - *nettles, cleavers, red clover*
- **Drug and Liver detoxification** - *milk thistle seed*

Note: Certain foods may interfere with medications. Dairy foods and iron supplements interfere with some antibiotics. Acid fruits (oranges, pineapples and grapefruit) may inhibit the action of penicillin and aspirin. Avocados, bananas, cheese, chocolate, colas and fermented foods interfere with monoamine oxidase (mao), an anti-depressant, hypertension drug. Avoid fatty foods before and after surgery; they slow nutrient assimilation.

Clean the body and vital organs, to counteract infection. Include daily for one month:
—High potency, multi-culture compound such as DOCTOR DOPHILUS, or Natren TRINITY with meals.
—Crystal Star LIV-ALIVE™ capsules, tea or extract.
—Crystal Star GINSENG/REISHI MUSHROOM extract to clear toxicity and provide deep body tone.
—Bovine cartilage capsules 6 daily, or colloidal silver, 1 teasp. for 1 week, then $^1/_2$ teasp., to fight infection.
—Enzyme therapy such as Rainbow Light DETOX-ZYME or Prevail VITASE.
—Fresh carrot juice, or one can of BE WELL juice daily.

Build up the body tissues. Include daily for one month:
—Crystal Star SYSTEMS STRENGTH™ drink, and BODY REBUILDER™ with ADR-ACTIVE™ caps.
—Vitamin C with bioflavonoids and rutin 500mg only, with pantothenic acid 1000mg.
—Carnitine 250mg with CoQ-10, 60mg 3x daily as antioxidants.
—Zinc 30-50mg, Futurebiotics VITAL K potassium, or Flora VEGE-SIL to help rebuild tissue.
—Co-enzymate B complex sublingual, 1 tablet 3x daily, or Nature's Bounty B_{12} INTERNASAL GEL.
—Enzymatic Therapy LIQUID LIVER capsules, or Crystal Star CHLORELLA-GINSENG extract.
—AloeLife ALOE SKIN GEL or Crystal Star ANTI-BIO™ gel to heal skin and scars.

Other recovery and recuperation information:
—If you are taking antibiotics, take them with bromelain 750mg for better effectiveness, and supplement with B Complex, Vitamin C, Vitamin K and calcium.
—If you are taking diuretics, add Vitamin C, potassium and B complex, to strengthen kidneys.
—If you are taking aspirin, take with vitamin C for best results.
—If you are taking antacids, supplement with Vitamin B_1 and/or calcium.
—If your surgery involved bone and cartilage, take Crystal Star MINERAL SPECTRUM™ capsules 4 daily.
—If you smoke, add Vitamin C 500mg, E 400IU, beta-carotene 50,000IU and niacin 100mg.
—If you are considering chelation therapy, remember that it works in your body like a magnet collecting heavy metals and triglycerides. It is not recommended if you have weak kidneys; too many toxins are dumped into the elimination system too fast, causing stress on a healing body. Consider FORMULA 1 by Golden Pride.

Normalize Your Body After Chemotherapy & Radiation

Chemotherapy and radiation treatments are widely used by conventional medicine for several types, stages and degrees of cancerous growth. While some partial successes have been proven, the effects of both treatments are often worse than the disease in terms of healthy cell damage, body imbalance, and reduced immunity. Doctors and therapists recognize the drawbacks to chemotherapy, but under current government and insurance restrictions, neither they nor their patients have alternatives.

Amazingly even with all the new information on alternative methods, new procedure success stories and even new drugs, surgery, chemotherapy, radiation and a few extremely strong drugs are still the only protocols approved by the FDA in the United States for malignant disease. The cost for these treatments is beyond the financial range of most people, who, along with physicians and hospitals must rely on health insurance to pay the expense. Medical insurance will not reimburse doctors or hospitals if they use other healing methods. Thus, exorbitant medical costs and special interest regulations have bound medical professionals, hospitals, and insurance companies in a vicious circle where no alternative or new measures may be used to control cancer. Everyone, including the patient, is caught in a political web where it comes down to money instead of health. This is doubly unfortunate, since there is advanced research and health care choice easily available in Europe and other countries to which Americans are denied access.

Scientists admit that current treatments have been pushed to their limits. But new testing and research are extremely expensive. Even today, the vast majority of funds provided by the National Cancer Act support research to improve the effectiveness of *existing* therapies — radiation, surgery and chemotherapy. This practice is easier and cheaper, but it leaves patients with the same three therapies, just a more precise use of them. Even when a new treatment is substantiated, there is no reasonable investment certainty that government (and therefore health insurance) approval can be obtained through the maze of red tape and politics.

Some of this is changing as cancer patients refuse to become victims of their medical system as well as the disease. The American people are demanding access, funding and insurance approval for alternative health techniques and medicines. Slowly, state by state, especially in the western states, legislators and regulators are listening, health care parameters are expanding, and insurance limitations are becoming more inclusive.

Conventional medicine rarely treats cancer as a systemic illness, defining it only by location and symptomology. It's the way lab science and our left brains work, breaking things down into one-for-one causes and effects, assaying, isolating, identifying.... in consequence, hardly ever looking at the whole person or the whole picture.

By contrast, alternative healers regard cancer as an unhealthy body whose defenses can no longer destroy abnormal cells. Naturopaths believe that a healthy body with strong immune response does not develop cancer, and that cancer is a reflection of the body as a whole rather than a localized disease in one part. Alternative therapists seek to strengthen the immune system of the cancer patient, and generally shun highly toxic modalities like radiation and chemotherapy. They use a multifaceted, non-toxic approach, incorporating treatments which rely on bio-chemistry, metabolic, nutritional and herbal therapies, and immune enhancement.

You can help your body clean out drug residues, minimize damage to healthy cells, rebuild strength after chemotherapy and radiation, and get over the side effects.

For three months after chemotherapy or radiation, take the following daily:
—Crystal Star SYSTEMS STRENGTH™ broth — 1 TB. in 8-oz. hot water.
—CoQ_{10} capsules, 60mg 3x daily, and/or germanium 150mg daily.
—Vitamin C crystals with bioflavonoids, $1/4$ teasp. in liquid every hour, about 5 to 10,000 mg daily.
—GINSENG/REISHI MUSHROOM extract 2x daily, or 2 cups Crystal Star GINSENG 6 SUPER™ tea.
—800mcg folic acid to normalize DNA synthesis, especially if methotrexate was used in your treatment.
—Ashwagandha 30 drops daily (extract) to rebuild immune white blood cells.

—Floradix HERBAL IRON, 1 teasp. 3x daily, or Crystal Star ENERGY GREEN™ drink to counteract the anemia that causes such extreme fatigue after chemo treatments.
—An herbal anti-inflammatory as needed for swelling —turmeric (curcumin), or Crystal Star ANTI-FLAM™.
—HAWTHORN or GINKGO BILOBA extract, 30 drops daily under the tongue as a circulatory tonic.
—Aloe vera concentrate, like AloeLife ALOE GOLD for detoxification and to ease nausea.
—A liver support capsule or tea, like Crystal Star LIV-ALIVE™ tea or capsules.
—Co-enzymate B complex sublingual, 1 tablet 3x daily for hair regrowth.
—Keep your diet about 60% fresh foods for the first month after chemotherapy.
—Exercise with a morning sun walk and some stretches on rising and retiring.

Facial Surgery Healing Program

We all want to look great at every age. The plastic surgery industry is booming! Face lifts are now the most commonly performed procedure in cosmetic surgery — fifty-three percent of total surgery procedures are for Americans between 51 and 64 years of age.

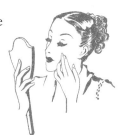

PRE-OP: daily - 2 to 3 weeks before surgery:
—Bromelain 1500mg
—Evening Primrose oil caps 1000mg
—Royal Jelly/Siberian ginseng combination, (best in an extract or tea)
—Ester C - 5000mg with bioflavonoids 500mg
—Vitamin K, sea greens and-or plenty of alfalfa sprouts
—Crystal Star ZINC SOURCE™ extract, POTASSIUM-IODINE and GINSENG SUPER 6 capsules
—Brown rice and a green salad every day
No aspirin or alcohol 1 week before or 2 weeks after surgery. They increase bleeding tendency and reduce healing ability.

POST-OP: pre-suture removal, daily for 1 week: (Apply ice packs every hour to reduce swelling for 3 days)
—Crystal Star ANTI-FLAM™ capsules as needed, for pain relief or swelling
—Bromelain 750 with quercetin 250mg 2x daily, to reduce bruising
—Co-Q10, 60mg 3x daily, for enzyme therapy tissue repair
—Centella Asiatica capsules (gotu kola), for nerve damage repair and reducing numbness
—Ester C - 5000mg w. bioflavonoids for new collagen production, tissue tightening, capillary healing
—Evening Primrose oil caps 1000mg daily, for essential fatty acids
—Royal Jelly-Siberian ginseng combination, for amino acids (protein for healing)
—Vitamin K, sea greens or plenty of alfalfa sprouts, (for bruising and bleeding)
—Brown rice and a green salad every day, for B vitamins (skin) and chlorophyll healing (blood)

POST-OP: post-suture removal, daily for 3 weeks:
—Bromelain 1500mg with Ester C - 5000mg with bioflavonoids daily
—Evening Primrose oil caps 1000mg
—Apply Crystal Star BEAUTIFUL SKIN™ gel and/or AloeLife SKIN GEL, for scar and scab healing
—Royal Jelly-Siberian ginseng tea combination
—CoQ10, 60mg 2x daily and *Centella Asiatica* (gotu kola), capsules by Solaray for nerve restoration
—Brown rice and a green salad every day. Add sea vegetables for skin tone and texture

2 Months later:
—Use a seaweed-aloe vera gel mask if you have had a full face lift: *1 tsp. kelp granules in 1 TB aloe vera gel.*

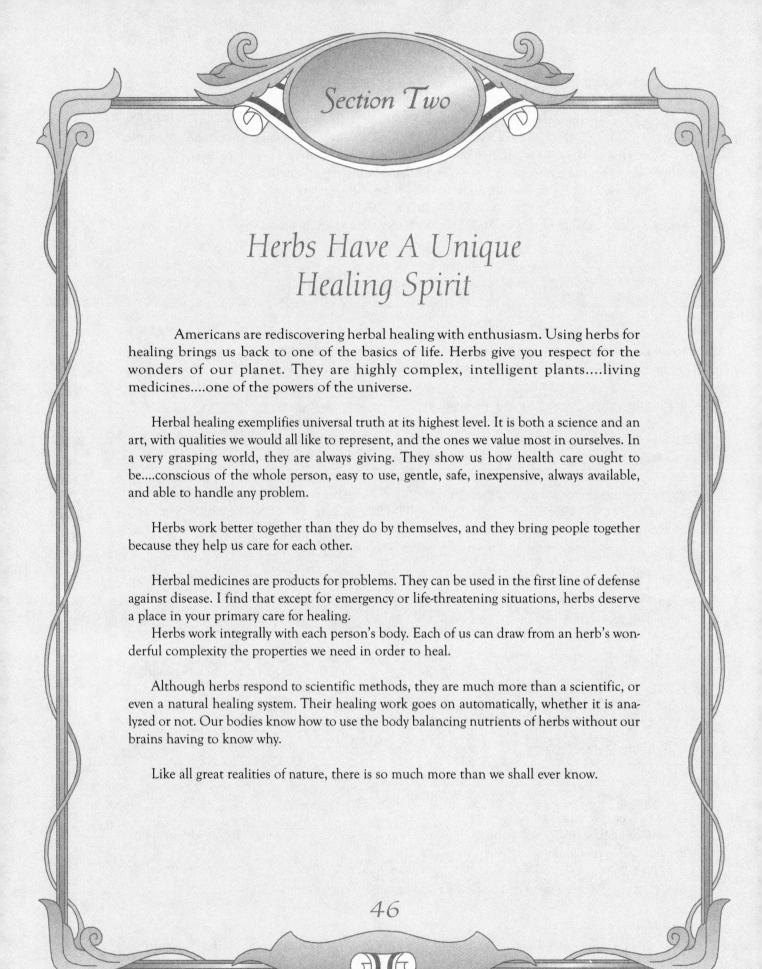

Herbs Have A Unique Healing Spirit

Americans are rediscovering herbal healing with enthusiasm. Using herbs for healing brings us back to one of the basics of life. Herbs give you respect for the wonders of our planet. They are highly complex, intelligent plants....living medicines....one of the powers of the universe.

Herbal healing exemplifies universal truth at its highest level. It is both a science and an art, with qualities we would all like to represent, and the ones we value most in ourselves. In a very grasping world, they are always giving. They show us how health care ought to be....conscious of the whole person, easy to use, gentle, safe, inexpensive, always available, and able to handle any problem.

Herbs work better together than they do by themselves, and they bring people together because they help us care for each other.

Herbal medicines are products for problems. They can be used in the first line of defense against disease. I find that except for emergency or life-threatening situations, herbs deserve a place in your primary care for healing.

Herbs work integrally with each person's body. Each of us can draw from an herb's wonderful complexity the properties we need in order to heal.

Although herbs respond to scientific methods, they are much more than a scientific, or even a natural healing system. Their healing work goes on automatically, whether it is analyzed or not. Our bodies know how to use the body balancing nutrients of herbs without our brains having to know why.

Like all great realities of nature, there is so much more than we shall ever know.

Herbal Healing Today

Medical science is changing fast. How does the tradition of herbal healing fit in? Herbal medicines have been meeting people's medical needs for thousands of years. Clearly, American consumers are enthusiastically increasing their use of herbs as natural complements to drugs and drugstore medicines.

In many ways in America, and indeed around the world, we are in a time of paradigm shift....especially in the global approach to healing. As our world grows undeniably smaller, people are interacting more, and changing long-held beliefs.

We are coming to see the Earth as an intelligent being, evolving and growing. Mankind is also evolving and growing. Unfortunately pathogenic organisms that cause disease, are changing, too — often replicating at enormous rates. Both organisms and diseases are becoming more virulent, and our immune defenses are becoming weaker.

The latest chemical drugs aren't the answer. In fact, it seems that new drugs are becoming less effective against pathogens like powerful viruses, instead of more effective. Recent research shows that even the newest, most powerful antibiotics hardly survive a year before the microbe they were designed to arrest, develops, mutates and grows stronger against them.

It's a good example of a non-living agent like a drug trying to control a living thing.

While we must be respectful of all ways of healing, most of us don't realize we have a choice. All the advances made by modern medicine still don't address chronic sickness or disease prevention very well.

I call today's allopathic medicine "heroic medicine" because it was developed largely in wartime for wartime emergencies. But this type of medicine often hits our systems with a heavy hammer, preventing us from being able to rebuild against slow-growing, degenerative diseases. Drugs can't help our bodies stimulate immune response either. In fact, most drugs, and all surgeries, create body trauma along with their corrective benefits.

Immune strength is where natural, complementary medicines, like herbs and homeopathic compounds are important. Each of us is so individual; our healing supports need to be able to work with us in a personal way for permanent health. Natural remedies involve the cooperation of our own bodies in the healing that takes place. **Herbs let your body do its own work better.**

Herbal medicines are part of a larger wellness picture too, because they are worldwide, alive, big enough and intelligent enough to grow along with us.

I have long believed that herbs are a path to the universe — an eye of the needle through which we can glimpse the wonders of creation and what it's really all about. God shows us his face in herbs, because they seem almost miraculous in their benefits to mankind.

Herbs can perhaps point out a path for us on how we might grow and change in a big world that is becoming a global village. We know we can count on the safety and efficacy of herbs in ways that the latest drug can never achieve. We know that they reach out to us with their marvelous complexity and abilities to help us address the health problems of today, just as they addressed ancient ones. Herbs may be our best hope to bring the balance back between the healing forces and diseases.

Herbs are without a doubt...UNIVERSAL. They do not discriminate, but embrace humans of all sorts and animals of all kinds, with their benefits. While it seems, on a day-to-day basis that we are hopelessly divided — in the end we are all one. Our hopes and dreams are the same.

Herbs help us care for each other. Today, in the natural healing world, I see an astonishing thing happening. Herbs may indeed be a force to bring us together. We may be able to use the diverse, worldwide herbal healing knowledge for the good of us all. Herbal medicines of the old traditions, such as the Ayurvedic philosophy, Native American herbs and rainforest medicines, long thought to work only for the people of their own cultures, are beginning to be used by grateful people everywhere. Even the strong tribal traditions, once so entirely separate, are sharing and combining their knowledge and their herbs.

Integration is most seen in herbal formulas rather than in the ancient traditional practices. Rainforest culture herbs and Native American formulas are good examples. Native American cleansing herbs and techniques such as herbal smudging and therapeutic sweating are also being used to help relieve modern pollution problems.

The West is beginning to use Chinese and Rainforest herbs successfully for Western diseases, even though the healing tradition that originally used them comes from a different viewpoint. Western herbalists are learning how to use time-honored Ayurvedic herbs, in combination with our own herbs, and for our own health problems.

On a recent trip to the Orient, I could see that herbal ideas and formulas are going both ways, as Western herbs flow east to Oriental healers. (Still, I was also surprised to see that many of the Chinese pharmacies, even in the large cities, carry no drugs. According to workers in the pharmacies, their customers don't believe in drugs — only herbs and fortifying animal extracts.)

If man, an intelligent being, is changing, might not herbs, intelligent plants, be changing, too?

Herbs are highly complex, and filled with such long memory. They have intelligently adapted to the Earth's changes as we have, and over the millennia, they have always interacted with man.

Perhaps they are moving along the universal continuum with us.... always available for us, with a highly complex structure able to match our own increasing complexity of need.

Where is herbal healing going from here?

The winds of change are blowing once more as we sit before the new millennium. There is clearly an enormous rebirth of interest in the ways of Nature and holistic healing.

It is not a new idea. As you can see from this short discussion of the world's herbal philosophies, the holistic approach is the prevalent one in all societies except our own. Western herbal thought has taken a detour through technology. Yet useful knowledge has surfaced that otherwise might not have been found. We live in a time when holistic medicine can be supported by scientific studies, and scientific analysis can be validated by its relevance to human lifestyles.

We must put aside the greed and politics that surround our health care, I believe we are at another beginning where modern medical technology and the holistic approach can come together for the good of mankind.

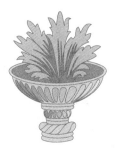

Traditional Chinese Medicine

Traditional Chinese herbal medicine has a 5,000 year legacy. From its earliest history, Chinese medicine has been bound up with nature — the earth and sea, the seasons and climate, plants and animals. Because of the strongly held Chinese belief that the human body is a microcosm of the grand cosmic order, and the forces at work in man are the same as those at work in the universe, all the elements of the earth are significant in traditional Chinese healing. Unity with nature is actually a belief held by all world civilizations up to the time of modern, scientific thought, which sees everything as separate and unrelated, instead of all one.

The basic premise of Chinese herbal medicine revolves around the belief in an essential life-force, called qi. Qi (pronounced "chee") is an ineffable, but vital energy in all things, including man. The food and drink we consume and the air we breathe are the most important factors for human qi. Digestion and breathing extract qi from food and air and transfer it to our bodies. When these two forms of qi meet in the bloodstream, they make human-qi, which circulates through the body as vital energy. The quality, quantity and harmonious balance of your qi determines your state of health and span of life.

Conditions which can upset the balance of qi are climatic factors, emotions, phlegm congestion and stagnant blood. Since variables that affect qi, like the weather and seasonal changes are not controlled by man, paramount importance is placed on diet and breathing exercises, variables that man *can* control. Qi is further affected by the condition of the organs which absorb it. If the stomach and lungs are not functioning properly, they cannot extract and absorb qi's vital energy in sufficient quantity, so the entire body suffers. When a person falls ill, Chinese herbal doctors first look to the patient's lifestyle and habits for things that might affect qi. Many qi-deficient conditions can be corrected with the powerful tools of lifestyle, breathing and hygiene changes.

Demystifying Chinese herbology by learning and understanding how the herbs are used, gives us new opportunities to obtain more healing tools. Chinese herbal healers learn largely from empirical observation, with little faith in rigid systems drawn from abstract theories, like those we have in the West. They look to observation by sight, hearing and smell, to touch and to questioning the patient for diagnosis confirmation. Disease is viewed as an imbalance of two opposing energies, yin and yang, in the major body systems. Disease factors fit into conformations and stages for better understanding and control.

Chinese herbal medicine also recognizes qi as an important part of medicinal plants. Herbs are thought to possess specific parallel characteristics with humans. The qi energy of certain herbs has a natural affinity for certain parts of the human body and the ability to work effectively with them to restore vital energy. Body balance is the goal as natural functions are steered back toward the direction of harmony. Chinese herbal treatment always works with the opposite herb characteristic to the human problem. For example, a fever is treated with cooling herbs, a cold is treated with heating herbs.

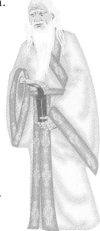

Modern drugs treat "excess syndromes," usually by inhibiting a physiologic function. Chinese herb formulas resolve "deficiency syndromes," usually by promoting physiologic functions.

Although most of the bio-chemical constituents of Chinese herbs have long been known, the real healing ability of an herbal medicine depends on the integration and complexity of its components. A prescription for a Chinese remedy may contain four to twelve herbs, or more. The complex aspects of the formulas make them hard to understand for the Westerner, used to the "one solution for one problem" principle. But traditional Chinese herbal formulas aim for broad spectrum healing and normalizing results — to balance hormones, regulate blood components, enhance immune function, reduce inflammation and improve digestion.

Need to find a good practitioner? Call the American Assn. of Oriental Medicine. (888) 500-7999.

49

Ayurveda

Ayurveda, "the science of life," is considered the world's most ancient existing medical system. Practiced for 6,000 years, it is even older than traditional Chinese herbalism. Originating on the Indian sub-continent, Ayurveda is a holistic legacy that emphasizes body-mind synergy and spiritual health. It is a scientific art for optimizing energy and developing greater powers of awareness as well as for healing. It has been called the first form of preventive medicine.

As in Chinese medicine, Ayurveda believes in universal life energy force, or prana (qi in Chinese). The force is expressed in bi-polar terms, yin-yang in Chinese medicine, and Shiva-shakti in Ayurveda. Diseases, medicinal herbs, diet elements and therapies are also classified as balancing opposites— warm or cool, strong or weak, etc. Still widely practiced in India, Ayurveda is enjoying a strong revival in the West.

Its chief aim is longevity and a rejuvenative quality of life, by optimizing energy balance and the body's own self-repair mechanisms. Its method of healing seeks mind-body harmony, and relies on detoxification, diet, natural therapies and herbs depending on body type. An Ayurvedic treatment includes music, yoga, herbs, massage, steams, facials and aromatherapy.

Ayurveda is a highly personalized system; each individual's health requirements are seen as unique and ever changing. Healing is accomplished by determining the balance of energy patterns that exist in each person's nature, along with the specific imbalances that arise due to time and circumstances, like the effects of age, climate or lifestyle.

Ayurvedic medicine is much more than just a reaction to disease using natural remedies. It stresses disease prevention through health-promoting substances, and addresses emotional, intellectual and spiritual well-being as well as physical health.

The key elements of Ayurveda healing are body typing, herbal therapy, diet and lifestyle.

Body Typing according to the tri-dosha is the most fundamental principal of Ayurvedic healing. Ayurveda considers that each person is a unique balance of physical, emotional, spiritual and mental traits called doshas, expressed in three great elements – water (Kapha), fire (Pitta), and air (Vata). Each dosha regulates functions in the mind-body system, and most people are not just one type, but have elements of each, even though one of the doshas predominates at birth. Changes in the doshas occur with age and season, the interrelating balance of the three dosha forces, and transformations of the three forces by the food, water, sunlight and air that a person takes in. Disease results when the balance of the doshas (especially the dominant dosha) is disturbed.

Here's how each dosha works:

—**Vata** represents the elements of space and air. Vata controls movement in the body like blood circulation, digestion, breathing, nerve impulses, etc. Vata people are usually taller or shorter than average, are thin and have difficulty holding weight. They tend to run dry and cold, with high activity but low stamina. Digestion and metabolism are average. They are mentally creative, restless, nervous and moody. They are often prone to fear and anxiety. Their greatest strength is quick response and adaptability.

—**Pitta** represents the elements of water and fire, which governs metabolism and biochemical processes, like transforming food, air, and water into the body. Pitta types are usually average height and build, with ruddy, or lustrous complexions. They have strong appetites, good digestion and circulation, and warmer body temperature than other people. They are intelligent, sharp, aggressive and ambitious. They are prone to anger and irritability. Their strength is courage and fearlessness.

—**Kapha** represents the elements of earth and water. Kapha influences the structure of tissues, muscles, bones, and sinews. Kapha types are usually large-boned and stocky. They put on weight easily, have slow digestion and metabolism, with slow, steady movements and responses. Psychologically they are prone to attachment. Their strength is calm, contentment and stability.

Herbal therapy is a key to the success of Ayurvedic healing. Much of its vast herbal legacy has been scientifically validated. The drugs reserpine for hypertension, digitalis for heart stimulation, and aloe vera stem from Ayurveda. Research continues on herbals for tumor reduction, and on *Boswellia* compounds for arthritis.

The aim is always for body balance. Herbal formulas are prescribed to balance body types, rather than just making use of the properties of the herb. Ayurveda believes that people are prone to the diseases corresponding in nature to their predominant element. For example: air-types may suffer from nervousness, pain or bone diseases; fire-types may suffer from fever, infection and blood disorders; water-types may develop congestive disorders with an excess of watery mucus.

Some well-known Ayurvedic herbals you can find in health food stores:

–*Triphala* - a laxative formula consisting of the fruit of three tropical trees is one of the best aids for restoring the tone of the colon. It is less likely than other herbal laxatives to cause dependency.

–*Guggul* - a resin like myrrh, is used for coronary heart disease, reducing cholesterol and weight control. It is also widely used for arthritis, diabetes and for chronic fevers.

–*Ashwagandha* - "Indian ginseng," is used to reduce anxiety, give strength and improve sexual function. Although energizing, ashwagandha also helps promote sleep, calming the nerves.

–*Gotu Kola* - an Ayurvedic nervine counters nerve pain, clears the senses, combats negative emotions, cleanses the liver, and removes toxins from the blood. It is an important aid to mental clarity and calm.

–*Chyavan Prash* - an herbal jelly based on the Amla fruit, the highest natural source of vitamin C, strengthens the blood and counters debility. It is recommended for all types as a general tonic.

–*Gymnema sylvestre* - A blood glucose regulator, gymnema blocks blood sugar absorption preventing blood sugar elevation in diabetics. Even helps repair damage to the kidneys, liver and muscle.

–*Sida cordifolia* - an herb with much of the broncho-dilating and thermogenic effects as ephedra, but without the strong heart palpitation effects some people feel from ephedra.

–*Neem* - NIH tests find neem stimulates immune response against the AIDS virus. Since early tests show neem lowers testosterone, researchers in India have a patent for a contraceptive neem oil product for men.

–*Arjuna* - an Ayurvedic heart tonic comparable to hawthorn in many ways. Increases circulation, regulates blood pressure; used to treat angina and arrhythmia. Especially effective for congestive heart failure.

Diet is thought to be a primary means of transforming body balance. Ayurveda recommends a highly nutritive, vegetarian diet, including whole grains, beans, cooked vegetables, nuts and dairy products, with combinations of spices like Indian curries. It does not recommend raw food diets except for short periods of body cleansing. Iced foods and drinks should be avoided. Foods are classified by their effects on the doshas, and diets are tailored to the patient's body type and personal imbalances.

Further: • Vata, air-types, need heavier, richer foods with sweet, sour and salty tastes, with nuts, dairy products, grains like wheat and oats, and spices for good digestion. • Pitta, fire-types need cooling foods with sweet, bitter and astringent tastes, including some raw food, and limiting the amount of salt, spices and sour foods. • Kapha, water-types do best on a light diet with pungent, bitter and astringent tastes, using lots of spices, and many vegetables, but avoiding sugar, dairy, nuts and oily foods.

Lifestyle recommendations include detoxification as a key part of treatment. An Ayurvedic physician may prescribe panchakarma, a program of internal purification therapies and oil massages. After a cleansing regimen, patients follow daily and seasonal routines to help them better integrate with the biological rhythms of nature. (See DETOXIFICATION, by Linda Page for more information on panchakarma.)

Native American Herbalism

Native Americans have always lived close to nature. From earliest times they have successfully relied on healing plants for daily health. Native Americans were almost disease-free before the arrival of the Europeans. They had a firm understanding of the science of illness, and many of their traditional medical practices were as good as or better than those of their European counterparts.

Native Americans understood that true healing takes time. They had a keen knowledge of anatomy; they practiced personal hygiene and sophisticated childbirth methods. They understood the antiseptic value of plant juices and oils, tied off arteries to prevent blood loss, pulled teeth, and used complex herbal pain killers. Health care was a normal part of life, and all family members were taught first aid techniques and how to cure common ailments from herbs stored at home. If these were not enough, tribal healers, who had a greater knowledge of plant medicines and supernatural powers, could be easily accessed as specialists to deal with life-threatening emergencies and serious problems, including advanced psychotherapy. Even today, Native American healing techniques have a strong spiritual strength that allows them to deal with the hardship of illness.

Native Americans had no word for medicine as we know it. The general concern of health care was for over all well-being, but it was believed health was a gift from supernatural powers, and an outcome of correct living. Medicine, therefore involved many healing practices, not just remedies.

Native Americans believed that health was holistic, that well-being, medicine, and religion were all intertwined. Everything depended on everything else; and the spirit world connected living and non-living environments in a giant circle that flowed together. Native American medicine is often symbolized by large, round medicine wheels or sacred circles.

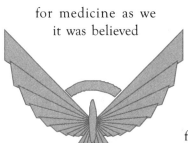

Healing was believed to occur as a result of the dual power of spirit and mind, and the relationship between the healer and the patient. Treatment of physical symptoms was never isolated from the spirituality of the patient. Medicine men and women were really shaman healers, powerful intermediary figures between man and the forces of nature who publicly demonstrated their powers in awe-inspiring ways. They cured the sick, controlled the weather, foretold the future, brought success in war and hunting, communicated with and received news about those who were far away, found and restored those who were lost or captured by enemies, and overthrew witches and evil spirits.

Native Americans healers also used medicinal herbs, acupuncture (the Cherokee used porcupine quills or thorns), guided imagery, and massage therapy in their healing traditions.

Many drugs we use today came from our Native American's heritage. Their contribution to present-day medicines includes salicin (the major ingredient in aspirin), syrup of ipecac (an emetic), quinine, morphine, curare, cocaine, atropine, scopolamine and hyoscyamine.

Most herbal healing compounds were complex and far-reaching.... in order to address different parts of a problem and its cause and effect. A Stomach Tea from the famous Chief Two Moons Meridas, for example, had thirteen herbs: *senna, coriander seed, gentian root, juniper berry, centaury, calamus root, buckthorn bark, ginger, cascara sagrada, pale rose buds, anise seed, lavender flowers and fennel seed.*

Chief Two Moons Female Tea contained *squaw vine, motherwort, chamomile, cramp bark, uva ursi, ginger, helonias root, celery seed, aletris, Mexican saffron, cascara sagrada, cornflowers and black haw bark.*

His Rheumatism Tea used eleven herbs: *wintergreen, yellow dock, black cohosh, uva ursi, birch bark, bittersweet twigs, cascara bark, buckbean, coriander seed, burdock root and buchu leaves.*

His Tonic Tea contained *fennel seed, dandelion root, licorice root, sarsaparilla, senna, cascara sagrada, sassafras bark, clover, juniper berries, chamomile, Mexican saffron, elder flowers, blue malva flowers and calendula.*

Today, modern herbalists are turning to many of these time-honored formulas with success.

Rainforest Herbal Healing

The New Science Of Ethnobotany

The last 20 years have witnessed a remarkable rediscovery in the West of plants as a source of pharmaceuticals. Interest started as a grassroots movement, with a huge rise in demand for herbal remedies in Europe and the Americas.... a demand that changed the focus of drug companies almost overnight. Today, over half of the top 250 pharmaceutical companies in the world, compared with almost none 15 years ago, have active research programs investigating the plant world for potential new drugs.

The search for powerful medicinal plants centers on the rainforests, where almost half of the world's flowering plants live. The rainforests of Central America are pre-eminent because they contain the largest plant pharmacopoeia. To western medical science, the rainforest is a treasure box just beginning to be opened. The huge variety of rainforest plants are still a great mystery for orthodox medicine. Rainforest herbs are so rich that often 6 or 7 biochemical drugs can be extracted from just one plant! Both western herbalists and medical science are beginning to see that living medicines from rainforest herbs are one of the best answers for true, non-invasive healing.

Yet rainforest conservation remains a critical issue. More and more rainforests, the "Earth's lungs," are being destroyed for economic development. Everyone realizes that the health of the entire planet, and all its inhabitants is at risk. Many native medicines have already been wiped out, and native healers know their heritage is threatened — by the erosion of their cultural traditions, and by the destruction to their environment. Education and information are the keys to the preservation of each.

Understanding life and its relationship with humans in the rainforest is not only crucial to its preservation, but also to the health of over 80% of the world's population which still depends on plants for its primary health care.

How can the ethnobotanical approach help all sides? Ethnobotany, the study of how native peoples use plants, is a complex mixture of sociology, anthropology, botany, ecology, and medicine. Western scientists are often amazed at the pharmacological knowledge of indigenous peoples. Traditional Shamanic medicine is more than just folklore and superstition. It is one the oldest forms of healing through mind-body communication. Shaman healers have been able for centuries to treat illnesses from colds to cancer.

Shamanic healers have incredible knowledge of the rainforest's ecosystem. When they discovered a remedy, it usually worked extremely well, and remained an integral part of their healing tradition for hundreds of years. The remedy was not tainted by the financial forces of modern medicine, nor was it subject to a constantly changing belief system like ours. This profound knowledge is still largely unknown to modern science; fortunately some wise traditional healers are starting to teach western doctors, pharmacists and botanists in an effort to benefit, perhaps even to save, humanity.

Everyone feels that time is running out. We must shorten the period required to make a botanical drug available. Western drug research takes a decade or more to reach the market. We must respect native healers who have known the plants intimately for centuries. If traditional rainforest healers agree to share their vast knowledge with western botanists, not only is understanding about the healing properties of various plants increased, but an enormous amount of time is saved without the trial and error of mass screenings. The shaman's information, in effect, "prescreens" the plants, identifying the best drug candidates without time-consuming random collection. Rainforest peoples will benefit as well, because their healing plants will become more economically valuable than real estate development. Everybody wins, including the rainforest and our planet.

Herbal Healing In Europe & The West

The medical path of herbal medicine in the west has been a twisted one — influenced by religion, kicked around by politics, distorted by societal philosophies and directed by vested interests. Today, some truths stand firm, and the ageless wisdom behind many old remedies has withstood the tests of time. Still, most medical policies are controlled by politics and power. Although we think the great conflict of orthodox and alternative medicine is recent, the struggle between the two has been long and bloody.

Western herbalism seems always to have been bound up with science.

Hippocrates, a physician during Greece's Golden Age, stood at the beginning of western medicine as we know it. His system of medicine had one foot in scientific reason and the other in the power of Nature. Hippocrates theorized that the human body had four humors; blood, phlegm, yellow bile (choler), and black bile. He assumed illness resulted when one humor was out of balance with another. He believed that the healing resources of nature were all-powerful, and that the task of the physician was to help the healing process along rather than to take it over. Hippocrates' beliefs continued in mainstream medicine until the late 19th century — 2,300 years after he presented them.

Western medical herbalism first seems to have come from a surgeon in the Roman armies of Nero, Dioscorides, who compiled the medicinal knowledge of the day into a volume known as *De Materia Medica*, still considered the prototype of herbal and pharmacopoeia materia medicas.

In the second century A.D., Galen, another Greek physician, brought a classification system to Hippocrates' concept of the four humors, evaluating plant remedies in terms of their reaction *with* the body's humors. He theorized that after a humor imbalance was diagnosed, the proper medication could easily be prescribed to counteract it. **Thus, the key to healing in the west became diagnosis** - the fitting of every health problem into a classification box. It is so today.

Galen's philosophy became the cornerstone for an elaborate, rigid system of medicine, where only a doctor had healing knowledge. The concept of "heroic medicine," man fighting against and overcoming disease, and intervening in body processes, began in Galen's time. Over the years, procedures were used with increasing intensity to "whip" an illness. Galen also believed that the more complex a remedy, the better it was. He favored elaborate medicines compounded of dozens of ingredients rather than simple teas of two or three herbs.

Amazingly, the 500 year period of Europe's Dark Age for literacy wasn't dark at all for herbal healing. Great medical advances were introduced by the Arabs who brought both alchemy and pharmacies into Western practice. Indeed, from the 12th century on, apothecaries swept over Europe, along with many new ointments, elixirs, pills, tinctures, suppositories, purgatives, cathartics and inhalations. In the 16th century, Paracelsus, a doctor today seen as the founder of chemical pharmacology, taught that alchemy and chemistry together were a way to unlock the secrets of Nature's healing plants. Paracelsus began the distillation of isolates — extracting the so-called "active principle" of the plant — claiming that the process was more potent and effective than the whole plant while still remaining safe. Indeed the alchemists of his day and the chemists of ours, adhere to this belief. Pharmacies have been proven wrong on the safety of isolates more times than not, but isolates remain popular with drug companies today because their manufacture can be patented and rigorously controlled.

As early as the 17th century, the battle began over using costly, imported drugs rather than local plant remedies. Nicholas Culpeper, an English apothecary, tiring of the fact that virtually all plant medicines that existed in England were imported, created his own herbal handbook, the *English Physician*, in the 1650's. It became a popular herbal text then and is still popular today. (In 1990, there were some 42 different current editions on record.) Culpeper detailed the practical use of herbs rather than the theoretical, and gave a big boost to herb usage in England.

American herbalism, like America itself, is a melting pot of European and Native American herbs and traditions, with an overlay of American science and technology. The first European settlers learned much from the native Americans, with great gratitude for their traditions. Yet, early in our history, the influence of science started medical practices which became very specialized and steered away from natural healing. The American colonies also relied heavily on imported medicines. By the 1800s, both American and European medical schools favored prescription medicines. Herbal medicine was not taught, nor was there room for nature's healing powers. Most doctors were also apothecaries, and drug sales were often the only way they could keep solvent.

The medical debate raged on for almost a century, between alternative healers, who relied as they do today, on the healing power of nature and years of empirical experience, and orthodox doctors who proceeded from theory to practice without stopping to consider the real results. Because alternative or "irregular" doctors undertook to restore body balance through detoxification procedures like sweating, vomiting and elimination, they were called "puke and steam doctors."

The name calling stopped in 1805, when an epidemic swept through the region of an herbalist named Samuel Thompson. He sweated his patients and gave them healing herbs. Conventional doctors bled their patients and administered calomel, a mercury derivative. Thompson lost none of the patients that he attended. The regular physicians lost over half of theirs to the epidemic.

Amazing results like this turned the debate in favor of herbal medicines and natural healing. Homeopathy (page 18), and the Eclectic movement were introduced during this time. Eclectic physicians believed that medicines should be gentle, should consist of the direct action of single drugs, uncombined with others, and that there should be no "heroic" shocks to the system, no violent cathartics, emetics or blisters. Eclectic chemists worked to ensure that medicines remained pure and they engaged in the most detailed botanical studies ever performed, putting the Eclectics on the cutting edge of herbal medicine for more than 50 years.

The popularity of "irregular" medical schools and movements, particularly the enthusiasm for the new homeopathic movement, forced conventional doctors to form the American Medical Association (AMA), in 1847. It was underwritten by the pharmaceutical companies, who had a great deal to gain from its philosophy. The whole vast, expanding medical-pharmaceutical industry of the United States formally turned its back on the plant world and looked to synthetic chemicals as its future.

By the turn of the 20th century, overwhelmed by the advancing growth of the AMA, herbal medicine went into a predictable decline. Chemists learned to synthesize some active plant constituents in the laboratory, standardizing and sterilizing drug doses to stabilize supplies. Surgery advanced, along with the discovery of antibiotics, especially during the emergency needs of the two World Wars.

Today, orthodox medicine's greatest accomplishments are still technical ones, involving incredibly sophisticated orthopedics, burn treatment, cesarean section, resuscitation, microsurgery to attach severed limbs, heart-valve replacements and extraordinary feats like open-heart surgery. But, there is a dark side to the coin. Even with the best of intentions, modern medical intervention produces an astonishing amount of dysfunction, disability and pain. The most rapidly spreading epidemic of the twentieth century is iatrogenic, or drug/doctor-caused disease. Its victims are more numerous than traffic and industrial accidents combined every year.

Americans take $19 billion worth of drugs annually. An expensive river of chemicals courses through our national veins. Many of these drugs are dangerous; many are ineffective in curing the condition for which they are prescribed. More than one million people a year (almost 5% of hospital admissions) end up needing hospital care as a result of bad reactions to drugs. It is now common knowledge that X-rays increase cancer risk.

Radiation from diagnostic X-rays contributes to blood disorders, tumors, diabetes, stroke and cataracts. (In some cases, where the tissue being X-rayed is very delicate, such as the breasts, fibroids have been found in as little as three months.) Yet over 300 million of X-rays are ordered yearly as standard procedure, even without a specific medical need.

Basic belief systems in modern medicine are at the root of some of its problems.
—That a disease must be "interrupted" by surgical intervention or by drugs to restore health.
—That dietary habits are not related to symptoms or illnesses... a belief that is changing, yet is still held by many, especially scientists who maintain that the body identifies and uses the nutrients it needs, regardless of the source of the nutrients.
—That a doctor's primary work must be arresting and dealing with symptoms instead of addressing the cause of the problem.

Western medicine must evolve to do more good and less harm. Alternative or holistic medicine has been rediscovered to meet this need. Nothing about a human being works in a vacuum. A weakness in the heart may also express a weakness of the other organs. An infection in a finger may indicate pollutants throughout the body. Improving nutrition and tonifying the body regularly leads to the improvement of many different symptoms. Holistic health recognizes that our individual body parts are components of an integrated physical being, who has social, emotional, and spiritual levels, all affected by our lifestyle.

Man is an integral part of Nature. He is governed by all of Nature's laws. His health and vitality depend on his harmony with the forces of the earth.
The well-being of every individual, every nation and the whole of humanity will always be in direct proportion to man's observances of Nature's laws.
Unity with Nature is the foundation of man's existence on the planet - of all his economic systems, of all his social relationships, of all his science.
Unless there is unity with Nature, our civilization, like those of the past, will decline and decay.

Using Herbs Safely: A Practical Guide

Herbal medicines have been meeting humanity's medical needs for thousands of years. Although today, we think of herbs as natural drugs, they are really foods with medicinal qualities. They combine with our bodies as foods do, so they are able to address both the symptoms and causes of a problem.

As nourishment, herbs offer the body nutrients it may not always receive, either because of poor diet, or environmental deficiencies in the soil and air. As medicine, herbs are essentially body balancers that work with the body functions, so that it can heal and regulate itself.

Herbs work like precision instruments in the body, not like sledge hammers.
Herbal medicines can be broad-based for overall support, or specific to a particular problem.

Most herbs, as edible plants, are as safe to take as foods. Herbs provide a rich variety of healing agents with almost no side effects. Occasionally a mild allergy-type reaction may occur as it might occur to a food. This could happen because an herb has been adulterated with chemicals in the growing or storing process, or in rare cases, because incompatible herbs were used together. Or, it may be just a personal adverse response to a certain plant. The key to avoiding an adverse reaction is moderation, both in formulation and in dosage. Anything taken to excess can cause negative side effects. Common sense, care, and intelligence are needed when using herbs for either food or medicine.

Two-thirds of the drugs on the American market today are based on medicinal plants.
—**But modern herb-based drugs are not herbs; they are chemicals.** Even when a drug is derived from an herb, it is so refined, isolated and purified that only a chemical formula remains. Chemicals work in our bodies far differently than herbs. Chemical drugs cause many effects — only some of which are positive. Eli Lilly, a pharmaceutical manufacturer, once said "a drug isn't a drug unless it has side effects."
—**Herbs in their whole form are not drugs.** Do not expect the activity or response of a drug, which normally treats only the symptoms of a problem. In general, you have to take more and more of a drug to get continuing therapeutic effect.
—**Herbal medicines work differently.** Herbs are foundation nutrients. They nourish the body's deepest, basic elements, like the brain, glands and hormones. Herbs work to normalize, balance and support at the cause of a problem, for a more permanent effect. Results seem to take much longer. Even so, some improvement from herbal treatment can usually be felt in three to six days. Chronic or long standing problems take longer, but herbal remedies tend to work more quickly with each new infection, and cases of infections grow fewer and further between. **A traditional rule of thumb is one month of healing for every year of the problem.**

Balance is the key to using herbs for healing. Herbal combinations are not addictive, but they are powerful nutritional agents that should be used with care. It takes a little more attention and personal responsibility than mindlessly taking a prescription drug, but the extra care is worth far more in the results you can achieve for your well-being.

As with other natural therapies, there is sometimes a "healing crisis" in an herbal healing program. This is known as the "Law of Cure," and simply means that you seem to get worse before you get better. The body may eliminate toxic wastes heavily during the first stages of a cleansing therapy. This is particularly true in the traditional three to four day cleansing fast that many people use to begin a serious healing program. Temporary exacerbation of symptoms can range from mild to fairly severe, but usually precedes good results. Herbal therapy without a fast works more slowly and gently. Still, there is usually some weakness as disease poisons are released into the bloodstream to be flushed away. Strength shortly returns when this process is over. Watching this phenomenon allows you to observe your body at work healing itself.....an interesting experience indeed.

Herbs work better in combination than they do singly.
Like the notes of a symphony, herbs work better in harmony than standing alone.

Here's why herbs work better in combination:
—Each formula contains two to five primary herbs for specific healing purposes. Since all body parts, and most disease symptoms, are interrelated, it is wise to have herbs which can affect each part of the problem. For example, in a prostate healing formula, there would be herbs to dissolve sediment, anti-inflammatory herbs, tissue-toning and strengthening herbs, and herbs with antibiotic properties.

—A combination of herbal nutrients encourages body balance rather than a large supply of one or two focused properties. A combination works to gently stimulate the body as a whole.

—A combination allows inclusion of herbs that can work at different stages of need. A good example of this is an athlete's formula, where there are herbs for short term energy, long range endurance, muscle tone, glycogen and glucose use, and reduction of lactic acid build-up.

—A combination of several herbs with similar properties increases the latitude of effectiveness, not only through a wider range of activity, but also by reinforcing herbs that were picked too late or too early, or grew in adverse weather conditions.

—No two people, or their bodies, are alike. Good response is augmented by a combination of herbs.

—Finally, certain herbs, like *capsicum, lobelia, sassafras, mandrake, tansy, Canada snake root, wormwood, woodruff, poke root, and rue* are beneficial in small amounts and as catalysts, but should not be used alone.

Herbs work better when combined with a natural foods diet. Everyone can benefit from an herbal formula, but results increase dramatically when fresh foods and whole grains form the basis of your diet. Subtle healing activity is more effective when it doesn't have to labor through excess waste material, mucous, or junk food accumulation. (Some congested people carry around over 10 pounds of excess density.)

Interestingly, herbs themselves can help counter the problems of "chemicalized foods." They are rich in minerals, the basic elements missing or diminished in today's quick-grow, over-sprayed, over-fertilized farming. Minerals and trace minerals are a basic element in food assimilation, providing not only the healing essences to support your body in overcoming disease, but also the foundation minerals that allow it to take them in!
Your body has its own unique, wonderful mechanism. It has the ability to bring itself to its own balanced and healthy state. Herbs simply pave the way for the body to do its own work, by breaking up toxins, cleansing, lubricating, toning and nourishing.

Herbs promote elimination of waste matter and toxins from the system by simple natural means.
They support nature in its fight against disease.

Here's how to take herbs for the most benefit:

Herbs are not like vitamins. I see herbs as healers and vitamins as insurance policies.
—The value of herbs is in their wholeness and complexity, not their concentration.

Herbs should not be taken like vitamins. Herbs are nutrients, and nutrients always work best as a team.
—Vitamins are usually taken on a maintenance basis to shore up nutrient deficiencies. Except for some food-grown vitamins, vitamins are partitioned substances. They do not combine with the body in the same way as foods or herbs do; excesses are normally flushed from the system. Vitamins work best when taken with food.

Herbs are foods; it is not necessary to take herbal formulas with food. They combine and work with the body's enzyme activity as foods do. Herbs have their own plant enzymes that work with yours.

—Taking herbs all the time is like eating large quantities of a certain food all the time. The body tends to have imbalanced nourishment from nutrients that are not in that food. This is also true of multiple vitamins. They work best when strengthening a deficient or weak system, not as a substitute for a good diet. However, superfood plants like green grasses, sea plants, aloe, and green algae, and adaptogen tonics like ginsengs and bee products can be taken for longer periods of body balancing.

—Unlike vitamins, herbs provide their own digestive enzymes for the body to take them in. In some cases, as in a formula for mental acuity, the herbs are more effective if taken when body pathways are clear, instead of concerned with food digestion.

Therapeutic herbs work best when used as needed.
Dosage should be reduced and discontinued as the problem improves.

Herbal effects are often specific; take the best formula for your particular goal at the right time — rather than all the time — for optimum results. Rotating and alternating herbal combinations according to your changing health needs allows your body to remain responsive to their effects. Reduce dosage as the problem improves. Allow your body to pick up its own work and bring its own vital forces into action. If you are taking an herbal remedy for more than a month, discontinue for one or two weeks between months to let your body adjust and maintain your personal balance.

Achieve best results by taking herbal capsule combinations in descending strength: 6 the first day, 5 the second day, 4 the third, 3 the fourth, 2 the fifth, and 2 the sixth for the first week. Rest on the 7th day. When a healing base is built in the body, decrease to the regular dose recommended for the formula. Most combinations should be taken no more than 6 days in a row without a break.

Take only one or two herbal combinations at the same time. Address your worst problem first. Take the herbal remedy for that problem — reducing dosage and alternating on and off weeks as necessary to allow the body to thoroughly use the herbal properties. One of the bonuses of a natural healing program is the frequent discovery that other conditions were really complications of the first problem, and often take care of themselves as the body comes into balance.

Herb effectiveness usually goes by body weight, especially for children. Child dosage is as follows:

$^1\!/_2$ *dose for children 10-14 years* $^1\!/_4$ *dose for children 2-6 years*
$^1\!/_3$ *dose for children 6-10 years* $^1\!/_8$ *dose for infants and babies*

Herbs are amazingly effective in strengthening your body's immune response. But the immune system is a fragile entity. It can be overwhelmed instead of stimulated. Even when a good healing program is working, and obvious improvement is being made, adding more of the medicinal agents in an effort to speed healing can aggravate symptoms. Even for serious health conditions, moderate amounts are the way to go, mega-doses are not. Much better results can be obtained by giving yourself more time and gentler treatment. It takes time to rebuild health.

Your Herbal Medicine Choices
Whole-Herb Healing or Standardized Plant Constituents

Clearly, American health care consumers are increasing their use of herbs as natural alternatives to drugs. Standardizing separate herbal constituents for potency is popular today as herbal manufacturers enter drug-oriented health care markets.

What do we sacrifice when herbal constituents are "standardized"?

Government regulations and orthodox medicine are trying make herbal medicines fit into a laboratory drug mold. Americans need safe, effective, alternative medicines. But to meet the demand with herbs means working with incredibly intricate, living medicines.... medicines whose value lies in their complexity, in their ability to combine with the human body — not in their concentration or the potency of any one constituent.

Standardization methods use chemicals to peel away one or two so-called "active ingredients" out of hundreds of constituents that make up an herb. The result is an overly refined product that misses the full range of benefits offered by the whole herb.

As a naturopath and traditional herbalist, I believe that standardization short-changes the full spectrum of whole-herb healing. Throughout the 6,000 year tradition of herbal healing, in every culture, herbalists have effectively used whole herbs for whole bodies. The immense success of herbs rivals modern day allopathic medicine. There is tremendous value in the knowledge gained through empirical observation and interpretive understanding of real people with real problems and natural solutions.

In today's health care world, laboratory yardsticks are the only measurements science understands or government approves. Herbal healing fell out of favor not because it was ineffective, or even because something better was discovered, but because science and technology had little understanding of nature. Medical market economics had no incentive to investigate herbs, because no one could "patent a plant."

Standardizing an active ingredient in a drug-like approach neglects one of the main benefits of whole herbs. Herbs have the unique ability to address multiple problems simultaneously. In most cases, the full medicinal value of herbs is in their internal complexity. Even though the business of standardizing herbs is less than a decade old, new research is showing that the chosen "active ingredient" to be standardized may have been the wrong one, or not the best choice, or the most powerful. It's almost impossible to chase the intricate principles that really make herbs heal.

An herb is rarely ever known for just a single function. Each herb has dozens of biochemical constituents working synergistically. Many of the constituents within a whole herb are unknown — even to modern science — and internal chemical reactions within and among herbs are even less understood.

Can we integrate herbal healing into scientific methods to make it available to everybody? It's a question that's splitting herbal product providers apart. Standardization is seen by some companies, especially those whose main focus has been vitamins or other partitioned supplements, as a way for herb products to challenge the monopoly of drug companies, by measuring and assuring some "active constituents" of a plant. Standardization is also considered a way to deal with FDA regulations that require drug measurability, and FDA guidelines that require active ingredients to be stated on product labels. As herb companies begin to use structure, function and potency health claims, a way must be found to work with regulations that were never intended to deal with the complexities or broad-based effects of herbal healing.

Standardizing potency for only one or two extracted "active ingredients" attempts to use limited laboratory procedures to convince the AMA, the FDA and medical scientists of the value of herbal therapy. We must not fall into the same wrong-headed, self-defeating pit of forty years ago, when the regulations for standardizing drugs nearly killed all herbal medicine.

Yet, quality and consistency are a major concern in considering herbal effectiveness. Somehow, herbalists and herbal product suppliers must integrate herbal traditions, ethical commitments, FDA regulations and consumer concerns.

Herbs have rejuvenative, tonic qualities entirely missed by standardization. Herbal healing is due not just to herbal bio-chemical properties, but also to their unique, holistic effects, and significantly, to their interaction with the human body.

Here's what we lose when we try to standardize a complex medicinal plant.
Herbs have a unique healing spirit. Herbs are intelligent plants – even thoughtful healers. They give our bodies a wealth of healing essences from which to choose. Science can only quantify, isolate and assay to understand. When we say that the standardized constituents are all there is to herbal healing, we lose. Herbs respond to scientific methods but an herbal compound is much more than the sum of its parts. Herbs are a healing art that can teach your body how to keep you well.

—**Standardization attempts to isolate "active constituents" for limited functions.** Using a standardized herb is like using a "natural drug," with one property for one problem. Potentizing a single property only gives you part of the picture. For example, ginseng is a popular ingredient in many herbal products. One laboratory test identified two of its 22 known constituents (called Rb1 and Rb2), in an attempt to isolate ginseng's functions as an antioxidant that lowers cholesterol. Yet thousands of years of world-wide, well-documented experience show that ginseng has dozens of other actions that control disease and promote wellness, functions entirely missed by this test. Should we deny people the ultimate value and effectiveness of ginseng's activity simply because a laboratory hasn't tested, or understood, every one of its functions yet?

—**Standardization fails to take advantage of the synergistic power of herbs in combination.** Standardizing one constituent within an herbal combination is risky because the whole balance of the compound is lost or altered. The plant's ability to work with other herbs is also lost. As an herbalist, I have been creating combination formulas since 1978. Combinations in most instances work more efficiently with multiple body functions. To make use of the full spectrum of healing possibilities, we combine ginseng, for example, with licorice. The resulting extract has synergistic benefits – exceptional body cleansing, nutrient assimilation support, and a significant role in balancing body sugar levels – **more than the action of either of these herbs used alone.**

Since all body parts, and most disease symptoms, are interrelated, it is wise to have herbs which can affect each part of the problem. Whole herb combinations offers a wide latitude to work with several aspects and stages of a problem, and allows each person to draw benefits from the complexity of the whole combination.

For example, Crystal Star's prostate healing formula contains herbs that help dissolve sediment, herbs with anti-inflammatory and antibiotic properties, and herbs to strengthen tissue. The combination encourages overall body balance in contrast to the limited goal of a "standardized" supply of one or two constituents.

A good herbal combination contains much more than even the **primary** whole herbs. It includes **secondary herbs** to soothe and repair; **catalysts and transporter herbs** to carry active constituents into the body; **complementary herbs** to address side effects related to the main problem and balance body chemistry.
The interaction of a single herb's constituents is much like the supportive roles that the primary, secondary catalyst and complementary perform in a good herbal combination.

Is there a way to assure ourselves that the herbs we buy have the medicinal qualities we want? Are the herbs on the label in there? Will the herbs work?

The evidence of your senses and common sense work with herbs. Here are some checkpoints to use:
√ Buy organically grown or wildcrafted (grown in their natural state) herbs whenever available. Buy fresh-dried, locally grown herbs whenever possible, to assure the shortest transportation time and freshest quality.

√ When choosing unpackaged, loose herbs, rub a sample between your fingers, smell it and look at its color. Even in a dried state, the life and potency of an herb are easily evident.

√ Buy the best herbs available. The experience and quality control methods in the growing-gathering-storage part of the herbal medicine chain are more costly, but they increase its healing abilities.

√ Choose packaged herb products from a company that specializes in herbs. Herb companies live and breathe herbs and are generally regarded as having the highest level of herbal integrity. Ask the supplement buyer at your local natural food store for herbal product manufacturers who have earned the trust of consumers.

√ Be sure the product is tightly sealed and away from light and heat. Also, check the expiration date.

The second part of the answer involves what I have come to trust.

A wise man once said that trust could settle every problem in the world right now. But, we're not talking about blind trust, or pie-in-the-sky trust. We're talking about common sense trust. All of us have to trust experts every day, to advise and inform us about things we don't know. We don't have to become physicists to use products that come from physics research, or mechanics in order to drive a car. Nor do we have to become herbal experts to avail ourselves of herbal medicines. It has been my experience that there are three things you can trust when you buy an herbal product in America today.

1: You can trust the herb or herbal combination to do what its centuries old tradition says it will do.

2: You can trust the vast majority of herbal product suppliers, most of whom are dedicated people, pledged to herbal excellence. In my opinion, their herbal knowledge and standards are worth more than chemical lab assays, many of which are incomplete, poorly done and expensive. A testimonial to this comes from a third party, non-profit lab that buys and tests health products for efficacy and quality. They inform me that almost 100% of the herbal products they review from open market samples contain what they say they contain.

3: Finally, you can trust your natural food store. The typical herbal expert in a natural food store is in the job largely because of a commitment to natural medicines, and a desire to share that commitment.

Just like you can't cheat an honest man, you can't cheat the honesty of herbs. They put out their truth no matter what. To get the whole truth, I believe you have to use the whole herb. Here's why:

—The so-called active constituent of a plant is only a part of the whole. Herbs are complex foods that combine with your body's enzyme activity. When your body tries to use an isolated constituent, a powerful but unbalanced reaction takes place, similar to eating refined sugar or taking a drug which works by overwhelming. Herbs are living medicines. Just like our own bodies, they work best in their natural balance.

—I don't believe any laboratory can quantify all that whole natural plants have to offer us. They can make tomatoes in a lab today. But are they a food, or a fabrication? I've tasted these tomatoes. The resemblance to an earth and sun grown tomato is pale. Herbal medicines are so much more than a laboratory creation.

—Standardization procedures allow the use of sub-standard materials. Since only one "active constituent" is measured, that constituent may be boosted with a concentration or isolate to reach the required standard, regardless of the quality of the herb itself. No one constituent, no matter how worthwhile, can do its healing job without the right stuff from the rest of the herb.

—Herbs are safer in their whole form. Like foods, herbs nourish the body with little danger of toxicity. Potentizing an herb to reach a certain standard makes it more drug-like, without the protection of the plant's natural balance — a safety factor that means herbs can be used by everybody, not just herbal experts, without having to worry about harmful interactions. This is a consideration in today's litigious marketplace, where powerful substances carry more risk of abuse and consumer misuse. The slower, long term action of whole herbs is preferable for self-treatment.

—Finally, standardization leaves no room for excellence, either in source of supply or in skillful preparation.

Herbs & Anatomy
Which Part Of Your Body Do You Want To Work On?

Herbal medicines work for every body system, every body function and every body structure. There are even herbs for the mind and spirit. The ANATOMY & HERB CHARTS in this section graphically show just how all-encompassing herbs can be for your health and well-being. Herbs are also quite specific; you can pinpoint a small body area as easily as a large one. The charts on these pages let you see at a glance which herbs to use for the body part or system you want to work on.

In general, herbs are very gentle, very subtle and very safe. A number of herbs listed on these charts can often be used together if two or more body areas have the same problem. Keep your combinations simple and direct if you decide to use more than one herb.

Blood

Bones

Blood Cleansing

Burdock Root
Pau d'Arco
Sarsaparilla
Chaparral
Licorice Root
Red Clover
Green Tea

Circulatory Stimulation

Ginkgo Biloba
Hawthorn
Siberian Ginseng
Capsicum
Ginger Root
Blessed Thistle
Motherwort

Normalizing Blood Make-Up

Dandelion
Alfalfa
Sea Greens
Yellow Dock Rt.
Marshmallow
Chlorella
Barley Grass
Barberry Bk.

Bone Strength

Wild Yam
Horsetail
Oatstraw
Sarsaparilla
White Oak Bk.
Comfrey
Marshmallow
Alfalfa
Black Cohosh
Barley Grass
Plantain
Dandelion
Sea Greens

Healing Broken Bones

Horsetail Herb
Nettles
Goldenseal
Chlorella
Sarsaparilla Root
Black Cohosh
Alfalfa
Wild Yam Root
Sea Greens
Comfrey
Barley Grass
Propolis
Arnica Montana

63

Muscle System

Muscle Tone

Sarsaparilla Root
Siberian Ginseng
Bee Pollen
Royal Jelly
Barley Grass
Suma
Sea Greens
Rosemary
Saw Palmetto
Damiana
Licorice Root
Alfalfa
Gotu Kola
Fo-Ti
Panax Ginseng
Scullcap
Horsetail
Spirulina
Evening Primrose
Chlorella
Bilberry
Wild Yam
Yarrow
Ginger Root
Capsicum

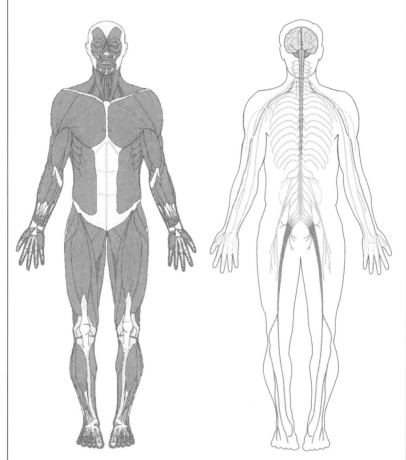

Nerve System

Nerve Health

Gotu Kola
Scullcap
Oatstraw
Kava Kava
Black Cohosh
Chamomile
Rosemary
Siberian Ginseng
Barley Grass
Catnip
Euro. Mistletoe
Lobelia
Barley Grass
Dandelion
Pau d'Arco
Evening Primrose
Peppermint
Reishi Mushroom
Wood Betony
Black Haw
Nettles
Parsley Rt. & Lf.
Bee Pollen
Valerian Root
Watercress

Cardio-Pulmonary System

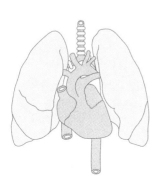

Cardio-Pulmonary Health

Hawthorn
Siberian Ginseng
Garlic
Capsicum
Sea Greens
Barley Grass
Chlorella
Bilberry
Ginger Root
Ginkgo Biloba
Motherwort
Evening Primrose
Scullcap

Respiratory & Lung Health

Marshmallow
Mullein
Ephedra
Fenugreek
Sarsaparilla Root
Pau d' Arco
Echinacea
Aloe Vera Juice
Royal Jelly
Lobelia
Barley Grass
Pleurisy Root
Comfrey

Respiratory Sinus System

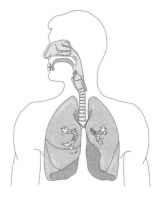

Digestive System

Elimination Systems

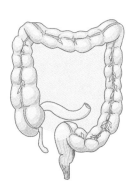

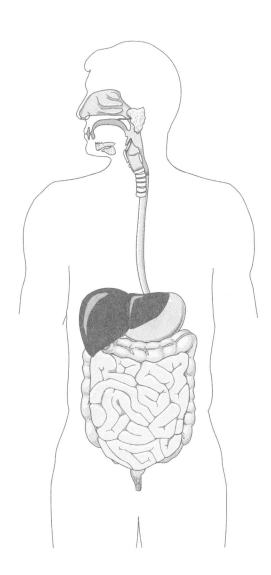

Colon Health

Aloe Vera
Fennel Seed
Kelp/Sea Greens
Marshmallow
High Chlorophyll Herbs
Licorice Root
Butternut Bark
Flax Seed

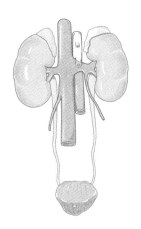

Digestive Health

Ginkgo Biloba
Fenugreek Seed
Barley Grass
Goldenseal Root
Garlic
Ginger Root
Alfalfa
Licorice Root
Fennel Seed
Catnip
Capsicum
Kelp/Sea Greens
Slippery Elm

Urinary Health

Dandelion
Uva Ursi
Parsley
Cornsilk
Watermelon Seed
Cleavers
Barley Grass
Alfalfa
Oregon Grape Root

Liver & Gallbladder

Heart & Arteries

Liver
Health

Chlorella
Milk Thistle Seed
Licorice Root
Gotu Kola
Sea Greens
Barley Grass
Goldenseal Root
Garlic
Dandelion
Yellow Dock
Siberian Ginseng
Panax Ginseng
Alfalfa
Barberry Bark
Astragalus
Royal Jelly
Reishi Mushroom
Evening Primrose
Fennel Seed

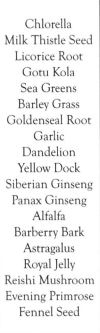

Heart
Health

Ginkgo Biloba
Hawthorn
Cayenne
Barley Grass
Panax Ginseng
Siberian Ginseng
Garlic
Ginger Root
Bee Pollen
Licorice Root
Wild Cherry Bk.

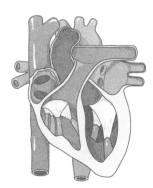

Kidneys

Kidney
Health

Dandelion
Uva Ursi
Parsley
Cornsilk
Nettles
Juniper Berry
Barley Grass
Alfalfa
Burdock Root
Garlic
Goldenseal Root
Green Tea
Ginger Root

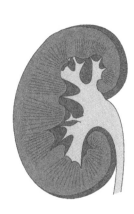

Spleen System

Spleen
Health

Licorice Root
Panax Ginseng
Siberian Ginseng
Yellow Dock Root
Burdock Root
Oregon Grape Root
Dandelion

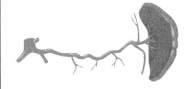

Lung System

Lung
Health

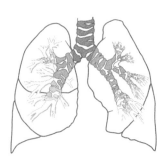

Ginkgo Biloba
Sea Greens
Rosemary
Chlorella
Aloe Vera juice
Garlic
Thyme
Echinacea Root
Fenugreek Seed
Oregano Oil
Bee Pollen
Chaparral
Pau d'Arco
Marshmallow

HERBS FOR YOUR GLANDS

Adrenals

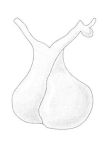

Adrenal Health

Bee Pollen/Roy. Jelly
Licorice Root
Hawthorn
Astragalus
Sea Greens
Siberian Ginseng
Gotu Kola
Sarsaparilla Root

Ovaries

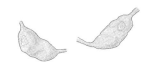

Ovary Health

Dong Quai Root
Damiana
Ashwagandha
Wild Yam Root
Burdock Root
Sea Greens
Vitex
Sarsaparilla Root

Pituitary

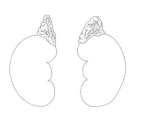

Pituitary Health

Royal Jelly
Sarsaparilla
Damiana
Dong Quai
Barley Grass
Horsetail
Alfalfa
Burdock Root
Licorice Root

Thymus

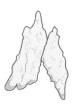

Thymus Health

Bee Pollen/Roy. Jelly
Evening Primrose
Panax Ginseng
Echinacea
Barley Grass
Fenugreek
Thyme
Burdock Root
Licorice Root

Lymph

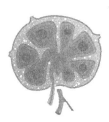

Lymph Health

Echinacea
Barberry Bark
Goldenseal Root
Garlic
Panax Ginseng
Burdock Root
Licorice Root
Green Tea

Thyroid

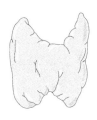

Thyroid Health

Sea Greens
Chlorella
Siberian Ginseng
Evening Primrose
Barley Grass
Mullein-Lobelia
Parsley
Sarsaparilla Root

Pancreas

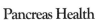

Pancreas Health

Juniper Berries
Dandelion
Licorice Root
Horseradish Root
Garlic

Testes

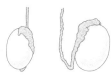

Testicle Health

Panax Ginseng
Damiana
Licorice Root
Dandelion Root
Sarsaparilla

Mind & Spirit

Mind/Spirit Balance

Ginkgo Biloba
Gotu Kola
Panax Ginseng
Sea Greens
Chlorella
Evening Primrose
Royal Jelly
Bee Pollen
Siberian Ginseng
Alfalfa
Rosemary
Sage

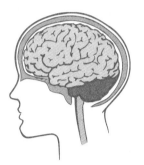

Skin System

Skin Health

Evening Primrose
Dandelion
Rose Hips
Chamomile
Royal Jelly

Skin Healing

Bee Pollen
Barley Grass
Horsetail
Panax Ginseng
Aloe Vera Gel

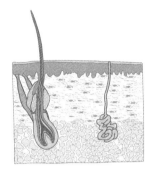

Vision System

Eye Health

Eyebright
Bilberry
Parsley Root
Aloe Vera
Calendula
Chaparral
Ginkgo Biloba
Burdock Root
Hawthorn
Yellow Dock Root
Barley Grass
Sea Greens

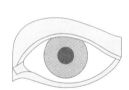

Hair Health

Hair Health

Rosemary
Jojoba Oil
Reishi Mushroom
Sea Greens
Sage

Hair Growth

Horsetail
Oatstraw
Cayenne

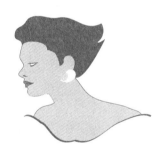

Hearing System

Ear Health

Mullein
Ginkgo Biloba
Turmeric
Yellow Dock Rt.
Garlic
Sea Greens
Spirulina
Echinacea Root
Yarrow
Bayberry Bark
Lobelia

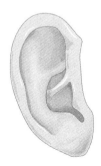

Nail Health

Nail Health

Horsetail
Nettles
Rosemary
Sage
Sea Greens
Oatstraw
Pau d' Arco
Evening Primrose
Garlic
Chamomile
Royal Jelly

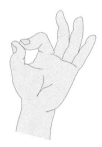

Herbal Preparation & Delivery Methods

Today, hundreds of herbs are available at all quality levels. Worldwide communications and improved storage allow us to simultaneously obtain and use herbs from different countries and different harvests, an advantage ages past did not enjoy. However, because of the natural variety of soils, seeds, and weather, every crop of botanicals is unique. Every batch of a truly natural herbal formula is slightly different, and offers its own unique benefits and experience.

There must be a firm commitment to excellence from growers and suppliers, because herbal combinations are products for problems. For therapeutic success, herbs must be BIO-ACTIVE and BIO-AVAILABLE.

If you decide to make your own herbal preparations, buy the finest quality you can find. There is a world of disparity between fairly good herbs and the best. Superior stock must go into a medicinal formula so that the herbal product can do its job correctly. Superior plants cost far more than standard stock, but their worth in healing activity is a true value for the health care customer.

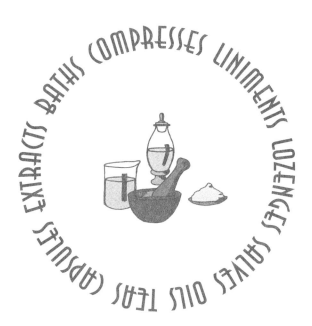

Which preparation form should you choose?

Whichever herbal preparation form you choose, it is generally better to take greater amounts at the beginning of your program, to build a good internal healing base, and to stimulate your body's vital balancing force more quickly. As the therapeutic agents establish and build, and you begin to notice good response, reduce your dose gradually, finally reducing to long range preventive amounts.

"Parts" are a good way to set a common denominator for building an herbal compound. For personal use, one tablespoon is adequate as one part when using powdered herbs for filling capsules; one handful is common as one part for cut herbs in a tea or bath blend. (See HOW TO MAKE AN HERBAL EXTRACT for quantity information for an extract or tincture.)

Herbs can be applied to almost any necessity of life. It's simply a matter of knowing their properties, how they work together and how to use them correctly. Herbs are foods, and your body knows how to use them. Give them time. Give yourself a good diet, some rest and relaxation for the best results.

Herbal teas are the most basic of all healing mediums — easily absorbed by the body as hot liquid. They are the least concentrated of all herbal forms, but many herbs are optimally effective when steeped in hot water. The hot brewing water releases herbal potency and provides a flushing action that is ideal for removing toxic loosened wastes. Although teas have milder, more subtle effects than capsules or extracts, they are sometimes the only way for a weakened system to accept therapeutic support, and often work synergistically with stronger medicinal forms to boost their value.

NOTE 1: Volatile essential oils are lost during cutting of herbs for tea bags. For best results, buy cut herbs or crumble leaves and flowers, and break roots and barks into pieces before steeping for best results.

NOTE 2: Medicinal teas may have bitter tasting properties. Where taste is unpleasant, I add mint, lemon peel, spices, or stevia (sweet herb) to improve taste without harming therapeutic qualities.

Tips on taking herbal teas:

1: Use 1 packed small teaball to 3 cups of water for medicinal-strength tea. Use distilled water or pure spring water for increased herbal strength and effectiveness.

2: Bring water to a boil, remove from heat, add herbs and steep covered off heat; 10 to 15 minutes for a leaf-flower tea; 15 to 25 minutes for a root-bark tea. Keep lid down during steeping so volatile oils don't escape.

3: Use a teapot of glass, ceramic or earthenware, not aluminum. Aluminum can negate the effect of the herbs as the metal dissolves into the hot liquid and gets into the body.

4: Drink medicinal teas in small sips throughout the day rather than all at once. One-half to 1 cup, taken 3 or 4 times over a day allows absorption of the tea, without passing before it has a chance to work.

An infusion is a tea made from dried or powdered herb. Use directions above, or pour 1 cup of boiling water over 1 tablespoon of fresh herb, 1 teaspoon of dried herb, or 4 opened capsules of powdered herb. Cover and let steep 10 to 15 minutes. Never boil. A cold infusion can be made by simply allowing the herbs, especially powders, to stand in cool water for an hour or more.

A decoction is a tea made from roots and barks. Use directions above, or put 2 tablespoons of cut herb pieces into 1 cup cold water. Bring to a light boil, cover, and simmer gently for 20 to 30 minutes. Strain. For best results, repeat the same process with the same herbs. Strain again and mix both batches.

Sun tea is a cold infusion where herbs are put in a covered jar and allowed to stand in the sun.

Herbal broth, rich in minerals and enzymes, are made by grinding dry ingredients in a blender. Simply mix 2 TBS. of dry mix to 2 cups hot water. Let flavors bloom for 5 minutes. Add 1 teasp. BRAGG'S LIQUID AMINOS to each broth for a flavor-nutrient boost if desired. Sip over a half-hour period for best assimilation.

Herbal capsules are generally four times stronger than teas, more concentrated, yet bypass any herbal bitterness and convenient to take. Capsules make both oil and water soluble herbs available through stomach acid and enzyme alteration. Freeze-dried powdered herbs, with all the moisture removed, are also available in capsules, and are four times more concentrated than regular ground herbs. As noted with herbal teas above, grinding herbs into powders creates facets on the whole herb structure causing potential loss of volatile oils. Effective potency for powdered herbs is six months to a year. (See page 59 for more information on how to take herbal capsules.)

Herbal extracts are 4 to 8 times stronger than capsules. They are effective used as a spray where all the mouth receptors can be brought into play, or as drops held under the tongue, bypassing the digestive system's acid-alkaline breakdown. Their strength and ready availability make extracts reliable emergency measures. Small doses may be used repeatedly over a period of time to help build a strong base for restoring body balance.

For treatment during the first week of an acute condition, hold an extract dose in the mouth for 30 seconds, 3 or 4 times daily. After the first week, the vital force of your body will often be sufficiently stimulated in its own healing ability, and the dose may be reduced so your system can take its own route to balance. As with other herbal preparations, take extracts 6 days in a row with a rest on the seventh day before resuming. As the body increases its ability to right itself, the amount, frequency and strength of the dosage should be decreased.

Herbal tinctures are also extractions, are made using a 25% alcohol and water mixture as the solvent. Tinctures are generally extracted from individual herbs rather than compounds. When a commercial compound is made, each separately prepared tincture is added rather than made from the beginning as a compounded extract. Commercial tinctures use ethyl alcohol, and may even be formed from fluid extracts, but diluted spirits are suitable for home use; vodka is ideal.

Extracts are more concentrated than tinctures, because they distill or filter off some of the alcohol. A tincture is typically a 1:10 or 1:5 concentration (10 or 5 units of extract come from 1 unit of herbs), while a fluid extract is usually 1:1.

Even stronger, *a solid or powdered extract* has the solvent completely removed. Powdered extracts are at least 4 times as potent as an equal amount of fluid extract, and 40 times as potent as a tincture. One gram of a 4:1 solid extract is equivalent to $1/7$ of an ounce of a fluid extract, and $1^1/_2$ ounces of a tincture.

Note: Homeopathic liquid formulas are not the same as herbal tinctures or extracts, and their use is different.

To make a simple herbal extraction:

Alcohol, wine, apple cider vinegar, and vegetable glycerine are common mediums for extracting herbal properties. Alcohol releases the widest variety of essential herbal elements in unchanged form, and allows the fastest sublingual absorption. Alcohol and water mixtures can resolve almost every relevant ingredient of any herb, and also act as a natural preserver for the compound. Eighty to one hundred proof (40-50%) vodka, is an excellent solvent for most plant constituents. It has long term preservative activity and is easily obtainable for personal use. The actual amount of alcohol in a daily dose is about $1/_{30}$ oz., but if alcohol is not desired, extract drops may be placed in a little warm water for 5 minutes to allow the alcohol to evaporate before drinking. Most extracts are formulated with 1 gram of herb for each 5ml of alcohol.

Extract directions:
1: Put about 4-oz. dried chopped or ground herb, or 8-ounces of fresh herb, into a quart canning jar.
2: Pour about one pint of 80 to 100 proof vodka over the herbs and close tightly.
3: Keep the jar in a warm place for two to three weeks, and shake well twice a day.
4: Decant liquid into a bowl; then pour slurry residue through several layers of muslin or cheesecloth into the bowl. Strain all the liquid through the layers once again to insure a clearer extract.
5: Squeeze out all liquid from cloth. (Sprinkle solid residue around your houseplants as herb food. I have done this for years, and they love it.)
6: Pour the extract into a dark glass bottle. Stopper, seal tightly, and store away from light. An extract made in this way will keep its potency for several years.

Herbal wine infusions are a pleasant, effective method of taking herbs, especially as digestive aids with meals. Take as warming circulatory tonics by-the-spoonful in winter. The alcohol acts as a transport medium and stimulant to the bloodstream.

To make a simple wine infusion, use fresh or dried herbs:

—Method 1: For a warming winter circulation and energy tonic, pour off $1/_4$ cup of a fortified wine, such as madeira, cognac or brandy. Place chosen herbs and spices in the wine and recork the bottle. Place in a dark cool place for a week or two. Strain off the solids, and combine the medicinal wine with a fresh bottle. Mix well, and take a small amount as needed for energy against fatigue.

—**Method 2:** For a nerve and brain tonic, steep fresh or dried herbs in a bottle of either white or red wine for about a week. Strain off herbs, and drink a small amount as needed.

Herbal syrups are well accepted by children, and can greatly improve the taste of bitter herbal compounds. They are also excellent treatment forms for throat coats and gargles, or bronchial, chest-lung infections. Syrups are simple and quick to make.

Two simple ways to make an herbal syrup:
—**Method 1:** Boil $\frac{3}{4}$ lb. raw or brown sugar in 2 cups of herb tea until it reaches syrup consistency.
—**Method 2:** Make a simple syrup with $\frac{3}{4}$ lb. raw sugar in 2 cups of water, boiling until it reaches syrup consistency. Remove from heat, and while the syrup is cooling, add an herbal extract or tincture — one part extract to three parts of syrup.

Herbal pastes and electuaries (mediums that mask the bitter taste of medicinal herbs) are made by grinding or blending herbs in the blender with a little water into a paste. The paste is then mixed with twice the amount of honey, syrup, butter, or cream cheese for taste. Other good electuaries include fresh bread rolled around a little of the paste, or peanut butter.

Herbal lozenges are an ideal way to relieve mouth, throat, and upper respiratory conditions. Make them by combining powdered herbs with sugar and a mucilage herb, such as marshmallow or slippery elm, or a gum, such as tragacanth or acacia. Both powdered herbs and essential herbal oils may be used. Proper mucilage preparation is the key to successful lozenges.

To make an herbal lozenge:
1: Soak 1-oz. powdered mucilage herb (listed above) in water; cover for 24 hours; stir occasionally.
2: Bring 2 cups of water to a boil and add the mucilage herb.
3: Beat to obtain a uniform consistency and force through cheesecloth to strain.
4: Mix with enough powdered herb to form a paste and add sugar to taste. Or, mix 12 drops essential peppermint oil (or other essential oil) with 2-oz. of sugar and enough mucilage to make a paste.
5: Roll on a board covered with arrowroot or sugar to prevent sticking. Cut into shapes and leave exposed to air to dry. Store in an airtight container.

External use preparations:
The skin is the body's largest organ of ingestion. Topical herbal mediums may be used as needed for all over relief and support.

Herbal baths provide a soothing gentle way to absorb herbal therapy through the skin. In essence, you soak in a diluted medicinal tea, allowing your skin to take in the healing properties instead of your mouth and digestive system. The procedure for taking an infusion bath is almost as important as the herbs themselves.

Two good therapeutic bath techniques:
—**Method 1:** Draw very hot bath water. Put the bath herbs in an extra large tea ball or small muslin bath bag (sold in natural food stores). Steep in the bath until the water cools slightly and is aromatic, about 10 to 15 minutes.
—**Method 2:** Make a strong tea infusion on the stove as usual with a full pot of water. Strain and add directly to the bath. Soak for at least 30 to 45 minutes to give your body time to absorb the herbal properties. Rub all over your body with the solids in the muslin bag while soaking for best herb absorbency.

Herbal douches are an effective method of treating simple vaginal infections. Simply steep the herbs as for a strong tea, strain, and pour the liquid into a douche bag. Sit on the toilet, insert the applicator, and rinse the vagina with the douche. Use one full douche bag for each application. Most vaginal conditions need douching three times daily for 3 to 7 days. If the infection does not respond in this time, see a qualified health professional.

Herbal suppositories and boluses are an effective way to treat rectal and vaginal problems, acting as carriers for the herbal medicine. Herbal suppositories generally serve one of three purposes: to soothe inflamed mucous membranes and aid the healing process; to help reduce swollen membranes and overcome pus-filled discharge; and to work as a laxative, stimulating normal peristalsis to overcome chronic constipation.

To prepare a simple suppository:

Mix about a tablespoon of finely powdered herbs with enough cocoa butter to make a firm consistency. Roll into torpedo shaped tubes about an inch long. Place on wax paper, and put in the freezer to firm. Remove one at a time for use and allow to come to room temperature before using. Insert at night.

Herbal ointments and salves are semi-solid preparations, that allow absorption of herbal benefits through the skin. They may be made with vaseline, UN-Petroleum Jelly or cocoa butter for a simple compound; or in a more complex technique with herbal tea, oils and hardening agents like beeswax, lanolin or lard.

To prepare a simple ointment or salve:

—**Method 1:** Warm about 6 oz. of vaseline, petroleum jelly or lanolin in a small pan with 2 TBS. of cut herbs; or stir in enough powdered herbs to bring the mixture to a dark color. Simmer gently for 10 minutes, stirring. Then filter through cheesecloth, pressing out all liquid. Pour into small wide-mouth containers when cool but still pliable.

—**Method 2:** This method is best when a carrier base is needed for volatile herbal oils, such as for chest rubs or anti-congestive balms, where the base itself is not to be absorbed by the skin. Steep herbs in water to make a strong tea. Strain off the liquid into a pan. Add your chosen oils and fats, such as almond, sesame, wheat germ, or olive oils, and cocoa butter or lanolin fats (about 6-oz. total) to the strained tea.

Simmer until water evaporates, and the herbal extract is incorporated into the oils. Add enough beeswax to bring mixture to desired consistency; use about 2-oz. beeswax to 5-oz. of herbal oil. Let melt and stir until well blended. Add 1 drop of tincture of benzoin (available at most pharmacies) for each ounce of ointment to preserve the mixture against mold.

Herbal compresses and fomentations draw out waste and waste residue, such as cysts or abscesses, via the skin or release them into your body's elimination channels. Compresses are made by soaking a cotton cloth in a strong herbal tea, and applying it as hot as possible to the affected area. The heat enhances the activity of the herbs, and opens the pores of the skin for fast assimilation.

—Use alternating hot and cold compresses to stimulate nerves and circulation. Apply the herbs to the hot compress, and leave the cold compress plain. Cayenne, ginger and lobelia are good choices for the hot compress.

To make an effective compress:

Add 1 teasp. powdered herbs to a bowl of very hot water. Soak a washcloth and apply until the cloth cools. Then apply a cloth dipped in ice water until it reaches body temperature. Repeat several times daily.

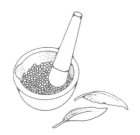

Green clay compresses, for growths, may be applied to gauze, placed on the area, and left for all day. Simply change as you would any dressing when you bathe.

Herbal poultices and plasters are made from either fresh herbs, crushed and blended in a blender with a little olive or wheat germ oil, or dried herbs, mixed with water, cider vinegar or wheat germ oil into a paste. Either blend may be spread on a piece of clean cloth or gauze, and bound directly on the affected area. The whole application is then covered with plastic wrap to keep from soiling clothes or sheets, and left on for 24 hours. There is usually a great deal of throbbing pain while the poultice is drawing out the infection and neutralizing the toxic poisons. This stops when the harmful agents are drawn out, and signals the removal of the poultice. A fresh poultice should be applied every 24 hours.

To make a plaster:

Spread a thin coat of honey on a clean cloth, and sprinkle it with an herbal mixture such as cayenne, ginger, and prickly ash, or hot mustard or horseradish. The cloth is then taped directly over the affected area, usually the chest, to relieve lung and mucous congestion.

Herbal liniments are used as warming massage mediums to stimulate and relieve sore muscles and ligaments. They are for external use only. Choose heat-inducing herbs and spices such as cayenne, ginger, cloves and myrrh, and drops of heating oils such as eucalyptus, wintergreen and cajeput. Steep in rubbing alcohol for two to three weeks. Strain and decant into corked bottles for storage.

Herbal oils are used externally for massage, skin treatments, healing ointments, dressings for wounds and burns, and occasionally for enemas and douches. Simply infuse the herb in oil instead of water. Olive, safflower or almond oil are good bases for an herbal oil.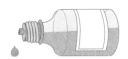

To make an herbal oil for home use:

—**Method 1:** Cut fresh herbs into a glass container and cover with oil. Place in the sun and leave in a warm place for three to four weeks, shaking daily to mix. Filter into a dark glass container to store.

—**Method 2:** Macerate dried, powdered herbs directly into the oil. Let stand for one or two days. Strain and bottle for use.

Hugging can keep you healthy.

It cures depression, it boosts immune response.

It reduces stress, it induces relaxation and sleep,
it's invigorating, it's rejuvenating.

It has no unpleasant side effects.

Hugging is a miracle drug.

The Herbal Medicine Garden

Growing your own herbal medicines is becoming increasingly popular as people get "back to the roots" of healing. Perhaps you've already grown culinary herbs for your kitchen needs. Many culinary herbs also have healing value. Most herbs are easy to grow and require minimal care. They grow in tiny spaces, (almost every herb can grow in a window box), and most are so potent that a little goes a long way. The majority of herbs are drought resistant, evergreen or herbaceous perennials.

A few tips on growing, harvesting and storing your own fresh medicinal herbs:

Herbs can help you get back to the basics, if you take care of their basics first. Fertile soil structure is extremely important to the potency of herbal medicines, both for mineral and enzyme concentrations. If you don't have good soil, enrich it before you plant. Add plenty of humus to either clay or sandy soil to improve soil structure and increase its fertility.

Most herbs are best planted in the fall, before the ground freezes, so they can establish a good root system in loose, well drained soil. If you live in a cold climate, where temperatures drop to and stay near zero, plant most herbs in early spring as soon as the ground can be worked. (I usually recommend window boxes for cold climates, and for basil anywhere because you can extend your growing season much longer.)

Carrot family herbs, like dill, fennel, chervil, coriander (cilantro) and parsley are easy to grow from seeds. Plant them directly into the garden or pot in which they are going to grow — they don't like being transplanted.

Annual herbs like borage, and non-woody perennials like lemon balm, feverfew, chives, elecampane, pennyroyal or violet usually reseed themselves.

Woody perennials, like lavender, rosemary and thymes don't self-seed well and produce far fewer offspring.

Mints and tarragons don't come up true from seed. They can only be propagated from cuttings or divisions. I purchase these from a good nursery.

Herbs are wonderful companion plants, not only for each other, but for other plants in your garden. They act as natural pesticides, enhance the growth and flavor of vegetables and help keep soil rich.

—Plant *basil* with tomatoes to improve flavor and growth, and to repel flies and mosquitoes.
    Don't plant basil near rue.
—Plant *hyssop* with cabbage and grapes to deter cabbage moths. Don't plant near radishes.
—Put a fresh *bay leaf* in storage containers of beans or grain to deter weevils and moths.
—Plant *borage* near tomatoes, squash and strawberries to deter tomato worms.
—Plant *caraway* to loosen compacted soil.
—Plant *catnip* to keep away flea beetles.
—Plant *chamomile* with cabbage and onions to improve flavor.
—Plant *chervil* with radishes to improve growth and flavor.
—Plant *chives* with carrots to improve growth and flavor.
—Plant *dill* with cabbage, but not near carrots.
—Plant *gopher purge* around your garden to deter burrowing pests.
—Plant *horseradish* in a potato patch to keep out potato bugs.
—Plant *bee balm* with tomatoes to improve growth and flavor.
—Plant *lovage* to improve health of most plants.
—Plant *garlic* near roses to repel aphids.
—Plant *marjoram* for more flavor of all vegetables.
—Plant *mint* for healthy cabbage and tomatoes, and to deter white cabbage moths.
—Plant *peppermint* to deter moths and carrot flies.
—Plant *nasturtiums* to deter white flies, cabbage moth and squash bugs.

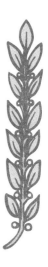

—Plant *rue* with roses and raspberries to deter Japanese beetles.
—Plant *sage* to deter cabbage moths, beetles and carrot flies. Don't plant near cucumbers.
—Plant *summer savory* with beans and onions to improve flavor and deter cabbage moths.
—Plant *tansy* to deter flying insects, Japanese beetles, cucumber beetles, squash bugs and ants.
—Plant *thyme* to deter cabbage worms.
—Plant *wormwood* as a border to keep animals out of your garden.

You can harvest the leaves of medicinal herbs any time during the growing season as long as they look, smell and taste fresh. Avoid harvesting from plants that have begun to discolor, are buggy or diseased. Herbal flowers are best harvested before they are in full bloom.

Harvest roots like burdock, dandelion and comfrey in the spring and fall when they are full of sap. Wait for a dry spell during rainy seasons because wet roots are difficult to dry and are not as concentrated in medicinal qualities. Look for roots that are fleshy, but not old-looking, woody or fibrous. Roots have to be fully developed, though; immature roots don't have vital nutritional properties. I don't recommend harvesting roots or corms unless you are something of an expert, because drying and storing techniques are much more difficult, and roots may be contaminated or moldy inside without your being aware of it.

Harvest barks when you harvest roots in the spring and fall when the sap is moving up and down the plant. Sassafras, birch, willow, oak and witch hazel are common tree barks valued for medicinal qualities.

Harvest seeds late in the day, after a few days of dry weather, to ensure that all plant parts are dry. Most herb seeds are brown or black when they're ready to harvest. Look for flower stalks that are dry and brown, and seed pods that have turned to brown, gray, or black. Cut off the entire seed head and place it in a large paper bag, cardboard box, or wooden bowl. Place only one kind of seed in each container, and label each container. Set seeds in a dry, warm place with good air circulation. Give them a few weeks of open-air drying before removing the seeds out of the pods or heads; then store them in airtight containers. Check seeds periodically for mold.

Drying herbs is the time-honored way of preserving their medicinal qualities. Harvesting herbs in the traditional way means cutting the stems with leaf, flower and all, tying the stalks in bundles and hanging them upside down in an attic or drying shed. I think a food dehydrator is by far the best way to dry herbs today. It provides you with a clean, thoroughly dried product, and it doesn't take up much space.

Once dry, put the herbs in airtight, glass containers away from light and heat. I don't recommend either metal canisters or paper bags for medicinal herbs, because the qualities are either changed or lost.

Freezing your fresh dried herbs retains their medicinal qualities well. Here's how to do it.
—Rinse the herbs and let them drain until dry. I usually strip the leaves off the stems, and snip them with kitchen shears for better storage and later use in teas. Lay the herb pieces in a single layer on baking sheets and freeze til rigid, about an hour. Pour the rigid herbs into small freezer plastic bags, press out air, seal, and return to the freezer.
—To use, simply take out what you need, reseal, and return the rest to the freezer. It's so easy.

In California,
the Earth is so kind that you just
tickle her with a hoe
and she laughs with a harvest.

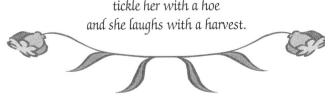

Herbal First Aid For Your Medicine Chest

An herbal first aid kit is a safe way to cope with everyday healing problems, temporary or non-serious health conditions. It can handle many problems immediately and simply, save you hundreds of dollars in doctor bills, and keep you from a traumatic, time consuming visit to a medical clinic.

The choices in this kit are easy to use, inexpensive, gentle enough for children, effective for adults.

—**For colds, flu and chest congestion:** *elder-yarrow-peppermint* tea for sniffles; *mullein oil* for earaches, *lavender* or *eucalyptus* steams or hot *ginger* compresses for chest congestion; an *echinacea-goldenseal-myrrh* combination as a natural antibiotic.

—**For coughs, and sore throat:** *loquat* syrup or *licorice-wild cherry-slippery elm* tea for coughs, Crystal Star ZINC SOURCE HERBAL THROAT SPRAY for sore throat, Zand herbal throat drops, *aloe vera juice* or *tea tree oil* gargle.

—**For cuts, wounds, scrapes and scars:** *ginseng* skin repair gel, *pau d'arco-calendula* gel, *witch hazel* compresses, *comfrey-aloe* salve, *aloe vera* gel, Deva Flowers FIRST AID REMEDY extract, *tea tree oil*.

—**For fungal infections like athlete's foot, ringworm and nail fungus:** *tea tree* oil, *grapefruit seed* extract, *black walnut* extract, *goldenseal-myrrh* solution, *pau d'arco-dandelion-gentian* gel.

—**For minor bacterial and viral infections:** *echinacea-golden seal-myrrh* combination, *white pine-bayberry* capsules for first aid; *osha root* tea, *usnea* extract, *St. John's wort-lomatium* extract.

—**For rashes, itching, swelling from insect bites or other histamine reactions:** antihistamine *marshmallow-bee pollen-white pine* capsules, *calendula-pau d'arco* gel, *comfrey-plantain* ointment, *tea tree* oil, aloe vera gel, *echinacea-St. John's wort-white willow* capsules.

—**For pain, cramping and headache relief:** *lavender* compresses, *black cohosh-scullcap* extract, *peppermint oil* rubs, *comfrey* compresses, *rosemary* tea or steam, *ginkgo biloba* or *feverfew* extract.

—**For strains, sprains and muscle pulls:** *White willow-St. John's wort* capsules or salve, Tiger Balm analgesic gel, Chinese *white flower oil*, *tea tree* or *wintergreen-cajeput oil*, and *Fo-Ti* (ho-shu-wu).

—**For periodic constipation and diarrhea:** fiber and herbs *butternut-cascara* capsules, *senna-fennel* laxative tea, *milk thistle seed* extract to soften stool, Ayurvedic *Triphala* formula, *aloe vera* juice.

—**For sleep aids for insomnia:** *rosemary-chamomile-catnip*, or *passion flower-spearmint* tea, *hops-rosemary* sleep pillow, *wild lettuce-valerian* extract, *ashwagandha-black cohosh-scullcap* capsules.

—**For calming stress and tension:** *ginseng-licorice* extract, *rosemary-chamomile* tea; Bach Flower RESCUE REMEDY drops, *lemon balm-lemongrass* tea, *valerian-wild lettuce* extract, *chamomile* aromatherapy.

—**For indigestion, gas and upset stomach relief:** *ginger* tea or capsules; *catnip-fennel* tea; mixed *mint* tea or extract, *comfrey-pepsin* capsules; *aloe vera juice* with herbs, or a *cinnamon-nutmeg-ginger* spice mix.

—**For eye infections and inflammations:** *aloe vera juice* wash, *eyebright-parsley-bilberry* capsules or wash, *echinacea-goldenseal* wash, *chamomile-elder* compress, *witch hazel-rosemary* solution.

—**For toothaches and gum problems:** *tea tree oil*, or apply *clove oil* directly onto tooth or gums.

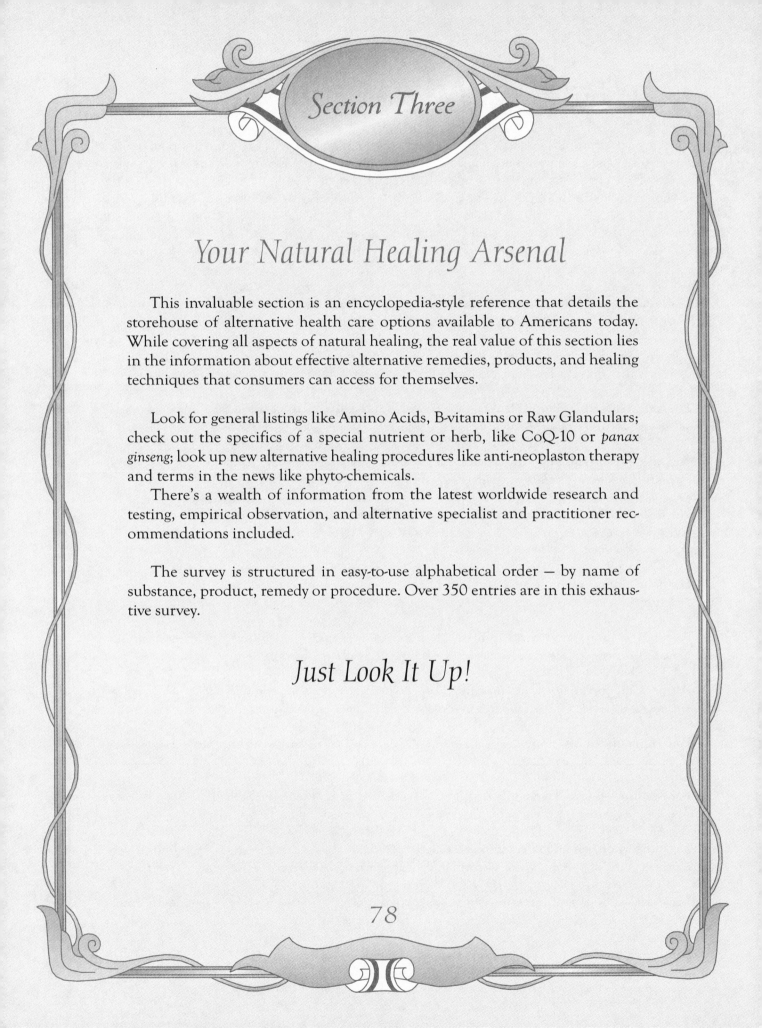

Your Natural Healing Arsenal

This invaluable section is an encyclopedia-style reference that details the storehouse of alternative health care options available to Americans today. While covering all aspects of natural healing, the real value of this section lies in the information about effective alternative remedies, products, and healing techniques that consumers can access for themselves.

Look for general listings like Amino Acids, B-vitamins or Raw Glandulars; check out the specifics of a special nutrient or herb, like CoQ-10 or *panax ginseng*; look up new alternative healing procedures like anti-neoplaston therapy and terms in the news like phyto-chemicals.

There's a wealth of information from the latest worldwide research and testing, empirical observation, and alternative specialist and practitioner recommendations included.

The survey is structured in easy-to-use alphabetical order — by name of substance, product, remedy or procedure. Over 350 entries are in this exhaustive survey.

Just Look It Up!

The Alternative Health Care Arsenal
Look It Up!

The alternative arsenal is an updated, exhaustive survey of the health care options available to Americans today. The value of this section lies in its quick reference data on effective alternative remedies, products and healing procedures that consumers can access for themselves. Information from worldwide studies, empirical observation, as well as natural healers and practitioners is included.

The survey is structured in alphabetical order as an easy-reference guide. Access it by name of substance, product, remedy or procedure.

ACEROLA: derived from the ripe fruit of the cherry-like fruit of *Malpighia Glabra*, acerola is a rich source of vitamin C and bioflavonoids. Used as an antioxidant and for its ascorbic acid content.

• **ACIDOPHILUS CULTURE COMPLEX:** like *lactobacillus, bulgaricus, and bifida bacterium*, are beneficial bacteria that synthesize nutrients in the intestinal tract, counteract pathogenic micro-organisms and maintain a healthy intestinal environment. Use for digestion and for friendly flora restoration after long drug use.

• **ACONITE:** a homeopathic remedy for children's earaches. Helps the body deal with the trauma of sudden fright or shock. See HOMEOPATHIC REMEDIES on page 19.

• **ACUPUNCTURE AND ACUPRESSURE:** see ALTERNATIVE HEALING TECHNIQUES, page 31.

• **AGAR:** a fibrous thickener in foods and cosmetics; derived from *Gelidiella Acerosa,* a sea algae.

• **ALANINE:** a non-essential amino acid which helps maintain blood glucose levels, particularly as an energy storage source for the liver and muscles. See also Amino Acids.

• **ALGAE, GREEN & BLUE-GREEN:** *phyto-plankton.* See GREEN SUPERFOODS, pg 135.

• **ALLANTOIN:** a cosmetic ingredient from the comfrey plant used as a skin protector and softener.

• **ALOE VERA,** *Aloe Barbadensis:* See HEALING POWERHOUSES OF THE DESERT, pg. 183.

• **ALPHA HYDROXY ACIDS (AHA'S):** naturally occurring substances found in foods like apples, grapes, citrus fruit, sugarcane and sour milk, as well as in the body. AHAs work by dissolving the glue-like lipids holding cells together and can penetrate deep into the skin to loosen clingy bonds that clog and roughen skin. When top layers of skin are loosened and released they reveal a smoother complexion. Not all AHAs work the same. Glycolic acid from sugar cane acts fastest and deepest, but is also one of the most irritating. Lactic acid from sour milk is often the AHA of choice because it doesn't penetrate as deeply so is not as irritating. Tartaric acid from grapes, malic acid from apples, citric acid from citrus, and new synthetics, work only on or near the skin surface. They take longer to show improvement, but do not sting or redden the skin. Products advertised with high AHA's don't necessarily work better — only faster. The real difference is in the pH level of the product. Quicker results can be achieved from a product lower on the pH scale (2.5pH) than a product higher on the pH scale (4.5pH). Products between 3pH and 4.5pH have more moisturizing effects.

• **ALPHA-LINOLENIC ACID (LNA):** See FATS & OILS, page 158.

• **ALPHA TOCOPHEROL (vitamin E):** found in wheat germ, nut and seed oils, eggs, organ meats, oats and olives, vitamin E boosts fertility, improves circulation, promotes longevity, prevents blood clots, strengthens capillary walls, helps our bodies use vitamin A, maintains cell membrane health, and contributes to healthy skin and hair. Alpha tocopherol is an antioxidant proven in preventing heart disease, and protecting healthy cells from free radical destruction.

• **AMLA BERRY,** (Indian gooseberry) *Emblica Officinalis:* is one of the richest natural sources of bioflavonoids and vitamin C; each amla fruit contains up to 700mg of vitamin C. It is a natural ascorbate, synergistically enhanced by both bioflavonoid and polyphenols. Amla is revered for its anti-aging, immune enhancing properties. It has been used since ancient times for anemia, asthma, bleeding gums, diabetes, colds, chronic lung disease, hyperlipidemia, hypertension, yeast infections, scurvy and cancer. Studies show that amla protects against chromosome damage from heavy metal exposure.

• **AMINO ACIDS:** the building blocks of protein in the body — absolutely necessary to life, growth and healing. Protein is composed of, and depends upon the right supply of amino acids. There are 29 of them known, from which over 1600 basic proteins are formed, comprising more than 75% of your body's solid weight of structural, muscle and blood protein cells. Amino acids are an important part of body fluids, antibodies to fight infection, and hormone-enzyme systems responsible for the growth, maintenance and repair of our bodies throughout our lives. Amino acids are sources of energy with a vital role in brain function, acting as neurotransmitters for the central nervous system. They are critical to rapid healing, and good acid-alkaline balance.

The liver produces about 80% of the amino acids it needs; the remaining 20% must be obtained from our foods. But poor diet, unhealthy habits and environmental pollutants mean that the "essential amino acids" (those we need but our bodies can't produce), may not be sufficient to produce the "non-essentials" (those formed by metabolic activity). We can correct this situation by increasing intake of protein foods or supplementation. A food-source, pre-digested supplement may often be used more quickly than dietary amino acids.

Specific amino acids produce specific pharmacological effects in the body, and can be used to target specific healing goals. Amino acids work well with other natural healers, like herbs, minerals and anti-oxidants.

The main amino acids are *Alanine, Arginine, Aspartic Acid, Branch Chain Aminos, Carnitine, Cysteine, Cystine, GABA, Glutamic Acid, Glutamine, Glutathione, Glycine, Di-methyl-glycine, Histidine, Inosine, Lysine, Methionine, Ornithine, Phenylalanine, Taurine, Threonine, Tryptophan, Tyrosine.* SEE REFERENCE BY NAME IN THIS SURVEY.

Tips for taking amino acids effectively:
1: Take amino acids with extra water or other liquid for optimum absorption by the body.
2: If using a single free form amino acid, take a full spectrum amino acid compound sometime during the same day for increased absorption and results.
3: Free form aminos compete for uptake; take free forms separately from each other for best results.
4: Take single free form amino acids with their nutrient co-factors for best metabolic uptake.
5: Take free form amino acids, except those for brain stimulation, before meals.

Note: Amino acid names may be preceded by the letters "D," "L," or "DL." The prefixes are needed because many biological compounds exist in nature in two identical forms, except that they are mirror images of each other (like your right and left hands). In most cases, only one form is active in the body. "D" stands for dextro (right), "L" stands for levo (left). Sometimes the "D" form is active – D-glucose or D-alpha-tocopherol, sometimes the "L" form is active – L-carnitine or L-lysine, sometimes the "DL" form is active – DL-Phenylalanine. Only the active form is usually available for sale, so even if the initial isn't stated, the product is the active form.

• **AMINOPHYLLINE:** a theophylline-type extract of *ephedra*, is the primary ingredient in some spot reducing creams. Here's how aminophylline works: fat cells are covered with switches called beta-receptors. When the body needs energy, beta-receptors are stimulated to release a substance that activates fat for fuel. But, the type of cells for long term storage, that reside in a woman's thighs and upper arms and on a man's belly, have only a few beta-receptors, so they hang on to their fat stores. Prolonging fat release activity in these cells can result in one to two inches of fat loss from fat storage depots. Aminophylline's role in this process is to keep the fat releasing substance activated to prolong the mechanism of fat loss.

• **ANDROSTENEDIONE:** a steroid hormone, naturally produced in both male and female gonads and the adrenal glands, a metabolite of DHEA, Andro is one step away from testosterone. Testosterone is a major player in the development of male sex organs, muscles, body hair and also in maintaining strength and energy. Serum levels of testosterone start rising about 15 minutes after oral administration of Andro (a precursor of testosterone) and stay elevated for up to 3 hours. Andro became a popular sports supplement in the summer of 1998, when baseball superstar, Mark McGwire revealed to the world he was taking androstenedione. Andro is found in the pollen of Scotch pine trees — the current supplement source.

Is Andro safe? It's a powerful hormone stimulant, so it shouldn't not be taken casually. We know very little about its long-term effects on health and hormone balance.

—In some men, Andro boosts testosterone levels too much and too fast, causing too much testosterone production, as well as aggressive behavior and acne.

—A study published in the June 1999 Journal of the American Medical Association finds that Andro may not always increase blood levels of testosterone as previously believed, but can actually convert into estrogen. This especially concerns men — Andro's target market. Excess estrogen in men's bodies can increase risk for pancreatic cancer and heart disease. It also can cause side effects like enlarged breasts or water retention!

—For women, Andro may cause facial whiskers, chest hair growth or voice deepening.

New information shows more serious concerns.....

—After long-term Andro use, your body may perceive abnormal amounts of the hormone and may shut down natural testosterone production as happens with melatonin, another steroid hormone.

—Teens should be especially warned — abnormally high testosterone levels in kids can stunt growth and cause permanent heart and liver damage.

—Andro is contraindicated if there are hormone-related problems like prostate enlargement or cancers of the breast, prostate or testes.

—Avoid Andro if you have acne, liver disease, heavy menstruation or Cushing's syndrome.

• **ANTI-NEOPLASTON THERAPY:** a relatively new cancer treatment developed by Dr. Stanislaw Burzynski. Antineoplastons consist of small peptides, components of protein, and peptide metabolites that are given orally or intravenously. They work by entering the cell and altering specific functions of the genes; some activate the tumor suppressor genes that prevent cancer, while others turn off the oncogenes that force the cancer cell to divide uncontrollably. Antineoplastons cause cancerous cells to either revert to normal or die without dividing. Burzynski first isolated the natural compounds from blood and urine in the early 1970's. He now synthesizes them at his own FDA regulated pharmaceutical lab. For complete information write to P.O. box 1770, Pacific Palisades, CA 90272.

• **ANTIOXIDANTS:** Increasing evidence shows that people live more vigorous, less-diseased lives when antioxidants are a part of their nutritional program. This is especially true if a person shows signs of premature aging, reduced immune response, allergies, or is regularly exposed to environmental pollutants. Antioxidants unite with oxygen, protecting the cells and other body constituents like enzymes from being destroyed or altered by oxidation. Antioxidant mechanisms are selective, acting against undesirable oxygen reactions but not with desirable oxygen activity. Although oxygen is vital to our body functions, the presence of either too much or too little oxygen creates toxic by-products called free radicals. These highly reactive substances can damage cell structures impairing immunity, even altering DNA codes — the result is degenerative disease and premature aging. Specifically, free radical attacks are the forerunners of heart attacks, cancer, and opportunistic diseases such as HIV infection, candidiasis or chronic fatigue syndrome. Antioxidants "scavenge" or quench free radical fires, neutralize their damage and render them harmless. A poor diet, inadequate exercise, illness and emotional stress result in a reduction of the body's system antioxidants. See also Free Radicals, page 95.

Some anti-oxidants you can use for protective health care and healing:

—**Pycnogenol:** an active bioflavonoid extract of pine bark. Fifty times stronger than vitamin E, 20 times stronger than vitamin C, it is one of the few antioxidants that crosses the blood-brain barrier to directly protect brain cells.

—**CoQ-10:** an essential catalyst co-enzyme for cellular energy in the body. Supplementation provides wide ranging therapeutic benefits. See Enzymes & Enzyme Therapy, pg.127 for complete information.

—**Germanium:** A potent antioxidant mineral (germanium sesquioxide), that detoxifies, blocks free radicals and increases production of natural killer cells. An interferon stimulus for immunity and healing.

—**Ginkgo Biloba:** combats the effects of aging, especially boosting memory acuity and circulation. Helps protect cells against free radical damage. Reduces blood cell clumping leading to congestive heart disease.

—**Glutathione Peroxidase:** an antioxidant enzyme that scavenges and neutralizes free radicals by turning them into stable oxygen and H_2O_2, then into oxygen and water. See Enzyme Therapy, pg. 127.

—**SOD, Superoxide Dismutase:** an antioxidant enzyme that works with catalase to scavenge and neutralize free radicals. See Enzymes & Enzyme Therapy, pg. 127.

—**Astragalus:** an herbal immune stimulant and body tonic that enhances adrenal function. Vasodilating properties lower blood pressure, increase metabolism and improve circulation.

—**Methionine:** a free radical deactivator; a lipotropic that keeps fats from accumulating in the liver and arteries. Protective against chemical allergic reactions.

—**Cysteine:** an antioxidant amino acid that works with vitamins C, E, and selenium to protect against radiation toxicity, cancer carcinogens, and free radical damage to skin and arteries. Stimulates immune white cell activity. Aids in the body's uptake of iron. *Note:* Take vitamin C in a 3:1 ratio to cysteine for best results.

—**Egg lipids, egg yolk lecithin:** a powerful source of choline and phosphatides. Used in treating AIDS and immune-deficient disease. Refrigerate; take immediately upon mixing with water to retain potency.

—**Octacosanol:** a wheat germ derivative; boosts energy and increases oxygen use during exercise.

—**L-Glutathione:** an antioxidant amino acid that works with cysteine and glutamine to balance blood sugar; neutralizes radiation, inhibits free radicals; a blood cleanser from chemotherapy, X-rays and liver toxicity.

—**Wheat Germ Oil:** a wheat berry extract; rich in B vitamins, proteins, vitamin E, and iron. One tablespoon provides the anti-oxidant equivalent of an oxygen tent for 30 minutes.

—**GLA, Gamma Linoleic Acid:** from evening primrose oil, black currant oil and borage seed oil. A source of cell energy, electrical insulation for nerves, a precursor of prostaglandins which regulate hormones.

—**Shiitake Mushrooms:** produce a virus that stimulates interferon for stronger immune function. Used in Oriental medicine to prevent high blood pressure and heart disease, and to reduce cholesterol.

—**Reishi Mushrooms** (*Ganoderma*): a tonic that increases vitality, enhances immunity and prolongs a healthy life. Helps reduce the side effects of chemotherapy for cancer.

—**Tyrosine:** an amino acid formed from phenylalanine — a GH stimulant that helps build the body's store of adrenal and thyroid hormones. A source of quick energy, especially for the brain.

—**Di-Methyl-Glycine** (*known as* B_{15})**:** an energy stimulant, used chiefly by athletes for endurance and stamina. Sublingual forms are most absorbable. For best results, take before sustained exercise. *Note:* Too much DMG disrupts the metabolic chain and causes fatigue. The proper dose produces energy; overdoses do not.

Some foods are also rich in antioxidants:

—**Selenium:** a component of glutathione; protects the body from free radical and heavy metal damage. Food sources: bran, brewer's yeast, broccoli, cabbage, celery, corn, cucumbers, garlic, mushrooms, onions, wheat germ and whole grains.

—**Vitamin E:** a fat soluble antioxidant and immune stimulant whose activity is increased by selenium. Neutralizes free radicals against aging; an effective anticoagulant and vasodilator against blood clots and heart disease. Food sources: almonds, soy, walnuts, apricots, corn, safflower oil, peanut butter, wheat germ.

—**Beta-carotene:** a vitamin A precursor, converting to vitamin A in the liver as needed. A powerful anti-infective and antioxidant for immune health, protection against pollutants, early aging and allergy control. Food sources: yellow - orange fruits and vegetables, and sea greens.

—**Vitamin C:** a primary preventer of free radical damage, and immune strengthener. Protects against infections, safeguards against radiation, heavy metal toxicity, environmental pollutants and early aging. Essential to formation of new collagen tissue, supports adrenal and iron insufficiency, especially when you're under stress. Food sources: broccoli, lemons, grapefruit, bell peppers, kale, kiwi, oranges, potatoes, strawberries.
Note: Take vitamins A, C, E, selenium and beta carotene together for the most cancer-fighting potential.

• **ANTI-CARCINOGENIC NUTRIENTS**: anticarcinogens are any substances that prevent or delay tumor formation and development. Some herbs and foods anti-carcinogens: *panax ginseng, soy foods, garlic, echinacea, goldenseal, licorice, black cohosh, wild yam, sarsaparilla, maitake mushroom and cruciferous vegetables.*

• **ANTI-PARASITIC NUTRIENTS:** parasites are extremely common and persistent around the globe. Parasites have adapted and become stronger in order to survive, developing defenses against drugs designed to kill them. In fact, most drugs commonly used to treat parasites not only lose effectiveness against new parasite strains, but also cause a number of unpleasant side effects in the host. Herbal remedies, however, have been successfully used for centuries as living medicines against parasites, with few side effects. Natural antiparasitic herbs include *black walnut hulls, garlic, pumpkin seed, gentian root, wormwood, butternut bark, fennel seed, cascara sagrada, mugwort, slippery elm* and *false unicorn.*

• **APIS:** a homeopathic remedy of macerated bee tincture. Relieves stinging after bee sting or insect bite See HOMEOPATHIC REMEDIES, page 19.

• **ARGININE:** a semi-essential amino acid, used for growth hormone and immune response. For athletes and body builders, increases muscle tone while decreasing fat. Promotes wound healing, blocks tumor formation and increases sperm motility. Helps lower blood serum fats, and detoxifies ammonia. Curbs appetite, and helps metabolize fat for weight loss. Herpes virus and schizophrenia can be checked by "starving" them of arginine foods like nuts, peanut butter or cheese. Take with cranberry or apple juice for best results.

• **ARNICA:** a homeopathic remedy for pain relief and to speed healing, especially from sports injuries, like sprains, strains and bruises. May be used topically or internally. See HOMEOPATHIC REMEDIES page 19.

• **AROMATHERAPY:** see ALTERNATIVE HEALING TECHNIQUES, pg. 37.

• **ARROWROOT:** powdered cassava herb, used as a thickener for sauces. Arrowroot works without the digestive, elimination and vitamin loss cornstarch can cause.

• **ARSENICUM ALBUM:** a homeopathic remedy for food poisoning accompanied by diarrhea; for allergic symptoms such as a runny nose; for asthma and colds. See HOMEOPATHIC REMEDIES page 19.

• **ASPARTAME:** FDA has received more complaints about adverse reactions to aspartame than any other food ingredient in the agency's history. See SUGAR & SWEETENERS IN A HEALING DIET, page 174.

• **ASPARTIC ACID:** a non-essential amino acid, abundant in sugar cane and beets; used mainly as a sweetener. A precursor of threonine, it is a neurotransmitter made with ATP that increases your resistance to fatigue. Clinically used to counteract depression and in drugs to protect the liver.

• **ASTRAGALUS:** a prime immune enhancing herb, it is a strong antiviral agent, working to produce extra interferon in the body. Astragalus counteracts immune-suppressing effects of cancer drugs and radiation. Vasodilating properties help significantly lower blood pressure, reduce fluid retention and improve circulation. Chinese research shows that astragalus is an anti-clotting agent in preventing coronary heart disease. Nourishes exhausted adrenals to combat fatigue. Effective in normalizing the nervous system and hormone balance.

BARLEY GRASS: See GREEN SUPERFOODS, page 136.

• **BEE POLLEN:** collected by bees from male seed flowers, mixed with bee secretions, and formed into granules. A highly bio-active, tonic nutrient rightly known as a superfood. Completely balanced nutrients — vitamins, minerals, proteins, fats, enzyme precursors, and all essential amino acids. Bee pollen is a full-spectrum rejuvenative food, especially beneficial for the extra nutritional and energy needs of athletes and those recuperating from illness. A pollen and spore antidote during allergy season, bee pollen relieves respiratory symptoms like bronchitis, sinusitis and colds. Like royal jelly, pollen helps balance the endocrine system, with specific benefits for menstrual and prostate problems. Enzymes in bee pollen normalize chronic colitis and constipation-diarrhea syndromes. Research shows that pollen counteracts early aging effects increasing both mental and physical capability. Two teaspoons daily is a usual dose. Use only unsprayed pollen for therapy.

• **BEE PROPOLIS:** collected by bees from the resin under tree bark, propolis is the first line of defense against beehive infections. It is a natural antibiotic, antiviral and antifungal. In humans, propolis stimulates the thymus gland to enhance resistance to infection, and like all bee products, has strong antibiotic effects. It is also a powerful anti-viral, effective against pneumonia and similar viral infections. Propolis is rich in bioflavonoids and amino acids, is a good source of trace minerals and high in B vitamins, C, E and beta-carotene.

Propolis has a wide range of healing uses: it treats stomach and intestinal ulcers; it speeds the healing of broken bones; and accelerates new cell growth. It is part of almost every natural treatment for gum, mouth and throat disorders. Research on propolis and serum blood fats confirms its reputation for lowering high blood pressure, reducing arteriosclerosis and lessening risk of coronary heart disease. Tests show healing effects on some skin cancers and melanomas. Propolis is available as a concentrated tincture for warts, herpes lesions or other sores, a lighter blend to mix with liquids and take internally, and chewable lozenges for mouth and gum healing. Normal dosage is 300mg daily.

• **BENTONITE:** a natural clay substance used for internal cleansing and externally as a poultice or mask.

• **BELLADONNA:** a homeopathic remedy for sudden fever or sunstroke; for childhood fevers, stomach spasms or restless sleep. See HOMEOPATHIC REMEDIES, page 19.

• **BETA CAROTENE:** a vitamin A precursor, converting to vit. A in the liver as needed. A powerful anti-infective and antioxidant for immune response, protection against environmental pollutants, the aging process, and allergy control. Supplements protect against respiratory diseases and infections. Beta carotene helps prevent lung cancer, and in developing anti-tumor immunity. Food sources: green leafy vegetables, green pepper, carrots and other orange vegetables, dandelion greens and sea vegetables. See Vitamins.

• **B COMPLEX VITAMINS:** the B complex vitamins are essential to almost every aspect of body function, including metabolism of carbohydrates, fats, amino acids and energy production. B Complex vitamins work together. While the separate B vitamins can and do work for specific problems or deficiencies, they should be taken as a whole for broad-spectrum activity. See Vitamins.

• **BIOFEEDBACK:** see ALTERNATIVE HEALING TECHNIQUES, page 23.

• **BIOFLAVONOIDS:** part of the vitamin C complex, bioflavonoids prevent arteries from hardening, and enhance blood vessel, capillary and vein strength. They protect connective tissue integrity, and control bruising, internal bleeding and mouth herpes. Bioflavs lower cholesterol and stimulate bile production. They are anti-microbial against infections and inflammation. One major study shows that bioflavonoids, when combined with enzymes and vitamin C, perform as well as anti-inflammatory drug prescriptions in reducing swelling. They retard cataract formation, and guard against diabetic retinopathy. The body does not produce its own bioflavonoids; they must be obtained regularly from the diet. The strongest supplementary form is quercetin.

Food sources include: blueberries, cherries, turmeric, ginger, alfalfa, the white part under the skin of citrus fruits and certain herbs. See Vitamins.

• **BIOTIN:** a member of the B Complex family, necessary for metabolism of amino acids and essential fatty acids, and in forming immune anti-bodies. Needed for the body to use folacin, B_{12} and pantothenic acid. Naturally made from yeast, biotin supplements show good results in controlling hair loss, dermatitis, eczema, dandruff and seborrheic scalp problems. Improves glucose tolerance in diabetics. Research shows enhanced immune response for Candida Albicans and CFS. Those taking long term antibiotics require extra biotin. Food sources include: poultry, raspberries, grapefruit, tomatoes, tuna, brewer's yeast, salmon, eggs, organ meats, legumes and nuts. See Vitamins.

• **BITTERS:** herbs or substances with a bitter taste that promote the secretion of bile and hydrochloric acid. Bitters tone the muscles of the digestive tract, and improve nutrient absorption and waste elimination. They also enhance immune response, increasing levels of antibodies and improving gut resistance to infections. Beneficial for inflammatory bowel disease, chronic constipation, liver problems, lethargy and low energy. Best used in liquid preparations before meals. Examples of herbal bitters include: *gentian, lemon peel, goldenseal, dandelion and Oregon grape.*

• **BORON:** a mineral which enhances the use of calcium, magnesium, phosphorus and vitamin D in bone formation and structure. Stimulates estrogen production to protect against the onset of osteoporosis. A significant nutritional deterrent to bone loss for athletes. Food sources: most vegetables, fruits and nuts.

• **BOSWELLIA:** *Boswellia glabra, Boswellia serrata -* an anti-inflammatory in Ayurvedic healing. Boswellia suppresses the proliferating tissue of inflamed areas and also prevents breakdown of connective tissue. Boswellia is effective in treating rheumatoid arthritis, osteoarthritis, low back pain, myositis and fibrocystitis.

• **BOVINE TRACHEAL CARTILAGE:** BTC is used to treat cancer, arthritis, rheumatism, acute and chronic skin allergies, and to accelerate the healing of wounds. BTC is a biological response modifier which activates and increases the ability of macrophages (white blood cells) to destroy bacteria and viruses. Paradoxically, BTC is a normalizer, stimulating the immune system to resist cancer and viruses, but suppressing it in rheumatoid diseases. Standard dosage of BTC is 9 grams daily.

• **BRANCH CHAIN AMINO ACIDS:** Leucine, Isoleucine, Valine (BCAAs) are essential amino acids called the stress amino acids; they must be taken together in balanced proportion. Easily converted into ATP, critical to energy and muscle metabolism, they aid hemoglobin formation, help stabilize blood sugar and lower elevated blood sugar levels. BCAAs show excellent results in tissue repair from athletic stress, rebuilding the body from anorexia deficiencies, and in liver restoration after surgical trauma.

• **BREWER'S YEAST:** (Nutritional Yeast) See PROTEINS AND A HEALING DIET, page 134.

• **BROMELAIN:** an enzyme derived from pineapple stems. Popular nutritional therapy, it is widely used to relieve painful menstruation and to treat arthritis. Bromelain inhibits blood-platelet aggregation (clotting) without causing excess bleeding. It is an effective internal sports injury medicine to reduce bruising, relieve pain and swelling, and promote wound healing. It may also be used externally, as a paste applied to stings, to deactivate the protein molecules of insect venom. I highly recommend bromelain before and after surgery of all kinds to accelerate healing. Typically, it is taken with meals, or 30 minutes before or 90 minutes after a meal to help treat sports injuries. See also ENZYMES & ENZYME THERAPY, pg. 127.

• **BRYONIA:** a homeopathic remedy for the swelling and inflammation of arthritis when the symptoms are worse with movement and better with cold. Also for flu infections. See HOMEOPATHIC REMEDIES, page 19.

- **BUCKWHEAT:** a non-wheat grain, acceptable for candida diets. Known as kasha when roasted.

- **BURDOCK:** a hormone-balancer and strong liver purifier, burdock is a significant anti-inflammatory, antibacterial, antifungal and antitumor herb. A specific for blood cleansing, detoxification, immune enhancing combinations, it has special value for skin, arthritic and gland problems.

CALCIUM: the body's most abundant mineral, every cell needs calcium to survive. Calcium is necessary for synthesis of vitamin B_{12} and uses vitamin D for absorption. It works with phosphorus to build teeth and bones, and with magnesium for cardiovascular health and skeletal strength. It helps blood clotting, lowers blood pressure, prevents muscle cramping, maintains nerve health, deters colon cancer and osteoporosis, controls anxiety and depression, and insures quality rest and sleep. Aluminum-based antacids, aspirin, cortisone, chemo-therapy agents, calcium channel blockers and some antibiotics all interfere with calcium absorption. Antibiotics and cortico-steroids increase calcium needs. Calcium citrate has the current best record of absorbability. Good food sources: green vegetables, dairy foods, sea greens, tofu, molasses and shellfish.

—**Calcium glucarate:** A natural compound found in alfalfa sprouts, apples, grapefruits and broccoli. Best known as a cancer preventive, calcium glucarate (the supplement D-Glucarate is a derivative of calcium glucarate) stimulates glucuronidation, a cleansing process of the body that helps detoxify carcinogens. Used primarily to prevent cancers of the breast (for high risk women) and lungs in smokers. Also found to lower cholesterol levels in animal tests. Currently being tested as a possible prostate cancer preventive.

- **CALCAREA FLUOR:** a homeopathic cell salt used to treat weak blood vessels, as found in hemorrhoids, varicose veins, hardened arteries and glands. See HOMEOPATHIC CELL SALTS, page 21.

- **CALCAREA PHOS:** a homeopathic cell salt used to strengthen bones and build blood cells. Deficiency results in anemia, emaciation, poor digestion and slow growth. See HOMEOPATHIC CELL SALTS, page 21.

- **CALCAREA SULPH:** calcium sulphate found in bile; promotes continual blood cleansing. When deficient, toxic build-up occurs in the form of skin disorders, respiratory clog, boils and ulcerations, and slow healing. Commonly used as a homeopathic cell salt. See HOMEOPATHIC CELL SALTS, page 21.

- **CAMPHOR OIL:** a mild antiseptic from the *cinnamonium camphora* tree, used in oily skin preparations.

- **CANOLA OIL:** See FATS & OILS, pg. 158.

- **CAPRYLIC ACID:** a short-chain fatty acid long known for its antifungal effects. Effective against all *candida* species, caprylic acid helps restore and maintain a healthy yeast balance. Caprylic acid is not absorbed in the stomach, making it an excellent choice for candida of the gut. Occurs naturally as a fatty acid in sweat, in cow's and goat's milk, and in palm and coconut oil.

- **CAPSICUM (cayenne):** increases thermogenesis for weight loss, especially when combined with caffeine herbs or ephedra. Works on the central system; gives the system a little cardiovascular lift by increasing circulation. Works as a catalyst to enhance the performance of other herbs in a formula.

- **CANTHARIS:** a homeopathic remedy for bladder infections and genito-urinary tract problems, especially if there is burning and urgency. Also good for burns. See HOMEOPATHIC REMEDIES, page 20.

- **CAROB POWDER:** a sweet powder with 45% natural sugars, made from the seed pods of a Mediterranean tree. It has a flavor similar to chocolate, but contains less fat and no caffeine.

• **CARNITINE:** an amino acid, vitamin-like nutrient is synthesized in the liver and kidney, and found principally in meat (hence the name carnitine). Carnitine's primary function is to facilitate fat metabolism by transporting long chain fatty-acid molecules into the mitochondria of cells where they are "burned" to produce energy. L-Carnitine enzymatically connects to the fatty acids, enabling them to cross the mitochondria membrane for fat breakdown. Although there are two forms, the D and L-isomers (mirror images of each other) only L-Carnitine is naturally found in nature and is biologically effective.

Carnitine reduces ischemic heart disease by preventing fatty build-up. Its role in fat use helps prostaglandin metabolism and improves abnormal cholesterol-triglyceride levels. Carnitine speeds fat oxidation for weight loss, and increases the use of fat for energy. Further, high protein weight-loss diets cause ketosis, the accumulation of fat waste ketones in the blood. Uncontrolled, ketosis in this type of weight-loss diet or in diabetes can be life-threatening. Carnitine prevents ketone build up. Consider it if you are on the "zone" protein diet.

Acetyl-L-carnitine (ALC) is gaining a reputation as a nootropic (a brain nutrient) which can reduce age- related mental decline. Available in Italy since 1986, ALC specifically increases alertness and attention span, improves learning and memory, and boosts eye-hand coordination.

• **CAT'S CLAW,** (*Una de Gato, uncaria tomentosa*)**:** a valuable rainforest botanical with a wide spectrum of therapeutic applications. It contains an immune stimulating oxindole alkaloid, *isopteropodine* that enhances the phagocyte (eater) ability of white blood cells and macrophages. A standardized compound with isolated active carboxyl-alkyl-esters been found to also enhance the DNA repair process and lymphocyte function. Cat's claw helps cleanse the intestinal tract and heal numerous intestinal disorders, such as ulcers, Crohn's disease, diverticulitis, leaky bowel syndrome and colitis. Rich in antioxidant polyphenols and several plant steroids like beta-sitosterol, cat's claw is effective for cardiovascular health and hormone imbalances like prostate swelling and PMS. Additional conditions which benefit from cat's claw include: arthritis, rheumatism, cancer, allergies, candidiasis, genital herpes, herpes zoster, HIV, bladder infections and environmental toxin poisoning.

• **CHAMOMILLA:** a homeopathic remedy for calming fussy children, when they are crying because of pain, especially for teething pain. An aid in drug withdrawal. See HOMEOPATHIC REMEDIES, page 20.

• **CHARCOAL, ACTIVATED:** a natural agent that relieves gas and diarrhea. An antidote for almost all poisons. ***Note:* For any case of severe poisoning, phone the Poison Control Center in your state.

• **CHLORELLA:** See GREEN SUPERFOODS, page 135.

• **CHLORINE:** naturally-occurring chlorine stimulates the liver, bile and smooth joint-tendon operation. An electrolyte, it helps maintain acid/alkaline balance. Good food sources: seafoods, sea greens and salt.

• **CHOLINE:** a lipotropic, B complex family member, choline works with inositol to emulsify fats. A brain nutrient and neurotransmitter that aids memory and learning, and helps retard Alzheimer's disease and neurological disorders. It is used as part of a program to overcome alcoholism, liver and kidney disorders. Research shows success in cancer control. Helps dizziness, lowers cholesterol and supports liver function.

• **CHONDROITIN SULFATE A (CSA):** an anti-inflammatory agent from bovine cartilage. May be used both topically and internally for a wide range of problems — anti-aging, anti-stress and anti-allergen uses, especially for arthritic symptoms, circulatory and orthopedic therapy. Also effective for cardiovascular disease.

• **CHROMIUM:** an essential trace mineral needed for glucose tolerance and sugar regulation. Chromium deficiency means high cholesterol, heart trouble, diabetes or hypoglycemia, poor carbohydrate and fat metabolism and premature aging. Supplementation can reduce blood cholesterol levels, increase HDL cholesterol levels, and diminish atherosclerosis. Most effective as a biologically active form of GTF (chromium, niacin and glutathione), it helps control diabetes through insulin potentiation. For athletes, chromium is a safe way to convert body fat to muscle. For dieters, chromium curbs appetite as it raises metabolism. Good food sources: brewer's yeast, clams, honey, whole grains, liver, corn oil, grapes, raisins.

   —Chromium picolinate is an exceptionally bio-active source of chromium. It is a combination of chromium and picolinic acid, a substance secreted by the liver and kidneys. Picolinic acid is the body's best mineral transporter, combining with elements like iron, zinc and chromium to move them efficiently into the cells. Chromium plays a vital role in sensitizing the body to insulin. Excess body weight in the form of fat tends to impair insulin sensitivity, making it harder to lose weight. Chromium picolinate helps build muscles without steroid side effects, promotes healthy growth in children, speeds wound healing and decreases proneness to arterial plaque accumulation. 200mcg of chromium picolinate seems to be the best dose.

• **COBALAMIN:** See Vitamin B$_{12}$. Cyanocobalamin may be made from sugar beets, molasses or whey.

• **COBALT:** an integral component mineral of vitamin B$_{12}$ synthesis. Aids in hemoglobin formation. Good food sources: green leafy vegetables and liver.

• **COCONUT OIL:** See Fats and Oils, page 164.

• **Co-ENZYME-A:** a metabolic enzyme critical to both aerobic and anaerobic energy metabolism. For example, co-enzyme-A is essential to the aerobic tricarboxylic acid cycle (the ATP, or Krebs cycle) which produces most of the body's energy, and also helps release energy anaerobically from blood glycogen. Coenzyme-A is critical to fatty acid metabolism which helps your body maintain cholesterol and triglyceride levels. A coenzyme-A deficiency means fatty acids cannot be converted into energy. Coenzyme-A starts the manufacture of acetylcholine in the brain and steroid hormones in the adrenal glands. Coenzyme-A activates white blood cells for immune response, contributes to hemoglobin formation and helps the body repair damaged RNA and DNA. Coenzyme-A helps make important components of connective tissue, like chondroitin sulfate and hyaluronic acid to keep joints flexible.

• **Co-ENZYME Q-10:** a vital enzyme catalyst in the creation of cellular energy, it is synthesized in the liver. The body's ability to assimilate Co-Q$_{10}$ declines with age. Co-Q$_{10}$ supplementation has a long history of effectiveness in immune enhancement, raising cardiac strength against angina, promoting natural weight loss, inhibiting aging and overcoming periodontal disease. Co-Q$_{10}$ is crucial in preventing and treating congestive heart and arterial diseases. It can reduce high blood pressure without other medication. The newest research at doses of 300mg for breast and prostate cancer protection and treatment is extremely encouraging. Food sources: rice bran, wheat germ, beans, nuts, fish and eggs. Consider supplementing with Co-Q$_{10}$ if you are taking drugs to lower cholesterol because these drugs can deplete Co-Q$_{10}$. Co-Q$_{10}$ is synergistic in combination with vitamin E.

• **COLEUS FORSKOHLII:** an Ayurvedic herbal medicinal used for allergic conditions such as asthma and eczema. Forskolin in coleus forskohlii boosts the enzyme adenylate cyclase involved in smooth muscle relaxation, particularly helpful in relaxing bronchial muscles in asthmatics. New studies also point to coleus in the treatment of psoriasis. Coleus seems to normalize out-of-whack cell division in psoriasis to reduce symptoms. Used frequently in extracts, coleus can be used alone or in conjunction with drug treatments.

• **COLLAGEN:** the most abundant protein of the body, is responsible for maintaining the integrity of vein walls, tendons, ligaments and cartilage. Collagen is similar to elastin and is the chief constituent in connective tissue. Connective tissue is dependant on nutrients from blood, so a healthy circulatory system aids in healthy skin, ligaments and tendons. (This is why smoking, a blood vessel constrictor, is so detrimental to connective tissue.) Exercise, a healthy diet and herbs like *ginkgo biloba, cayenne* and *garlic* help keep circulation healthy. *Horsetail herb*, high in silica, is an important trace mineral for connective tissue. Vitamin C complex, especially with PCO flavonoids, supports collagen growth and structure, and prevents collagen destruction. PCOs have the unique ability to reinforce the natural cross-linking of the collagen matrix of connective tissue.

• **COLLOIDAL SILVER:** pure metallic ionic silver held in suspension by the minute electrical charge of each particle. Probably the most universal natural antibiotic substance, colloidal silver is not produced by a chemical process. It is tasteless, nonaddictive and nontoxic. Many forms of bacteria, viruses and fungi utilize a specific enzyme for their metabolism. Colloidal silver acts as a catalyst to disable the enzyme. It has proven toxic to most fungi, bacteria, parasites, and many viruses. Most important, the bacteria, fungi and viruses do not seem to develop an immunity to silver as they do to chemical antibiotic agents.

• **COLOSTRUM:** a mammary secretion in Mother's milk. It is rich in natural immune agents, *Immunoglobins IgG, IgA and IgM, Cytokines, Interferon, Nucleotides, Gamma Interferon, Orotic Acid, Lactobacillus bifidus acidophilus,* Enzymes and Vitamin A, E and B-12. It also contains *lactoferrin* and growth-enhancing factors. It triggers over 50 immune and growth processes in newborns. Colostrum supplements are obtained from bovine colostrum, with a higher concentration of IGF-1 (insulin growth factor 1) but a chemical structure virtually identical to that of humans. Studies using bovine colostrum show significant fitness improvements in stamina, muscle tone and growth, and shortened recovery time for athletes. It appears to increase bone density and returns elasticity to the skin. In adults, colostrum supplements help regulate immune response and inhibit the growth of a wide array of harmful pathogens. *Note: Choose a product from pasture-fed cows that are free of pesticides, antibiotics and hormones.*

• **COPPER:** a mineral that helps control inflammatory arthritis-bursitis symptoms. Aids in iron absorption, protein metabolism, bone formation and blood clotting. Helps prevent hair from losing its color. SOD (superoxide dismutase) is a copper-containing enzyme that protects against free radical damage. Copper deficiencies can be caused by mega-dose zinc therapy, or excessive amounts of refined sugar. Deficiencies result in high cholesterol, anemia, heart arrhythmias and nervousness. Excess copper can result in mental depression.

• **CORDYCEPS SINENSIS:** a mushroom-fungus used in traditional Chinese medicine as a tonic and energizer. Research suggests that cordyceps enhances immunity, increasing activity of helper T-cells and natural killer cells, accelerates spleen regeneration, increases SOD (superoxide dismutase) activity, enhances oxygen uptake to the heart and brain, possesses testosterone-like effects, improves libido and sperm count, and is effective in reducing uterine fibroid tumors. Cordyceps took the spotlight in 1993 when a group of Chinese runners, previously considered mediocre, took a cordyceps-based tonic formula and broke nine world records.

• **CREAM of TARTAR:** is tartaric acid, a leavening agent used in baking to incorporate egg whites. $1/2$ teasp. cream of tartar and $1/2$ teasp. baking soda can be substituted for 1 teasp. baking powder.

• **CREATINE** (*methyl guanidine-acetic acid*): is made naturally in the human liver, as creatine phosphate. Creatine is also found in red meat and fish. Creatine monohydrate supplements, with more weight of material than any other form, are popular with athletes today who want to gain weight and muscle mass, and increase their stamina. While research shows that using creatine along with an exercise program does increase lean body mass and muscle strength faster, creatine supplementation may cause an electrolyte imbalance. Creatine draws on water from other parts of the body. When using, drink lots of water.

• **CURCUMIN:** a constituent of *curcuma longa*, curcumin is a turmeric extract, the yellow spice used in curry. Curcumin is anti-inflammatory, it relieves arthritic symptoms, inhibits platelet aggregation; its fibrinolytic activity controls excess buildup of fibrin in blood vessels which can lead to blood clots. Curcumin increases bile secretion and protects against blood cholesterol rise from eating fatty foods. It is a powerful, oil-soluble antioxidant which can fight viruses. Curcumin inhibits tumor necrosis factor (TNF), a cytokine that increases HIV replication in T-cells. Numerous studies show the anti-tumor effect of turmeric and curcumin.

• **CYSTEINE:** a semi-essential antioxidant amino acid that works with vitamins C, E and selenium to protect against radiation, cancer carcinogens and free radical damage to skin and arteries. Stimulates immune white cell activity. Helps heal burns and surgery wounds, and renders toxic chemicals in the body harmless.

Taken with *evening primrose oil*, cysteine protects brain from alcohol and tobacco effects (highly effective in preventing hangover). Used for hair loss, psoriasis, dental plaque prevention and skin dermatitis. Relieves bronchial asthma by breaking down mucous plugs. *Note: Take vitamin C in a 3:1 ratio to cysteine for best results.*

—N-acetyl-cysteine, NAC: an antioxidant amino acid, a more stable, bio-available form of L-cysteine, converted in the body to glutathione, a prime immune T-cell enhancer (especially for people with HIV who have low glutathione. NAC detoxifies from alcohol, heavy metals, X-rays and radiation damage, treats viral diseases, protects the liver, and breaks up pulmonary-bronchial mucus. *Note: NAC is a powerful chelator of zinc and copper, capable of removing enough of these minerals from the body to produce deficiencies unless supplies are adequate.*

• **CYSTINE:** a semi-essential amino acid, cystine is the oxidized form of cysteine, and like it, promotes white blood cell activity and heals burns and wounds. The main constituent of hair, essential to formation of skin. Cystine can sometimes be harmful to the kidneys, and should generally not be used clinically.

DEAD SEA SALTS: obtained from the Dead Sea in Israel, are composed of potassium, chlorine, sodium, calcium and magnesium salts, and sulfur and bromine compounds. Used in detoxifying baths.

• **DHEA,** *dehydro-epiandro-sterone:* an abundant hormone produced from cholesterol by the adrenals, with smaller amounts made by female ovaries. It is part of an important cascade that ends in the making of estrogen and/or testosterone. DHEA helps maintain muscle and skin tone, and bone health. It stimulates immune defenses and T-cells to fight infections, interferes with immune suppression and monitors over-reactions (like lupus or rheumatoid arthritis) that attack the body. Research shows that HIV progression can be predicted by monitoring DHEA levels. (Full-blown AIDS does not develop until adrenal output of DHEA drops.)

DHEA is effective therapy for menopause symptoms much the same as estrogen replacement, and for post-menopausal women with osteoporosis who are low in DHEA. *Pre*-menopausal women who have low levels of DHEA may develop breast cancer. Breast cancer risk associated with synthetic estrogen replacement therapy (ERT) is apparently reduced when DHEA is used, and may even be prevented by DHEA's immune support. (Animal studies show that mice susceptible to breast cancer do not develop it when treated with DHEA.)

DHEA is of enormous interest as an anti-aging substance that lowers serum cholesterol, and as a promoter of energy and libido. Yet, hormone activity is highly individual, so hormone test results are often inconclusive or contradictory. For example, a U.C. San Diego Medical study shows that DHEA *does* act as a kind of youth drug, because the older subjects who took it had more energy and muscle tone and better heart health. Another study shows that men with high DHEA levels have half the heart disease as those with low levels. But, women with high DHEA have a *higher* risk of heart disease. Follow-up studies were even more contradictory, and didn't bear out long term DHEA benefits.

DHEA has few side effects, but if you take too much, it suppresses your body's ability to make its own. People who get good results usually have to take it for the rest of their lives to continue the results. Adult acne is a common side effect, as is excess facial and body hair. DHEA dosage falls between 5-15mg for women and 10-30mg for men. Most physicians today give it with a combination of estrogen, progesterone, and testosterone.

DHEA supplements are synthesized from *wild yam* sterols. Unable to unravel all the actions of this complex plant, researchers currently disregard the idea that wild yam acts as a precursor to DHEA. But the fact that wild yam is used to manufacture both synthetic DHEA and synthesized progesterone show that it works well for women's hormone problems that involve progesterone.

• **DLPA, DL-PHENYLALANINE:** an amino acid which is a safe, effective pain reliever and anti-depressant with an endorphin effect for arthritis, and lower back and cerebro-spinal pain. Increases mental alertness, and improves the symptoms of Parkinson's disease. Normal therapeutic dose is 500-750mg. Contra-indications: avoid DLPA if you have high blood pressure, are pregnant, or diabetic. See Amino Acids for more.

• **DMAE:** a naturally occurring nutrient that *stimulates the production of choline.* Choline is a building block of acetylcholine, a neurotransmitter involved in memory and learning. By providing a feeling of mild stimulation, DMAE has also been found to elevate mood. DMAE is the precise salt of a substance called Deaner (*DMAE p-acetamidobenzoate*). In Europe, deaner is used for schizophrenia, phobias, low spirits and problems with learning and concentration. The FDA removed deaner from US citizens in 1983 because it was judged that although deaner was very safe, the drug was of no use for hyperactivity in children, its approved use.

• **DNA,** *deoxyribonucleic acid*: the substance in cell nuclei that genetically codes amino acids and determines the life form into which a cell develops. Derived from fish sperm, commercial DNA is used as a skin revitalizer to boost circulation and oxygen uptake. Repeated exposure to radiation causes DNA breakdown. Drastic medical treatments like chemotherapy help destroy cancers but also tend to mutate normal cell DNA.

EDTA, *ethylenediamine tetra-acetic acid*: used in chelation therapy to remove toxic, clogging minerals from the circulatory system — particularly those that impair membrane function and contribute to free radical damage. EDTA puts these minerals into solution where they can be excreted by the kidneys.

• **EGG OIL:** fat-soluble emollients and emulsifiers extracted from eggs. Provides protection against dehydration and has lubricating, anti-friction properties when rubbed on the skin. —**Egg replacer** is a combination of starches and leavening used to give qualities of eggs in baking. It is a vegetarian product, cholesterol free.

• **ELASTIN:** protein in connective tissue, similar to collagen and the chief constituent in connective tissue. Collagen and elastin give the skin its strength and elasticity. Elastin is also found in the artery walls. The skin is made up of 79% collagen, 11% lipids, 7% mucopolysaccharides, 2% elastin, and 1% carbohydrates. Elastin is used as an emollient in cosmetics to prevent water loss. *Horsetail herb*, high in silica, is an important trace mineral for connective tissue. Vitamins A (and-or beta-carotene), B, C, and D are essential for connective tissue health. Smoking harms connective tissue because it constricts the blood vessels.

• **ELECTROLYTES:** the ionized salts in blood, tissue fluids and cells, that transport electrical operating energy throughout the body. Electrolyte salts include sodium, potassium and chlorine. They are essential to cell function and body pH balance, but are easily lost through perspiration, so regular replacement is necessary from drinking electrolytic fluids. When electrolytes are low, we tire easily. When they are adequate, we experience more energy. Electrolyte drinks are especially beneficial for athletes and those doing hard physical work.

• **EMOLLIENTS:** a mixture of oils, help soften and smooth the skin, reduce roughness, cracking and skin irritation, and retard the fine wrinkles - coating the skin with a film and retarding evaporation of water. Glycerine, an emollient, actually attracts water to the skin. Seaweeds are some of Nature's best plant emollients.

• **ENERGIZERS and STIMULANTS, NATURAL:** natural energizers and stimulants increase the action of a body system or process to create a sense of well-being, exhilaration and self-confidence, and to relieve fatigue and drowsiness. In battling fatigue, natural energizers have great advantages over chemically processed stimulants. They have more broad-based activity so that they don't exhaust an organ or body system. They can be strong or gentle for individual needs. At correct dosage, they are supportive rather than depleting. The downside to many stimulants (even some natural ones), is tolerance, dependency and nervousness, with difficulty in concentrating or after-effect headaches. Increasing the strength of a stimulant can increase the toxicity and-or dependency potential. Taken too often, even natural stimulants can drive a body system to exhaustion.

Specific remedies for fatigue can be classified under central nervous system stimulants, metabolic enhancers, and adaptogens. The following list takes a quick look at natural stimulants and what they do. See individual nutrient entries for more information about their properties, activity and benefits.

—**Central Nervous System (CNS)** stimulants act by affecting the cerebral cortex and the medulla of the brain. Most contain either natural caffeine, naturally-occurring ephedrine, or certain free-form amino acids. CNS stimulators promote alertness, energy, and more rapid, clearer flow of thought. They also act as respiratory stimulants. Most central nervous system stimulants should be used for short-term energy needs. Long term use can result in a net loss of energy to the system. Most stimulants, even natural ones, should also be avoided during pregnancy. The tiny body of the fetus cannot handle the systemic excitation.

Examples of food and herb source central nervous system stimulants:

Coffee and caffeine: America's most popular stimulant. See CAFFEINE, page 151.

Guaraña: a rich, natural source of rainforest *guaranine*, for long, slow endurance energy without coffee's heated hydrocarbons that pose health problems.

Glutamine: converts readily into 6-carbon glucose - an excellent brain nutrient and energy source. Improves memory recall, sustained concentration and alertness. Improves mental performance in cases of retardation, senility and schizophrenia. Increases libido and helps overcome impotence. See Amino Acids.

Kola Nut: a natural caffeine without heated hydrocarbons. Allays hunger; combats fatigue.

L-Phenylalanine: a tyrosine precursor that works on the central nervous system with vitamin B-6 as an antidepressant and mood elevator. Successful in treating manic, post-amphetamine and schizophrenic depression. Aids in learning and memory retention. A thyroid stimulant that helps curb the appetite by increasing the body's production of CCK. See Amino Acids.

Tyrosine: builds adrenaline and thyroid stores. Rapidly metabolized as an antioxidant in the body; effective as a quick energy source, especially for the brain. Safe therapy for depression, hypertension, in controlling drug abuse and aiding drug withdrawal. Increases libido. A growth hormone stimulant. See Amino Acids.

Yerba Maté: a South American herbal that naturally lifts fatigue and provides broad range nutrition to body cells. Rich in vitamins A, E, C and B (especially pantothenic acid), with measurable amounts of chlorophyll, calcium, potassium, iron and magnesium. Protects against stress effects. Helps open respiratory passages to overcome allergy symptoms. Yerba maté is a catalyst that increases the healing effects of other herbs.

Ephedra: a CNS stimulant that contains the biochemicals *ephedrine* and *pseudoephedrine*. Acts as an energy tonic to restore body vitality. A natural bronchodilator and decongestant for respiratory problems. Used in many weight loss formulas for its ability to increase thermogenesis. Ephedra is also a cardiac stimulant and should be used with caution by anyone with high blood pressure. See also Ephedra.

Ginkgo Biloba: a primary brain and mental energy stimulant. Increases both peripheral and cerebral circulation through vasodilation. A good stimulant choice for older people who suffer from poor memory and other aging-related CNS problems. Causes an increase in acetylcholine levels, and therefore the ability to better transmit body electrical impulses. Best results are achieved from the extract. See Ginkgo Biloba.

Damiana: a mild aphrodisiac, synergistic with other energy herbs in stimulating libido. A specific in a combination to treat frigidity in women and impotence in men. Also a mild anti-depressant tonic.

Yohimbe: A strong aphrodisiac affecting both male impotence and female frigidity. Stimulates the sympathetic nervous system which results in more rapid penile erections. An effective bodybuilding and athletic formula herb. *Note: Avoid if there is high blood pressure or heart arrythmia.*

—**Metabolic Enhancers** improve the performance of biochemical pathways by providing catalysts and co-factors for system support. They do not stress or deplete the body. Examples of metabolic enhancers include co-enzyme factors like B vitamins, fat mobilizers like L-carnitine, electron transporters like CoQ-10, lactic acid limiters like inosine and gamma oryzonal (GO), and tissue oxygenators like *Di-Methyl-Glycine* (B_{15}).

Examples of food and herb source metabolic stimulants:

Ginger: a warming circulatory stimulant and cleansing herb, useful in all formulas where circulation to the extremities is needed, such as arthritis. Ginger helps in lung-chest clearing combinations, in digestive stimulants and stomach alkalizers for clearing gas, in promoting menstrual regularity and cramping relief, and for all kinds of nausea, motion sickness and morning sickness. It may be used directly on the skin as a compress to stimulate venous circulation. Other uses include: catalytic action in nervine and sedative formulas, as a gargle and sore throat syrup, as a diaphoretic to remove wastes, and to stimulate kidney activity.

Capsicum: increases thermogenesis for weight loss, especially when used with xanthine herbs like guarana or kola nut. A central system catalyst that enhances cardiovascular function, increases circulation and enhance the performance of other herbs in a formula.

Bee Pollen: an energizing, nutritive "superfood." See Bee Pollen and Royal Jelly, page 183-184.

Royal Jelly: supplies key nutrients for energy, mental alertness and a general feeling of well-being. Enhances immunity and deep cellular health. One of the world's richest sources of pantothenic acid to combat stress, fatigue and insomnia. See Bee Pollen and Royal Jelly, page 184.

Green Tea: rich in flavonoids with antioxidant and anti-allergen activity. A beneficial fasting tea, providing energy support and clearer thinking during cleansing. Contains polyphenols (not tannins as commonly believed) that act as antioxidants, yet do not interfere with iron or protein absorption. Like other plant antioxidants, such as beta carotene and vitamin C, green tea antioxidants work at the molecular level, combatting free radical damage to protect against degenerative diseases. See Tea, page 154.

Lipoic Acid: a unique antioxidant, able to quench free radicals in both fat and water mediums. A potent promoter of glutathione and an important co-factor in energy metabolism. See Lipoic acid, page 103.

Rosemary: an anti-oxidant herb and strong brain and memory stimulant. A circulatory toning agent, and effective nervine for stress, tension and depression.

CoQ-10: an essential catalyst co-enzyme for cellular energy in the body. Supplementation provides wide ranging therapeutic benefits. See ENZYMES & ENZYME THERAPY, pg. 128.

DMG: *Di-Methyl-Glycine,* B-15: a powerful antioxidant and energy stimulant. DMG is a highly reputed energizer and stimulant whose effects are attributed to its conversion to glycine. See Amino Acids.

—**Adaptogens** are herbal regulators tonics that help the body handle stress, build strength and maintain vitality. They are more for longterm revitalization than immediate energy — rich sources of strengthening nutrients such as germanium, and steroid-like compounds that provide concentrated body support. They increase the body's overall immune function with broad spectrum activity rather than specific action. They promote recovery from illness and may be used synergistically with other tonic herbs to restore and normalize.

Examples of adaptogen herbs:

Panax Ginseng: including Oriental red and white, and American Ginseng, is the most broad spectrum of all adaptogenic herbs. Stimulates both long and short term energy, especially rain and memory centers, ginseng has measurable amounts of germanium, helps to lower cholesterol and regulate sugar use in the body, promotes regeneration from stress and fatigue, and rebuilds strength. Panax is rich in phytohormones for both men and women's problems, thought to be responsible for its long tradition as an aphrodisiac. Studies show that ginseng may be a source of phytotestosterone for men, and may be a protective factor for breast cancer in women because of its phytoestrogen content. Ginseng benefits are cumulative in the body. Taking panax for several months is more effective than short term doses. See Panax Ginseng.

Siberian Ginseng, *(Eleuthero):* a long-term energy tonic for the adrenal glands and circulatory health.

Schizandra: synergistic with eleuthero against stress, weight gain and sports fatigue. Supports sugar regulation, and liver function and strength. Helps correct skin problems through better digestion of fatty foods.

Gotu Kola: a brain and nervous restorative, especially effective as a toner after illness or surgery.

Astragalus: a superior tonic and strong immune enhancing herb. Provides therapeutic support for recovery from illness or surgery, especially from chemotherapy and radiation. Nourishes exhausted adrenals to combat fatigue. Helps normalize nervous, hormonal and immune systems. See Astragalus.

Suma: an ancient herb with modern benefits for overcoming fatigue and hormonal imbalance. Used to rebuild the system from the ravages of cancer and diabetes.

Fo-Ti, *(Ho-Shou-Wu):* a flavonoid-rich herb with particular success for longevity. A cardiovascular strengthener, increasing blood flow to the heart.

Reishi: an adaptogen mushroom for deep immune support, anti-cancer and anti-oxidant protection, liver regeneration and blood sugar regulation. Excellent for recovery from illness. See Reishi Mushroom.

Germanium, *(organic sesquioxide):* a potent adaptogen that detoxifies, blocks free radicals and increases killer cell production. An interferon stimulus for immune strength and healing. See Germanium.

Burdock: a hormone balancer with antibacterial, antifungal and antitumor properties. A specific in all blood cleansing and detoxification combinations; an important anti-inflammatory and anti-infective.

• **ENFLEURAGE:** the time-consuming, expensive technique of making essential oils from delicate flowers, such as roses and orange blossoms that cannot be steam distilled. Glass trays are lined with fat and scattered with fresh flowers. The next day the flowers are removed from the fat and replaced with fresh ones. The cycle is repeated for 4 to 5 weeks. The lard is then scraped from the trays and mixed with alcohol. When the alcohol is removed by distillation, a highly scented essential oil, or "absolute," is left behind.

• **ENZYMES:** see ENZYMES & ENZYME THERAPY, page 127.

• **EPHEDRA,** *Ma Huang:* used in Traditional Chinese Medicine for more than 5,000 years, cultivated for its therapeutic properties longer than any other medicinal plant, few herbs have been as misunderstood as Ma Huang. A wonderful bronchodilator for colds, coughs and flu, fever, headache, edema, bronchial asthma, nasal congestion and aching joints. Some uses for ma huang are approved by the FDA in over-the-counter (OTC) drugs, but Western manufacturers also use it for energy and diet products which are not FDA approved. Concerns over the potency and safety of ma huang, especially its isolated alkaloids have prompted increased regulatory scrutiny. Ma huang contains a total of 0.5 to 2.5 percent of several ephedra alkaloids, with ephedrine comprising between 30 and 90% of total alkaloids. Ephedrine is a potent isolate; it produces effects similar to adrenaline, raising blood pressure. In large doses, ephedrine causes nervousness, insomnia, dizziness, palpitations and skin flushing. *The whole ephedra plant, which most knowledgeable herbalists use instead of the isolate, is safe, especially combined with other herbs, as an anti-asthmatic, bronchodilator, hypertensive and peripheral vasoconstrictor.*

• **ESCIN:** a saponin occurring in the seeds of the horse chestnut tree, *Aesculus hippocastanum.* Used externally to reduce swelling and increase skin tissue tone by increasing circulation and encouraging flexibility.

• **ESSENTIAL FATTY ACIDS:** See FATS & OILS, page 160.

• **ESSIAC:** an herbal tea formula of the Ojibway Indians, made famous by Rene Caisse for treating cancer, being popularly rediscovered today. The name "Essiac" is an anagram of her last name "Caisse." Her formula consists of *sheep sorrel, burdock root, turkey rhubarb and slippery elm bark.*

• **ESTROGEN:** natural estrogens are conjugated hormones, including estradiol, estrone and estriol, thought to be formed through the adrenals and the pituitary, especially after menopause.
    –Estradiol: produced by the ovaries, possessing estrogenic properties; taken orally, converted to estrone.
    –Estrone: an estrogen produced by the ovaries and by conversion of estradiol; linked to breast cancer.
    –Estriol: believed to be a "good" estrogen (non-cancer-facilitating). Phytoestrogens (plant estrogens) are thought to be close in chemical makeup to human estriol.

FERRUM PHOS: a homeopathic cell salt used to treat colds and flu, inflammation and nausea. A remedy for first stage inflammations and infective wounds. See HOMEOPATHIC CELL SALTS, page 21.

• **FLAX SEED OIL:** see ESSENTIAL FATTY ACIDS & OMEGA-3 OILS, page 160.

• **FLUORIDE:** new research shows that fluoride is more poisonous than lead, just slightly less poisonous than arsenic. The difference between calcium fluoride (naturally occurring) and other forms is the higher availability of free fluoride ions in sodium-fluoride, and in fluoride from hydrofluosilicic acid. Fluoride is linked to cancer, Alzheimer's, poor child brain development and nervous system health, and fluorosis (fluoride poisoning of cells that form tooth enamel). Where calcium fluoride occurs naturally in the water, people age before their time, suffer from bone disease, tooth disorders, and premature hardening of the arteries. Disastrous effects are more apparent in elderly populations, in people with low calcium-magnesium or vitamin C levels and people with cardiovascular and kidney problems. Postmenopausal women in fluoridated areas are at increased risk of fractures. As little as 0.7 parts per million fluoride in the water has been associated with skeletal fluorosis.

• **FOLIC ACID,** *Folacin:* a B vitamin that plays an important role in the synthesis of DNA, enzyme production and blood formation. Essential for division and growth of new cells, it is an excellent supplement during pregnancy (400mcg daily) to guard against spina bifida and neural tube defects. It prevents anemia, helps control leukemia and pernicious anemia, and is effective against alcoholism, even some precancerous lesions. It is critical in overcoming the immuno-depression state following chemotherapy with MTX. Folic acid can reduce high homocysteine levels. Homocysteine tends to thicken the blood and facilitates the conversion of LDL (bad cholesterol) into free radical particles. Aluminum antacids, oral contraceptives, alcohol, long-term antibiotics and anti-inflammatory drugs increase the need for folic acid. Good food sources: green leafy vegetables, organ meats, peas, brewer's yeast, broccoli, fruits, soy foods, chicken, brown rice, eggs and whole grains.

• **FREE RADICALS:** unstable fragments of molecules produced from oxygen and fats in cells. Free radicals result when high energy chemical oxidation reactions in the body get out of control. Atoms and molecules consist of protons, neutrons and electrons, which normally come in pairs. Electron pairs form chemical bonds which hold all molecules together. A free radical contains an unpaired electron. In this unbalanced state, the free radical is stimulated to combine with other molecules, and the combination may destroy an enzyme, a protein or a complete cell. The destruction causes chain reactions that result in the release of thousands more free radicals, stimulating age pigment, damaging protein structures and impairing fat metabolizing enzymes.

The body normally produces some free radicals in its ordinary metabolic breakdown of organic compounds. Indeed, some are released to fight bacteria during immune response. But as with most activities in nature, the body also produces the necessary substances (in this case the antioxidant enzymes superoxide dismutase, catalase, and glutathione peroxidase) to deactivate them. Free radicals can be caused by exposure to radiation, rancid oils, food additives and chemicals, heavy metal pollutants, UV sunlight and fast foods.

Specific antioxidant depleters are:
—Infections from viruses, bacteria, or parasites.
—Trauma from surgery, injury, inflammation, and wound healing.
—Burns, and exposure to excessive heat or cold.
—Smoking or passive exposure to cigarette smoke. Excessive alcohol and/or addictive drug intake.
—Exposure to toxic chemicals, pesticide residues, nitrites, nitrates and other food additives.
—Exposure to radiation, including excessive UV rays from sunlight.
—Cytotoxic drugs, such as the anticancer drug Adriamycin.
—Oxidant drugs that steal electrons, such as acetaminophen (Tylenol).
—Dietary lack of antioxidant-rich foods.

Some foods make free radicals more likely to occur. Polyunsaturated fats, in sunflower, corn and soy oils, and junk foods can lead to excessive free radical production. A low-fat diet reduces the damage of oxidation by free radicals. Iron and copper, okay in small quantities, increase free radical production in large amounts.

Cell damage, partially responsible for the effects of aging, is involved in cancer, triggers some forms of heart disease and is an integral part of eye diseases like cataracts and macular degeneration. Antioxidants block excess oxidation to prevent these conditions. However, our polluted environment means it is doubtful that our bodies receive enough antioxidants in our food intake to meet our needs. Supplements like zinc, carotenes and B vitamins work synergistically with antioxidants. Vitamins C and E, and the protein glutathione act as antioxidants themselves. Herbs like *garlic, ginkgo biloba, rosemary* and *ginsengs* are rich in antioxidants.

• **FRUCTOSE:** See SWEETENERS IN A HEALING DIET, page 171.

GABA, *Gamma-Aminobutyric Acid:* a non-essential amino acid useful in treating brain and nerve dysfunctions, such as anxiety, depression, nerves, high blood pressure, insomnia, schizophrenia, Parkinson's and Alzheimer's diseases, and ADD in children. GABA acts as a natural tranquilizer, improves libido, and along with glutamine and tyrosine, helps overcome alcohol and drug abuse. Used with niacinamide, it is a relaxant.

• **GARLIC:** a therapeutic food with antibiotic, antifungal, antiparasitic and antiviral activity. Used extensively for disease prevention; internally against infection of all kinds; externally for eye, ear, nose and throat infections; and because of its thiamine content, to prevent mosquito and insect bites. Garlic has measurable amounts of germanium, an antioxidant for endurance and wound healing.

• **GELSEMIUM:** a homeopathic remedy for chronic lethargy. See HOMEOPATHIC REMEDIES, page 20.

• **GENISTEIN:** a phytohormone constituent of soy. See SOY FOODS IN A HEALING DIET, page 142.

• **GERMANIUM,** *(organic sesquioxide)*: an anti-oxidant mineral. Acts as an anticancer agent, particularly where there is tumor metastasis, by activating macrophages and increasing production of killer cells. An interferon stimulus for immune strength. Facilitates oxygen uptake, detoxifies and blocks free radicals. Effective for viral, bacterial and fungal infections, osteoporosis, arthritis, heart, blood pressure and respiratory conditions. Studies show success with leukemia, HIV, and brain, lung, pancreatic and lymphatic cancers. Good food sources: chlorella, garlic, tuna, oysters, green tea, reishi mushroom, aloe vera, ginseng, leafy greens.

• **GINGER:** a flavorful, aromatic, spicy herb. Both fresh and dried ginger root have therapeutic properties for digestion, hypertension, headaches and other problems. It's easy to have fresh ginger on hand. Peel fresh roots, chop in the blender, put in a plastic bag and freeze. Ginger thaws in less than 10 minutes, ready for use.

• **GINKGO BILOBA:** the leaf extract of an ancient Chinese tree, used therapeutically to combat the effects of aging. It improves circulation throughout the body, sends more blood and oxygen to the brain for better memory and mental alertness, and protects the brain against mental disorders. Ginkgo is effective for vertigo, dizziness and ringing in the ears. A potent antioxidant, it protects cells against free radical damage and reduces blood cell clumping which can lead to congestive heart disease. Helps return elasticity to cholesterol-hardened blood vessels. Reduces inflammation in the lungs leading to asthmatic attack.

• **GINSENG, PANAX:** the most effective adaptogen of all tonic herbs, *Panax ginseng,* and its American brother, *Panax Quinquefolium* are intensely studied today by science. Scientific research is incredibly expensive — the wealth of testing on ginseng gives you an idea of its importance in the minds of researchers around the world. *Fortunately, even while scientific experiments go on, we can buy and use this safe remedy during its testing, something impossible with drugs. Taking ginseng for several months to a year is far more effective than short term doses.*

A small sampling of modern scientific validation of the benefits of this ancient healing plant:
—**Ginseng** aids treatment for cardiovascular disorders, including heart attack, and heart disease. In clinical trials on patients with high blood pressure, ginseng tea helped produce a steady, consistent reduction in blood pressure. The average drop was 23 in the blood pressure of patients with a systolic pressure above 140.
—**Ginseng** benefits deep hormone balance for both men and women, an explanation for its long reputation as an aphrodisiac. Amazingly, it works with the needs and qualities of the opposite male and female systems.

For men, ginseng has a long tradition as a reproductive restorative. While ginseng won't make a man a SUPERMAN, recent tests show that it is the only herb to clinically test as a source of phyto (plant) testosterone. Ginseng seems to increase sperm count and seminal vesicle weight, and supports key gland functions like the adrenals and prostate. Ginseng's antioxidant qualities help cardiovascular performance not only for sexual energy, but for sports and workouts... important for a man's outlook.

For women, ginseng helps normalize hormones, notably those that guard against breast cancer, endometriosis, and hormone driven problems. Ginseng has an estrogen-like effect due to the chemical similarity of ginsenosides and female steroidal hormones. It exerts the estrogen effect on the vaginal mucosa, to prevent thinning of the vaginal walls after menopause, and also to prevent general menopause discomfort. It affects a woman's mental energy through hypothalamus stimulation.... a factor in turning a woman's attention to lovemaking. Ginseng also has distinct, antioxidant cardiovascular benefits for women.

—**Ginseng** polysaccharides protect against gastric ulcers induced by hard alcohol. Ginseng is a good preventive medicine choice for anyone regularly drinking hard liquor with a damaged stomach lining.

—**Ginseng** demonstrates an insulin-like effect on sugar regulation, stimulating sugar removal.

—**Ginseng** shows therapeutic activity against recurrent, severe viral infections and syndromes, like HIV and other immune deficient diseases, according to recent Russian studies.

—**Ginseng** has powerful, intercellular antioxidant substances, particularly in regard to its anti-aging capabilities, free radical neutralization and immune enhancement.

—**Ginseng** stimulates RNA synthesis in bone marrow cells, and has anti-toxic effects against radiation, heavy metals, and airborne pollutants.

—**Ginseng** stimulates many parts of the immune system, including phagocyte action, antibody response and natural killer cell activity. It modifies cytokine production, strengthens the immune properties of cellular connective tissue, enhances interleukin and balances red and white blood cell count.

—**Ginseng** plays a role in normalizing skin cancer cells and protects against aging skin and early wrinkling. This may be a boon to all the world as the ozone layer thins, exposing all of us to harmful UV rays.

—**Ginseng** offers longterm mental and psychological benefits. Ginseng is regularly recommended for depression and insomnia in Europe where experiments with ginseng and the elderly show clear improvement for mental outlook, optimistic spirits and improving attitude.

—**Ginseng** assists memory, concentration, alertness and improved learning ability. It is currently being tested for Alzheimer's disease, and I myself have seen evidence that ginseng helps in Alzheimer's cases.

—**Ginseng** is the quintessential herb for stress — the very thing people need to handle the growing pressure in their lives today. Stress is anything that lessens vitality, and it's the single greatest factor in the development of health problems. Beyond its specific abilities, ginseng *superbly* helps us to deal with stress.

—**Ginseng** is being tested for its ability to inhibit the growth and formation of liver cancer cells, one of the most difficult cancers to overcome. Tests show that ginseng stimulates protein synthesis and converts cancer cell characteristics both functionally and morphologically to those resembling normal liver cells, a process induced in the cells by a **single ginsenoside**!

• **GLA,** *Gamma Linoleic Acid:* obtained from evening primrose oil, black currant, and borage seed oil. A source of energy for the cells, electrical insulation for nerve fibers, a precursor of prostaglandins which regulate hormone and metabolic functions. Therapeutic use is wide ranging — from control of PMS and menopause symptoms, to help in nerve transmission for M.S. and muscular dystrophy.

• **GLANDULAR EXTRACTS, RAW**: the organs and glands communicate biochemically with our bodies through micro-nutrients and polypeptides. Gland therapy is based on the premise that glandular substance is biologically active in humans, and that "like cells help like cells." Research shows that it is valid, effective and safe. Only minute amounts of raw animal glandulars are needed to support and normalize a particular organ or gland. For serious diseases, such as cancer, that debilitate organs and glands, this type of cell therapy is helpful in augmenting the body's own gland substance so that it can better heal itself.

Predigested gland tissue provides many benefits of whole fresh glands. Freeze-dried, de-fatted, dehydrated concentrates are also effective. Highest quality preservation is essential, since heat or salt precipitation render the glands useless. Every gland works with a particular amino acid, so a combination of a raw glandular and a harmonizing amino acid provides the human gland with more ability to produce its hormone secretions.

The most essential glandulars:

—**Raw Adrenal:** stimulates and nourishes exhausted adrenals. Reduces inflammation and increases endurance without synthetic steroids. Helps protect against chronic fatigue syndrome and candida albicans by normalizing metabolism. Increases resistance to allergic reactions and infections associated with poor adrenal function. Works to control both hypoglycemic and diabetic reactions, and menopause imbalance symptoms.

—**Raw Brain:** improves brain chemistry. Helps prevent memory loss, chronic mental fatigue and senility onset. Encourages better nerve stability and restful sleep. Beneficial support during alcoholism recovery.

—**Raw Female Complex,** (including ovary, pituitary, uterus): re-establishes hormonal balance, especially between estrogen and progesterone. Helps regulate the menstrual cycle and stimulates delayed or absent menstruation. Normalizes PMS symptoms and controls cramping. Indicated for low libido and infertility.

—**Raw Heart:** improves heart muscle activity and reduces low density lipoproteins in the blood.

—**Raw Kidney:** aids in normalization of waste filtering function and kidney-urinary disorders. Helps normalize blood pressure, body fluid and acid-alkaline balance.

—**Raw Liver:** helps restore the liver after abuse, disease and exhaustion. Improves metabolic activity and filtering of wastes and toxins like alcohol and chemicals. Aids fat metabolism. Increases healthy bile flow and glucose regulation. Raw liver is effective for jaundice, hepatitis, toxemia and alcoholism.

—**Raw Lung:** supports the lungs against asthma, emphysema, congestion, bronchitis and pneumonia.

—**Raw Male Complex,** (contains raw orchic, pituitary, and prostate), re-establishes hormonal balance of testosterone-progesterone-estrogen. Helps normalize functions of diseased or damaged male organs. Supports male body growth and fat distribution, improves sperm count, virility, and chances of fertilization.

—**Raw Mammary:** helps heal breast-nipple inflammation. Controls profuse menstruation, period pain, and normalizes too-frequent cycles, especially at onset of menopause. Supports scant milk during lactation.

—**Raw Orchic:** helps increase male sexual strength and potency by stimulating testosterone production and sperm count. Raw orchic can bring noticeable improvement in male athletic performance.

—**Raw Ovary:** normalizes estrogen-progesterone balance. Helps correct endometrial misplacement and overgrowth, PMS symptoms and cramping. Supports hormone production slow down during menopause.

—**Raw Pancreas:** the pancreas is a triple function gland producing pancreatin for digestion, and insulin and glucagon for glucose metabolism and balanced blood glucose levels. Raw pancreas supports enzyme secretions for fat metabolism, hormone balance, food assimilation, and intestinal immune response.

—**Raw Pituitary:** the "master gland," stimulates overall body growth through electrolyte metabolism in the ovaries, testes, adrenals and skin. Plays a major role in reproduction, estrogen secretion, blood sugar metabolism, kidney function, skin pigmentation, water retention and bowel movements. Helps overcome hypoglycemia and infertility. Effective for athletes in controlling body stress, sugar balance and fatigue.

—**Raw Spleen:** aids in the building and storage of red blood cells to promote strength and tissue oxygenation. Filters harmful substances from the bloodstream and enhances immune function by increasing white blood cell activity. Increases absorption of calcium and iron.

—**Raw Thymus:** stimulates and strengthens immune response against foreign organisms and toxins. Raw thymus helps activate T-cells in the spleen, lymph nodes and bone marrow. Minimizes aging symptoms as the thymus gland shrinks with age. Use with zinc to help regenerate thymic tissue.

—**Raw Thyroid:** supports energy production, helps regulate metabolism and circulation, and controls obesity and sluggishness caused by thyroid deficiency. Helps mental alertness, hair, skin and reproductive-sexual problems. Works synergistically with tyrosine and natural iodine. *Note: use a thyroxin-free compound.*

—**Raw Uterus:** helps menses dysfunctions like amenorrhea, habitual abortion, infertility and irregular periods. Acts as a preventive against inflammation and infection of the cervical canal and vagina. Aids in calcium use for bone and muscle. Improves tissue growth and repair. Helps overcome birth control side effects.

• **GLUCOSAMINE SULFATE:** a proteoglycan, or amino sugar that promotes tissue elasticity and cushioning. Glucosamine stimulates manufacture of glycosaminoglycans, important cartilage components that help the body repair damaged or eroded cartilage. Glucosamine thus stimulates proper joint function and joint repair. Glucosamine sulfate is the form used because sulfur takes part in forming cartilage. The commercial supplement is derived from chitin (exoskeleton of shrimp, lobsters or crabs). *Note: GS may thin the blood. Avoid if taking other blood thinning drugs.*

• **GLUTAMIC ACID:** a non-essential amino acid, important for nerve health and metabolism of sugars and fats. Over 50% of the amino acid composition of the brain is represented by glutamic acid and its derivatives. It is a prime brain fuel because it transports potassium across the blood-brain barrier. Helps correct mental and nerve disorders, like epilepsy, muscular dystrophy, mental retardation and severe insulin reactions.

• **GLUTAMINE:** a non-essential amino acid that converts readily into 6-carbon glucose, a prime brain nutrient and energy source. Supplements rapidly improve memory retention, recall, concentration and alertness. Glutamine helps mental performance in cases of retardation, senility, epileptic seizure and schizophrenia. It reduces alcohol and sugar cravings, protects against alcohol toxicity, and controls hypoglycemic reactions.

• **GLUTATHIONE:** a non-essential amino acid that works with cysteine and glutamine as a glucose tolerance factor and anti-oxidant to neutralize radiation toxicity and inhibit free radicals. Assists white blood cells in killing bacteria. A prime immune booster that helps detoxify from heavy metal pollutants, cigarette smoke, alcohol and drug (especially PCP) overload, and from the effects of chemotherapy, X-rays and liver toxins. Works with vitamin E to break down fat and protect against stroke, kidney failure and cataract formation. Stimulates prostaglandin metabolism. Food sources: watermelon, asparagus, avocados, oranges, peaches.

• **GLYCERINE, VEGETABLE:** a naturally-occurring substance, metabolized in the body like a carbohydrate, not a fat or oil, today extracted from coconut, and used in natural cosmetics as a smoothing agent.

• **GLYCINE:** a non-essential amino acid which releases growth hormone when taken in large doses. Converts to **creatine** to retard nerve and muscle degeneration, so therapeutically effective for myasthenia gravis, gout, and muscular dystrophy. A key to regulating hypoglycemic sugar drop, especially when taken upon rising.
—**Di-Methyl-Glycine, DMG,** once known as B-15, is a powerful antioxidant and energizer. Used successfully to improve Down's Syndrome and mental retardation, and to curb craving in alcohol addiction. DMG's highly reputed energy effects can be attributed to its conversion to glycine. Successfully used as a control for epileptic seizures, with notable therapeutic results for atherosclerosis, rheumatic fever, rheumatism, emphysema and liver cirrhosis. For best results, take sublingually before exercise. *Note:* Too much DMG disrupts the metabolic chain and causes fatigue. The *proper* dose produces energy, overdoses do not.

• **GRAPEFRUIT SEED EXTRACT:** a multipurpose, natural antibiotic, for bacterial, viral and fungal infections; works against yeast infections like candida albicans and vaginal infections, moderate parasitic infestations, dysentery, infected cuts, gingivitis, strep and sore throat, ringworm, ear infections, nail fungus, dandruff and warts.

• **GREEN TEA:** See BLACK & GREEN TEAS & HEALING BENEFITS, page 154.

• **GUAR GUM:** an herbal product that provides soluble digestive fiber and absorbs undesirable intestinal substances. Used therapeutically to lower cholesterol and to flatten the diabetic sugar curve.

• **GUM GUGGUL:** an Indian gum resin herb from the mukul myrrh tree, it is used as a natural alternative to drugs for reducing cholesterol. In Ayurvedic healing, it is used for rheumatism, nervous diseases, tuberculosis, urinary disorders and skin diseases. Guggulipid, an extract of guggul, is credited with the ability to lower both cholesterol and triglyceride levels because it increases the liver's metabolism of LDL cholesterol. Guggulipid prevents the formation of atherosclerosis and aids in regressing pre-existing atherosclerotic plaques. It also helps inhibit platelet aggregation, promotes fibrinolysis, and may also prevent development of a stroke or embolism. A successful treatment for acne.

• **GUIDED IMAGERY:** See ALTERNATIVE HEALTH CHOICES, page 28.

• **GYMNEMA SYLVESTRE:** See SUGAR & SWEETENERS IN A HEALING DIET, page 172.

HDLs and LDLs (*High and Low Density Lipoproteins*): water-soluble, protein-covered bundles that transport cholesterol through the bloodstream, and are synthesized in the liver and intestinal tract. Bad cholesterol (LDL) carries cholesterol through the bloodstream for cell-building needs, but leaves excess behind on artery walls and in tissues. Good cholesterol (HDL) helps prevent narrowing of the artery walls by removing the excess cholesterol and transporting it to the liver for excretion as bile.

• **H_2O_2, HYDROGEN PEROXIDE, Food Grade:** Much controversy has surrounded the use of food grade hydrogen peroxide for therapeutic, anti-infective and antifungal health care. Our experience with this source of nascent oxygen has been successful in many areas, but a great deal of that success is predicated on the *way* H_2O_2 is used. Proper medicinal directions are very specific as to dosage and ailment. Read the bottle label carefully before embarking on a program that includes H_2O_2. Food grade H_2O_2 is available in two refrigerated forms: hydrogen dioxide (hydrogen peroxide), mainly for external use or magnesium dioxide (magnesium peroxide), for internal use. The internal product is formulated by Dr. Donsbach and can be purchased at health food stores or by calling 800-423-7662. It contains less oxygen but is much more palatable and more stable.

Both compounds form a stable substance we know as oxygen. The 3% dilute solution may be used internally for asthma, emphysema, arthritis, candida albicans, and degenerative conditions like chronic fatigue syndromes and HIV infections. Other applications for a 3% solution include fungal infections, as a douche for vaginal infections, and as an enema solution for detox cleansing. It may be used as a mouthwash, skin spray, or on the skin to replace the skin's acid mantle that has been removed by soap.

Oxygen baths are valuable detoxifying agents, and noticeably increase body energy. About 1 cup H_2O_2 per bath produces significant effect for 3 to 7 days. Oxygen baths are stimulating rather than relaxing. Therapeutic benefits include body pH balance, reduction of skin cancers, clearing of asthma and lung congestion, arthritis and rheumatism relief, and conditions where increased body oxygen can prevent and control disease. Add $1/_2$ cup sea salt and $1/_2$ cup baking soda for extra benefits.

Here are some common guidelines: *See* HOME HEALING PROCEDURES *page 543 for how to use H_2O_2 safely.*

—H_2O_2 is not for health maintenance use. It should be taken only if there is a specific need. Once improvement is noticed, the use of H_2O_2 should be discontinued. If you need to take H_2O_2 for more than 12 days orally or more than 60 days externally, contact a holistic physician for a custom protocol.

—Like many antibiotics, H_2O_2 also kills friendly bacterial culture in the digestive tract. When taking H_2O_2 orally, replace the intestinal flora (*acidophilus, bifidus, and bulgaricus*) by eating cultured foods, or take a supplement culture 2 hours after taking H_2O_2. If you experience nausea or bloating, discontinue use.

—Do not use H_2O_2 if you have had a heart or liver transplant.

• **HERBAL WRAPS:** the best European and American spas use herbal wraps as restorative body-conditioners. Wraps are also good body cleansers that alkalize and release body wastes quickly. They should be used in conjunction with a short cleansing program and 6-8 glasses of water a day to flush out loosened fats and toxins. Crystal Star's ALKALIZING ENZYME™ WRAP replaces and balances important minerals, enhance metabolism and alkalizes body chemistry. (Enzyme wraps are an important part of every spa program in Japan.)

• **HESPERIDIN:** a bio-chemical present in orange and lemon peel; increases capillary strength.

• **HISTIDINE:** a semi-essential amino acid in adults, essential in infants. Histamine is formed from histidine, a precursor to good immune response, to effective defense against colds, respiratory infections, and for countering allergic reactions. It has strong vasodilating and hypotensive properties for cardio-circulatory diseases, anemia and cataracts. Abundant in hemoglobin and a key to the production of both red and white blood cells. Synthesizes glutamic acid, aids copper transport through the joints, and removes heavy metals from the tissues, making it successful in treating arthritis. Histidine raises libido in both sexes. See Amino Acids.

• **HUPERZINE A:** the active alkaloid extracted, then standardized, from *Huperzia serrata*, a rare Chinese club moss. Huperzine A is a potent *blocker* of the enzyme acetylcholinesterase (AChE) that helps break down acetylcholine, the neurotransmitter essential for memory and brain function. The *inhibition* of AChE helps to enhance thinking, concentration and memory. Alan Kozikowski, Ph.D, the scientist who first synthesized Huperzine A extract, says the product is effective for decreasing deterioration of brain cells by increasing the brain's levels of acetylcholine and other neurotransmitters. It appears to be effective for Alzheimer's disease.

• **HGH, Human Growth Hormone** (also called *somatotrophin*) is produced by the pituitary gland. HGH promotes the growth of bone and regulates height, stimulates the breakdown of body fat to produce energy, and the synthesis of collagen for cartilage, tendons and ligaments. HGH helps increase muscle mass, hence its promise to the sports community and as an anti-aging therapy.

HGH supplements are synthetic HGH produced from bacterial suspension and contain an additional methionine amino-acid terminal. Side effects of the synthetically produced product include carpal tunnel syndrome, aching joints; increased risk of diabetes and severe fluid retention. Animal studies have shown shorter life spans, not longer. Some amino acids and vitamins that can stimulate the natural release of growth hormone in the body: arginine, lysine, glutamine, ornithine, glycine and niacin.

• **HYDROLYZE:** the decomposing of a compound into a simpler compound by water. Hydrolysis occurs during digestion — proteins in the stomach react with water and enzymes to form peptones and amino acids.
　—Hydrolyzed animal elastin: the hydrolyzed animal connective tissue used in emollients and creams.
　—Hydrolyzed milk protein: moisturizer made of protein extracted from milk.
　—Hydrolyzed vegetable protein: the hydrolysate (liquefaction) of vegetable protein.

• **HYPERTHERMIA, CLINICAL:** see Overheating Therapy, page 225.

• **HYPNOTHERAPY:** see ALTERNATIVE HEALTH CHOICES, page 30.

• **HYPOALLERGENIC:** a term for cosmetics meaning less likely to cause an allergic reaction. Hypoallergenic cosmetics are made without the use of common allergens that most frequently cause allergic reactions. However, some people may still be sensitive to these products.

IGNATIA: a homeopathic female remedy to relax emotional hypertension; especially during times of great grief or loss. See HOMEOPATHIC REMEDIES, page 20.

• **INOSINE:** a non-essential amino acid that stimulates ATP energy and helps provide muscle endurance when the body's glycogen reserves run out. Take on an empty stomach with an electrolyte drink before exercise.

• **INOSITOL:** part of the B-complex family, a sugar-like crystalline substance found in the liver, kidney and heart muscle, and in most plants. Deficiency is related to loss of hair, eye defects and growth retardation.

• **IODINE:** a mineral which exerts antibiotic-like action and also prevents toxicity from radiation. A key component of good thyroid function and proper metabolism, necessary for skin, hair and nail health, and for wound healing. White blood cells absorb iodine from the blood and use it to enhance their pathogen killing capacity. Iodine also prevents mucous buildup. Iodine deficiency results in goiter, hypothyroidism, cretinism, confused thinking and menstrual difficulties. Good food sources: seafoods and sea vegetables.

• **IPRIFLAVONE:** a semi-synthetic isoflavonoid, ipriflavone and isoflavonoids have a chemical structure that resembles estrogen. Ipriflavone's estrogen-like effect helps to reduce bone loss, giving it the title of the "new bone builder." Studies suggest that ipriflavone and its metabolites protect bones by inhibiting bone resorption (bone-degrading osteoclast activity). Ipriflavone also appears to activate bone-building cells called osteoblasts. Three different Italian studies show that 200mg of ipriflavone 3 times a day reduces postmenopausal bone loss.

• **IRON:** a mineral that combines with proteins and copper to produce hemoglobin to carry oxygen throughout the body. Iron deficiency means fatigue, muscle weakness and anemia. Iron strengthens immunity, helps wound healing, and is important for women using contraceptive drugs and during pregnancy. It keeps hair color young, eyes bright, the body strong. However, free, un-bound iron is a strong pro-oxidant, and can be toxic at abnormally high levels. Iron overload is linked to some cancers, heart disease, diabetes, arthritis and gland malfunction. Using herbal or food source iron supplements avoids the problem. Food sources: molasses, cherries, prunes, leafy greens, poultry, liver, legumes, peas, eggs, fish and whole grains. Vitamin C-rich foods like tomatoes, citrus juice and vinegar greatly enhance iron absorption. Herbal sources: *alfalfa, bilberry, burdock, catnip, yellow dock root, watercress, sarsaparilla and nettles.*

JOJOBA OIL: oil extracted from the bean-like seeds of the desert shrub, *Simondsia Chinensis.* A liquid wax used as a lubricant and a substitute for sperm oil, carnauba wax and beeswax. Mexican and American Indians have long used the jojoba bean wax as a hair conditioner and skin lubricant.

KALI MUR: potassium chloride, a homeopathic remedy for inflammatory arthritis. Deficiency results in glandular swelling, skin scaling, and excess mucous discharge. See HOMEOPATHIC CELL SALTS, page 21.

• **KALI PHOS:** potassium phosphate, (a body deficiency is characterized by intense odor from the body). A homeopathic remedy to treat mental problems such as depression. See HOMEOPATHIC CELL SALTS, page 21.

• **KALI SULPH:** potassium sulphate, a homeopathic cell salt that oxygenates the skin. Deficiency causes tongue deposits, and slimy nasal, eye, ear and mouth secretions. See HOMEOPATHIC CELL SALTS, page 21.

• **KEFIR:** a cultured milk product, it comes plain or fruit-flavored, and may be taken as a liquid or used like yogurt or sour cream. Kefir provides friendly intestinal flora. Use the plain flavor, cup for cup as a replacement for whole milk, buttermilk or half and half; fruit flavors may be used in sweet baked dishes.
—**Kefir Cheese:** a good cultured replacement for sour cream or cream cheese in dips and other recipes, kefir cheese is low in fat and calories, and has a slightly tangy-rich flavor that really enhances snack foods. Use it cup for cup in place of sour cream, cottage cheese, cream cheese or ricotta.

• **KOMBUCHA MUSHROOM:** actually a colony of yeast and bacteria. Proponents of kombucha claim that it is a panacea for almost any disease. People use kombucha for weight loss because it contains caffeine, and helps both liver and gallbladder work efficiently. Others say it helps bronchitis, asthma and muscle aches. One study shows the tea contains a strong antibacterial, effective against antibiotic-resistant strains of *staphylococcus.*
A mixture of black tea and sugar is brewed and a Kombucha "mother" (starter) is added. The B vitamin-rich environment allows the bacteria to convert to a type of vinegar, which is really an amino acid and enzyme-rich, digestive "tea." To use kombucha tea, start with about 2-oz. a day; do not exceed 8-oz. a day. People with uric acid problems or gout should limit use, since the active yeasts contain significant amounts of nucleic acid which increases uric acid in the blood. Diabetic use is controversial because kombucha contains 3-4% simple sugars. If mold is floating on the surface, or the mushroom falls apart when handled, discard the tea entirely.

• **KUZU:** a powdered thickening root for Japanese dishes and macrobiotic diets. Superior for imparting a shine and sparkle to stir-fried foods and clear sauces. A dairy alternative in cooking.

LACHESIS: a homeopathic remedy for premenstrual symptoms that improve once menstrual flow begins. For menopausal hot flashes. See HOMEOPATHIC REMEDIES, page 20.

• **LACTIC ACID:** a by-product of the metabolism of glucose and glycogen, present in blood and muscle tissue. Also present in sour milk, beer, sauerkraut, pickles, and other foods made by bacterial fermentation. It is used in cosmetics to exfoliate skin.

• **LACTASE:** an enzyme normally produced in the small intestine, lactase supplements can be taken before or with meals that include dairy to aid in digestion. When there is insufficient lactase, unabsorbed lactose (milk sugar) migrates to the colon, where it ferments causing gastrointestinal problems.

• **LACTOBACILLUS:** there are several types of lactobacilli, including *L. acidophilus, L. bifidus, L. caucassus, and L. bulgaricus,* all beneficial bacteria that synthesize intestinal tract nutrients, counteract pathogenic microorganisms and maintain intestinal health. Lactobacillus organisms are readily destroyed by noxious chemicals and drugs, particularly chlorine and antibiotics. In fact, a single long course of antibiotics can destroy most bowel flora, leading to the overgrowth of yeasty pathogenic organisms, like candida albicans, which are resistant to antibiotics. Even eating antibiotic-laced meats and dairy products leads to an insidious decline in the number of Lactobacillus organisms within the human body. Skin disorders, chronic candidiasis, irritable bowel syndrome and other intestinal disorders, hepatitis, lupus and heart disease are all associated with a *Lactobacillus* deficiency. Top food sources: yogurt, kefir, miso, tempeh and uncooked sauerkraut.

• **LANOLIN:** also known as wool fat or wool wax is a product of the oil glands of sheep. Chemically, a wax instead of a fat, lanolin is a natural emulsifier that absorbs and holds water to the skin.

• **LECITHIN:** a phospholipid (fat-like substance) produced in the liver, and present in some foods. Lecithin consists mostly of phosphatidyl choline. There is a high concentration of lecithin in heart cells and in the sheathing around the brain, spinal cord and nerves. Lecithin is a source of phosphatidyl choline for brain and nerve function. Choline is recognized as the direct precursor of acetylcholine, the neurotransmitter essential for memory. Acetylcholine deficiency is associated with Alzheimer's disease and senile conditions that involve memory and neurological abnormalities. Lecithin supplements significantly increase choline levels.

Lecithin supplements come from high phosphatide soy or eggs, are low in fat and cholesterol and help thicken recipes without using dairy foods. Lecithin may be substituted for $\frac{1}{3}$ the oil in recipes. Add two teaspoons daily to almost any food to increase phosphatides, choline, inositol, potassium and linoleic acid. Lecithin is a natural emulsifier, breaking down fat particles, an action essential to control of cholesterol and triglyceride levels. Lecithin reduces dangerous LDL cholesterol, and elevates healthier HDL particles.

• **LEDUM:** a homeopathic remedy for bruises. May be used following arnica treatment to fade the bruise after it becomes black and blue. See HOMEOPATHIC REMEDIES, page 20.

• **LEMON,** *Citrus Limon:* rich in vitamin C and potassium, a traditional tonic for increasing salivary and gastric secretions, currently used to dissolve gallstones, and now showing promising anticancer properties.

• **LINOLEIC ACID:** See FATS & OILS, page 160.

• **LIPOIC ACID:** (alpha lipoic acid or thioctic acid) is a unique, "universal" antioxidant, both lipid and water soluble, able to quench free radicals in both fat and water mediums. Lipoic acid is a potent promoter of glutathione and an important co-factor in energy metabolism, especially during stress conditions. It also increases the effectiveness of other antioxidants, like vitamins C and E. Lipoic acid is among the most powerful liver detoxifiers ever discovered. It shows great promise for heart disease (especially stroke recovery and atherosclerosis), diabetes (approved in Europe for diabetic retinopathy), neuro-degenerative diseases, such as Parkinson's and Alzheimer's, inflammatory diseases like arthritis and irritable bowel syndromes, HIV and AIDS, cataracts, heavy-metal toxicity and detoxification support.

• **LITHIUM:** an earth's crust trace mineral used clinically as *lithium arginate.* Successful in treating manic-depressive disorders, ADD in children, epilepsy, alcoholism, drug withdrawal and migraine headaches. Research shows therapy success with malignant lymphatic growths, arteriosclerosis and chronic hepatitis. Overdoses can cause palpitations and headaches. Good food sources: mineral water, whole grains and seeds.

• **LUTEIN:** a carotenoid nutrient like alpha-carotene, beta-carotene, cryptoxanthin, lycopene and zeaxanthin. Carotenoids are found in spinach, kale and other fruits and vegetables. Lutein is not converted to vitamin A like beta-carotene, but it does serve as a potent antioxidant. Of all the carotenoids, lutein and zeaxanthin lend the most support to the eyes. Lutein and zeaxanthin make up the yellow retinal pigment and appear to specifically protect the macula. A Harvard study reports that people eating the most lutein and zeaxanthin foods are most likely to have healthy retinas and maculae.

• **LYCOPODIUM:** a homeopathic remedy that helps to increase personal confidence. Also favored by estheticians to soothe irritated complexions and as an antiseptic. See HOMEOPATHIC REMEDIES, page 20.

• **LYSINE:** an essential amino acid; a primary treatment for the herpes virus. May be used topically or internally. High lysine foods — corn, poultry and avocados should be added if there are recurrent herpes breakouts. Helps rebuild muscle and repair tissue after injury or surgery. Important for calcium uptake for bone growth, and in cases of osteoporosis, reduces calcium loss in the urine. Helps the formation of collagen, hormones and enzymes. Supplements are effective for Parkinson's disease, Alzheimer's and hypothyroidism.

MSM *(methylsulfonylmethane)*: a dietary sulfur, MSM contains 34% sulfur important in body elements like hormones, enzymes, antibodies, antioxidants, in tissues and body proteins. Four major amino acids, methionine, cysteine, cystine, and taurine depend heavily on sulfur. MSM contributes to healthy hair and nails, to skin softness and pliability, and encourages repair of damaged skin by stimulating the production of collagen. It increases blood circulation and maintains acid-alkaline balance. It boosts both natural detoxification and immune functions by helping the body to produce immunoglobulins (antibodies). MSM is often used for muscle and joint pain stopping pain impulses before they reach the brain. It relieves constipation, and helps heal burns and scars. The supplement is derived from a naturally produced form of DMSO (dimethyl sulfoxide).

• **MAGNESIUM:** a critical mineral for osteoporosis and skeletal structure. Necessary for good nerve and muscle function, healthy blood vessels, balanced blood pressure and athletic endurance. Important for tooth formation, heart and kidney health, and restful sleep. Counteracts stress, irregular heartbeat, emotional instability and depression. Calms hyperactive children. Supplements help alcoholism, diabetes and asthma. Deficiency means muscle spasms, cramping, stomach disturbances, sometimes fibromyalgia. Magnesium is readily absorbed from dark green vegetables, seafood, whole grains, dairy foods, nuts, legumes, poultry and hot spices.

• **MAGNESIUM PHOS:** a homeopathic remedy for abdominal cramping or spasmodic back pain; particularly for menstrual cramps. See HOMEOPATHIC REMEDIES, page 20.

• **MAGNETS:** Static-magnetic-field-therapy, although used even centuries ago is currently undergoing a surge of new research for its pain relieving potential. Scientific studies show magnets increase blood and oxygen circulation, aid nutrient flow through the blood, balance body pH, speed up calcium, help to heal nerve tissue and bones, affect endocrine glands, and stimulate enzyme activity. Although the answers aren't in for the reasons magnets relieve pain, study after study is showing that magnets do work.

• **MANGANESE:** a mineral that nourishes brain and nerve centers, and aids in sugar and fat metabolism. Manganese is synergistic with calcium in nourishing bones. Some enzymes also need manganese to work properly. SOD (superoxide dismutase), a powerful free radical quenching enzyme, is solely dependent on manganese for its immune enhancing activity. Manganese also helps eliminate fatigue, nervousness and lower back pain. It reduces seizures in epileptics. Deficiencies result in poor hair and nail growth (white spots on nails), hearing loss, blood pressure disturbances, impotence, latent diabetes, and poor muscle-joint coordination. **Tranquilizer drugs deplete manganese.** Manganese supplements protect nerves from adverse effects of tranquilizers. Good food sources: blueberries, ginger, rice, eggs, green vegetables, legumes, nuts and bananas.

• **MELATONIN:** an antioxidant hormone secreted cyclically by the pineal gland to keep us in sync with the rhythms of the day and the seasons. Melatonin helps us recover from the effects of jet lag faster.

Certain protective functions give it an anti-aging reputation: 1: Melatonin helps protect the body from free radical damage. 2: Reduced immune function is an aging factor, as the thymus shrinks reducing our ability to generate T-cells. Melatonin slightly reverses thymus shrinkage, enabling it to produce more infection-fighting T-cells and enhances immune antibody production. 3: Studies show that a nightly melatonin supplement can boost the performance of immune systems compromised by age, drugs or stress, during sleep.

Melatonin facts:

—Breast and perhaps prostate cancer, hormone driven cancers, may indicate a deficiency of melatonin.

—Melatonin dampens release of estrogen. High melatonin levels can even temporarily shut down the reproductive system (the theory basis for a new contraceptive combining high dose melatonin with progestin).

—Melatonin decreases the size of the prostate gland. (A melatonin deficiency allows it to grow.) This is good news for older males with enlarged prostate. But melatonin supplements can greatly decrease sex drive and actually shrink gonads — certainly an unwanted effect.

—Melatonin may be indicated in low-tryptophan diseases, like anorexia, hypertension, manic depression, Cushing's disease, schizophrenia, and psoriasis, because tryptophan is the raw material for melatonin.

—If you supplement melatonin longterm, the body tends to shut down its own melatonin production.

—Melatonin is not recommended for people under 40 except short-term, or for a specific purpose, like a sleep disorder or jet lag. Unless you have a sleep disorder, melatonin may actually disrupt sleep patterns.

—High levels of melatonin can be found in delayed puberty, narcolepsy, obesity, and spina bifida.

—Beta blockers suppress melatonin. Serotonin stimulants, like 5-HTP or chlorpromazine (an antipsychotic), raise melatonin levels.

Consider carefully longterm melatonin supplements. Hormones are incredibly delicate substances with long-ranging effects we don't fully understand. I believe taking a hormone contraceptive drug that eventually shuts down the reproductive system is asking for trouble. If you decide to take melatonin as a protective measure against breast or prostate cancer, a small protective dose...about .1 to .3 mg at night, gives your body a chance to use the supplement yet still make its own hormone. You can always resume if needed. Other immune protective choices that don't carry the hormone risk of melatonin, are *panax ginseng, ginkgo biloba or garlic.*

• **METHIONINE:** an essential amino acid; an antioxidant and free radical deactivator. A major source of organic sulphur for healthy liver activity, lymph and immune health. Protective against chemical allergic reactions. An effective "lipotropic" that keeps fats from accumulating in the liver and arteries, thus keeping high blood pressure and serum cholesterol under control. Effective against toxemia during pregnancy. An important part of treatment for rheumatic fever. Supports healthy skin and nails, and prevents hair loss.

• **MINERALS and TRACE MINERALS:** the building blocks of life, minerals are the most basic of nutrients, the bonding agents between you and food — allowing your body to absorb nutrients. Minerals are especially necessary for athletes and people in active sports, because you must have minerals to run. Your body's minerals comprise only about 4% of your body weight, but they are keys to major areas of your health. Minerals keep your body pH balanced — alkaline instead of acid. They are essential to bone formation and bone health. They regulate the osmosis of cellular fluids, nerve electrical activity and most metabolic functions. They transport oxygen, govern heart rhythm, help you sleep, and keep you emotionally balanced. Trace minerals are only .01% of body weight, but even deficiencies in these micro-nutrients can cause severe depression, PMS and other menstrual disorders, hyperactivity in children, hypoglycemia and diabetes, nervous stress, high blood pressure, premature aging, memory loss and poor healing.

Minerals are important. Hardly any of us get enough. Your body doesn't synthesize minerals=; they must be regularly obtained from our foods. Minerals from plants and herbs are higher quality and more absorbable than from meat sources. Today's diet of chemicalized foods inhibits mineral absorption. High stress lifestyles that rely on tobacco, alcohol, steroids and antibiotics contribute to mineral depletion. Many minerals are no longer even sufficiently present in our fruits and vegetables. They have been leached from the soil by the

105

chemicals and pesticide sprays used in commercial farming. Even foods that show good amounts of minerals have less than we believe, because measurements were done decades ago when pesticides were not as prolific as they are now. Plant minerals from earth and sea herbs are one of the most reliable ways to get mineral benefits. Herbal minerals are whole foods that your body easily uses. Unlike chemically-formed supplements, they can be used as healing agents and to maintain body nutrient levels. **Minerals can really give your body a boost.** Eat organically grown produce whenever possible, and take a good herb or food-source mineral supplement.

• **MOCHI:** is a chewy rice "bread" made from sweet brown rice. It is baked very hot, at 450° and puffs up to a crisp biscuit that can be used in a variety of delicious ways. It is acceptable for candida albicans diets.

• **MOLYBDENUM:** a metabolic mineral, necessary in mobilizing enzymes. New research shows benefits for esophageal cancers and sulfite-induced cancer. Molybdenum amounts are dependent on good soil content. Good food sources: whole grains, brown rice, brewer's yeast and mineral water.

• **MUCOPOLYSACCHARIDES:** See polysaccharides.

• **MUSHROOMS:** There are four main mushroom species with specific healing properties:
  —**Shiitake:** usually sold dry, these mushrooms are linked to cures for cancerous tumors. They produce a virus which stimulates interferon. Use them frequently — just a few each time. A little goes a long way.
  —**Reishi:** a rare mushroom from the Orient, now cultivated in America. Reishi, or ganoderma, increases vitality, enhances immunity and prolongs a healthy life. It is a therapeutic antioxidant used for a wide range of serious conditions, including anti-tumor and anti-hepatitis activity. It reduces the side effects of chemotherapy. Research shows success against chronic fatigue syndrome. Reishi helps regenerate the liver, lowers cholesterol and triglycerides, reduces coronary risk and high blood pressure, and alleviates allergy symptoms.
  —**Poria Cocos:** regulates excess fluid buildup; purifies body fluids and prevents build-up of toxins.
  —**Maitake:** contains a polysaccharide that boosts immunity against hormone-driven cancers. Maitake may also help CFS, diabetes, hepatitis, HBP, HIV infections, obesity and arthritis.
  —**Cordyceps:** a tonic and energizer that enhances immunity and oxygen uptake to the heart and brain, possesses testosterone-like effects, improves libido and sperm count, and reduces fibroid tumors.

NADH (*nicotinamide adenine dinucleotide*): a potent antioxidant coenzyme involved in the synthesis of ATP (*adenosine triphosphate*), enhances cellular energy in the brain and body. Brain and muscle cells contain the highest amounts of NADH. Although NADH is in every living animal and plant cell, the first supplement was derived from yeast in 1993 (although the finished product is yeast free), by George Birkmayer, M.D., Ph.D.. NADH enhances the immune system by its "metabolic burst" step that leads to the destruction of a cytotoxic invader. It also repairs DNA, enhances the two brain neurotransmitters, dopamine and norepinephrine and has anti-aging potential. Studies promise hope for Alzheimer's and Parkinson's disease, chronic fatigue syndrome and depression. Recommended dosage for energy enhancement is 2.5 to 5mg daily.

• **NEEM OIL,** *Azadirachta Indica*: a tropical tree related to mahogany, used medicinally for centuries, now being rediscovered by alternative healers. Recent science validates the traditional uses of neem, including skin care, treatment of bacterial and viral infections and immune system enhancement. Numerous studies show neem to be versatile, effective against skin and dental disease, fungi, viruses, bacteria and parasites, fever, allergies, inflammation, ulcers, tuberculosis, cardiovascular problems; it's even used as a spermicide.

• **NATRUM MUR,** *sodium chloride*: regulates moisture within cells. Deficiency causes fatigue, chills, craving for salt, bloating, profuse sweating, tearing, salivation and watery stools. HOMEOPATHIC CELL SALTS, page 21.

• **NATRUM PHOS,** *sodium phosphate*: regulates pH balance. Imbalance is indicated by a coated tongue, itchy skin, sour stomach, loss of appetite, diarrhea and flatulence. See HOMEOPATHIC CELL SALTS, page 21.

• **NATRUM SULPH,** *sodium sulphate*: imbalance produces tissue edema, dry skin with watery eruptions, poor bile and pancreas activity, headaches and gouty symptoms. See HOMEOPATHIC CELL SALTS, page 21.

• **NONI** (*Morinda Citrifolia*), also known as nonu, has been used by Polynesian islanders as a main adaptogen medicine for more than 1,500 years, for arthritis, heart disease, digestive disorders, colds, flu, sinus infections, headaches, infections, menstrual problems, injuries, pain relief, type II diabetes, skin disorders and more.
Research documents antibacterial properties against *M. pyrogenes, Ps. aeruginosa,* even *E. coli.* Noni has anti-tumor activity, anti-inflammatory effects, pain relieving properties, cell repair and regeneration effects and stimulates the immune system. Noni contains vitamins, minerals, trace elements, enzymes and co-enzymes, plant sterols, antioxidants, phytonutrients, and bioflavonoids. Many believe the synergistic effect of all these nutrients is what gives it its powerful punch. Look for a freeze-dried product that uses only the whole fruit for best results.

• **NUX VOMICA:** a homeopathic remedy for gastrointestinal problems. A prime remedy for hangover, recovering alcoholics, drug addiction and migraine prevention. See HOMEOPATHIC REMEDIES, page 20.

O CTACOSANOL: a wheat germ derivative, used to counteract fatigue and increase oxygen use during exercise and athletic performance. Antioxidant properties are helpful for muscular dystrophy and M.S.

• **OLIVE LEAF EXTRACT:** is a potent herbal antibacterial, antiviral, antifungal, antiparasite and antioxidant. It stimulates the immune system by phagocyte production, restores energy and boosts stamina. Olive leaf's powerful punch comes from its oleuropein and oleuropein's hydrolysis. Oleuropein is a member of the iridoid group, a uniquely structured chemical class in which one member has the capability to transfer into another group, a biogenetic characteristic which gives oleuropein its antimicrobial power.
Clinical research and experience have shown that olive leaf extract has a wide range of successes against viral, bacterial, fungal, and protozoan infections, particularly for treatment of herpes I and II, human herpes virus 6 and 7, HIV-AIDS, flu, the common cold, meningitis, Epstein-Barr virus, encephalitis, shingles, chronic fatigue, hepatitis B, pneumonia, tuberculosis, gonorrhea, malaria, severe diarrhea, blood poisoning, and dental, ear, urinary tract and surgical infections. Lab tests done by Upjohn Co. find that olive leaf extract kills 56 pathogens. Tests from East Park Research finds that olive leaf extract treats as many as 120 illnesses.

• **OMEGA-3 and OMEGA-6 FATTY ACIDS:** See FATS & OILS, page 161.

• **OREGANO OIL:** is rich in polyphenolic flavonoids, two of which, carvacrol and thymol are potent antiseptics. (Note: Both oregano and thyme contain the active ingredients carvacrol and thymol. Carvacrol is the predominant polyphenol in oregano; thymol the predominant in thyme.) Oregano oil contains over 50 compounds with antimicrobial actions that inhibit candida yeast, bacteria, viruses and parasites. Oregano oil is also a powerful antioxidant. Direct contact of oregano essential oil can cause mild burns — avoid irritation by mixing with olive oil. Oregano oil can be used externally or internally (in a capsule).

• **OREGON GRAPE CREAM** (*Mahonia aquifolium*): has a direct action on the skin when applied topically. Tests show it's over 80% effective in relieving psoriasis, eczema, dermatitis, dandruff, acne and dry scaly skin. Alkaloids extracted from the root and bark have strong anti-microbial and anti-fungal properties, and are potent antioxidants which neutralize skin damaging free radicals, reduce inflammation, and inhibit abnormal skin cell growth (as in psoriasis). Although used extensively by early American physicians, Oregon grape has been replaced by cortisone preparations. Today, herbs like Oregon grape are again popular as people learn the debilitating side effects of drugs. An Oregon grape cream called PRIMADERM is by Prime Pharmaceutical Corp.

• **ORNITHINE:** a non-essential amino acid that works with arginine and carnitine to metabolize excess body fat; with the pituitary gland to promote growth hormone, muscle development, tissue repair, and endurance. A good aid to fat metabolism through the liver; builds immune strength; helps scavenge free radicals.

• **OPCs,** *Oligomeric Proanthocyanidin Complexes*: a class of bioflavonoids composed of polyphenols. Generally extracted either from grape seeds or white pine bark, these potent antioxidants destroy free radicals, activity widely accepted in slowing the aging process and enhancing immune response. Free radicals also weaken cell membranes, cause inflammation, genetic mutations, and contribute to major health problems like cancer and cardiovascular disease. Increasing evidence shows that people live less-diseased lives when OPCs are a part of their nutritional program. This is especially true for premature aging, immune deficiency, allergies or exposure to environmental pollutants. A "side effect" of proanthocyanidin activity is the inhibition of histamine production, which allows the body to better defend against LDL-cholesterol.

Vitamin C activity is vastly increased with all OPCs, especially strengthening collagen in blood vessels, and increasing capillary resiliency. German studies show OPCs have a unique ability to bind to collagen structures and to inhibit collagen destruction. Blood vessel strength is enhanced by as much as 140% after OPC supplementation. Capillaries become more elastic, circulation noticeably improves. Easy bruising and varicose vein tendency lessens. New tests on grape seed extract indicate that its properties were the primary anti-carcinogen in the world famous "grape cure" against cancer widely used in the early part of this century.

—**Pycnogenol:** a trade name for pine bark OPCs, is a highly active bioflavonoid. It helps the body resist inflammation and free radical damage to blood vessels and skin. It strengthens the entire arterial system. Pycnogenol is used in Europe as an "oral cosmetic," because it stimulates collagen-rich connective tissue against atherosclerosis and helps joint flexibility. It is used against diabetic retinopathy, varicose veins and hemorrhoids. It is one of the few dietary antioxidants that crosses the blood-brain barrier to directly protect brain cells.

—**Grape seed extract:** highly bio-available proanthocyanidin bioflavonoids....a prime antioxidant. Studies show PCOs from grape seed extract scavenge free radicals 50% more effectively than vitamin E, and 20% more effectively than vitamin C. Vitamin E scavenges harmful free radicals in fatty environments of the body; vitamin C scavenges free radicals in the watery environments. Grape seed extract scavenges free radicals in both environments, and does so more efficiently.

OPCs from herbs in particular do more than protect, they also help repair, reducing capillary fragility, and restoring skin smoothness and elasticity.

The demonstrated benefits from OPC's from herbs include:
—potent free radical scavengers, with tumor inhibiting properties
—an arteriosclerosis antidote, strengthening capillary/vein structure
—reduces vein fragility to help prevent bruising, varicose veins, restless legs and lower leg blood volume
—anti-allergy properties, protective against early histamine production
—specifically aids vascular fragility associated with diabetic retinopathy
—improves skin elasticity, enhances circulation, fights inflammation and improves joint flexibility
—helps PMS symptoms

• **OSCILLOCOCCINUM:** a homeopathic remedy for flu. See HOMEOPATHIC REMEDIES, pg. 20.

• **OVERHEATING THERAPY** (*Hyperthermia*): See page 225. *Note: simple overheating therapy may be used in the home. It stimulates the body's immune mechanism without the stress of fever-inducing drugs.*

• **OXALIC ACID:** a component of chard, spinach and beet greens that binds to calcium and iron in the body, thus preventing their absorption. To reduce oxalic acid in these foods, lightly cook them until they turn bright green and slightly tender. In addition, consider a Japanese variety of spinach called "Toyo" which is reported to contain less oxalic acid than regular spinach.

PABA, *Para-Aminobenzoic Acid*: a B Complex family member and component of folic acid, PABA has sun-screening properties, is effective against sun and other burns, and is used in treating vitiligo, (depigmentation of the skin). Successful with molasses, pantothenic and folic acid in restoring lost hair color. New research shows success against skin cancers caused by UV radiation (lack of ozone-layer protection). Good food sources: brewer's yeast, eggs, molasses and wheat germ. See Vitamins.

- **PANTOTHENIC ACID:** See vitamin B-5

- **pH:** the scale used to measure acidity and alkalinity. pH is hydrogen, or "H" ion concentration of a solution. "p" stands for the power factor of the H ion. pH of a solution is measured on a scale of 14. A neutral solution, neither acidic nor alkaline, such as water, has a pH of 7. Acid is less than 7; alkaline is more than 7.

- **PHENYLALANINE:** an essential amino acid; a tyrosine precursor that works with vitamin B-6 on the central nervous system as an anti-depressant and mood elevator. Successful in treating manic, post-amphetamine, and schizophrenic-type depression (check for allergies first). Aids in learning and memory retention. Relieves menstrual, arthritic and migraine pain. A thyroid stimulant that helps curb the appetite by increasing the body's production of CCK.
  Contra-indications: phenylketonurics (elevated natural phenylalanine levels) should avoid aspartame sweeteners. Pregnant women and those with blood pressure imbalance, skin carcinomas, and diabetes should avoid phenylalanine. Tumors and cancerous melanoma growths have been slowed by reducing *dietary intake* of tyrosine and phenylalanine. Avoid if blurred vision occurs when using.

- **PHOSPHORUS:** the second most abundant body mineral. Necessary for skeletal structure, brain oxygenation and cell reproduction. Increases muscle performance while decreasing muscle fatigue. Excessive antacids deplete phosphorus. Good food sources: eggs, fish, organ meats, dairy foods, legumes, nuts and poultry.

- **PHOSPHATIDYL CHOLINE:** a natural component of lecithin, phosphatidyl choline is an essential component of cell membranes, maintaining fluidity of the membranes and playing a critical role in all membrane-dependent metabolic processes. Its emulsifying action controls cholesterol and triglyceride levels, and is often used to increase the absorption of fat-soluble vitamins and herbs.

- **PHOSPHATIDYL SERINE,** (PS): a brain cell nutrient that rapidly absorbs and readily crosses the blood-brain barrier. PS helps activate and regulate proteins that play major roles in nerve cell functions and nerve impulses. Studies show that PS helps maintain or improve cognitive ability — memory and learning, especially for Alzheimer's victims. PS effectively helps individuals maintain mental fitness, with benefits persisting even for weeks after PS is stopped. Common foods have insignificant amounts of PS, and the body produces only limited amounts. Until recently, concentrated PS was available only as a bovine-derived product with potential safety problems. A new concentrated, safe-source PS is derived from soybeans.

- **PHYTOCHEMICALS:** the natural constituents in plants that have specific pharmacologic action. Also known as neutraceuticals, the actions of phytochemicals are predictable in much the same way as pharmaceuticals, but they are foods. To use phytochemicals best, ingest the plant source in its whole form.
  —**Anticarcinogens:** phytochemicals that prevent or delay tumor formation. Some herbs and foods with known anticarcinogens include: ginseng, some soy products, garlic, echinacea, goldenseal, licorice, black cohosh, wild yam, sarsaparilla, maitake mushroom and cruciferous vegetables.
  —**Phytohormones:** many plants contain substances with hormonal actions. Plant hormone phyto-chemicals are very similar to human hormones and capable of binding to hormone receptor sites in the human body. Unlike synthetic hormones, plant hormones show little or no adverse side effects. Some food plants and herbs with phytohormone activity: soy, *licorice, wild yam, sarsaparilla root, dong quai, damiana and black cohosh.*
    Phytoestrogen: plant estrogenic hormones remarkably similar to human estrogen hormones. Especially important in hormone-driven cancers, phytoestrogens bind to estrogen receptor sites in the body without the negative side effects of synthetic estrogens or even excess body estrogens. Recent studies show phytoestrogens inhibit the proliferation of both estrogen-receptor positive and negative breast tumor cells. Some plants with phytoestrogenic activity: *dong quai, panax ginseng, licorice, fennel, alfalfa and red clover.*
    Phytoprogesterone: plant progesterone hormones similar to human progesterone. Progesterone participates in almost every physiological process. Biochemically, it provides the material out of which all the

other steroid hormones (such as cortisone, testosterone, estrogen and salt-regulating aldosterone) can be made. Progesterone's simple molecular structure allows it to balance either an excess or deficiency of other hormones. As a precursor to estrogen, its tremendous increase during pregnancy serves to stabilize the hormone adjustment and growth of both mother and child. This is especially visible in muscle tissue, such as the uterus, the heart, the intestines and bladder. Less visibly, progesterone normalizes gland processes for both men and women. When progesterone is deficient, there tends to be hypoglycemia, often accompanied by obesity. Some plants with a long tradition of phytoprogesterone activity: *sarsaparilla, licorice root and wild yam.*

Phyto-testosterone: plant testosterone similar to the androgen or male hormone found in both men and women. Accelerates tissue growth and stimulates blood flow, as well as the balance of secondary sexual characteristics. Testosterone is essential for normal sexual behavior and male erections. Yet, few people realize that testosterone determines sex drive in both sexes. The body's production of testosterone decreases and in some cases, changes its structure with age. Ginseng is the only herb tested so far to stimulate testosterone production in the body.

• **PHYTOSOMES:** a new form of botanical technology, the phytosome process enhances and intensifies the power of certain herbal compounds. A phytosome is created by binding flavonoid molecules from herbs to molecules of phosphatidyl choline from lecithin. The union becomes a new molecule that is better used by the body. Phytosomes are similar to the liposomes composed of phosphatidyl choline widely used in cosmetics.

About phytosome absorbability: Phytosomes can deliver liposomes from plants directly into the body. The phytosome process works synergistically, both providing extra phosphatidyl choline and magnifying the power of an herbal compound in its absorption through the skin.

• **PODOPHYLLUM:** a homeopathic remedy that helps diarrhea. See HOMEOPATHIC REMEDIES, page 20.

• **POLYSACCHARIDES:** long chains of simple sugars, plant polysaccharides have long been used in healing, particularly in stimulating the immune system. Aloe, green tea, echinacea, astragalus and maitake mushroom contain large amounts of polysaccharides.

—**Mucopolysaccharides:** polysaccharides that form chemical bonds with water. An important constituent of connective tissue, supporting and binding together the cells to form tissues, and the tissues to form organs. Mucopolysaccharides, especially in the form of Chondroitin Sulphate A (CSA), are beneficial for prevention and reversal of coronary heart disease. CSA is also anti-inflammatory, antiallergenic, and antistress. It is used successfully in treating osteoporosis and in accelerating recovery from bone fractures.

• **POTASSIUM:** an electrolyte mineral in body fluids, potassium balances the acid-alkaline system, transmits electrical signals between cells and nerves, and enhances muscle performance. It works with sodium to regulate the body's water balance, and protects the heart against hypertension and stroke (people who take high blood pressure medication are vulnerable to potassium deficiency). Potassium helps oxygenate the brain for clear thinking and controls allergic reactions. Stress, hypoglycemia, diarrhea and acute anxiety or depression generally result in potassium deficiency. A vegetable potassium broth (page 215) is one of the greatest natural healing tools available for cleansing and restoring body energy. Good sources: fresh fruits, especially kiwis and bananas, potatoes, sea greens, spices like coriander, cumin, basil, parsley, ginger, hot peppers, dill weed, tarragon, paprika and turmeric, lean poultry and fish, dairy foods, legumes, seeds and whole grains.

• **PROBIOTICS** (meaning "for life"): dietary supplements consisting of beneficial microorganisms. Friendly bacteria have a profound influence on our health. Most health professionals recommend a blend of varying species of *lactobacillus* and *bifidophilus*. The intestine is home to hundreds of species of microorganisms, both friendly and unfriendly, and competition for survival is fierce. When friendly microorganisms are plentiful and flourishing, they inhibit the growth of pathogenic organisms, boost the immune system, manufacture important vitamins (vitamin K and B vitamins - including B12), improve digestion, combat vaginal yeast infections, maintain the body's vital chemical and hormone balance and keep our bodies clean and protected from toxins.

• **PROSTAGLANDINS:** a vital group of hormone-like substances derived from essential fatty acids (EFA's) that regulate body functions electrically. EFA's control reproduction and fertility, inflammation, immunity and communication between cells. Prostaglandins supplement and balance the body's essential fatty acid supply. Foods like ocean fish, sea foods, olive, safflower or sunflower oils, and herbs like evening primrose and flax oils benefit prostaglandin balance. Conversely, excess saturated fats in the body, especially from fatty animal foods, inhibit both prostaglandin production and proper hormone flow.

• **PSYLLIUM HUSKS:** a lubricating, mucilaginous, fibrous herb with cleansing, laxative properties. A "colon broom" for constipation; effective for diverticulitis; a lubricant for ulcerous intestinal tract tissue.

• **PULSATILLA:** homeopathic remedy for child allergies or infections. HOMEOPATHIC REMEDIES, page 20.

• **PYCNOGENOL:** a trade name for pine bark OPC's. See OPC's.

• **PYRIDOXINE:** see vitamin B-6.

• **PYRUVATE:** Pyruvic acid is a natural element in the human body, a by-product of energy metabolism of a sugar or starch. As a supplement pyruvic acid is stabilized with calcium, sodium or potassium to form pyruvate. The popular attention to pyruvate is for its potential as a weight loss and fat loss enhancer. Tests show pyruvate supplements elevate the body's resting metabolic rate and enhance lean muscle mass. Researcher Ronald Stanko, M. D. of University of Pittsburgh Medical School found pyruvate supplements increase weight loss by 37% and fat loss by 48%. Studies also find pyruvate boosts endurance, reduces fatigue and increases energy levels. As a potent antioxidant it inhibits free radicals, lowers cholesterol level, and is heart-healthy because it helps the heart pump more blood with less oxygen use. Results are obtained from doses as low as 5 grams a day.

QUERCETIN: a powerful bioflavonoid cousin of rutin, quercetin is isolated from blue-green algae. Its primary therapeutic use is in controlling allergy and asthma reactions, since it suppresses the release and production of the two inflammatory agents that cause asthma and allergy symptoms — histamines and leukotrienes. Take quercetin with bromelain for best bioavailability and synergistic anti-inflammatory activity.

• **QUINOA:** an ancient Inca supergrain, containing complete protein from amino acids, and good complex carbohydrates. It is essentially gluten-free, light and flavorful, and can be used like rice or millet.

REFLEXOLOGY: see YOUR ALTERNATIVE HEALTH CARE CHOICES, page 35.

• **RETIN-A:** a prescription drug for treating acne, fine lines and hyperpigmentation, Retin-A is a vitamin A derivative, available, through prescription in five strengths and in cream, gel or liquid form. Retin-A works by decreasing the cohesiveness of skin cells, causing the skin to peel. Because it is a skin irritant, *other* irritants (like extreme weather, wind, cosmetics, or soaps) can cause severe irritation. Many people are sensitive to Retin-A.
Note: Alpha Hydroxy Acids (AHAs) are an alternative, but should be used cautiously. See Alpha Hydroxy Acids.

• **RIBOSE:** a simple sugar found naturally in all body cells, a vital part of the metabolic process for ATP energy, the number one fuel used by cells. Maintaining an adequate level of ATP is vital in providing peak energy to the heart and muscles. People with cardiovascular disease, or athletes who experience diminished heart and skeletal muscle nucleotides following high-intensity exercise are the best candidates for ribose. Ischemia, a heart condition of poor blood flow which causes a lack of sufficient oxygen to reach the cells decreases ATP levels by 50 percent or more. Studies with ribose showed that the heart was able to recover 85 percent of its ATP levels within 24 hours. Athletes who experience anoxia (when muscles use oxygen faster than the bloodstream can supply), enhance energy recovery in the muscle cells with ribose.

• **RHUS TOX:** a poison ivy derivative; used homeopathically for pain and stiffness in the joints and ligaments when the pain is worse with cold, damp weather. See HOMEOPATHIC REMEDIES, page 20.

• **RIBOFLAVIN:** see vitamin B-2.

• **ROYAL JELLY:** the milk-like secretion from the head glands of the queen bee's nurse-workers. RJ is a powerhouse of B vitamins, calcium, iron, potassium and silicon. It has enzyme precursors, a sex hormone and all eight essential amino acids. In fact, it contains every nutrient necessary to support life. It is a natural antibiotic, stimulates immune response, supplies key nutrients for energy and mental alertness, promotes cell longevity, and is effective for wide ranging health benefits. It is one of the world's richest sources of pantothenic acid, known to combat stress, fatigue and insomnia, and is a necessary nutrient for healthy skin and hair. It has been found effective for gland and hormone imbalances that reflect in menstrual and prostate problems. The highest quality royal jelly products are preserved in their whole, raw, "alive" state, which promotes ready absorption by the body. As little as one drop of pure, extract of fresh royal jelly can deliver an adequate daily supply.

SALICYLIC ACID: occurs naturally in wintergreen leaves, sweet birch, and white willow. Synthetically prepared, it is used in making aspirin, and as a preservative in cosmetics. It is antipyretic (anti-itch) and antiseptic. In medicine, it is used as an antimicrobial at 2 to 20% concentration in ointments, powders, and plasters. It can be absorbed by the skin, but large amounts may cause abdominal pain and hyperventilation.

• **SAMBUCUS NIGRA,** (*Black Elderberry*): has been used in herbal medicine since the days of Hippocrates. Dr. Madeleine Mumcuoglu, Ph.D., Pharm, has found that elderberry extracts successfully and consistently defeat the flu virus, accelerating flu recovery by two to four days compared with a placebo. Viruses have tiny protein spikes with H and N antigens. The H antigen of the virus binds to healthy cell receptors and punctures the cells walls - thus enabling it to reproduce. Active substances in black elderberry disarm the virus's tiny protein spikes of the H antigen, preventing the virus from reproducing itself, thus stopping the virus infection. Besides key antiviral components elderberry contains high anthocyanin (antioxidant) content.

• **SAMe,** (S-Adenosyl Methionine): prescribed for two decades in 14 countries, SAMe has finally hit the US market. SAMe is normally produced in the brain from the amino acid methionine. It becomes an *active methionine* in the body by the combining of the amino acid L-methionine with ATP (primary energy molecule). The stable supplement form of SAMe is made by first producing the amino acid L-methionine by a micro-fermentation processes followed by an artificial means of zapping it with ATP.

SAMe is an important donor of methyl groups in a process called methylation, important to the biochemical pathway of cellular DNA. Methylation affects everything from fetal development to brain function. Neurotransmitters such as L-dopa, dopamine and related hormones are the products of methylation reactions.

SAMe is useful for:
—**Depression:** Widely prescribed in Italy, clinical studies show that SAMe is an effective natural antidepressant. Synthesis of SAMe is impaired in depressed patients. Supplementing with SAMe results in increased levels of serotonin and dopamine, and improved binding of neurotransmitters to receptor sites. SAMe has a quicker onset of action and is better tolerated than tricyclic antidepressants.
—**Osteoarthritis pain:** SAMe relieves the pain of osteoarthritis by aiding chemical processes that control pain and inflammation. The U.S. Arthritis Foundation states that SAMe "provides pain relief."
—**Liver disease:** Studies show that SAMe helps cirrhosis, hepatitis, cholestasis (blockage of bile ducts), and may prevent liver damage caused by some drugs. Alcohol harms the liver partly by depleting SAMe.
—**Fibromyalgia:** Helps relieve pain, improves mood and activity levels.
—**Migraine headaches:** provides pain relief.
—**Alzheimer's disease:** studies show its neurotransmitter improvement helps enhance memory centers.

Common dosage: 200 to 400mg — therapeutic doses are higher. SAMe is extremely safe, but people with bipolar (manic) depression should consult a physician. Include B vitamin complex when taking SAMe. When a SAMe molecule loses its methyl group, it breaks down to become homocysteine. Homocysteine is toxic to cells if it builds up. Vitamin B-6, B-12 and folic acid convert homocysteine into the antioxidant glutathione.

• **SAUNA HEAT THERAPY:** a sauna is another way to use overheating therapy. A long sauna not only induces a healing, cleansing fever, but also causes profuse therapeutic sweating. The skin, in overheating therapy, acts as a "third kidney" to eliminate body wastes through perspiration. Professional saunas are available in every health club and gym as part of the membership, and the new home-installed models are not only adequate but reasonable in price. For optimum skin cleansing and restoration, take a sauna once or twice a week.

Some of the health benefits of a dry sauna: 1: speeds up metabolism; 2: inhibits the replication of pathogenic organisms; 3: stimulates activity of all vital organs and glands; 4: supports the body's immune system and accelerates its healing functions; 5: dramatically increases detoxifying capacity of the skin; 6: a proven jump-start technique for a weight loss program, especially for sugar cravers.

Note: Although induced fever is a natural, constructive means of biological healing, advice from an expert practitioner is recommended. A heart and general vitality check is advisable. Some seriously ill people lose the ability to perspire; this should be known before using overheating therapy. Reduce time in the sauna if there is redness or skin irritation that persists over a week. See page 226 for more about saunas.

• **SEA GREENS:** including *arame, bladderwrack, dulse, hijiki, kelp, kombu, nori, sea palm, and wakame* are foods with superior nutritional content. They are rich sources of proteins, carbohydrates, antioxidants, minerals and vitamins, especially healing carotenes. They are good alkalizers for the body, and can be used in place of salt or other seasonings. Sea vegetables are the mainstay of iodine therapy for wide ranging health needs. See ABOUT SEA GREENS & IODINE THERAPY, pg. 178 for more information on their healing properties.

• **SELENIUM:** a component of glutathione and powerful antioxidant, selenium protects the body from free radical damage and heavy metal toxicity. An anticancer substance and immune stimulant, it works with vitamin E to prevent cholesterol accumulation, protects against heart weakness and degenerative disease. It enhances skin elasticity. Deficiency results in aging skin, liver damage, hypothyroidism and sometimes in digestive tract cancer. The most effective supplement is organic seleno-methionine. Food sources: brewer's yeast, sesame seeds, garlic, tuna, sea greens, wheat germ, oysters, fish, organ meats, vegetables, nuts and mushrooms.

• **SEPIA:** a homeopathic remedy for treating herpes, eczema and hair loss. See HOMEOPATHY, page 20.

• **SEROTONIN:** a neurotransmitter which has widespread and often profound implications. It plays a role in sleep, mood, depression, appetite, memory, learning, body temperature, sexual behavior, cardiovascular function, muscle contraction, and endocrine regulation. Serotonin is a precursor to the neurohormone, melatonin. Serotonin has a number of functions in the central nervous system, blood vessels and intestines. About 2% of all serotonin is located in the brain.

• **SHARK CARTILAGE:** contains a biologically active protein that strongly inhibits development of new blood vessel networks (angiogenesis). Angiogenesis is a primary cause of rheumatoid arthritis and tumor growth in cancers. Other health conditions dependent on angiogenesis blood supply may be corrected somewhat by shark cartilage: eye diseases like diabetic retinopathy, macular degeneration and neo-vascular glaucoma; lupus erythematosus; inflammatory bowel diseases like Crohn's disease; scleroderma; yeast diseases like candida enteritis; cancers like Kaposi's sarcoma and solid tumors; skin disorders such as eczema and psoriasis.

Note: Because of its efficient inhibition on the formation of new capillary networks, there are some contraindications: a pregnant woman should not supplement with shark cartilage because she wants capillary growth for the fetus. If you have heart disease or peripheral vascular disease, avoid shark cartilage since new capillaries are desirable. Shark cartilage is unsuitable if you suffer from liver dysfunction or disabling kidney disease. Large amounts of shark cartilage can cause gastric upset — take smaller dosages throughout the day.

Daily dosage is between 20 and 90 gm daily; the course of therapy often runs from six to nine months.

• **SILICA,** *silicon dioxide:* a chemical compound of silicon and oxygen, silica comprises a large percent of the earth's crust and mantle, rocks and sand. Quartz consists solely of silica. There is some confusion between *silica* and *silicon.* Both are available in health food stores. Silicon is the elemental silicon mineral that is found in man, animals and plants. Silica is generally silicon dioxide, the most abundant silicon compound.

Silica gel contains hydrogen, oxygen and silicon, one form of which is an agent used to absorb moisture (as in containers for certain foods and in the bottles of our supplements). Silica gel is derived from quartz crystals. Some silica supplements are water-soluble extracts of the herb horsetail. Others are derived from purified algae. In addition to its benefits for healthy hair, skin and nails, and for calcium absorption in bone formation, silica/silicon maintains flexible arteries and plays a significant role in cardiovascular health. Beneficial food sources: grain husks (particularly barley, oats, millet, wheat), seeds, green leafy vegetables, red beets, asparagus, Jerusalem artichokes, parsley, bell peppers, sunflower seeds and horsetail herb.

—**Silicon:** a mineral responsible for connective tissue growth and health. Prevents arteriosclerosis. Necessary for collagen synthesis. Regenerates body infrastructure, including skeleton, tendons, ligaments, cartilage, connective tissue, skin, hair and nails. Silicon supplements may bring about bone recalcification. Silicon counteracts the effects of aluminum on the body, and is important in the prevention of Alzheimer's disease and osteoporosis. Silicon levels decrease with aging and are needed in larger amounts by the elderly. Beneficial food sources: whole grains, horsetail herb, well water, bottled mineral water and fresh vegetables.

• **SILICEA,** *(silica):* a homeopathic cell salt essential to the health of bones, joints, skin and glands. Deficiency produces respiratory system catarrh, pus discharges from the skin, slow wound healing and offensive body odor. Very successful in the homeopathic treatment of boils, pimples and abscesses, for hair and nail health, blood cleansing, and rebuilding the body after illness or injury. See HOMEOPATHIC CELL SALTS, page 21.

• **SODIUM:** an electrolyte mineral that helps regulate kidney and body fluid function. Involved with high blood pressure only when calcium and phosphorous are deficient in the body. Works as an anti-dehydrating agent. Beneficial food sources include: celery, seafoods, sea vegetables, cheese, dairy products.

• **SORBITOL:** a humectant that gives a velvety feel to skin. Used as a replacement for glycerin in emulsions, ointments, embalming fluid, mouthwashes, toothpastes, and cosmetics. Used in foods as a sugar substitute. First found in the ripe berries of the mountain ash, it also occurs in other berries and in cherries, plums, pears, apples, seaweed and algae. Medicinally used to reduce excess body water and for intravenous feedings. If ingested in excess, it can cause diarrhea and gastrointestinal disturbances.

• **SOY:** see SOY FOODS & THERAPEUTIC BENEFITS, page 142.

• **SPIRULINA:** see GREEN SUPERFOODS, page 135.

• **STEVIA REBAUDIANA,** *(sweet herb):* see SUGAR & SWEETENERS IN A HEALING DIET, page 171.

• **SULPHUR:** the "beauty mineral" for smooth skin, glossy hair, hard nails and collagen synthesis. It is critical to protein absorption. Good food sources: eggs, fish, onions, garlic, hot peppers and mustard.

• **SUPER OXIDE DISMUTASE (SOD):** an enzyme, SOD prevents damage caused by the toxic oxygen molecule known as superoxide. Manganese and zinc, in particular, stimulate production of SOD. Many experts do not believe that antioxidant enzyme levels in cells can be increased by taking antioxidant enzymes like SOD orally. Human tests with SOD supplements do not appear to increase the levels of SOD in the blood or tissues. See also Antioxidants.

TAURINE: a non-essential amino acid, taurine is a potent anti-seizure nutrient. A neurotransmitter that helps control hyperactivity, nervous system imbalance after drug or alcohol abuse, and epilepsy. Normalizes irregular heartbeat, helps prevent circulatory and heart disorders, hypoglycemia, hypothyroidism, water retention and hypertension. Lowers cholesterol levels. Found in high concentrations in bile, mother's milk, shark and abalone. Supplementation is necessary for therapy.

• THIAMINE: see Vitamin B-1.

• THREONINE: an essential amino acid that works with glycine to aid in overcoming depression, and neurologic dysfunctions such as genetic spastic disorders and M.S. Works with aspartic acid and methionine as a lipotropic to prevent fatty build-up in the liver. Helps to control epileptic seizures. An immune stimulant and thymus enhancer. Important for the formation of collagen, elastin and enamel.

• THUYA: a homeopathic remedy for warts and sinusitis. See HOMEOPATHIC REMEDIES, page 20.

• TOCOTRIENOLS: compounds related to the vitamin E tocopherols. Tocotrienols lower cholesterol, and have potent antioxidant and anti-cancer properties. Studies show tocotrienols are more effective than tocopherols in decreasing both total and LDL cholesterol levels. Although tocotrienols and tocopherols both offer significant protection against damage to the arterial wall - tocotrienols have a stronger lipid lowering effect. Vitamin E supplements containing natural mixed tocopherols, including the tocotrienols, offer the best choice.

• TRYPTOPHAN: an essential amino acid; a precursor of the neurotransmitter serotonin, involved in mood and metabolism regulation. It is a natural, non-addictive tranquilizer for restful sleep. Used successfully, through blood vessel dilation, to decrease hyperkinetic, aggressive behavior, migraine headaches, and schizophrenia. Counteracts compulsive overeating, smoking and alcoholism. An effective anti-depressant, it raises abnormally low blood sugar, and reduces seizures in *petit mal* epilepsy. Produces nicotinic acid (natural niacin) which is being tested to counteract the effects of nicotine from cigarettes. *Note: At the time of this writing L-Tryptophan supplements are still not allowed as over-the-counter nutrients by the FDA. It now appears in many prescription sleep-aid drugs, and is a safe nutrient sleep aid and relaxant.*
　　—5-HTP *(L-5-Hydroxytryptophan):* plays an important role in the serotonin story. Tryptophan is plays a role in the synthesis of serotonin in our bodies. 5-HTP is the step between tryptophan and serotonin. Once tryptophan is taken up into a nerve cell, it is converted into 5-HTP with the help of the enzyme tryptophan hydroxylase. 5-HTP is then converted to serotonin. 5-HTP extracted from *Griffonia* seed, is available as a supplement to boost serotonin. Many researchers consider 5-HTP to be the safest tryptophan alternative available, and successful studies using 5-HTP show that it alleviates serotonin-deficiency by elevating brain serotonin.

• TYROSINE: a semi-essential amino acid and growth hormone stimulant formed from phenylalanine, tyrosine helps to build the body's natural store of adrenaline and thyroid hormones. It rapidly metabolizes as an antioxidant throughout the body, and is effective as a source of quick energy, especially for the brain. It converts to the amino acid L-Dopa, making it a safe therapy for depression, hypertension, and Parkinson's disease, helps control drug abuse and aids drug withdrawal. It appears to increase libido and low sex drive. It helps reduce appetite and body fat in a weight loss diet. It produces melanin for skin and hair pigment. *Note: Tumors, cancerous melanomas and manic depression are slowed through dietary reduction of tyrosine and phenylalanine.*

UMEBOSHI PLUMS: pickled Japanese apricots with alkalizing, bactericide properties; part of a macrobiotic diet.

• UREA, *carbamide:* used in yeast food and wine production, also to "brown" baked goods such as pretzels. Commercial urea consists of colorless or white odorless crystals that have a cool, salty taste. Widely used as an antiseptic in antiperspirants and deodorants, mouthwashes, shampoos, lotions and other such products.

VANADIUM: a mineral cofactor for several enzymes. Deficiency is linked to heart disease, poor reproductive ability and infant mortality. Good food sources: whole grains, fish, olives, radishes, vegetables.

• **VINEGAR:** brown rice, balsamic, apple cider, herb, raspberry, ume plum — vinegars have been used for 5000 years as healthful flavor enhancers and food preservers. As condiments, like relishes or dressings, they help digest heavy foods and high protein meals. The most nutritious vinegars are not overly filtered, and still contain the "mother" mixture of beneficial bacteria and enzymes in the bottle. They look slightly cloudy.

• **VITAMINS:** organic micro-nutrients that act like spark plugs in the body, keeping it "tuned up" and functioning at high performance. You can't live on vitamins; they are not pep pills, substitutes for food, or components of body structure. They stimulate, but do not act as, nutritional fuel. As catalysts, they work on the cellular level, often as co-enzymes, regulating body metabolic processes through enzyme activity, to convert proteins and carbohydrates to tissue and energy. Most vitamins cannot be synthesized by the body, and must be supplied by food or supplement. Excess amounts are excreted in the urine, or stored by the body until needed.

Even with their minute size and amounts in the body, vitamins are absolutely necessary for growth, vitality, resistance to disease, and healthy aging. It is impossible to sustain life without them. Even small deficiencies can endanger the whole body. Unfortunately, it takes weeks or months for signs of most vitamin deficiencies to appear because the body only slowly uses its supply. Even when your body is "running on empty" in a certain vitamin, problems may be hard to pinpoint, because the cells usually continue to function with decreasing efficiency until they receive proper nourishment or suffer irreversible damage.

Vitamin therapy does not produce results overnight. Vitamins fill nutritional gaps at your body's deepest levels. **Regenerative changes in biochemistry may require as much time to rebuild as they did to decline.** In most cases, after a short period of higher dosage in order to build a good nutrient foundation, a program of moderate amounts over a longer period of time brings about better body balance and more permanent results.

Vitamin RDA's were established by the National Academy in the 1950's as a guideline to prevent severe deficiency diseases. Today, poor dietary habits, over-processed foods, and agri-business practices show health professionals that supplements are needed for adequate nutrition. Even as basic as the RDA recommendations are, not one dietary survey has shown that Americans consume anywhere near the RDA amounts in their normal diets. A recent large USDA survey of the daily food intake of 21,500 people over a three day period showed that not a single person got 100% of the RDA nutrients. Only 3% ate the recommended number of servings from the four food groups. Only 12% got the RDA for protein, calcium, iron, magnesium, zinc or vitamins A, C, B_6, B_{12}, B_2, and B_1. The study concluded that trying to change long-held dietary habits and ignoring vitamin supplements as an option left much of the American population at nutritional risk.

People most affected by vitamin deficiencies include:
　　1: Women with excessive menstrual bleeding who may need iron supplements.
　　2: Pregnant or nursing women who may need extra iron, calcium and folic acid.
　　3: The elderly, many of whom do not even get two-thirds of the RDA for calcium, iron, vitamin A or C. (Note: The elderly take more than 50% of all medication prescriptions in the U.S. Since 90 out of the 100 most prescribed drugs interfere with normal nutrient metabolism, it is a sad fact that many older people don't absorb even very much of the nutrition that they do eat.)
　　4: Everyone on medications that interfere with nutrient absorption, digestion or metabolism.
　　5: People on weight loss diets with extremely low calorie intake.
　　6: People at risk for heart and circulatory blockages, and those at risk for osteoporosis.
　　7: People who have recently had surgery, or suffer from serious injuries, wounds or burns.
　　8: People with periodontal disease.
　　9: Vegetarians, who may not receive enough calcium, iron, zinc or vitamin B_{12}.

Vitamins help us go beyond average health to optimal health. Here's what vitamins do for you:
　　—**VITAMIN A:** is a fat soluble vitamin, requiring fats, minerals (especially zinc) and enzymes for absorp-

tion. Available in both plants and animals, plants contain the beta carotene form while animal sources contain retinol. Vitamin A counteracts night blindness, weak eyesight, and strengthens the optical system. Supplementation lowers risk of many types of cancer. Retinoids inhibit malignant transformation, and reverse pre-malignant changes in tissue. Vitamin A is particularly effective against lung cancer. It is also an anti-infective that builds immune resistance. It helps develop strong bone cells, a major factor in the health of skin, hair, teeth and gums. Deficiency results in eye dryness and the inability to tear, night blindness, rough, itchy skin, poor bone growth, weak tooth enamel, chronic diarrhea and frequent respiratory infections. Vitamin A is critical to adrenal and steroid hormone synthesis, and is a key to preventing premature aging. Good food sources: fish liver oils, seafood, sea greens, dairy foods, yellow fruits and vegetables, dark leafy greens, yams, sweet potatoes, liver, watermelon and canteloupe, and eggs. *Note: Avoid high doses of Vitamin A during pregnancy.*

—**VITAMIN B-1**, *(Thiamine)*: known as the "morale vitamin" because of its beneficial effects on the nerves and mental attitude. Promotes proper growth in children, aids carbohydrate utilization for energy and supports the nervous system. Enhances immune response. Helps control motion sickness. Wards off mosquitos and stinging insects. Pregnancy, lactation, diuretics and oral contraceptives require extra thiamine. Smoking, heavy metal pollutants, excess sugar, junk foods, stress and alcohol all deplete thiamine. Deficiency results in insomnia, fatigue, confusion, poor memory and muscle coordination. Food source thiamine is sensitive to heat and chlorine. Avoid washing or cooking thiamine-rich foods in chlorinated water if you suspect you are thiamine deficient. A high sugar diet or too much alcohol also increases your thiamine needs. Good food sources: asparagus, brewer's yeast, brown rice, beans, nuts, seeds, wheat germ, organ meats and soy foods.

—**VITAMIN B-2**, *(Riboflavin)*: a vitamin commonly deficient in the U.S. diet. Necessary for energy production, and for fat and carbohydrate metabolism. Helps prevent cataracts and corneal ulcers, and generally benefits vision. Promotes healthy skin, especially in cases of psoriasis. Helps protect against drug toxicity and environmental chemicals. Pregnancy and lactation, excess dairy and red meat consumption, prolonged stress, sulfa drugs, diuretics and oral contraceptives all require extra riboflavin. Deficiency is associated with alcohol abuse, anemia, hypothyroidism, diabetes, ulcers, cataracts and congenital heart disease. Good food sources: almonds, brewer's yeast, broccoli, green leafy veggies, eggs, mushrooms, yogurt, organ meats and caviar.

—**VITAMIN B-3**, *(Niacin)*: a vitamin involved with energy production, sex hormone synthesis and good digestion, boosting production of hydrochloric acid in the stomach. Niacin is highly effective in improving joint function, strength and endurance in patients with osteoarthritis. Niacin can lower cholesterol. A study at Wayne State University reveals niacin combined with chromium can lower blood cholesterol by as much as 30%! Niacin promotes healthy skin and nerves, relieves diarrhea and gastrointestinal conditions, migraines and vertigo. Deficiency results in dermatitis, headaches, gum disease, sometimes high blood pressure and schizophrenic behavior. However, because niacin can rapidly open up and stimulate circulation, (a niacin flush is evidence of this), it can act quickly to reverse deficiency disorders. Niacin works with chromium to regulate blood sugar for diabetes and hypoglycemia. Good food sources: almonds, avocados, brewer's yeast, fish, legumes, bananas, whole grains, cheese, eggs and sesame seeds.

—**VITAMIN B-5**, *(Pantothenic Acid)*: an antioxidant vitamin vital to proper adrenal activity, pantothenic acid is a precursor to cortisone production and an aid to natural steroid synthesis. It is important in preventing arthritis and high cholesterol. It fights infection by building antibodies, and defends against stress, fatigue and nerve disorders. It is a key to overcoming postoperative shock and drug side effects after surgery. Pantothenic acid inhibits hair color loss. Deficiency results in anemia, fatigue and muscle cramping. Individuals suffering from constant psychological stress have a heightened need for B$_5$. Good food sources include: brewer's yeast, brown rice, poultry, yams, organ meats, egg yolks, soy products and royal jelly.

—**VITAMIN B-6**, *(Pyridoxine)*: a key vitamin in red blood cell regeneration, and protein metabolism, and carbohydrate use. A primary immune stimulant with particular effectiveness against liver cancer. Supplementation inhibits histamine release in treating allergies and asthma. Supports all aspects of nerve health including neuropsychiatric disorders, epilepsy and carpal tunnel syndrome. Works as a natural diuretic, especially in premenstrual edema. Controls acne, promotes beautiful skin, relieves morning sickness and is an anti-aging factor. Protects against environmental pollutants, smoking and stress. Oral contraceptives, thiazide diuretics, penicillin and alcohol deplete B-6. Deficiency results in anemia, depression, lethargy, nervousness, water retention and skin lesions. Good food sources: bananas, brewer's yeast, buckwheat, organ meats, fish, avocados, legumes, poultry, nuts, rice bran, brown rice, wheat bran, sunflower seeds and soy foods.

—**VITAMIN B-12,** (*Cyano Cobalamin*): an anti-inflammatory analgesic that works with calcium for absorption. Critical to DNA synthesis and red blood cell formation; involved in all immune responses. A specific for sulfite-induced asthma. New research shows some success in cancer management, especially in tumor growth. Energizes, relieves depression, hangover and poor concentration. Supplied largely from animal foods, B-12 may be deficient for vegetarians, and a deficiency can take five or more years to appear after body stores are depleted. Deficiency results in anemia, nerve degeneration, dizziness, heart palpitations and excess weight loss. Long use of cholesterol drugs, oral contraceptives, anti-inflammatory and anti-convulsant drugs deplete B-12. Good food sources: cheese, poultry, sea greens, yogurt, eggs, organ meats, brewer's yeast and fish.

—**VITAMIN C,** (*Ascorbic Acid*): a primary factor in immune strength and health. Protects against cancer, viral and bacterial infections, heart disease, arthritis and allergies. It is a strong antioxidant against free radical damage. Safeguards against radiation poisoning, heavy metal toxicity, environmental pollutants and early aging. Accelerates healing after surgery, increases infection resistance, and is essential to formation of new collagen tissue. Vitamin C controls alcohol craving, lowers cholesterol, and is a key factor in treating diabetes, high blood pressure, male infertility, and in suppressing the HIV virus. Supports adrenal and iron insufficiency, especially when the body is under stress. Relieves withdrawal symptoms from addictive drugs, tranquilizers and alcohol. Aspirin, oral contraceptives, smoking and tetracycline inhibit vitamin C absorption and deplete C levels. Deficiency results in easy bruising, receding gums, slow healing, fatigue and rough skin.
—**Ester C™,** a metabolite form of vitamin C, is biochemically the same as naturally metabolized C in the body. It is both fat and water soluble, and non-acid. Ester C is absorbed twice as fast into the bloodstream and excreted twice as slowly as ordinary vitamin C. Good food sources: citrus fruits, green peppers, papaya, tomatoes, kiwi, potatoes, greens, cauliflower and broccoli.

—**VITAMIN D:** a critical fat soluble vitamin, D works with vitamin A to utilize calcium and phosphorus in building bones and teeth. Although we call it a vitamin, D is really a hormone produced in the skin from sunlight. Cholesterol compounds in the skin convert to a vitamin D precursor when exposed to UV radiation. Twenty minutes a day of early morning sunshine make a real difference to your body's vitamin D stores, especially if you are at risk for osteoporosis. Vitamin D helps in all eye problems including spots, conjunctivitis and glaucoma. Helps protect against colon cancer. Deficiency results in nearsightedness, psoriasis, soft teeth, muscle cramps and tics, slow healing, insomnia, nosebleeds, fast heartbeat and arthritis. Good food sources: cod liver oil, yogurt, cheese, butter, herring, halibut, salmon, tuna, eggs and liver.

—**VITAMIN E:** a fat soluble antioxidant and important immune stimulating vitamin. An effective anticoagulant and vasodilator against blood clots and heart disease. Retards cellular and mental aging, alleviates fatigue and provides tissue oxygen to accelerate healing of wounds and burns. Works with selenium against the effects of aging and cancer by neutralizing free radicals. Beneficial for chronic, so-called incurable diseases like arthritis, lupus, Parkinson's disease and MS. Improves skin tone and texture; helps control alopecia and dandruff. Deficiency results in muscle and nerve degeneration, anemia, skin pigmentation. Good food sources: almonds, leafy vegetables, seafoods and sea greens, soy, wheat germ, wheat germ oil and organ meats.

—**VITAMIN K:** a fat soluble vitamin necessary for blood clotting and may be taken as a guard against too-easy bleeding. Vitamin K is easy to get from the normal diet and is stored in the body. Deficiency occurs from poor nutrient absorption, from conditions like celiac disease, intestinal worms or chronic colitis. Antibiotic overload contributes to many cases of vitamin K deficiency because these drugs deplete and destroy friendly intestinal flora. Vitamin K reduces excessive menstruation, helps heal broken blood vessels in the eye, aids in arresting bone loss and post-menopausal brittle bones. Vitamin K is an integral part of liver function and is a good source of help for cirrhosis and jaundice of the liver. Good food sources: seafoods, sea greens, dark leafy vegetables, liver, molasses, eggs, oats, crucifers and sprouts.

WHEAT GERM and WHEAT GERM OIL: wheat germ is the embryo of the wheat berry — rich in B vitamins, proteins and iron. It goes rancid quickly. Buy only in nitrogen-flushed packaging. Wheat germ oil is a good vitamin E source and body oxygenator. One tablespoon provides the anti-oxidant equivalent of an oxygen tent for 30 minutes.

• **WHEAT GRASS:** See GREEN SUPERFOODS, page 136.

ZINC: a mineral that acts as a co-factor of SOD to protect against free radical damage, is essential to the formation of insulin, immune strength, gland, sexual and reproductive health. Helps prevent birth defects, enhances sensory perception, accelerates healing. Zinc is a brain food that helps control mental disorders and promotes mental alertness. A high stress lifestyle depletes zinc, impairing immune response and the ability to heal. People who get little sleep, work a 16-hour day (or more than one job), or those recovering from injury need to increase zinc levels in their diet. The picolinate form is highly absorbable. Good food sources: crab, herring, liver, lobster, oysters, turkey, poppy, sunflower, pumpkin and caraway seeds, brewer's yeast, eggs, mushrooms and wheat germ.

Illness is a form of searching.

Health is the manifestation of inner peace.

Food & Diet Choices That Affect Healing

Clearly, your diet is the basis for good health and optimum healing.

Recent research on nutraceuticals and phytonutrients in our foods shows a wealth of evidence to support the fact that our diets can heal as well as nourish us.

Diet improvement is a major weapon against disease, from the common cold to cancer. Whole food nutrition allows the body to use its built-in restorative and repairing abilities. A healthy diet can intervene in the disease process at many stages, from its inception to its growth and spread.

However, foods aren't equal in their healing abilities, and certain foods don't contribute to healing activity at all. This section can help you sort out the facts about foods, especially the foods and food categories that are making news today.

Diet options that affect the healing process:

—**Fruits, vegetables, and chlorophyll for plant enzyme therapy**
—**Is a vegetarian diet better? What's the truth about red meat?**
—**Protein: how much do you need for healing?**
—**Green superfoods and healing mushrooms for faster healing**
—**Macrobiotics for serious healing: balancing your body chemistry**
—**Soy foods and cultured foods for probiotics**
—**Water is essential for healing**
—**Caffeine in a healing diet? What about green and black teas?**
—**Does wine fit into a healing program?**
—**Fats and oils: there's good news and bad news**
—**Dairy foods in a healing diet? Are butter and eggs okay?**
—**Sugar and sweeteners: are they all bad?**
—**Low salt or no salt?**
—**Sea greens and iodine therapy**
—**Powerhouses of the desert: bee nutrients, jojoba, aloe vera**

Fresh Fruits, Vegetables & Juices

Fruits and vegetables top the list of healing foods! Massive research is validating what natural healers have known for decades. The more fruits and vegetables you eat, the more nutrition you get and the less your risk of disease.

Fresh fruits and vegetables do what natural healers do best..... work with your body so it can use its built-in restorative abilities. Even if your genetics and lifestyle are against you, your diet still makes a tremendous difference in your health and healing odds. Fresh fruits and vegetables accelerate body cleansing, and help normalize body chemistry. I emphasize a detoxification fresh juice diet as part of almost every healing program.

Fruits and vegetables are full of nutraceuticals, the natural chemicals in plants with pharmacologic action. Scientists are enthusiastically embracing the healing possibilities of plant nutrients in fresh foods. Green leafy vegetables, for example, have almost 20 times more essential nutrients, ounce for ounce than any other food. What's more, the nutrients in greens make the nutrients in other foods work better for our health.

The preventive medicine possibilities are astounding. Studies show that people who eat plenty of vegetables have half the cancer risk of people who eat few vegetables. Even moderate amounts of vegetables make a big difference. For instance, eating fresh vegetables twice a day, instead of twice a week, cuts the risk of lung cancer by 75%, even for smokers. One National Cancer Institute spokesman said it is almost most mind-boggling that common foods can be so effective against a potent carcinogen like tobacco!

There's more. Certain body chemicals must be "activated" before they can initiate cancer cell growth. Fresh foods can block the activation process, because food chemicals in cells can determine whether a cancer-causing virus, or a cancer promoter like excess estrogen, will turn tissue cancerous.

Fruits and vegetables may intervene even if you already have cancer. When cells mass into tumors, food compounds in cruciferous vegetables can restrain further growth by flushing certain carcinogens from the body or shrinking patches of precancerous cells. Antioxidant foods can snuff out carcinogens, nip free radical cascades in the bud, even repair some cellular damage.

Although less powerful at later stages, good foods can help prolong your life even after cancer takes hold. Fresh foods foster a healthy environment that deters wandering cancer cells from attaching to unhealthy tissues. The evidence is so overwhelming that researchers are starting to view fruits and vegetables as powerful preventative that might wipe out cancer — an about-face for cancer study!

Fresh fruits are Nature's smiles.

Fruits are wonderful for a quick system wash and cleanse. Their natural water and sugar content speeds up metabolism to release wastes rapidly. Fresh fruit has an alkalizing effect in the body. Its easily convertible natural sugars transform to give us quick energy and speed up the calorie burning process.

But these advantages are only true of fresh fruits. The way that you eat fruit is as important as what fruit you eat. Fruits have their best healing and nutrition effects when eaten alone or with other fruits, as in a fruit salad, separately from grains and vegetables. With a few exceptions, both fruits and fruit juices should be taken before noon for best energy conversion and cleansing benefits.

Cooking fruits changes their properties from alkalizing to acid-forming in the body. This is also true of sulphured, dried fruit, and combining fruits with vegetables or grains. When you eat fruit in any of these ways, digestion slows down because the fruits stay too long in the stomach; gas forms, because the fruit sugars become concentrated, resulting in fermentation instead of assimilation.

New studies on fruits show more amazing benefits. Citrus fruits possess fifty-eight known anti-cancer compounds, more than any other food! Some researchers call citrus fruits a total anti-cancer package because they have every class of nutrient — carotenoids, flavonoids, terpenes, limonoids, coumarins, and more — known to neutralize chemical carcinogens. **Yet, citrus fruits act more powerfully as a whole than any of the separate anti-cancer compounds they contain.** One phytochemical, for example, in oranges, is the potent antioxidant glutathione, a confirmed disease combatant. Commercially processed orange juice, unlike whole oranges, lose its glutathione concentration. Oranges are also rich in beta-carotene and vitamin C, and the highest food in glucarate, a powerful cancer-inhibitor.

Eat organically grown fruits whenever possible. The pesticides from sprayed fruits can enter your body very rapidly because of quick fruit sugar metabolism.

Fresh vegetables are Nature's superfoods.

The healing power of vegetables works both raw and lightly cooked. It is not always true that raw vegetables are better. Some fragile anti-cancer agents, like indoles and vitamin C, are destroyed by heat, but a little heat makes beta-carotene more easily absorbed. The action of lightly cooked vegetables is gentler, especially if your digestion is impaired.

What is a serving of fresh fruits or vegetables? One serving is about $1/2$ cup of cooked, chopped veggies; 1 cup of raw leafy vegetables; 1 medium piece of fruit, or 6-oz. of fruit or vegetable juice. Only 10 percent of Americans eat that much every day.

Here's a short recap of the astounding new studies which show that the same phytochemicals that protect plants from pests and disease may also protect our bodies from cancers and heart disease.
See my new book, FOOD IS YOUR PHARMACY for all the details on these studies.

1: Organic sulphur compounds, like the allylic sulfides in garlic and onions contain more than 30 different anti-carcinogens — like quercetin and ajoene that can block the most feared cancer-causing agents like nitrosamines and aflatoxin, linked specifically to stomach, lung and liver cancer. Ajoene in garlic is three times as toxic to malignant cells as to normal cells. Interleukin in garlic boosts macrophages and T-lymphocytes, your immune agents responsible for destroying tumor cells.
—**Allylic sulfides** in garlic also provide cardiovascular protection. Garlic suppresses cholesterol synthesis in the liver, lowering serum cholesterol by reducing LDL cholesterol, but maintaining good high density lipoproteins at normal levels. Garlic may even reverse arterial blockages caused by atherosclerosis.
—**Sulforaphane,** a sulphur compound in cruciferous vegetables, mustard and horseradish, induces protective phase II enzymes, which detoxifiy carcinogens. Sulforaphane delays onset of cancer, and inhibits the size and numbers of tumors.

2: Antioxidants in foods like wheat germ, soy, yellow and green vegetables, green tea, citrus fruits and olive oil help normalize pre-cancerous cells, by snuffing out carcinogens and nipping free radical cascades in the bud.
—**Allylic sulfides** (see above) are also powerful antioxidants, defending cells against damage by oxidizing toxins. Allylic sulfides in garlic and onions inhibit the growth of a wide spectrum of bacteria and viruses, including staphyloccus, streptoccocus and salmonella. Garlic particularly fights funguses and parasites, making it a specific for candida albicans yeast overgrowth and HIV related conditions.
—**Green leafy vegetables** exhibit extraordinary broad cancer protective powers, largely because they are so rich in antioxidants. Alpha, beta and other carotenes, folic acid and zeaxanthin in greens offer potent cancer protection. (Lutein, a little known antioxidant, is **more** potent than beta-carotene against cancer.) The darker green the vegetables, the more cancer-inhibiting carotenoids they have. I recommend a green salad every day!

3: Organic acids, metabolic compounds with significant antioxidants and far reaching anti-cancer effects.

—**Phytic acid,** an antioxidant compound from rye, wheat, rice, lima beans, sesame seeds, peanuts and soybeans, appears to prevent colon cancer and enhance immune killer cell activity. It may be a better antioxidant than vitamin C, because it naturally chelates both iron and zinc to help prevent heart disease.

—**Folic acid,** a B vitamin in wheat, wheat germ, leafy vegetables, beets, asparagus, fish, sunflower seeds, and citrus fruits is critical to normal DNA synthesis — so healthy cells stay healthy. Folic acid reduces the risk of two birth defects, lowers the risk of atherosclerosis and, potentially, cancer. Folic acid is also seen as a weapon against heart disease because it reduces homocysteine levels.

Note: While folic acid is seen as a cancer protector after menopause, excess folate can be tumor promoting. The key is getting plenty of folic acid from your food instead of just taking supplements. For example, people who eat lots of leafy greens have a low incidence of lung cancer. People who merely take folic acid supplements but do not eat leafy greens still lack protective folic acid in their lungs.

—**Vitamin C,** an antioxidant from citrus fruits, cherries, tomatoes, green peppers, strawberries, leafy greens, hot red peppers and broccoli, reduces both LDL cholesterol and triglyceride levels. Vitamin C's antioxidants also promote wound healing and boost interferon for immune response and T-cell production. Antioxidants in C, E and carotenoids lower the common cataract risk of oxidative stressors like ultraviolet light. Vitamin C also improves blood sugar levels in non-insulin dependent diabetics. Some scientists believe that America's high rates of asthma are a result of a marked decrease in vitamin C antioxidants.

4: Bioflavonoids, initially called vitamin P (for their rapid permeability), are a significant part of the vitamin C complex for healing. Biolfavs help vitamin C keep your collagen (the boy's intercellular "cement") healthy. Bioflavonoids strengthen capillaries, connective tissue and blood vessel walls to reduce hemorrhages and ruptures which lead to spider and varicose veins and bruise marks. The first signs of deficiency in vitamin C and bioflavonoids is a tendency to bruise easily, varicose veins, or noticeable purplish spots on the skin. Find bioflavs in the skins and pulp of citrus fruits, grapes, cherries and many berries. Good herb sources: buckwheat greens, peppers, yellow dock, elder, hawthorn, horsetail, rosehips, shepherd's purse, sea plants and nettles.

Here are some of the benefits bioflavonoids have for you:
• bioflavs help build a protective antibiotic barrier against infections and boost immune response
• bioflavs have potent anti-inflammatory action without the side effects of aspirin
• bioflavs help prevent allergies and asthma
• bioflavs reduce excessive internal bleeding, and promote healing of cuts and bruises
• bioflavs help detoxify carcinogenic chemicals, radiation and heavy metals
• bioflavs assist in preventing cardiovascular disease
• bioflavs act much like estrogens to curtail menopausal symptoms
• bioflavs help prevent cataracts and macular degeneration

5: Genistein, a flavonoid in soy and cruciferous vegetables like broccoli, impedes angiogenesis (the growth of blood vessels that feed tumors), and deters cancer cell development by inhibiting enzymes that promote tumor formation. New tests on genistein from soy show that it promotes the positive effects of estrogen while preventing many of estrogen's bad effects, especially hormone-driven cancers like breast and ovarian cancers.

6: Quercetin, a flavonoid in garlic, dark berries and superfoods like chlorella, is one of the strongest anti-cancer food agents known. Quercetin blocks cell changes that initiate cancer, and stops malignant cells from clumping together to become tumors. An antioxidant, quercetin inhibits free radicals to prevent them from oxidizing LDL cholesterol. Quercetin also controls sticky blood, a risk factor for arteriosclerosis and coronary atery disease, by preventing platelet build-up and removing excess iron in the blood. Quercetin is one of Nature's most powerful protectors against allergy attacks. It is a powerful natural antihistamine and anti-inflammatory. Quercetin works best when a healing base is allowed to build up in the body.

7: Carotenoids, found mainly in fruits, vegetables and sea plants, are critical to your successful healing program. Carotenoids are present in virtually every cell of the human body. Most of us have heard of beta-carotene, but there are over 600 other carotenoids, some even more important in decreasing degenerative disease and boosting immune response. New studies on carotenes like alpha-carotene, lycopene, lutein, zeaxanthin, and beta-cryptozanthin show a 3 to 1 reduction in strokes and other heart risks when they're added to your diet.

Some of the newest healing benefits attributed to carotenes:
- Cataracts — eating less than 3 servings of carotene-rich foods increases risk of cataracts.
- Immune system — carotenes enhance both infection-fighting functions and immunity against tumors.
- Heart disease — drops almost 50% in men who take beta-carotene every other day for five years.

Note: Carotenes are most effective when working together as they do in nature. Different body organs selectively store different carotenoids depending on need. There is mounting evidence that high doses of one carotenoid can result in depressed levels of other carotenoids. Too much supplementation of any one carotene may reduce the protective level of other carotenes.

—**Lycopene,** a carotene in tomatoes, red grapefruit, apricots and watermelon protects plants from the harmful effects of UV rays. It protects the human body in the same way. Lycopene, the body's most common carotene, is concentrated in the prostate gland and is used successfully as a preventative for prostate cancer. Lycopene also protects against cancer of the mouth, lung, stomach, pancreas, bladder, colon and rectum. Lycopene is 56% more powerful than beta-carotene and 100 times more efficient than vitamin E as a free radical scavenger. Lycopene is fat-soluble, so when lycopene-rich tomatoes are cooked with oil, as in spaghetti sauce, their bio-availability improves.

—**Lutein** is the most abundant carotenoid in fruits and vegetables, especially dark leafy greens like spinach, kale and broccoli, and in egg whites. Lutein and zeaxanthin are potent antioxidants, especially concentrated in the macula of the eye, responsible for detailed vision. The macula is covered by a layer of two carotenes, lutein and zeaxanthin, natural sunscreens which selectively filter out visible blue light. If blue light is allowed to reach the retina, it can cause photodamage that contributes, over time, to degeneration of the macula. Lutein and zeaxanthin help protect against retinal damage and strengthen blood vessels that supply the macular region.

—**Beta carotene,** in red, yellow and dark green vegetables and fruits, and sea plants, protects against cancer, heart disease, cataracts, enhances immune response and lowers cholesterol. Beta carotene reduces tumor cell proliferation and free radical activity in the tumor. Even after they form, studies show tumors exposed to beta carotene are substantially smaller than tumors not exposed. Harvard studies say that beta carotene acts like a chemotherapy agent on squamous carcinoma tumor cells. Tufts University studies show that beta carotene changes into a subtance called retinoic acid which can treat bladder cancer with considerable success.

—**Alpha carotene,** found in apricots, carrots, peaches and sweet potatoes, is 30% more powerful than beta carotene in preventing cancer. Alpha carotene studies show it especially inhibits tumor growth.

—**Canthaxanthin,** a carotene in mushrooms which can decrease skin cancer risk and boost immunity.

8: Plant polyphenols are a form of bioflavonoids. Active polyphenols appear in grapes, pomegranates, raspberries, huckleberries, strawberries and green tea. Some experts believe that polyphenols in the famous "Grape Cure" for cancer in the early 1900's were factors in its success. Polyphenols inhibit the growth of cancerous tumors, and lower the risk of heart attack by decreasing the likelihood of blood clots and cholesterol plaques.

–**Catechin,** the most abundant plant polyphenol breaks up free radical cell chains of fats, prevents DNA damage, helps block carcinogens, protect against digestive and respiratory infections.

–**Green tea catechins** show excellent antioxidant effects on fatty foods. Antioxidant properties of green tea catechins are 30 times more powerful than vitamin E and 50 times more potent than this in vitamin C.

Note: Don't miss these benefits from Green Tea, page 154.

9: Ellagic acid, a phenol found in walnuts, berries, grapes, apples, tea and pomegranates is an antimutagen against nictoine-induced lung tumors, an anticarcinogen for skin tumors and for chemically-induced cancers.

10: Saponins are abundant steroids in plants like beans, spinach, tomatoes, potatoes, oats, and alfalfa and sea foods. They are significant in many herbs, like panax ginseng and licorice root. Ginseng saponins lower cholesterol by binding to cholesterol in the gastrointestinal tract. Saponins fight infections by forming disease-specific antibodies. They effectively ward off microbial and fungal infections, even viruses. Saponins biochemically stimulate the immune system to help the body protect itself from cancerous growths.

11: Glycyrrhizin, a hormone-like saponin in licorice root, is effective for normalizing menopausal hormone levels. It appears to deter hormone-driven tumors (like those of breast cancer) by its action as a natural estrogen blocker. Glycyrrhizin has anti-viral properties — for example, it is able to slow progression of the HIV virus by inhibiting cell infection and inducing interferon activity for immune response. Glycyrrhizin encourages production of hydrocortisone for anti-inflammatory acitvity. Like cortisone, but without the side effects, it relieves arthritic and allergy symptoms, including those that accompany candida albicans yeast infections.

12: Indoles, like indole-3 carbinole from broccoli, cabbage, radishes, turnip or mustard greens are natural antioxidants with tumor preventing activity. Indole-3-carbinole also prevents cancer in two other amazing ways:
　　–Indoles improve the enzyme pathways through which our bodies get rid of cancer-causing agents. Indole-3-carbinole changes the metabolism of carcinogenic toxins by producing phase 1 and phase 2 detoxification enzymes. The enzymes make toxins water soluble. But since oil and water don't mix, water soluble toxins can be stored in fatty body tissues. Your body can rid itself of them more easily, reducing the risk of cancer. The same detox enzymes also lessen the ability of certain carcinogenic materials to bind with DNA. When the material cannot attach to DNA, cancer can't get started. In one of Nature's miracle pathways, the by-products formed when indole-3-carbinole reacts with stomach acids are more bioactive than indole-3-carbinole itself. The by-products even help clear the body of bad cholesterol.
　　–Indoles improve estrogen metabolism and our ability to eliminate excess estrogens, especially from exogenous estrogen sources like pesticides and synthetic hormones. Women who eat plenty of vegetables containing indole-3-carbinole lower their risk of breast cancer. Men who eat plenty of vegetables containing indole-3-carbinole have a substantially lower risk of colon cancer compared to men who eat little or none.
　　–Indoles also alleviate some symptoms of fibromyalgia and related chronic fatigue syndrome.

13: Isoprenoids are fat soluble antioxidants that neutralize free radicals by anchoring themselves to fatty membranes. They quickly grab free radicals that attach to the membranes and pass them to other antioxidants.
　　–Vitamin E, from almonds, wheat germ, wheat germ oil, leafy veggies, salmon, soy foods, and organ meats, is an antioxidant isoprenoid. There's a clear correlation between vitamin E, a lower risk of heart disease and Alzheimer's, and better body balance for women during menopause or menstrual difficulties. I believe the best vitamin E comes from dietary sources — foods and herbs. Many doctors say synthetic vitamin E may increase hemorrhaging during surgery; they don't recommend it for a pre-op or post-op nutritional program. I have found this not to be a problem for dietary vitamin E, which is safe before and after surgery.
　　–CoQ-10, an isoprenoid also known as ubiquinione or uniquinol, is available mainly through protein sources like fish, meats, sea vegetables and some of the green superfoods. CoQ-10 is an extremely important antioxidant enzyme that does a lot more than just protect us from free radical damage. It actually targets particular diseases with its powerful brand of enzyme therapy. CoQ-10 is highly successful against gum disease, ulcers and is even effective against some AIDS related diseases. It strengthens your cardiovascular system against coronary atery disease, especially if you've had a previous heart attacks. It helps lower high cholesterol levels and high blood pressure. It helps overcome fatigue. It reduces the risk of breast and prostate cancers; I have seen myself that it can even reduce the rate of tumor growth once the cancer has begun.
　　Note: for more about CoQ-10, see Enzymes & Enzyme Therapy, page 128.

Chlorophyll is a key to Healing from Green Vegetables

Green foods are power plants for humans. Our body chemistry comes from plant nutrients because plant chlorophyll (one of the most powerful nutrients on Earth) transmits the energies of the sun and the soil to our bodies. The sun is the energy source of the Earth — plants constitute the most direct method of conserving the energy we receive from the sun. Fruits, vegetables, grains and grasses reach out to us on branches and stems, making themselves beautiful and nourishing to attract us. Plants have no fear of being eaten as animals do. The life energy of plants simply transmutes into higher life form of mankind.

Chlorophyll offers amazing healing benefits for humans. The most therapeutic ingredient in green foods is chlorophyll, the basic component of the "blood" of plants. Chlorophyll is the pigment that plants use to carry out photosynthesis - absorbing the light energy from the sun, and converting it into plant energy. This energy is transferred into our cells and blood when we consume fresh greens. Chlorophyll is in all green plants, but is particularly rich in green and blue-green algae, wheat grass, parsley, and alfalfa.

Our blood has a unique affinity to chlorophyll. The chlorophyll molecule is remarkably similar to human hemoglobin in composition, except that it carries magnesium in its center instead of iron. Eating chlorophyll-rich foods helps our bodies build oxygen-carrying red blood cells. To me, eating green foods is almost like giving yourself a little transfusion to help treat illness and enhance immunity.

–Chlorophyll is a better tonic than Geritol for tired blood. It calms the nerves, so it's helpful for insomnia, exhaustion and nervous irritability. It's beneficial for skin disorders, helps you cope with deep infections, and dental problems like pyorrhea. Its anti-bacterial qualities are a proven remedy for colds, ear infections and chest inflammation.

–Chlorophyll detoxes your liver. It helps neutralize and remove drug deposits, and purifies the blood. Even the medical community sees chlorophyll as a means of removing heavy metal buildup, because it can bind with heavy metals to help remove them. A new U.S. Army study reveals that a chlorophyll-rich diet doubles the lifespan of animals exposed to radiation. Since the days of Agent Orange and Gulf War Syndrome, chlorophyll is even being considered as protection against some chemical warfare weapons.

–Chlorophyll is rich in vitamin K, necessary for blood clotting. Naturopathic physicians use chlorophyll for women with heavy menstrual bleeding and anemia. Vitamin K helps form a compound in urine that inhibits growth of calcium oxalate crystals, so chlorophyll helps with kidney stones. Vitamin K also enhances adrenal activity, so chlorophyll-rich foods help maintain steroid balance for a more youthful body.

Tucked away in a quiet corner of every life are wounds and scars.

If they were not there, we would not need Healers.

Nor would we need one another.

Plant Enzymes Offer Built-In Enzyme Therapy

Enzymes are the cornerstones of healing because they are the foundation elements of the immune system, providing active antioxidants that fight free-radical destruction.

Enzymes operate on both chemical and biological levels. Chemically, they are the workhorses that drive metabolism to use the nutrients we take in. Biologically, they are our life energy. Without enzyme energy, we would be a pile of lifeless chemicals.

Each of us is born with a battery charge of enzyme energy at birth. As we age our internal enzyme stores are naturally depleted. A new study shows that a 60 year old has 50% fewer enzymes than a 30 year old. Enzyme depletion, lack of energy, disease and aging all go hand in hand. Unless we stop the one-way-flow out of the body of enzyme energy, our digestive-eliminative capacities weaken, obesity and chronic illness set in, lifespan shortens. The faster you use up your enzyme supply —the shorter your life.

There are three categories of enzymes:

1: Metabolic enzymes repair cells and stimulate enzymatic activity. Metabolic enzymes like proteases help us heal faster by repressing inflammation and breaking up debris in the injury area. They stimulate without repressing immune response (unlike cortisone or hydrocortisone drugs).

Note: If you take enzyme supplements between meals without food, they absorb directly into your body and function as metabolic enzymes in the repair and healing process.

2: Human digestive enzymes assimilate our food nutrients. Digestive enzymes are stronger than any other enzymes in human beings and more concentrated than any other enzyme combination in nature. A very good thing, since our processed, over cooked, nutrient-poor diets demand a great deal of enzymatic work!

3: Fresh plant enzymes start food digestion, and aid our own digestive enzymes. All foods contain the enzymes required to digest them. The best food sources of plant enzymes for humans are bananas, mangos, sprouts, papayas, avocados and pineapples.

There are three interesting facts about food enzymes:

—All food, whether plant or animal, has its own enzymes that serve it in life. When eaten, these become the property of the eater, are now its food enzymes, and begin immediately to work for the eater's digestive benefit.

—All animals have the proteolytic enzyme, cathepsin, which comes into play after death, and becomes the prime factor for autolysis. In other words, the food helps its own breakdown for the good of the eater.

—Only enzymes from whole foods give the body what it needs to work properly. Our bodies cannot independently absorb food; we must have the help of the food itself.

How does enzyme therapy work to heal? Enzyme therapy uses metabolic enzymes to stimulate immune response. The link between enzymes and immunity comes from lymphocytes, or white blood cells which circulate through the body to attack foreign invader cells. When toxins are detected, white blood cells attack them by secreting enzymes on their surfaces. Some diseases, like cancer, leukemia, anemia and heart disease can even be diagnosed by measuring the amount and activity of certain enzymes in the blood and body fluids.

Some enzymes clean wounds, dissolve blood clots, and control allergic reactions to drugs. Proteolytic enzymes (proteases) are used as anti-inflammatories to reduce swelling and pain. Enzyme therapy allows respiratory vessels to unclog, helps degenerative diseases like heart disease, regulates blood sugar, and relieves stomach and colon pain. Bromelain from pineapples is a good example of a rapid recovery enzyme for these things.

Do you have enough enzymes? The first signs of enzyme deficiency are fatigue, premature aging and weight gain. Most nutrient deficiency problems as we age result not from the lack of the nutrients themselves, but from our lack of enzymes to absorb them.

Nature has designed an interlocking digestive program for us. When our foods don't have enough enzymes for us to digest them, reserve enzymes for metabolic processes get pulled from their normal work to digest food. The pancreas and liver have to use their enzyme stores, too. But these substitute measures don't make up for the missing food enzymes because we need those enzymes to break down and actually deliver the nutrients.

Low enzymes mean we end up with undigested food in our blood. So, white blood cell immune defenses are pulled from their jobs to take care of the undigested food, and the immune system takes a dive. It's a perfect envionment for disease.

Enzyme rich foods take care of this unhealthy cascade of reactions before it ever starts. Fresh foods have the most plant enzymes. As you increase your fresh foods, your enzymatic activity also increases. If you don't get enough fresh foods, or you need extra enzyme concentration for healing, plant-based enzyme supplements are the next best choice, especially from herbs and superfoods. If you can't make them, take them.

Can we maximize daily enzyme benefits?
Enzymes are extremely sensitive to heat. Heat above 120° F. completely destroys them. Even low degrees of heat can greatly reduce your digestive ability. Enzymes are also affected by tobacco, alcohol, caffeine, fluorides, chlorine in drinking water, air pollution, chemical additives and many drugs. Enzyme protection and enzyme therapy are dramatically reduced by the use of a microwave oven.

What about Co-enzyme Q-10?

Co-enzymes work as catalysts in biochemical reactions. I call CoQ-10 the "holistic enzyme" because it's found in every body cell, especially the heart, brain, liver and kidneys. All living foods contain a form of Co-enzyme Q-1 to Q-10.

CoQ-10 is one of the most powerful antioxidants known. It has a long history of boosting immune response and cardiac strength, reversing high blood pressure, promoting weight loss, slowing aging, and healing gum disease. Specific enzyme therapy treatments of CoQ-10 include: congestive heart failure, angina, ischemic heart disease, cardiomyopathy, mitral valve prolapse, diabetes, tumors and candida albicans. CoQ-10 can alleviate toxic effects of drugs commonly used to treat cancer and hypertension.

Like other anti-oxidant co-enzymes like glutathione peroxidase, and superoxide dismutase, (SOD) for example, CoQ-10 scavenges and neutralizes free radicals by turning them into stable oxygen and H_2O_2, and then into oxygen and water.

How much CoQ-10 should you take? As little as 30 mg a day of CoQ-10 is an effective dose. Some cancer patients take up to 400mg a day. CoQ-10 is a fat soluble nutrient, so your body assimilates it better if taken in conjunction with fatty acids like Omega-3 oils or evening primrose oil. CoQ-10 is only effective as long as it is taken; once discontinued, the illness can return. This is especially true in cancer treatment. After 35, the age at which people begin to notice a decline in their energy levels, the ability to synthesize CoQ-10 declines. Take CoQ-10 for one to three months to saturate deficient tissues.

What reduces healthy CoQ10 levels? An overactive thyroid, aging, some cholesterol lowering drugs, some antidepressants and beta blockers deplete CoQ10.

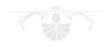

Is a Vegetarian Diet Better?

Vegetarian eating is seen today as a practice of enlightenment, of increased understanding of responsibility for mankind's place on the Earth, perhaps even of higher consciousness.

As we try to explain the horrors on our daily news, we start to shrink from every kind of violence. Killing of any kind doesn't seem right. It is reserved for our "enemies." But who, as our world grows smaller, and we see people everywhere just like us in distress, is our enemy? Certainly not the Earth's animals. Our views of our ancient ancestors is changing as our view of ourselves changes, too. The stereotype of early humans as "Man the hunter" is more accurately seen as "Man the gatherer."

Today's vegetarian culture is not the first. Vegetarianism was widely practiced by the ancient Greeks and Romans. But, the fall of Rome led to a "dark ages" in vegetarian thought as it did in the arts. Scientific rationale dominated western thought. Animals were killed, eaten, and exploited under the argument that animals were placed on earth for the convenience and use of humans. Vegetarianism was not practiced by the general populace for over 1500 years. The Christian abbeys of the time, however, kept vegetarian diet principles alive.

Then Darwin's theory of evolution challenged the philosophical justification for eating animals. He believed that both humans and animals were part of a continuum of life, only separated in degree, not in kind. His work began the vegetarian "renaissance" of the late 18th and 19th centuries.

What is a vegetarian? It's a legitimate question. When we try to apply the different social foundations and ideas from around the world to vegetarianism, an easy definition becomes incredibly confusing if not impossible. Food and diet are inextricably intertwined in both the religion and culture to which they belong. Different kinds of foods are seen differently by different peoples.

Here are some ways vegetarians are classified today.
- Semi vegetarian: eats poultry, fish, eggs and dairy foods, but not red meats or pork
- Pesco vegetarian: eats fish, eggs and dairy foods, but not poultry, red meats or pork
- Lacto ovo vegetarian: eats eggs and dairy foods, but no animal food that "has eyes"
- Ovo vegetarian: eats eggs, but no other animal food product
- Vegan: excludes all animal derived foods

What are the benefits of a vegetarian diet? Becoming a vegetarian affects both body and mind. As their diet changes, people find their point of view about life changes. Nutrition awareness and knowledge increases. Most vegetarians support a "green" lifestyle as their consciousness of the planet heightens.

–A vegetarian diet is low in fat, so it's heart smart. Vegetarians have a well documented history of lower risk for high blood pressure, heartburn, obesity, diabetes, osteoporosis and several types of cancer.
–Vegetarians are energetic. Energy comes from carbohydrates and fats from grains, legumes, fruits and vegetables. Energy also comes from vitamins, minerals and amino acids, plentiful in plant foods.
–Vegetarians report better body balance, especially in terms of protein intake. Vegetable protein abounds in grains, legumes like beans and lentils, potatoes, green vegetables, nuts and seeds, pasta and corn.
–Vegetarians are better hydrated from the high water content of fresh foods.
–Being a vegetarian is easier on your pocket book that a meat-based diet.

Does it take long to become a vegetarian if you've been a lifelong meat-eater? Transition time varies widely. Only 30% of newly converted vegetarians stop eating meat immediately; 70% eliminate meat from their diets over months or even years. Make the transition a new adventure in eating. Vegetarian cuisine is incredibly diverse and interesting. Get a new cookbook or two and tantalize your taste buds!

What's the Truth About Red Meat?

I believe eating red meats puts us a step away from environmental harmony. The human digestive system is not easily carnivorous. Our bodies have to struggle to use red meat energy. Eating red meat is a lot like extracting oil out of the ground. It may cost more to get the oil out than it's worth on the market. Meat protein, which the body can use, is often cancelled out by lengthy digestion time and after-dinner lethargy, because a disproportionate amount of energy goes to the task of assimilation. Further, too much of the highly concentrated protein in red meat can create toxicity from unused nitrogens — hard for your kidneys to cope with. Kidney stones are far more frequent in heavy red meat eaters.

Animals are closer to us on the bio-scale of life. They experience fear when killed. They don't want to be eaten. When we eat plants, there is an uplifting transmutation of energy. When we eat red meats, our bodies become denser, with more internal fermentation and body odor. Commercial red meats today are shot through with hormones and slow-release antibiotics (stock yard animals are often sick and over-medicated), and preserved with nitrates or nitrites. These substances are passed into us at the dinner table.

Red meat is our biggest diet contributor of excess protein and saturated fat levels. No one argues that less fat in the diet is healthier, or that saturated fats are the most harmful. Knowing this, livestock growers and butchers have made some changes. Beef now has 27%, and pork 43% less trimmable fat than cuts sold in the supermarket in the 1970s and 1980s. (There's still a lot of saturated fat in the meat marbling, however.)

Cooked red meats are acid-forming in the body; when red meat is cooked to well-done, chemical compounds are created that are capable of causing many diseases.

Finally, meat eating promotes more aggressive, arrogant behavior — a lack of gentleness in personality. From a spiritual point of view, red meat eating encourages ties to life's material things, expansion of territory, and the self-righteous intolerance that makes adversaries.

Most of us eat more meat than we really need. A 100 gram serving of meat is the size of a deck of cards, smaller than your computer mouse. A small can of salmon or tuna is two servings. Half a chicken breast, a drumstick, or a small hamburger patty is one serving. A small boneless roast weighing a kilogram (just over 2 pounds) provides 10 servings.

About Red Meat and a Healing Diet

Many recent scientific studies find that eating red meat increases the risk of degenerative diseases like heart disease, stroke and cancer. The American Heart Association, American Cancer Society, National Academy of Sciences, and American Academy of Pediatrics are just a few of the scientific organizations recommending less consumption of red meat and other animal foods, and a shift to a more vegetarian diet.

I don't believe red meat should be part of a healing diet. Here's why:

Health implications begin when meat is killed because it immediately starts to decompose. Although salt preservation and refrigeration retard spoilage, even slight putrefaction produces toxins and amines that accumulate in your liver, kidneys, and intestines, destroy friendly bacteria cultures (especially those that synthesize B vitamins), and degrade small intestine villi where food is absorbed into the blood. Saturated animal fats accumulate around organs and blood vessels, leading to cysts, tumors, cholesterol build-up and clogged arteries. Experts say that excess absorption of meat proteins may overstimulate immune response, resulting in immune tolerance.

Meat is significantly harder to digest than plant foods, taking 4 to 4 $\frac{1}{2}$ hours to be absorbed in the intestines versus 2 to 2 $\frac{1}{2}$ hours for grains and vegetables. Meat digestion requires more oxygen in the bloodstream.

Beef contains the highest concentration of herbicides of any food in America. The National Research Council (NRC) of the National Academy of Sciences cites pesticide-tainted beef as nearly 11 percent of the total cancer risk to consumers from pesticides. Eighty percent of all herbicides used in the U.S. are sprayed on corn and soy beans, which are used primarily as feed for cattle. The chemicals accumulate in the cattle and are passed onto consumers in finished cuts of beef.

Unfortunately, there's even more recent bad news about red meat.

—Irradiation: Tainted meats are now so wide-spread in America, the FDA has approved irradiation of red meat to destroy deadly bacteria like *E. coli*. Advocates of the move say that for a few cents a pound, hamburger or sausage can be zapped with radiation that kills pathogens by altering the genetic make up of the harmful bacteria. Irradiated meat is exposed to the equivalent of 10 to 70 million chest X-rays, and there are no long term studies to prove that food irradiation is safe. Benzene, a potent carcinogen, is created when red meat is exposed to irradiation. Just one molecule of benzene absorbed into the body is enough to cause cancer.

—Hormones: More than 95 percent of all feedlot-raised cattle in the U. S. receive growth hormones, antibiotics or other drugs. (Europe rejects our hormone-injected beef.) In order to speed weight gain and time-to-market, hormone levels are increased two to five times through anabolic steroids. Time-release synthetic estradiol, testosterone and progesterone slowly seep into the animal's blood. These hormones then become part of the hormone assault on people now implicated in increased cancer risk and other hormone-driven diseases.

—Antibiotics: In 1990, more than 15 million pounds of antibiotics were given to U.S. livestock to fight the diseases which were running rampant in cramped feedlots and contaminated pens. The beef industry says it has discontinued automatic use of antibiotics in beef cattle, but antibiotics are still given to dairy cows, which account for 15% of the beef eaten in the America. Veal calves become so sick in their tiny pens that antibiotics are routinely used to keep them alive until slaughter. Contrary to veal industry claims, no drugs have been approved by the U.S. FDA for formula-fed veal calves. Some of the drugs used routinely, like sulfamethazine are carcinogenic and residues may be present in consumer veal.

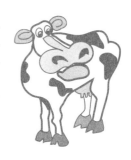

—Inadequate inspections: Since 1985, the National Academy of Sciences reported that federal meat inspections were inadequate to protect the public from meat-related diseases. Recommended corrective steps were never adopted. Instead, an experimental inspection system to increase online meat production by up to 40 percent was developed. It virtually eliminated the federal meat inspector and placed responsibility for carcass inspection on packing house employees. Thousands of carcasses pass through inspection with pneumonia, measles, peritonitis, abscesses, fecal or insect adulteration, and contaminated heads (called "puke heads"), on their way to American dinner tables.

—Disease: There appears to be a new link between cattle diseases and disease in humans. Bovine leukemia virus (BLV), an insect-borne retrovirus that causes malignancy in cattle, is found in 20% of cattle and 60% of U.S. herds. It may cause some forms of leukemia, since BLV antibodies have been found in leukemia patients. Bovine immunodeficiency virus (BIV), widespread in American cattle herds since the 1980's, genetically resembles the human HIV virus, and like HIV in humans, appears to suppress the immune system in cattle. At least one study suggests that BIV "plays a role in either malignant or slow viruses in humans."

We've seen the down side of a meat-based diet, especially for a healing diet.
Are there enough benefits in red meat to add it back to your diet after healing?

Red meat has complete protein and all the amino acids. In order to build human protein, we need 22 amino acids. Our bodies make amino acids, except for the eight essential amino acids that must be obtained from our foods. Plant proteins havemore amino acids, but no plant on its own has enough of the essential amino acids.

Can vegetarians get enough amino acids for protein building?

Plant protein combinations are good choices — like beans with rice or corn, tofu with whole grains, and legumes like peanuts and beans with whole wheat or corn. Bee pollen and sea plants contain all the amino acids and are considered complete foods by many vegetarians.

Red meat is the best source of food iron. Hemoglobin, the plasma of red blood formation, is part of red meat tissue, and delivers from 2 to 10 times more iron than any other source. Yet, new research shows us that body absorption of red meat iron may not be very efficient, because vegetarians have almost the same levels of iron in their blood as people who eat one or more servings of meat daily.

Can vegetarians get enough absorbable iron? Legumes, whole grains, nuts, spinach, clams, asparagus, poultry, prunes, raisins, pumpkin seeds, beets and soy foods all provide easy-to-use iron. Most iron supplements are not as well absorbed as food iron and are constipating, especially for children and pregnant women. I recommend herbal iron in combinations that include yellow dock root, dandelion, alfalfa, sea greens and nettles.

Red meat is a good source of zinc, needed for growth and immunity.

Can vegetarians get enough zinc for proper growth? Food sources include: chicken, seafood, whole wheat and wheat germ, lima beans, legumes, soy foods, nuts and eggs.

Red meat is a good source of B complex vitamins like riboflavin, thiamine and niacin. B vitamins help muscle tissue utilize food energy, so it's not surprising that animal muscle is a good source.

Can vegetarians get enough B vitamins? Whole grains and sea greens are primary sources of B vitamins.

Red meat is a good source of B-12, responsible for the growth and repair of body cells. A deficiency can take a long time to notice and can cause serious health problems.

Can vegetarians get B-12 from their diet? Its role is essential new red blood cells. Vitamin B-12 is in sea greens, soy foods, cereals and supergreens like chlorella, spirulina and barley grass. If you do not include these foods in your vegetarian diet, take a vitamin B-12 supplement.

Red meat and dairy foods are a good source of calcium for strong teeth and bones.

Can vegetarians get enough calcium? Calcium is plentiful in root vegetables, broccoli, nuts and seeds, leafy greens, legumes like peas and beans, soy foods, whole grains, and supergreens like chlorella and spirulina.

Note: If you decide to include red meat in your diet, you might consider ostrich meat as a healthier red meat in America. Ostrich meat tastes, looks and feels like beef. It is comparable to beef in iron and protein content. But ostrich meat has less than half the fat of chicken and two-thirds less fat and calories than beef and pork.

I believe vegetarians play a key, ac- tive role in conserving precious water, top-soil, and our Earth's energy resources that are wasted by an animal-based diet. Avoid-ing red meats may become one of most important things you can do for your own health and that of the plant.

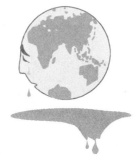

Protein: How Much Do You Need?

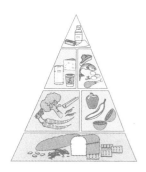

You must have protein to heal. Next to water, protein is your body's most plentiful substance, its primary source of building material for muscles, blood, skin, hair, nails, and organs like the heart and brain. All body tissues depend on protein. Blood can't clot without protein. Protein and its precursors, amino acids, work at hormonal levels to control basic functions like growth, sexual development and metabolism. The enzymes for immune and antibody response are formed from protein.

The human body doesn't make protein, it must be obtained through diet. But since protein is available from a wide range of sources, usually only people with severe malnutrition are protein deficient. Even people in less industrialized countries, get plenty of protein from foods like lentils, tofu, nuts, peas, seeds and grains. In children, protein deficiency leads to growth abnormalities. In adults, protein deficiency means low stamina, mental depression, low immune resistance and slow wound healing. Surgery, wounds, or prolonged illness are stresses that use up protein fast. At times of high stress, you'll want to take in extra protein to rebuild worn-out tissues.

The heart of the debate between a vegetarian diet and a meat-based diet is protein. How much protein do you need? There's no agreement among experts about how much protein is best. Protein requirements differ according to your health, body size and activity level. The American Journal of Clinical Nutrition says adults need 2.5% of their calorie intake in protein. World Health sets adult protein needs at 4.5% of calorie intake. The National Academy of Sciences recommends 6%. The National Research Council recommends 8%. The FDA says protein should make up 10% of your total daily calories. A 2,000-calorie diet allows for 50 grams of protein. The official RDA for adult men and women is 0.8g for each kg of body weight per day (about 55 grams of protein for 150 pound person). American's average consumption of protein is about 90 grams daily.

The rule of thumb is to simply divide your body weight by 2; the result is the approximate number of grams of protein you need each day. An easy way to translate protein grams into your diet is to eat an amount of protein food that covers the palm of your hand at each meal; vegetarians double the amount to two palmfuls.

The problem with too much protein.

Experts say that Americans eat too much protein for good health. Unlike carnivorous animals, whose digestive and metabolic systems are adapted to a meat-based diet, humans who consume more than half their calories as meat protein are at risk for protein poisoning (a serious watch word for dieters on the new extra high-protein "zone" diets). The National Academy of Sciences now recommends that Americans reduce their protein intake by 12 to 15 percent and switch from animal to plant protein sources.

Protein is the least efficient of the body's cellular engines — fats, carbohydrates and protein; to burn it the body must boost its metabolic rate by 10%, straining the liver's ability to absorb oxygen. Protein does not burn cleanly, leaving behind nitrogen waste that your body must eliminate, a taxing process on your kidneys. It's why excessive protein consumption is linked to urinary tract infections. For diabetics, the extra workload increases the risk of serious kidney disease. John's Hopkins Hospital now treats and cures severe kidney disease with a very low protein diet and amino acid supplements.

—**Too much protein is linked to high cholesterol levels.** Protein that is not used for building tissue or energy may be converted by the liver and stored as fat.

—**Too much protein irritates the immune system,** keeping it in a state of overactivity.

—**Too much protein may cause fluid imbalance,** so calcium and other minerals are lost through the urine.

—**Too much animal protein actually contributes to osteoporosis,** heart disease and cancers like renal cancer and lympho-sarcoma through loss of critical minerals.

Does your body know the difference between animal and vegetable protein? Does your body work differently depending on the type of protein you eat? Amazingly enough, it appears that it does.

Animal source proteins have been considered superior in the past because they are:
1: high in protein. Actually they have too much protein, which is then stored in the body as toxins or fat.
2: complete protein, supplying necessary amino acid. But they also include unhealthy inorganic acids.
3: supply larger iron and zinc amounts off-set by the cholesterol, fat and calories that meat also supplies.

Scientific opinion about protein is changing. One important study by Baylor College of Medicine in Houston showed men on diets high in soy protein had a drop in cholesterol, compared to men on diets high in animal protein. The study concluded that men should replace up to 50% of meat protein with vegetable protein.

Research shows that eating lots of high protein animal foods may cause the body to extract calcium from the blood and excrete it, a cause of osteoporosis. Osteoporosis is rare in Chinese people with a plant-based protein diet. It only appears in Chinese cities where people are living more western lifestyles. In contrast, Eskimos, who have a meat-based diet, with twice the RDA of calcium, have the highest rate of osteoporosis in the world.

Other research in China shows that when animal protein in the diet increases, so does the risk of coronary heart disease, arteriosclerosis, kidney stones, arthritis, cataracts, and cancer.

Women may need more protein per pound of body weight than men to attain the same level of health. Cases of depression, PMS, menopause symptoms and chronic fatigue have disappeared when protein was increased. But protein from meat tends to be high in fat, so women's protein consumption should lean in favor of seafoods, whole grains, beans and other legumes.

Can vegetable protein satisfy your body's needs?
Protein is formed from combinations of the 22 amino acids. There is an amino acid pool in our blood, so protein from food is slowly released into the bloodstream allowing for maximum utilization of amino acids. Early nutritional opinion held that vegetable proteins had to be carefully combined so that all essential amino acids and proteins were available at each meal to create a complete protein. Later research shows that this is not necessary. Since the body breaks proteins down into amino acids and redistributes them, food combinations with incomplete proteins have the same effect as a complete protein.

Plant foods also team up to make complete proteins in a process called protein complementarity. Beans and rice are an example. Many beans like soy and black beans contain equal or more protein than beef. Eating a wide variety of plant protein foods is the secret. Vegetarians typically eat less protein than meat eaters, but their diets still meet or exceed the protein RDA.

Good vegetable protein sources to consider for your healing diet:
–Whole grains, nuts, seeds, legumes, and soy foods are good sources of protein and essential fatty acids.
–Dark green, leafy vegetables, like kale and chard, and cruciferous vegetables, like broccoli, cabbage and cauliflower, have easily absorbed protein (about 8%) plus EFA's.
–Other good plant protein sources include the blue-green algae, spirulina and chlorella.
–Brewer's yeast is an excellent source of protein, B vitamins, amino acids and minerals. It is a key immune-enhancing food. Chromium-rich, brewer's yeast can be a key food for improving blood sugar metabolism, for substantially reducing cholesterol and top speed wound healing by boosting production of collagen.
–Sprouts are a natural source of protein and almost every other nutrient (vitamins, enzymes, essential fatty acids, antioxidants and minerals that strengthen immune response and protect from toxic chemical buildup.)
–Flax, sesame, sunflower, pumpkin (lots of zinc), almonds, and chia are my favorite nuts and seeds for protein. Roasting or healing deactivates enzyme inhibitors that may make them hard to digest.

Nature's Superfoods Can Help You Heal Faster

Green "superfoods" are superior sources of essential nutrients — nutrients we need but can't make ourselves. We may all be adding more salads and vegetables to our diets, but concern for the quality of foods grown on mineral-depleted soils makes green superfoods like chlorella, spirulina, barley and wheat grass popular. They are nutritionally more potent than regular foods, and are wonderful food antioxidants for healthy healing.

Green, and blue-green algae (phyto-plankton), are almost perfect superfoods.
They have rich high quality protein, fiber, chlorophyll, vitamins, minerals and enzymes. Use them therapeutically to stimulate immune response, accelerate healing and tissue repair, help prevent degenerative disease and promote longer life.
- They are the most potent source of beta carotene available in the world today.
- They are the richest plant sources of vitamin B-12.
- Their amino acids are virtually identical to those needed by the human body.
- Their protein yield is greater than soy beans, corn or beef.
- They are the only food source, other than mother's milk, of GLA, an essential fatty acid.
- They are natural detoxifiers to protect against chemical pollutants and radiation.

Chlorella alone has a higher concentration of chlorophyll than any known plant.
It is a complete protein food, with all the B vitamins, vitamin C and E, and many minerals high enough to be considered supplemental amounts. The list of chlorella benefits is long and almost miraculous, from detoxification to energy enhancement, to immune system restoration.

- Chlorella's cell wall material is especially beneficial for intestinal and bowel health, detoxifying the colon, stimulating peristaltic activity, and promoting friendly bacteria.
- Chlorella eliminates heavy metals, like lead, mercury, copper and cadmium.
- Chlorella is an important source of carotenes in healing tumors.
- Chlorella strengthens the liver, your body's major detoxifying organ, to rid you of infective agents.
- Chlorella reduces arthritis stiffness.
- Chlorella normalizes blood pressure.
- Chlorella relieves indigestion, hiatal hernia, gastritis and ulcers.
- Chlorella is effective in weight loss programs. It has cleansing ability, rich nutrition that keeps energy up during dieting, and maintains muscle during lower food intake.
- Chlorella's most important benefits come from a unique biochemical combination of molecules called the Controlled Growth Factor, a composition that provides noticeable increase in immune health.

Spirulina is the original green superfood. It's an ecological wonder because it grows in both ocean and lake waters and can be cultivated in extreme environments useless for conventional agriculture. It grows in such a variety of climates and conditions that some consider it the nutrition answer for whole populations on the brink of starvation. Amazingly prolific, spirulina doubles its bio-mass every two to five days.

Acre for acre, spirulina yields 20 times more protein than soybeans, 40 times more protein than corn, and 400 times more protein than beef. It is a complete protein, with all 22 amino acids, the entire vitamin B-complex, including B-12, carotenes, minerals, and essential fatty acids. Digestibility is high, for both immediate and long range energy.

Big business isn't necessary for spirulina. Small scale community farms are spirulina's biggest producers. Researchers say that spirulina alone could double the protein available to people on a fraction of the world's land, while helping restore the environmental balance of the planet.

Green grasses are some of the lowest-calorie, yet nutrient-rich edibles on the planet.

Green grasses are the only plants on earth that can give sole nutritional support to an animal throughout life. Yet they are some of the most underused.

Grasses have the extraordinary ability to transform inanimate elements from soil, water and sunlight into living cells with energy. Grasses contain all the known minerals and trace minerals, balanced vitamins and hundreds of enzymes. The small molecular proteins and chlorophyllins in grasses are absorbed directly through our cell membranes.

Their rich chlorophyll helps humans, as it does plants, to resist the destructive effects of air pollution, carbon monoxide, X-rays and radiation. Studies on barley, wheatgrass and alfalfa show capacity for a wide range of health problems: high blood pressure, diabetes, gastritis, ulcers, liver disease, asthma, eczema, hemorrhoids, skin infections, anemia, constipation, body odor, bleeding gums, burns, even cancer. Good sources of vitamin K, green grasses are effective for bone strength and varicose veins, too.

Barley grass has highly concentrated vitamins, minerals, enzymes, proteins and chlorophyllins — eleven times more calcium than cow's milk, five times more iron than spinach, and seven times more vitamin C and bioflavonoids than orange juice. Its significant contribution to a vegetarian diet is 80mcg of vitamin B-12 per 100grams of powdered juice.

Barley grass research shows results for DNA damage repair and delaying aging. Barley juice has anti-viral activity and neutralizes heavy metals like mercury. Barley is an ideal anti-inflammatory for healing gastrointestinal ulcers, hemorrhoids and pancreatic infections. Dr. Kubota of Tokyo Pharmacy Science says, "barley grass has effects measurably stronger than either steroid or non-steroid drugs, and few if any side effects."

Alfalfa is one of the world's richest mineral-source foods, pulling up earth minerals from root depths as great as 130 feet! Alfalfa's high chlorophyll content and rich plant fiber make it a good spring tonic, infection fighter and natural body deodorizer. It is a restorative in treating cases of narcotic and alcohol addiction. It is a specific therapy for arthritis, skin disorders and liver problems. Because of its high vitamin K content, herbalists use alfalfa to encourage blood-clotting. It is also used to treat bladder infections, colon disorders, anemia, hemorrhaging and diabetes. Alfalfa's recognized phytohormones are effective in normalizing estrogen production.

Wheat grass liquid has curative powers for cancerous growths, with particular success as rectal implants in colon cancer cases. As with all the green grasses, its ability to provide protection from carcinogens comes from chlorophyll's capacity to strengthen cells, detoxify the liver and blood, and biochemically neutralize pollutants. Wheat grass ointment is used uccessfully for disorders like skin ulcers, impetigo and itching.

Fifteen pounds of fresh wheat grass has the nutritional value of 350 pounds of vegetables with all their enzyme activity. Wheat grass also normalizes the thyroid gland to stimulate metabolism, which may be helpful in correcting obesity problems.

Medicinal mushrooms boost your resistance to toxic chemicals, bacteria and viruses.

Maitake mushrooms are the strongest tumor growth inhibitors of all the healing mushrooms. They are also highly effective against hormone driven cancers like breast, prostate and endometrial cancer, even high mortality cancers like lung, liver, pancreas and brain cancer. Maitake has a most unusual synergistic effect with chemotherapy. Most natural therapies do not co-exist well with either chemotherapy or radiation, but patients taking maitake along with chemotherapy report a lessening of side effects such as loss of appetite and nausea. Maitake also appears to protect healthy cells from becoming cancerous, and prevent the spread of cancer once it has taken hold.

Maitake chemical structure stands apart from other mushrooms. Known as D-fraction, researchers say it's Nature's most effective agent for targeting foreign substances and stimulating cell immune response. For example, studies confirmed by the Japan National Institute for Health and the U.S. National Cancer Institute, show that maitake works rapidly to prevent the destruction of T-cells by HIV. Almost 40% of AIDS patients develop Kaposi's Sarcoma, a malignant skin cancer. Conventional medicine has not developed an effective treatment. Naturopaths report improvement in just a few days when maitake extract is applied to KS lesions.

Researchers document anti-diabetes, anti-hypertension, anti-obesity and anti-hepatitis activity, as well as success against Chronic Fatigue Syndrome for maitake.

Maitake is effective taken orally, an advantage over other mushrooms where extracts often need to be injected, or where the therapeutic benefit is lost when taken orally.

Reishi mushrooms (*ganoderma*) **are in the highest class of adaptogen tonics for promoting longevity.** They have strong antioxidant protection and free radical scavenging activity for deep immune support. They are especially effective for recovery from serious illness. Reishi is an excellent cardiotonic, even significantly lowering blood pressure in those individuals with hypertension who were unresponsive to ACE inhibitors.

Reishi may also be used therapeutically against fatigue, to relieve allergy symptoms, liver toxicity (especially hepatitis), bronchitis and carcinoma. New research shows success against chronic fatigue syndrome. Reishi may be used daily to lower cholesterol and triglycerides, induce sound sleep and increase resistance to infections.

Shiitake mushroom extracts can protect the body from cancer risk, even help shrink existing tumors. An immense amount of research has been done on two components of shiitake, lentinan and lentinula edodes mycelium (LEM) which have shown strong anti-tumor power. These constituents work by bolstering the body's own ability to eliminate the tumor rather than by attacking the tumor cells themselves. One Japanese study found that chemotherapy patients who also received lentinan injections twice a week survived significantly longer with less tumor growth, than patients who received chemotherapy alone.

Shiitakes are especially effective in treating systemic conditions related to early aging and sexual dysfunction. Renowned in Japan and China as both food and medicine for thousands of years, shiitake helps lower cholesterol levels, reduces blood pressure and fights viruses and bacteria. Shiitakes stimulate immunity by producing a virus that stimulates our body's interferon.

Studies with HIV patients show that LEM may be more effective at preventing the spread of the HIV virus in the body than AZT, the most commonly prescribed single drug in the treatment of AIDS — possibly because LEM works by blocking the initial stages of HIV infection, while AZT merely slows replication of the virus, and generally becomes less effective over time. LEM also shows results for hepatitis and chronic fatigue syndrome.

Add shiitakes frequently to your diet, just a few each time. A little goes a long way.

Poria cocos has a unique ability to balance body chemistry, especially mineral balances. Poria is a mushroom amphoteric (with both alkaline and acidic properties). A Traditional Chinese medicine herb, poria cocos works on the heart, spleen, and kidney meridians, and is used to remove spleen dampness when indicated by poor appetite, diarrhea and lethargy. TCM specialists believe that poria replenishes the spleen, thus strengthening the body against dizziness, and fluid elimination problems.

American naturopaths use poria to reduce excess water retention, balance body fluids and prevent toxic build-up. Poria cocos is used in herbal remedies for insomnia, restlessness, fatigue, sleep disorders, tension, and nervousness.

Cordyceps sinensis (*caterpillar mushroom*) is used in Traditional Chinese Medicine as a tonic and energizer. Chinese runners who broke nine world records in 1993 first brought Cordyceps into the modern spotlight. Research shows that cordyceps also enhances immunity by increasing activity of helper T-cells and natural killer cells, accelerates spleen regeneration, increases SOD (*superoxide dismutase*) activity, enhances oxygen uptake to the heart and brain, possesses testosterone-like effects, improves libido and sperm count, and is effective in reducing uterine fibroids.

Macrobiotics: A Choice For Serious Healing

In America, macrobiotics has become a popular, purifying diet approach for serious, degenerative illness. It is an effective technique because it works to normalize body chemistry, not only to remove toxins, but also to rebuild healthy blood and cells.

Most notably, macrobiotics is seen an against cancer and has for most of this cen- for cancer. Macro-biotic (or long life), stems the seasons, climate, traditional culture, and ing how to eat. A macrobiotic regimen en- ity is achieved through living in harmony quires the realization that we create our

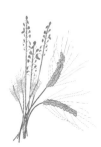

effective method of improving body chemistry tury, been part of the natural healing tradition from the Oriental philosophy that considers a person's health and activity level in determin- courages body harmony by teaching that vital- with the universe. A macrobiotic way of life re- health through our lifestyle choices.

One of the principles of macrobiotics is that it adapts to individual needs. There is no single macrobiotic diet. Still, the macrobiotic way of eating is low in fat, non-mucous-forming, and rich in plant fiber and protein. It stimulates the heart and circulation through emphasis on Oriental foods like miso, green tea and shiitake mushrooms. It is alkalizing with umeboshi plums, sea greens and soy foods. It is nutrient rich — especially high in potassium, natural iodine, other minerals, and B-complex vitamins.

For most Americans, becoming macrobiotic requires a major shift in the way we look at life; indeed, it is usually a complete lifestyle change. For this reason, I usually recommend making the change to a macrobiotic diet slowly.

1: The first diet change is to eat organic whole foods whenever possible. This is often a greater change than it might seem, because it means seeking these foods out, changing shopping habits and-or grocery stores to find new sources. One of the cornerstones of macrobiotic body balancing is eating with the seasons. Yet, America's world-wide, market driven culture stands at the opposite end of this principle. We import all foods any time of the year without regard to our own seasons. Buying organically grown produce is good way to ensure this fundamental element of macrobiotics.

2: The next change is to gradually eliminate foods not at ease in a macrobiotic diet, like fried foods, highly processed, chemicalized foods, frozen, packaged and canned foods, and foods with colorants and preserv- ers. Most animal protein and fat should be avoided, including dairy products (except fertile eggs). Eliminate white sugar foods. Use sweeteners like rice syrup and barley malt in small amounts instead. Refrain from sweet, tropical fruits, carbonated sodas and caffeine. Hot spices, artificial vinegar and strong alcoholic beverages should also be eliminated.

3: The third change is learning to prepare foods in their whole form, a change that takes some attention for people who are used to pre-prepared foods. It means buying fresh foods, and simply preparing them to keep the greatest value of the nutrients.

4: The fourth change is to include foods that are in harmony with macrobiotic principles, and to begin eating them in the macrobiotic way. The most apparent difference between macrobiotics and other diet approaches is its reliance on whole grains. In macrobiotics, at least half of the daily food intake is whole grains — brown rice, whole wheat, oats, barley, millet, buckwheat, rye, amaranth, kamut and corn. Cooking grains with a little seasalt is recommended; my favorite way to season is with the mineral salts of sea greens. Don't use processed grains like pastas and non-yeasted breads.

Vegetables, both raw and cooked, are the second most important foods for macrobiotics, comprising about 30% of the diet. Steam, sauté in olive or sesame oil, parboil or bake them. Good vegetables to include for healing are: green cabbage, dark leafy greens, broccoli, cauliflower, parsley, burdock root, carrots, squash and scallions. Vegetables like potatoes, tomatoes, eggplant, peppers, spinach, beets and zucchini are not recommended for a serious healing diet because they are thought to aggravate body acidity.

Beans and sea greens are considered supplementary, rather than daily foods, comprising about 5 to 10 percent of a macrobiotic diet. Yet, for Americans used to more protein in their diet, I find that eating beans makes an easier change to macrobiotics. I recommend black beans, chickpeas, soy and lentils. Sea greens such as kombu, dulse, kelp, sea palm, wakame, hijiki, arame, mekabu and nori can be used with grains, beans, and vegetables, especially in soups. Soups may make up 10 to 15% of the initial macrobiotic diet. A daily bowl of miso soup starts the alkalizing, immune-boosting process right away.

Other foods in order of their importance in a macrobiotic diet are vegetable oils, nuts, fruits, fish and occasional fertile eggs. Although many macrobiotic followers prefer to avoid all animal foods, macrobiotics is not a vegetarian system. White meat fish, like flounder, cod, sole and halibut are recommended 2 to 3 times a week. Fruits are eaten only occasionally as desserts or snacks 2 to 3 times a week. Nuts and seeds, like pumpkin, sesame and sunflower seeds are occasional snacks. Therapeutic foods, like green tea, shiitake, maitake and reishi mushrooms, raw sauerkraut, and umeboshi plums should be included regularly.

5: The fifth change is learning to chew your food well - about 50 times per bite for the best nutrition absorption. Chewing is the cornerstone of a grain-based macrobiotic diet because grains are by nature acidic; saliva which is alkaline, counteracts the acid. The acid - alkaline balance of your body's blood is crucial to your all body functions including mood and emotion, and to your body's healing ability. Americans, who generally lead fast-paced, high stress lives, sometimes find this change the hardest to make.

Is there a way to tell if your macrobiotic changes are helping your healing program? Here is the usual sequence for normalizing body chemistry: It usually takes ten days for plasma to recycle, so improvements beome noticeable after ten days. It takes 30 days for white blood cells to renew, so immune function begins to improve after a month. It takes 120 days for red blood cells to renew, so it is then that true healing begins. Most people say they notice results in healthier emotional and mental patterns around this time as well.

Even in its strict form, a macrobiotic diet is nutritionally balanced with adequate protein and low fat. The majority of the foods are from the center of the food spectrum – vegetables and whole grains – with a minimum of foods from the extremes; fruits and sugars are more cooling, meat and dairy foods are more stimulating. Some herbs and spices, like garlic, onions, and cayenne are considered too stimulating.

Harvard's School of Public Health analyzed the standard recommendations of a macrobiotic diet. The results showed that the diet exceeded the recommended daily nutrient allowances of both the FDA and the World Health Organization, without having to take extra protein, vitamins or minerals. From a macrobiotic perspective, it is not desirable to take supplements other than whole herbs, since it is thought that they interfere with the nutrients in the whole foods themselves.

Is macrobiotics for you?
A macrobiotic diet's greatest benefit is that it is cleansing and strengthening at the same time. I view macrobiotics a little differently than the traditional Oriental model. I see macrobiotics not as a "no deviation" regimen, but as a way of life based on a whole foods diet and an active lifestyle in harmony with nature.

A strict macrobiotic diet used over a long period of time, can be too stringent for a person living a busy, stressful life in today's polluted environment. I normally recommend a strict macrobiotic diet for three to six months, then a gradual move to a modified macrobiotic diet which doesn't follow rigid rules, but rather emphasizes the principles of macrobiotics with the flexibility of each person's needs.

Cultured Foods Offer Healing Probiotics

What are probiotics? Why are they so important for your healing diet? Probiotics are beneficial microorganisms like Lactobacillus, Bifidobacteria, and Streptococcus in your intestinal tract. They manufacture vitamins, especially B vitamins like biotin, niacin, folic acid and B-6, that detoxify chemicals and metabolize hormones. They empower enzymes that maximize food assimilation and digestion.

I see probiotics (as opposed to antibiotics), as an amazing fighting force that competes at a basic level with disease-causing microorganisms in your body.

—First, probiotics prevent the growth of undesirable bacteria by depriving them of nourishment.

—Second, probiotics attack specific pathogens by changing your body's acid/alkaline balance to an antibiotic environment. (Probiotic activity against vaginal yeast infections is a good example of this.) If you are taking long courses of drug antibiotics, remember that they kill all bacteria, both bad and good. All intestinal flora are severely diminished. For most people, poor digestion, diarrhea or constipation, flatulence, bad breath, bloating, tiredness, migraines, even acne are a result of long antibiotic treatment.

It doesn't matter how good your diet is if your body can't use it. Your body ecology must maintain an ecological balance of bacteria to protect intestinal and immune function. But our modern lifestyle destroys normal body balance. Stress, alcohol, chemicalized foods, environmental pollutants, antibiotic and steroid drugs all adversely affect our ability to use nourishment. When unfriendly bacteria get the upper hand in the balance, the door opens to infections and allergy reactions. Probiotic organisms prevent disease, even treat infections by restoring microorganism balance in your intestinal tract.

The best way to get probiotics in your diet? Add them through foods like yogurt, kefir or raw sauerkraut.

I see probiotic supplements as a health insurance policy. Most supplements have lactobacillus acidophilus (which attaches in the small intestine), bifidobacterius (which attaches in the large intestine), and lactobacillus bulgaricus (three protective strains of flora). Together they produce hydrogen peroxide, a byproduct that helps maintain protective microbial balance and protects against pathogens.

Here's what probiotics can do for you:

—Probiotics boost immune response by inhibiting growth of pathogenic organisms

—Probiotics detoxify the intestinal tract by protecting intestinal mucosa levels

—Probiotics develop a barrier to food-borne allergies

—Probiotics neutralize antibiotic-resistant strains of bacteria

—Probiotics reduce cancer risk

—Probiotics reduce the risk of inflammatory bowel disease (IBS) and diverticulosis

—Probiotic synthesize needed vitamins for healing

—Probiotics prevent diarrhea by improving digestion of proteins and fats

Important new discoveries about probiotics:

Probiotics play a key role in the prevention of osteoporosis. Bone loss is one unfortunate result of a lack of friendly microorganisms in the gastrointestinal tract. Vitamin K, a vital building block to healthy bones, is a byproduct of lactobacilli.

New research shows new benefits for acidophilus. *Lactobacilli acidophilus,* part of the normal flora in your urinary tract and vaginal tissue, helps you digest dairy foods, prevents most yeast infections and restores intestinal balance especially for traveler's and antibiotic-induced diarrhea. Acidophilus is highly successful for children's diseases. Children have naturally strong immune systems and may only need the gentle body balancing of friendly flora instead of a harsh drug or chemical antibiotic.

Important note: Experience with many people has shown me that acidophilus is very effective as a healing medicine when it is sprinkled directly on food..... particularly for low immune response conditions, like candida albicans, eating disorders and HIV infection where nutrient assimilation is seriously compromised.

Acidophilus benefits:
   —helps synthesize B vitamins and produces essential enzyme stores
   —helps overcome lactose intolerance by digesting milk sugars
   —reduces blood fat and cholesterol levels
   —improves elimination — contributing to sweet breath and normal body odor
   —kills harmful bacteria that contribute to cancer; helps block tumor development
   —inactivates some harmful viruses
   —helps detoxify the gastrointestinal tract and improves G.I. health
   —prevents yeast infections
   —prevents urinary tract infections

As beneficial as they are, not everyone can use probiotics. Each person's digestive system is highly individual, like the immune system to which it is a gateway. Many experts question whether single strain probiotic supplements can survive the digestion process. Digestion, even though it offers some protection from unfriendly bacteria, is not able to differentiate between good and bad bacteria.

Prebiotics like FOS are a more practical approach. Prebiotics feed the beneficial bacteria you already have in your gastrointestinal tract. Fructo-oligo-saccharides (FOS) are naturally-occurring carbohydrates in vegetables like artichokes, bananas, onions, garlic, barley and tomatoes. The FOS saccharides can't be digested by humans, but are easily used by our intestinal flora. Competition for food and attachment sites in our intestines is fierce between hundreds of microorganisms, both good and bad. Research shows that FOS supplements give your friendly bacteria a competitive edge and actually increase your body's population of beneficial bacteria.

Cultured foods add natural friendly flora to your healing diet

Soyfoods are nutritional powerhouses. Even if soy isn't a magic bullet for preventing heart disease or curing cancer, it possesses amazing health benefits. Soy protein compares in quality to animal protein — it's a good alternative to meat or dairy foods. Soy foods are rich in other essential nutrients, too, like calcium, iron, zinc and B vitamins.

What can cultured soy foods do for you?
1: Soy protein helps lower your cholesterol. Numerous studies show that when animal protein in the diet is replaced by soy protein, there is significant reduction in both total blood cholesterol and LDL (bad) cholesterol. Adding as little as 25 to 50 grams of soy protein daily to your diet for one month can result in a cholesterol drop.
2: Soy amino acids can lower high insulin levels. Low insulin levels mean= your liver makes less cholesterol.
3: Soy antioxidants help control atherosclerosis by preventing oxidative damage to LDL cholesterol.
4: Soy possesses rich diet sources of five known anticancer agents:
   a. protease inhibitors that hinder development of colon, lung, liver, pancreatic and esophageal cancers.
   b. compounds that block formation of nitrosamines leading to liver cancer.
   c. phytosterols that inhibit cell division and proliferation in colon cancer.
   d. saponins that slow the growth of cancerous skin cells.
   e. isoflavones that slow osteoporosis and lower risk of hormone-related cancers, like breast and prostate cancer. (One study finds that pre-menopausal females who rarely eat soy foods have twice the risk of breast cancer as those who frequently eat soy foods. The test showed that just one serving a day of soy protein led to

significant lengthening of the menstrual cycle, suppressing the midcycle surge of gonadotrophins and luteinizing hormones — effects that decrease the risk of breast cancer.) The Japanese, with low rates of hormone-driven cancers, eat five times more soy products than Americans. The typical U.S. diet yields 80 milligrams of phytosterols a day, the Japanese eat 400 milligrams a day. Western vegetarians eat about 345 milligrams a day.

Soy contains genistein.
　—**Genistein** - an abundant isoflavone in soy which work much like human estrogen. Genistein helps balance your body's estrogen supply, acting both as an estrogen and as an estrogen blocker, depending on your need. Like many phytohormone herbs, it promotes the positive actions of estrogen, while preventing many of its bad effects by competing for both estrogen and progesterone receptors to prevent their availability for tumor growth.
　—**Genistein** - also has benefits for men's health. Research on 8,000 Hawaiian men found that the men who ate the most tofu had the lowest rates of prostate cancer, kidney disease and diabetes complications.
　—**Genistein** - also inhibits angiogenesis, the formation of new blood vessels that nourish tumors.

Soy foods that benefit a healing diet:

• **Tofu,** made from cooked, curdled soybean milk, water and nigari, a mineral-rich seawater precipitate, is the soy food highest in both total isoflavones and genistein. Tofu is a nutritionally balanced healing food. Cooked, it is easy to digest, full of fiber, and a non-mucous-forming way to add richness and creamy texture to recipes. Ironically, nearly all the soybeans raised in the U.S. go into animal feed. Most of the rest is shipped to Japan. Tofu, combined with whole grains, yields a complete protein, providing dairy richness without the fat or cholesterol, yet with all the calcium and iron.

As tofu's popularity has risen in America, so have its culinary talents. Fresh tofu has a light, delicate character that can take on any flavor, from savory to sweet. It comes firm-pressed in cubes, in a soft, delicate form, or with a custard-like texture. It is smoked or pre-cooked in seasonings for more flavor. It comes in deep-fried pouches called age (pronounced "ah-gay") for stuffing. It is both aseptically packaged and freeze-dried to be stored at room temperature and reconstituted for later use, camping and travel.

Tofu by the numbers:
　—Tofu is low in calories. Eight ounces has only 164 calories.
　—Tofu provides organic calcium. 8-oz. supplies the same amount of calcium as 8-oz. of milk, about 12% of the adult calcium RDA, with more absorbability.
　—Tofu is high in iron. 8-oz. supplies the same amount of iron as 2-oz. of beef liver or 4 eggs.
　—Tofu has almost 8% quality protein. Eight ounces supplies the same amount of protein as $3\frac{1}{4}$ oz. of beef, $5\frac{1}{2}$ oz. of hamburger, $1\frac{2}{3}$ cups of milk, 2-oz. of cheese, or 2 eggs; it is lower in fat than all of these. Unlike most animal protein, cooked tofu is easy to digest, with a digestion rate of 95%.
　—Tofu contains all 8 essential amino acids.
　—As little as 4-oz. of tofu a month offers women breast cancer prevention benefits.

• **Miso,** a tasty food made from fermented soybean paste, is body alkalizing, lowers cholesterol, represses carcinogens, helps neutralize allergens and pollutants, lessens the effects of smoking, and provides an immune-enhancing environment, even to the point of rejuvenating damaged cells. Miso also attracts and absorbs environmental toxins like radioactive elements in the body and helps to eliminate them.

Miso has even stronger antioxidant effects than soy itself. As miso ages, its color turns deep brown from melanoidine. Melanoidine suppresses the production of fat peroxide in the body. Fat peroxides (oxidized fats) become free radicals, which destroy normal cell functions and are a cause of aging.

Miso's essential fatty acid, linoleic acid, stimulates sebaceous glands for baby soft skin texture. LA also significantly inhibits the production of melanin, the pigment that causes dark spots on the skin, by repressing synthesis of the enzyme tyrosinase that synthesizes melanin.

Miso's fatty acid, ethyl linoleate, has an anti-mutagenic effect against carginogens found in scorched foods like charcoal barbecued meats and French roasted coffee.

Miso's linoleic acid, plant sterols and vitamin E work synergistically to suppress cholesterol, inhibiting cholesterol absorption in the small intestine and promoting excretion of serum cholesterol. Vitamin E, a component of HDL (good cholesterol), helps transport harmful cholesterol and increase HDL levels.

Miso is a healthy substitute for salt or soy sauce. There are many kinds, strengths and flavors of miso, from chickpea (light and mild) to hatcho (dark and strong). Delicious natto miso is a sweet mix of soybeans, barley and barley malt, kombu, ginger and sea salt.

Miso is naturally fermented for your healing diet. Miso is still a living food, with its active enzymes and beneficial microorganisms intact to aid digestion.

Miso is highly concentrated; use $^1/_2$ to 1 teasp. of dark miso, or 1 to 2 teasp. of light miso per person. Dissolve in a small amount of water to activate the beneficial enzymes before adding to a recipe. Omit salt from the recipe if you are using miso.

• **Tamari** is a wheat-free soy sauce, lower in sodium and richer in flavor than regular soy sauce. Bragg's Liquid Aminos, an energizing protein broth sold in health food stores, is of the tamari family, but unfermented, even lower in sodium, with all 8 essential amino acids.

• **Soy milk,** nutritious, smooth, delicious, and versatile, is simply made by pressing ground, cooked soybeans. It's lactose and cholesterol free, with less calcium and calories than cow's milk, but more protein and iron. Use it cup for cup like milk in cooking. It adds a slight rise to baked goods. Soy milk formulas are excellent for infants allergic to cow's milk. It's often used in treatment diets for diabetes, anemia and heart diseases.

• **Soy cheese,** made from soy milk, is lactose and cholesterol free. (A small amount of calcium caseinate, milk protein, is added to allow soy cheese to melt.) Mozzarella, cheddar, jack and cream cheese types are widely available. Use it cup for cup in place of any low-fat or regular cheese.

• **Soy ice cream, frozen desserts and yogurt** are also widely available.

• **Soy mayonnaise** has the taste and consistency of regular mayonnaise.

• **Tempeh** is a meaty, Indonesian soy food, with complete protein and all essential amino acids. It has a robust texture and mushroom-like aroma. Tempeh is an enzyme-active, predigested cultured food, making it highly absorbable. It's rich in B vitamins (especially B-12), low in calories and fat, and cholesterol free. Tempeh differs from tofu - it has a denser firmer texture, and is higher in fiber. Tempeh has the highest quality protein of any soyfood, with 19.5% protein (about as much as beef and chicken), and 50% more protein than ground beef.

• **Kombucha,** although known as a "mushroom," is not a mushroom at all, but a symbiotic culture of yeast and microorganisms. It is a popular natural tonic of Russian origin, for lowering blood pressure, raising immune T-cell counts and increasing vitality. It is noted for its dramatic antibiotic and detoxifying activity.

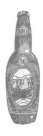

—To make kombucha tonic, place a small amount of kombucha culture into sweetened black or green tea. The culture feeds on the sugar and like a tiny biochemical factory, produces glucuronic acid, glucon acid, lactic acid, vitamins, amino acids, antibiotic substances, and more to make it a healthful cultured drink.

I recommend buying Kombucha tea from the refrigerated section of your health food store. I have personally known several cases where making kombucha culture at home was unsuccessful, and became contaminated with unsafe organisms.

The benefits of kombucha culture tonic:
      —helps the liver bind up toxic substances so they can be eliminated from the body
      —cleanses the colon, relieves constipation and colitis, arrests simple diarrhea
      —relieves arthritis pain and carpal tunnel syndrome
      —helps return gray hair to its natural color; thickens hair and strengthens nails
      —relieves bronchitis and asthma
      —helps overcome candida albicans yeast infections
      —reduces menopausal hot flashes, headaches and migraines
      —reduces cravings for fatty foods
      —improves eyesight, cataracts and floaters
      —relieves acne, eczema and psoriasis
      —vitalizes flagging libido and sexual energy

• **Vinegar** is an ancient, but still excellent, cultured food, full of beneficial organisms that help digest heavy foods and high protein meals. Brown rice, balsamic, apple cider, herbal, raspberry, ume plum and wine vinegars have been used for 5000 years as health enhancers. The most nutritious vinegars are not overly filtered (they look slightly cloudy) and still contain the "mother" mix of bacteria and enzymes in the bottle.

Vinegar has an array of health benefits:
— loaded with gallbladder enhancing enzymes and essential acids that aid digestion
—assists in killing infections, both bacterial and fungal
—a powerful remedy for resolving liver stagnation and indigestion
—a vinegar hair rinse treats dandruff and seborrhea
—remarkable effects in the treatment of arthritis, osteoporosis and memory loss
—high potassium helps balance body sodium, encourages bowel regularity and sustains nerve health
—large amounts of pectin and potassium help a healthy, relaxed heartbeat and blood pressure
—diluted vinegar eardrops can ward off and gently relieve children's ear infections
—a vinegar footbath softens hard callouses, and a footbath is an effective treatment for athlete's foot

A warm water vinegar drink has remarkable detoxifying effects. Mix 1 tsp. apple cider vinegar, 1 tsp. honey or maple syrup, and warm water. Drink a half hour before each meal. A regular drink like this can help ease heartburn and chronic indigestion, soothe throat irritation, halt hiccups, and for many people, improve memory.

• **Yogurt** is an intestinal cleanser that helps balance and replace friendly flora in the G.I. tract. Yogurt is nutrient-dense, providing a wealth of proteins, vitamins, and minerals (more protein and calcium than milk). The culturing process makes yogurt a living food. Most yogurt contains the beneficial bacteria *lactobacillus bulgaricus* and *streptococcus thermophilus*; some have extra *lactobacillus acidophilus*. Yogurt is dairy in origin, but is far better tolerated than regular dairy foods, because yogurt itself stimulates lactase activity. Bacterial fermentation elements in yogurt actually substitute for the missing enzyme lactase.

Yogurt has wide-ranging health benefits:
—helps lower bad cholesterol and raise protective lipoprotein levels (HDL's)
—boosts blood levels of gamma interferon to rally killer cells to fight infections
—enzymes in yogurt cultures help lessen intolerance for lactase-deficient people
—a good source of absorbable calcium, yogurt strengthens against osteoporosis
—helps decrease diarrhea in children, especially when exacerbated by antibiotics
—yogurt lactic acid bacteria lower enzymes responsible for developing colon cancer
—spoonable yogurt with fruit (or even veggies) is well adapted for older infants (after three months) through
    toddlers. Introduce it gradually into the diet when the child begins to eat solid foods, usually between
    four and six months.

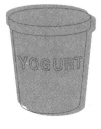

• **Yogurt cheese** is delicious, creamy, meltable, widely available in health food and gourmet stores. It's easy to make from regular plain yogurt, is much lighter in fat and calories than sour cream or cream cheese, but has the same richness and consistency.

—To make yogurt cheese: Spoon about 16-oz of plain yogurt onto a piece of cheesecloth or into a sieve-like plastic funnel (available from kitchen catalogs or hardware stores). Hang the cheesecloth over a kitchen sink faucet, or put the funnel over a large glass. It takes 14 to 16 hours for yogurt whey to drain out. Store in a covered container in the refrigerator; it keeps well for 2 to 3 weeks.

• **Low-fat cottage cheese** is a cultured dairy product, but okay for those with a slight lactose intolerance. It is a good substitute for ricotta, cream cheese, and chemical-filled cottage cheese foods. Mix with non-fat or low-fat plain yogurt to add the richness of cream or sour cream to recipes without the fat.

• **Kefir,** a Bedouin drink originally made with camel's milk, is today made from kefir grains or mother cultures prepared from grains. Kefir is a complete protein. It's full of biotin, B vitamins, especially B-12, calcium, magnesium and the amino acid tryptophan, for natural calm. In Russia, kefir is used medicinally as part of the treatment for metabolic and gastric disorders, tuberculosis, atherosclerosis, allergies, even cancer.

Kefir replenishes beneficial intestinal bacteria, producing lactic acid which balances stomach pH. Kefir is acidic when made, but becomes alkaline once ingested. Kefir's friendly bacteria contain partially digested proteins along with the minerals which contribute to the assimilation of proteins essential to healing.

—**Kefir cheese** is a delicious cultured food, low in fat and calories, similar to sour cream. Kefir cheese has a slighty tangy rich flavor that really enhances snack foods and raw vegetables like celery, cauliflower and carrots. Use it cup for cup in place of sour cream, cottage cheese, cream cheese or ricotta.

• **Cultured vegetables,** commonly called sauerkraut, from the Austrian words sauer (sour) and kraut (greens), are fresh veggies changed by fermentation into one of the richest food sources of lactobacilli and enzymes. They're loaded with vitamin C and minerals. Cultured vegetables improve digestion (especially for animal proteins and grains), and re-establish your inner ecosystem. The enzymes in cultured vegetables boost your own enzymes, especially those essential to cell rejuvenation, toxin elimination and immune response.

Raw cultured vegetables are pre-digested and alkaline-forming for better body balance. The lactobacilli in cultured veggies are star players in beating Candida albicans yeast overgrowth and controlling the cravings for sugary foods so common in candidiasis. Sauerkraut is also effective in treating peptic ulcers, ulcerative colitis, colic, various food allergies, cystitis, vaginal infections, constipation and digestive disorders.

However, the healing power of sauerkraut's probiotics and enzymes is only in unpasteurized sauerkraut. The sauerkraut that most Americans find on supermarket shelves is highly salted and pasteurized, with its lactobacilli and enzymes destroyed. Find effective cultured veggies instead at your health food store (in the refrigerated section) from Rejuvenative Foods, P.O. Box 8464, Santa Cruz, CA 95061, 408-462-6715.

If you can't find cultured veggies, here's how to make your own:

Cabbage is the main element of unheated, fresh sauerkraut. You can use green cabbage alone, or make a half-and-half blend of green and red.

For mixed cultured vegetables: chop or shred a small head of green cabbage and set aside. Use a food processor or blender for finer consistency. Chop a blend of other vegetables — like 1 beet, 2 carrots and 1 green bell pepper. Or make a Kim Chee blend of carrots, onions, red or yellow bell pepper, some fresh grated ginger and a little chili pepper. Place the veggies in a sanitary glass or stainless steel pot (never use plastic) and let sit for about 7 days at a moderate room temperature (59° to 71°). The naturally present enzymes, lactobacillus acidophilus, lactobacillus plantarum, and lactobacillus brevi in the vegetables proliferate, transforming the sugars and starches in the vegetables into lactic and acetic acids.

Refrigerate your cultured vegetables and eat them within six months. They'll hold their flavor, enzymes and lactobacillus cultures.

145

Water Is Essential For Healing

Your body goes down fast without water. Water is second only to oxygen in importance for health and just a few short days without water can be fatal! Making up almost three-fourths of the body, every cell is regulated, monitored and dependent on an efficient flow of water. Messages in the brain cells are transported on "water-ways" to the nerve endings. Water transports minerals, vitamins, proteins and sugars around the body for assimilation. Water maintains your body's equilibrium and temperature, lubricates tissues, flushes wastes and toxins, hydrates the skin, acts as a shock absorber for joints, bones and muscles, and adds needed minerals.

When your body gets enough water, it works at its peak. Fluid retention decreases, gland and hormone functions improve, the liver breaks down and releases more fat, hunger is curtailed. Dehydration plays a role in elimination ailments like chronic constipation and urinary tract infections, peripheral vascular problems like hemorrhoids and varicose veins, kidney stones, even many degenerative diseases like arthritis.

Experts tell us that thirst is an evolutionary development designed to indicate severe dehydration. Drinking only if you're thirsty may not be enough to keep your skin moist and supple, your brain sharp or your elimination systems regular. There's another side to the body water story. Many Americans have reduced their intake of fats (including the good Omega-3 fats and other essential fatty acids) to the point that their bodies don't hold and use the water they do take in. It's one of the reasons I regularly recommend adding sea greens to your diet for moister skin, shining eyes and lustrous hair.... a quality of sea plants known since ancient Greek times.

Water quality is poor in many areas of fluoridated, and treated to the point where instead of a healthful drink. City tap water ease-causing bacteria, viruses and para- tion of aluminum from deodorants, cern for Alzheimer's dementia. their way into our ground water, add- without the enormous effort our ingested enough of them to turn us people from drinking tap water. Keep hooked to your fridge will make your the U.S. Most tap water is chlorinated, it can be an irritating, disagreeable fluid may contain as many as 500 different dis- sites. Fluoridated water increases absorp- pots and pans, etc. by 600%, a possible con- Chemicals used by industry and agriculture find ing more pollutants. Some tap water is so bad, that bodies exert to dispose of these chemicals, we would have to stone by the time we were thirty! These concerns keep many plenty of bottled water near at hand. Purifiers or a purifier tap water more drinkable.

Should you drink more water? Here's how your body uses it up every day. Your kidneys receive and filter your entire blood supply 15 times each hour! If you become overheated, your 2 million sweat glands perspire to cool your skin and keep your internal organs at a constant temperature, using 99% water. You use a small amount of water during breathing and through tear ducts that lubricate the upper eyelids 25 times per minute. Crying and hearty laughter release water from your eyes and nose. Even normal activity uses up at least 3 quarts of replacement water each day. Strenuous activity, a hot climate or a high salt diet increases this requirement.

What happens when you don't get enough water? A chain reaction begins.
1: a water shortage message is sent from your brain;
2: your kidneys conserve water by urinating less (constipation and bloating occur);
3: at 4 percent water depletion, muscle endurance diminishes — you start to get dizzy;
4: at 5 percent water loss, headaches from mild to quite severe begin — you get drowsy, lose the ability to concentrate and get unreasonably impatient;
5: at 6 percent water loss, body temperature is impaired — your heart begins to race.
6: at 7 percent body water depletion, there is a good possibility of collapse.

To tell whether or not you're drinking enough water, check your urine. The color should be a pale straw and you should urinate every few hours. If your urine color is dark yellow, start drinking more water!

Other common signs that you might be dehydrated:
- —unexplained headaches (mild to severe), usually with some dizziness
- —unexplained irritability, impatience, restlessness and difficulty sleeping
- —unusually dry skin and loss of appetite along with constipation
- —dull back pain that is not relieved by rest
- —unexplained weight gain and swollen hands and-or feet (from water retention)

Gradual loss of body water is an aging factor. It is a major complication in illness. Dehydration is reportedly one of the top 10 causes of hospital stays among the elderly. Some studies show thirst-impaired seniors do not even seek water when they need it because their sense of thirst is so impaired. For many elderly people, fear of urinary incontinence makes them drink less liquid — doubly unfortunate because water hydration at all levels, from body cleansing to skin beauty is a protection against accelerated aging.

Water is critical for an effective detoxification program because it dilutes and eliminates toxin accumulations in the bloodstream, and cleanses the kidneys. Add half a squeezed lemon to each glass of water for the best cleansing effects. The best time to detoxify is at night, while you sleep.

Water is your most important catalyst in losing weight and keeping it off. It naturally suppresses appetite and helps your body metabolize stored fat. Low water intake causes fat deposits to increase — more water intake actually reduces fat deposits. If you are overweight, the more body fat you have, the less system water you have. Larger people have larger metabolic loads — they need more water.

Thirst is not a reliable signal that your body needs water.

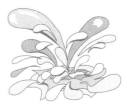

By the time you feel thirsty, you are probably already suffering from some degree of dehydration. Thirst is an evolutionary development, controlled by a part of the fore-brain called the hypothalamus, (which also controls sleep, appetite, satiety, and sexual response) designed to alert us to severe dehydration. So you can easily lose a quart of water during activity before thirst is even recognized.

Solving the dehydration problem: Human bodies have some strange anomalies. We have to plan for our water supply. From an early adult age our thirst sensation begins to fail, putting us inexplicably at risk for dehydration. Even more strange, our thirst signal shuts off before we have had enough for well-being.

Where does your body get its daily replacement water? Plain or carbonated cool water is the best way to replace body fluids but other healthy liquids beside water count as replenishment. Unsweetened fruit juices diluted with water or seltzer, and vegetable juices should be considered. Foods provide up to $1^1/_2$ quarts. Fruits and vegetables are more than 90% water. Even dry foods like bread are about 35% water. Digestive processes yield as much as a pint a day for metabolism.

Remember:
- —Alcohol and caffeine drinks are counter-productive for water replacement because they are diuretic.
- —Drinks loaded with dissolved sugars or milk increase water needs instead of satisfying them.
- —Commercial sodas leach several important minerals from your body.

Even though most of us don't get enough water today, drinking too much water can have some adverse health effects. It can severely depress electrolytes, imperative to vibrant energy, pH balance and mineral uptake. Purified water, such as distilled or reverse osmosis techniques compound the problem.

It sounds like a lot, but eight to ten 8-ounce glasses of water daily is a sufficient amount. If you are physically active or working under hot weather conditions, you'll need more. Replace lost electrolytes with electrolyte drinks like Alacer EMERGEN-C, or supplement drinks like Bragg's LIQUID AMINOS.

Are you worried about retaining too much water, or getting water logged? Believe it or not, drinking more water is the best treatment against retaining fluid!

When you don't get the water you need, your body holds onto the water it has. Diuretics are only a temporary solution because you'll end up ravenously thirsty as your body tries to replace the water that the diuretics flush out. (See "What happens when you don't get enough water," previous page.) Diuretics also have a compromising effect on important nutrients like potassium. Overcome a water retention problem by giving your body what it needs — **plenty of water**. When your body has the right amount, it will naturally release the excess.

Hydrate before, during and after exercise. You may not be pushing yourself to the brink of collapse, but even 30 minutes of exercise can put you at risk for dehydration. Humans sweat more than any mammal; normal exercise causes a loss of one to two quarts of fluid every hour of a workout. Sweat acts as your body's air conditioner, keeping your muscles (which generate 8 to 10 times more heat during exercise), cooled. Take in water, juice or an electrolyte drink during your workout to maintain fluid needs.

If you're exercising in hot weather, drink about 20-ounces of fluid two hours before your workout, even if you aren't thirsty. This gives your body time to absorb what it needs. Drink another 8-oz. about 15 minutes before you exercise. During exercise, drink 8-oz. of water or an electrolyte drink every 20 minutes. Don't wait until you feel thirsty. You may already be one or two quarts low. When your workout is over, weigh yourself. The scale may show some weight loss, but it's not fat loss — it's water. Conditioned athletes drink a pint of water for every pound lost during a workout.

For a healing program, several types of water are worth consideration.
—**Mineral water** comes from natural springs with varying mineral content and widely varying taste. The natural minerals are beneficial to digestion and regularity. In Europe, bottled mineral water has become a fine art, but in the U.S., it isn't tested for purity except in California and Florida.

—**Distilled water** can be from a spring or tap source; it is "de-mineralized" so that only oxygen and hydrogen remain. Distilling is accomplished by reverse osmosis, filtering or boiling, then converting to steam and recondensing. It is the purest water available.

—**Sparkling water** comes from natural carbonation in underground springs. Most bottles are also artificially infused with CO_2 to maintain a standard fizz. This water aids digestion, and is excellent in cooking to tenderize and give lightness to a recipe.

—**Artesian well water** is the Cadillac of natural waters. It always comes from a deep uncontaminated source, has a slight fizz from bubbling up under rock pressure, and is tapped by a drilled well.

Water fluoridation's tainted history

Historically, water fluoridation is mandated by governments but rejected by citizens. The controversy has raged since fluoride was introduced in 1945. Most developed countries have banned fluorides in their water. Japan has rejected fluoridation. Europe is 98% fluoridation-free, with active opposition in Britain, Australia and New Zealand. Yet, today in the U.S. , the federal government continues to push for the mass fluoridation of the American water supply.

Even many in our government don't think it's a good idea. On July 2, 1997, the union representing all toxicologists, chemists, biologists and other professionals at the Environmental Protection Agency in Washington, D.C., went on record against the practice of adding fluoride to public drinking water, stating "As the professionals who are charged with assessing the safety of drinking water, we conclude that the health and welfare of the public is not served by the addition of fluoride to the public water supply."

The fluoridated water controversy affects every city and county in America.

If you're like most people, finding out the truth about our public water supply is a shock. After extensive research into the history of fluoride use and its results over the last two decades, as well as many conversations with scientists and knowledgeable, holistic dentists, I feel that no other substance added to food or water poses the health risks that fluoride does. Fluoride is in almost all commercial toothpastes and regularly added to over 60% of public drinking water. Today, mandatory water fluoridation throughout the U.S. is either about to begin or has already been instituted.

We need to dispel the myths about fluoride. It could mean your health....

Fiction: Fluoride is safe for humans.

Fact 1: Fluoride is more toxic than lead, and even in minute doses, is damaging to brain/mind development of children. In areas where fluorosis (fluoride poisoning) is prevalent, a higher concentration of fluoride is found in fetal brain tissue of unborn children.

Fact 2: Some studies show that fluoride is linked to Alzheimer's and senile dementia. One link appears to come through a fluoride-aluminum combination in the brain. A new study shows fluoride increases the body's absorption of aluminum from deodorants, or pots and pans by over 600%! The aluminum concentration in the brains of Alzheimer's patients is 15 times higher than in healthy individuals.

Fact 3: Hip fracture rates are much higher in people living in fluoridated communities. Fluoride's cumulative effect on bone density is devastating.

Fact 4: Postmenopausal women, people over 50, people with nutrient deficiencies and people with cardiovascular and kidney problems are especially affected by fluoride exposure. Our own U.S. Dept. of Health and Human Services stated in its Toxicological Profile (1993) that "postmenopausal women and elderly men in fluoridated communities may be at increased risk for bone fractures."

Fiction: Calcium fluoride found naturally in water is safe.

Fact 1: All forms of fluoride are poisonous. The most toxic forms are those with a higher solubility of free fluoride ions such as in hydrofluosilicic acid, a hazardous waste product of the phosphate fertilizer which is the substance routinely added to fluoridate water.

Fiction: Fluoride reduces tooth decay.

Fact 1: National survey data by the National Institute of Dental Research shows that children who live in fluoridated areas have tooth decay rates almost identical with those who live in non-fluoridated areas. Even large-scale studies show no difference in decay rates of permanent teeth in fluoridated and non-fluoridated areas. In fact, in a recent study by the New York Department of Health, children who drink fluoridated water have more cavities and tooth discoloration than children who drink non fluoridated water.

Fact 2: The U.S. National Research Council admits that dental fluorosis (fluoride poisoning causing teeth to become brittle and chip easily) affects from 8% to 51% of children drinking fluoridated water. Dental fluorosis has steadily increased since the introduction of fluoride to drinking water in 1945.

Fiction: Mandatory water fluoridation is safe for the American population.

Fact 1: Evidence from animal and human epidemiology studies links fluoride exposure to cancer, genetic damage, nervous system dysfunction and bone diseases. Fluoride exposure is also linked to low IQ in children.

Fiction: Fluoride toothpaste is safe and prevents cavities.

Fact 1: A University of Arizona study finds that the more fluoride a child drinks, the more cavities appear.

Fact 2: The poison control center receives over 11,000 calls a year for poisoning from ingesting fluoride toothpaste. In 1997, the FDA even mandated a poison warning label on fluoride toothpaste! Small children, who tend to swallow toothpaste are most at risk. Signs of fluoride poisoning include vomiting and muscle cramps. Look for non-fluoridated toothpastes like Nature's Gate SPEARMINT or CINNAMON TOOTHPASTE at your health food store. My own favorite is the Ayurvedic herb peelu (literally "tree for tooth care"). Peelu is a natural antibacterial that removes tartar and has natural chlorine to help whiten teeth.

As we enter the millennium our country's water supply is in a grave situation. Americans need to work hard to stop mandatory water fluoridation before it's too late. It isn't just the water we drink, it's the food we eat, too. Crops watered with fluoridated water mean fluoride is leeched into our fruits and vegetables. Not even organic produce is safe from fluoride in the water supply.

After forced fluoridation by its public health service, the city of Natick, Mass mailed its water bills with a warning that pregnant women, parents of children under 3 years, and anyone with fluoride sensitivity should consult their physicians before drinking city water. Santa Cruz, California became the first city in California (following the state fluoridation mandate of Oct. 1995) to pass an ordinance to prevent its waters from being fluoridated. Other California cities are jumping on the "no fluoridation" bandwagon as their citizens become aware and alarmed about water safety.

Massive fluoridation in our water, food, beverages, and dental products may cause massive fluoride poisoning in the U.S. population. I equate it to something like the widespread lead poisoning that decimated the health of Romans, especially the children, 2000 years ago.

If you want to help stop mandatory water fluoridation, contact David C. Kennedy, D.D.S. @ Citizens for Safe Drinking Water 2425 3rd Ave, San Diego, CA 92101, 888-728-3833.

or E-mail: davidkennedy-dds@home.com- jgreen@abac.com

For more information about fluoride, check the internet: www.sonic.net/~kryptox/fluoride.htm; or www.cadvision.com/fluoride.

—No one deserves the right to lead without first perservering through pain and heartache and failure.

—People who are really worth following have paid their dues. They have come through the furnace melted, beaten, tempered and re-shaped.

Caffeine In A Healing Diet?

Like most of mankind's other pleasures, there is good news and bad news about caffeine. Moderate use of caffeine has been hailed for centuries for its therapeutic benefits. Every major culture uses caffeine in some food form to overcome fatigue, handle pain, open breathways, control weight and jump-start circulation.

Caffeine is a plant-derived nutraceutical — it's a food with medicinal attributes. Coffee, black tea, colas, sodas, chocolate and cocoa, analgesics like Excedrin, and over-the-counter stimulants like Vivarin, all contain caffeine. Taking regular aspirin or an herbal pain reliever with a caffeine drink increases the pain relieving effects.

Caffeine absorbs rapidly into the bloodstream. In just a few minutes, it enters all organs and tissues. Within an hour after ingestion, it is distributed in body tissues in proportion to their water content. Caffeine remains in the body for only about three hours and is then excreted in the urine; it does not accumulate in body tissue.

Caffeine is an effective short-term energy booster. It mobilizes fatty acids into the circulatory system, allowing greater energy production, endurance and work output. It has a direct potentiating effect on muscle contraction for both long and short-term sports and workout activity.

Caffeine shows solid evidence of its effects on clearer mental performance and shortened reaction times. Caffeine stimulates serotonin, a brain neurotransmitter produced by tryptophan, that increases the capacity for intellectual tasks and alertness by releasing adrenaline into the bloodstream. The net effect also decreases drowsiness and improves mood.

Caffeine's benefits for weight loss have long been known. Caffeine promotes weight control because it enhances thermogenesis, the conversion of stored body fat to energy. Oftentimes, overweight dieters don't burn enough calories to produce normal heat during dieting. When caffeine is added to their diet, obese and post-obese people respond with greater thermogenesis.

Even relatively small, commonly consumed doses of caffeine significantly influence calorie burning. Caffeine actually raises metabolic rate, and the rise lasts for several hours, far beyond its direct stimulation.

One study shows that a single dose of 100mg. of caffeine (the amount in one cup of coffee) increased metabolic rate 4% for up to three hours! When the same amount of caffeine was consumed at two-hour intervals for 12 hours, metabolic rate increased between 8 to 11%. These metabolic increases seem small, but over several months there is steady, substantial weight loss.

The same study shows that low doses of caffeine help weight control after initial weight loss because caffeine blocks appetite while keeping calorie-burning efficient.

Caffeine stimulates the nervous system and heart action, relaxes smooth muscles in the digestive tract and blood vessels, increases urine flow, enhances stomach acid secretion and boosts muscle strength. New research in India reports that caffeine, taken with antioxidant supplements, provides powerful protection against DNA damage caused by free radicals by altering the behavior of a gene-damaging chemical. The DNA-protective effect was stronger with the combined coffee-antioxidant regimen than with either coffee or antioxidants alone.

Olfactory hallucinations are an unexpected effect of the new caffeine research. When given caffeine intravenously, sleeping volunteers awoke recalling smells of wet hay, dirty socks and ammonia from their childhood.

Caffeine's health problems are also well known. *In excessive amounts,* caffeine has drug-like activity, causing jumpiness, nerves and heart palpitations. *In excessive amounts,* caffeine can produce oxalic acid in the system, causing health problems waiting to become diseases. It can lodge in the liver, restricting proper function, and constrict arterial blood flow. It leaches B vitamins from the body, particularly thiamine, which is needed for stress control. It depletes essential minerals, including calcium and potassium.

Like any addictive substance, caffeine is difficult to overcome, but if you have caffeine-related health problems, it is worth going through the temporary withdrawal symptoms. Improvement in the health condition is often noticed right away.

Decide for yourself. Here are the caffeine links to specific health concerns:
• **Caffeine and Bone Health:** excessive caffeine causes calcium depletion increasing risk of osteoporosis. (Moderate amounts do not cause calcium depletion or contribute to bone loss.)

• **Caffeine and Fertility:** caffeine seems to affect women's health more than men's. Some experts say the more coffee a woman drinks the less likely she is to conceive, but new studies show there is no relationship between a morning cup of coffee and infertility.

• **Caffeine and Pregnancy:** avoid caffeine during pregnancy. Like alcohol, it can cross the placenta and affect the fetus' brain, central nervous system and circulation.

• **Caffeine and PMS:** reduce, rather than avoid caffeine during menses. Caffeine causes congestion through cellular overproduction of fibrous tissue and cyst fluids. Yet low-dose caffeine intake improves memory and alertness during menses.

• **Caffeine and Breast Disease:** the link between caffeine and breast fibroids isn't official, but there is almost immediate improvement when caffeine is decreased or avoided.

• **Caffeine and Menopause:** caffeine is a trigger for hot flashes in menopausal women, and can provoke night time panic attacks in some women.

• **Caffeine and Sleep:** caffeine consumed late in the day or at night disrupts brain wave patterns. You'll take longer to get to sleep.

• **Caffeine and Severe Blood Sugar Swings:** caffeine causes the liver to release glycogen which triggers insulin release, and a sharp blood sugar drop within 1 to 2 hours.

• **Caffeine and Exhausted Adrenal Glands:** excessive caffeine exhausts the adrenals by releasing too much adrenaline, so you have less resistance to stress and are more vulnerable to hormone imbalances that affect health in both men and women.

• **Caffeine and Cancer:** studies on caffeine and cancer, particularly bladder and organ cancers, show a link but no definite causal relationship. Further, the carcinogenic effects blamed on caffeine are now thought to be caused by the hydrocarbon roasting process used in making coffee, since decaffeinated coffee is also implicated in some organ cancers. I believe the acidic body state promoted by caffeine is not beneficial to the healing process as the body works to normalize its chemistry during healing.

• **Caffeine and Heart Disease:** heavy coffee drinking (more than 4 cups a day), has been directly implicated in heart disease. New research shows caffeine may increase homocysteine, an amino acid whose high levels contribute to heart disease. Moderate caffeine does not appear to increase heart disease risk.

• **Caffeine and High Blood Pressure:** excessive caffeine can elevate blood pressure significantly and produce nervous anxiety. Watch out when caffeine is combined with phenyl-propanolamine, the appetite suppressant in most commercial diet pills.

• **Caffeine and Ulcers:** caffeine is not linked to gastric or duodenal ulcers, but it stimulates gastric secretions, sometimes leading to a nervous stomach or heartburn. On the good side, caffeine is a "bitter" food, stimulating bile secretion for good digestion.

• **Caffeine and Headaches:** caffeine causes headaches in some people — and withdrawal headaches when eliminated after regular use. Strangely enough, coffee is a niacin-rich healing remedy for temporary relief of migraine headaches (the niacin content of coffee increases when the beans are roasted).

• **Caffeine and Asthma:** caffeine reduces asthma symptoms by dilating lung and nasal passages. Regular caffeine consumption reduces wheezing considerably. Some researchers believe this is why asthma symptoms decrease when children become adults.

Caffeine in common foods: (a pharmacologically active dose of caffeine is about 200 mg)

CAFFEINE FOOD	APPROXIMATE CAFFEINE
Coffee — 5-oz. cup Decaf	4mg
Coffee — 5-oz. cup Instant	65mg
Coffee — 5-oz. cup Percolated	110mg
Coffee — 5-oz. cup Drip	135mg
Tea — 5-oz. cup Bag, brewed 3 minutes	45mg
Tea — 5-oz. cup Loose, black, brewed 3 minutes	55mg
Tea — 5-oz. cup Loose, green, brewed 3 minutes	35mg
Tea — 5-oz. cup Iced	30mg
Cola — 12-oz. glass	45mg
Chocolate/Cocoa — 5-oz. cup	10mg
Milk chocolate — 1-oz	10mg
Bittersweet Chocolate — 1-oz	30mg

You can break the caffeine habit with herb teas, caffeine-free coffee substitutes, and energy supportive herbal pick-me-ups with no harmful stimulants of any kind. Use green tea and kola nut as bio-active forms of caffeine for weight loss and mental clarity. Neither has the heated hydrocarbons of coffee.

Tea And Your Healing Diet

Black and green teas have caffeine. Is it different than the caffeine in coffee or chocolate? All black, green and Oolong teas come from one plant, *thea sinensis*, an incredibly productive shrub that ranges from the Mediterranean to the tropics. Tea leaves can be harvested every 6 to 14 days for 25 to 50 years!

Tea is defined by the way its leaves are processed. For green tea, the first tender leaves of spring are picked, rolled, steamed, crushed and dried with hot air. Green tea leaves are not fermented. Oolong tea leaves are semi-fermented for one hour. Black tea is fermented for 3 hours, then often scented with spices to strengthen aroma and reduce bitterness.

How does tea fit into a healing diet? Both green tea and black tea have enzymes that promote digestion and help our bodies resist harmful bacteria, like *Staphylococcus aureus*. High flavonoids in both teas reduce harmful blood clotting linked to heart attacks. Both contain polyphenols (not tannins as commonly believed) that act as antioxidants, yet do not interfere with iron or protein absorption. The natural, bioactive caffeine contained in both black tea (50 to 80mg per cup) and green tea (about 30mg per cup) helps combat mental fatigue.

But far more health benefits lie in green tea. It contains larger amounts of healing nutrients, including twice as much vitamin C, more than twice the amount of bioflavonoid activity (two cups a day of green tea can meet your body's daily needs for bioflavonoids), and six times the antioxidant properties of black tea. Green tea is highly enzyme-active for weight loss. It is a good fasting tea, providing energy support and clearer thinking during cleansing. Green tea is a vasodilator and smooth muscle relaxer with theophylline for bronchial dilation against asthma.

Should you be drinking a daily cup of green tea for better health? Science validates green tea's health benefits. Most studies center around the over 200 different catechin polyphenol compounds that comprise up to 35% of green tea. The polyphenols lower cholesterol, and protect against cancer by thwarting nitrosamines that produce cancer-causing substances. Research at the American Health Foundation in N.Y. shows that green tea's anticarcinogens are anti-mutants "preventing activation of carcinogens so that free radicals never even form."

One green tea compound, EECG (epigallocatechin-3 gallate), has formidably high levels of free-radical-scavenging activity. Green tea's EECG is 30 times more powerful than vitamin E against DNA-destroying attacks. Black tea loses its EECG and other beneficial polyphenols entirely during fermentation.

Scientists also believe EECG is the substance that inhibits the enzyme urokinase, crucial for cancer growth and metastasis. EECG attaches to urokinase and prevents it from invading cells to form tumors. Some cancer tests show that EECG may even engender a process called apoptosis, in which cancer cells shrivel and die.

More amazing, research shows that green tea's caffeine may be the synergistic delivery system for therapeutic catechins like EECG. A cup of green tea contains 100-200mg of EGCG. Scientists believe two to four cups per day could provide cancer protection.

Green tea has an astounding catalog of curative applications.
—Green tea is antibacterial, a quality known for 5,000 years ago by the Chinese, who used it to purify water. Green tea polyphenols have wide-ranging antimicrobial action against food poisoning, and *streptococcus mutans*, a mouth bacterium that causes tooth decay and may cause serious illness if it establishes in the heart valve. Tea polyphenols bind to mouth bacteria as a shield to strengthen tooth enamel against plaque.

Note: Don't add milk to green tea. Milk inhibits absorption of the protective polyphenols.

—Green tea also provides a protective effect against both esophageal and oral cancers, according to the American National Cancer Institute. *Note: To fully benefit from green tea's anti-cancer properties, pour hot, not boiling water over the tea leaves.*

—A dual study by the Shanghai Cancer Institute and the U.S. National Cancer Institute shows that drinking green tea once a week for six months means less risk for colon and pancreatic cancers, with benefits stronger for women. (The same study showed that green tea increased female fertility through its body-balancing effects.)

—Green tea may reduce the risk of several forms of environmentally induced cancers. Research in Japan on stomach, skin and lung cancers (where people drink large amounts of strong green tea) show a low incidence of these cancers. The large Japanese study recorded that drinking several cups of green tea on a daily basis was effective in reducing lung cancer death rates even in men who smoked two packs of cigarettes a day. Smoking is far more prevalent in Japan than in the U.S., but the instance of lung cancer is much lower, indicating to researchers that green tea protects against lung cancer.

—Green tea may protect our skin against radiation damage. As the ozone layer thins and UV radiation increases, skin cancers have risen throughout the world. In a Rutgers University study, green tea showed good results against skin cancer when it was taken before and during exposure to UV rays.
Green tea is an antimicrobial skin refresher. Acne, cuts, sunburn and athlete's foot all benefit from a cool green tea bath.

—Green tea is a significant heart health protector. Its catechins are potent inhibitors of blood clumping which leads to atherosclerosis. The catechins also suppress the formation of the angiotensin I conversion enzyme which contributes to high blood pressure.

—Green tea stabilizes and increases elimination of harmful blood lipids to prevent the oxidation of LDL cholesterol. University of Kansas research shows that green tea is over 100 times more effective than vitamin C at protecting cells from damage from heart disease, and is 25 times more effective than vitamin E as a heart protecting antioxidant.

—Green tea helps dieters because it pro-   motes fat burning, regulates blood sugar and insulin, and has a satiating and tension calming effect during dieting.

Tea nomenclature can be confusing. Names like oolong, black or jasmine tea refer to how the tea leaf process. Names like Assam, Darjeeling or Ceylon, etc., refer to country or region where the tea is grown. Names like pekoe, orange pekoe, etc., refer to leaf size.

- **Green tea (bancha)** - tender spring leaves of the Japanese tea plant. (See above.)
- **Green tea (kukicha)** - made from roasted twigs rather than the leaves of the tea plant. Kukicha is a favorite in macrobiotic diets for its blood cleansing qualities, high available calcium and mellow, smooth flavor.
- **Darjeeling** - the finest, most delicately flavored of the black Indian teas.
- **Earl Grey** - a popular, hearty, aromatic black tea scented with bergamot oil.
- **English Breakfast** - a connoisseur's rich, mellow, fragrant black tea.
- **Ceylon** - a tea grown in Sri Lanka with an intense, flowery aroma and flavor.
- **Irish Breakfast** - a combination of Assam and Ceylon flowery orange pekoes.
- **Jasmine** - a black tea scented with white jasmine flowers during firing.
- **Lapsang Souchong** - a fine black tea with a strong, smoky flavor.
- **Oolong** - a complex, delicate tea, semi-fermented, fired in baskets over hot coals.

Does Wine Fit Into A Healing Diet?

Naturally fermented wine is still a living food. It is a complex biological fluid possessing definite physiological values. Records dating back 4,000 years refer to wine as a food, a medicine, a part of religious ceremonies and a pleasing element in social life.

Wine is much more than an alcoholic beverage — vastly more complex than beer or spirits; it is never boiled, so its biologically active compounds are not destroyed or altered by heat. Many small, family owned wineries make chemical-free, additive-free wines that retain their nutrients, including B vitamins, and minerals like potassium, magnesium, calcium, organic sodium, iron and phosphorus.

Wine has significant health benefits. In moderation, it is a mild tranquilizer for the heart and blood pressure. U.C. Davis research on wine tannins shows that a glass or two of wine a day may cut coronary heart disease risk by 50%, help prevent blood clot formation, and considerably reduce stress. Tannin-rich red wine reduces blood platelet stickiness, increases good cholesterol levels, and lowers dangerous cholesterol levels to protect against heart disease.

Wine is a cultured food. It mented foods. Wine boosts circulation, production. It is superior to tranquiliz-portant in a weight loss program, be-relaxed, you tend to eat less.

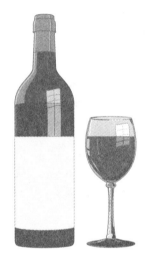

helps digestion like yogurt and other fer-relieves pain and reduces excess body acid ers or drugs for nervous tension. It is im-cause a glass of wine relaxes. When you are

Wine is full of antioxidants. is rich in polyphenols, powerful anti-which damage DNA and alter body its carotenes like lutein and zeaxanthin, new study reveals that just drinking 2 to macular degeneration (the leading cause percent. A study of wine antioxidants by polyphenols even help prevent hepatitis

Studies at U.C. Berkeley show that red wine oxidants that help neutralize free radicals chemistry. Wine antioxidants, along with are significant protectors for the eyes. A 4 glass of wine a month can cut the risk of of blindness in people over 60) by over 20 the journal Epidemiology shows that its A virus replication.

Wine is a more powerful anti-microbial against common bacteria than some drugs. It can, for example, reduce the growth of some harmful stomach bacteria colonies within 20 minutes. Bismuth salicylate, a pharmaceutical remedy for traveller's diarrhea, takes two hours to do the same job. The latest research shows wine can successfully address the food and water-borne micro-organisms that cause digestive havoc and upset tummies referred to as "Delhi belly" and "Montezuma's revenge."

There's much more...

—**Quercetin,** an antioxidant flavonoid in red wine may be one of the most powerful anticancer agents ever discovered. Early results show that quercetin reverses tumor development by blocking the conversion of normal body cells to cancer cells. Quercetin activity is boosted by the wine fermentation process and by friendly flora in our intestinal tracts. Quercetin also normalizes insulin release levels, so it prevents some complications of diabetes like cataracts, diabetic retinopathy (blindness), neuropathy (nerve damage) and nephropathy (kidney damage). Doctors use quercetin in wine as a potent free radical scavenger against HIV infection, because wine also relieves AIDS pain and stress.

—**Resveratrol,** a compound in red grape skins, is a key to wine drinkers' healthy cholesterol levels. Resveratrol also seems to prevent blood platelet aggregation, and reduce blood clotting in arteries narrowed by years of heavy fat consumption. In nature, **resveratrol** fights off fungal disease for the grape plants. In animal tests, resveratrol stops production of abnormal cells, like cancer cells at three separate stages of development — inhibiting the enzyme cyclo-oxygenase that stimulates tumor growth.

Are sulfites in wine really a health hazard? Sulfur dioxide (SO_2) is a naturally occurring sulfite that protects the wine's character by inhibiting the growth of molds and bacteria. Wine yeasts naturally produce up to 20 parts per million of SO_2 during fermentation. (Human bodies produce about 1,000mg of sulfites a day in our normal biochemical processes.) Top European winemakers have counted on sulfur dioxide to prevent wine spoilage for centuries. In a method used since Roman, even Egyptian times, today's winemakers use mined SO_2 heated into a liquid, to protect wine from oxidizing.

What is organic wine? The health dangers of pesticides on grapes mean that wines made from organically grown grapes are increasingly popular in both Europe and California. To a purist, organic wine means wine made from organically-grown grapes, without using sulfites, yeast, bentonite, egg whites, gasses like N_2 or CO_2 in the process. To most people an "organic" wine label signifies only whether sulfites have been added or not.

In 1988, following a food-borne sulfites scare, the U.S. ATF required alcoholic beverages of all kinds, both imported and domestic, to carry a "CONTAINS SULFITES" label if there were more than 10 parts per million sulfites in the beverage, regardless of whether sulfites had actually been added. This hasty ruling became, and still is, a major problem for winemakers, especially when wine has naturally-occurring sulfites at this level.

Are both red and white wines healthy? Research shows that phenol compounds in both red and white wine reduce LDL oxidation, platelet formation and fat buildup in your arteries. Both white and red wines seem to be protective for women against heart disease.

Note: I don't recommend liquor other than wine, even for cooking, during a healing program. Although most people can stand a little hard liquor without undue effect, and alcohol burns off in cooking, concentrated sugar residues won't help a recovering body.

America's motto is live free or die....
not live free or whine.

The American Constitution says the
pursuit of happiness....
not the department of happiness,
or happiness therapy,
or happiness stamps.

Fats & Oils In A Healing Diet

The debate about fat has filled the American media for more than a decade, but much of the information is contradictory and inaccurate. Most people know today that there is a direct relationship between the quantity of fat we consume and the quality of health we can expect. **Yet, in the last half of the 20th century, Americans have increased their intake of fat calories (especially omega-6 fats) by over 33%.**

The link between high salt and fat intake on health has also become clear. **Too much salt inhibits the body's capacity to clear fat from the blood.** Yet, in the last thirty years, Americans have consumed more salt than ever before, largely because we eat almost 50% more restaurant and pre-prepared foods than our parents did. Much of this food is fried and salty, or salt-preserved (animal foods), and full of spicy or salty condiments.

But not all fats are alike. We need to clear up the confusion about fats and oils, so you can make the best choices for your healing diet. Regardless of its "bad press," our bodies need fat to keep warm, protect body tissues and organs, and supply us with energy. Fat is the most concentrated source of energy in our diets, providing nine calories per gram of energy compared to four calories per gram from carbohydrates or protein. Fat even helps us use carbohydrates and proteins more efficiently by slowing down digestive processes.

Fat supplies essential fatty acids, (see page 160.) We need fat for healthy skin, to metabolize cholesterol and for prostaglandin balance. Fat releases a hormone in the stomach called cholecystokinin that sends the brain a "full" message when we have satisfied hunger so we don't overeat. We need fat in order to absorb critical fat-soluble vitamins A, D, E and K. Fats elevate calcium levels and transport calcium for strong bones and elastic muscles.

What is the difference between saturated, poly-unsaturated and mono-unsaturated fats?
The difference is in molecular structure. All fat molecules are composed of carbon and hydrogen atoms. A saturated fatty acid has the maximum possible number of hydrogen atoms attached to every carbon atom — hence the term "saturated." An unsaturated fatty acid is missing one pair of hydrogen atoms in the middle of the molecule — a gap called an "unsaturation." A fatty acid with one gap is said to be "monounsaturated." Fatty acids missing more than one pair of hydrogen atoms are called "polyunsaturated."

Animal foods have more saturated fat, and except for palm and coconut oil, plant foods have more unsaturated fats. Saturated fats, like butter, meat and dairy fats, shortening and lard, are solid at room temperature. They are the culprits that clog the arteries, and lead to heart disease. Saturated fats tend to thicken the blood, causing blood pressure to rise and increasing the work load on your heart. They also promote blood stickiness, exaggerate plaque build up on the arteries and reduce oxygen availability to your heart muscle. Unsaturated fats, both mono and poly-unsaturated, like seafood, plant or nut oils, are liquid at room temperature. Although research supports unsaturated fats as helping to reduce cholesterol, just switching to unsaturated fats without increasing dietary fiber will not bring about health improvement. For the best benefits, eat moderate amounts of unsaturated fats along with a high fiber diet.

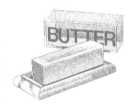

Is there a health difference between polyunsaturated and monounsaturated fats?
—Mono-unsaturated fats, in seafoods, avocados, nuts, olive oil, canola and peanut oil, are considered the healthiest fats. Mono-unsaturated oils are rich in fatty acids and important for normalizing prostaglandin levels. Tests show that eating moderate amounts of unrefined, mono-unsaturated oils also considerably lower allergic reactions.

—Polyunsaturated fats, in seafoods, walnuts and vegetable oils, are healthier than saturated fats, but not as healthy as monounsaturated fats. Poly-unsaturated vegetable oils are good sources for "essential fatty acids" (linoleic, linolenic and arachidonic) necessary for cell membrane function, balanced prostaglandin production and metabolic processes. Good poly-unsaturates include: sunflower, safflower, sesame oil, and flax oil.

Are all plant oils unsaturated fats? All plant oils are cholesterol-free, but commercial oils go through several processing stages to prevent rancidity.

—Refined oils are degummed, de-pigmented through charcoal or clay, clarified by deodorizing under high heat, and chemically preserved. Unfortunately, processing also destroys healthy antioxidants and forms hazardous free radicals. Refined oils are clear, odorless..... and almost totally devoid of nutrients.

—Unrefined vegetable oils are the least processed and most natural. They are mechanically pressed and filtered (cold pressing applies only to olive oil). They have small amounts of sediment, and taste and smell like the nut, seed or fruit they came from.

—Solvent-extracted oil is a second pressing from the first pressing residue. The petroleum chemical hexane is generally used to get the most efficient extraction; even though minute amounts of hexane remain, it is still considered an unrefined oil.

Note 1: Vegetable oils are traditionally seen as top dietary sources of essential fatty acids. New research shows this to be true only of cold pressed oils. Commercial oils contain such a large number of contaminants and are so heavily processed that they can no longer be regarded as good sources of EFAs.

Note 2: Heat and air exposure easily cause unrefined oils to spoil, so store them in an air-tight container in a cool dark cupboard (65°F) or the fridge. Purchase small bottles if you don't use much oil in your cooking.

What are hydrogenated fats?

All fats, especially unsaturated fats, tend to break down when exposed to air. To delay rancidity, hydrogenation bubbles hydrogen molecules through a poly-unsaturated oil to reconstruct its chemical bonds for more stability. For example, hydrogenation converts liquid corn oil to a semi-solid form — margarine. Some tests show that these altered fats are comparable to animal fats in terms of saturation and effects by the body.

What are trans fats? Why are they such a problem for our health?

Trans fatty acids are byproducts of hydrogenation. When hydrogen molecules are added back to a polyunsaturated fatty acid, some of the hydrognated fatty acids take on a "straight" structure, and become trans fatty acids. While originally only used for foods like shortening and margerine, today trans fats are part of most snack foods, pastries and desserts. Some researchers think they may be real villains in health problems.

Here's why:

Trans fatty acids have proven to raise blood cholesterol almost as much as saturated fat. They may even be worse. Where saturated fats increase both LDL and HDL cholesterol levels, trans fats *increase* LDL cholesterol (bad), and *decrease* HDL cholesterol, the good cholesterol which actually helps clear arteries. Trans fats have been linked to increased cancer risk, premature skin aging and lowered immune response from impaired prostaglandin and cell functions. Most significant, they interfere with the metabolism of natural fats and with your body's ability to use essential fatty acids.

How do you know if trans fats are part of the foods you buy?

You don't. Trans fats are neither saturated, monounsaturated, or polyunsaturated, so food labels don't have to disclose how much a food contains. Foods with "partially hydrogenated oil" in their ingredient lists do contain trans fats, but some foods have only slightly hydrogenated oils with tiny amounts of trans fats. Other foods contain heavily hydrogenated oils. FDA limits the saturated fat in foods labeled "no-cholesterol" or "low-cholesterol." But there is no label requirement or limit on the trans fats allowed in those same foods.

What about margarine. We used to think it was healthier than butter. Is it?

Margarine products today are lower in calories, total fat, saturated fat and trans fats than ever before. Many are made from soy oil, so they are cholesterol-free and contain vitamin E. Most are sold in a squeeze tube, soft and liquid, meaning thay have low amounts of trans fatty acids. Yet margarine manufacturerers are allowed to omit trans fats from their labels (presumably because the amounts are small). Since margarine is a main source of polyunsaturated fats in the American diet, hopefully this consumer information problem can soon be solved.

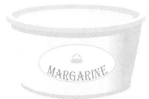

A good, low saturated fat alternative to margarine or shortening is a combination of equal amounts of warm butter and vegetable oil.

What are essential fatty acids?

1: Essential fatty acids (EFA's), are the healthy fats that protect our bodies from degenerative disease and boost our brain power. EFA's help us maintain energy, insulate our body, and protect our tissues and organs.

2: Essential fatty acids and the essential amino acids from which protein is made form lipoproteins, the organic compounds that make up our bodies. They are indispensable to each other and work synergistically.

3: Essential fatty acids like other essential nutrients, are nutrients your body needs, but cannot make for itself. Fatty acids include AA-arachidonic acid, ALA-omega 3, LA-omega 6, DHA-docosahexaenoic acid, EPA-eicosapentaenoic acid and GLA-gamma linolenic acid. A healthy body can make GLA from linoleic acid (LA), the most common fatty acid in foods, but that ability is impaired if your body is deficient in zinc, magnesium and vitamins A, B_6, B_3 and C. Conversion is also blocked if the diet is high in saturated fats or hydrogenated oils.

4: Essential fatty acids are major components of hemoglobin production and cell membranes; without them the membranes would become stiff and lose their ability to function.

5: Essential fatty acids are significant components of nerve cells, part of the "hormone-prostaglandin cascade" converting the cells into hormone-like messengers known as prostaglandins that are instrumental in energy production, essential to circulatory health, and integral to good metabolism. Low EFA's disconnect the hormone-prostaglandin cascade.

6: Essential fatty acids play an important role in regulating blood trigylceride levels.

7: EFA's impact our growth, vitality, and mental state, by connecting oxygen, electron transport, and energy in the body's vital oxidation processes.

An amazing amount of scientific research has been done on the effects of essential fatty acids on specific ailments. Here are some of the positive results:

—EFA's are a big part of your brain. 60% of your brain is made up of fatty material! If you aren't getting enough of these good fats in your diet, your brain suffers first, in terms of learning impairment and recall capacity. Recent studies find high EFA's in breast milk even increases IQ in children. Conversely, a lack of essential fatty acids appears to be a regular problem of children with attention deficit hyperactive disorder.

—EFA's inhibit harmful blood clots in the arteries, and help prevent cardiovascular damage through significant antioxidant and anti-bacterial activity.

—EFA's reduce the risk of breast and colon cancer and inhibit tumor growth.

—EFA's show remarkable results in reducing the inflammation of rheumatoid arthritis and osteoarthritis as well as that found in Parkinson's and M.S.

—EFA's are significant for healthy skin and hair. In fact, EFA deficiency is involved in most serious skin diseases like eczema, dermatitis, psoriasis, acne and hair loss.

—EFA's reduce irritability and depression associated with PMS and menopause through their involvement in the hormone-prostaglandin cascade process.

—EFA's, especially linoleic acid, CLA (conjugated linoleic acid) and LNA, fight fat. They protect against damage from hard fats, because they repel their stickiness and disperse them in the body. The more saturated fats you eat, the more EFA's you need.

Scientific research continues. EFA treatment shows promise for many health problems including:
- Autoimmune disorders — chronic fatigue syndrome, Lupus (SLE) and fibromyalgia
- Hypertension and high blood pressure
- Certain cases of schizophrenia and autism
- Childhood infections, especially recurrent respiratory problems like asthma
- Neurologic conditions like multiple sclerosis or Guillaume Barre syndrome
- Reynaud's disease (unexplained colds hands and feet)
- Chronic headaches especially from drug, caffeine or alcohol withdrawal symptoms
- Less incidence of anaphylactic shock and allergic reactions
- Colon and bowel inflammatory conditions like Crohn's disease and I.B.S.
- Adult onset diabetes
- Scleroderma

Do you have enough essential fatty acids? The first signs of deficiency are usually in the form of dermatitis — red, dry, scaly skin that appears first on the face, clustered near the oil-secreting glands (in the folds of the nose, lips, forehead, eyes and cheeks). Dry, rough areas may also appear on the forearms, thighs and buttocks. If you experience reduced vision and unexplained mood swings, you may be suffering from an EFA deficiency. A diet rich in plant foods results in low levels of saturated fat and relatively higher levels of essential fatty acids.

Warning: If you're on a serious weight loss diet, a very low-fat diet may cause a deficiency in EFAs.

We hear a lot about Omega-3 and Omega-6 health oils today. What are they?

Omega oils contain a family of fatty acids — EPA (eicosapentaenoic acid), DHA (docosahexenoic acid), CLA (conjugated linolenic acid), LNA (alpha linolenic acid) and GLA (gamma linoleic acid). Omega oils are in walnut, canola and wheat germ oil, dark greens like spinach, and herbs like evening primrose oil, ginger and flax, but the richest Omega oils come from the sea. Omega oils are synthesized by plankton at the base of the ocean food chain. They are in the tissues of all sea life, both plant and animal.

Omega-3 and Omega-6 fatty acids differ in bio-chemical structure, but both are important in proper body fat balance. They are equally important in the development and levels of prostaglandins, the essential hormone-like substances that control reproduction, inflammation reactions, immunity and cell communications.

Clinical results show a long list of benefits for Omega oils:

—Omega oils mean smoother skin, smoother muscle action and better digestion. Their PGE 3 prostaglandins enhance lymph function for immune response, and protect against cancer growth by suppressing malignant cell division. Health problems like PMS and rheumatoid arthritis improve with omega fatty acids.

—Omega oils are an effective diet remedy for the 30% of America's population who need to lower their cholesterol levels. Omega-3 oils are precursors for series 3 prostaglandins (PGE 3), which help balance cholesterol by raising HDLs and decreasing triglycerides. In fact, recent research shows that they reduce excess blood fats of all kinds — slowing down the rate at which the liver produces harmful triglycerides.

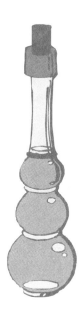

—Omega oils help prevent artery blood clots, by inhibiting excess production of thromboxane which promotes clotting. They inhibit platelet aggregation to fight atherosclerosis, improve circulation by vasodilation allowing more blood to reach the muscles, and increase oxygen supply. Enhanced blood flow is important in lowering high blood pressure, may even repair some damage caused by clogged arteries, and relieve the chest pain of coronary heart disease.

Omega-3 oils are abundant in cold water fish and sea greens, flaxseed oil, perilla oil and purslane (the number one dark green vegetable containing omega 3's). Omega-3 fatty acids increase your metabolism, rid your body of excess fluids and increase your energy.

Omega-6 fatty acids are found in black currant seed, borage, flaxseed, walnut, chestnut, soy, hemp and primrose oil. Omega-6 oils are precursors for series 1 prostaglandins (PGE1) needed for T-lymphocyte immune function, kidney health, tumor protection, low cholesterol and inhibiting blood platelet stickiness.

Here's a closer look at some of the beneficial fatty acids in omega oils.

The Omega-3 fatty acids, **DHA and EPA,** are naturally found in fish, sea vegetables, marine algae and eggs; they are synthesized from **LNA** in the body. Experts have known for years that fish eaters suffer less heart disease and have lower cholesterol and triglyceride levels than those who don't eat fish. Both DHA and EPA support coronary health. EPA, however, especially from salmon and herring, is given the major medical credit for heart protection, improving cholesterol levels, and thinning the blood to prevent re-clogging of arteries after balloon angioplasty. EPA treatment is most promising for the elderly who regularly experience re-clogging within 6 months of an angioplasty.

DHA is the most predominant EFA in our brain tissue. DHA is a large part of the retina of the eye and is needed for good eye function. DHA is the most abundant fatty acid in breast milk (see page 238). Unfortunately, recent studies show that American women have the lowest levels of DHA in the world and pregnancy depletes stores even further.

Much media attention has surrounded treating non-insulin dependent diabetes with fish oil EPA. There's also a lot of controversy. EPA may seem like a good choice for diabetics who suffer from high blood fat levels and are at high risk of heart disease, but studies are conflicting. Early 90's studies showed that supplemental fish oil might raise blood sugar levels, (a health risk for type II diabetes or clinical hypoglycemia), and that large doses of fish oil supplements might even lead to insulin resistance. Newer data in the American Journal of Clinical Nutrition report that fish oil supplements are NOT linked to higher blood sugar or insulin. More information is needed. If you have blood sugar disturbances, use fish oil supplements under professional supervision.

More EPA-DHA news: both EFA's help overcome food allergies. Both help clear skin inflammatory diseases like ezcema and psoriasis. Both benefit inflammatory rheumatoid arthritis. Both have significant effect on normalizing high cholesterol and triglyceride levels. Deficiencies of both are linked to mental problems like depression, memory loss, attention deficit/hyperactivity disorders, hostility, Alzheimer's disease, and senility. Current studies show that both DHA and EPA help protect against Alzheimer's and promote clearer thinking. New studies are currently being done on the ability of EPA and DHA to eliminate binging and food addiction during dieting and to help burn fats. Our body's ability to make both EPA and DHA decreases as we age.

CLA is a relatively new discovery getting a lot of media attention.

CLA (*conjugated linoleic acid*) occurs naturally in dairy products like cheese, lamb, sunflower oil and beef. (Its discovery occurred during scientific studies on the cancer-causing substances in beef where it was found to actually inhibit cancer growth.) It plays a role in muscle growth and nutrient-energy conversion. CLA's ability to convert the most energy from the least amount of food makes it popular among athletes for increasing muscle mass and burning fat. Like other fatty acids CLA contains powerful antioxidants for immune health and shows remarkable results for lowering cholesterol.

CLA studies were the first to show that fats can help you lose fat. CLA especially inhibits the body's mechanism for storing saturated fat by boosting its ability to use fat reserves for energy. The more saturated fat you eat, the more CLA you need. Since Americans are eating more vegetable oils, chicken and fish, and reducing their dairy and meat intake, CLA consumption has dropped in our diets over the last 20 years. Some researchers speculate that the marked increase in body fat in the American population may be due to CLA decrease.

Is GLA the most bioactive fatty acid? My healing observations indicate that it is.

GLA (Gamma Linoleic Acid - an omega-6 fatty acid) is made in the body from LA (linoleic acid). LA itself is an omega-6 fatty acid found abundantly in most vegetable oils. GLA can also be obtained from evening primrose oil (perhaps the most bio-active), black currant and borage seed oil.

GLA is a source of cellular energy and helps the body burn fat instead of storing it. It's part of the team of structural fats that form the brain, bone marrow, cell membranes and muscles. It acts as electrical insulation for nerve fibers, is regarded as an anti-coagulant and has anti-inflammatory qualities. GLA is significant as a precursor of prostaglandins which regulate hormone and metabolic functions.

GLA is therapy for breast tenderness during PMS, for vaginal dryness during menopause, for better nerve transmission in M.S. cases, for weight loss, for pain and morning stiffness of arthritis, chronic fatigue syndrome, heart health, diabetes, eczema, hyperactivity in children, schizophrenia and skin or hair dryness.

What about hemp seed oil? Experts say it has the most broad spectrum, most remarkable fatty acid profile we know of. It has GLA, absent from the fats we normally eat. Hemp contains a perfect balance of omega and gamma fatty acids — a ratio of 3:1. Hemp has been used for thousands of years as a valuable resource of edible seeds and oil, as a medicine and as fiber for clothes and rope. It's popularity is rising again as people learn about its rich nutritional properties. Hemp seeds contain 25% high quality protein and 40% fat with high amounts of EFA's — Omega-6, (Linoleic Acid- 58%), Omega-3, (Alpha-Linolenic Acid-20%), Omega-9, (Oleic Acid-11%), Saturated Fatty Acids- 9% and GLA, (Gamma Linolenic Acid- 2%).

Research shows that hemp oil has anti-inflammatory properties, so it's useful as a topical first aid for wounds and burns. It stimulates the growth and health of the skin, hair and nails. Many of today's cosmetic manufacturers are using hemp's rich EFA's as a primary ingredient in skin products.

Hemp is not good for cooking because it shouldn't be heated above 120ºF/49ºC. But it has a distinct, nutty flavor and is good in salad dressings, spreads, dips and baked potato mixed with fresh herbs. Keep hemp oil refrigerated. Buy unrefined, unfumigated, residue-free oil like Omega Nutrition VIRGIN HEMP SEED OIL.

Does hemp seed oil alter your consciousness? Hemp seed oil DOES NOT contain the psychoactive marijuana compound, THC (tetra-hydrocannabinol), in the resin produced by the flowering tops of female plants before the seeds mature. Hemp seed *oil* is perfectly legal and not psychoactive. Canada passed an Industrial Hemp Act in 1998 so that this remarkable plant could be used for its nutritional benefits. Unfortunately, hemp is still illegal to grow in the U.S.

What about coconut oil, palm oil and other tropical oils?

Coconut oil, a much maligned tropical oil, long under attack by the American Soybean Association, is making a comeback for its taste and therapeutic value. The sponsored studies were used to promote polyunsaturated oils and replace the use of tropical oils. Coconut oil was falsely accused. Scientists now know that the studies were flawed and the conclusions of the studies were incorrect. The true villains were actually found to be hydrogenated oil products along with a lack of healthy EFA's in the diet. For more than forty years, however, the negative publicity caused a coconut oil scare and set fire to the foundation of its popularity.

You may have heard that coconut oil is over 90% saturated fatty acids (SFA), and believe you should avoid it as an unhealthy oil. The truth is there are two kinds of saturated fats — long chain and medium chain. Long chain saturated fats (LCT's) are associated with "bad" cholesterol, medium chain saturates or triglycerides (MCT's) are found in coconut oil. Medium chain triglycerides provide energy, are easily digested and do not clog arteries like the long chain group. MCT's help your body metabolize fat efficiently, so that the fats provide energy instead of being stored. MCT's are easily digested so coconut oil is useful for people who have trouble digesting fat. Natural practitioners use a formula with coconut oil MCT's for patients with malabsorption problems, like those with eating disorders. Infant formula with coconut MCT's can be a lifesaver for premature babies.

Common misconceptions of coconut oil are that it raises blood cholesterol, causes heart disease and obesity. However, coconut oil does not cause heart disease nor raise blood cholesterol in a normal diet. Studies show coconut oil has a neutral effect on blood cholesterol. Polynesian islanders, who have gotten most of their fat calories from coconut oil for centuries have an exceedingly low rate of heart disease. Coconut oil is actually a good choice if you are a dieter, body builder or athlete concerned about weight and body fat. It's less likely than other oils to cause obesity, because the body easily converts its calories into energy rather than body fat.

Coconut oil is one of the few plant sources of *lauric acid* (almost 50% of its fatty acid content), a rare disease fighting fatty acid. It is naturally found in mother's milk and protects an infant from viral and bacteria infection. For example, natives who live in the tropics, an ideal environment for parasites, are protected from infections. *Lauric acid* has proven effective for immune-compromised conditions like HIV infection, fibromyalgia and lupus, respiratory infections like chronic bronchitis, pneumonia or severe flu, and as an immune booster.

Coconut oil is a good cooking oil with a sweet, tropical flavor. Compared to flax oil, which has alpha-linolenic acid easily oxidized by heating, the SFA's of coconut oil are 300 times more resistant to oxidation. It is a healthy alternative to refined oils and hydrogenated vegetable oils, like margarine. It may be used in place of butter - use three-quarters the amount of coconut butter to obtain the same baking results. Try Omega Nutrition COCONUT BUTTER — 100% organic, unrefined coconut oil.

Coconut oil is still one of the best kept nutritional secrets. Forty years of false dietary information have taken their toll in the marketplace. But the general public is catching on to the truth. New, more balanced information will help this healthy oil to rise out of the ashes of unfair publicity and take its place in our healing pantheon.

Is palm oil okay? It's another tropical oil that's received a great deal of negative publicity, falsely accused under the same series of polyunsaturated oil tests. Once again, all the evidence wasn't taken into account. Like coconut oil, palm oil is high in saturated fats, but no discernment was made between the two kinds of saturated fats — long chain and medium chain. (See previous page.) Palm oil, too, was accused of hiking blood cholesterol levels and contributing to clogging of the arteries. (Several new studies show that even a diet high in palm oil doesn't boost cholesterol in people with normal levels.)

In fact, of all the commonly used vegetable oils, palm oil is the most versatile. Even after refining, palm oil doesn't need hydrogenation — the big health culprit, for its use. Palm oil is a rich source of beta carotene and vitamin E. Still, it is usually heavily refined (coconut oil is not) which depletes its nutrient value and makes it harder for the body to digest. For this reason, I recommend avoiding palm oil in a healing diet.

How do you maintain the right balance of fats in your diet? As we fight the battle of the bulge in America we have seriously disrupted our fat balance. We've cut back on saturated fat from meats and dairy foods and increased our intake of omega-6's from corn and soybean oils. In the U.S., we eat the highest amount of omega-6 fatty acids of any population on Earth! And the animals we eat are fed a diet high in omega-6 oils, so we get even more omega 6's when we eat them.

A good ratio of omega 6 to omega 3 fatty acids may be about 1:1, (the ratio our primitive forebears lived on), but diet amounts for modern man are 10 to 20 parts Omega-6 oils to 1 part Omega-3's, a highly imbalanced ratio. Americans are eating 10:1 to even 40:1! The result for health? Experts believe that an overload of Omega-6 fatty acids leads to body chemistry changes that increase our risk for heart disease. Further, an overload of Omega 6's causes the body to overproduce prostaglandins that have pro-inflammatory and pro-clotting effects!

Take a look at your diet. If you eat a lot of vegetable oils and animal foods, you may be getting too many Omega 6's. Reduce your ratio of these foods for better fat balance.

It's easy. Simply increase your intake of omega-3 fatty acid foods like fish, flaxseed and green vegetables. They help your body compete with the production of omega 6 prostaglandins and reduce their adverse effects.

Dairy Foods In A Healing Diet

I believe you should avoid dairy foods during a cleansing diet, especially a mucous cleansing diet. Dairy products interfere with the cleansing-healing process because their density and high saturated fats challenge both digestion and metabolism. Dairy foods are tremendous mucous producers that burden the respiratory, digestive and immune systems. Cow's milk in particular has clogging properties for many people. Pasteurized milk is a relatively dead food as far as nutrition is concerned. Even raw milk can be difficult to assimilate for someone with respiratory problems.

One-quarter of Americans have dairy intolerance. They experience allergy reactions, poor digestion and mucous build-up. Besides a lactose sensitivity, many people process some proteins in cow's milk poorly, throwing off excess from cheeses, cream, ice cream and milk. In humans, milk-digesting lactase levels are at their highest immediately after birth, decreasing after weaning. So dairy foods become harder to digest as we age, accumulating strain and mucous clogs on eliminative organs. Even people without great sensitivity to dairy foods report an energy rise when they reduce their dairy intake.

Children can be especially susceptible to dairy reactions. Besides childhood allergies, cow's milk can cause loss of iron and hemoglobin in infants by triggering blood loss from the intestinal tract. Heavy consumption of milk, especially by small children, may result in vitamin D toxicity. Some research shows that iron absorption is blocked by as much as 60% after dairy products are eaten in a meal. Studies in the New England Journal of Medicine show that children who are not given cow's milk products during infancy have a dramatically lower risk of diabetes. The culprit appears to be a cow's milk protein — bovine serum albumin, which differs just enough from human proteins to cause an anti-body reaction. The antibodies attack and destroy insulin producing beta cells in the pancreas, increasing the chance of childhood diabetes.

When dairy foods are removed from the diet of mucous clogged children, enlarged tonsils and adenoids shrink, a clear sign of immune system relief. Doctors who put children on dairy-free diets often report a marked reduction in colds, flu, sinus and ear infections.

Women do not handle dense, building foods like dairy products, as well as men. Their systems back up more easily, so less dairy (especially cheese) usually means easier bowel movements for women. Female problems, like fibroids, bladder and kidney ailments can also be improved by avoiding dairy. A sugar in dairy products, galactose, may even be fatal to a woman's eggs, impacting her level of fertility. When a women is having trouble getting pregnant, I usually recommend that she reduce her dairy consumption first.

Isn't calcium from dairy foods good for us? Contrary to advertising, dairy products are not a very good source of calcium for people. We don't absorb dairy calcium well because of pasteurizing and processing, high fat content, and an unbalanced ratio with phosphorus. Even in cattle tests, calves given their own mother's milk that had first been pasteurized, didn't live six weeks!

Hormone residues, pesticides and additives used in modern cattle-raising also inhibit absorption of calcium and other minerals. In contrast, calcium from dark green leafy vegetables is easily absorbable. A recent study compared the absorption of calcium from a vegetable source, kale, with the absorption from cow's milk. The absorption amount of calcium from kale was 41%, compared with 32% from milk.

Besides leafy greens, other vegetables, nuts, seeds, fish and soy foods have measureable amounts of absorbable calcium, along with minerals like magnesium, potassium and zinc that are easy for us to assimilate. Herbs, like sea plants, borage seed, pau d'arco, valerian, wild lettuce, nettles, burdock and yellow dock offer healing concentrations of calcium.

Dairy foods aren't a very usable source of protein for humans, either. Cow's milk contains proteins that are harmful to our immune systems, (see previous page). Repeated exposure to these proteins disrupts normal immune response. Fish and poultry proteins are much less damaging; plant proteins pose the least hazard.

I use soy milk and cheese, tofu and nut milks in place of dairy foods. At the least, use low-fat or non-fat products, and goat's milk, raw milk and raw cheeses instead of pasteurized. Kefir and yogurt, although made from milk, don't have the absorption problems of dairy foods. Unless lactose intolerance is severe, cultured foods don't cause a lactose reaction, and their friendly flora cultures help you heal without the downside of dairy.

For long range diets, consider most dairy products as good for taste, but questionable for nutrition. **A little is fine — a lot is not.** Small changes in your cooking habits and point of view are all it takes - mostly a matter of not having dairy products around the house, and substituting dairy-free alternatives in your recipes. (See FOOD EXCHANGES section pg. 271.) Reducing your dairy intake usually means some weight loss, too, with lower blood pressure and cholesterol levels. Soon, you won't feel deprived at all, just delighted.

Here's how specific dairy foods can affect your healing diet:

What about butter? Surprise! Butter is okay in moderation. Although a saturated fat, butter is relatively stable, and like raw cream, it is a whole, balanced food, used by the body better than its separate components. When butter is needed, use raw, unsalted butter, not margarine or shortening. Don't let it get hot enough to smoke. If less saturated fat is desired, use the new butter-yogurt blends or clarified butter. Simply melt the butter and skim off the top foam. Let it rest a few minutes and spoon off the clear butter for use. Discard whey solids that settle to the bottom, and the foam. Soy margarine is a vegan alternative for baking.

There's good news about eggs! "Eggsperts" are finally realizing what many of us in the whole foods world have long known. Although high in cholesterol, eggs are also high in balancing lecithins and phosphatides, so they don't add to the risk of atherosclerosis. Nutrition-rich fertile eggs from free-run chickens are a perfect food. The difference in fertile eggs and eggs from commercial egg factories is remarkable; the yolk color is brighter, the flavor fresher, the workability in recipes better. The distinction is most noticeable in poached and baked eggs, where the yolks firm up and rise higher. Cook eggs lightly for the best nutrition — poached, soft-boiled, hard boiled or baked, never fried. Eggs are concentrated protein; use them with discretion.

The saturated fats in cheese make it hard for a healing diet to succeed.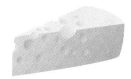
Commercial cheeses, even when labeled "natural," contain bleaches, coagulants, emulsifiers, moisture absorbants, mold inhibitors and rind dyes that visibly leak into the cheese itself. Many restaurant and pizza cheeses add synthetic flavors, colors and preservatives. Processed cheese foods (like Velveeta) get their texture from hydrogenated fats rather than natural fermentation. Even if you're not on a healing diet, limit your cheese consumption to small amounts of low-fat or raw cheeses that provide usable proteins with good mineral ratios. Low sodium, low fat cheeses are easy to find today, and are a better choice for a healing program. Raw cheeses are superior in taste and health value to pasteurized cheeses, which have higher salts and additives.

Options to make your cheese choice healthier:

—**Rennet-free cheeses** use a bacterial culture, instead of calves' enzymes to separate curds and whey. Rennet, the dried extract of the enzyme rennin, is derived from the stomach of a suckling calf or a lamb. It speeds up the separation process of cheese making.

—**Goat cheese (chevre) and sheep's milk cheese (feta)** are both lower in fat than cow's milk cheeses, and more easily digested. There is a world of difference in taste.

—**Rice cheese,** made from cultured rice milk is the newest entry into the healthy "cheese" market. It's meltable and delicious.

—**Real mozzarella cheese** is from buffalo or sheep's milk - low fat, and delicious!

—**Raw cream cheese** is light years ahead of commercial with gums, fillers and thickeners.

—**Lowfat cottage cheese,** is a good substitute for ricotta, cream cheese and processed cottage cheese foods that are full of chemicals. Usually okay for those with a slight lactose intolerance, cottage cheese mixes with non-fat or low-fat plain yogurt to add the richness of cream or sour cream to recipes without the fat.

—**Yogurt cheese** is easy to make, lighter in fat and calories but with all the richness of sour cream or cream cheese. See page 145 for how to make fresh yogurt cheese. It's also widely available in gourmet stores.

—**Kefir cheese** is an excellent replacement for dairy foods in dips and other recipes. (I like it better.) Available in health food stores, kefir cheese is low in fat and calories and has a slightly tangy, rich flavor that really enhances snack foods. Use it cup for cup in place of sour cream, cottage cheese, cream cheese or ricotta.

—**Tofu** is a white digestible cheesy curd made from fermented soybeans. Tofu is a good replacement for cheese, in texture, taste and nutritional content. It is high in protein, low in fat, extremely versatile, and may be used in place of sour cream, cheese, milk and cottage cheese in cooking. Tofu can even be used in place of eggs in quick breads, cakes, custard-based dishes, quiches and frittatas.

—**Soy cheese,** made from soy milk, is a non-dairy cheese free of lactose and cholesterol. A minute amount of calcium caseinate (milk protein) is added for melting. Mozarella, cheddar, jack and cream cheese are available. Use it cup for cup in place of cheese.

Apart from how dairy foods affect healing ability, there are controversial issues surrounding the manufacture of dairy foods that influence your health.

There is a whirlwind of controversy about rBST (recombinant bovine somatotrophin) and rBGH (recombinant bovine growth hormone). The hormones increase milk production, but since America always has a surplus milk supply and long-standing dairy subsidies, it's hard to see why an American dairy farmer would use a potentially harmful hormone in order to produce even more surplus milk. We know little about the long-term effects of these hormones. We do know they increase mastitis infections in treated cows, leading to increased use of antibiotics to treat the mastitis. This leads to higher levels of antibiotics in the milk, widely questioned by scientists and concerned consumers alike.

Modern medicine is losing the battle against the onslaught of new drug-resistant pathogens. **Some researchers believe that even moderate use of antibiotics in an animal's feed can result in antibiotic resistance in the animal's bacteria, and a transfer of that resistance to human bacteria.** A 1997 study in the International Journal of Health Services, suggests that genetically engineered rBGH may promote breast and colon cancer, acromegaly, hypertension, diabetes and breast growth in men. Even the milk itself from hormone-treated cows is not as wholesome. It has less protein and higher levels of saturated fat.

More worrisome news:

—Pesticides seem to concentrate in the milk of both farm animals and humans. A study by the Environmental Defense Fund found widespread pesticide contamination of human breast milk among 1,400 women in forty-six states (1997). The levels of contamination were twice as high among meat-and-dairy-eating women as among vegetarians.

—Ovarian cancer rates parallel dairy-consumption patterns around the world. The culprit is galactose, a milk sugar from lactose. Women with ovarian cancer often have trouble breaking down galactose. In tests, animals fed galactose develop ovarian cancer. Unlike lactose intolerance, there are no clear signs of digestive upset, but a new series of enzyme tests can tell you whether you lack the proper enzymes.

—Cow's milk is associated with insulin-dependent diabetes. The milk protein bovine serum albumin (BSA) somehow leads to an autoimmune reaction in the pancreas impairing its ability to produce insulin. Exposure to large amounts of cow's milk in the diet may lead to juvenile diabetes.

—Dairy proteins may play a major role in the development of non-Hodgkin's lymphoma, a cancer of the immune system. A 1989 study and a growing consensus among scientists shows that high levels of the cow's milk protein beta-lactoglobulin are found in the blood of lung cancer patients as well.

—Bovine leukemia virus is found in 3 out of 5 dairy cows in the U. S.! In about 80% of U.S. dairy herds, a large percentage is contaminated when the milk is pooled for distribution. Pasteurization, if done correctly, kills the virus, but the issue continues to haunt, because the percentage of cattle with the virus is so large.

Are you lactose intolerant? Do you have gas, bloating, cramps, nausea or diarrhea from 30 minutes to 2 hours after eating dairy foods?

Here are some good dairy substitutes.
—**Kefir** is a cultured food made by adding kefir grains (natural milk proteins available at health food stores), to milk and letting the mixture incubate overnight at room temperature to milkshake consistency. Kefir has 350mg of calcium per cup. Use the plain flavor cup for cup as a replacement for whole milk; buttermilk for half and half; use fruit flavors in sweet baked dishes.

—**Soy milk** is nutritious, versatile, smooth and delicious. It is lactose and cholesterol free, (substituting soy milk for dairy milk in your diet can help reduce serum cholesterol). Soy milk contains less calcium and calories than milk, but more protein and iron. It adds a slight rise to baked goods. Use it cup for cup as a milk replacement in cooking — plain flavor for savory dishes, vanilla for sweet dishes or on cereal.

—**Almond milk** is a rich, non-dairy liquid. Use it 1 to 1 in place of milk in baking, sauces, gravies, cream soups and protein drinks. For 1 cup almond milk: place 1 cup blanched almonds in a blender; add 2 to 4 cups water, depending on consistency desired. Add 1 tsp. honey; whirl until smooth. Other nut milks are okay; I like almond the best.

—**Sesame tahini** is rich, creamy, ground sesame seed butter. Use tahini as a dairy replacement in soups, dressings or sauces without the cholesterol yet with all the protein. Mix tahini with water to milk consistency as a milk substitute in baking. Use it in healthy candies and cookies, and on toast in place of peanut butter. Mix tahini with oil and seasonings for an excellent salad topping to greens and salad ingredients.

—**Yogurt** helps balance and replace friendly flora in the G.I. tract. Yogurt's culturing process makes it a living food. Yogurt contains more bioavailable protein and easily absorbed calcium than milk, a good thing for people at risk for osteoporosis. Even if you have a lactase enzyme deficiency, bacterial fermentation elements in yogurt actually substitute for the missing enzyme to help you digest lactose. Yogurt also kills the bacteria which causes most ulcers and gastritis. Yogurt boosts blood levels of gamma interferon, a component of the immune system that rallies killer cells to fight infections. The lactic acid bacteria in yogurt lowers levels of enzymes responsible for the development of colon cancer.
Yogurt is a remarkably good food treatment for children with diarrhea, especially if the child's diarrhea is aggravated by antibiotics. Many parents introduce spoonable yogurt to their children early — after between four and six months of age, as soon as the child begins to eat solid food.

What's really low-fat? Here's the strange low-down on low-fat milk.
—Two percent (reduced fat) milk is actually 35% fat.
—One percent (low-fat) milk is actually 25% fat by calories.
—Skim milk is called "fat free" or "non-fat."

Sugar & Sweeteners: Are They All Bad?

Is the bad health rap on sugar too extreme?

Sugar in America is synonymous with fun, good times and snacking. Our culture instills the powerful urge for sweetness from an early age. Americans eat sugar to "cope" in times of stress and tension.

For the average American, almost 20% of daily calories come from refined white sugar. That works out to about 150 pounds of sugar per year — a substantial amount when you realize that sugar often replaces more nutritious foods in our diets.

Today, sugar qualifies as America's favorite but most poorly understood drug, easily the most addictive because it affects so many body systems and is so highly concentrated. (Did you know it takes 16 feet of 1-inch diameter sugar cane to produce 1 teaspoon of refined sugar?) In fact, refined sugar first appeared as a "military drug," medicinal in The War of 1812 — a light-weight energy source for Napoleon's army. (Interestingly, he lost his first battle.) Sugar only entered into our food supply at the turn of the last century.

There's some good news about sugar. It offers quick energy, helps metabolism and "closes" our digestive processes. A little sugar can actually suppress appetite, reducing the likelihood of overeating. It's the reason we traditionally eat sweet things at the end of a meal. Sugar can also improve the taste of complex carbohydrate foods which are better for you than fatty foods. New research shows that some of the caveats about sugar have been overstated. In regard to weight gain, for instance, the sugar in most snacks and desserts is a less-fattening culprit than fat. Fat not only contributes more calories, but the calories are metabolized differently in the body, causing more weight gain than sugar.

But sugar interferes in a healing program. Refined sugar is sucrose, the ultimate naked carbohydrate — stripped of all nutritional benefits. Sugars available include: white, raw, brown and turbinado, yellow D and sucanat. All sugars can be addictive, most add nothing but calories to your body. Like a drug or alcohol, sugar affects your brain first, offering a false energy lift that eventually lets you down lower than when you started.

Large amounts of sugary foods raise your insulin production resulting in problems like diabetes and hypoglycemia, high triglycerides and high blood pressure.

Raised insulin is also the body's signal to store fat. Sugar needs insulin for metabolism. Eating a lot of sugar means some of those calories become fat instead of energy. Excess metabolized sugar is transformed into fat globules, and distributed over body storage areas like the stomach, hips and chin.

Too much sugar upsets mineral balances like magnesium and zinc. Sugar especially drains calcium, which advances aging and overloads your body with acid-ash residues responsible for much of arthritic stiffening. Sugar ties up and dissolves B vitamins, producing over-acid conditions that become gout, nerve, gum and digestive problems.

You raise your risk for infection because a high sugar diet provides a breeding ground for staph and yeast infections. Bacteria, fungi and parasites thrive on sugary foods.

Excess sugar depresses immune response. It's linked to high cholesterol, heart disease and coronary thrombosis. New data implicates sugar in nearsightedness and skin problems like eczema, psoriasis and dermatitis. A study at the University of Alabama shows that people suffering from depression have less symptoms when sugar is removed from their diets. Other research shows that when women switch from a diet high in sugar to a sugar-free, high nutrient diet, their food addictive behavior stopped.

Unfortunately, it doesn't stop there.
Personality-changing, mental and emotional signs of too much sugar:
—irritability, irrational mood swings
—chronic or frequent bouts of depression with manic-depressive tendencies
—difficulty concentrating, forgetfulness or absentmindedness
—lack of motivation, loss of enthusiasm for plans and projects
—increasing undependability, inconsistent thoughts and actions
—moody personality changes with emotional outbursts

Physical effects of eating too much sugar:
—anxiety episodes and panic attacks
—bulimia eating disorder
—candidiasis and chronic fatigue syndrome
—diabetes and-or hypoglycemia
—food addiction with loss of B-vitamins and minerals
—menopausal mood swings and unusual low energy periods
—obesity
—high cholesterol and triglycerides leading to risk of atherosclerosis
—excessive emotional swings and food cravings, especially before menstruation
—tooth decay and gum disease

Foods that affect your sugar balance have a major impact on your healing program. Glucose is the main sugar in the blood and brain. Under ideal conditions, glucose is released into the bloodstream slowly to maintain balanced blood sugar levels. Small blood sugar fluctuations disturb one's feeling of well being. Large blood sugar fluctuations cause feelings of depression, anxiety, mood swings, fatigue and even aggressive behavior. Today, the inability to use glucose correctly affects millions of Americans. At least twenty million of us suffer from diabetes (high blood sugar) or hypoglycemia (low blood sugar).

Hypoglycemia, often called a "sugar epidemic," in America is widespread in every industrialized country today. It's a direct effect of too much sugar and refined carbohydrates coupled with low fiber foods. The pancreas reacts to too much sugar by producing too much insulin. The excess insulin lowers blood sugar too much as the body strives to achieve normal glucose-insulin balance. Hypoglycemia results.
Hypoglycemia is marked by dozens of unpleasant symptoms, especially in the way the brain functions. The brain requires glucose as an energy source to think clearly, and is the most sensitive organ to blood sugar levels. Worst case scenario reactions of hypoglycemia can even range to unconsciousness or death.

Diabetes, another "civilization" disease, also results from too much sugar, refined carbohydrates and caffeine. Chronic hypoglycemia often precedes diabetes. When your body doesn't use carbohydrates correctly, it may produce too little insulin, so blood sugar levels stay too high. The pancreas can't work properly; glucose can't enter the cells to provide energy. Instead, it accumulates in the blood, resulting in serious symptoms from mental confusion to uncontrollable obesity, blindness, even coma.

While seeming to be opposite problems, diabetes and hypoglycemia really stem from the same cause — an imbalance between glucose and oxygen in the body. Poor nutrition, the common cause of both disorders, can be improved with a high mineral, high fiber diet, adequate protein, small frequent meals, and regular mild exercise. If you have either condition, there must be diet and lifestyle change for there to be a real or permanent cure. Alcohol, caffeine, refined sugars and tobacco must be avoided.
Note: Even though poor sugar metabolism is the cause of both diabetes and hypoglycemia, the different effects of each problem call for specific modifications. Get better body response by addressing low blood sugar and high blood sugar separately. See DIABETES and HYPOGLYCEMIA DIETS, pages 367 and 427 in this book.

There are many healthy alternatives to refined sugar.

Just because you follow a sugar-free diet doesn't mean you have to give up good taste or sweet comforts. Whole food sweeteners like honey, molasses, maple syrup, fruit juice or barley malt can satisfy your sweet tooth. Your body metabolizes them easily. Clinical tests on crystalline fructose, and the herbs *stevia rebaudiana* and *gymnema sylvestre*, show good news for sugar disorders. These natural sweeteners are heros in the effort to control sugar balance and sugar cravings. But they do not eliminate hypoglycemia or diabetes. Only a better diet and regular exercise can make a permanent difference.

Note: Always look for the least processed sweetener. Most commercial sweeteners bear no resemblance to their natural counterpart. For example, before sugar cane (the worst culprit), is refined and bleached, it is rich in vitamins and minerals.

Here are some sweet choices to consider for your healing diet:

—**Crystalline fructose** is a commercial sugar with the same molecular structure as that found in fruit. It is called fruit sugar, but it's usually made from corn starch. It has a low glycemic index, releasing its glucose into the bloodstream slowly. Fructose produces liver glycogen rapidly making it a more efficient energy supply than other sweeteners. It is almost twice as sweet as sugar, so less is needed for the same sweetening power.

Fructose may be the sweetener of choice in a weight loss diet. In clinical tests before meals, subjects who drank liquids sweetened with fructose ate 20 to 40% fewer calories than normal, more than compensating for the 200 calories in the fructose. Those who drank liquids sweetened with table sugar ate 10 to 15% fewer calories; those who drank liquids sweetened with NutraSweet, Equal or aspartame ate the same amount of calories as normal. Fructose also helps people pick foods with less fats. In dental health studies, dentists reported less plaque and tarter with fructose than with sugar.

Fructose is as common in prepared foods as sucrose. Does it have drawbacks? Data on fructose chemical stucture shows that its highly reactive molecules bind to protein molecules, sometimes altering the structure of enzymes and their proteins. The protein-fructose interaction may cause major organ damage in diabetics.

Lack of critical information is another problem. Products labeled fructose can be pure fructose, 90% fructose or high fructose corn syrup (55% fructose with a high percentage of glucose needing insulin for metabolism). Fructose also inhibits the absorption of copper, essential to the production of hemoglobin and linked to coronary problems. New information indicates it may also stimulate high cholesterol levels.

Bottom line? There are advantages to fructose, but if you are hypoglycemic or diabetic, fructose is still sugar and should be avoided.

—**Stevia rebaudiana** (sweet herb), is a South American sweetening leaf. It is non-caloric, and about 25 times sweeter than sugar when made as an infusion with 1 tsp. leaves to 1 cup of water. *Two drops* of the infusion equal 1 tsp. of sugar in sweetness. In baking, 1 tsp. finely ground stevia powder equals 1 cup of sugar.

Tests show stevia can regulate blood sugar. In South America, stevia is sold as an aid to people with diabetes and hypoglycemia. Stevia helps lower high blood pressure but does not affect normal blood pressure. Stevia users claim it inhibits tooth decay, aids mental alertness, counteracts fatigue and improves digestion.

Stevia has been used as a natural sweetener in South America for over 1500 years; clinical studies indicate it is safe even in cases of severe sugar imbalance. In the 1970's, the Japanese refined the sweet glycosides from stevia to make a product called Stevioside, 300 times sweeter than sugar. Stevioside is currently used as a non-calorie sweetener in South America and the Orient where it enjoys a 42% share of the food sweetener market. While Stevioside does not affect blood glucose levels and is a good sweetener for both diabetics and hypoglycemics, it does not retain the extraordinary healing benefits of whole stevia leaves and extract.

Unlike other sweeteners, stevia is effective for weight control because it contains no calories, yet significantly increases glucose tolerance. New research indicates that stevia may block fat absorption, too. People whose weight loss problems stem from sugar cravings benefit most from stevia, reporting that they experience reduced desire for sugary foods. Most stevia users also say they have less desire for tobacco and alcohol.

Today, stevia is back on the market after a long FDA ban, heavily influenced by Nutrasweet™ competition politics. Experts say that stevia may soon be regarded as one of the Earth's good-for-you sweeteners.

—**Gymnema sylvestre** is an herb that reduces blood sugar levels after sugar consumption. Gymnema's molecular structure, similar to that of sugar, can block absorption of up to 50% of dietary sugar calories. Both sugar and gymnema are digested in the small intestine, but the larger molecule of gymnema cannot be fully absorbed. Thus, taken before sugar, the gymnema molecule blocks the passages through which sugar is normally absorbed, so fewer sugar calories get assimilated. A person who eats a 400 calorie, high sugar dessert only absorbs 200 of the sugar calories. The remaining sugar is eliminated as waste. Gymnema also helps curb cravings for sweet foods. Gymnema has obvious uses for diabetes. Studies show gymnema may enhance endogenous insulin production in both Type I and Type II diabetics to regenerate pancreatic cells destroyed in the course of diabetes. Take with GTF Chromium for best results.

You can take the gymnema taste test. Taste something sweet, then swish a sip of gymnema sylvestre tea in your mouth. Now taste something sweet again. You will not be able to taste the sugar, because gymnemic acid prevents the taste buds in your mouth from being activated by sugar molecules in the food. Gymnema blocks the taste of the sugar in your mouth in the same way it blocks sugar in digestion.

—**Fructo-oligo-saccharides (FOS)** are compounds, only half as sweet as sugar, found naturally in foods like bananas, onions, garlic, artichokes, barley, tomatoes, rye, honey, and asparagus. FOS are not digested in the stomach, they pass untouched into the large intestine where friendly intestinal flora consume them as nourishment. More significant, the by-products of FOS consumption are healthy EFA's, which are absorbed by the walls of the large intestine and used for energy. Studies show no harmful links for FOS. They do not affect DNA nor promote cancer. Available in health food stores.

The advantages of FOS:
—FOS feeds beneficial bacteria, while starving harmful bacteria
—FOS relieves constipation
—FOS stops antibiotic-induced yeast
—FOS lowers cholesterol and triglyceride levels
—FOS inhibits formation of cavities
—FOS lowers blood sugar levels in diabetics

Note: FOS can be used as a partial replacement for sugar in recipes. Too much (more than 40 grams) can cause loose stools, since FOS are not digested. I suggest FOS as a nutritional enhancement rather than a complete replacement.

—**Agave Nectar** is a new, high fructose sweetener. It's 90% solids, a percentage much greater than traditional high fructose corn syrup. (This amount of fructose may aggravate a copper deficiency linked to serious coronary problems.) Agave may cause disintegration of red blood cells, irritate the skin and the lining of the gastrointestinal tract, depress the central nervous system, and immune response, and may cause miscarriage. More testing must be done, but agave nectar is likely a sweetener to look for soon.

—**Amazake** is a pudding-like, whole-grain sweetener made from organic brown rice. The rice is cooked, then injected with koji, the Aspergillus enzyme culture used in miso and shoyu. Amazake is about 21% sugar, mainly glucose and maltose, and is high in nutrients, including available B complex and iron.

—**Barley malt and brown rice syrups** are mild, natural sweeteners made from barley sprouts, or cultured rice and water cooked to a syrup. Only 40% as sweet as sugar, barley malt's blood sugar activity is a slow, complex carbohydrate release that does not upset insulin levels.

—**Blackstrap molasses** is the liquid sludge after sucrose is extracted from the cane sugar refining process. Rich in minerals and vitamins, molasses has more calcium, ounce for ounce, than milk, more iron than eggs, and more potassium than any other food. The amounts of B vitamins, pantothenic acid, iron, inositol and vitamin E make it an effective treatment for restoring thin and fading hair.

—**Sorghum molasses** is concentrated sorghum juice, a grain related to millet. It is similar to molasses but with lighter, milder flavor. Sorghum is made by crushing the plant stalks then boiling the juice into a syrup.

—**Corn syrup** is commercial glucose made from chemically purified cornstarch with everything removed except the starch. Most corn syrup has sugar syrup added to it because glucose is only half as sweet as white sugar. It is highly refined and absorbed into the bloodstream very quickly.

—**Turbinado sugar** is raw sugar refined by washing in a centrifuge so that surface molasses is removed. It goes through the same refining process as white sugar, just short of the final extraction of molasses, and is essentially the same as white sugar.

—**Date sugar** is ground, dried dates. It is the least refined, most natural sweetener. It has the same nutrient values as dried dates — about half as sweet as sugar. Use like brown sugar. In baking, mix with water before adding to the recipe to prevent burning, or add as a sweet topping after removing your dish from the oven.

—**Fruit juice concentrate** is a highly refined product with about 68% soluble sugar. It contains measureable levels of fiber, vitamins and minerals, and promotes slower digestion. Refined sugars raise serotonin levels in the brain, which can make you feel drowsy. Unrefined fruit sweeteners have less impact on brain chemistry because natural fruit sugars do not affect serotonin levels.

—**Honey** is a mixture of sugars formed from nectar in the bodies of bees by the enzyme invertase. A natural sweetener with bioactive, antibiotic and antiseptic properties, honey contains all the vitamins, minerals and enzymes necessary for proper metabolism and digestion of glucose and other sugars. Still, honey is almost twice as sweet as sugar. Avoid it if you have candidiasis or diabetes; use it with great care if you are hypoglycemic.

—**Maple syrup** is made from sugar maple tree sap. It takes 30 to 40 gallons of sap to make one gallon of syrup. Unless labeled pure maple syrup, it may be mixed with corn syrup or other additives to cut its cost. —Maple sugar is crystallized maple syrup.

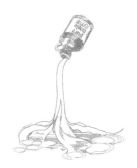

—**Sucanat,** (an acronym from sugar cane natural) is the trade name for a sweetener made from dried granulated cane juice, available in health food stores. Its average sugar content is 85%, with complex sugars, vitamins, minerals, amino acids and molasses retained. Use 1 to 1 in place of sugar. It is still a concentrated sweetener; use carefully if you have sugar balance problems.

The following chart helps you convert your favorite recipes from sugar to natural sweeteners. If you have serious blood sugar problems, like diabetes or hypoglycemia, consult the appropriate diet pages in this book or your healing professional, about the kind and amount of sweets your body can handle.

Sweetener substitution amounts are for each cup of sugar:

Substitute Sweetener	Amount	Reduce Liquid in the Recipe
• Fructose	$1/3$ to $2/3$ cup	....
• Maple Syrup	$1/3$ to $2/3$ cup	$1/4$ cup
• Honey	$1/2$ cup	$1/4$ cup
• Molasses	$1/2$ cup	$1/4$ cup
• Barley or Rice Syrup	1 to $1 1/4$ cups	$1/4$ cup
• Date Sugar	1 cup	....
• Sucanat	1 cup	....
• Apple/Pear Juice	1 cup	$1/4$ cup

What about aspartame, and its brand names, Nutrasweet and Equal?

The FDA has received more complaints about adverse reactions to aspartame than any other food ingredient in the agency's history! Yet we get an incredible amount of these chemical sweeteners in our food today. At least 30% of the U.S. population is sensitive to even moderate doses of aspartame and may suffer several symptoms.

Health problems related to synthetic sweeteners are nothing new. They've been a market-submerged health risk for decades. Saccharin has been used for 100 years, even though its involvement in bladder cancer from the 50's to the 70's was undeniable. NutraSweet and Equal have taken the place of saccharin in pre-prepared foods and drinks. Americans are consuming more of these sweeteners than ever.

—Aspartame, 200 times sweeter than sugar, is a combination of two amino acids with neurotransmitter activity — phenylalanine and aspartic acid. PKU seizures (phenylketonuria) result when the body can't effectively metabolize phenylalanine. High levels of the amino acid phenylalanine in body fluids can cause brain damage in anyone. All aspartame products include a warning that the sweetener contains phenylalanine.

Aspartame is clearly linked to blood sugar use problems — high blood pressure, insomnia, hypoglycemia, diabetes, ovarian cancer and brain tumors. (A recent study shows that the more NutraSweet consumed, the more likely tumors are to develop.) Aspartame is also associated with brain damage in fetuses.

There are immediate, serious reactions to aspartame..... severe headaches, extreme dizziness, throat swelling, allergic effects, and retina deterioration, generally attributed to methyl-alcohol, a substance released when aspartame breaks down.) Dangerous side effects are worse when NutraSweet is used hot or cooked, as it is in pre-prepared foods. Adverse effects are reversible when NutraSweet consumption is stopped.

Avoid aspartame sweeteners if you have sugar sensitivities, if you have genetic PKU, advanced liver disease, are allergy-prone (especially children) or are pregnant.

Despite a huge health outcry, the synthetic sweetener problem isn't going away. It's just changing. Here's how the next generation of sweeteners can affect you.

—**Acesulfame K,** acesulfame potassium, an organic salt, entered the U.S. market in 1988, under the brand names Sunette, Sweet One and Swiss Sweet table sweeteners. It is 200 times sweeter than sugar and boosts the sweetening effect of other sweeteners. It passes through the human digestive system unchanged, and therefore is non-caloric. Ninety studies on its safety were submitted to the FDA.

—**Sucralose,** chlorinated sucrose, is 400 to 800 times sweeter than sugar. It was approved in Canada in 1991 for baking; approval is pending in the U.S. I feel it would be treacherous to try and convert this concentrated sweetener to sugar amounts in baking. Sucralose is seen as a chemical by your body, not as a carbohydrate, so it has no effect on insulin secretion or carbohydrate metabolism. Absorption of sucralose is limited; most of it passes through the body unchanged. The small amount that is absorbed is not metabolized for energy, which makes sucralose non-caloric. Over 100 studies were submitted to the FDA showing that sucralose is not carcinogenic and does not cause genetic change, birth defects, brain or nerve damage, or other health risks. Forty studies indicate it is biodegradable, safe for plant and aquatic life.

—**Alitame,** brand name ACLAME, is formed from the amino acids l-aspartic acid and L-alanine, chemically similar to aspartame. It is 2,000 times sweeter than sucrose. Alitame is hydrolyzed to release aspartic acid, metabolized normally in the body, then excreted in urine and feces. Fifteen studies indicate that alitame is safe at a dose of 100 mg/kg per day. However, the FDA, bowing to the negative side effects publicity from aspartame (alitame is even more concentrated), is delaying approval in the U.S. pending further tests.

Chemical sweeteners on today's food labels. Beware if you have sugar-related health problems:

—**Dextrose,** a plant monosaccharide, often synthetically derived from cornstarch.

—**Lactose,** milk sugar, a di-saccharide sweetener mainly in infant foods and baked goods. May cause gastrointestinal disturbances in lactose intolerant people.

—**Xylitol,** from birchwood chips, may reduce cavities by neutralizing mouth acids.

—**Maltose,** malt sugar, a disaccharide often synthetically derived from corn syrup. It does not normally stimulate insulin production.

—**Sorbitol,** derived from corn, is absorbed slowly. It is used in diabetic safe foods because it needs little insulin. It does not promote tooth decay, but can cause diarrhea.

—**Saccharin,** made from petroleum and toluene, a solvent used to stop knocking in gasoline engines, is 300 times sweeter than sugar and calorie free, but is linked to bladder cancer. The FDA tried to ban saccharin in 1977, but relented under industry pressure. It is now sold with a warning label, but has largely been replaced by Nutrasweet and Equal. It does not metabolize, is excreted quickly and does not build up in the body.

—**Raw sugar,** a granulated, evaporated sugar cane juice product. It is 98% sucrose.

Is there a healthy diet that won't stimulate over-production of insulin but will allow normal blood sugar activity? Can we keep hunger under control all day, and manage our weight without starving?

A low glycemic diet is a good answer, both for blood sugar regulation and for a sugar craver's weight control.

What is a low glycemic diet? It's a diet that keeps insulin levels low meaning fewer calories are turned into fat and more are burned for energy, resulting in weight loss. A low-glycemic diet is low in fats and total calories, largely vegetarian, with most proteins from vegetable sources. It includes mono-unsaturated oils like olive or canola oil.

Whole foods, especially whole grains and fresh vegetables, have a low-glycemic index. They don't elevate blood sugar after a meal like sugary, high-glycemic index foods, which put blood sugar on a roller coaster and elevate it too rapidly. Insulin responds immediately to stimulate fat production. Too much insulin also causes too much sugar storage, which then results in low blood sugar. Low blood sugar causes stress-hormone release, fatigue and ultimately ravenous hunger. The process begins all over again.

Plant fiber from whole foods also regulates digestion for more balanced blood sugar levels. Plant fiber binds with most fats to prevent their absorption. In addition, plant fiber foods speed up bowel transit time to take stress off your liver so it can metabolize fats efficiently. Eat whole grains, fresh fruits and vegetables, seafood, sea greens, soy foods and brown rice frequently. They are high fiber foods that will help stabilize blood sugar swings and lessen cravings for sugar. Some spices like cinnamon, clove and bay leaf also help control both blood sugar levels and sugar cravings.

By combining low glycemic foods, like high fiber foods, along with exercise and certain nutritional supplements that help balance your blood sugar, you can optimize brain biochemistry. You'll feel more comfortable while dieting and can diet without binging.

Nutrients that help reduce sugar cravings and withdrawal are B vitamins, vitamin C, zinc, trace minerals, the amino acid L-glutamine and chromium. Chromium helps insulin work more efficiently at removing sugar from the blood. Glutamine is used directly by the brain and is helpful in reducing sugar craving.

For longer life and better health, use sugar sparingly, on special occasions.

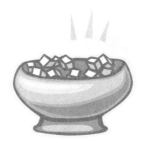

A Low Salt Diet & Healing

In the past generation, Americans have consumed more NaCl than ever before — too much restaurant food, too many refined foods and too many animal foods. Heart disease, hypertension and high blood pressure have increased correspondingly, so most people are aware that excessive salt is a diet problem. Too much salt constricts circulation, and causes kidneys to retain fluid and migraines to occur frequently. Like too much sugar, salt is a cause of hyperactivity and aggressive behavior. The average American adult consumes between 8,000 and 10,000mg of sodium a day.

Nutrition and medical studies are replete with the negative effects of salt. Yet, sodium is undeniably a necessary nutrient for good health; indeed, it is essential to human existence. In ancient times, salt was so valuable that men traded it for its weight in gold. Today's sound-byte media medicine teaches us that salt is dangerous and that the public should avoid it. But, while certain individuals who are salt-sensitive must curb their intake, most Americans do not suffer ill effects when they use salt sensibly in their diets.

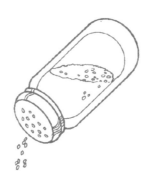

Sodium occurs naturally in foods. sium, sodium regulates blood pressure, muscle activity. Together, sodium and po- nourish, and drain waste products out tassium relationship also helps maintain fluid or get dehydrated.

We need salinity for good body tone contract. It is needed for strong blood — cium. Sodium helps keep body pH bal- pulses. It keeps glands and organs we can digest our food. Too little sodium of clear thinking, because the brain de-

Accompanied by its partner mineral, potas- transmits nerve impulses and maintains tassium pump nutrients into the cells to of them to clean the cells. The sodium-po- fluid balance, so you don't retain excess

because sodium is necessary for muscles to without sodium, the body cannot use cal- anced. It transports nutrients and nerve im- healthy, and produces hydrochloric acid so leads to low vitality, stagnate blood and loss pends on good fluid circulation.

Your body's salt balance is important. Diseases like congestive heart failure, kidney diseases (healthy kidneys control sodium levels), gastrointestinal disease and diabetes all affect salt balance.

Sodium is critical to blood pressure balance. Table salt is 40% sodium and 60% chloride; it's the sodium that affects blood pressure. A sodium-restricted diet for hypertension ranges from 1,000 to 3,000mg a day. Our bodies need about 500 milligrams ($1/4$ teaspoon) of sodium to help regulate the distribution of body fluids. Sodium restriction has no effect on the blood pressure of people who have normal blood pressure.

What are signs that you have too little salt? Signs of sodium deficiency include flatulence, diarrhea, and unexplained nausea. Tissue dehydration causes wrinkles and sunken eyes. Poor fluid circulation in the brain causes confusion, irritability, heightened allergies and low blood pressure. Diuretics, excessive sweating, fever, diarrhea, heat, even exercise can cause severe sodium imbalance, and make your body lose too much salt.

What are the signs that your body has too much salt? PMS symptoms like breast tenderness and bloating, constipation, headaches and dizziness, aggravated asthma, fatigue, ringing in the ears and body weakness. Beyond eating extra salty food, excess use of cortisone drugs or anabolic steroids causes us to build up salt.

Where does the extra salt in our diets come from?

It is a common myth that table salt is the major source of sodium in the average American diet. Ten percent of the sodium in the average diet occurs naturally in food, 15 percent comes from salt you personally add to your food, (one teaspoon of salt = about 2,000mg of sodium). Most sodium today is added during food processing - up to 4,000 milligrams of sodium a day. **A whopping 75 percent is added to food during processing.**

Junk and fast foods are the worst offenders. A steady diet of these foods along with high blood pressure is an explosive health situation. We get salt from medicines, too. Over-the-counter drugs like antacids, laxatives, and sleeping aids contain generous amounts of sodium. Effervescent antacid tablets, for example, contain 276mg sodium per tablet and Instant Metamucil has 250mg sodium per package. Read labels carefully.

Sodium-containing ingredients that you may not recognize on a label include: *sodium caseinate, monosodium glutamate, trisodium phosphate, sodium bicarbonate and sodium sterol lactate.*

The Average American consumes 8000 - 10,000mg of salt a day.
1: Ten hard, salted pretzel twists........................ 2400mg
2: 1 large dill pickle... 1700mg
3: 1 cup Campbell's Tomato-Rice soup.............. 1480mg
4: 1 tablespoon tamari soy sauce........................ 960mg
5: Stouffer's Chicken Stir-Fry with Vegetables... 630mg
6: 1 cup canned French cut green beans............ 780mg
7: One shake of the salt shaker........................... 250mg
8: 6 large black olives.. 230mg

Note: Fat-free foods usually have even more salt to compensate for the lack of flavor from fat. Fat-free mayonnaise, margerine and cream cheese, for example, can have double the sodium content of their fattier counterparts.

There are many good ways to get the good salts that your body needs:
1: Sea greens' salty taste is really a balanced mineral chelate.
2: Herb salts and seasonings provide plant enzymes to make salts absorbable.
3: Sea salt is a rich source of iodine, potassium and many minerals besides sodium.
4: Tamari is a wheat-free soy sauce, lower in sodium and richer in flavor than soy sauce.
5: Umeboshi plums are highly alkalizing, excellent for a macrobiotic diet.
6: Naturally fermented foods like pickles, relishes, olives are also healthy cultured foods.
7: Bragg's LIQUID AMINOS is an energizing protein broth, with valuable amino acids.
8: Miso is a salty-tasting soy paste made from cooked, aged soybeans.
9: Gomashio blends sesame seeds and sea salt, a delicious staple in oriental cooking.

A salt-free diet may be desirable for someone who eats too much salt. However, once the body's salinity normalizes, some salt should be brought back into the diet quickly.

LOW SALT, NOT NO SALT, is best for a permanent way of eating. Don't worry about sodium deficiency; even a low sodium diet has 2,400mg.

The moments of happiness we enjoy take us by surprise. We do not seize them. They seize us....

—*Ashley Montagu.*

Sea Greens & Iodine Therapy

Sea greens have superior nutritional content. They transmit the energies of the sea to your body as a rich source of nutrients. Ounce for ounce, along with herbs, they are higher in vitamins and minerals than any other food. Sea greens are one of nature's richest sources of vegetable protein, and they provide full-spectrum concentrations of beta carotene, chlorophyll, enzymes, amino acids and fiber. The distinctive salty taste is not just "salt," but a balanced, chelated combination of sodium, potassium, calcium, magnesium, phosphorus, iron and trace minerals.

Sea greens help re-mineralize us. eral salts that combine with amino ac- get usable nutrients for structural essary trace elements for life, many They convert inorganic ocean min- ids. Our bodies use this combination as an ideal way to building blocks. In fact, sea greens contain all the nec- of which are depleted in the Earth's soil.

Our body fluids have the same ments that circulate in the ocean position is so close to human efit from sea greens is promoting as the ocean's purifiers, and they for our bodies. Their rich antioxi- for detoxification. Sea greens help alkalize and normal- modern diet. They strengthen us against disease, and chemical composition as sea water. The same 56 ele- course through our veins. Sea plant chemical com- plasma, that perhaps the greatest ben- our internal rebalance. Sea greens act perform many of the same functions dant qualities are effective toxin scavengers ize our bodies from the over-acid effects of a reduce excess stores of fluid and fat.

Sea greens are some of our most powerful healers. They have anti-inflammatory, antiviral, antimicrobial, antifungal, and anticancer activity. Modern science validates many of the traditional benefits of sea plants, especially their algin, the element thought to be responsible for sea plant's success in treating obesity, asthma and atherosclerosis. Algin absorbs toxins from our digestive tracts in much the same way that a water softener removes the hardness from tap water. Less toxins enter our bloodstream because of algin's activity.

Sea greens are the most nutritionally dense plants on the planet. They have access to all the nutrients in the ocean, acquiring nourishment across its entire surface through wave action and underwater currents. Sea greens are rich in fiber and packed with vitamins, with measureable amounts of vitamins K, A, D, B, E and C, and a broad range of carotenes. Sea greens are almost the only non-animal source of vitamin B-12 for our cell development and nerve function. They are full of amino acids, up to 20% protein, active enzymes and essential fatty acids to rejuvenate us. **They contain 10 to 20 times the minerals of land plants,** and beyond their mineral quantities, their mineral balance is a natural stabilizer for building sound nerve structure and good metabolism. Sea plant iodine, for example, helps control and prevent gland disorders like breast and uterine fibroids, prostate inflammation and adrenal exhaustion.

Here are some of the things sea greens can do for you:

1: Sea greens and our destructive environment: Sea plants can protect us from a wide range of toxic elements in the environment, including heavy metals (most dental fillings still contain them) and radiation byproducts, converting them into harmless salts that our bodies can eliminate. The natural iodine in sea greens can reduce by almost 80% the radioactive iodine-131 absorbed by the thyroid. Still, although seaweeds contain the compounds that directly counteract carcinogens, most researchers believe that their success is in boosting the body's immune system so it can combat the carcinogens itself.

Sea greens contain powerful antioxidant and anti-cancer properties, to arrest the proliferation of cancer cells. Some experts consider them more potent than the drugs used to treat breast and prostate cancer, especially as interceptive measures. Japanese studies show that a diet with as little as 5% sea greens inhibits cancer growth, even causing remission of some active tumors.

2: Sea greens and breast cancer: Iodine deficiency and hypothyroidism are clearly involved with a higher incidence of breast cancer. Japanese women have less than one-sixth the breast cancer rate of American women of similar age. Japanese women who live in rural areas have a much lower breast cancer rate than Japanese women in urban areas. The determining factor seems to be diet. The rural Japanese women routinely eat sea plants — a food uncommon in the diets of American and urban Japanese women who eat many processed foods. In animal studies, rats exposed to chemicals known to cause breast cancer were fed sea greens and were protected against getting cancer.

Women with low iodine levels often have cervical hyperplasia and breast fibroids, too. In clinical trials, hyperplasia lesions have been corrected by sea plants. My own experience with sea plant iodine shows that it reduces both breast and uterine fibroids, with significant anti-inflammatory and anti-scarring effects.

3: Sea greens and bone health: Sea greens have high magnesium, essential for the absorption of calcium. Magnesium stimulates production of calcitonin, the hormone which increases calcium in the bones. Sea greens are a good source of natural vitamin D, also essential for calcium absorption, bone health and muscle function. Many people don't store vitamin D very well; our indoor lives don't let us get out in the sun as much as in times past. Forty percent of Americans (especially women) are deficient in this nutrient. Even many who take vitamin D supplements show a deficiency.

4: Sea greens and your thyroid: In our era of processed foods and iodine-poor soils, sea greens and sea foods stand alone as potent sources of natural, balanced iodine. Iodine is essential to life; the thyroid gland cannot make thyrozin, the enzyme that regulates metabolism, without it. Iodine is an important element of alertness and rapid brain activity, and a prime deterrent to arterial plaque.

Thyroid hormones are made from iodine and the amino acid tyrosine. Thyroglobulin, the mixture of tyrosine and iodine stored in the thyroid gland, is transformed into hormones that regulate our metabolism, protein, carbohydrate and carotene use, and cholesterol (sea greens help lower cholesterol). The amount of thyroid hormone released into the bloodstream determines the body's basic energy level and along with the adrenal glands, the rate that sex hormones are made. Sea plants nourish an underactive thyroid and normalize adrenal functions to trigger increased libido.

Goiter, a thyroid disorder, develops when the pituitary gland stimulates the thyroid to make more hormones but the thyroid can't do it because of an iodine deficiency. It enlarges in the attempt and goiter develops. The rate of goiter in the U.S. is still relatively high — 6% of the population in some areas. It's a strange situation, because few people in the U. S. are iodine deficient (the average American intake of iodine is estimated at over 600 micrograms daily from iodized salt). Since the recommended adult allowance for iodine is quite small, 150 micrograms, experts believe that at least some of the high rates of goiter are really connected to too much sugar, alcohol, fats and caffeine, or to eating a lot of goitrogen foods, which block iodine absorbtion.

Goitrogen foods are cruciferous vegetables like broccoli, cauliflower or cabbage, legumes like beans, peas and peanuts, beets, and nuts like almonds, which may cause a mild hypothyroid state when eaten raw. Cooking neutralizes the thyroid-blocking components. If you have a tendency to goiter or hypothyroidism, cook these healthy foods lightly.

5: Sea greens and pregnancy: Iodine deficiency has a profound effect on the health of the fetus early in conception. I recommend that a woman who wants to become pregnant consider adding sea greens to her diet while she is trying to conceive, rather than waiting until she realizes that she is pregnant. Most American women get enough iodine from fish and seafood, but in developing, landlocked countries, where iodine is not plentiful in food, infants are often born with cretinism which results in stunted growth, mental deficiency, puffy facial features and lack of muscle coordination, all signs of low iodine.

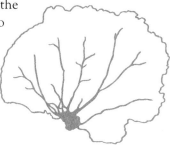

Sea greens in a pregnant woman's diet help the health of the mother, too.
—Hemoglobin counts rise from 65% to 83%
—Colds decrease in number and severity; arthritic conditions improve
—Hair color and quality improve; fingernails grow stronger
—Skin texture improves; capillary strength increases, so there is less bruising
—Eye conditions improve, especially if there is eye redness or inflammation
—Constipation lessens and a sense of well-being increases
—Stretch marks are less during pregnancy and skin heals better afterwards

6: Sea greens are a valuable treatment for candida albicans. Their high mineral, especially selenium content, builds up immunity against candida. Enzymes use the rich iodine in seaweeds to produce iodine-charged free radicals, which deactivate yeasts. Other immune-compromised diseases like chronic fatigue, HIV infection, arthritis and allergies respond to sea plant treatment, too.

7: Sea greens and vaginal infections: Iodine-rich sea plants are effective against a wide range of harmful organisms like trichomonas, candida and chlamydia. A douche solution with 1 tablespoon dried sea vegetables to 1 quart of water, used twice daily for 7 to 14 days, is effective against most of these pathogens.

8: Nutrition studies show that sea plants effectively lower blood pressure and cholesterol, help deter arteriosclerosis and reduce toxins in the liver and kidneys.

9: Sea greens boost weight loss and deter cellulite build-up. Virtually fat-free (mostly healthy EFA's), with low calories, sea plants help your thyroid normalize metabolism, especially as you age. Sea plant fiber and algin lower bowel transit time to aid weight loss. Sea plant antioxidants increase your body's fat-burning ability.
The detoxifying qualities of sea plant algin stimulate lymphatic drainage to discourage cellulite. Seaweed helps your skin tissue and fat cells absorb minerals. The minerals act like electrolytes to break the chemical bond that seals the fat cells. The fat cells open temporarily to allow trapped wastes to escape into the lymph system and be eliminated by the kidneys and bladder. Both eating sea greens and bathing in them helps reduce cellulite. The best spas apply a sea plant solution as part of a body wrap or bath to do this very thing. It's called thalasso-therapy, and it's been used for centuries to speed up metabolism and increase circulation to cellulitic areas.

10: Sea greens are a beauty treatment: Seaweeds add amazing luster to the skin. The sea-loving Greek culture said that Aphrodite, the goddess of love who rose out of the foaming sea, owed her supple skin, shiny hair, and sparkling eyes to the plants of the sea. A seaweed face mask increases circulation, stimulates lymphatic drainage and dilates capillaries to tone your skin. Seaweed returns mineral salts to your skin that stress and pollution deplete. Skin cells hold moisture better when they absorb the mineral salts, making the skin more supple and elastic. By retaining moisture, the skin plumps, removing the look of dry skin, lines and wrinkles. Many women report smoother skin and better skin texture after a seaweed treatment. Amino acid, mineral and vitamin content help nourish the skin, too. Certain types of seaweeds possess molecules similar to collagen.

A seaweed bath is a great way to get the benefits of sea plants all over your body.
Seaweed baths are Nature's perfect body-psyche balancer, and they're a good way get natural iodine.
Remember how good you feel after a walk in the ocean? Seaweeds purify and balance the ocean; they can do the same for your body. Noticeable rejuvenating effects occur when toxins are released from your tissues. A hot seaweed bath is like a wet-steam sauna, only better, because the sea greens balance body chemistry instead of dehydrating it. The electrolytic magnetic action of the sea plants releases excess body fluids from congested cells and dissolves fatty wastes through the skin, replacing them with depleted minerals, particularly potassium and iodine. As the natural iodine boosts thyroid activity, food fuels are used before they can turn into fatty deposits. Vitamin K, a fat-soluble vitamin in seaweeds, aids adrenal regulation, so a seaweed bath also helps maintain hormone balance for a more youthful body.

If an ocean near you has unpolluted waters, you can collect your own sea greens. Gather them from the water, (not the shoreline), in buckets or clean trash cans, and carry them home to your tub. If you don't live near the ocean, buy dried sea greens in health food stores.

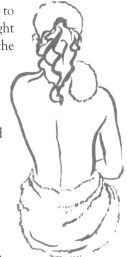

Whichever form you choose, run very hot water over the seaweed in a tub, filling it to the point that you will be covered when you recline. The leaves will turn a beautiful bright green. The water will turn rich brown as the plants release their minerals. As you soak, the gel from the seaweed transfers onto your skin. This coating increases perspiration to release toxins from your system, and replaces them by osmosis with minerals. Rub your skin, especially cellulite areas with the sea leaves during the bath to stimulate circulation, smooth and tone the body, and remove wastes coming out on the skin surface. When the sea greens have done their work, the gel coating dissolves and floats off the skin, and the leaves shrivel — a sign that the bath is over.

Each bath varies with the individual, the seaweeds used, and water temperature, but the gel coating release is a natural timekeeper for the bath's benefits. Forty-five minutes is usually about right to balance the acid-alkaline system, encourage liver activity, cellulite release and fat metabolism. Skin tone, color, and better circulation are almost immediately noticeable. To get the most from a seaweed treatment, dry brush cellulitic skin before your seaweed bath or wrap to exfoliate dead skin, and open up pores for waste elimination and blood flow to the affected area.

Note: A hot seaweed bath is one of the most effective treatments in natural healing, but use it with care. If you are under a doctor's care for heart disease or high blood pressure, check with your physician to see if a seaweed bath is okay for you.

Sea plants come in green, brown, red and blue-green algae. A quick profile:

—**Kelp** (*laminaria*) contains vitamins A, B, E, D and K, is a main source of vitamin C, and rich in minerals. Kelp proteins are comparable in quality to animal proteins. A brown marine plant, kelp contains sodium alginate (algin), an element that helps remove radioactive particles and heavy metals from the body. Algin, carrageenan and ager are kelp gels that rejuvenate gastrointestinal health and aid digestion. Kelp works as a blood purifier, relieves arthritis stiffness, and promotes adrenal, pituitary and thyroid health. Kelp's natural iodine can normalize thyroid-related disorders like overweight and lymph system congestion. It is a demulcent that helps eliminate herpes outbreaks. Kelp is rich — a little goes a long way.

—**Kombu** (*laminaria digitata, setchelli, horsetail kelp*), has a long tradition as a Japanese delicacy with great nutritional healing value. It is a decongestant for excess mucous, and helps lower blood pressure. Kombu has abundant iodine, carotenes, B, C, D and E vitamins, minerals like calcium, magnesium, potassium, silica, iron and zinc, and the powerful skin healing nutrient germanium. Kombu is a meaty, high-protein seaweed. It is higher in natural mineral salts than most other seaweeds. Add a strip of kombu to your bean pot to reduce gas.

—**Hijiki** is a mineral-rich, high-fiber seaweed, with 20% protein, vitamin A, carotenes and calcium. Hijiki has the most calcium of any sea green, 1400mg per 100gr. of dry weight.

—**Nori** (*porphyra, laver*) is a red sea plant with a sweet, meaty taste when dried. It contains nearly 50% balanced, assimilable protein, higher than any other sea plant. Nori's fiber makes it a perfect sushi wrapper. Nori is rich in all the carotenes, calcium, iodine, iron, and phosphorus.

—**Arame** (*Eisenia bycyclis*), is one of the ocean's richest sources of iodine. Herbalists use arame to help reduce breast and uterine fibroids, and through its fat soluble vitamins and phytohormones, to normalize menopausal symptoms. Arame promotes soft, wrinkle-free skin, enhances glossy hair and prevents its loss.

—**Sea Palm** (*Postelsia Palmaeformis*), American arame, grows only on the Pacific Coast of North America. One of my favorites, it has a sweet, salty taste that goes especially well as a vegetable, rice or salad topping.

—**Bladderwrack** is packed with vitamin K — an excellent adrenal stimulant. It is still used today by native Americans in steam baths for arthritis, gout and illness recovery.

—**Wakame** (*alaria, undaria*) is a high-protein, high calcium seaweed, with carotenes, iron and vitamin C. Widely used in the Orient for hair growth and luster, and for skin tone.

—**Dulse** (*palmaria palmata*), a red sea plant, is rich in iron, protein, and vitamin A. It is a supremely balanced nutrient, with 300 times more iodine and 50 times more iron than wheat. Tests on dulse show activity against the herpes virus. It has purifying and tonic effects on the body, yet its natural, balanced salts nourish as a mineral, without inducing thirst.

—**Irish moss** (*chondrus crispus, carrageen*) is full of electrolyte minerals — calcium, magnesium, sodium and potassium. Its mucilaginous compounds help you detoxify, boost metabolism and strengthen hair, skin and nails. Traditionally used for a low sex drive.

Preventive measures may be taken against iodine deficiency problems or disease risk by adding just 2 tablespoons of chopped, dried sea greens to your daily diet.

Sea greens are tasty. Crush, chop, snip or crumble any mix of dry sea greens you like into soups and sauces, pizzas or focaccias, casseroles, rice and salads. Roast them into anything you cook. If you add sea veggies, no other salt is needed, an advantage for a low salt diet. Sundried, they are convenient to buy, store, and use as needed. Store them in a moisture proof container and they keep indefinitely. A wide variety of sea greens is available today.

"The greatest work that we do is not at the desk in the office, but when we are wandering in the woods or sitting quietly relaxed.
At such times there flash into our minds those ideas that direct and mould our lives. For growth and health a sufficient amount of leisure and rest is essential."
—*Dr. Philip Welsh*

Healing Powerhouses of the Desert

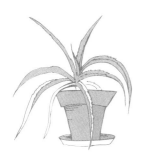

Aloe vera, the lily of the desert, is a unique, potent healing superfood with a wealth of new research. Over seventy-five healing compounds have been identified in aloe, including steroids, antibiotic and anti-carcinogenic agents, amino acids, minerals and enzymes (one enzyme has been isolated to treat burns). It has excellent transdermal properties, allowing it to penetrate deep skin levels.

Aloe gel has been used since Egyptian times as a skin lubricant and healer for cuts, sunburn, bruises, insect bites, sores, acne, eczema and burns. New research shows healing results for skin cancers, hemorrhoids and varicose veins. Aloe is recommended in the medical world for post-op healing, because it is a natural antiseptic, astringent and stimulates lymphatic circulation to boost antibody formation against infections.

Aloe juice is widely popular today because it boosts the body's self-cleansing action – balancing rather than causing harsh irritant effects. Aloe juice has anti-inflammatory EFA's that help the stomach and colon. Aloe juice alkalizes digestive processes to prevent overacidity, a common cause of indigestion, acid reflux, digestive tract irritations like IBS, colitis, Crohn's disease and ulcers. Ulcer patients taking aloe juice show up to 80% reduction in the number of ulcers being formed. Even after the formation of ulcers, healing is three times faster.

Aloe is a core healer in the alternative arsenal with unique nutritional and body balancing properties. It helps normalize fat metabolism to reduce cholesterol and triglycerides. New research shows it effective for immune disorders like candida, parasite invasions, fatigue syndromes like fibromyalgia, allergies, arthritis, eczema and psoriasis.

I call aloe vera an intelligent plant, because it can differentiate between normal cells, mutated cells (cancer) or diseased cells (HIV). It stimulates normal cell growth, while inhibiting cancer cell division (even lymphocytic leukemia) and virus spread. Aged aloe vera juice is widely used in AIDS treatment to block the HIV virus movement from cell to cell. Acemannan, an aloe derivative with powerful anti-viral effects, shows promise against herpes viruses.

Aloe vera is loaded with mucopolysaccharides, phytochemicals with profound healing qualities. Mucopolysaccharides are credited with aloe's immune enhancement qualities, antiviral and antibacterial activity, and its ability to eliminate toxic wastes. Rich in organic silicon, MPS's are a vital component of cell and artery walls, mucous membranes, and the connective tissues of bones, teeth and cartilage. They link with collagen and elastin to maintain tissues and organs, alleviate joint problems and rebuild degenerating cartilage. Essentially mucopolysaccharides and collagen hold our tissues together. MPS's also reduce inflammation and blood clotting time, lessening the risk for cardiovascular disease.

Nature's most energizing superfoods come from high desert beehives.

—**Royal jelly** is a nutritional powerhouse containing every nutrient necessary to support life. No other food source compares nutritionally to royal jelly, and it can't be duplicated in a lab. The exclusive food of the queen bee, royal jelly transforms a "cinderella" worker bee into a queen bee. Her life expectancy rises to an astounding 6 years, compared to a worker bee's 6 week life span — an amazing result of her royal jelly diet!

Royal jelly's rejuvenative powers have been seen for centuries as a fountain of youth for us, too. Herbalists say royal jelly is a fabulous nutrient for skin and hair, nourishing the skin to ease wrinkles, dryness, even adult acne. It is effective for gland and hormone imbalances that mean menstrual, menopause and prostate problems. Chinese herbalists advocate royal jelly as a natural antibiotic, for liver disease, arthritis and anemia.

Royal jelly has extraordinary powers to strengthen the human immune system. It is a rich source of B vitamins (especially B-5, pantothenic acid), minerals, sex hormones, enzyme precursors and all eight essential amino acids. Success stories show royal jelly is effective against fatigue, stress, insomnia and depression.

Royal Jelly is quite difficult to harvest and commands high prices because of its scarcity and consumer demand. The highest quality royal jelly products are preserved in their whole, raw, "alive" state for the best body absorption. As little as one drop of pure, extracted fresh royal jelly can deliver a daily supply.

I find that panax ginseng and royal jelly in a health drink is one of the best ways to take these two dynamos for a healing diet. The attributes of ginseng and royal jelly have synergistic activity in combination.

—**Propolis** is one of the most powerful antibiotics in nature. Bee hives have been called "the most antiseptic places in nature," because propolis neutralizes harmful organisms that enter the hive. Bees are prone to bacterial and viral infections; propolis protects the bees from these infections. The powerful antibiotic properties of propolis can also protect humans — specifically against *staphylococcus aureus*, a bacteria that causes serious infections, blood poisoning and a type of pneumonia. (Interestingly, *staph. a.* has become resistant to all but one pharmaceutical antibiotic.) New studies show that propolis inhibits the streptococcal bacteria that causes strep throat and dental cavities. Propolis even works well with two anti-staph drugs, streptomycin and cloxacillin, because it performs much like a prescription antibiotic — preventing bacteria cell division and breaking down bacteria cell structure. Even better, propolis works against viruses, something that antibiotics cannot do.

Bees collect the base for propolis from the leaf buds on the bark of trees, then convert it with bee enzymes to a sticky material of 50-55% resin and balsam, 30% wax and 10% pollen. Rich in immune defense vitamins, minerals and amino-acids (all 22 of them), bees paste a propolis shield on the inner hive walls to guard against harmful microorganisms as well as to patch holes or cracks in the hive. Nature is incredibly efficient.

Propolis creates a natural antibiotic shield for humans too. Research shows that taking propolis during high risk "cold and flu" seasons reduces colds, coughing, and inflammation of mouth, tonsils and throat membranes. Look for a supplement that contains propolis, vitamin C and zinc for the best results. Further, propolis is rich in flavonoids and B-vitamins that work both internally and externally to heal scars, bruises and blemishes.

—**Bee pollen** is called Nature's perfect food because it's nutritionally complete. It has all 22 amino acids, 27 minerals, the full span of vitamins, complex carbohydrates, essential fatty acids, enzymes and co-enzymes. Bee pollen has 5 to 7 times more protein than beef! Bee pollen is so nutrient rich, it's been used worldwide for centuries to rejuvenate and rebuild the body after illness. I've experienced this healing ability myself.

The West discovered pollen's long life benefits by accident during a 1950's investigation of native Russian bee keepers who regularly lived past 100 years of age, and who ate raw honey, rich in bee pollen, every day.

Pollen is a valuable aid to weight control. It's ability to normalize body metabolism and stoke metabolic fires helps keep calories burning and weight stable. Bee pollen also acts as a natural appetite suppressant through its amino acid phenylalanine (for people who need to gain weight, phenylalanine produces the opposite effect).

There's more. Bee pollen also:
—increases energy levels and strength for athletes
—helps the body normalize from diarrhea and constipation
—tranquilizes without side effects
—increases blood hemoglobin
—rids the body of toxins from drugs, alcohol, smoking, and chemicalized food
—chelates and flushes out artery-clogging biochemical deposits
—reduces the negative effects associated with radiation
—protects against skin dehydration and stimulates growth of new skin tissue

Note: Bee pollen has shown great effectiveness for the relief of allergy symptoms. However, a small percentage of the population may be allergic to bee products.

Jojoba benefits are attracting more and more Americans.

Desert plants are always full of natural, long-lasting moisturizers. For us, this means they are wonderful cosmetics as well as soothing healers. The jojoba plant is no exception. Jojoba nut oil has been used by Native Americans for hundreds of years — treating sores, cuts, bruises, and burns. As a diet supplement and appetite suppressant, they roasted the nuts to make a coffee-like beverage when food was scarce. As a skin conditioner, it was used to soothe and heal the skin after sun or wind burn. As a hair restorative oil, it was an effective scalp treatment.

Jojoba oil is actually like a liquid wax with rich antioxidant properties to keep it from turning rancid. For people, this means that jojoba oil is a natural mimic of sebum oil secreted by the human skin. So it is an effective lubricant and protector in protecting human skin from aging and wrinkling.

Fortunately for the world's sperm whale population, jojoba oil is virtually identical to sperm whale oil, with a melting temperature close to that of the human body. It is an ideal natural base for the cosmetics in which whale oil was used until the mid 1950's.

Jojoba oil is rapid, penetrating, hypo-allergenic skin therapy. Besides moisturizing and soothing skin, jojoba gives your skin a healthy glow because it restores natural pH balance. Studies show that just one hour after application, jojoba oil increases skin softness by as much as 37 percent, reducing superficial lines and wrinkles, especially around the eyes, by as much as 25 percent! Because of its purity and antioxidant freshness, herbal healers use jojoba to treat skin problems like adult acne, psoriasis, and neurodermatitis which are not responsive to chemical medicines.

Jojoba oil is the most effective natural scalp cleaning substance discovered so far. As it did in Native American medicine, jojoba helps restore non-hereditary hair loss that is linked to dandruff and clogged scalp follicles. Each single hair is lubricated by sebum, manufactured by sebaceous glands that lie next to the hair follicles. Healthy hair grows about one half inch per month for 2 - 4 years unless there is sebum imbalance, a vitamin or diet deficiency, illness or excessive stress. When too much sebum collects, hair follicles clog, resulting in unhealthy hair, poor hair growth and shortened hair life. Jojoba dissolves excess sebum deposits, opens up hair follicles and encourages healthy hair growth.

Jojoba's natural appetite suppressing activity comes from a constituent called *simmondsia*. A highly versatile weight control aid, jojoba can be made into anything from a tasty candy bar to a chocolate-y beverage.

Admiration becomes the carbon paper that transfers character qualities by the rubbing of one life against another.

A Special Guide To Detoxification

Body purification has been a part of mankind's rituals for health and well-being for thousands of years. Cleansing is a rich tradition that has helped humans through all ages and cultures. It is at the foundation of every great healing philosophy.

Today, we see how important detoxification is becoming once again — for everybody. No one is free from the enormous amount of environmental toxins assaulting us in the world today. No one is immune to every unhealthy lifestyle option. How do we remain healthy in a destructive environment?

This chapter answers your questions about body cleansing. It discusses detoxification in detail. It defines a good detoxification program, how it works in the body, and the benefits you can expect. It includes visible signs that your body needs a good cleansing, and the types of detox programs you can use to best suit your needs.

Step by step instructions are included for the initial diets, supplements, and herbs you'll need, along with tips that can give you the best results.

Detoxification programs are included for:
  1: Colon and bowel cleansing
  2: Bladder and kidney cleansing
  3: Lung and mucous congestion cleansing
  4: Liver and organ cleansing
  5: Lymphatic cleansing
  6: Skin cleansing
  7: Blood cleansing — for heavy metal toxicity, alcohol and drug addictions

For more information, see my new book, DETOXIFICATION ©1999, a comprehensive book on all aspects of cleansing for safe, effective personal detox programs. Over 250 pages, it includes delicious green cuisine cleansing recipes, detox plans for specific health problems, and extensive detox charts for easy use.

Understanding Detoxification

What is detoxification? Our bodies naturally do it every day. Detoxification is a normal body process of eliminating or neutralizing toxins through the colon, liver, kidneys, lungs, lymph and skin. In fact, internal detoxification is one of our body's most basic automatic functions. Just as our hearts beat nonstop and our lungs breathe continuously, so our metabolic processes continuously dispose of accumulated toxic matter. But in our world today, body systems and organs that were once capable of cleaning out unwanted substances are now completely overloaded, so much toxic material stays in our tissues. Our bodies try to protect us from dangerous material by setting it aside, surrounding it with mucous or fat so it won't cause imbalance or trigger an immune reaction. **(Our bodies store foreign substances in fatty deposits — a significant reason to keep your body fat low. Some people carry around up to 15 extra pounds of mucous that harbors this waste!)**

We mourn yesterday's pollution-free environment, whole foods and pure water. But, since humans are born with a "self-cleaning system," this ideal probably never existed. Today, we control our environment even less. The best thing is to keep pollutants to a minimum and to periodically get rid of them through detoxification.

Does a detox program work if our self-cleaning system is overwhelmed?

Detoxification through special cleansing diets may be the missing link to disease prevention, especially for immune-compromised diseases like cancer, arthritis, diabetes and fatigue syndromes like candida albicans. Our chemicalized-food diet, with too much animal protein, too much fat, too much caffeine and alcohol radically alters our internal ecosystems. Even if your diet is good, a body cleanse can restore your vitality against environmental toxins that pave the way for disease-bearing bacteria, viruses and parasites.

A detox program aims to remove the cause of disease before it makes us ill. It's a time-honored way to keep immune response high, elimination regular, circulation sound, and stress under control, so your body can handle the toxicity it encounters. In the past, detoxification was used either clinically for recovering alcoholics and drug addicts, or as a once-a-year personal "spring cleaning" for general well-being. Today, a regular detox program two or three times a year makes a big difference not only for health, but for the quality of our lives.

Should you detoxify?

Today, Americans are exposed to chemicals of all kinds on an unprecedented scale. Industrial chemicals and their pollutant run-offs in our water, pesticides, additives in our foods, heavy metals, anesthetics, residues from drugs, and environmental hormones are trapped within the human body in greater concentrations than at any other point in history. Every system of the body is affected, from tissue damage to sensory deterioration.

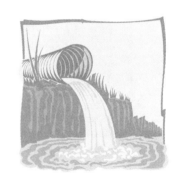

Many chemicals are so widespread that we are unaware of them. But they have worked their way into our bodies faster than they can be eliminated, and are causing allergies and addictions in record numbers. **More than 2 million synthetic substances are known, 25,000 are added each year, and over 30,000 are produced on a commercial scale.** Only a tiny fraction are ever tested for toxicity. A lot of them come to us from developing countries that have few safeguards in place. This doesn't even count the second-hand smoke, caffeine and alcohol overload, or daily stress that is an increasing part of our lives.

The molecular structure of some chemical carcinogens interacts with human DNA, so long term exposure may result in metabolic and genetic alteration that affects cell growth and behavior. World Health Organization research implicates environmental chemicals in 60 to 80% of all cancers. Hormone-disrupting pesticides and pollutants are linked to hormone problems, psychological disorders, birth defects, still births and now breast cancer.

As toxic matter saturates our tissues, antioxidants and minerals in vital body fluids are reduced, so immune defenses are thrown out of balance. Circumstances like this are the prime factor in today's immune compromised diseases like candidiasis, lupus, fibromyalgia, and chronic fatigue syndrome.

Chemical oxidation is the other process that allows disease. The oxygen that "rusts" and ages us also triggers free radical activity, a destructive cascade of incomplete molecules that damages DNA and other cell components. And if you didn't have a reason to reduce your animal fat intake before, here is a critical one: **oxygen combines with animal fat in body storage cells and speeds up the free radical process.**

Almost everyone can benefit from a cleanse. It's one of the best ways to remain healthy in dangerous surroundings. Not one of us is immune to environmental toxins, and most of us can't escape to a remote, unpolluted habitat. In the last few decades, technology has become seriously able to harm the health of our entire planet, even to the point of making it uninhabitable for life. We must develop our culture further and take larger steps of cooperation. Mankind and the Earth must work together — to save it all for us all. It starts with us. We can keep our own body systems in good working order so that toxins are eliminated quickly.

We can also take a closer look at our own air, water and food, and keep an ever watchful eye on the politics that control our environment. Legislation on health and the environment follows two pathways in America today.... the influence of business and profits, and the demands of the people for a healthy habitat and responsible stewardship of the Earth. (See "Fluoridation — An unnecessary poison in our drinking water," page 148).

Is your body becoming toxic? Body signs can tell you that you need to detoxify.

We all have different "toxic tolerance" levels. Listen to your body when it starts giving you those "cellular phone calls." If you can keep the amount of toxins in your system below your toxic level, your body can usually adapt and rid itself of them.

Do you have:
—Frequent, unexplained headaches, back or joint pain, or arthritis?
—Chronic respiratory problems, sinus problems or asthma?
—Abnormal body odor, bad breath or coated tongue?
—Food allergies, poor digestion or chronic constipation with intestinal bloating or gas?
—Brittle nails and hair, psoriasis, adult acne, or unexplained weight gain over 10 pounds?
—Unusually poor memory, chronic insomnia, depression, irritability, chronic fatigue?
—Environmental sensitivities, especially to odors?
Laboratory tests like stool, urine, blood or liver tests, and hair analysis can also shed light on the need for a detox.

What benefits can you expect from a good detox?

A detox cleans out body waste deposits, so you aren't running with a dirty engine or driving with the brakes on. After a cleanse, the body starts rebalancing, energy levels rise physically, psychologically and sexually, and creativity begins to expand. You start feeling like a different person — because you are. Your outlook and attitude change, because through cleansing and improved diet, your actual cell make-up has changed.

1) You'll clean your digestive tract of accumulated waste and fermenting bacteria.
2) You'll clear excess mucous and congestion from the body.
3) You'll purify the liver, kidney and blood, impossible under ordinary eating patterns.
4) You'll enhance mental clarity, impossible under chemical overload.
5) You'll be less dependent on sugar, caffeine, nicotine, alcohol or drugs.
6) You'll turn around bad eating habits; your stomach will have a chance to reduce to normal size for weight control.
7) You'll release hormone secretions that coupled with essential fatty acids from fresh plant sources can stimulate and strengthen your immune system.

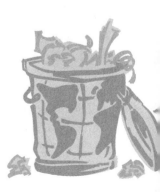

You've decided your body needs a cleanse. What are the steps in a good detox program?

How long can you give out of your busy lifestyle to focus on a cleansing program so that all the processes can be completed? 24 hours, 2 or 3 days, or up to ten days? The time factor is important — you'll want to allocate your time ahead of time, to prepare both your mind and your body for the experience ahead.

A good detox program is in 3 steps — cleansing, rebuilding and maintaining.

Years of experience with detoxification have convinced me that if you have a serious health problem, a brief 3 to 7 day juice cleanse is the best way to release toxins from the system. Shorter cleanses can't get to the root of a chronic problem. Longer cleanses upset body equilibrium more than most people are ready to deal with except in a clinical environment. A 3 to 7 day cleanse can "clean your pipes" of systemic sludge — excess mucous, old fecal matter, trapped cellular and non-food wastes, or inorganic mineral deposits that are part of arthritis.

A few days without solid food can be an enlightening experience about your lifestyle. It's not absolutely necessary to take in only liquids, but a juice diet increases awareness and energy availability for elimination. Fresh juices literally pick up dead matter from the body and carry it away. Your body becomes easier to "hear," telling you via cravings what foods and diet it needs — for example, a desire for protein foods, or B vitamin foods like rices or mineral from greens. This is natural biofeedback.

A detox works by self-digestion. During a cleanse, the body decomposes and burns only the substances and tissues that are damaged, diseased or unneeded, such as abscesses, tumors, excess fat deposits, and congestive wastes. Even a relatively short fast accelerates elimination, often causing dramatic changes as masses of accumulated waste are expelled.

You will know your body is detoxing if you experience the short period of headaches, fatigue, body odor, bad breath, diarrhea or mouth sores that commonly accompany accelerated elimination. However, digestion usually improves right away as do many gland and nerve functions. Cleansing also helps release hormone secretions that stimulate immune response and encourages a disease-preventing environment.

What about a water fast? I don't recommend it. Here's why:

Juice cleansing is a better evolution in detoxification methods. Detoxification experts agree that fresh vegetable and fruit juice cleansing is superior to water fasting. Fresh juices, broths and herb teas help deeply cleanse the body, rejuvenate the tissues and guide you to a faster recovery from health problems than water fasting.

A traditional water fast is harsh and demanding on your body, even in times before huge amounts of food and environmental toxins were part of the picture. Today, it can even be dangerous. Deeply buried pollutants and chemicals from our tissues are released into elimination channels too rapidly during a water fast. Your body is essentially "re-poisoned" as the chemicals move through the bloodstream all at once. Sometimes, the physical and emotional stress of a water fast even overrides the healing benefits.

Vegetable and fruit juices are alkalizing, so they neutralize uric acid and other inorganic acids better than water, and increase the healing effects. Juices support better metabolic activity, too. Metabolic activity slows down during a water fast as the body attempts to conserve dwindling energy resources. Juices are very easy on digestion — easily assimilated into the bloodstream. They don't disturb the detoxification process.

Step one: elimination. You'll clean out mucous and toxins from the intestinal tract and major organs. Everything functions more effectively when toxins, obstructions and wastes are removed.

Step two: rebuilding healthy tissue and restoring energy. With obstacles removed, your body's regulating powers are activated to rebuild at optimum levels. Eat only fresh and simply prepared, vegetarian foods during the rebuilding step. Include supplements and herbal aids for your specific needs.

Step three: keeping your body clean and toxin-free. Modifying lifestyle habits is the key to a strong resistant body. Rely on fresh fruits and vegetables for fiber, cooked vegetables, grains and seeds for strength and alkalinity, lightly cooked sea foods, soy foods, eggs and low fat cheeses as sources of protein, and a little dinner wine for circulatory health. Include supplements, herbs, exercise and relaxation techniques.

What Type of Cleanse Do You Need?

Cleanses come in all shapes and sizes. You can easily tailor a cleanse to your individual needs. Unless you require a specific detox for a serious illness, or recovery from a long course of drugs or chemical therapy, I recommend a short cleanse twice a year, especially in the spring, summer or early autumn when sunshine and natural vitamin D can help the process along.

A "Spring Cleanse" is a breath of fresh air for your body after a long winter.

A mild spring cleanse is an important, annual vitality technique no matter how healthy you are. Even though you may exercise during the winter to keep trim, most people still feel at an energy low during the cold, dark seasons. Our bodies still reflect the ancient seasonal need to harbor more fat for warmth and survival. In a time when people were closer to Nature than we are today, the great majority farmed the land from spring to fall, and lived lives of demanding physical labor. Winter was a time of inactivity, with a natural tendency towards rest. Harvested food supplies stored in the autumn lost much of their nutrition value through the winter, so people had to eat denser foods, and more of them to receive the same nutrients. Even in modern times, many days without sunshine and vitamin D mean that our bodies are less able to utilize nutrients properly.

Cold weather prompts people to consume heavier, fattier, comfort foods. Old winter "hibernation" patterns also mean that metabolism slows, sometimes by as much as 10%. So, much to the dismay of many of us, fall and winter are the most difficult times of the year to control body weight.

Nature has designed the perfect time for a spring cleanse. Winter weather illnesses like colds and flu leave us with accumulated toxins. Heavy winter clothing, especially thick waterproof coats, hinders normal breathing and perspiration of our skin. When spring finally arrives, new green leafy vegetables liven up our metabolism. Cleansing, antioxidant-rich herbs promote a feeling of new life and restored well-being. Nature starts chuckling in the spring. (Laughter is a good cleanser for people, too. It boosts our beta endorphins for a sense of euphoria.) Warmer weather lowers our appetite needs, prompts more activity and movement, and stimulates cleansing.

A "spring cleanse" is actually a very light diet, focusing on digestion and the intestines to help eliminate accumulated wastes, and improve body functions. A good length for a spring or summer cleanse is 2 or 3 days or a long weekend. A weekend is enough time to fit comfortably into most people's lives, and it doesn't become too stressful on the body. The best way is to start on Friday night with a pre-cleansing salad, then follow with a cleansing diet like the one in this book, and end with a light Monday morning fruit bowl. Amplify the purifying effect with a stimulating, circulation bath or sauna and steam baths.

What body signs show that you need a Spring Cleanse?
—Do you feel bloated, constipated and congested? (a sign that your diet is heavier and richer than usual)
—Have you gained unwanted pounds even though you aren't eating more food? (a sign of winter fat storage)
—Do you feel slow and low energy most of the time? (a sign of cold weather body slowdown)
—Has your digestion worsened? (a sign your body isn't using its nutrients well)
—Do your lungs feel clogged and swollen? (a sign of shallower breathing, and perhaps a low-grade infection)

What benefits can you expect from a Spring Cleanse?
—Your digestive tract gets a "wash and brush" of accumulated waste.
—Your liver, kidney and blood are purified, impossible under ordinary eating patterns.
—Your mental clarity receives a boost, impossible under an overload of food chemicals.
—You'll relieve dependency on habit-forming sugars, caffeine, nicotine, alcohol or drugs.
—Bad eating habits get a break..... with a new chance to improve your diet patterns.
—Your stomach has a chance to reduce its size for weight loss and better weight control.

Spring Cleanse Detox Plan

Start with this 3‑day nutrition plan: Focus on fresh plant foods: 1) high chlorophyll plants for enzymes; 2) fruits and vegetables for fiber; 3) cultured foods for probiotics; 4) eight glasses of water a day.

The evening before your spring cleanse.....
—Have a light salad with plenty of greens. Take your choice of gentle herbal laxatives.

The next day....
—**On rising:** take a cleansing and flushing booster product, or 1 heaping teaspoon of a fiber drink in juice. Add 1000mg vitamin C with bioflavonoids 3x a day to raise glutathione levels, an important detox compound.
—**Breakfast:** take your choice of fruit juices.
—**Mid-morning:** take a small glass of potassium broth (pg. 215), or 2 TBS. aloe juice concentrate in juice or water, or a superfood green drink (see suggestions below); or a cup of green tea.
—**Lunch:** a fresh carrot juice; or raw sauerkraut or a seaweed salad (in natural or Oriental food stores)
—**Mid-afternoon:** take a glass of fresh apple juice; or an herbal cleansing tea.
—**About 5 o' clock:** take another small potassium broth, a fresh carrot or vegetable juice (page 218), or a superfood green drink (suggestions below).
—**Supper:** take miso soup with 2 TBS dried sea vegetables (dulse, nori, etc.) snipped over the top.
(Note: Finish your cleanse with a small green salad with fresh sprouts on the last night.)
—**Before Bed:** repeat the herbal cleansers that you took on rising, and take a cup of mint tea.

Spring cleanse supplement suggestions: Choose 2 or 3 cleansing boosters.
•**Gentle herbal laxatives:** HERBALTONE TABLETS, Crystal Star LAXATEA, AloeLife ALOE GOLD. After your initial juice detox, Zand Herbals QUICK CLEANSE KIT for the intestinal tract and the liver.
•**Cleansing boosters:** Crystal Star DETOX™ caps with goldenseal; Planetary Formulas RIVER OF LIFE.
•**Cleansing, flushing boosters:** Nature's Secret SUPERCLEANSE; Crystal Star FIBER & HERBS COLON CLEANSE™.
•**Chlorophyll-rich plants — spring's great gift to us:** Sun Wellness CHLORELLA; Green Foods GREEN ESSENCE; Crystal Star ENERGY GREEN™; NutriCology PRO-GREENS; Nature's Secret ULTIMATE GREEN.
•**Enzyme support:** Transformation Enzyme RELEASEZYME; Herbal Products POWER-PLUS ENZYMES.
•**Electrolyte boosters help detoxify cells:** Nature's Path TRACE-LYTE MINERALS; Arise & Shine ALKALIZER.
•**Probiotics replenish healthy bacteria:** Prevail INNER ECOLOGY; Prof. Nutrition DOCTOR-DOPHILUS+FOS.
•**Antioxidants defeat pollutants:** Biotec Food CELL GUARD; NutriCology ANTIOX FORMULA II; Rainbow Light MULTI CAROTENE COMPLEX; Enzymatic Therapy GREEN TEA ANTIOXIDANT.
•**Fiber:** All One WHOLE FIBER COMPLEX; Crystal Star CHO-LO FIBER TONE™ drink; AloeLife FIBERMATE.

Spring cleanse bodywork suggestions: Choose techniques to accelerate and round out your cleanse.
Irrigate: Take an enema the first, second and the last day of your spring cleansing program.
Exercise: take a walk for ten minutes the first day of your cleanse. Each day increase by five minutes.
Sauna: Take a hot sauna or a long warm bath with a rubdown, to stimulate circulation. Dry brush your body before your sauna to help release toxins coming out through the skin.
Massage therapy: get one good lower back and pelvis massage during your cleanse
Aromatherapy bath: add 8 to 10 drops of essential oil to a bath. Stir water briskly to disperse. Lavender and chamomile are good choices. Try Nature's Alchemy AROMATHERAPY HERBAL MINERAL BATHS.
Deep Breathing Exercise: Remove stress, increase energy, compose your mind, improve your mood: Take a deep breath. Exhale slowly.... slowly. Take another deep breath. Release slowly. And again. Maintain a quiet rhythm, exhaling more slowly than you inhale. Close your eyes. As you exhale, visualize toxins dislodging and leaving your body. As you inhale, visualize nutrients rebuilding your vibrancy.

A "24-Hour Cleanse" is an invaluable healing tool.

Put this cleanse into action as soon as you realize you aren't feeling well. It's a special jewel to pull out of your pocket at the first signs of unexplained low energy, poor skin or congestion. It's one of the best ways I know to turn around (and get quick recovery) from a cold or flu. It's also an easy first step before making a significant diet improvement or change. A 24-hour cleanse is a good answer if you need a cleanse, but even a short cleanse seems like too much time.

A 24-hour detox is a juice and herbal tea cleanse that lets you go on with your normal activities, and "jump start" a healing program. Even though it's quick, without the depth of vegetable juices needed for a major or chronic problem, it's often enough, is definitely better than no cleanse at all, and it will make a difference in the speed of healing. Even if your program is only going to consist of lifestyle changes aimed at better health, a 24 hour cleanse can point you in the right direction.

Is your body showing signs that it needs a twenty four hour cleanse?
—Do you feel "toxic"? Are you tired a lot for no reason?
—Are you starting to feel congested? Do you have the first signs of a cold or flu? (Go right into this cleanse.)
—Is your skin dry or flaky? Is your skin tone sallow? Is your hair dull, dry and brittle?
—Are the soles of your feet or your palms often peeling?
—Do you frequently get mouth herpes? yeast infections? urinary tract infections? unusual allergy reactions?

24-Hour Detox Plan

The evening before you begin... have a green leafy salad to give your bowels a good sweeping. Dry brush your skin before you go to bed to open your pores for the night's cleansing eliminations. Take an herbal laxative.

The next day... the next 24 hours take fresh juices, herbal drinks, water, and a long walk.
—**On rising:** take 2 TBS. fresh lemon or lime juice, 1 TB. maple syrup and 1 pinch cayenne in water.
—**Breakfast:** a fresh juice with 1 pear, 2 apples, 4 oranges and 1 grapefruit; or cranberry juice from concentrate.
—**Mid-morning:** have a Zippy Tonic: 1 handful dandelion greens, 3 fresh pineapple rings and 3 radishes; or a cleansing, energizing tea with antioxidants like Crystal Star GREEN TEA CLEANSER™.
—**Lunch:** juice 4 parsley sprigs, or a handful of dandelion greens, 3 tomatoes, $\frac{1}{2}$ green bell pepper, $\frac{1}{2}$ cucumber, 1 scallion, 1 lemon wedge; or a glass of apple juice with 1 packet chlorella granules dissolved.
—**Mid-afternoon:** take a cup of Crystal Star CLEANSING & PURIFYING™ TEA or MEDITATION™ TEA.
—**Dinner:** take a glass of papaya-pineapple juice for enzymes; or try this high mineral broth: 7 carrots, 7 celery stalks, beet tops from 1 bunch, 2 potatoes, 1 onion, 4 garlic cloves, 3 zucchini, 1 handful of parsley. Place in a large soup pot, cover with water, bring to a boil and simmer 30 minutes. Remove and discard veggies.
—**Before Bed:** have a cup of mint tea, or I teasp. Sovex NUTRITIONAL YEAST BROTH or miso soup.

24-Hour cleanse supplement suggestions:
- **Cleansing boosters:** Crystal Star CLEANSING & PURIFYING™ TEA or Crystal Star LIV-ALIVE™ caps.
- **Electrolyte boosters for removal of toxic body acids:** Nature's Path TRACE-LYTE LIQUID MINERALS.
- **Probiotics:** Wakunaga of America KYO-DOPHILUS; New Chapter ALL-FLORA.
- **Vitamin C:** Take 1,000mg of vitamin C 3x per day with bioflavonoids.

Pointers for best results from your twenty four hour cleanse:
—Drink 8 to 10 glasses of water a day to hydrate and flush wastes and toxins from all cells.
—Focus on chlorophyll-rich foods (leafy greens, sea greens) and juices (super green foods like chlorella, barley grass or spirulina). Chlorophyll is the most powerful cleansing agent in nature.

Do you need an overall body stress cleanse?

You change the oil in your car to make it run smoother and last longer. You plunge into spring cleaning to rid your home of dirt and germs that might threaten your health. You buy air and water filters to clean your environment of toxins. You sink into a hot bath to cleanse your body's exterior.

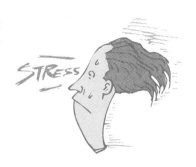

If you stop there, you've left an important part of the cleansing job unattended. Cleansing on the inside improves everything on the outside. A whole body stress detox is the key to revitalizing your body, mind and spirit. A stress cleanse focuses on your entire body. Rather than targeting a specific body system or problem, this cleanse reflects broad spectrum, mild body refreshment. It clears the "junk" out of body pathways so that wholesome nutrients can get in quickly to rebuild energy and strength.

You may have been struggling with the low nutrition of a Standard American Diet (SAD) for decades. Many people do not recognize that much of the "food" in America's supermarkets doesn't really have very much that your body can translate into usable nutrients. Some "foods" like designer fake fats may even contribute to illness.

Here's what a really healthy diet is.
—It's fresh fruit and vegetable juices several times a week.
—It's a fresh salad once a day, and steamed, stir-fried or baked veggies for at least one other meal.
—It's adding sea greens at least once a week for their superior nutrition. (Six pieces of sushi are fine.)
—It's adding cultured foods for good intestinal flora (like raw sauerkraut, yogurt, kefir or cottage cheese). Raw sauerkraut, rich in acidophilus, is especially good at deterring infectious bacteria.
—It's plenty of water — at least eight 8-oz. glasses a day.
—It's whole grains, nuts, seeds and beans for protein and essential fatty acids.
—It's healthy fats, like omega-3 oils and EFAs from cold water fish, flax and canola oil, and seafood to enhance thyroid and metabolic balance; and from sea greens, spinach and herbs like ginger and evening primrose oil. It's just as important to include healthy fats as it is to eliminate unhealthy fats, like hydrogenated fats.
—It's superfoods like bee pollen, royal jelly and aloe vera; or green superfoods like chlorella and spirulina.
—It means less meat and dairy foods. You'll feel better if you eat them in moderation.

Is your body showing signs that it needs an overall body stress cleanse?
—Is your immune response low? Are you catching every bug that comes down the pike?
—Are you unusually tired? Do you feel like you need a pick-me-up?
—Have you had unusual body odor or bad breath lately?
—Do you feel mentally dull?
—Have you gained weight even though your diet hasn't changed?

Benefits that you may notice as your body responds to a body stress cleanse:
• Your digestion noticeably improves as your digestive tract is cleansed of accumulated waste.
• You'll feel lighter (most people lose about 5 pounds on this cleanse) and more energized.
• You'll feel less dependent on habit-forming substances like sugar, caffeine, nicotine, alcohol and drugs as your bloodstream purifies.
• You'll feel healthier. Most people have noticeably better resistance to common colds and flu.
• You'll feel more mentally alert, less space-y, more emotionally balanced. Creativity begins to expand.
• You'll feel energized as your body rebalances. Energy levels rise physically, psychologically and sexually.

Stress Cleanse Detox Plan

Start with a 3 day juice-liquid diet and follow with 1 to 4 days of a diet of all fresh foods. Eat plenty of fresh vegetables and fruits. Choose foods high in fiber like whole grains and beans. Especially avoid unhealthy fats, like partially hydrogenated oils. But make a point to get plenty of essential fatty acids from sea vegetables, and herbs like ginger, ginseng or evening primrose oil. Don't forget to drink plenty of daily water.

—**On rising:** take a glass of 2 fresh squeezed lemons, 1 TB. maple syrup and 8-oz. of pure water.
—**Breakfast:** have a nutrient-dense Kick-Off Cleansing Cocktail: juice 1 handful fresh wheat grass or parsley — extremely rich in chlorophyll and antioxidants, 4 carrots, 1 apple, 2 celery stalks with leaves, $1/2$ beet with top.
—**Mid-morning:** have a glass of fresh carrot juice or fresh apple juice. Add 1 TB. of a green superfood like Crystal Star ENERGY GREEN™ drink mix; Green Kamut GREEN KAMUT; Vibrant Health GREEN VIBRANCE.
—**Lunch:** have a Salad-In-A-Glass: juice 4 parsley sprigs, 3 quartered tomatoes, $1/2$ green or red pepper, $1/2$ cucumber, 1 scallion, 1 lemon wedge.
—**Mid-afternoon:** have a cup of Crystal Star CLEANSING & PURIFYING™ tea, green tea or mint tea.
—**Dinner:** have a warm Potassium Essence Broth (page 215), for mineral electrolytes. Or try Super Soup, with antioxidants, antibiotic properties and immune boosters: 1 cup broccoli florets, 1 leek (white parts, a little green), 2 cups fresh peas, $1/2$ cup sliced scallions, 4 cups chard leaves, $1/2$ cup diced fennel bulb, $1/2$ cup fresh parsley, 6 garlic minced cloves, 2 tsp. astragalus extract (or $1/4$ cup broken pieces astragalus bark), 6 cups vegetable stock, a pinch of cayenne, 1 cup diced green cabbage, $1/4$ cup snipped sea vegetables. Bring all ingredients to a boil, then simmer for 10 min. Let sit for 20 minutes. Strain and use broth only.

Stress cleanse supplement suggestions: Choose 2 or 3 cleansing boosters.
•**Cleansing boosters:** Crystal Star DETOX™ caps with goldenseal stimulates the body to eliminate wastes rapidly or Crystal Star CLEANSING & PURIFYING™ tea.
•**Cleansing support formulas:** New Chapter LIFE SHIELD; Futurebiotics OXY-SHIELD protects the body against oxidative damage. When solid food is again introduced, use Nature's Secret ULTIMATE CLEANSE.
•**Enzyme support:** Prevail DETOX ENZYME FORMULA; Transformation EXCELLZYME.
•**Antioxidants help remove toxins:** Biotec CELL GUARD; Rainbow Light MULTI CAROTENE COMPLEX.
•**Probiotics:** Professional Nutr. DOCTOR-DOPHILUS+FOS; Wakunaga KYO-DOPHILUS; Prevail INNER ECOLOGY.
•**Electrolytes dramatically boost energy levels:** Nature's Path, TRACE-LYTE LIQUID MINERALS.
•**Green superfoods:** Crystal Star ENERGY GREEN™ drink; Vibrant Health GREEN VIBRANCE.
•**Detoxing flower remedies:** Natural Labs STRESS/TENSION; Nelson Bach RESCUE REMEDY.

Stress cleanse bodywork suggestions: Choose techniques to accelerate and round out your cleanse.
—**Enema:** Enemas can be a best friend to your cleansing program. Flushing your colon on the first, the second and the last day of your stress detox gives your body a giant step forward in releasing toxins.
—**Especially helpful:** Guided imagery, biofeedback and aromatherapy techniques.
—**Exercise:** Do this body stretch daily during your cleanse. Repeat this at least 5 times. Stand tall — raise your hands above your head. Stretch your arms and fingers to reach for the sky — move your hands and fingers as if you are trying to climb up into the sky. As you reach, inhale deeply through your nostrils while rising on your toes. Exhale slowly; gradually return to your starting position, arms hanging loosely at your sides. Follow your stretch with a brisk walk.
—**Deep Breathing Exercise:** Deep, relaxed breathing takes away stress, induces relaxation, composes the mind, improves mood and increases energy levels. 1. Take a deep, full breath. Exhale, slowly. Slowly. 2. Take another deep, full breath. Release slowly. 3. And again. 4. Maintain a quiet rhythm, exhaling more slowly than you inhale.
—**Massage:** Have a massage therapy treatment to further remove toxins and stimulate circulation.

Do you need a mucous congestion cleanse?

Your body needs some mucous. We tend to think of body mucous as a bad thing because it obstructs our breathing during a sinus infection, asthma or a cold. But that same mucous is also a needed body lubricant and an important body safeguard. Human beings take about 22,000 breaths a day, and along with the oxygen, we take in dirt, pollen, disease germs, smoke and other pollutants. Mucous gathers up these irritants as they enter the nose and throat to protect the mucous membranes that line the upper respiratory system. Mucous build-up may be a sign that your body is trying to bring itself to health. The problems start when your body holds on to too much. Some of us carry around as much as 10 to 15 pounds of excess mucous!

Your body systems work together, of course. Extra pressure of disease or heavy elimination on one body part puts extra stress on another. Supporting your kidneys, for example, takes part of the waste elimination load off your lungs so they can recover faster. Similarly, promoting respiratory health also helps digestive and skin cleansing problems. The lungs, though, are on the front line of toxic intake from viruses, allergies, pollutants, and mucous-forming congestives.

A program to overcome any chronic respiratory problem is usually more successful when begun with a short mucous elimination diet. This allows the body to rid itself first of toxins and accumulations that cause congestion before an attempt is made to change eating habits. Foods that putrefy quickly inside your body are the same foods that spoil easily in the air — like meat, fish, eggs and dairy products. These same foods are the ones most likely to produce excess mucous, too, which in turn slows down transit time through your gastrointestinal tract and colon.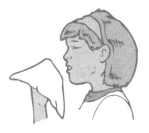

Is your body showing signs that it needs a mucous cleanse? Any respiratory system congestion, a cold or flu is a sure sign of excess mucous in the body, especially in the colon and intestinal tract. A mucous cleanse helps to release excess mucous in the respiratory system and in the colon.

Pointers for best results from your mucous cleanse:
—Herbal supplements are a good choice for a mucous congestion cleanse. They act as premier bronchodilators and anti-spasmodics to open congested airspaces. They can soothe bronchial inflammation and coughs. They have the ability to break up mucous. They are expectorants to remove mucous from the lungs and throat.
—Drink 8 to 10 glasses of water daily to thin mucous and aid elimination.
—Take 10,000mg ascorbate vitamin C crystals with bioflavonoids daily the first three days; just dissolve $\frac{1}{4}$ teasp. in water or juice throughout the day, until the stool turns soupy, and tissues are flushed. Take 5,000mg daily for the next four days.
—Take a brisk, daily walk. Breathe deeply to help lungs eliminate mucous.
—Take an enema the first and last day of your fasting diet to thoroughly clean out excess mucous.
—Apply wet ginger-cayenne compresses to the chest to increase circulation and loosen mucous.
—Take a hot sauna or a long warm bath with a rubdown to stimulate circulation.

Benefits you'll notice as your body responds to a mucous congestion cleanse.
—You'll start to see congestion clear right away as the non-mucous forming cleansing diet with supportive supplements go to work.
—If there is bronchial inflammation and/or cough it will give way to relief as the cleanse progresses.
—Mucous from the lungs and throat will break up and be eliminated from the body.
—Mucous from the colon may also be expelled from the body.
—Symptoms like discomfort from colds or flu, allergies or asthma will clear faster as the cleanse speeds up recovery.

Mucous and Congestion Cleanse Detox Plan

The night before your mucous cleanse...
—Mash 4 garlic cloves and a large slice of onion in a bowl. Stir in 3 TBS. honey. Cover, let macerate for 24 hours; remove garlic and onion and take only the honey-syrup infusion — 1 teasp. 3x daily.

The next day....
—**On rising:** take 2 squeezed lemons in water with 1 TB. maple syrup.
—**Breakfast:** take a glass of grapefruit, pineapple, or cranberry-apple juice.
—**Mid-morning:** have a glass of fresh carrot juice; or a cup of congestion clearing tea, like Crystal Star X-Pect™, an expectorant to aid mucous release, or Crystal Star Respr Tea™, an aid in oxygen uptake.
—**Lunch:** have a vegetable juice like V-8, or a potassium broth (page 215); or make this Mucous Cleansing Tonic by juicing: 4 carrots, 2 celery stalks, 2-3 sprigs parsley, 1 radish and 1 garlic clove.
—**Mid-afternoon:** have a veggie drink (page 218), or a packet of Sun Wellness Sun Chlorella granules in water; or a greens and sea vegetable drink like Crystal Star Energy Green™ drink.
—**Dinner:** apple or papaya/pineapple juice.
—**Before Bed:** take a hot vegetable broth, add in 1 TB. nutritional yeast. Have a small fresh salad on the last night of the cleanse.
—**The next day...** begin with small simple meals. Have toasted muesli or whole grain granola for your first morning of solid food, with a little yogurt or apple juice; a small fresh salad for lunch with lemon/oil dressing; a fresh fruit smoothie during the day; a baked potato with butter and a light soup or salad for dinner.

Mucous cleanse supplement suggestions: Choose 2 or 3 cleansing boosters.
• **Deep body cleanser for intestinal tract and lungs:** Use Nature's Way 5 System Cleanse caps after juice cleansing to help pull intestinal mucous and clear mucous congestion from the respiratory system.
• **Mucous cleansers:** Use Crystal Star X-Pect-Tea™ to aid mucous release; Herbs Etc. Lung Tonic to loosen and remove mucous; Herbs Etc. Respiratonic to loosen mucous and clear lung congestion.
• **Herbs to relieve mucous:** mullein loosens and expels mucous; slippery elm removes excess mucous, soothes mucous membranes; sage helps mucous discharge; white pine, an antioxidant expectorant, reduces mucous.
• **Better oxygen uptake:** Crystal Star Respr™ Tea; NutriCology Germanium.
• **Enzyme support:** Prevail Digestion Formula; Herbal Products and Development Power-Plus Enzymes; Transformation Enzyme Gastrozyme relieves bouts of mucous congestion.
• **Electrolyte boosters help digestive efficiency up to 80%:** Nature's Path Trace-Lyte Liquid Minerals.
• **Probiotics maintain proper mucous levels:** Nature's Path Flora-Lyte; Ethical Nutrients Intestinal Care.

Mucous cleanse bodywork suggestions: Choose techniques to accelerate and round out your cleanse.
—**Enema:** Take an enema the first, second and last day of your juice fasting to help thoroughly clean out excess mucous. Or, irrigate: have a colonic for a more thorough colon cleanse.
—**Exercise:** Take a brisk walk each day of your cleanse. Breathe deep to help the lungs eliminate mucous.
—**Massage therapy with percussion:** a rubdown loosens mucous. Most people have several congestion-releasing bowel movements and expectoration incidences within 24 hours after a massage therapy treatment.
—**Compress:** Apply wet ginger-cayenne chest compresses to increase circulation and loosen mucous.
—**Essential oil support:** Eucalyptus (inhale) — antiviral action loosens mucous. Tea tree oil (inhale) — antiviral, antibacterial decongestant. Oregano oil (inhale) — antiviral, antibacterial helps eradicate lung infection.
—**Visualize your detox:** Close your eyes — inhale and exhale long and slowly. As you exhale, visualize mucous dislodging and leaving your lungs and also your colon. As you inhale, visualize oxygen and nutrients renewing all your cells.
—**Bathe and Sauna:** long warm baths and saunas help loosen mucous congestion. Add to your bath 5 drops of eucalyptus, tea tree oil or oregano oil.

A brown rice diet is a good 7-Day cleanse for weight loss.

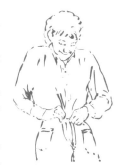

A brown rice cleanse is especially useful for dropping a few quick pounds, and it's a great way to transition from an unhealthy diet into a better diet. A brown rice cleanse is based on macrobiotic principles for body balance. A brown rice diet is cleansing, yet filling. You don't feel like you're on a cleanse at all, yet it does the trick. It's a diet that uses rice as a nutrient building food, and vegetables and vegetable juices as concentrated cleansing supplements. A brown rice cleanse is high in potassium, natural iodine, and other minerals, so most people notice improvement in their hair, skin texture and nail growth.

A brown rice diet is the best cleansing diet for colder times of the year. Brown rice adds a building, warming factor to a cleanse, making your meals more satisfying, ensuring that you get plenty of fiber and minerals. It's an effective option to a juice cleanse and much easier to fit into your lifestyle.

Almost everybody loses some weight during this cleanse. Most people experience about a 2 to 5 pound weight drop. Most people notice an improvement in vitality and energy levels right away, too. People with heart problems regularly notice a more stable heartbeat and better circulation. A fiber-rich cleansing diet with sea vegetables, that eliminates meat and dairy protein, almost invariably lowers the risk of cardiovascular problems.

Is your body showing signs that a brown rice cleanse would do you some good?
   —Is your immune response low?
   —Do you feel like you need to clear cobwebs from your brain? Are you feeling logy and out-of-sorts?
   —Do you need to lose about 10 pounds?

7-Day Brown Rice Detox Plan

The night before your brown rice cleanse....
A green leafy salad for dinner sweeps your bowels. Take an herbal enema the night before your cleanse.

The next day....
—**On rising:** take a glass of 2 fresh squeezed lemons, 1 TB. maple syrup and 8-oz. of pure water.
—**Breakfast:** have an energy green drink: 6 carrots, 1 beet, 8 spinach leaves and $^1/_4$ cup fresh parsley leaves.
—**Mid-morning:** take a cup of Crystal Star CLEANSING & PURIFYING™ TEA or DAILY DETOX by M.D.
—**Lunch:** have a veggie juice like Super V-7: 2 carrots, 2 tomatoes, a handful of spinach leaves and parsley, 2 celery ribs, $^1/_2$ cucumber, $^1/_2$ green bell pepper. Add 1 TB. green superfood, like Crystal Star ENERGY GREEN™, Body Ecology VITALITY SUPERGREEN, or Ethical Nutrients FUNCTIONAL GREENS.
—**Mid-afternoon:** have a glass of carrot juice.
—**Dinner:** have steamed brown rice and mixed steamed vegetables. Sprinkle with sea vegetables (like dulse or kelp, easily purchased in flakes or granules). Use 1 TB. flax or olive oil, and 1 TB. Bragg's LIQUID AMINOS.
—**Before Bed:** have a cup of herbal tea such as peppermint, spearmint or chamomile.
—**The next 6 days:** have 2 to 3 glasses of any blend of mixed vegetable juices throughout the day. Don't eat any solid food during the day. Have steamed brown rice and mixed vegetables for an early dinner each evening. Either steamed or raw vegetable salads can be used. Enzymes in raw vegetables provide greater cleansing quality.

7-day brown rice cleanse supplement suggestions: Choose 2 or 3 cleansing boosters.
   •Cleansing boosters: Crystal Star FIBER & HERBS COLON CLEANSE™ caps stimulate the body to eliminate wastes rapidly; Nature's Secret ULTIMATE CLEANSE helps detoxify all five channels of elimination.
   •Cleansing teas: Crystal Star CLEANSING & PURIFYING™ TEA; DAILY DETOX by M.D. is a mild cleanser, gentle enough to take on a daily basis, yet stimulates all the major elimination organs.
   •Enzyme support, a dieter's best friend: Transformation Enzyme DIGESTZYME.

Do you need a pollutant or heavy metal cleanse?

Chemical pollutants and toxic by-products affect every facet of our lives, from our water and food supply to the workplace and our homes. Heavy metal poisoning and pollutant toxicity are major health problems of the American culture. We have moved from fetid air to undrinkable water to severe allergy reactions and serious diseases caused by pollution. There seems to be no way to avoid toxic exposure. The main effect of an unhealthy environment is reduced immune response, especially in the way that our filtering organs, the liver and kidneys, are impacted. Periodic detoxification needs to be a part of life to keep our bodies able to defend us.... against yet more pollutants. (An astounding twenty-five thousand NEW chemicals enter our society every year.) A hair analysis can help you determine nutrient deficiencies and which heavy metals are lodged in your body.

Is your body showing signs that it needs a pollution/heavy metal cleanse?
—Are you far more sensitive to odors like perfumes and strong cleansers than most people?
—Do you have an unusually small tolerance for alcohol?
—Are there medications you can't take, or some vitamins or other supplements that make you feel worse?
—Do you have small black spots along your gum line? Unusually bad breath or body odor?
—Is your reaction time when driving noticeably poorer in city traffic?
—Do you have unexplained seizures, memory failure or psychotic behavior?
—Have you become infertile or impotent?

7-Day Chemical Pollution Detox Plan
Note: A heavy metal, pollutant detox is one of the most likely cleanses for a "healing crisis" to occur. You may feel head-achy, with a slight upset stomach as toxins are released. The feelings should pass quickly, usually within 24 hours. But I don't recommend an all-liquid diet if you're trying to release heavy metals or chemicals. They may enter the bloodstream too fast and heavily for your body to handle safely. Eat solid cleansing foods instead to release the toxins more slowly and safely.

—**On rising:** 2 TBS. cranberry concentrate in water with $1/2$ tsp. vitamin C crystals; or Crystal Star GREEN TEA CLEANSER™; or blend 2 tsp. lemon, 1 tsp. honey, 1 cup water and 1 tsp. acidophilus in 8-oz. aloe vera juice.
—**Breakfast:** have a glass of fresh carrot juice with 1 TB. green superfood like Crystal Star ENERGY GREEN™ or Green Foods GREEN MAGMA, and whole grain muffins or rice cakes with kefir cheese; or a cup of soy milk or plain yogurt blended with a cup of fresh fruit, walnuts, and $1/2$ teasp. acidophilus) in 8-oz. aloe vera juice.
—**Mid-morning:** take a cup of green tea, with $1/2$ teasp. ascorbate vitamin C crystals; or a fresh vegetable juice with 1 TB. green superfood such as Nutricology PRO-GREENS or Wakunaga KYO-GREEN.
—**Lunch:** have a leafy salad with lemon-flax oil dressing; or a cup of miso soup with brown rice; or steamed veggies with brown rice; and green tea with $1/2$ teasp. vitamin C and $1/2$ teasp. acidophilus powder.
—**Mid-afternoon:** have a carrot juice with 1 TB. green superfood like Crystal Star ENERGY GREEN™.
—**Dinner:** have a baked potato with Bragg's LIQUID AMINOS and a fresh salad with lemon-flax dressing; or a black bean or lentil soup; or a Chinese steam/stir fry with vegetables, shiitake mushrooms and brown rice.
—**Before Bed:** an 8-oz. glass of aloe vera juice with $1/2$ teasp. vitamin C and another carrot juice.

7-day chemical-pollutant cleanse supplement suggestions:
• **Pollutant/Heavy Metal cleansers:** Crystal Star HEAVY METAL CLEANZ™ caps.
• **Enzyme support:** Protease binds to heavy metals, sparing metabolic enzyme destruction. Transformation Enzyme PUREZYME (high doses effective in lowering blood mercury toxins).
• **Liver enhancers:** Crystal Star LIV-ALIVE™ caps/tea; MILK THISTLE SEED extract; dandelion extract.
• **Antioxidants defeat pollutants:** Alpha Lipoic Acid is among the most powerful liver detoxifiers ever discovered. Jarrow Formulas ALPHA LIPOIC ACID or ALPHA-LIPOIC ACID by MRI; NutriCology ANTIOX FORMULA II.
• **Oral Chelation cleanses heavy metals:** Hayestown TRICARDIA; Golden Pride FORMULA ONE w/ EDTA.

Which Body System Do You Need To Cleanse?

You can target your detox to focus on a specific body system. Each body system has tell-tale signs when it becomes overloaded with pollutants or congestion. Directing your detox to the body system that needs it most often goes to the heart of a problem right away, and frequently clears up other related conditions as well. This chapter details the seven body systems that make a noticeable difference in your health after a cleanse.

Do you need a colon cleanse?

A colon elimination cleanse is a cleanse most of us need. The latest estimates show that over 90% of disease in America is directly or indirectly attributable to an unhealthy colon. As the solid waste management organ for the entire body, your colon is also the easiest breeding ground for putrefactive bacteria, viruses and parasites. (A nationwide survey reveals that one in every six people has parasites living somewhere in the body.)

Health problems like headaches, skin blemishes, bad breath, fatigue, arthritis and heart disease are linked to a congested colon. Colon and bowel malfunctions are one of the biggest factors in accelerated aging, too. When colon health is compromised, waste backs up, becomes toxic, and releases the toxins from the bowel into the bloodstream. Cleansing your colon lightens the toxic load on every other part of your body.... even your mind (mental dullness is a sign of colon congestion). In fact, hardly any healing program will work without a colon cleanse as part of it. Real healing takes place at the deepest levels of your body, your cells. All your cells are fed by your blood. The nutrients that reach your blood get there by the way of the colon. So a clogged, dirty colon means toxins in your blood.

Is your colon toxic? Here are some questions to ask yourself:

Is your elimination time slow? Bowel transit time should be approximately twelve hours. Slow bowel transit time allows wastes to become rancid. Blood capillaries lining the colon absorb these poisons into the bloodstream, exposing the rest of your body to the toxins.

Do you eat a lot of highly processed, chemicalized food, fast foods or synthetic foods? A clean, strong system can metabolize or eliminate many pollutants, but if you are constipated, they are stored in your body. As more and different chemicals enter your body they tend to inter-react with those that are already there, forming second generation chemicals more harmful than the originals. Colon cancer, now the second leading cancer in the United States (only slightly behind lung cancer in men and breast cancer in women), is a direct result of accumulated toxic waste. Colitis, irritable bowel syndrome, diverticulosis, ileitis and Crohn's disease, are all signs of waste congestion. They're on the rise, too. Over 100,000 Americans have a colostomy every year! An incredible fact.

Is your digestion poor? The most common sign of toxic bowel overload is poor digestion. If you're eating too many acid-forming foods — rich, red meats and cheeses, refined-flour bread, sugary, salty foods or fried foods, they're robbing your body of critical electrolytes and they have almost no fiber for digestion. A high fiber diet is both cure and prevention for waste elimination problems. Eating high fiber means you're moving food through your digestive system quickly and easily. A low residue diet causes a gluey state — your intestinal contractions can't work efficiently. You can picture this if you remember the hard paste formed by white flour and water when you were a kid. A lot of the food we eat today is simply crammed into the colon, never fully excreted.

So much media attention has been focused on high fiber foods, you'd think everybody in America would have changed their diet to a more colon-health oriented pattern. This is simply not the case. Most diet attention has been targeted at reducing fat at all costs, often at the expense of a fiber-rich diet. Even a gentle, gradual change from low fiber, low residue foods helps almost immediately. In fact, a gradual change is better than a sudden, drastic about-face change, especially when the colon is inflamed.

Check your fiber. The protective level of fiber in your diet is easily measured:
—The stool should be light enough to float.
—Bowel movements should be regular, daily and effortless.
—The stool should be almost odorless, signalling decreased bowel transit time.
—There should be no gas or flatulence.

Is your body showing signs that it needs a colon cleanse?
—Are you constipated most of the time? (a colon cleanse softens and removes clogging colon congestion)
—Do you feel heavy and logy? (a colon cleanse helps you lose colon congestive weight)
—Do you have gas or bloating after you eat? (a colon cleanse removes gluey materials impairing digestion)
—Do you catch a cold, or flu every few weeks? (a colon cleanse releases excess mucous that harbors viruses)
—Are you tired for no real reason? (a colon cleanse boosts immune and liver response for more energy)
—Do you have a coated tongue, bad breath or body odor? (a colon cleanse clears rancidity that causes smells)
—Do you feel mentally slow and tired? (a colon cleanse lets more blood circulation get to your brain)
—Is your skin unusually sallow and dull? (a colon cleanse removes toxin that come out through your skin)
—Do you have a degenerative disease like cancer, arthritis or lupus? (a colon cleanse removes toxic elements)
—Are your cholesterol numbers too high? (a colon cleanse increases absorption of cholesterol-lowering foods)

Colon Elimination Detox Plan

Start with this 3 to 5 -day nutrition plan: The 4 keys: 1) high chlorophyll plants for enzymes; 2) fruits and vegetables for fiber; 3) cultured foods for probiotics; 4) eight glasses of water a day.

The night before your colon cleanse...
—Take your choice of gentle herbal laxatives.
—Soak dried figs, prunes and raisins in water to cover; add 1 TB. molasses, cover, leave over night.

The next day...
—**On rising:** take a cleansing booster product, or 1 heaping teaspoon of a fiber drink in juice or water. Take 1000mg vitamin C with bioflavonoids to raise body glutathione levels.
—**Breakfast:** discard dried fruits from soaking water and take a small glass of the liquid.
—**Mid-morning:** take 2 TBS. aloe juice concentrate in a glass of juice or water and 1000mg vitamin C.
—**Lunch:** take a small glass of potassium broth (page 215); or a glass of fresh carrot juice.
—**Mid-afternoon:** take a large glass of fresh apple juice; or an herbal colon cleansing tea.
—**About 5 o' clock:** take a small glass of potassium broth, or fresh carrot juice, or a vegetable drink (page 218).
—**Supper:** take a glass of apple or papaya juice and 1000mg vitamin C. (Note: Finish your cleanse with a small raw foods salad on the last night.)
—**Before Bed:** repeat the herbal cleansers that you took on rising, and take a cup of mint tea.

Colon cleanse supplement suggestions: Choose 2 or 3 cleansing boosters.
• **Gentle herbal laxatives:** HERBALTONE TABLETS, Crystal Star LaxaTea, M. D. Labs DAILY DETOX TEA. Note: If you have a sensitive colon or irritable bowel disease (IBS), heal your colon before you cleanse. Avoid products with senna or psyllium. Use a gentle herbal cleansing formula, with peppermint oil, like Crystal Star BWL TONE I.B.S.™ to lessen inflammation and irritation of bowel mucosa which make the bowel more permeable to toxins.

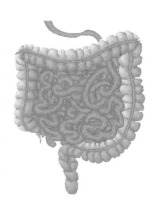

• **Cleansing and flushing boosters:** Nature's Secret SUPERCLEANSE tabs; Crystal Star FIBER & HERBS COLON CLEANSE™; *una da gato* extract drops in water.

• **Chlorophyll sources:** Sun Wellness SUN CHLORELLA; Futurebiotics COLON GREEN; Crystal Star ENERGY GREEN™ drink.

• **Enzymes:** Transformation Enzyme DIGEST-ZYME.
• **Electrolyte boosters speed up the cleanse:** Nature's Path TRACE-LYTE LIQUID MINERALS; Arise and Shine ALKALIZER.
• **Probiotics replenish healthy bacteria:** Professional Nutrition DOCTOR-DOPHILUS+FOS; Nature's Path FLORA-LYTE; Arise and Shine FLORA GROW.
• **Antioxidants defeat pollutants:** Country Life SUPER 10 ANTIOXIDANT; NutriCology ANTIOX FORMULA.
• **Fiber support:** All One FIBER COMPLEX; Crystal Star CHO-LO FIBER TONE™ drink; AloeLife FIBERMATE.

Note 1: Drugstore laxatives aren't really body cleansers. They offer only temporary relief, are usually habit-forming and destructive to intestinal membranes, and don't even get to the cause of the problem. The bowels tend to expel debris simply because the colon becomes so irritated by the laxative that it expels whatever loose material is around.

Note 2: Bowel elimination problems are often chronic, and may require several rounds of cleansing. Space out more than one colon cleanse by alternating it with periods of eating a healthful diet

Colon cleanse bodywork suggestions: Choose techniques to accelerate and round out your cleanse.
    —**Irrigate:** a colonic irrigation is a good way to start a colon/bowel cleanse. (See how to take a colonic, page 540.) Grapefruit seed extract (15 to 20 drops in a gallon of water) is effective, especially if there is colon toxicity along with constipation. Or, take a catnip or diluted liquid chlorophyll enema every other night during the cleanse. *Note:* Enemas may be given to children. Use smaller amounts according to size and age. Allow water to enter very slowly; let them expel when they wish.
    —**Exercise:** take a brisk walk for an hour every day to help keep your elimination channels moving.
    —**Bathe:** take several long warm baths during your cleanse. A lower back and pelvis massage and dry skin brushing will help release toxins coming out through your skin. Lemon Detox Bath: add into warm bath — 5 drops lemon and 2 drops geranium essential oil.
    —**Massage therapy: get one good lower back and pelvis massage during your cleanse.**
    —**Visualize your detox:** Close your eyes and inhale and exhale long and slowly. As you exhale, visualize toxins dislodging and leaving your colon. As you inhale, visualize pure, nourishing nutrients rebuilding your vibrancy.

Note: After the initial cleanse above, the second part of a colon health system is rebuilding healthy tissue and body energy. This stage takes 1 to 2 months for best results. It emphasizes high fiber from fresh vegetables and fruits, cultured foods to replenish healthy intestinal flora, green foods for enzyme production, and alkalizing foods to prevent irritation while healing. Avoid refined foods, saturated fats, fried foods, red meats, caffeine and pasteurized dairy foods.

*Your soul would have
no rainbows*

*if your eyes had
no tears.*

Do you need a bladder/kidney cleanse?

Kidney function is vital to health. The kidneys are largely responsible for the elimination of waste products from protein breakdown (such as urea and ammonia). If the movement of salts, proteins or other bio-chemicals goes awry, a whole range of health problems arises, from mild water retention, to major kidney failure, and mineral loss. Concentrated protein wastes can cause chronic inflammation of the kidney filtering tissues (nephritis), and can overload the bloodstream with toxins, causing uremia.

But your bladder and kidneys do more than just remove water wastes. Channeling pollutants and chemicals out of our systems before they build up in the tissues and contaminate our cells is obviously crucial to the body's internal hygiene. The bladder and kidneys are primary removal sites for toxic and potentially toxic chemicals in the bloodstream.

The urinary system is also part of a complex process that maintains your body's fluid stability. Urinary controls are involved with the brain, hormones, and receptors all over the body. They are smart controls that register what your body needs for fluids. Sometimes, they remove very little salt or water; at other times, they remove a lot. By the way.... dehydration is the most common stress on the kidneys. Natural medicine emphasizes the importance of ample, high-quality water for kidney health.

Is your body showing signs that it needs a bladder/kidney cleanse?
Do you have chronic lower back pain, irritated urination, frequent unexplained chills, fever, or nausea or unusual fluid retention? If you do, a gentle, natural, three to five day cleansing course might be just the thing to keep you from getting a full-blown, painful bladder infection.

Bladder-Kidney Detox Plan

Start with this 3-day nutrition plan: Water is the key. Drink 8 to 10 glasses of water each day. Bladder and kidneys operate efficiently only if there is sufficient water volume flowing through them to carry away wastes. Avoid dietary irritants on the kidneys, such as coffee, alcohol, and excessive protein.

Note: Avoid commercial antacids during healing. Some NSAIDS drugs have been implicated in kidney failure cases.

The night before your bladder cleanse....
—One cup of bladder cleansing herb tea, like Crystal Star BLDR-K TEA™. Add $\frac{1}{4}$ tsp. non-acidic C crystals.

The next day....
—**On rising:** take 1 lemon squeezed in a glass of water, with 1 teasp. acidophilus liquid; or 3 tsp. cranberry concentrate in a small glass of water, add $\frac{1}{4}$ teasp. non-acidic vit. C crystals. (Cranberry juice reduces ionized calcium in the urine by over 50% to create an unfavorable environment for urinary tract infections.)

—**Breakfast:** have a glass of watermelon juice or cranberry juice with $\frac{1}{4}$ tsp. non-acidic vitamin C crystals or a glass of organic apple juice with $\frac{1}{4}$ tsp. acidophilus powder.

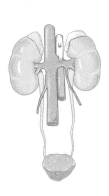

—**Mid-morning:** take 1 cup watermelon seed tea. (grind seeds, steep in hot water 30 minutes, add honey); or a potassium broth (page 215) with 2 tsp. Bragg's LIQUID AMINOS; or an herbal bladder cleansing tea.

—**Lunch:** have a carrot-beet-cucumber juice, or a chlorophyll-rich drink, or a glass of carrot juice.

—**Mid-afternoon:** a cup of bladder herb tea, (parsley/oatstraw, plantain, watermelon seed tea or cornsilk).

—**Dinner:** have a carrot juice, add 1 tsp. spirulina powder; or another cranberry juice, add $\frac{1}{4}$ teasp. ascorbate vitamin C crystals.

—**Before Bed:** take a glass of papaya or apple juice with $\frac{1}{4}$ tsp. acidophilus powder.

Bladder-Kidney cleanse supplement suggestions: Choose 2 or 3 cleansing boosters.

Liquid supplements are best with this cleanse. Herbal supplements provide excellent support for a kidney cleanse. Take them as liquids (drinks or teas) for best results.

•**Supergreen foods:** Take a liquid green supplement each day of your cleanse – Green Foods GREEN ESSENCE; Sun Wellness CHLORELLA drink; Crystal Star ENERGY GREEN™ drink; spirulina powder in juice.

•**Bladder/kidney cleansers:** Crystal Star BLDR-K™ tea; cornsilk tea; Nature's Apothecary DETOX.

•**Antibiotic-anti-infective-anti-inflammatory:** Crystal Star ANTI-BIO™; marshmallow tea; vitamin C-1,000mg 3x a day; Nature's Answer BLADDEX or Nature's Plus AQUAACTIN.

•**Enzyme support:** Transformation Enzyme EXCELL-ZYME (kidney antioxidant), and PUREZYME (a protease supplement that breaks apart protein-based viscid matter that cements salts into stones).

•**Bladder/kidney healing tonics:** Crystal Star GREEN TEA CLEANSER™; Herbs Etc. KIDNEY TONIC; Gaia Herbs PLANTAIN/BUCHU SUPREME; Nature's Apothecary KIDNEY SUPPORT; dandelion tea; parsley tea.

•**Electrolyte mineral support:** Nature's Path TRACE-LYTE LIQUID MINERALS; Arise & Shine ALKALIZER.

•**Probiotic support:** Professional Nutrition DOCTOR-DOPHILUS + FOS; Wakunaga KYODOPHILUS.

•**Fiber supplements reduce risk of stones:** All One FIBER COMPLEX; Nature's Secret ULTIMATE FIBER.

Bladder cleanse bodywork suggestions: Choose techniques to accelerate and round out your cleanse.

—**Exercise:** Take a daily brisk walk to keep kidney function flowing.

—**Enemas:** Take a spirulina or catnip enema at least one day of your kidney cleanse to help release toxins. See enema instructions (page 539) in this book.

—**Heat therapy:** Hot saunas release toxins and excess fluids, and flush acids out through the skin.

—**Compresses:** Apply wet and hot to lower back to speed cleansing. Combine your choice – ginger and oatstraw, or cayenne and ginger, or mullein and lobelia. Or, take alternating hot and cold sitz baths.

—**Massage therapy:** Have at least one massage during your cleanse to stimulate circulation.

—**Bladder-Kidney Baths:** Add 8-10 drops of essential oils to your bath – a combination of two or three oils, like juniper, cedarwood, sandalwood, lemon, chamomile, eucalyptus or geranium. Stir the water to disperse. (Or use about 15 drops essential oil in 4-oz of jojoba oil and rub on kidney area).

Note: After your cleanse, add sea foods and sea vegetables, whole grains and vegetable proteins. Continue with a morning green drink or Crystal Star GREEN TEA CLEANSER™. Kidney healing foods include garlic and onions, papayas, bananas, watermelon, sprouts, leafy greens and cucumbers. Take these frequently for the rest of the month. Avoid heavy starches, red or prepared meats, dairy foods (except yogurt or kefir), and salty, fatty and fast foods. They all inhibit kidney filtering.

Improvement signs show that your body is responding to the cleanse:
• The flow of urine is increased.
• Bladder infections and-or irritated urination abate.
• You'll feel lighter and cleaner as your kidney do their detoxification duties free of congestion.

*Everything is a blessing in disguise.
Even bad news can be fortuitous from another vantage point.*

Your liver is your most important organ of detoxification.
Do you need a liver cleanse?

Your life depends on your liver. To a large extent, the health of your liver determines the health of your entire body. The liver is really a wonderful chemical plant that converts everything we eat, breathe and absorb through the skin into life-sustaining substances. The liver is a major blood reservoir, forming and storing red blood cells, and filtering toxins at a rate of a quart of blood per minute. It manufactures natural antihistamines to keep immune response high.

More than any other organ, the liver enables us to benefit from the food we eat. Without the liver, digestion would be impossible and the conversion of food into living cells and energy nonexistent. It is the primary metabolic organ for proteins, fats and carbohydrates. It synthesizes and secretes bile, a substance that not only insures good food assimilation but also is critical to the excretion of toxic material from the gastrointestinal tract. Blood flows directly from the gastrointestinal tract to the liver, where it deals with toxic substances from our food before they are distributed through our blood. Blood also keeps returning to the liver, processing toxins again and again through the lymph system until they are excreted by the bile or kidneys.

Liver congestion and exhaustion interfere with these vital functions. Unfortunately, since the common American diet is high in calories, fats, sugars and alcohol, with unknown amounts of toxins from preservatives, pesticides and nitrates, almost everybody has liver malfunction to some extent. Health problems occur after many years of abuse, when the liver is so exhausted it loses the ability to detoxify itself. Still, your liver also has amazing rejuvenative powers, continuing to function when as many as 80% of its cells are damaged. More remarkable, the liver can regenerate its own damaged tissue, so that even in life-threatening situations, such as cirrhosis, hepatitis, acute gallstone attacks, mononucleosis or pernicious anemia, the liver can be rejuvenated, and major surgery or even death averted. You can help your liver take a "deep cleansing breath"... something I've found you can almost feel as its miraculous powers of recovery begin to flow.

A liver detox is often the first vital step for the body to begin to heal itself. Gland function and digestion often improve right away. You will notice this in terms of fewer instances of swollen glands during cold and flu season, and less lower back fatigue (adrenal swelling). Weight and cellulite control difficulties may be solved, especially if you notice unusual stomach distension, a clear sign of a swollen liver. Both gallstone and kidney stone accretions lessen. Drug and alcohol cravings reduce. Most women notice that PMS and other menstrual difficulties like endometriosis are far less severe. Seemingly unrelated problems like breast and uterine fibroids or infertility, even osteoporosis may be corrected. Male impotence is normally improved. Inflammatory conditions like shingles flare-ups, neuritis pain, and herpes outbreaks are helped. Brown skin spots and spots before the eyes (signs that the liver is congested and eliminating poisons by other body avenues) begin to fade.

Is your body showing signs that it needs a liver cleanse?
—Unexplained fatigue, listlessness, depression or lethargy, lack of energy; numerous allergy reactions
—Unexplained weight gain and the appearance of cellulite even if you are thin
—A distended stomach even if the rest of your body is thin
—Mental confusion, spaciness
—Sluggish elimination, general constipation alternating to diarrhea
—Food and chemical sensitivities, accompanied by poor digestion, and
    sometimes unexplained nausea
—PMS, headaches and other menstrual difficulties; bags under the eyes
—A yellowish tint to the skin and/or liver spots on the skin; poor hair
    texture and slow hair growth; skin itching and irritation
—Anemia and large bruise patches indicate severe liver exhaustion

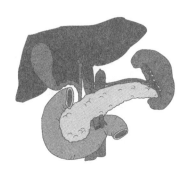

Liver Detox Plan

I recommend a short liver detox twice a year in the spring and fall, using the extra vitamin D from the sun to help. Your liver is probably the most stressed in the spring and early summer (one of the reasons that people with skin problems get more flare-ups in the spring). As upward energy movement in the spring is mirrored in the human body, outgoing energy more readily rids us of wastes accumulated during the fall and winter.

Start with this 3-day nutrition plan:
Drink 8 glasses of water each day. Add $1/4$ tsp. vitamin C crystals to each drink you take. It's a natural chelator of heavy metal toxins that deteriorate liver function. Have a dark green leafy vegetable salad every day.

The night before your liver cleanse...
—Take a cup of miso soup with sea greens snipped on top.
—Make a liver tonic tea: 4-oz hawthorn berries, 2-oz. red sage, and 1-oz. cardamom seeds. Steep 24 hours in 2 qts. water. Add honey. Take 2 cups daily.

The next day....
—**On rising:** take 1 lemon squeezed in a glass of water; or 2 TBS. cider vinegar in water with 1 teasp. honey.
—**Breakfast:** take a potassium broth, (page 215) or carrot-beet-cucumber juice; or Crystal Star SYSTEMS STRENGTH drink™. Add 1 teasp. spirulina to any drink.
—**Mid-morning:** take a green veggie drink (page 218); or a green superfood powder mixed in water or vegetable juice (superfood choices: Green Foods GREEN MAGMA, Crystal Star ENERGY GREEN or NutriCology PRO-GREEN).
—**Lunch:** have a glass of fresh carrot juice, or organic apple juice, or a cup of liver tonic tea (above).
—**Mid-afternoon:** have a cup of peppermint tea, green tea, or Crystal Star LIV-ALIVE TEA™.
—**Dinner:** have another carrot juice or a mixed vegetable juice; or have a hot vegetable broth.
—**Before Bed:** a pineapple/papaya juice with 1 tsp. royal jelly.
   Note: Keep fat low in your nutrition plan. It's crucial to liver regeneration and vitality. Beets, artichokes, radishes and dandelions are good liver foods because they promote the flow of bile, the major pathway for chemical release from the liver. A permanent diet for liver health should be lacto-vegetarian, low in fats, rich in vegetable proteins, with plenty of vitamin C foods for good iron absorption. A complete liver renewal program can take from 3 to 6 months.

Liver cleanse supplement suggestions: Choose 2 or 3 cleansing boosters.
   • **Bitters herbs stimulate liver and bile flow:** Crystal Star BITTERS & LEMON CLEANSER™; Floradix HERBAL BITTERS; Solaray turmeric caps; dandelion tea.
   • **Liver cleansers:** Crystal Star LIV-ALIVE™, or GREEN TEA CLEANSER™; Nature's Apothecary LIVER CLEANSE.
   • **Liver tonics and vitality support:** Milk thistle seed extract (accelerates liver regeneration by a factor of four); Enzymatic Therapy SUPER MILK THISTLE COMPLEX WITH ARTICHOKE; Herbs Etc. LIVER TONIC.
   • **Enzyme support:** Transformation Enzyme DIGESTZYME.
   • **Lipotropics prevent fatty accumulation:** Phos. Choline or choline 600mg, or Solaray LIPOTROPIC PLUS; sea greens (any kind) every day; dandelion tea; gotu kola or fennel seed tea.
   • **Liver antioxidants:** ALPHA-LIPOIC ACID by MRI. (Lipoic acid is one of the most powerful liver detoxifiers ever discovered); CoQ$_{10}$ 60mg 3x daily; Solaray ALFA-JUICE caps; Transformation Enzyme EXCELLZYME.

Liver cleanse bodywork suggestions: Choose techniques to accelerate and round out your cleanse.
   —**Get adequate rest:** the liver does some of its most important work while you sleep!
   —**Enema:** take a coffee enema (1 cup coffee to 1 qt. water) the first and last day of your liver cleanse.
   —**Massage therapy:** Have a massage to stimulate circulation.

Improvement signs show that your body is responding to the cleanse. Many skin conditions trace back to liver problems, so skin conditions show signs of clearing and skin becomes more radiant. Stiff, aching muscles experience relief. Warmth may return to cold hands and feet. Recurring headaches or migraines may disappear.

Do you need a lung-respiratory cleanse?

Lung and respiratory diseases of all kinds have increased dramatically in just the last decade. Air, water and environmental pollutants may have finally reached an overload point on the general population where having a congestive "cold" is more common than breathing free. During high risk seasons, almost a third of Americans have a cold every two or three weeks. Cold symptoms are frequently your body's attempt to cleanse itself of wastes and toxins that have built up to the point where natural immunity cannot handle or overcome them.

Your glands are always affected, (since the endocrine system is on a 6 day cycle, a cold usually runs for about a week) as the body works through all its detoxification processes.

Your lungs are on the front line of toxic intake from viruses, allergies, pollutants, and mucous-forming congestants. An occasional lung cleanse supports your respiratory system in releasing pollutant-caused infections. But your body works together. Extra pressure of disease or heavy elimination on one part of the body puts extra stress on another. Cleansing your kidneys, for example, takes part of the waste elimination load off your lungs so they can recover faster. Similarly, promoting respiratory health through a lung cleanse also helps digestive and skin problems.

Any program to overcome a chronic respiratory problems is usually more successful when begun with a short mucous elimination plan like a lung cleansing diet. This allows the body to first rid itself of toxic accumulations that cause congestion before an attempt is made to change eating habits that support better health.

Is your body showing signs that it needs a lung and respiratory cleanse?

Do you have a chronic phlegmy cough? Do you wheeze with asthma? Is your head stuffy with congestive allergies? Do you have bronchitis or severe sinusitis? Are you highly sensitive to chemicals and pollutants? Do you have a runny nose in any weather? Are you a cigarette smoker?

Lung and Respiratory Detox Plan

Alkalize your body during a lung cleanse. Acid-forming foods tend to aggravate or prolong colds and other respiratory problems. Use alkalizing foods like fresh fruits, high chlorophyll greens and sea greens, and non-gluten grains like brown rice or millet in a ratio of about 4:1 over acid-forming foods during a lung detox. Begin with a 3 day juice/liquid diet and follow with 1 to 4 days of a diet of 100% fresh foods. Drink plenty of non-dairy fluids, like water, juices, herb teas or broth, to hydrate and flush the body. Milk congests and constipates.

The night before your lung cleanse....
—Take your choice of gentle herbal laxatives.

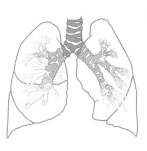

The next day....
—**On rising:** take 2 squeezed lemons in water with 1 TB. maple syrup.
—**Breakfast:** have a water-diluted grapefruit juice with 1 TB. of a green superfood, like Transitions EASY GREENS or Nature's Secret ULTIMATE GREEN; or water-diluted pineapple juice as a natural expectorant — add one TB. of a green superfood powder.
—**Mid-morning:** take a carrot juice or mixed fresh vegetable juice such as Personal Best V-8 (page 218).
—**Lunch:** have a Potassium Juice (page 215).
—**Mid-afternoon:** have a cup of mucous cleansing tea like Crystal Star X-PEC™ tea with mullein, marshmallow, comfrey, pleurisy root, rose hips, calendula, boneset, ginger, peppermint and fennel seed.
—**Dinner:** have a warm Potassium Essence broth (page 215); or try this broth, rich in zinc, vitamin A, C, potassium and magnesium electrolytes: In 2 $\frac{1}{2}$ cups water, cook 1 $\frac{1}{2}$ cups fresh mixed vegetables with 1 TBS. miso. Strain and take broth. Blender blend veggies, broth and 4 TBS sunflower seeds for a hearty version.
—**Before Bed:** have cranberry or celery juice.

Lung cleanse supplement suggestions: Choose 2 or 3 cleansing boosters.

• **Lung cleansers:** Creation's Garden LNG-1 (assists respiratory ailments settling in the lungs) and LNG-3 (clears lung congestion, bronchial inflammation).

• **Lung anti-infectives:** NutriCology PROLIVE WITH ANTIOXIDANTS (olive leaf extract); oregano oil for lung conditions like cough, asthma, colds, flu, bronchitis and pneumonia. (Oregano oil has antiviral and anti-bacterial properties that help eradicate lung infection. Also thins mucous and stops excessive mucous secretion.) Tea Tree has decongestant, antiviral and antibacterial properties. Herbs Etc. LUNG TONIC supports lung cleansing; Crystal Star X-PECT-TEA™, an expectorant to aid mucous release.

• **Chlorophyll-rich super green foods:** like chlorella, spirulina and barley grass speed up lung cleansing, increase oxygen in the body and help treat respiratory tract infection; Solgar EARTH SOURCE GREENS & MORE.

• **Lung superfoods:** Country Life SHIITAKE/REISHI COMPLEX.

• **Enzyme support:** Transformation Enzyme GASTRO-ZYME (mucous congestion); PUREZYME (immunity).

• **Electrolytes increase oxygen uptake:** Nature's Path TRACE-LYTE LIQUID MINERALS.

• **Probiotics inhibit harmful organisms:** Source Naturals LIFE FLORA; Nature's Path, FLORA-LYTE.

• **Antioxidants linked to better lung function:** Vit. C 1,000mg 3x day raises body's glutathione levels to protect the lungs; Source Naturals PROANTHODYN.

Lung cleanse bodywork suggestions: Choose techniques to accelerate and round out your cleanse.

—**Deep Breathing Exercise:** Do this deep breathing exercise often during your cleanse to remove stress, compose your mind, improve your mood and increase your energy: Take a deep, full breath. Exhale it slowly... slowly. Take another deep, full breath. Release slowly. And again. Maintain a quiet rhythm, exhaling more slowly than you inhale.

—**Exercise:** If you are cleansing your lungs and not ill with a cold, flu, or other respiratory infection, take a brisk, daily walk on each day of your cleanse. Breathe deep to help the lungs eliminate mucous.

—**Compress:** Apply wet ginger/cayenne compresses to chest to increase circulation and loosen mucous.

—**Essential oil support:** To assist your lung cleanse, use oregano, tea tree, and eucalyptus oils (singly or in combination). Put a total of 15 drops essential oils in 1-oz of a carrier oil (such as jojoba) and rub on the chest. As an inhalant: add 6 drops of the essential oils to one quart hot water — inhale the steam. Eucalyptus especially has antiviral action to loosen mucous, and treat asthma, bronchitis and sinusitis.

—**Bathe-Sauna:** Take a hot 20 minute bath or sauna at the onset of a cold, flu or beginning of a respiratory cleanse to stimulate your body's defenses and increase toxin elimination.

Note: Consciously steer clear of air pollution. Environmental and heavy metal pollutants, like chlorofluorocarbons and tobacco smoke (even secondary smoke) contribute greatly to respiratory problems and can undo all your hard cleansing work.

Today's opportunities are like lettuce— crisp and beautiful today, but brown and wilted tomorrow. Go for it today.

Do you need a blood purifying cleanse?

Your blood is your river of life. The health of your blood is critical. The blood must supply oxygen to your body's sixty trillion cells, transport nutrients, hormones and wastes, warm and cool the body, ward off invading microorganisms, seal off wounds and much more. It is your body's chief neutralizing agent for bacteria and toxic wastes. Toxins ingested in sublethal amounts can eventually add up to disease-causing amounts. For example, slow viruses like those that lead to MS, a nerve disease, can enter the cells and remain dormant for years, feeding on toxic wastes, then reappearing in a more dangerous form. While the body has a self-purifying complex for maintaining healthy blood, the best way to protect yourself from disease is to keep those cleansing systems in good working order. A blood purifying diet may be followed for 1 to 2 months, or longer if your body is still actively cleansing, or needs further balancing. You can return to a blood cleansing regimen as needed.

Cautionary note for people who suffer from severe blood toxicity:
Most immune deficient diseases are the result of blood toxins and can benefit from a blood purifying diet to boost compromised immunity. However, in serious degenerative conditions like AIDS, lupus, chronic fatigue syndrome or fibromyalgia, there are usually large amounts of toxins and pollutants in the blood. When this is the case, *an all-liquid fast is not recommended*. It is often too harsh for an already weakened system, and in fact may dump more toxins out into the bloodstream than the body can handle. The initial diet in these severe cases, should be as pure as possible in order to be as cleansing as possible — totally vegetarian — free of all meats, dairy foods, fried, preserved and refined foods and saturated fats.

Is your body showing signs that it needs a blood cleanse?
—a simple blood-color test monitors blood improvement. Make a small, quick, sterilized razor cut on your finger. If the blood is a dark, bluish-purplish color, it is not healthy. Healthy blood is a bright red color.
—a deep, choking, chronic cough
—depression, memory loss or unusual insomnia, schizophrenic behavior, seizures, periodic black-outs
—sexual impotence or dysfunction
—black spots on the gums, bad breath or body odor, unusual, severe reactions to foods and odors
—loss of hand/eye coordination, especially in driving

Blood Cleansing Detox Plan
Begin with a 3 day juice/liquid diet; follow with 1 to 4 days of 100% fresh solid and liquid foods.

The night before your blood cleanse.....
—Take your choice of gentle herbal laxatives or Gaia Herbs SUPREME CLEANSE.

The next day....
—**On rising:** Take 2 to 3 TBS. cranberry concentrate in 8-oz. water with $^1/_2$ teasp. ascorbate vitamin C crystals, or use a green tea formula like Crystal Star GREEN TEA CLEANSER™; or cut up a half lemon with skin and blender blend with 1 teasp. honey, and 1 cup water; or $^1/_2$ teasp. Natren TRINITY in 8-oz. aloe vera juice.
—**Breakfast:** a glass of fresh carrot juice; or an 8-oz. aloe vera juice with $^1/_2$ teasp. Natren TRINITY.
—**Mid-morning:** take a potassium broth (page 215), add $^1/_2$ teasp. ascorbate vitamin C crystals; and another fresh carrot juice, or pau d'arco tea.
—**Lunch:** have a glass of fresh PERSONAL BEST V-8 juice (page 218) or a carrot or apple juice. Mix in 1 TB. of a green superfood such as Crystal Star ENERGY GREEN™ or NutriCology PRO-GREENS.
—**Mid-afternoon:** a vegetable juice: handful spinach, 4 romaine leaves, 4 sprigs parsley, 6 carrots, $^1/_4$ turnip.
—**Dinner:** a cup of miso soup with 2 TBS. dried sea greens (any kind) snipped over the top.
—**Before Bed:** an 8-oz. glass aloe vera juice with $^1/_2$ teasp. ascorbate vitamin C, and $^1/_2$ teasp. Natren TRINITY.

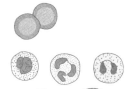

Blood cleanse supplement suggestions: Choose 2 or 3 cleansing boosters.
Note: Vegetable and fruit juices stimulate rapid, heavy waste elimination, a process that can generate mild symptoms of a "healing crisis." A slight headache, nausea, bad breath, body odor and dark urine occur as the body accelerates release of accumulated toxins. If you are detoxifying from alcohol or drug overload, 5,000 to 10,000mg. of ascorbate vitamin C is recommended daily during serious cleansing, to help keep the body alkaline and encourage oxygen uptake. In addition, sprinkle $^{1}/_{2}$ tsp. lactobacillus powder over any food for body chemistry improvement.

Note 2: One of the most potent blood cleansing formulas available is Crytal Star's DETOX™ capsule blend, with blood cleansing herbs: *red clover, dandelion, burdock, yellow dock, echinacea, Oregon grape root, sarsaparilla, astragalus, pau d'arco, goldenseal root, garlic and cayenne.* This formula has been used successfully for over two decades to rebalance blood and body chemistry. It is strong and fast-acting. Should you decide to use it, take it alone.... not with other herbal formulas, or even vitamins other than vitamin C.

  • **Herbal blood cleansers:** Crystal Star GREEN TEA CLEANSER™ and LIV-ALIVE™ capsules; M.D. Labs DAILY DETOX II tea; Herbal Magic COL-LIV HERBAL BASE; Planetary Formulas COMPLETE PAU D'ARCO PROGRAM; Nature's Way DANDELION WITH GOLDEN SEAL.
  • **Blood purifiers with immune stimulants:** HEMATONIX-Nature's Answer; RIVER OF LIFE by Planetary.
  • **Enzyme support:** Transformation Enzyme PUREZYME, breaks down protein invaders in the blood supply leaving them vulnerable to destruction by the immune system; Rainbow Light ADVANCED ENZYME SYSTEM.
  • **Electrolytes establish healthy blood and strengthen immunity:** Arise & Shine ALKALIZER; Nature's Path TRACE-LYTE LIQUID MINERALS.
  • **Probiotics provide nutrients for building blood:** Arise & Shine FLORA GROW; Source Naturals LIFE FLORA; or Premier Labs MULTI-DOPHILUS.
  • **Chlorophyll enhances blood cleansing:** SUN CHLORELLA by Sun Wellness; New Chapter CHLORELLA.
  • **Antioxidants strengthen white blood and T cells:** Schiff PHYTOCHARGED ANTIOXIDANT; Solgar ADVANCED ANTIOXIDANT FORMULA; Jarrow COENZYME Q_{10}; Enzymatic Therapy GRAPE SEED PHYTOSOME 100.
  • **Antioxidant blood cleansers:** germanium, 100 to 150mg; Vitamin E 1000IU with selenium 200mcg; CoQ_{10} 180mg daily; Vit. C-1,000mg w. bioflavs. 3x daily; Quercetin and bromelain 500mg 3x daily, for autoimmune reactions; shark cartilage 750-1200mg to stimulate interferon, interleukin and lymphocytes.

Blood cleanse bodywork suggestions: Choose techniques to accelerate and round out your cleanse.
  —**Enema:** Take an enema (page 539) the first, second and the last day of your blood cleansing program.
  —**Irrigate:** Take a colonic or Nature's Secret SUPERCLEANSE once a week to remove infected feces.
  —**Exercise:** Exercise daily in the morning, if possible.
  —**Massage therapy:** Have a massage to stimulate blood circulation.
  —**Bathe or sauna:** Take several saunas or long hot baths if possible during a blood cleanse for faster, easier detoxification. Add 15 drops of essential oil, rosemary, cypress and vetiver to your bath to assist your blood cleanse. Stir the water briskly to disperse evenly.

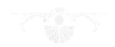

Do you need a lymph cleanse?

The lymphatic system includes lymphatic vessels and nodes, thymus gland, tonsils and spleen. It's really a network of tubing that drains waste products from tissues, produces disease-fighting white blood cells (lymphocytes) and antibodies, and carries the bulk of the body's waste from the cells to the elimination organs. Experts call the lymphatic system a secondary circulatory system, because it assists the bloodstream throughout the body to collect tissue fluid not needed by the capillaries or skin and return it to the heart for recirculation. Your lymph system is also a key to your body's immune defenses, because special filtering lymph nodes along the lymph ducts remove infective organisms.

Liver health is a key to lymphatic health. The liver produces the majority of lymph in the body. Lymph is a major route for nutrients from the liver and intestines, so it's rich in fat-soluble nutrients, especially protein. The integrity of the lymph system depends on special immune cells that filter out harmful bacteria and yeasts.

The spleen is the largest mass of lymphatic tissue. It destroys worn-out red blood cells, and serves as a healthy blood reservoir for fresh red blood. During times of demand, such as a hemorrhage, the spleen can release its stored blood and prevent shock from occurring.

Here's an even more amazing fact: **Physical exercise and diaphragmatic deep breathing are critical to healthy lymph and to immune response.** The valves of the lymph system transport waste-filled fluids to be flushed and filtered. But since there is no pump, as there is with the heart, lymph circulation depends solely upon breathing and muscle movement.

Is your body showing signs that it needs a lymph cleanse?
If you are under chronic stress; if you are constantly tired (indicating liver exhaustion); if your skin is very pale; if you are extremely thin; if your memory is noticeably failing; if you have low immune response with frequent colds, a revitalizing lymph cleanse can make a difference. If your body looks uncharacteristically soft and pudgy or has newly noticeable cellulite (indicating too many saturated fats and sugary foods), you probably need a lymph-draining cleanse.

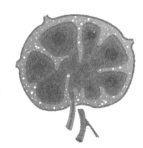

Lymph Cleansing Detox Plan
Nutrient deficiency is the most frequent cause of sluggish lymph. Immune-boosting vegetables are cabbage, kale, carrot, bell pepper, collards and garlic. Lymph-enhancing fruits are apple, pineapple, blueberry and grape.
Start your lymph cleanse: with a 4 to 7 day cleanse; follow with 1 to 4 days of a diet of 100% fresh foods.

—**On rising:** take a glass of lemon juice and water regularly in the morning for lymph revitalization.
—**Breakfast:** have a fresh mixed vegetable lymph juice builder: handful parsley, 1 garlic clove, 5 carrots, and 3 celery stalks. Add 2 TBS green superfood: Solgar EARTH SOURCE GREENS & MORE or Wakunaga KYO-GREEN.
—**Mid-morning:** have 2 cups of Crystal Star LIV-ALIVE™ tea for liver and lymph cleansing, or a lymph tea blend of *white sage, astragalus, echinacea root, Oregon grape root and dandelion root.*
—**Lunch:** have a vitamin A/carotene/C drink: 3 broccoli flowerets, 5 carrots, 1 garlic clove, 2 celery stalks and $1/_2$ green pepper. Add 2 TBS green superfood: Vibrant Health GREEN VIBRANCE or Arise & Shine POWER UP.
—**Mid-afternoon:** a glass of apple or grape juice.
—**Dinner:** have a Potassium Essence Broth (page 215), for mineral electrolytes. Or try a broth rich in zinc, vitamin A and C, potassium and magnesium electrolytes: In $2 1/_2$ cups water, cook $1 1/_2$ cups mixed carrots, broccoli, dark leafy greens, celery and parsley and 1 teasp. miso. Strain and use broth. Hearty version: blend warm broth and vegetables. Add 4 TBS. sunflower seeds.
—**Before Bed:** have a glass of papaya juice.

Dietary pointers for best results from your lymph cleanse:
　—Drink 8-10 glasses of bottled water each day of your cleanse.
　—Include potassium-rich foods regularly — sea vegetables, broccoli, bananas and seafood.
　—Avoid caffeine, sugar, dairy foods and alcohol during your cleanse. They add to lymphatic stagnation.
　—Spicy foods like natural salsas, cayenne pepper, horseradish and ginger boost a sluggish lymph system.

Lymph cleanse supplement suggestions: Choose 2 or 3 cleansing boosters.
　•**Lymphatic cleansers:** Crystal Star ANTI-BIO™ caps for white blood cell formation-lymph purifying; Herbs Etc. LYMPHATONIC - with *echinacea* to reduce lymphatic congestion; *red root*, a powerful lymphatic cleanser, synergistic with echinacea and ocotillo to flush lymph congestion; Nature's Apothecary LYMPH CLEANSE; Enzymatic Therapy LYMPHO-CLEAR; Gaia Herbs ECHINACEA RED ROOT SUPREME a lymphatic and liver cleanser. Note: Echinacea extract and astragalus extract are highly successful deep lymph cleansing single herbs.
　•**Herbal lymph immune support:** Crystal Star REISHI/GINSENG™ extract.
　•**Immune support:** Silica decisively increases phagocytes to strengthen immune response. Eidon SILICA MINERAL SUPPLEMENT; Flora VEGE-SIL.
　•**Supporting lymph nutrients:** Vitamins A, C, E, B-complex, carotenes, iron, zinc and selenium.
　•**Enzyme support:** Protease is a powerful lymph immune booster. Transformation Enzyme PUREZYME; shark cartilage - 1400mg for leucocyte production.
　•**Electrolyte boosters:** Mineral electrolytes play a major role in detoxifying the lymph glands, helping to remove acid crystals. Nature's Path TRACE-LYTE LIQUID MINERALS.
　•**To overcome lymph deficiencies:** Protein and vitamin B-12.

Lymph cleanse bodywork suggestions: Choose techniques to accelerate and round out your cleanse.
　—**Irrigate:** take a colonic irrigation or a Sonné BENTONITE CLAY CLEANSE once a week to remove lymph congestion and infected feces from the intestinal tract.
　—**Exercise:** exercise is critical to lymphatic flow. To stimulate lymph flow activate muscles with regular exercise and stretching. Start every exercise period with deep, diaphragmatic breathing. Mini-trampoline exercise clears clogged lymph nodes.
　—**Massage therapy:** elevate feet and legs for 5 minutes every day, massaging lymph node areas.
　—**Lymph supporting therapies:** acupuncture and acupressure have both been successful.
　—**Essential oil support:** use geranium, juniper and black pepper. Use one or a combination of all three oils. Put a total of 15 drops essential oil in 1-oz. of a carrier oil (such as jojoba) and rub on the skin.
　—**Shower:** take an alternating hot and cold hydrotherapy treatment at the end of your daily shower to stimulate lymph circulation.
　—**Bathe:** a lymph-cleansing mineral bath — add 1 cup Dead Sea salts, 1 cup Epsom salts, $\frac{1}{2}$ cup regular sea salt and $\frac{1}{4}$ baking soda to a tub; swish in 3 drops lavender oil, 2 drops chamomile oil, 2 drops marjoram oil and 1 drop ylang ylang oil.
　—**Eliminate aluminum:** cookware, food additives, alum-containing foods like relishes and commercial condiments, and deodorants.

Improvement signs show that your body is responding to the lymph cleanse:
　—Most people notice an increase in their daily energy.
　—You'll no longer catch every cold that comes your way; illnesses you do get won't last as long.
　—Most people notice far fewer stress reactions as body chemistry normalizes.
　—You'll notice better weight control, especially if you were overweight; with less cellulite formation as congestion lessens.

Do you need a skin cleanse?

Your skin is the surest mirror of your lifestyle. Almost everything that's going on inside you shows on your skin. Your skin is your body's largest organ of elimination and detoxification. The skin acts as a backup for every other elimination organ. When your colon becomes overloaded and stagnant with toxins, or your liver cannot efficiently filter the impurities coming from the digestive tract, your skin will try to compensate by releasing toxins from your body. It sweats them out, or throws them off through rashes or boils. Your skin is the essence of renewable nature.... it sloughs off old, dying cells every day, and gives the body a clean, new start.

Your skin is also your body's largest organ of absorption and ingestion — both for nutrients and toxins. Good dietary care and habits show quickly. By the same token, chemicalized food toxins and nutritional deficiencies from a poor diet show up first on your skin. For example, toxins eliminated through the oil glands in the skin, show up as acne. The skin mirrors our emotional state and our hormone balance, too. So, stress reactions and hormone disruption show up as poor skin texture, or spots and blemishes.

Is your body showing signs that it needs a skin cleanse?
—Do you have sallow skin? Poor skin coloring may indicate build-up from liver wastes or drug residues.
—Do you have age spots? Brown mottled spots on the hands or face may reflect liver waste accumulation.
—Do you have adult acne, or uneven skin texture? Waste build-up from environmental pollutants, poor diet, liver exhaustion and stress allow increased free radical formation which attack skin cell membranes.
—Do you have wrinkles, or sagging skin contours? Free radical activity also affects skin collagen and elastin proteins, resulting in wrinkling and dry skin. Poor skin tone is a sign of antioxidant deficiency.
—Do you have puffy or swollen eyes, dark circles under your eyes, or crusty, mucous formations in your eyes?
—Is your breath bad? Do you have body odor? They're pretty solid signs your body is overloaded with wastes.
—Do you have a skin disorder? Psoriasis, dermatitis and seborrhea all indicate its time for a skin cleanse.
—Do you have skin sores or rashes that aren't healing? or hard skin bumps? Your body may be overloaded with wastes you're not eliminating.
—Do you have unusually oily skin? or scaly, itchy skin? or chronically chapped and red skin?
—Is your circulation poor with cold hands and feet, and swollen ankles? Your body lacks tissue oxygen uptake.

Benefits you may notice as your body responds to skin cleansing:
—Most people experience noticeable appearance improvement in about 3 weeks.
—Your face will look rested, rejuvenated and revitalized.
—Your skin's natural glow will return as capillary circulation and lymphatic drainage improve.
—Skin blemishes, blotches and spots diminish or disappear.
—The whites of your eyes will become whiter; dark circles will disappear.
—Your skin texture will appear smoother and softer; fine lines will appear less noticeable.

Skin Cleansing Detox Plan

1: Your diet is the quickest way to change your looks. Soft smooth skin depends on a diet rich in fresh fruits and vegetables. Skin tissues need a rich, oxygen blood supply, and plenty of mineral building blocks. Silica, sulphur, calcium and magnesium are specific minerals for your skin. Plants are the most absorbable way for your body to get them.

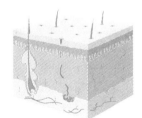

2: Beautiful skin tone needs vitamin A, vitamin C, minerals and vegetable protein foods for collagen and interstitial tissue health. Eliminate or limit sugary foods, fried foods and trans-fats, like those in milk and dairy foods, margarine, shortening and hydrogenated oils. Avoid red meats and refined foods of all kinds.

3: Drink at least 8 glasses of bottled water each day of your cleanse — herbal "skin" teas are fine, too. Water keeps your body flushed so wastes and toxins won't be dumped out through the skin as blemishes or rashes. Fluoridated water may leach vitamin E out of your body.

Begin your skin cleanse with a 3-day liquid diet and follow with 4 days of a diet of fresh foods.

—**On rising:** take a glass of lemon juice and water; add New Moon GINGER WONDER syrup if desired.

—**Breakfast:** make a Complexion Booster: juice 2 slices of pineapple and 2 apples. Add 1 TBS. Crystal Star BIOFLAV, FIBER & C SUPPORT™, 1 teasp. brewer's yeast and 1 teasp. wheat germ oil.

—**Mid-morning:** have watermelon juice when available (rich in natural silica), or a skin tonic drink: juice 1 cucumber, 1 handful fresh parsley, 1 4-oz. tub fresh sprouts and sprigs of fresh mint. Or, have a superfood green drink, like Crystal Star ENERGY GREEN™ or Transformation EASY GREENS.

—**Lunch:** have a fresh carrot juice; or a skin drink: juice 5 carrots, 2 apples, add 15 drops GINGER EXTRACT.

—**Mid-afternoon:** have a carrot/beet/cucumber juice once a week for the next month for a clean liver .

—**Dinner:** have a warm POTASSIUM ESSENCE BROTH (page 215) for mineral electrolytes. Or, make a high luster skin broth: In 2 $\frac{1}{2}$ cups water cook 2 cups chopped fresh mixed vegetables, add 1 tsp. miso and 2 TBS chopped dried sea vegetables. Vegetable protein aids faster healing for damaged skin.

—**Before Bed:** have Crystal Star BEAUTIFUL SKIN™ Tea or Japanese green tea for skin support; or a pineapple-papaya, papaya or apple juice; or VEGEX yeast broth for high B-complex vitamins.

Skin cleanse supplement suggestions: Choose 2 or 3 cleansing boosters.

• **Deep skin-blood cleansing:** Creations Garden TOTAL BODY CLEANSE, Crystal Star SKIN THERAPY #1™ and SKIN THERAPY #2™ CAPS; sage or burdock root tea. Include a green superfood daily during your skin cleanse.

• **Smoothing/hydrating herbs for skin:** Crystal Star BEAUTIFUL SKIN™ CAPS for blemishes and skin maintenance; Nature's Apothecary SKIN SUPPORT - blood purifiers and mineralizers; Herbs Etc. DERMATONIC - stimulates waste elimination; burdock root normalizes production of the skin's beneficial oils; chamomile tea or CamoCare FACIAL THERAPY; lavender aromatherapy oil to reduce puffiness.

• **Skin vitamins and minerals:** Diamond HERPANACINE for superior skin support; Futurebiotics HAIR, SKIN & NAILS - results in just 2 weeks; Crystal Star MINERAL SPECTRUM™ caps.

• **Antioxidants are critical for skin health:** Beta carotene protects against sun's free radicals; vitamin E protects against the lipid peroxidation caused by UV rays; Bioflavonoids improve vascularization of the skin.

• **Essential fatty acid deficiency reflected by skin dehydration and wrinkling:** Crystal Star EVENING PRIMROSE; Spectrum ORGANIC ESSENTIAL MAX EFA OIL.

• **Enzyme support:** Protease heals skin disorders; Transformation Enzyme PUREZYME.

• **Silica:** a mineral for collagen support, reduces dry, wrinkled skin. Eidon SILICA MINERAL SUPPLEMENT; Flora VEGESIL; Crystal Star SILICA SOURCE™.

• **MSM** (*Methyl Sulfonyl Methante*) **enhances tissue pliability and helps repair damaged, scarred skin:** Nature's Path MSM-LYTE.

Skin cleanse bodywork suggestions: Choose techniques to accelerate and round out your cleanse.

The healthiest skin needs some sunlight every day. Early morning sunlight on the body for natural vitamin D is a key. Exercise to get skin circulation flowing is another key.

—**Dry brushing:** Use a natural bristle brush. Start with the soles of your feet - brush vigorously making rotary motions and massage every part of your body — work up to the neck.

—**Facial massage:** Skin circulation for better tone.

—**Healing, beautifying skin application treatments:** Crystal Star BEAUTIFUL SKIN™ GEL — a cleansing, restorative phytotherapy gel. Beautiful Face tea: steep chamomile, calendula, rosehips, juice of 1 lemon and 2 teasp. rose water. Strain; apply with cotton balls to the face. Nature's Path SKIN-LYTE a liquid electrolyte spray.

—**Aloe vera:** Herbal Answers HERBAL ALOE FORCE GEL boosts circulation and stimulates new cell growth.

—**Fruit acid treatment:** Rub face with the insides of papaya or cucumber skins (natural AHA's) to neutralize wastes that come out on the skin.

—**Essential oil support:** Lavender, geranium, sandalwood and neroli. Use one or a combination of all three oils. Put a total of 15 drops essential oil in 2-oz of a carrier oil (such as jojoba) and rub on the skin.

—**Skin mineral bath:** Add 1 cup Dead Sea salts, 1 cup Epsom salts, $\frac{1}{2}$ cup regular sea salt and 4 TBS. baking soda to a tub; swish in 3 drops lavender, 2 drops geranium, 2 drops sandalwood and 1 drop neroli oil.

Detox Drinks

Detoxification drinks have a powerful effect on the body's recuperative powers because of their rich, easily absorbed nutrients. Fresh juices contain proteins, carbohydrates, chlorophyll, mineral electrolytes and healing aromatic oils. But most importantly, fresh juice therapy makes available to every cell in our bodies large amounts of plant enzymes, an integral part of the healing and restoration process.

Nothing gets done in our bodies without enzymes. They are the activity components of life. Digestive function, assimilation and elimination are all instigated or assisted by enzymes. Enzymes cause every chemical reaction in our bodies. They play a vital part in breaking down foreign matter (like toxins) as well as food. Enzymes and mineral electrolytes (which restore peristaltic bowel activity) are major contributors to moving toxins out of the body instead of building up and poisoning us. When your diet is full of cooked foods without enzymes, or low residue, processed foods (which have more tendency to stagnate and putrefy), the process of internal decay develops far more rapidly.

Our bodies are designed to be self-healing organisms. Healing is allowed to occur through cleansing. Cleansing foods and juices can optimize your detox program. In fact, they are crucial to its success in three ways:
• They keep your body chemistry balanced and your body processes stable while you detox, so you don't become uncomfortable. Don't forget that Mother Nature is cleaning house during a detox cleanse. You may eliminate accumulated poisons and wastes quite rapidly, causing headaches, slight nausea and weakness as your body purges. (These reactions are usually only temporary and disappear along with the waste and toxins.)
• They regulate the speed of your detox so your body doesn't cleanse too fast or dump too many toxins into your bloodstream all at once that your body can't handle. Green cuisine keeps you from re-poisoning yourself during the detox process.
• They support your nutrition and energy levels while you detox, so you don't become too hungry or too tired. New healthy tissue starts building right away when the detoxification juices are taken in. Gland secretions stimulate the immune system during a cleanse to set up a disease defense environment.

Should you get a juicer?

Juicers are expensive appliances, but they can really boost the nutrient power of your cleansing drinks. A good juicer essentially predigests fresh fruits and vegetables for almost immediate assimilation by your body. Juicer juices can accelerate your cleanse and notice-ably boost your energy level. A juicer can juice all of a fruit or vegetable (even rinds, stems, peels, seeds) to give you up to 95% of the plant's food and nutritive value.

Champion, JuiceMan and Acme are all good juicers for a detox program.

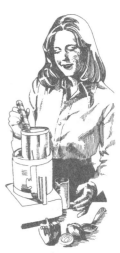

Cleansing foods should be organically grown and eaten fresh for best results. Only fresh foods and juices retain the full complement of nutrients and plant enzymes that Mother Nature offers.
• **Fruits and fruit juices** eliminate wastes quickly and help reduce cravings for sweets.
• **Fresh vegetable juices** carry off excess body acids, and are rich in vitamins, miner-als and enzymes that satisfy the body's nutrient requirements with less food.
• **Chlorophyll-rich drinks and green superfoods** like spirulina, chlorella, and bar-ley grass help stabilize and maintain the acid/alkaline balance of the body and also have anti-infective properties. Since chlorophyll has a molecular structure close to our own plasma, drinking them is like giving yourself a mini transfusion. They especially help clear the skin, cleanse the kidneys, and clean and build the blood.
• **Herb teas and mineral drinks** provide energy and cleansing at the same time, without having to take in solid food for fuel.

• **Sea greens** act as the ocean's purifiers and they perform much the same for the human body, also largely made up of salt water. Sea plant chemical composition is so close to human plasma, that it can help balance your body at the cellular level. Sea vegetables alkalize and purify the blood from the effects of a modern diet. They strengthen your body against illness caused by environmental toxins. Their benefits against serious disease rival the healing powers of their land-based cousins, broccoli and cabbage. They reduce stores of excess fluid and fat, and work to transform toxic metals (including radiation), into harmless salts that the body can eliminate. The natural iodine in sea greens reduces by almost 80% radioactive iodine-131 in the thyroid.

Sea vegetables have superior nutritional content. As one of Nature's richest sources of complex carbohydrates, minerals and vitamins, and a superior source of plant protein. They provide full-spectrum concentrations of all the carotenes, chlorophyll, enzymes, amino acids and fiber. They transmit those nutrients to your body. Ounce for ounce sea vegetables are higher in vitamins and minerals than any other food group except herbs. They are almost the only non-animal source of Vitamin B_{12}, necessary for cell development and nerve function. Their mineral balance is a natural tranquilizer for sound nerve structure and good metabolism. The distinctive salty taste is not just "salt," but a balanced, chelation of sodium, potassium, calcium, magnesium, phosphorus, iron and trace minerals. They convert inorganic ocean minerals into organic mineral salts that combine with amino acids — an ideal way for us to get body structural building blocks! In fact, sea vegetables contain all the necessary trace elements for life, many of which are depleted in the earth's land-based soil.

Remember these easy diet watchwords as you use the detox drinks:
—The day before you begin your detox, eat green salads and fresh fruits, and drink plenty of healthy liquids, so that the upcoming body chemistry changes will not be uncomfortable. A gentle herbal laxative taken the night before is beneficial.

—Avoid all dairy products and cooked foods during a cleansing detox.

—Drink six to eight 8-oz. glasses of bottled water daily to keep your body continually flushing out the toxins your tissues are releasing.

POTASSIUM JUICE

This is the single most effective juice for cleansing, neutralizing acids and rebuilding the body. It is a blood and body tonic that provides rapid energy and system balance.
For one 12-oz. glass:

Juice in a juicer 3 CARROTS, 3 STALKS CELERY, $\frac{1}{2}$ BUNCH SPINACH, 1 TB snipped, dry SEA GREENS, $\frac{1}{2}$ BUNCH PARSLEY. —Add 1 teasp. Bragg's LIQUID AMINOS if desired.

POTASSIUM ESSENCE BROTH

If you don't have a juicer, make a potassium broth in a soup pot. While not as concentrated or pure, it is still an excellent source of energy, minerals and electrolytes.
For a 2 day supply:

Cover with water in a soup pot 3 to 4 CARROTS, 3 STALKS CELERY, $\frac{1}{2}$ BUNCH PARSLEY, 2 POTATOES with skins, $\frac{1}{2}$ HEAD CABBAGE, 1 ONION, and $\frac{1}{2}$ BUNCH BROCCOLI, 2 TBS snipped, dry SEA GREENS.
—Simmer covered 30 minutes. Strain and discard solids.
—Add 2 teasp. Bragg's LIQUID AMINOS or 1 teasp. MISO. Store in the fridge, covered.

Cleansing Fruit Drinks

Fruit juices are like a quick car wash for your body. Their high water and sugar content speeds up metabolism to release wastes quickly. Their alkalizing effects help reduce cravings for sweets. Still, because of their fast assimilation, pesticides, sprays and chemicals on fruits can enter your body rapidly. So, eat organically grown fruits whenever possible. Wash fruit well if commercially grown. Fruits and fruit juices have their best nutritional effects when taken alone. Eat them before noon for best energy conversion and cleansing benefits.

BLOOD PURIFIER

For 4 large drinks:

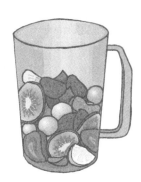

Juice 2 bunches GRAPES or 2 cups GRAPE JUICE, 6 ORANGES or 2 cups ORANGE JUICE, and 8 LEMONS peeled or 1 cup LEMON JUICE.
—Stir in: 2 cups WATER and $^1/_4$ cup HONEY.

EVER GREEN ENZYME DRINK

A personal favorite for taste, mucous release and enzyme action.
For 1 drink:

Juice 1 APPLE, cored, 1 tub (4 oz.) ALFALFA SPROUTS, $^1/_2$ FRESH PINEAPPLE, skinned/cored, 3 small handfuls FRESH MINT and 1 teasp. SPIRULINA GRANULES.

FRUIT & ALOE STOMACH & DIGESTIVE CLEANSER

For one 8-oz. glass:

Whirl in the blender, 1 APPLE cored, 2 TBS. ALOE VERA JUICE and $^1/_4$ teasp. GROUND GINGER.
—Add enough WATER to make 8-oz.

ENZYME CHOLESTEROL REDUCER

An intestinal cleanser to help lower cholesterol and allow better assimilation of foods.
For 2 large drinks:

Juice 1 APPLE, cored, or $^1/_2$ cup APPLE JUICE, 2 LEMONS, peeled, or $^1/_4$ cup LEMON JUICE, and 1 PINE-APPLE, skinned and cored, or $1^1/_2$ cups PINEAPPLE JUICE.

GINGER-LEMON CLEANSE FOR ALLERGIES

For 2 drinks (a day's supply):

1-inch slice FRESH GINGER ROOT, 1 FRESH LEMON, 6 CARROTS with tops, and 1 APPLE, seeded.

COLON-CONSTIPATION CLEANSER
For 1 drink:

Juice I firm PAPAYA, $1/4$- inch slice GINGER ROOT, 4 PRUNES and I PEAR.

FLUSHING DIURETIC MELON MIX
Take on an empty stomach, 3x daily for best results.
For 1 quart:

Juice 3 cups WATERMELON CUBES, 2 cups PERSIAN MELON CUBES, and 2 cups HONEYDEW CUBES.

BLADDER INFECTION CLEANSER
For 2 drinks:

Juice 3 to 4 APPLES, and $1/2$ cup CRANBERRIES and $1/4$ TEASP. GINGER POWDER or CRYSTALLIZED GINGER.

GINGER AID PROSTATE CLEANSER
For 2 drinks:

Juice $1/2$ LEMON, $1/2$-inch slice FRESH GINGER ROOT, and I bunch GREEN GRAPES
—Fill glass with SPARKLING WATER.

ACNE CLEANSER
For 1 drink:

Juice 2 slices PINEAPPLE with skin, $1/2$ CUCUMBER, $1/2$ APPLE, and $1/4$-inch slice GINGER ROOT.

MUCOUS CONGESTION APPLE CLEANSE
For 1 drink:

Juice 2 large APPLES, seeded, and $1/2$ teasp. grated HORSERADISH.

Note: Other good cleansing fruit juices include:
—black cherry juice for gouty conditions
—cranberry juice for bladder and kidney infections
—grape and citrus juices for high blood pressure
—celery for nerves
—canteloupe for allergies

Green Drinks, Vegetable Juices & Blood Tonics

I believe green drinks are critical to the success of every cleansing program. The molecular composition of chlorophyll is so close to that of human hemoglobin that these drinks can act as "mini-transfusions" for the blood, and tonics for the brain and immune system. They are an excellent nutrient source of vitamins, minerals, proteins and enzymes. They contain large amounts of vitamins C, B_1, B_2, B_3, pantothenic acid, folic acid, carotene and choline. They are high in minerals, like potassium, calcium, magnesium, iron, copper, phosphorus and manganese. They are full of enzymes for digestion and assimilation, some containing over 1,000 of the known enzymes necessary for human cell response and growth. Green drinks also have anti-infective properties, carry off acid wastes, neutralize body pH, and are excellent for mucous cleansing. They can help clear the skin, cleanse the kidneys, and purify and build the blood.

Green drinks and vegetable juices are potent fuel in maintaining good health, yet don't come burdened by the fats that accompany animal products. Those included here have been used with therapeutic success for many years. You can have confidence in their nutritional healing and regenerative ability.

Note: A high quality juicer is the best way to get all the nutrients from vegetable juices. A blender or food processor only gives moderate results but is better than not juicing at all. Use organically grown vegetables whenever possible.

(See my book DETOXIFICATION, ©1999, for a complete section of cleansing drinks and foods.)

PERSONAL BEST V-8

A high vitamin/mineral drink for normalizing body balance. A good daily blend even when you're not cleansing.

For 6 glasses:

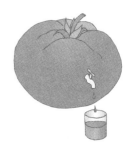

Juice 6 to 8 Tomatoes (or 4 cups Tomato Juice), 3 to 4 Green Onions with tops, 1/2 Green Pepper, 2 Carrots, 2 Stalks Celery with leaves, 1/2 Bunch Spinach, washed, 1/2 bunch Parsley, 2 Lemons, peeled, (or 4 TBS. Lemon Juice), 1 TB. snipped, dry Sea Greens (any kind).
—Add 2 teasp. Bragg's Liquid Aminos and 1/2 teasp. ground celery seed.

IMMUNE BOOSTER

For 2 drinks:

Juice 1/2 Bunch Parsley, 1 Garlic Clove, 6 Carrots, 3 Stalks Celery with leaves, 1 Large Tomato, 1 Red Bell Pepper, a dash of Hot Pepper Sauce (or Cayenne Pepper), 4 Romaine Leaves, 1 Stalk Broccoli.
—Add 1 teasp. Miso Paste mixed with a little water.

VIRGIN MARY GREEN DRINK

A virgin mary is really a healthy green drink when you make it fresh.
For 4 drinks:

Juice 3 cups water, 1/2 Green Bell Pepper, 2 Large Tomatoes, 2 Celery Stalks with leaves, 1 Green Onion with tops, and 1 handful Fresh Parsley.
—Add 1 TBS. crumbled, dry Sea Greens, (any kind), or 1 teasp. Kelp Powder.

DAILY CARROT JUICE CLEANSE

For 2 large drinks:

Juice 4 Carrots, ¹/₂ Cucumber, 2 Stalks Celery with leaves, and 1 TB. chopped Dry Dulse.

KIDNEY FLUSH

A purifying kidney cleanser and diuretic, with high potassium and other minerals.
For four 8-oz. glasses:

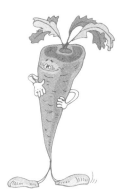

Juice 4 Carrots with tops, 1 Cucumber with skin, 4 Beets with tops, 1 handful Spinach Leaves, and 4 Celery Stalks with leaves.
—Add 2 teasp. Bragg's Liquid Aminos.

CANDIDA YEAST CLEANSER

For 2 drinks:

Juice 1 bunch Parsley, 2 Cloves Garlic, 6 Carrots, 2 Stalks Celery, and 3 Kale or Collard Leaves.
—Add 1 teasp. Miso Paste mixed with a little water.

PROSTATE SEDIMENT CLEANSER

For 2 large drinks (a day's supply):

Juice 2 large handfuls mixed dark green leaves, especially Spinach, Kale, Collards and Dandelion leaves, and 3 Large Tomatoes.

REMOVE THE COBWEBS BRAIN BOOSTER

For 1 large drink:

Juice 1 bunch Parsley, 4 Carrots, a 1-inch piece fresh or preserved Burdock or Ginseng Root, 2 Stalks Celery, and 1 teasp. snipped, dry Sea Greens for EFA's.

ARTHRITIS RELIEF DETOX

For 1 large drink:

Juice a large handful Spinach, a large handful Parsley, a large handful Watercress, 5 Carrots with tops, 3 Radishes, 1 teasp. snipped, dry Sea Greens (any kind).
—Add 1 TBS. Bragg's Liquid Aminos.

GENTLE CLEANSE FOR CROHN'S DISEASE & COLITIS
For 2 large drinks:

Juice 3 handfuls greens — 1 SPINACH, 1 PARSLEY, and 1 KALE or COLLARDS, 3 BEETS with tops, 5 CARROTS, $\frac{1}{2}$ GREEN PEPPER, and $\frac{1}{2}$ APPLE, seeded.

STRESS CLEANSE
For 1 drink:

Juice 1 small handful each PARSLEY and WATERCRESS, 2 STALKS CELERY, 1 CARROT, $\frac{1}{2}$ RED BELL PEPPER, 1 TOMATO and 1 teasp. GINGER POWDER or CRYSTALLIZED GINGER.

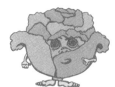

CONSTIPATION CLEANSE
For 2 large drinks (a day's supply):

Juice $\frac{1}{4}$ head GREEN CABBAGE, 3 stalks CELERY with leaves, and 5 CARROTS with tops.

PSORIASIS & ECZEMA CLEANSE
For 1 large drink:

Juice 1 TOMATO, 1 CUCUMBER, 2 STALKS CELERY, and 1 handful each: PARSLEY and WATERCRESS.

OVERWEIGHT DETOX
For 1 drink:

Juice 1 large handful dark greens like SPINACH, KALE or PARSLEY, 1 STALK CELERY with leaves, 1 CARROT, 1 BELL PEPPER, 1 TOMATO, and 1 BROCCOLI FLOWERET, 1 teasp. snipped, dry SEA GREENS (any kind).

REDUCE HIGH CHOLESTEROL
For 2 drinks:

1 large handful PARSLEY, 5 CARROTS with tops, 2 APPLES, and $\frac{1}{2}$ TUB ALFALFA SPROUTS.

MAGNESIUM MIGRAINE CLEANSE
For 2 large drink:

Juice 1 GARLIC CLOVE, 1 handful each WATERCRESS and PARSLEY, 5 CARROTS, 3 STALKS CELERY, with tops.

BLOOD CLEANSING TONIC

This is an amazingly simple, but effective Chinese medicine restorative for women after childbirth, people with anemia, or those suffering blood loss from surgery.

For 8 small drinks:

Simmer 35 Black Dates and 5 slices Fresh Ginger in 8 cups Water.
—Stir in 1 teasp. Royal Jelly (or 1 TBS. royal jelly mixed with honey) and 1 TBS. Sesame Tahini. Sip throughout the day for several weeks.

HEMORRHOIDS & VARICOSE VEINS DRINK

Vitamin C, calcium and bioflavonoids boost collagen for more elastic new tissue to form.

For 2 large drinks (a day's supply):

Juice 3 handfuls of dark greens — Kale Leaves, Parsley, Spinach, or Watercress, 2 teasp. snipped, dry Sea Greens (any kind), 5 Carrots with tops, 1 Green Bell Pepper and 2 Tomatoes.

SKIN CLEANSER

Deep greens to cleanse, nourish and tone skin tissue from inside.

For 1 drink:

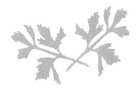

Juice 1 Cucumber with skin, $^1/_2$ bunch Fresh Parsley or 1 teasp. snipped, dry Sea Greens (any kind), one 4-oz. tub Alfalfa Sprouts, and 3 to 4 Sprigs Fresh Mint.

EXCESS BODY FLUID, WATER RETENTION CLEANSER

For 1 large drink:

Juice 1 Cucumber, 1 Beet, 1 teasp. snipped, dry Sea Greens (any kind), and 4 Carrots with tops.
—Add a 2-inch piece fresh Daikon Radish or soak a few slivers of dried Daikon and add.

HIGH BLOOD PRESSURE REDUCER

For 1 large calcium/magnesium drink:

Juice 2 Garlic Cloves, 1 handful Parsley, 1 Cucumber, 4 Carrots, and 2 Stalks Celery with leaves.

BLADDER INFECTION DETOX

For 2 drinks (a day's supply):

Juice 3 Broccoli Flowerets, 1 Garlic Clove, 2 Large Tomatoes, 2 Stalks Celery with leaves, and 1 Green Bell Pepper.

High Enzyme Therapy Drinks

Plant enzymes are the key to longterm results from detoxing with fresh juices. Plant enzymes allow our bodies to use the full array of plant nutrients, including the main components of anti-aging — antioxidants to fight free radicals and keep immunity strong.

VEGETABLE & VINEGAR STOMACH/DIGESTIVE CLEANSER
For one 8-oz. glass:

Juice $\frac{1}{2}$ Cucumber with skin, 2 TBS. Apple Cider Vinegar and $\frac{1}{4}$ teasp. Ground Ginger.
—Add enough Water to make 8-oz.

MINERAL-RICH AMINOS AND ENZYMES
Enough for 8 drinks:

Whirl ingredients in a blender, then mix about 2 TBS. of the powder into 2 cups hot water for 1 drink. Let flavors bloom for 5 minutes, then drink. Sip over a half hour period for best assimilation.
4 to 6 packets Miso Soup Powder (Edwards & Son Co. makes a good one), 1 TB. crumbled Dry Sea Greens (any type), $\frac{1}{2}$ cup Soy Protein Powder, 1 packet Instant Ginseng Tea, 2 TBS. Bee Pollen Granules, 1 teasp. Spirulina Granules, 1 TB. Brewer's Yeast Flakes, 1 teasp. Acidophilus Powder, 2 TBS. Fresh Parsley. —Add 1 teasp. Bragg's Liquid Aminos to each drink if desired.

SPRING CLEANING ENZYME SOUP
For 8 cups soup:

Simmer washed chopped greens: 2 cups Fresh Nettle Tops, 1 cup Fresh Watercress Leaves, $\frac{1}{2}$ cup Fresh Dandelion Leaves, in pot with 2 cups Water.
—Saute 1 large minced Onion in 2 TBS. Olive Oil. Add 2 Carrots diced, 2 Turnips diced, 3 TBS. Miso Paste and 6 cups Water. Simmer 30 min. Add 1 cup Sunflower Sprouts.

WEIGHT CONTROL ENZYME SOUP
A detox recipe for a weight loss liquid diet. Take 2 to 4 cups daily to eliminate congested fluids, break down blood fats and activate the intestines.

Tie herbs in a muslin bag: 2-oz. Astragalus, 2-oz. Poria, 12 to 18 pitted Red Dates, 2-oz. fresh chopped Ginger. Simmer with $\frac{1}{2}$ cup Barley for one hour in 7 cups Vegetable Stock.
—Add 3 Celery Stalks, diced with leaves, 3 Beets, sliced in matchstick, 3 Cloves Garlic, minced, 12 Shiitake Mushrooms, soaked and sliced, and simmer for another 20 minutes. Remove herb bag. Add $\frac{1}{2}$ cup Fresh Watercress Leaves or Sunflower Sprouts and serve.

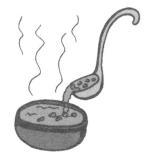

Herb Teas For Detoxification

Herbal teas are the most time-honored of all natural healing mediums. Herb teas during a cleansing diet provide energy and cleansing without having to take in solid proteins or carbohydrates for fuel. Essentially body balancers, teas have mild cleansing and flushing properties easily absorbed by your body. The important volatile oils in herbs are released by the hot brewing water. Taken in small sips throughout the cleansing process, they flood the tissues with concentrated nutritional support to accelerate regeneration, and release toxic waste. In general, herbs are more effective when taken together in combination than when used singly.

How to take herbal teas for best results in your detox program:

1) Use a glass, ceramic or earthenware pot. Stainless steel is acceptable, but aluminum negates the herbal effects, and the metal may wash into the tea and into your body.

2) Pack a small tea ball with loose herbs.

3) Bring 3 cups of cold water to a boil. Remove from heat. Add herbs, and steep covered (10 to 15 minutes for a leaf and flower tea, 20 to 25 minutes for a root and bark tea).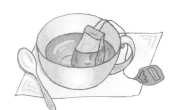

4) Keep lid tightly closed during steeping and storage. Volatile herbal oils are the most valuable part of the drink, and will escape if left uncovered.

5) Drink teas in small sips over a long period of time rather than all at once, to allow the tissues to absorb as much of the medicinal value as possible.

6) Take 2 to 3 cups of tea daily for best medicinal effects.

—**A tea combination for blood cleansing might include:** red clover, hawthorn, pau d' arco, nettles, sage, alfalfa, milk thistle seed, echinacea, horsetail, gotu kola and lemongrass.

—**A tea combination for mucous cleansing might include:** mullein, comfrey, ephedra, marshmallow, pleurisy root, rose hips, calendula, boneset, ginger, peppermint and fennel seed.

—**A tea combination for cleansing the bowel and digestive system might include:** senna leaf, papaya leaf, fennel seed, peppermint, lemon balm, parsley, calendula, hibiscus and ginger.

—**A tea combination for bladder flushing might include:** uva ursi, juniper berry, ginger and parsley.

—**A tea combination for clearing sinuses might include:** marshmallow, rose hips, mullein and fenugreek.

—**A tea combination for clearing a stress headache might include:** rosemary, spearmint or peppermint, catnip and chamomile.

—**A tea combination for removing chest and sinus congestion might include:** marshmallow root, mullein, rose hips and fenugreek seed.

—**A tea combination for warming against aches and chills might include:** wild cherry bark, licorice root, rose hips and cinnamon.

—**A tea combination for restoring bowel and colon regularity might include:** fennel seed, flax seed, fenugreek seed, licorice root, burdock root and spearmint.

—**A tea combination for loosening lung congestion might include:** ginger root, cinnamon, cloves, lemon peel and cardamom pods.

I think my favorite herb tea for a good detox is GREEN TEA, an unfermented tea rich in flavonoids with antioxidant and anti-allergen activity. Green tea has a long history in the Orient as a beneficial body cleanser. Its antioxidant polyphenols do not interfere with iron or protein absorption, and as with other plant antioxidants, like beta carotene and vitamin C, green tea polyphenols work at the molecular level, combatting free radical damage to protect against degenerative disease.

HOMEMADE GINGER ALE FOR CLEANSING & DIGESTION

This is an original nineteen-twenties home remedy tea for both children and adults. It works amazingly well to settle the stomach, and help elimination during a cold, flu or fever. I like it better than today's ginger ale. Use it as part if your liquid intake during a detox.

For 1 quart:

Bring 3 cups WATER to a boil and simmer for 5 minutes. Add 2 teasp. fresh grated GINGER ROOT, 1 teasp. dry RED RASPBERRY LEAVES, 1 teasp. dry SASSAFRAS ROOT, chopped, and 1 teasp. dry SARSAPARILLA ROOT, broken.

—Let steep for 15 minutes. Strain and add 1 cup SPARKLING WATER, like Evian or Calistoga just before serving. Add 3 fresh lemon slices if desired.

ROOTBEER REVITALIZER

Here's the old-fashioned version of a popular favorite. Decidedly delicious medicine for cleansing and digestion.

For 1 quart add 4 TBS. of the following dry blend:

Combine in a large pot: 3-oz. dry SASSAFRAS BARK, broken, 2 teasp. fresh grated GINGER ROOT, 2-oz. dry SARSAPARILLA ROOT, 1 TB. ground CINNAMON, 1-oz. dry DANDELION ROOT, 2 teasp. ORANGE PEEL, 1-oz. dry BURDOCK ROOT.

—Add 4 TBS. dry mixture. Simmer for 15 to 20 minutes.

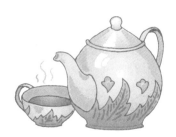

Bodywork Techniques For Detoxification

Detoxing is lifestyle therapy. Bodywork is a big part of body cleansing. This chapter includes step-by-step instructions for bodywork techniques you can do to acclerate and enhance your detox program.

Overheating therapy is an ancient cleansing technique

Overheating therapy, or hyperthermia as a healing technique, has been known throughout history. Ancient Greek physicians raised body temperature in healing centers as an immune defense against infection (I visited a center that still exists in Turkey). The Romans had elaborate bath complexes for cleansing and healing. American Indians used sweat lodges for spiritual and cleansing rituals. The Scandinavians used healing steam baths.

Ancient healers knew that a slight fever was a powerful healing tool against disease. Today, high heat procedures, like overheating baths, saunas and steam rooms are experiencing new popularity as people realize their enormous benefits for health. Modern health care professionals are finding that a non-life-threatening fever can do exceptional healing work. Slightly raising body temperature creates a natural defense and healing force by the immune system to rid the body of harmful pathogens... to literally burn out invading organisms.

Ancient herbalists used heat-producing herbs as protective healing measures against colds and simple infections, even against serious degenerative diseases like skin tumors. Today, alternative healing clinics use artificially induced fevers to treat infections like acute bronchitis, pneumonia, arthritic conditions like fibromyalgia and lupus, even cancers like leukemia. AIDS syndromes like cytomegalovirus respond to blood heating.

Despite skepticism by conventional medicine, supergerms like the HIV virus that have no effective counteractive drug therapies, mean that other methods must be tried. In 1997, CNN Health News reported on a blood heating procedure for AIDS in treating Kaposi's sarcoma, a cancer that produces severe skin lesions in HIV-infected patients. The sores vanished in about four months after the therapy, along with other symptoms. Since then, many AIDS sufferers with sarcoma have undergone hyperthermia with success. In some cases, the blood has even tested negative for the HIV virus! (Researchers warn that even if the blood tests free of HIV, the virus may still be in the bone and resurface.)

Here's how overheating therapy works as a detoxification mechanism:
When exposed to heat, blood vessels in the skin dilate to allow more blood to flow to the surface, activating sweat glands which then pour water onto the skin's surface. As the water evaporates from the skin, it draws both heat and toxins from the body, becoming a natural detoxification treatment as well as a cooling system.
Simple overheating therapy can be effectively practiced in your home, via either a dry sauna or an overheating bath. Both are able to stimulate the body's immune mechanism without the stress of fever-inducing drugs.

How to take an overheating bath:
1: Do not eat for two hours before treatment. Empty your bladder and colon if possible.
2: Get a good thermometer so that your water temperature can be correctly measured. I recommend monitoring bath temperature at all times.
3: Use a large tub if possible. Plug the emergency outlet to raise the water to the top of the tub. You must be totally immersed for therapeutic results — with only nose, eyes and mouth left uncovered. Start slowly running water at skin temperature. After 15 minutes raise temperature to 100°F, then in 15 minutes to 103°F. Even though the water temperature is not high, heat cannot escape from your body when you are totally covered, so body temperature will rise to match that of the water, creating a slight healing fever.
4: A therapy bath should be about 45 minutes. If you have any discomfort, sit up in the tub for 5 minutes.
5: Gentle massaging with a skin brush during the bath stimulates circulation, brings cleansing blood to the surface of the skin and relieves the heart from undue pressure.

A sauna is another way to use overheating therapy principles.

Today, alternative physicians and clinics use saunas as a easy, pleasant way to help people release toxins like pollutants and heavy metals. A 30 to 40 minute sauna raises body temperature enough to induce a mild, cleansing fever, and a healing, therapeutic sweat. A good sweat allows your skin to eliminate body wastes through perspiration. It dramatically increases the detoxification capacity of your skin and optimizes the skin's ability to normalize its protective mantle and pH.

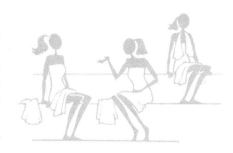

Finish each sauna with a cool shower and a brisk rubdown to remove toxins that are eliminated through the skin.

To use a sauna as a healing technique, and to enhance immune response, especially during high risk seasons, take a sauna once or twice a week. Like an overheating therapy bath, a sauna also inhibits the advance of infective organisms that cause diseases like flu and bronchitis. A sauna reaches deeper into body processes, boosting organs and gland activity and helping to regulate their functions. I personally have seen people with blood sugar disorders like hypoglycemia benefit dramatically from a bi-weekly sauna.

Cleansing benefits of a dry sauna:
—creates a fever that inhibits the replication of pathogenic bacteria and viruses.
—increases the number of leukocytes in the blood to strengthen the immune system.
—provides a prolonged, therapeutic sweat that flushes out toxins and heavy metals.
—accelerates cardiovascular activity and reduces high blood pressure.
—stimulates vasodilation of peripheral blood vessels to relieve pain and speed healing.
—promotes relaxation and a feeling of well-being.

Steam baths go back to the prehistoric hot springs of our first ancestors.

Early man, like primates today in both Japan and Russia, used hot springs to clean and warm himself, and to remove parasites. As with dry heat saunas, ancient Greeks and Romans used them to sweat for health. But the benefits of a steam bath are different than those of a sauna. Hot steam particularly helps respiratory diseases and rheumatic pain. The humid heat of a steam bath is ideal for skin tone and texture.

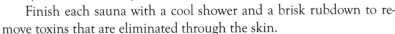

A steam bath works quicker than a sauna, too, cleansing the body in about 15 minutes compared to 30 to 40 minutes in a sauna. The powerful detoxification process of hyperthermia does not take place until the body reaches a temperature of 101-103° F. In a dry heat sauna, your body's cooling mechanism retards hyperthermia by natural evaporation. In a steam bath, evaporation is not possible so there is no loss of body heat. In fact, steam condensation actually becomes the heat transfer mechanism on the body.

Note: Overheating is one of the most effective treatments in natural healing. Inducing a "fever" is a natural, constructive means the body also uses to heal itself. Yet, heat methods are powerful and should be used with care. If you are under medical supervision for heart disease or high blood pressure, a heart vitality check-up is advisable. If you are, or have been recently ill, supervision is needed during an overheating bath, and reactions must be monitored closely. The pulse should not go over 130 or 140. Further, some people who are seriously ill lose the ability to perspire; this should be known before using overheating therapy. Check with your physician to determine if overheating therapy from a sauna or a seaweed bath is all right for you.

Water therapy helps your cleanse in almost every way

1: A detox bath is pleasant, easy and stress free.

Healing clinics and spas are famous all over the world for their therapeutic baths. They use mineral clays, aromatherapy oils, seaweeds and enzyme herbs to draw toxins out of the body through the skin, and to put restorative nutrients into the body through the skin. During a detox program, I recommend a daily therapy bath to remove toxins coming out on the skin. The procedure for taking an effective healing bath is important. In essence, you soak in an herbal tea, and your skin takes in the healing nutrients instead of the mouth and digestive system.

There are two good ways to take a therapeutic bath:
1: Draw very hot bath water. Put the herbs and seaweeds into a large teaball or muslin bath bag. Add mineral salts directly to the water. Steep until water is aromatic. Rub your body with the solids in the muslin bag during the bath.

OR

2: Make a strong tea infusion in a large teapot, strain and add to hot bath water. Soak as long as possible to give the body time to absorb the healing properties.

—Before your therapeutic bath, dry brush your body all over for 5 minutes with a natural bristle, dry skin brush to remove toxins from the skin and open pores for nutrients.
—After your bath, use a mineral salt rub, such as Crystal Star LEMON BODY GLOW™, a traditional spa "finishing" technique to make your skin feel healthy for hours.

2: Thalassotherapy uses the sea for cleansing and health.

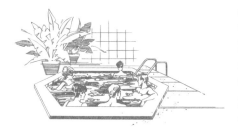

Thalassotherapy is an ageless, cleansing, health-restorative technique. Thalassa is the ancient Greek word for sea. The Greeks indeed used the sea for their well-being. I myself have seen 2500 year-old healing sites on the Greek islands of Rhodes and Corfu, and the ancient Greek healing center at Pergamum in what is now Turkey. Even judging by the therapeutic centers still known to us, much of the population of the ancient world soaked in sea water tubs and hot seaweed baths, drank and inhaled sea water for health, got sea water massages, had seaweed facials and and used sea water pools for hydrotherapy and detoxification. Today, we are learning once again, about the ability of the sea to reduce tension and de-stress us, detoxify our bodies, improve circulation, relieve allergies and congestion, and ease arthritis symptoms.

Seaweed baths are Nature's perfect body/psyche balancer. Remember how good you feel after an ocean walk? Seaweeds purify and balance the ocean — they can do the same for your body. A hot seaweed bath is like a wet-steam sauna, only better, because the sea greens balance body chemistry instead of dehydrating it. The electromagnetic action of the seaweed releases excess body fluids from congested cells, and dissolves fatty wastes through the skin, replacing them with minerals, especially potassium and iodine. Iodine boosts thyroid activity, so food fuels are used before they can turn into fatty deposits. Vitamin K in seaweeds boosts adrenal activity, meaning that a seaweed bath can help maintain hormone balance for a more youthful body.

A seaweed bath once a week stimulates lymphatic drainage and fat burning so you can keep off excess weight, reduce cellulite and rid your body of toxins.

How to take a hot seaweed bath:

If you live near the ocean, gather kelp and seaweeds from the water, (not the shoreline) in clean buckets or trash cans, and carry them home to your tub. If you don't live near the ocean, dried seaweeds are available in most health food stores. Crystal Star Herbal Nutrition (ph. 800-736-6015) packages dried seaweeds, gathered from the pristine waters around the San Juan islands, in a made-to-order HOT SEAWEED BATH™.

Whichever form you choose, run very hot water over the seaweed in a tub, filling it to the point that you will be covered when you recline. The leaves (whether dried or fresh) will turn a beautiful bright green. The water turns rich brown as the plants release their minerals. Add an aromatherapy oil if desired, to help hold the heat in and boost your cleansing program. Let the bath cool enough to get in. As you soak, the gel from the seaweed will transfer onto your skin. This coating increases perspiration to release system toxins, and replaces them with minerals by osmosis. Rub your skin with the seaweed during the bath to stimulate circulation, smooth the body, and remove wastes coming out on the skin surface. When the sea greens have done their work, the gel coating dissolves and floats off the skin, and the seaweeds shrivel — a sign that your bath is over. Each bath varies with the seaweeds used, but the gel coating release is a natural timekeeper for the bath. Forty-five minutes is usually long enough to balance body pH, encourage liver activity and fat metabolism. Skin tone, color, and circulatory improvement are almost immediately noticeable. After the bath, take a capsule of cayenne and ginger to assimilate the seaweed minerals.

Don't have time for a bath? Seaweed facials are great tonics for your skin.

The ancient Greeks said that Aphrodite, the goddess of love, rising out of the foaming sea, owed her supple skin, shiny hair and sparkling eyes to sea plants. Human body makeup is a lot like that of the ocean, so taking in things from the sea helps replace nutrients we may have lost. Seaweed contains minerals that stress and pollution deplete from our skin. The structure of seaweed cells allows our skin to easily absorb those minerals.

Most people report better skin texture after a seaweed treatment. If your skin has poor tone, a seaweed facial or mask stimulates lymphatic drainage and dilates capillaries. Seaweed also has mineral salts that help your skin hold its moisture better. When your skin retains moisture it plumps up, and smooths out fine lines. Seaweeds also have molecules similar to collagen that make the skin more supple and elastic, and add amazing luster.

Thalassotherapy seaweed wraps are premier restorative body conditioners.

Top European and American spas use seaweed wraps to rapidly cleanse the body of toxins, and to elasticize and tone the skin. As with all sea treatments, the sea herb and mineral solution easily penetrates through the millions of pores of your skin to break down and shrink unwanted fatty cells and cellulite deposits stored in the fluids between cells. Wraps are most successful when used along with a short detox program that includes 8 glasses of water a day to flush out the loosened fats and wastes.

I have seen almost miraculous benefits from thalassotherapy wraps during my work at a European spa. The results were so amazing I formulated a wrap for home use — Crystal Star (ph. 800-736-6015), ALKALIZING ENZYME™ wrap replace important minerals, enhance metabolism and balance system pH.

3: Hot and cold hydrotherapy stimulates your body's vital healing energies.

Alternating hot and cold showers increase lymph drainage, discharge toxins, improve blood flow, stimulate metabolic activity, relieve cramps, tone muscles, relax bowel and bladder tightness, and boost energy.

—Home hydrotherapy is easy and convenient. Begin with a comfortably hot shower for three minutes. Follow with a sudden change to cold water for 2 minutes. Repeat this cycle three times, ending with cold. Follow with a full or partial massage, or a brisk towel rub and mild stretching exercises for best results.

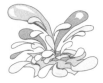

4: What are ozone pools? How do they help your body purify?

Ozone, or "activated oxygen" (O_3) is the fresh, clean scent you smell in the air after a thunderstorm. Ozone is the most powerful natural oxygenator available and one of the fastest, safest and most thorough methods of purification known. Professional spas use ozone pools in their detox treatments today to destroy water and airborne viruses, cysts, bacteria and fungi on contact.

Ozone pool baths are actually the next generation of oxygen baths that you can use in your own home detox plan. They noticeably increase energy and tissue oxygen uptake.

Take an oxygen bath once a day each day of your cleanse. Here's how:
Start with a food grade 35% hydrogen peroxide. Pour in about 1 cup per bath. Soak for about a half hour. Oxygen baths are stimulating rather than relaxing. Most people notice a significant energy increase within 3 days. Other therapeutic benefits include body balance and detoxification, reduction of skin cancers and tumors, clearing of asthma and lung congestion, and arthritis and rheumatism relief.
Note: Alternate bath - add $^1/_2$ cup food grade H_2O_2, $^1/_2$ cup sea salt, and $^1/_2$ cup baking soda to bath.

Certain herbs used in a bath supply oxygen through the skin. Rosemary is one of the best; peppermint and mullein are also effective. Pack a small muslin bath or tea bag with the herb, drop it into the tub or spa, and soak for 15 to 20 minutes. Use the bag as a skin scrub during the bath for skin smoothing and tone.

5: A baking soda alkalizing bath balances an over-acid system.

It is a simple but remarkable therapeutic treatment for detoxification. It is especially helpful if you suffer from too little sleep, high stress, too much alcohol, caffeine or nicotine, chronic colds or flu, or over-medication. Baking soda balances an over-acid system leaving you refreshed and invigorated, with extra soft skin.

Here's how to take a baking soda bath:
Fill the bath with enough pleasantly hot water to cover you when you recline. Add 8-oz. baking soda and swirl to dissolve. Soak for 20 to 30 minutes. When you emerge, wrap up in a big thick towel or a blanket and lie down for 15 minutes to help overcome any feelings of weakness or dizziness that might occur from the heat and rapid toxin release. Zia Wesley-Hosford of Z-Line Natural Cosmetics recommends this rest time for a face mask, since the hot water will have opened up the pores for maximum benefits.

6: An arthritis sweat bath releases a surprising amount of toxic material.

Inorganic sediment residues can aggravate your joints. Epsom salts or Dead Sea salts, and herbs with a diaphoretic action, can play a big part in the success of the bath.

Here's how to take the arthritis bath:
Make a tea of elder flowers, peppermint and yarrow. Drink as hot as possible before the bath. Then pour about 3 pounds of Epsom salts or enough Dead Sea salts for 1 bath into very hot bath water. Rub arthritic joints with a stiff brush in the water for 5 to 10 minutes; try to stay in the bath for 15 to 25 minutes. On emerging, do not dry yourself. Wrap up immediately in a clean sheet and go straight to bed, covering yourself with several blankets. The osmotic pressure of the Epsom salt solution absorbed by the sheet will draw off heavy perspiration. Your mattress should be protected with a sheet of plastic. The following morning the sheet will be stained with wastes excreted through your skin — sometimes the color of egg yolk. (This is a strong detox procedure and it happens relatively quickly. Take care if you have a weak heart or high blood pressure.)

Improvement after an arthritic sweat bath experience is notable. Repeat the bath once every two weeks until the sheet is no longer stained, a sign that the body is well cleansed. Drink pure water throughout the procedure to prevent dehydration and loss of body salts.

7: A sitz bath puts herbal help where you need it most.

A sitz bath is a healing technique for increasing circulation in the pelvic and urethral area. It's a good way to relieve anal and vaginal irritations, and improve the pelvic muscle tone if you suffer from incontinence (a fast growing group of people in America). The best sitz baths combine herbs with astringent, antiseptic, emollient, and hemostatic properties that assist the natural healing process. Sitz baths help women recover from hemorrhoids and vaginal infections. They help men strengthen the prostate, urinary and anal area.

How to take a sitz bath:
—For a cold sitz bath, use cool water at a temperature from 40° to 85°F. Make a strong, strained tea with your choice of herbs. A good combination includes herbs like *goldenseal root, marshmallow root, plantain, juniper berry, saw palmetto berry, slippery elm and witch hazel leaf.* Add the tea to 3" of water in a tub. Soak in the bath for 5 minutes with enough water to reach your navel, once a day for 5 minutes until healed. Use the strained herbs as a compress on the affected area.

OR

—For a hot sitz bath, start with water about 100° and increase the heat by letting hot water drip continuously into the tub until the temperature reaches about 112°. The water should cover your hips when seated. Place your feet at the faucet end of the tub so that they are soaking in slightly hotter water as the water drips in. Cover your upper body with a towel, and your forehead with a cool, wet washcloth. After 20 or 30 minutes, take a quick, cool rinse in the shower, or splash your body with cool water before drying off to further stimulate circulation. Add Epsom salts, Breh or Batherapy bath salts, ginger powder, comfrey or chamomile to the bath water for the best results.

Enemas use water flushing to cleanse your insides

Enemas are an important part of a congestion cleansing detox. They release old, encrusted colon waste, discharge parasites, freshen the G.I. tract and make the cleansing process easier and more thorough. Enemas accelerate any cleanse for better results. They are especially helpful during a healing crisis, after a serious illness to speed healing, or to remove drug residues. Migraines and skin problems like psoriasis are relieved with enemas. Adding herbs to the enema water serves to immediately alkalize the bowel area, control irritation and inflammation, and provide healing action to ulcerated or distended tissue.

Herbs for specific enemas. Use two cups strong brewed tea to 1-qt. water per enema.
—**Garlic** helps kill parasites, harmful bacteria, and cleanses mucous congestion. Blend 6 garlic cloves in 2 cups water and strain. For small children, use 1 clove garlic to 1 pint water.
—**Catnip** is effective for stomach and digestive conditions, and for childhood diseases. Use 2 cups of very strong brewed tea to 1-qt. of water.
—**Pau d'arco** normalizes body pH, especially against immune deficient diseases like chronic yeast and fungal infections. Use 2 cups of very strong brewed tea to 1-qt. of water.
—**Spirulina** helps detoxify both blood and bowels. Use 2 TBS. powder to 1-qt. water.
—**Wheat grass** boosts immune response; helps eliminate blood toxins; stimulates the liver and colon.
—**Lobelia** neutralizes food poisoning especially if vomiting prevents antidote herbs being taken by mouth.
—**Aloe vera juice enemas** heal tissues in cases of hemorrhoids, irritable bowel and diverticulitis.
—**Lemon juice enemas** rapidly neutralize an acid system, cleanse the colon and bowel.
—**Acidophilus enemas** relieve gas, yeast infections and candidiasis. Mix 4-oz. powder in 1-qt. water.
—**Coffee enemas** detoxify the liver, stimulating both liver and gallbladder to remove toxins, open bile ducts, increase peristaltic action, and produce enzyme activity for healthy red blood cell formation and oxygen uptake. Use 1 cup of regular strong brewed coffee to 1- qt. water. Also often effective for migraine headaches.

The procedure for an effective detox enema:

Place warm enema solution in an enema bag. Hang the bag about 18 inches higher than the body. Attach the colon tube, and lubricate its attachment with vaseline or vitamin E oil. Expel a little water to let out air bubbles. Lying on your left side, slowly insert the attachment about 3 inches into the rectum. Never use force. Rotate attachment gently to ease insertion. Remove kinks in the tubing so liquid will flow freely. Massage abdomen, or flex and contract stomach muscles to relieve any cramping. When all solution has entered the colon, slowly remove the tube and remain on the left side for 5 minutes. Then move to a knee-chest position with your body weight on your knees and one hand. Use the other hand to massage the lower left side of the abdomen for several minutes.

Massage loosens old fecal matter. Roll onto your back for 5 minutes, massaging up the descending colon, over the transverse colon to the right side and down the ascending colon. Then move onto your right side for 5 minutes, in order to reach each part of the colon. Get up and quickly expel into the toilet. Sticky grey-brown mucous, small dark crusty chunks or tough ribbony pieces are usually loosened and expelled during an enema. These poisonous looking things are obstacles and toxins interfering with normal body functions. An enema removes them from you. You may have to take several enemas until there is no more evidence of these substances.

Fresh wheatgrass juice enemas stimulate the liver to cleanse. Wheatgrass enema nutrients are absorbed by the hemorrhoidal vein, just inside the anal sphincter, then circulate to the liver where they increase peristaltic action of the colon, and attract waste and old fecal matter like a magnet to be eliminated from the body. Wheatgrass juice tones the colon and is absorbed into the blood, adding oxygen and energy to the body.

—Use pure water for an initial enema rinse of the colon.
—Then use about a cup of water to 4 ounces of fresh wheatgrass juice.
—Hold the juice for ten minutes while massaging colon area. Then, expel.

Herbal implants are concentrated enema solutions for more serious health problems, like colitis, arthritis or prostate inflammation. Prepare for an implant by taking a small enema to clear out the lower bowel. You'll be able to hold the implant longer.

Implant procedure: Mix 2 TBS. herbal powder like spirulina, or wheat grass in $\frac{1}{2}$ cup water. Lubricate the tip of a syringe with vaseline or vitamin E oil, get down on your hands and knees and insert the nozzle into the rectum. Squeeze the bulb to insert the mixture, but do not release pressure on the bulb before withdrawing, so the mixture stays in the lower bowel. Hold 15 minutes before expelling.

A colonic irrigation is a "super enema."

Both colonics and enemas are effective in detox programs. Benefits are matter of degree but they're dramatically different, both in terms of waste removed and body improvement. Your colon is over five feet long. If you want to cleanse all of it you need a colonic irrigation. Here's how a colonic works. A colonic irrigation uses special equipment and gravity (or oxygen for more control) to give your colon an internal bath.

To take a colonic, you lie on a special colema-board which is about three feet below the temperature-controlled water flow. A speculum is gently inserted in your rectum, and under the control of the practitioner, a steady flow of water gently flows from a small water tube. There is no discomfort, no internal pressure, just a steady gentle water flow in and then out of the colon through the evacuation tube, carrying with it impacted feces and mucous. Unlike an enema, a colonic irrigation does not involve the retention of water. As the water flows out of the colon the practitioner gently massages the abdomen to help the colon release its contents, recover its natural shape, and normalize peristaltic wave action. A view tube lets you see the colonic material being released — an edifying experience. You do nothing but lie back and relax while the entire colon is cleansed.

A colonic irrigation uses about 40 gallons of water and takes about forty-five minutes. The colonic procedure is not offensive, nor painful. The first things most people feel after a colonic irrigation is a sense of lightness, energy and an improved sense of well-being. Skin condition, digestion and immune response improve. Body odor and bad breath essentially disappear, as does belly distension.

Colonics are best done in the evening so that you can relax and retire for healing rest. For a best results take an herbal green drink before and after the colonic.

Bentonite Clay Colonic:

Bentonite clay is a mineral substance with powerful absorption qualities to pull out suspended impurities from body tissues. It helps prevent proliferation of pathogenic organisms and parasites, and sets up an environment for rebuilding healthy tissue. It is effective for lymph congestion, cellulitic fatty tissue, blood cleansing and reducing toxicity from environmental pollutants. It may be used orally, anally, or vaginally. It works like an internal poultice, drawing out toxic materials, then draining and eliminating them through evacuation. Bentonite clay packs are also effective applied topically to varicose veins and arthritic areas.

To take bentonite as an enema:
1: Mix $\frac{1}{2}$ cup clay to an enema bag of water. Use 5 to 6 bags for each enema set to replace a colonic. Follow normal enema procedure, or the directions with your enema apparatus.
2: Massage across the abdomen while expelling toxic waste into the toilet.

Exercise has significant influence on detoxification

—Exercise speeds up removal of toxins through perspiration. Sweating helps expel toxins through the skin, your body's largest organ of elimination. Exercising to the point of perspiration offers overheating therapy benefits, too. Tests show that when athletes sweat, for example, they excrete potential cancer causing elements, like heavy metals and pesticide PCBs from their bodies through perspiration.

—Exercise stimulates removal of toxins through deep breathing. Low impact aerobics help build a stronger diaphragm and elasticize your lungs.

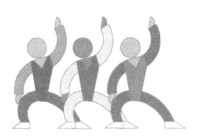

—Exercise stimulates metabolism, **especially before you eat,** to aid weight loss. Exercise uses up stored body fat. Calories are burned at a greater pace for several hours after you exercise.

—Exercise stimulates circulation, lowering blood pressure and preventing heart disease by increasing blood flow. Heart endurance tests show exercise strengthens your circulatory system right down to your capillaries.... even forming new ones!

—Exercise stimulates your lymphatic system. Blood is pumped through your body by your heart, **but lymphatic fluid depends solely on exercise for circulation.** Good lymph function is critical to your body's ability to cleanse itself.

—Exercise reduces stress by increasing body oxygen levels. It improves your mood while you purify. Endorphins, the body's "feel good" hormones, are released into the brain by vigorous exercise, explaining the "high" people often experience after exercise.

—Disease often results from an underactive body. Exercise transports oxygen and nutrients to your cells while it carries away toxins and wastes to your elimination organs.

Exercise recommendations for your cleanse:
1: During initial, heavy cleansing – simple, body-balancing, stretching exercises.
2: During the rest of your cleanse – low-impact, aerobic exercise, like a walk or an easy swim.
3: For your maintenance program, strengthening exercise, like daily walking for better circulation and lymph activity. An exercise program that raises your heart rate for 20 to 30 minutes offers the most benefits.

Your skin is a key organ for detoxification

Herbal compresses draw out waste and waste residues, such as cysts or abscesses, through the skin and release them into the body's elimination channels. Use alternating hot and cold compresses for best results. Apply the herbs to the hot compress, and leave the ice or cold compress plain. I regularly use cayenne, ginger and lobelia effectively for the hot compresses.

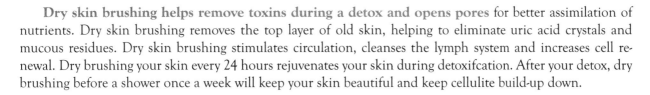

Effective herbal compresses I use:
1: Add 1 teasp. powdered herbs to a bowl of very hot water. Soak a washcloth and apply until the cloth cools. Then apply a cloth dipped in ice water until it reaches body temperature. Repeat several times daily.
2: Green clay compresses are effective toxin-drawing agents for growths. Apply to gauze, place on the area, cover and leave all day. Change as you would any dressing when you bathe.

Dry skin brushing helps remove toxins during a detox and opens pores for better assimilation of nutrients. Dry skin brushing removes the top layer of old skin, helping to eliminate uric acid crystals and mucous residues. Dry skin brushing stimulates circulation, cleanses the lymph system and increases cell renewal. Dry brushing your skin every 24 hours rejuvenates your skin during detoxifcation. After your detox, dry brushing before a shower once a week will keep your skin beautiful and keep cellulite build-up down.

Your technique for skin brushing can make all the difference to its success:
—Use a natural bristle brush, not synthetic — it scratches skin surface.
—Do not wet your skin. It stretches the skin and will not have the same effect.
—Especially brush the bottoms of your feet, nerve endings here affect the whole body.
—Do circular, counter-clockwise strokes on the abdomen; lighter strokes over and around the breasts.
—Dry brush before you bathe in the mornings (before bed, it can cause too much stimulation).
—Brush the whole body, for best results. Wash your brush every few weeks in water and let it dry.

Ear Coning for Ear Cleansing

Ear coning or candling is a comfortable way to clean out excess wax and other accumulations. It's an ancient healing process used by virtually every healing tradition. Chinese Traditional Medicine, Native American and Mayan societies, even the ancient Egyptians all used ear candling to gently remove ear wax, fungus, and yeast from ear canals. Ear coning was even considered a spiritual practice that also cleared the mind and senses.

Ear candles are strips of cotton muslin dipped into a mixture of wax and herbs with natural antibiotic, decongestant activity like *sage, cedar, spearmint, echinacea, goldenseal and rosemary*, then formed into a tapered cone. In the coning process, the narrow end of the candle is gently placed at the ear canal, while the opposite end is lit. The spiral design of the cone creates a vacuum which draws the soothing smoke into the ear canal. The smoke goes through the Eustachian tube into the lymphatic system, then by osmosis, it draws accumulations out into the cone. The process is soothing, and takes only about 45 minutes.

The benefits of ear coning:
—stimulates and detoxifies the lymph system.
—helps remove excessive wax and allows better hearing, usually immediately.
—clears "swimmers ear," where ear wax stops water clearing from the ear, allowing bacteria to fester.
—relieves pain and pressure from mucous blown into the ear from the Eustachian tube.
—helps clear itching mold caused by candida yeast allergy.
—helps remove parasites growing in the ear.

Give your body a detoxifying ascorbic acid flush

Vitamin C (ascorbic acid) accelerates detoxification, changing body chemistry to neutralize allergens, fight infections, promote more rapid healing and protect against illness.

Here's how:
1: Use a non-acidic vitamin C or Ester C powder with bioflavonoids for best results.
2: Take $\frac{1}{2}$ teasp. every 20 minutes until a soupy stool results. (Use $\frac{1}{4}$ teasp. every hour for a very young child; $\frac{1}{2}$ teasp. every hour for a child six to ten years old.)
3: Then, slightly reduce amount taken so that the bowel produces a mealy, loose stool, but not diarrhea. The body will still continue to cleanse. You will be taking about 8-10,000mg of vitamin C daily depending on body weight and make-up. Continue for one to two days for a thorough flush.

An herbal "vag pac" can detox the vaginal area

A cleansing herbal combination may be used as a vaginal pack by placing it against the cervix, or as a bolus inserted in the vagina. The pack acts as an internal poultice to draw out toxic wastes from the vagina, rectum or urethral areas. A "vag pac" is effective for cysts, benign tumors, polyps and uterine growths, and cervical dysplasia. It takes 6 weeks to 6 months for complete healing, depending on the problem and severity.

How to make a pack:
—Formula #1: Mix 1 part each with cocoa butter to form a finger-sized suppository: *squaw vine, marshmallow root, slippery elm, goldenseal root, pau d'arco, comfrey root, mullein, yellow dock root, chickweed, acidophilus powder.*

—Formula #2: Mix 1 part each with cocoa butter to form a finger-sized suppository: *cranesbill powder, goldenseal root, red raspberry leaf, white oak bark, echinacea root, myrrh gum powder.*

Place suppositories on waxed paper in the refrigerator to chill and harden slightly. Smear a suppository on cotton tampon and insert, or insert as is, and use a sanitary napkin to catch drainage. Use suppositories at night; rinse out in the morning with *white oak bark tea, or yellow dock root tea* to rebalance vaginal pH. Repeat for 6 days. Rest for one week. Resume and repeat of necessary.

Chelation therapy cleans out your arteries

Chelation therapy was developed in Germany in the early 1930's and introduced into the United States in 1948 as a method of preventing or reversing heart and artery pathology (hardening of the arteries) from diminished blood circulation. Today chelation is used by medical authorities around the world as a cleansing treatment for heavy metal and radiation toxicity, digitalis intoxication, lead and snake venom poisoning and heart arrhythmias. A chelating, synthetic amino acid, protein called EDTA, (ethylene-diamine-tetracetic acid) has the unique property of binding with divalent metals that are clogging arteries. When EDTA is injected, it flushes the cells of ionic minerals, especially calcium, and travels with them out of the body through the kidneys.

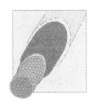

Oral chelation refers to specific foods and nutritional supplements that help cleanse the blood vessels of accumulated detritus (waste) and improve blood flow. While experience among chelating physicians indicates that oral chelates take about eight times longer to show health benefits than do IV chelates, oral chelation is successful in improving circulation, reversing heart disease, stroke and sexual impotency due to poor circulation. I use oral chelation as a protective against atherosclerosis and many degenerative diseases.

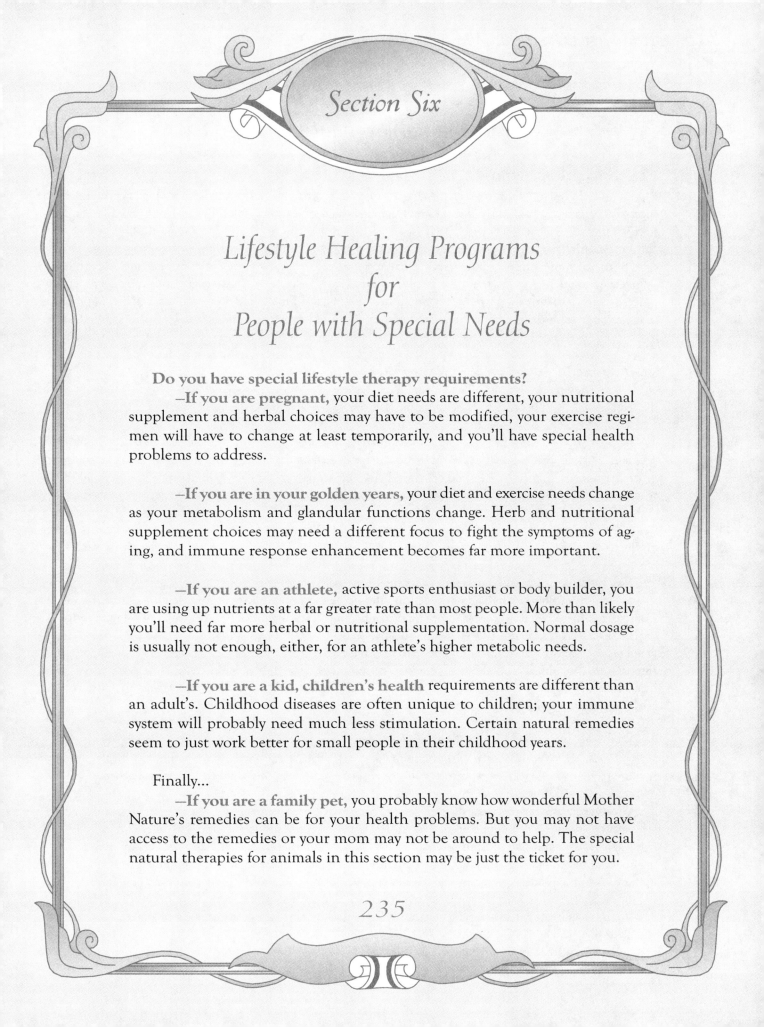

Lifestyle Healing Programs
for
People with Special Needs

Do you have special lifestyle therapy requirements?

—**If you are pregnant,** your diet needs are different, your nutritional supplement and herbal choices may have to be modified, your exercise regimen will have to change at least temporarily, and you'll have special health problems to address.

—**If you are in your golden years,** your diet and exercise needs change as your metabolism and glandular functions change. Herb and nutritional supplement choices may need a different focus to fight the symptoms of aging, and immune response enhancement becomes far more important.

—**If you are an athlete,** active sports enthusiast or body builder, you are using up nutrients at a far greater rate than most people. More than likely you'll need far more herbal or nutritional supplementation. Normal dosage is usually not enough, either, for an athlete's higher metabolic needs.

—**If you are a kid, children's health** requirements are different than an adult's. Childhood diseases are often unique to children; your immune system will probably need much less stimulation. Certain natural remedies seem to just work better for small people in their childhood years.

Finally...

—**If you are a family pet,** you probably know how wonderful Mother Nature's remedies can be for your health problems. But you may not have access to the remedies or your mom may not be around to help. The special natural therapies for animals in this section may be just the ticket for you.

Having A Healthy Baby
Optimal Pregnancy Choices

Pre-conception Planning:

In America today, one in six married couples of child-bearing age has trouble conceiving and completing a successful pregnancy. Poor nutrition and stress seem to be at the base of most fertility problems. For men, conception is affected by a zinc deficiency, a fast food diet, chronic infections and too much alcohol. For women, conception inhibitors are anxiety, emotional stress, severe anemia and hormone imbalance. New research implicates hormone mimics from pollutants, chemical residues in food, water and plastics to infertility in both sexes.

Note: If you're worried by the studies linking herbs like *St. John's wort, ginkgo biloba* and *echinacea* to fertility problems, know that the herbs were only tested in vitro (in a test tube) on hamster eggs. It is highly improbable that the same herbs used in a living animal or human would have the same effect. Herbs, as gentle healing foods, are processed by our enzymatic systems.... neutralizing, in the majority of cases, potential for toxicity.

Diet is a critical key to successful conception:

Nature tries in every way possible to insure the survival of a new life. I've seen over and over again that a good diet and lifestyle is imperative for at least six months before trying to conceive for both partners.

—Up to 40% of the time, the man is the infertile one in conception problems. A **"virility nutrition"** program for a man includes a short cleansing diet, then zinc-rich foods, healthy omega-3 fats, some meat and other protein rich foods, minimal sweets and dairy foods, and plenty of whole grains. Add natural vitamin E, 400IU to your diet. New studies show vitamin E significantly improves sperm motility and fertility in men. Tests show the amino acid L-carnitine, 500mg daily, boosts sperm quality in subfertile men. Unless you're grossly overweight, a weight loss diet may not be a good idea during preconception. Fasting or severe food limitation has a direct impact on the testicles. A man's fertility rise may take place in as little as 2 months after his diet improvements.

—A "fertility nutrition" program for a woman includes plenty of salads and greens, very low sugars, and a smaller volume of whole grains and nuts. Her diet should be low in saturated fats, but rich in essential fatty acids from sea greens and omega-3 oils. I recommend avoiding meats during pre-conception, except fish and seafoods, (unless certified organic, much of America's meat and poultry is antibiotic and hormone laced). Drink a cup of green tea every morning. A new study shows that women who drink a cup of green tea daily get pregnant faster! Important: Normalize your body weight before conception! Overweight women increase their risk of developing toxemia or high blood pressure during pregnancy. Severely underweight women may risk premature births or low birth weight babies. A woman's fertility rise may take 6 to 18 months after her diet change.

Both men and women should limit their saturated fat intake to about 10% of the diet. Especially reduce sugary foods (artificial sweeteners like aspartame are particularly hazardous for your unborn child) and meats that are regularly laced with nitrates and-or hormones, like red meats, and smoked, cured and processed meats.

Lifestyle habits are important.

Avoid or reduce consumption of tobacco, caffeine, and alcohol. (Moderate wine is ok until conception.) Get light exercise, and morning sunshine every day possible. Take alternating hot and cold showers or apply alternating hot and cold compresses to the abdomen or scrotum to increase circulation to the reproductive areas. Massage therapy sessions, and deep breathing exercises, especially during long walks together, are very beneficial.

Vitamins, minerals and herbs can help, too. There is a link between infertility and lack of vitamin C in both sexes. See my small book "Do You Want To Have A Baby?" for complete information and recommendations for both men and women trying to conceive a child.

Can't find a recommended product? Call the 800 number in Product Resources for the store nearest you.

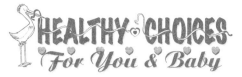

Optimal Eating For Two During Pregnancy

A woman's body changes so dramatically during pregnancy and childbearing that her normal daily needs change. The body takes care of some of its needs through cravings. During this one time of life, the body is so sensitive to its needs, that the cravings you get are usually good for you. We know that every single thing the mother does or takes in affects the child. Good nutrition for a child begins before it is born, even before it is conceived. New research shows that when a child reaches adulthood, his or her risk for heart disease, cancer, and diabetes can be traced to poor eating habits of the parents as well as genetic proneness. The nutritious diet suggestions in this section will help build a healthy baby, minimize the mother's discomfort, lessen birth complications and reduce excess fatty weight gain that can't be lost after birth.

A highly nutritious diet helps prevent miscarriage and high blood pressure, and supports your body against toxemia, fluid retention, constipation, hemorrhoids and varicose veins, anemia, gas and heartburn, morning sickness and hormone adjustment. After pregnancy, a good diet is important for sufficient breast milk, reducing post-partum swelling, and for healing tissues and stretch marks.

Promise yourself and your baby that at least during the months of pregnancy and nursing, your diet and lifestyle will be as healthy as you can make it. A largely vegetarian diet of whole foods provides optimum nutrition. The staples of a lacto-vegetarian, seafood and poultry diet are nutritional powerhouses. Base your pregnancy diet on whole grains, leafy greens, fish (avoid shark and swordfish, notorious for high mercury levels that can be dangerous to a developing fetus), turkey, eggs, legumes, nuts, seeds, green and yellow vegetables, nutritional yeast, bananas and citrus fruits for confidence that the baby is getting the best possible nutrition.

Your Diet Keys: **Eat small frequent meals instead of large meals.**

1: **Protein is important.** Most experts recommend 60 to 80 grams of protein daily during pregnancy, with a 10 gram increase every trimester. Focus on vegetable protein diet - whole grains, seeds and sprouts, with fish, seafood or turkey at least twice a week. Take a protein drink several times a week for optimal growth and energy.

The following drink is a proven example: *Mix $\frac{1}{2}$ cup raw milk, $\frac{1}{2}$ cup yogurt, juice of one orange, 2 TBS brewer's yeast, 2 TBS wheat germ, 2 teasp. molasses, 1 teasp. vanilla, and a pinch cinnamon.* Even though protein requirements increase during pregnancy, it's the quality of the protein, not the quantity that prevents and cures toxemia.

2: **Have a fresh fruit or green salad every day.** Eat plenty of soluble fiber foods like whole grain cereals and vegetables for regularity. Eat complex carbohydrate foods like broccoli and brown rice for strength.

3: **Drink plenty of healthy fluids** - pure water, mineral water, and juices throughout the day to keep your system free and flowing. Carrot juice at least twice a week is ideal. Include pineapple and apple juice.

4: **Eat folacin rich foods**, like fresh spinach and asparagus for healthy cell growth.

5: **Increase your essential fatty acids (EFA's)** from fish, spinach and arugula, and especially from sea greens (2 TBS per day of snipped dry sea greens do the trick.) for your baby's healthy brain and skin.

6: **Eat carotene-rich foods**, such as carrots, squashes, tomatoes, yams, and broccoli for disease resistance.

7: **Eat zinc-rich foods**, like pumpkin and sesame seeds for good body formation.

8: **Eat vitamin C foods**, like broccoli, bell peppers and fruits for connective tissue.

9: **Eat bioflavonoid-rich foods**, such as citrus fruits and berries for capillary integrity.

10: **Eat alkalizing foods**, such as miso soup and brown rice to combat and neutralize toxemia.

11: **Eat mineral-rich foods**, such as sea veggies, leafy greens, and whole grains for baby building blocks. Especially include silicon-rich foods for bone, cartilage and connective tissue growth, and for collagen and elastin formation; brown rice, oats, green grasses and green drinks.

Note: See my book COOKING FOR HEALTHY HEALING *for a complete, detailed pregnancy diet.*

Can't find a recommended product? Call the 800 number in Product Resources for the store nearest you.

237

There are important diet watchwords you should know during pregnancy and nursing:

—**Don't restrict your diet to lose weight.** Low calories often mean low birth weight for the baby.

—**Eat a wide range of healthy foods to assure the baby access to all nutrients.** Avoid cabbages, onions, and garlic. They sometimes upset body balance during pregnancy. Broccoli, cauliflower, cabbage, onion, milk and chocolate have all been found to aggravate colic in nursing babies. Avoid red meats.

—**Don't fast** - even for short periods where fasting would normally be advisable, such as constipation, or to overcome a cold. Food energy and nutrient content may be diminished.

—**Avoid chemicalized, smoked, preserved, colored foods.** Refrain from alcohol, caffeine and tobacco.

—**Avoid X-rays, chemical solvents, CFCs** such as hair sprays, and cat litter. Your system may be able to handle these things without undue damage; the baby's can't. Even during nursing, toxic amounts occur easily.

—**Avoid smoking and secondary smoke.** Your baby, like you, metabolizes the harmful cancer-causing residues of tobacco. The chance of low birth weight, SIDS and miscarriage is much more likely if you smoke. Smoker's infants have a mortality rate 30% higher than non-smoker's. Nursing babies take in small amounts of nicotine with breast milk, and become prone to chronic respiratory infections.

—**Avoid alcohol** to reduce risk of Fetal Alcohol Syndrome, disabilities, mental retardation and motor-skill problems.

More diet watchwords:

—During labor: Take no solid food. Drink fresh water, or carrot juice; or suck on ice chips.

—During lactation: Add almond milk, brewer's yeast, green drinks and green foods, avocados, carrot juice, goats milk, soy milk and soy foods, and unsulphured molasses, to promote milk quality and richness. *Fennel seed* tea has long been used to promote breast milk in lactating women. *Vitex* (chaste berry) extract also improves poor milk quality. Wayne State University studies show that exposure to pollutant PCBs from breast milk can lower a child's IQ score by as much as 6 points. Focus on organic foods to minimize exposure.

—During weaning: Drink papaya juice to slow down milk flow.

About Breast Feeding

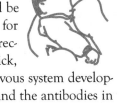

Mother's milk is best. Unless there is a major health problem, your breast milk should be the only food for your baby during the first six months of life. Despite all the claims made for fortified formulas, nothing can take the place of breast milk. Pediatricians now routinely recommend breast feeding your baby for up to a year for the most health benefits. The first thick, waxy colostrum is extremely high in protein, essential fatty acids needed for brain and nervous system development, and protective antibodies. A child's immune system is not fully established at birth, and the antibodies in breast milk are critical. They fight early infections and create solid immune defenses that prevent the development of allergies. The baby who is not breast fed loses Nature's "jump start" on immune response and may face health disadvantages that can last a lifetime.

Breast-fed babies have a lower bouts of colic and other digestion problems than bottle-fed babies. Breast milk is loaded with *bifidobacteria*, the beneficial micro-organisms that make up 99% of a healthy baby's intestinal flora — extremely important for protection against salmonella food poisoning and other intestinal pathogens.

Mother's milk is the best for boosting and balancing your baby's fats. Breast milk contains the full range of EFA's needed for proper development of a child's central nervous system, brain and eyes. A study published in the journal of Pediatrics shows that breast-feeding your baby may even make him or her smarter throughout life, giving your child an academic advantage! The determining factor seems to be the high content of DHA (*docosahexaenoic acid*) in breast milk, an essential fatty acid which comprises over 50% of the brain. DHA, particularly vital in infant development, increases 3 to 5 times in the last trimester of pregnancy and triples again in the first 12 weeks of life.

If there is simply no way to breast feed your baby, goat's milk is a better alternative than either chemically made formulas or cow's milk, both of which result in children with higher risk of allergy development.

Can't find a recommended product? Call the 800 number in Product Resources for the store nearest you.

Supplements Help Nutritional Deficiencies During Pregnancy

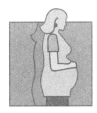

Illness, body imbalance, even regular supplements need to be handled differently than your usual healing approach during pregnancy, even if your method is holistically oriented. A mother's body is very delicately tuned and sensitive at this time; imbalances occur easily. Mega-doses of anything are not good for the baby's system. Dosage of all medication or supplements should almost universally be less (usually about half of normal), to allow for the infant's tiny system capacity. Ideal supplements should be food-source complexes for best absorbability.

Avoid all drugs during pregnancy and nursing — including alcohol, tobacco, caffeine, MSG, saccharin, X-rays, aspirin, Valium, Librium, Tetracycline and harsh diuretics. Even the amino acid L-Phenylalanine can adversely affect the nervous system of the unborn child.

Especially stay away from recreational drugs — cocaine, PCP, marijuana, meth-amphetamines, Quaaludes, heroin, LSD and other psychedelics.

Supplements that can help you during pregnancy:

—**A superfood green drink.** A green drink is a good nutrition "delivery system" during pregnancy because it is so quickly absorbed with so little work by the body. Crystal Star's ENERGY GREEN™ drink mix or capsules contains land and sea greens, grasses and herbs full of absorbable, potent chlorophyllins, complex carbohydrates, minerals, proteins, and amino acids. Other good ones: Body Ecology VITALITY SUPER GREEN, Morada Research Laboratories GOD'S GARDEN, Vibrant Health GREEN VIBRANCE.

—**A good prenatal multi-vitamin and mineral supplement**, especially starting six to eight weeks before the expected birth. Clinical testing shows that mothers who take nutritional supplements during pregnancy are far less likely to have babies with neural tube and other defects. Be sure your daily prenatal formula contains 350 to 500mg of magnesium. Body demands for magnesium increase during pregnancy. Pre-eclampsia (marked by elevated blood pressure, fluid retention and protein loss through the urine), premature labor and poor fetal growth are all tied to magnesium deficiency during pregnancy. New Chapter PERFECT PRENATAL.

—**A food source multi-mineral supplement** (not just calcium or iron) that can be absorbed well by both you and the baby. Nature's Path TRACE-MIN-LYTE or Crystal Star MINERAL SPECTRUM™ capsules offer good body building blocks. Studies show that beta-carotene 10,000mg, with vitamin C 500mg, niacin 50mg, and available plant iron are better for skeletal, cellular and connecting tissue development than calcium supplements.

—**Take extra folic acid**, 800mcg daily to prevent neural tube defects. Timing is essential. Supplementing folic acid *after* the first three months of fetal development cannot correct spinal cord damage.

—**Take vitamin B$_6$ 50mg** for bloating, leg cramps and nerve strength, as well as to prevent proneness to glucose intolerance and seizures in the baby.

—**Take bioflavonoids daily**. Tests show that over 50% of women who habitually miscarry have low levels of vitamin C and bioflavonoids. Part of the natural vitamin C complex, bioflavonoids also often occur naturally with vitamin A and rutin, so they're best known for enhancing vein and capillary strength, and for helping to control bruising and internal bleeding from hemorrhoids and varicose veins.

Support goes to even deeper body levels. Bioflavonoids are a "tissue tonic" because they support and maintain tissue integrity. Bioflavonoids tighten and tone activity for skin elasticity. They minimize skin aging and wrinkling due to pregnancy stretching. A good natural bioflavonoid compound will also be fiber-rich for regularity — a definite advantage during prenatal care! Take bioflavonoids 1000mg with vitamin C daily, or bioflavs from herbs, like Crystal Star BIOFLAVONOID, FIBER & C SUPPORT™ drink. Research shows bioflavonoids help control excess fatty deposits, too. Herbs and citrus fruits are some of the best sources for bioflavonoids. **BILBERRY EXTRACT** is one of the single richest sources of herbal flavonoids in the botanical world. It is especially helpful for pregnant women suffering from distended veins, hemorrhoids, weak uterine walls and toxemia. It is gentle for both mother and child at a time when strong supplements are inadvisable.

Can't find a recommended product? Call the 800 number in Product Resources for the store nearest you.

239

—**Take kelp tablets,** about 6 daily, or Crystal Star IODINE/POTASSIUM SOURCE™ capsules, for natural potassium and iodine. A lack of these minerals means mental retardation and poor physical development.

—**Take natural vitamin E,** 200-400IU, or wheat germ oil capsules, to help prevent miscarriage and reduce the baby's oxygen requirement, lessening the chances of asphyxiation during labor.

—**Take EFAs,** (omega-3 rich flax oil, borage seed or evening primrose oils), for baby's brain development.

—**Take calcium lactate** with calcium ascorbate vitamin C for collagen development.

—**Take zinc,** 10-15mg daily, (or get it from your pre-natal multi-mineral). Zinc deficiencies often result in poor brain formation, learning problems, low immunity, sub-normal growth and allergies in the baby.

Important Supplement Watchwords:

During the last trimester: Rub vitamin E or wheat germ oil on your stomach and around vaginal opening each night to make stretching easier and skin more elastic. Begin to take extra minerals as labor approaches.

During labor: Take natural vitamin E and calcium-magnesium to relieve pain and aid dilation.

During nursing: Nutritional supplements that you used during pregnancy, like iron, calcium, B vitamins or a prenatal multiple, should be continued during nursing. They may be slightly increased if you have not recovered normal strength. Breast milk is a filtered food supply that prevents the baby from overdosing on higher potencies. Apply vitamin E oil to alleviate breast crusting. Apply a *marshmallow* fomentation to relieve pressure in engorged breasts.

Herbs For A Healthy Pregnancy

Herbs have been used during pregnancy for centuries to ease the hormone imbalances and discomforts of stretching, bloating, nausea and pain without impairing the development or health of the baby. Herbs are concentrated mineral-rich foods that are perfect for the extra growth requirements of pregnancy and childbirth. They are easily-absorbed and non-constipating. Ideal supplementation that affects a developing child's body should be from food source complexes. Herbs are identified and accepted by the body's enzyme activity as whole food nutrients, lessening the risk of toxemia or overdose, yet providing gentle, easy nutrition for both mother and baby. Herbs are good and easy for you; good and gentle for the baby.

Important Note: Early pregnancy and later pregnancy must be considered separately with herbal medicinals. If there is any question, always use the gentlest herbs and consult with your health care professional.

HERBS YOU CAN TAKE DURING PREGNANCY:

—Many women prefer teas as a way to take in balancing nutrients during pregnancy. They are the gentlest way to overcome effects of morning sickness and hormone adjustment. Take two daily cups of red raspberry tea, high in iron, calcium and other minerals. Blends like Crystal Star MOTHERING TEA™ (a red raspberry blend), or Mother Love TEA FOR TWO also strengthen the uterus and birth canal, guard against birth defects, long labor and afterbirth pain, and have uterine toning properties for a quicker return to normal.

—Iodine-rich foods are a primary deterrent to spinal birth defects. Take kelp tablets, or Crystal Star IODINE/POTASSIUM SOURCE™ capsules or SYSTEMS STRENGTH™ drink mix, or a sea greens sprinkle, or Nature's Path TRACE-MIN-LYTE.

—Many pregnant women need extra calcium and iron. Herbal sources can be the best way to get these minerals because they absorb through the body's own enzyme system, and are rich in other nutrients that encourage the best uptake and use by the body. Herbal minerals provide the best bonding agent between your body and the nutrients it is taking in.

Can't find a recommended product? Call the 800 number in Product Resources for the store nearest you.

—Take a mineral-rich pre-natal herbal compound during the 1st and 2nd trimester, for gentle, absorbable minerals and toners to elasticize tissue and ease delivery. A broad spectrum herbal capsule compound, rich in extra minerals might include herbs like red raspberry, nettles, oatstraw, alfalfa, yellow dock root, fennel, rosemary and vegetable acidophilus. During the last trimester, I recommend a broad range herbal mineral compound, such as Crystal Star MINERAL SPECTRUM™ capsules, with highly absorbable, gentle plant minerals.

—Certain herbs are excellent sources of absorbable calcium and iron, minerals that are easily depleted during pregnancy. Take Crystal Star CALCIUM SOURCE™, a calcium-rich compound of herbs with magnesium for optimum uptake, and naturally-occurring silica to help form healthy tissue and bone; and SILICA SOURCE™, an organic silica from oatstraw and horsetail herb — a prime factor in collagen formation for connective and interstitial tissue, or Morada Research Labs BONES/CALCIUM. Crystal Star IRON SOURCE™ is an absorbable, non-constipating herbal iron source with measurable amounts of calcium and magnesium, along with naturally-occurring vitamins C and E for optimum iron uptake.

—Five weeks before the expected birth date, an herbal formula to help your body prepare for parturition, aid in hemorrhage control and uterine muscle strength for correct presentation of the fetus might contain herbs like *red raspberry, pennyroyal, false unicorn, black cohosh, cramp bark squaw vine, blessed thistle, lobelia leaf,* and *bilberry.*

HERBS YOU CAN TAKE DURING LABOR:
—Medicine Wheel LABOR-EASE drops, or Crystal Star CRAMP BARK COMBO™ extract ease contraction pain. Put 15 to 20 drops in water and take small sips as needed during labor. Take Crystal Star BACK TO RELIEF™ capsules for afterbirth pain, an analgesic formula for the lower back and spinal block area.

—For false labor, drink 4 to 6 cups *catnip-blue cohosh* tea to renormalize. If there is bleeding, take 2 capsules each, *cayenne* and *bayberry*, and get to a hospital or call your midwife.

HERBS YOU CAN TAKE DURING NURSING:
—Add 2 TBS. brewer's yeast to your diet, along with *red raspberry, marshmallow root,* or Crystal Star MOTHERING TEA™ to promote and enrich milk.
—Take *Vitex* extract or Mother Love MORE MILK to promote an abundant supply of mother's milk.
—*Fennel seed, alfalfa, red raspberry, cumin, or fenugreek* teas help keep the baby colic free.
—For infant jaundice, use Hyland's *BILIOUSNESS* tabs.

HERBS YOU CAN TAKE FOR WEANING:
—Take *parsley-sage* tea to help dry up milk.
— Amazake rice drink can help wean from breast milk.

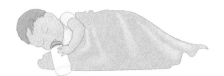

Safe herbs you can use during pregnancy:
I recommend herbs in the mildest way, as relaxing teas, during pregnancy.
• **Red raspberry:** the quintessential herb for pregnancy. An all around uterine tonic. It is anti-abortive to prevent miscarriage, antiseptic to help prevent infection, astringent to tighten tissue, rich in calcium, magnesium and iron to help prevent cramps and anemia. It is hemostatic to prevent excess bleeding during and after labor, and facilitates the birth process by stimulating contractions. Assists with plentiful milk production, too.
• **Nettles:** a mineral-rich herb, with vitamin K to guard against excessive bleeding. Improves kidney function and helps prevent hemorrhoids. Diminishes leg cramps and childbirth pain, too.
• **Peppermint:** use after the first trimester to help digestion, soothe the stomach and overcome nausea. Contains highly absorbable amounts of vitamin A, C, silica, potassium and iron.
• **Ginger root:** excellent for morning sickness; has lots of needed minerals.

Can't find a recommended product? Call the 800 number in Product Resources for the store nearest you.

241

- **Bilberry:** strong, gentle astringent, rich in bioflavonoids to fortify veins and capillaries. A hematonic for kidney function and a mild diuretic for bloating.
  - **Burdock root:** a mineral-rich, hormone balancer. Helps prevent water retention and baby jaundice.
  - **Yellow dock root:** improves iron assimilation; helps prevent infant jaundice.
  - **Dong quai root:** a blood nourisher, rather than a hormone stimulant. Use in moderation.
  - **Echinacea:** an immune system stimulant to help prevent colds, flu and infections.
  - **Chamomile:** relaxes for quality sleep, and helps digestive and bowel problems.
  - **Vitex:** normalizes hormone balance for fertility. Discontinue when pregnancy is realized.
  - **False unicorn, black and blue cohosh:** for final weeks of pregnancy only, to ease and-or induce labor.
  - **Wild yam:** for general pregnancy pain, nausea or cramping; lessens chance of miscarriage.
  - **Alfalfa:** highly nutritive, rich in enzymes, full of vitamin K to reduce postpartum hemorrhage.
  - **Dandelion:** a gentle diuretic that reduces pregnancy-related water retention.
  - Aromatherapy essential oils of lavender and chamomile alleviate nausea.
  - Aromatherapy essential oils of fennel seed and anise reduce heartburn.

HERBS TO AVOID DURING PREGNANCY: Medicinal herbs should always be used with common sense and care, especially during pregnancy. Some herbs are not appropriate.
Contra-indicated, cautionary herbs:
  - **Aloe vera:** can be too laxative. Dilute aloe vera juice with 4 parts water if you decide to use it.
  - **Angelica and rue:** stimulate oxytocin that causes uterine contractions.
  - **Barberry, buckthorn, rhubarb root, mandrake, senna and cascara sagrada:** too strong as laxatives.
  - **Black cohosh:** may stimulate uterine contractions. Blue cohosh also affects uterine sloughing. (Some health professionals use it to induce labor.)
  - **Buchu and juniper:** too strong diuretics.
  - **Coffee:** too strong a caffeine and heated hydrocarbon source - irritates the uterus. In extremely sensitive individuals who take in excessive amounts, may cause miscarriage or premature birth.
  - **Comfrey:** pyrrolizides (carcinogenic) cannot be commercially controlled for an absolutely safe source.
  - **Ephedra, Ma Huang:** too strong an anti-histamine if used in extract or capsule form. It is gentle enough as a tea to relieve bronchial and chest congestion.
  - **Horseradish:** too strong for a baby.
  - **Goldenseal, lovage, mugwort and wormwood:** emmenagogues that cause uterine contractions.
  - **Male fern:** too strong a vermifuge.
  - **Mistletoe, tansy and wild ginger:** emmenagogues that cause uterine contractions.
  - **Pennyroyal:** stimulates oxytocin that can cause abortion. May be used in the final weeks of pregnancy.
  - **Yarrow and shepherd's purse:** strong astringents and mild abortifacients.

PREVENTING SIDS, Sudden Infant Death Syndrome:

If your baby has a weak system, or poor lung tissue development (signs that he or she is a candidate for SIDS) give a weak ascorbate vitamin C, or Ester C with bioflavonoids solution in water daily. Routinely feeding babies iron-fortified weaning foods to prevent anemia may increase the risk of SIDS, according to the British Medical Journal. Evidence indicates that infant pillows filled with foam polystyrene beads cause babies to inhale toxic gases and suffocate. Just putting your child to sleep on his back cuts SIDS risk in half because it helps prevent accidental suffocation!

Smoking increases the risk of SIDS. Even when a baby is merely in rooms where smoking occurs, its risk of dying from SIDS can increase 800%! A newly identified SIDS risk is a heart abnormality called a prolonged QT interval which can be detected by an EKG and treated with up to 90% success rate. Some new research shows that low doses of carnitine (less than 100mg) during the last trimester can help protect the baby from SIDS. Evidence from seven different studies suggests that babies who use pacifiers have lower risk for SIDS. If your child is at risk, Georgia tech engineers have developed a high tech T shirt to monitor heartbeat and breathing.

Can't find a recommended product? Call the 800 number in Product Resources for the store nearest you.

Bodywork For Two

—Get some mild daily exercise, such as a brisk walk for fresh air, oxygen and circulation. Take an early morning, half hour sun bath when possible for vitamin D, calcium absorption and bone growth.

—Consciously set aside one stress-free time for relaxation every day. The baby will know, thrive, and be more relaxed itself.

—If you practice reflexology, do not press the acupressure point just above the ankle on the inside of the leg. It can start contractions.

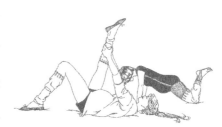

—Rub cocoa butter, vitamin E oil or wheat germ oil on the stomach and around the vaginal opening every night to make stretching easier and the skin more elastic.

—Get adequate sleep. The body energy turns inward during sleep for repair, restoration and fetal growth.

Special Problems During Pregnancy

Reduce standard dosage of any medication, orthodox or natural, to allow for the infant's tiny system.

AFTERBIRTH PAIN: take Crystal Star MOTHERING TEA™ or BACK TO RELIEF™ capsules, especially after a long labor, to tone and elasticize uterus; *una da gato* tea for quicker return to normal. For post-partum tears and to heal sore perineal muscles, use a sitz bath with *1 part uva ursi, 1 part yerba mansa rt., and 1 part each comfrey leaf and root.* Simmer 15 minutes, strain, add 1 teasp. salt, pour into a large shallow container; cool a little. Or use MOTHER LOVE'S SITZ BATH or Crystal Star CRAMPBARK COMPLEX. Sit in the bath for 15 to 20 minutes twice daily.

ANEMIA: take a non-constipating herbal iron, such as MONAS CHLORELLA, yellow dock tea, or Crystal Star IRON SOURCE™ caps. Have a green drink often, such as apple-alfalfa sprout-parsley juice, Green Foods BETA CARROT, or Crystal Star ENERGY GREEN™. Add vitamin C and E to your diet, and eat plenty of dark leafy greens.

BREASTS:
-**for infected breasts:** 500mg vitamin C every 3 hours, 400IU vitamin E, and beta-carotene 10,000IU daily. Get plenty of chlorophyll from green salads, green drinks, or super green supplements – Crystal Star ENERGY GREEN™ drink or Green Foods GREEN MAGMA.
-**for caked or crusted breasts:** simmer elder flowers in oil and rub on breasts. Wheat germ oil, almond oil and cocoa butter are also effective, or use Mother Love's PREGNANT BELLY SALVE.
-**for engorged breasts during nursing:** apply ice bags to the breasts to relieve pain; or use a marshmallow root fomentation with $\frac{1}{2}$ cup powder to 1 qt. water. Simmer 10 minutes. Soak a cloth in mixture and apply to breast.

CONSTIPATION: use a gentle fiber laxative, like Nature's Secret ULTIMATE FIBER, or Crystal Star CHO-LO FIBER TONE™, or an herbal laxative such as Nature's Secret ULTIMATE CLEANSE. Add fiber fruits, like prunes and apples to your diet.

FALSE LABOR: catnip tea or red raspberry tea will help. See also MISCARRIAGE pg. 455 in this book.

GAS and HEARTBURN: usually caused by an enzyme imbalance. Take papaya or bromelain chewables or papaya juice with a pinch of ginger. After meals, try a weak tea made with *fennel, dill or anise seeds*

HEMORRHOIDS: take BILBERRY extract, or Crystal Star HEMR-EASE™ capsules, or Mother Love's RHOID BALM (May also use any of these combinations effectively mixed with cocoa butter as a suppository.)

INSOMNIA: take Crystal Star CALCIUM SOURCE™ caps or Nature's Path CAL-LYTE. Nervine herbs like *scullcap, oats* and *passion flower* help. Or use *chamomile* tea. Crystal Star RELAX™ caps gently help within 25 minutes.

Can't find a recommended product? Call the 800 number in Product Resources for the store nearest you.

243

LABOR: for nausea during labor, take ginger tea or miso broth, or Alacer EMERGEN-C with a little salt added. For labor pain, take crampbark extract, or lobelia, scullcap or St. John's wort extract in water. For nerve pain, apply St. John's wort oil to temples and wrists; or use rosemary/ginger compresses. Acupressure treatments during labor reduce stress and increase dilation. For post-partum bleeding, take shepherd's purse or nettles tea. For sleep during long labor: use scullcap tincture. (Scullcap may be used throughout labor for relaxation.) Hydrate with cool drinks during labor even if there is nausea. Take bromelain to relieve pain and swelling after episiotomy.

MORNING SICKNESS: use homeopathic IPECAC and NAT. MUR, add vitamin B-6, 50mg 2x daily; sip mint tea whenever queasy. See MORNING SICKNESS program 464 in this book.

MISCARRIAGE: for prevention and hemorrhage control, drink raspberry tea every hour with $\frac{1}{4}$ teasp. ascorbate vit. C powder added, and take drops of hawthorn or lobelia extract every hour. See MISCARRIAGE program, page 455 for complete information.

According to John Lee M.D., transdermal progesterone 40 mg. per day can help prevent miscarriage caused by luteal phase failure. Ask your healthcare professional.

POST-PARTUM SWELLING and DEPRESSION: use homeopathic ARNICA. Make a post-partum cordial with 4 slices of dong quai rt., $\frac{1}{2}$ oz. false unicorn rt., 1 handful nettles, $\frac{1}{2}$ oz. St. John's wort extract, 1 handful motherwort herb, $\frac{1}{2}$ oz. hawthorn berries, and 2 inch-long slices of fresh ginger. Steep herbs in 1 pint of brandy for 2 weeks, shaking daily. Strain an add a little honey if desired. Take 1 teasp. daily as a tonic dose.

Depression is helped by B vitamins - Nature's Secret ULTIMATE B. Progesterone deficiency may be indicated. Consider progesterone balancing herbs like sarsaparilla and wild yam, or an herbal formula like PRO-EST™ BALANCE roll on.

STRETCH MARKS: apply wheat germ, avocado, sesame oil, vitamin E, or A, D & E oil. A *comfrey-calendula* beeswax salve also works well. Take vitamin C 500mg 3 to 4 times daily for collagen development. See STRETCH MARKS program pg. 501 in this book.

SWOLLEN ANKLES: use Nature's Apothecary BILBERRY extract in water.

TOXEMIA, Eclampsia: toxemia is caused by liver malfunction and disease. The liver cannot handle the increasing load of the progressing pregnancy. There is a marked reduction in blood flow to the placenta, kidneys and other organs. Severe cases result in liver and brain hemorrhage, convulsions and coma. Toxemia is indicated by extreme swelling, accompanied by high blood pressure, headaches, nausea and vomiting.

Take several green drinks such as apple-alfalfa sprout-parsley or Green Foods GREEN MAGMA for a "chlorophyll cleanout." Add vitamin C 500mg every 3 to 4 hours, 10,000IU beta-carotene, BILBERRY extract in water, and B Complex 50mg daily. Apply Transitions PROGEST CREAM as directed. Enzymatic Therapy MUCOPLEX and DGL have also been helpful, as has iodine therapy via daily kelp tablets.

UTERINE HEMORRHAGING: take bayberry/cayenne capsules, and get professional help immediately. Take bilberry extract daily with strengthening herbal flavonoids for tissue integrity. Use angelica tea for uterine contractions or Mother Love's SHEPHERD'S PURSE extract.

VARICOSE VEINS: take vitamin C 500mg with bioflavonoids and rutin, 4 daily; or bilberry extract 2x daily in water; or butcher's broom tea daily (also helpful for leg cramps during pregnancy). Take and apply Crystal Star VARI-TONE™ caps and VARI-VAIN™ roll-on gel directly to swollen veins.

Note: Baby diapers have been a huge cause for concern for mothers and families who are ecologically minded. Most diapers are still non-biodegradable, and most are impregnated with chemical polymer salts to absorb moisture. Use a diaper service, or your own washing machine, or use all-cotton Rmed TUSHIES.

Alternative Healing Options For Children

Healthy children develop powerful immune systems in infancy. Unless unusually or chronically ill, a child often needs only the subtle body-strengthening forces that nutritious foods, herbs or homeopathic remedies supply, rather than the highly focused medications of allopathic medicine which can have such drastic side effects on a small body.

Still, the undeniable ecological, social and diet deterioration in America during the last fifty years has had a marked effect on children's health. We see evidence of it in every aspect of their lives — declining educational performance, learning disabilities, mental disorders, obesity, drug and alcohol abuse, hypoglycemia, allergies, chronic illness, delinquency and violent behavior; they're all evidence of declining immunity and poor health.

 You can get a lot of help from the kids themselves in a natural health boosting program. Kids don't want to be sick, they aren't stupid, they don't like going to the doctor any more than you do. They often recognize that natural foods and therapies are good for them. Children are naturally immune to disease. A nutritious diet and natural health enhancer like herbs help keep them that way.

Diet Help For Childhood Diseases

Diet is your most important weapon in safeguarding your child's immunity defenses against disease. Pathogenic organisms and viruses are everywhere. But they aren't the major factor in causing disease if the body environment is healthy. Well-nourished children are usually strong enough to deal with infection in a successful way. They either don't catch the "bugs" that are going around, they contract only a mild case, or they develop strong healthy reactions that are short in duration, and get the problem over and done with quickly. This difference in resistance and immune response is the key to understanding children's diseases.

A wholesome diet can easily restore a child's natural vitality. Even children who have eaten a junk food diet for years quickly respond to a diet of fresh fruits, vegetables, whole grains, less dairy and sugar. I have noted substantial improvement in as little as a month's time. A child's hair and skin takes on new luster — they fill out if they are too skinny, and lose weight if they are fat. They sleep more soundly. Their attention spans markedly improve, and many learning and behavior problems lessen or disappear.

Keep it simple. Let kids help prepare their own food, even though they might get in the way and you feel like it's more trouble than it's worth. You'll be giving them a better understanding of good food (they're also more likely to eat the things they have a hand in making). Keep only good nutritious foods in the house. Children may be exposed to junk foods and poor foods at school or friend's houses, but you can build a good, natural foundation diet at home. For the time that they are at home, they should be able to choose only from nutritious choices.

Kids have extraordinarily sensitive taste buds. Everything they eat is very vivid and important to them. The diet program I offer in this section has lots of variety, so they can experiment and find out where their own preferences lie. There are plenty of snacks, sandwiches, fresh fruits, and sweet veggies like carrots — all foods children naturally like.

A healing diet for most common childhood diseases, including measles, mumps, chicken pox, strep throat and whooping cough, is fairly simple and basic. It's a therapy that starts with a short liquid elimination fast, followed by a fresh light foods diet in the acute stages.

Can't find a recommended product? Call the 800 number in Product Resources for the store nearest you.

245

A Short, Liquid Detox Cleanse For Childhood Diseases: *24 to 72 hours*

1: Start the child on cleansing liquids as soon as the disease is diagnosed to clean out harmful bacteria and infection. Give fruit juices such as apple, pineapple, grape, cranberry and citrus juices, or give Crystal Star FIRST AID TEA FOR KIDS™. The juice of two lemons in a glass of water with a little honey may be taken once or twice a day to flush the kidneys and normalize body chemistry.

2: Alternate fresh fruit juices throughout the day with fresh carrot juice, bottled water, and clear soups. A potassium broth or veggie drink (pages 215, 218) may be taken at least once a day. Encourage the child to drink as many healthy cleansing liquids as she or he wants. Light smoothies are favorites with kids. Avoid dairy products.

3: Offer herb teas throughout the cleanse. Children respond to herb teas quickly, and they like them more than you might think. Make them about half the strength. Add a little honey or maple syrup if the herbs are bitter.

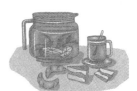

The following teas are effective for most childhood diseases:
—elder flowers with peppermint to induce perspiration
—catnip/chamomile/rosemary tea to reduce a rash
—mullein/lobelia or scullcap as relaxants
—catnip, fennel and peppermint for upset stomachs
—Crystal Star COFEX TEA™ for sore throats
—Crystal Star X-PEC-TEA™ to help bring up mucous
—Crystal Star FIRST AID™ TEA for warming against chills
—Echinacea drops in water every 4 hours to clear lymph glands and process out infective toxins

4: Acidophilus culture compounds are excellent for children. I always recommend them to get a child over the hump of a childhood disease. They keep friendly bacteria in the G.I. tract, especially if the child has taken a course of antibiotics. Acidophilus makes a big difference in both recovery time and immune response. Bifido-bacteria provides better protection for infants and children than regular acidophilus strains. Nutrition Now CHILDREN'S PB 8 (ages 1-4), RHINO ACIDOPHILUS (ages 4 and up), Solaray BABY LIFE, or DR. DOPHILUS powder work well for children. Use about $1/4$ teasp. at a time in a glass of water or juice three to four times daily.

Effective bodywork therapies for children:
—Give a gentle enema at least once during the detox cleanse to clear the child's colon of impacted wastes that hinder the body's effort to rid itself of diseased bacteria. A catnip tea enema is effective and safe for children.

—Oatmeal baths help neutralize rashes coming out on the skin. Herbal baths help induce cleansing perspiration, too, but the child should be watched closely all during the bath to make sure he or she is not getting too hot. Make up a big pot of *calendula* or *comfrey* tea for the bath water. Rub the child's body with *calendula* or *tea tree* oil, or Tiger Balm to loosen congestion after the bath.

—Apply hot ginger-cayenne compresses to affected or sore areas to stimulate circulation and defense response, to rid the body more quickly of infection. Alternate hot compresses with cold, plain water compresses.

—Clear your child's chest congestion with herbal steam inhalations. Use eucalyptus or tea tree oil, or Crystal Star RSPR TEA™ in a vaporizer help to keep lungs mucous free and improve oxygen uptake.

—Dab on with cotton balls, a water infusion of *golden seal, myrrh, yellow dock, black walnut, and yarrow,* or Crystal Star ANTI-BIO™ phyto-therapy gel to sores, scabs and lesions to help heal and soothe.

Fresh Foods Purification Diet For Children's Diseases: *A 3 day diet.*

Use this diet for initial, acute and chronic symptoms when a liquid detox is not desired, or after a liquid cleanse when the acute stage has passed. A fresh foods diet continues the cleansing activity while the addition of solid foods starts to rebuild strength. Dairy products, except for yogurt should be avoided. This diet should last about three days depending on the strength and condition of the child.

On rising: give citrus juice with a teaspoon of acidophilus liquid, or $1/4$ teasp. acidophilus powder;
　　or a glass of lemon juice and water with maple syrup.
Breakfast: offer a choice of favorite fresh fruits. Top with vanilla yogurt, Rice Dream or soy milk if desired.
Mid-morning: Give a vegetable drink, a potassium broth, (page 215) or fresh carrot juice.
　　Add $1/4$ teasp. ascorbate vitamin C or Ester C crystals with bioflavonoids.
Lunch: give fresh raw crunchy veggies with a yogurt dip; or a fresh veggie salad with yogurt dressing.
Mid-afternoon: offer a refreshing herb tea, such as licorice or peppermint tea,
　　or Crystal Star FIRST AID TEA FOR KIDS™ to keep the stomach settled and calm tension;
　　or another vegetable drink with $1/4$ teasp. vitamin C added.
Dinner: give a fresh salad, with avocados, carrots, kiwi, romaine and other high vitamin A foods;
　　and/or a cup of miso soup or other clear broth soup.
Before bed: offer a relaxing herb tea, like chamomile or scullcap tea, or Crystal Star GOOD NIGHT TEA™.
　　or a cup of miso broth for strength and B vitamins. Snip 1 teasp. dry sea greens on top if desired.

Note: The cleansing drinks and broths below are full of enzymes which I believe are critical to a child's health. Use them as a guide for highly nutritive vegetable juices. With your own variations they may be used as part of a nourishing diet as well as for purification. If you have a vegetable juicer, make the juices fresh.

BABY VEGGIE GREEN DRINK FOR KIDS

Kids like baby veggies. Make this in a juicer. Choose fresh veggies that your child likes most.

Choose green leafy vegetables like BABY SPINACH, SUNFLOWER GREENS **and** LETTUCES.
—Add BABY BOK CHOY, BABY CARROTS **and** SPROUTS.
—Don't forget sweet tasting veggies like CUCUMBERS, CELERY **and** TOMATOES.

ENERGY SOUP FOR KIDS

A liquid salad for kids. Make in the blender.

Blender blend: $1/2$ cup WATER, $1/4$ cup CELERY, $1/4$ cup FRESH PEAS, 1 cup SALAD GREENS, like BOK CHOY, DANDELION, LETTUCES **and** SPINACH.
—Add $1/2$ to 1 CUP SPOUTS like SUNFLOWER GREENS, ALFALFA **or** MUNG BEAN SPROUTS.
—Add half an avocado for creaminess; add tamari sauce or Bragg's LIQUID AMINOS for taste.

HEALING FRUIT SMOOTHIE

Always use fresh fruit (organic if possible) for this drink, not canned or frozen.

Blend 1 BANANA **and** 1 peeled ORANGE **with some unpasteurized apple juice. Add half a** PAPAYA **or** MANGO **if available, or one-quarter fresh** PINEAPPLE.

Can't find a recommended product? Call the 800 number in Product Resources for the store nearest you.

247

Supplements for your child's fresh foods diet. Continue to give them until the child is symptom free.
—A vitamin/mineral drink, such as 1 teasp. Floradix CHILDREN'S MULTIVITAMIN liquid in juice, Prevail CHILDREN'S MULTI-VITAMIN & MINERALS caps, or Nutrition Now RHINO CHEWY VITES.

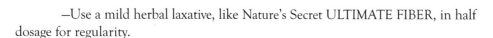

—Continue giving your acidophilus choice. Add vitamin A & D in drops if desired, and ascorbate vitamin C or Ester C crystals in juice.

—Continue the herbal tea choices you found effective during the liquid cleanse, especially Crystal Star FIRST AID TEA FOR KIDS™.

—Use a mild herbal laxative, like Nature's Secret ULTIMATE FIBER, in half dosage for regularity.

—Use garlic oil drops or open garlic capsules into juice for natural antibiotic activity; or give Crystal Star ANTI-BIO™ cap or extract in half dosage or Wakunaga KYOLIC liquid in juice.

Bodywork is a good choice for children throughout any illness.
—Continue with herbal baths, washes and compresses to cleanse toxins coming out through the skin. Give a soothing massage before bed. Get some early morning sunlight on the body every day possible .

When the crisis has passed, and the child is on the mend with a clean system, begin an optimal nutrition diet, like the one below, to prevent further problems, and increase general health and energy.

An Optimal Whole Foods Diet For Children:

We may live in the most affluent country in the world, but many of our children's basic nutritional needs are not met. The September 1997 issue of Pediatrics says only a tiny 1% of American kids meet the USDA requirements for all five food groups. Only 36% eat the recommended 2 to 4 servings of vegetables a day; only 30% get 3 to 5 vegetable servings a day. Instead fats and sugars supply an astounding 40% of American children's daily energy needs! Because much of our agricultural soils are depleted, and most of our foods are sprayed or gassed, many micronutrients like vitamins and minerals are no longer sufficiently present in our foods. The most common childhood nutrient deficiencies are calcium, iron, B-1, and vitamins A, B-complex and C.

The most protective diet for children is high in whole grains and green veggies for minerals, vegetable proteins for growth, and complex carbohydrates for energy. Offer organic foods to your child whenever possible. An Environmental Health Perspectives study shows children regularly exposed to pesticides experience serious problems — including low stamina, underdeveloped hand-eye coordination, and significantly poorer short-term memory. Make sure you tell, and graphically show your child what junk and synthetic foods are. I find over and over again that because of TV advertising and peer pressure, kids often really don't know what wholesome food is, and think they are eating the right way.

Use superfoods for kids! Superfoods are concentrated nutrients widely popular with adults today (check out the many superfoods listings in this book). They're just as good in healthy diet programs for kids. Mix them in or sprinkle them on other foods to increase the nutritional content of any meal. Superfood supplements can get some great nutrients into fussy eaters. Crystal Star SYSTEMS STRENGTH™ drink mix is a potent vegetarian blend of sea greens, herbs, and foods like miso, soy protein, brewer's yeast and brown rice. Add it to soups, sauces, even salad dressings. Green Foods BERRY BARLEY ESSENCE has natural raspberry and strawberry tastes. Kids like bee pollen, a highly bio-active superfood often called "nature's complete nutrition," because it is so full of balanced vitamins, minerals, proteins, carbohydrates, fats, enzymes, and essential amino acids. It has a sweet flavor which works well sprinkled on cereals or added to smoothies (about a half teaspoon).

Diet tips to help keep your child healthier and happier:

I know it's a lot easier said than done to change old dietary patterns to healthier eating.... for anybody, but especially for kids. A good way to start is to find something delicious to replace whatever is being taken away.

For example:

—If you want to include more wholesome foods, like fruits and vegetables, start with *food forms that children naturally go for* —like dried fruit snacks, and smoothies for fruits. Sandwiches, tacos, burritos and pitas can hold vegetables. Most kids like soup.... another good place to add vegetables. Let them add sauces or flavors they like.

—If you want to include whole grains in your child's diet, start by keeping only whole grains in the house. Kids love bagels, for instance.... and pastas, which come in a wide variety of whole grain options. Brown basmati rice is *much tastier than white rice* if your kid is a "rice kid." Stuffing is a big favorite — make sure it's whole grain. Popcorn is a healthy snack. Season it with tamari or a healthy season blend instead of gobs of butter and salt.

—If you want to add healthy cultured foods to your child's diet, start by keeping a good assortment of yogurt flavors with fruit for snacks in the fridge. Offer delicious kefir cheese for snack spreads instead of sour cream.

—To reduce the amount of sugar your child is getting, buy delicious, sugar-free snacks. Replace sugar-filled cereals with granola or oatmeal with healthy toppings. Offer dried fruit. Almost every kid likes raisins.

—If you want to reduce the amount of meat and heavy dairy proteins your child is eating, keep good plant protein available. Kids like tofu and grain burgers, especially with their favorite trimmings. Most kids like beans — look for healthy chili blends. Keep peanut butter, and nuts and seeds, like almonds, sunflower seeds and pumpkin seeds around the house for snacks. Recommend them as toppings for everything from soup or salad crunchies to smoothies and desserts. (Seeds and nuts give kids unsaturated oils and essential fatty acids, too.) Eggs are a good protein choice for kids.... one of Nature's perfect foods that's gotten a bad rap. Most kids like deviled eggs, and eggs are great in honey custards, another kid favorite.

—If you want to add more seafood to a child's diet, start with favorites like shrimp, tuna fish or salmon.

—If you want to encourage your child to drink more water instead of carbonated sodas or sweetened drinks, keep plenty of natural fruit juices and flavored mineral water around the house.

Your presence as a loving parental authority is a powerful influence. Gather your family together for a meal at least once a day to establish good eating habits for your kids.

Try this sample diet for optimal health for your child. It's been kid-tested for taste.

On rising: offer a protein drink such as NutriTech ALL-ONE, especially if the child's energy or school performance level is poor, or if the child seems to be constantly ill, (a child's body must have protein to heal), or 1 teaspoon liquid multi-vitamin in juice, such as Floradix CHILDREN'S MULTI-VITAMIN/MINERAL.

Breakfast: have a whole grain cereal with apple juice or a little yogurt and fresh fruit;
and/or whole grain toast or muffins, with a little butter, kefir cheese or nut butter;
add eggs, scrambled, baked or soft boiled (no fried eggs);
or have some hot oatmeal or puffed kashi cereal with maple syrup or yogurt.

Mid-morning: whole grain crackers with kefir cheese or dip, and a fruit juice;
or some fresh or dried fruit, or fruit leathers with yogurt or kefir cheese;
or fresh crunchy veggies with peanut butter or a nut spread;
or a sugar-free candy bar, or a healthy trail mix, stirred into yogurt.

Lunch: have a veggie, turkey, chicken or shrimp salad sandwich on whole grain bread, with low fat cheese.
Add whole grain or corn chips with a low fat dip;
or bean soup with whole grain toast, and a small salad or crunchy veggies with garbanzo spread;
or a baked potato with a little butter and kefir cheese, and a small green salad with dressing;
or a vegetarian pizza on a chapati or whole grain crust;
or whole grain spaghetti or pasta with a light sauce and parmesan cheese;
or a Mexican bean and veggie, or rice burrito with fresh salsa.

Can't find a recommended product? Call the 800 number in Product Resources for the store nearest you.

249

Mid-afternoon: have a sparkling juice and a dried fruit candy bar; or fresh fruit or fruit juice, or a kefir drink; or a hard boiled egg and some whole grain chips with a veggie or low fat cheese dip; or some whole grain toast and peanut butter or other nut butter.

Dinner: have a pizza on a whole grain, chapati or egg crust, with veggies, shrimp, and low fat cheese topping; or whole grain or egg pasta with vegetables and a light tomato/cheese sauce; or a baked Mexican quesadilla with low fat cheese and some steamed veggies or a salad; or roast turkey with cornbread dressing and a salad; or a tuna casserole with rice, peas and water chestnuts.

Before bed: a glass of apple juice or a little soy milk, Rice Dream or flavored kefir.

Note: See my book COOKING FOR HEALTHY HEALING for a complete Children's Diet for Disease Control, and for a Healthy Vegan Diet For Infants and Toddlers.

Extra supplements to optimize your child's nutritional health for the long term:
　　—Acidophilus – liquid or powder; give in juice 2 to 3x daily for good digestion and assimilation. DR. DOPHILUS, Nature's Path FLORA-LYTE, Nutrition Now RHINO ACIDOPHILUS, or Solaray BABY LIFE are excellent for children.
　　—Vitamin C, or Ester C in chewable or powder form with bioflavonoids; give in juice, $1/4$ teasp. at a time 2x daily. For chewable wafers, use 100mg, 250mg, or 500mg potency according to age and weight of the child.
　　—A sugar-free multi-vitamin and mineral supplement in either liquid or chewable tablet form. Some good choices are from Floradix, Prevail, Solaray and Mezotrace.

Exercise for kids is a primary nutrient for body and mind. US Public Health studies show a third of American children are unfit! Exercise is a key to health, growth and energy. Don't let your kid be a couch potato, or a computer junkie. Encourage outdoor activity, and make sure your child is taking P. E. classes in school.

About Herbal Remedies For Healing Children

A child's body responds well to herbal medicines. Children are born with naturally well-developed immune systems; this resistance ability is a key factor in understanding childhood diseases. Kids often only require the subtle, body strengthening forces that herbs or homeopathic medicines supply. Highly focused allopathic medications can have drastic side effects on a small body. I find that children will drink herbal teas, take herbal drops, syrups and homeopathic medicines much more readily than you might think. The remedies and methods listed in this section are building, strengthening and non-traumatic to a child's system.

Most herbal remedies may be taken as needed. Herbal effects can be quite specific; take the best formula for your particular need at the right time — rather than all the time — for optimum results. Rotating and alternating herbal combinations according to the changing health state of the child allows the body to remain most responsive to herbal effects. Reduce, then discontinue dosage as the problem improves — allowing the body to pick up its own work and bring its own vital forces into action.

Take only one or two herbal combinations at the same time when working with a child's system. Choose the herbal remedy that addresses the worst problem first. Alternate products to allow the body to thoroughly use the herbal properties. One of the bonuses of a natural healing program is the frequent discovery that other conditions were really complications of the first problem, and often take care of themselves as the body comes into balance.

Let herbs gently rebuild health. Even when a good healing program is working, and improvement is being made, adding more of the remedy in order to speed healing can aggravate symptoms and bring about worse results!

Herbal remedy dosage goes by body weight. Child dosage is as follows:
　　$1/2$ dose for children 10 - 14 years
　　$1/3$ dose for children 6 - 10 years
　　$1/4$ dose for children 2 - 6 years
　　$1/8$ dose for infants and babies

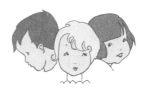

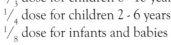

Can't find a recommended product? Call the 800 number in Product Resources for the store nearest you.

Special Remedies For Children's Problems

Note: Conditions not listed here have their own specific page in the AILMENTS section of this book.

ALLERGIES: (see how to determine specific allergies in the DIAGNOSTICS section of this book, page 526.)
General allergy diet guidelines:
—Common allergen foods: dairy, wheat, eggs, chocolate, nuts, seafood and citrus fruits. Try eliminating one at a time for a few weeks and watch to see if there is improvement. Eliminate dairy foods and cooked fats and oils because they thicken mucous and stimulate an increase in mucous production.
—Give lots of water to thin secretions and ease expectoration. Use Crystal Star ALLR-HST™ tea, or *fenugreek-thyme-nettles* tea, to help restore breathing and dry out sinuses. Use Crystal Star ADRN™ drops in water to support adrenals. Use an herbal combination of *echinacea, goldenseal and garlic* 2 times daily for 5 to 7 days to boost immunity and clear the lymph system. Use flaxseed oil for essential fatty acids to help regulate the inflammatory response. Mix into foods like salad dressing or in place of butter.
General supplement guidelines: (be sure to give in childhood amounts.)
—Beta-carotene to help heal irritated mucous membranes. One dose per day during allergy season.
—Vitamin C with bioflavonoids acts as an anti-inflammatory. One dose, 3x daily for two weeks.
—Calcium-magnesium for overreactive nerves. Use a ratio of 250mg calcium to 125mg magnesium.

ASTHMA: Use flax oil to help regulate inflammatory response, and Crystal Star ASTH-AID™ tea for bronchodilating effects. Use *lobelia* tea as a mild muscle relaxant. Use vitamin B-complex with extra pantothenic acid or 1 TB bee pollen granules, or Crystal Star ADRN™ extract in water for adrenal support, or Herbs Etc LUNG TONIC (alcohol free). Use milk thistle extract in water daily as a liver cleansing, bile stimulant. Vitamin B-12 deficiency is linked to some types of childhood asthma — check with a naturopathic physician and consider adding sea greens to the child's diet. *Astragalus* extract in water helps strengthen lungs — use for 2 weeks per month for six months after an asthma attack (except during a fever or infection). (See ASTHMA page 319.)

BITES and STINGS: (for mosquitoes, fleas, gnats, etc.) Seek immediate medical attention for bites from black widow spiders or other serious bites. Apply B &T STINGSTOP Insect Gel for pain and itch. (Also use as a repellent). Apply *tea tree oil* to the bite, and give vitamin C 100-500mg chewables every 4 hours to neutralize poison. Nature's Path CAL-LYTE helps relieve pain and calm nerves. Crystal Star GINSENG SKIN CARE™ gel is an anti-inflammatory. Use vitamin B-1 thiamine, as a natural insect repellent, 100mg 2x daily.

BRONCHITIS: go on a mucous cleansing diet to reduce congestion. See the short Liquid Elimination Cleanse in this section and the chapter on DETOXIFICATION for effective juices and broths. After the liquid diet, offer only fresh foods for a day. Avoid dairy foods, sweets and fried foods which continue mucous formation.
—Vitamin C with bioflavs for anti-inflammatory properties; beta-carotene to aid mucous membranes.
—Zinc to boost immune response (ZINC SOURCE™ drops from Crystal Star are especially effective.)
—Herbal remedies: *thyme, mullein or plantain* tea every 4 hours. *Chamomile-honey* tea for inflammation.
—Crystal Star BRNX™ extract encourages respiratory tract drainage and stimulates immune response.
—Prevail CHILDREN'S DEFENSE FORMULA, and B & T COUGH & BRONCHIAL SYRUP.

BRUISES: apply a cold compress (ice inside a towel) immediately. Leave on for 10 minutes — then off for 15 minutes. Repeat cycle 3 to 5 times to reduce swelling. Use vitamin C with bioflavonoids to restore integrity of blood vessel walls. Homeopathic *Arnica* 30x or 9c eases pain and prevents bruise from becoming larger. B & T ALPHA B & B makes black and blue marks go away faster.

BURNS (minor): seek medical assistance for a serious burn. Apply *tea tree oil* or Crystal Star ANTI-BIO GEL™ or Nature's Path BURN-AID to promote healing. Give vitamin C and bioflavonoids, beta-carotene, zinc, and B-complex 25 to 50mg to support healing.

Can't find a recommended product? Call the 800 number in Product Resources for the store nearest you.

251

CHEST CONGESTION: see BRONCHITIS, previous page for diet suggestions. Herbal steam inhalations with *eucalyptus oil, tea tree oil*, or Crystal Star RESPR™ TEA help keep lungs mucous free and improve oxygen uptake. Hydrotherapy baths with *calendula* flowers or strong *comfrey* tea infusions induce cleansing perspiration. Take *peppermint* and *raspberry* tea 2x daily. Apply a soothing chest rub with TIGER BALM, WHITE FLOWER or *calendula* oil to loosen congestion after a bath.

COLDS: Use Crystal Star BIOFLAV, FIBER & C SUPPORT™ drink for nasal congestion during the day, and 2 TBS <u>each</u> lemon juice and honey with 1 teasp. fresh grated ginger at night. Crystal Star ZINC SOURCE™ drops boost immune response. Zand ZINC LOZENGES arrest a nagging cough. Crystal Star COLD SEASON DEFENSE™ caps soften symptoms. If using antibiotic drugs, add acidophilus daily. See also COLDS page 353.

COLIC: if you are nursing, watch your diet carefully. Sometimes mother's milk is acidic from stress or diet. Avoid cabbage, brussels sprouts, onions, garlic, yeast breads, fried and fast foods. Avoid red meat, alcohol, sugary foods and caffeine until the child's digestion improves. Use goat's milk instead of cow's milk if the child is drinking milk. To promote healthy gastrointestinal flora, Solaray BABYLIFE for infants, Hyland's COLIC tabs, or Natren LIFE START $1/4$ teasp. in water or juice 2-3x daily. Give a dilute B Complex liquid in water once a week. Give papaya or apple juice, or small doses of papaya enzymes. Give the baby a morning sunbath for vitamin D. Give a *catnip* enema once a week for gas release. Never give honey to babies less than 1 year old. Effective weak teas include *chamomile* and *lemon balm*.

CONSTIPATION: increase the amount of fiber and fluid in the child's diet, with more fresh vegetable salads, fresh fruits, spring water, herbal teas, juices and soups. Soak raisins in senna tea and feed to young children for almost instant relief; use Crystal Star FIBER & HERBS CLEANSE™ for older children. Give weak *licorice* or *mullein* tea and molasses in water, 2 times daily. A gentle catnip enema will effectively clear the colon of impacted waste. See CONSTIPATION, page 357.

CRADLE CAP: if you are nursing, avoid refined sugar which supports bacteria and yeast. Use Nature's Path FLORA-LYTE, or BABYLIFE by Solaray for infants to foster healthy flora. Massage scalp with vitamin E or jojoba oil for 5 minutes. Leave on 30 minutes, then brush scalp with soft baby brush and shampoo with *tea tree* or *aloe vera* shampoo. Repeat twice weekly. Apply *comfrey root* tea to infant's scalp or dry skin area, and let air dry. Symptoms usually disappear within 10 days. Cradle cap may be a biotin deficiency. Take biotin 1000mcg while nursing; the baby will receive the necessary amount through breast milk.

CUTS: apply *tea tree oil* or Crystal Star ANTI-BIO GEL™ as an antiseptic. Use a *calendula* ointment, or AloeLife ALOE SKIN GEL or B & T CALIFLORA *calendula gel* every 2 or 3 hours. Use Crystal Star GINSENG SKIN REPAIR™ gel, then apply vitamin E oil at bedtime. Apply B & T ARNIFLORA GEL for swelling.

DIAPER and SKIN RASH: give plenty of water to help dilute urine acids. Mix *comfrey, goldenseal* and *arrowroot* powders with *aloe vera* gel and apply. Or use *calendula* ointment, liquid lecithin, or a vitamin A, D & E oil. Expose the child's bottom to morning sunlight for 20 minutes for vitamin D nutrients. Wash diapers in water with 1 teasp. of *tea tree* oil. Try Mother Love GREEN SALVE. Homeopathic remedies help, too: Sulfur, Rhux tox. Avoid petroleum jelly. Use talc-free powders from the health food store.

DIARRHEA: to prevent dehydration give frequent small sips of water, broths, diluted apple juice and herbal teas. To give intestines a chance to heal avoid dairy products during diarrhea and for two weeks. Use foods that are easily digested — pureed brown rice (B vitamins), bananas, dry cereal, crackers, toast, lightly cooked vegetables, grains and yogurt (friendly intestinal flora). Use Nature's Path FLORA-LYTE, Solaray BABYLIFE or Professional Nutrition DOCTOR-DOPHILUS +FOS to help restore healthy flora. Homeopathic remedies like *Arsenicum album* and *Podophyllum* relieve stress. Offer *slippery elm tea* or *peppermint tea* in a little juice twice daily. *Red raspberry, chamomile, thyme teas*, and Crystal Star FIRST AID TEA FOR KIDS™ are also helpful.

EARACHE: 80% of kids who take antibiotics for ear infections don't get better any sooner. Offer plenty of water, soups, herbal teas and diluted fruit juices. Avoid dairy foods which make it difficult for the ear to drain. Use *mullein* essence, or Mother Love MULLEIN FLOWER ear oil, or *garlic* oil (antibacterial) ear drops directly in the ear. Or mix vegetable glycerine and *witch hazel*, dip in cotton balls and insert in the ear to draw out infection. Give *lobelia* extract drops in water or juice for pain. Use an *echinacea-goldenseal* combination to clear infection. See also EAR INFECTIONS, page 373.

FEVER: a child's moderate fever is usually a body cleansing, healing process — a result of the problem, a part of the cure. (See a doctor if fever is high.) Diet should be liquids only - diluted fruit or vegetable juices, herb teas, like *peppermint* and *raspberry*, water and broth for at least 24 hours until fever breaks. *Catnip* tea and *catnip* enemas can help moderate a fever. Homeopathic remedies for fever, *Aconitum napellus*, *Camomilla* and *Bryonia alba* are effective for kids. Use *echinacea-goldenseal drops* for immune-boosting effects. See FEVER page 384.

FLU: during the acute stage give only liquid nutrients — fresh vegetable juices and green drinks, hot broths and chicken soup to stimulate mucous release. Refer to the Short Liquid Elimination Fast in this chapter. During the recuperation stage: follow a vegetarian, light diet, such as the Raw Foods Purification Diet For Children's Diseases in this chapter. Anti-viral herbal remedies include: *garlic, echinacea, yarrow, St John's wort, osha root, bee propolis* and *una de gato*. Use Crystal Star ANTI-VI™ to fight the flu virus, ZINC SOURCE™ extract for immune boosting zinc, and ANTI-BIO™ and vitamin C with bioflavonoids to help overcome inflammation. Silver has proven toxic to many viruses as well as bacteria, fungi and parasites. Use Nature's Path SILVER-LYTE.

GAS and FLATULENCE: unhealthy food choices, poor food combinations, eating too fast and not chewing food well are the main reasons for gas in kids. See the FOOD COMBINING CHART, page 555 and the Optimal Children's Diet (in this section). A plant based digestive enzyme, such as Prevail VITASE or Dr. Green's POWER-PLUS Food Enzymes by Herbal Products Development are helpful. Soak *anise, dill, caraway seed* or *chamomile* in water or juice and strain off. Give 1 to 2 TBS of liquid every 4 hours until digestion rebalances.

HEADACHES: add stress-busting lavender oil (about 10 drops) to a hot bath in the evening. Calcium and magnesium help calm muscles and relax blood vessels; Nature's Path CAL-LYTE, or Crystal Star ASPIR-SOURCE™ caps for pain, two at a time for children. *Feverfew* drops or *valerian-wild lettuce* drops in water help.

INDIGESTION: give *chamomile, fennel* or *catnip* tea, or a little ground *ginger* and *cinnamon* in water. Use soy milk or goat's milk instead of cow's milk for digestibility. Avoid fruit juice until discomfort passes. Give 1 teaspoon acidophilus liquid before meals.

JAUNDICE: mainly an infant condition — give a tiny amount of low-dose vitamin E oil on the tip of your finger, or a diluted lemon water with maple syrup.

MUMPS: the salivary and parotid glands swell and cause pain when chewing or swallowing. During acute stage give only liquid nutrients — fresh fruit and vegetable juices, except citrus, green drinks, chicken or vegetable soups. To alleviate pain in swallowing: heat 1 qt. apple juice with 8-10 *cloves*. Strain and cool. Anti-viral herbs include: *garlic, echinacea, yarrow, St John's wort* and *osha root*. Use Crystal Star ANTI-VI™ to fight the virus; Crystal Star ANTI-BIO™ extract in water or *burdock* tea every few hours to clear lymph glands, and help overcome infection. Make sure the child gets plenty of rest and sleep.

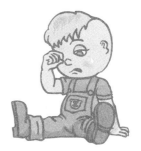

Supplements for childhood mumps include: (give in childhood amounts.)

—Extra vitamin C with bioflavonoids as an anti-inflammatory. One dose, 3x daily for two weeks.

—Colloidal or ionized silver helps fight the mumps virus. Use Nature's Path ionized SILVER-LYTE

Can't find a recommended product? Call the 800 number in Product Resources for the store nearest you.

253

PARASITES and WORMS: eliminate sugary foods and refined carbohydrates. (See Children's Optimal Whole Foods Diet in this chapter.) High fiber foods like grains, vegetables, especially greens help both treatment and prevention. Give probiotics like Nature's Path FLORA-LYTE, or Solaray BABYLIFE. Give raisins soaked in senna tea to cleanse the intestines or use Crystal Star FIBER & HERB CLEANSE™ capsules in child dosage. *Garlic* is a natural antiparasitic; use a *garlic* enema 2x a week. Give chlorophyll liquid, *wormwood* tea or herbal pumpkin oil tablets by Hain. Nature's Path SILVER-LYTE may also be effective. See PARASITES, page 476.

—**HEAD LICE:** *garlic* and *tea tree oil* fight head lice infestation. Use 25 drops in 1 pint of water. Rub the mixture onto the child's head 3 times daily; rinse hair after third application. *Goldenseal* tincture or strong *goldenseal* tea can be added as a rinse. Comb hair with a fine-toothed comb to remove lice and eggs.

—**RINGWORM:** apply *tea tree oil* on affected area until rash goes away. Use Crystal Star FUNGEX GEL™ or *black walnut* extract on affected area. Use the homeopathic remedy *Sulphur* 30x or 9c, three times daily, for 3 days. (Use at least one hour before or after using *tea tree oil* because the oil may affect the homeopathic remedy). Boost immune strength with an *echinacea-goldenseal-burdock root* combination 3x a day for ten days.

SINUS INFECTION: refer to the Short Liquid Elimination Fast in this chapter. See recipes for juices, broths, tonics, etc. in the general DETOXIFICATION chapter. A short three day cleansing liquid diet helps clear mucous congestion. Use Crystal Star ANTI-BIO™ drops or *goldenseal* liquid drops in the nose to overcome infection and inflammation, and FIRST AID CAPS™ for vitamin C and antioxidant activity 2x daily for a week. Use Crystal Star X-PEC-TEA™ to release mucous buildup in the head and chest.

SORE THROAT: give Crystal Star COFEX™ TEA as a throat coat at night for almost immediate relief. Zand ZINC LOZENGES or other zinc lozenges for coughing. Give *echinacea and goldenseal* or Crystal Star ANTI-VI™ or BIO-VI™ drops to fight infections. Give pineapple juice 2x daily for enzyme therapy. *Licorice* sticks or tea are effective. Give vitamin C with bioflavonoids to help ease throat inflammation and to fight infection.

SLEEPLESSNESS: avoid stimulants like sugary foods, chocolate or foods containing caffeine. Use Nature's Path CAL-LYTE™ or the calming Homeopathic Hylands CALMS FORTE; Crystal Star RELAX CAPS™ or GOOD NIGHT™ tea, *wild lettuce-valerian* extract in water, *passion flower, skullcap and chamomile* teas are effective.

TEETHING: rub gums with honey, *peppermint* oil, or drops of *lobelia* tincture. Give weak *catnip, fennel or peppermint* tea to soothe. Add a few daily drops of A, D & E oil to food. *Licorice root* powder (2 pinches) made into a paste soothes inflamed gums. Use B & T ALPHA TLC by for teething. (See TEETHING, page 510 for more.)

THRUSH FUNGAL INFECTION: Give probiotics like Nature's Path FLORA-LYTE or Natren LIFESTART (also use as a rectal suppository). Add vitamin C 100mg or Ester C chewable. Thrush is often caused by widespread antibiotic use. Give *garlic* extract in water, like Wakunaga KYOLIC, or squirt a pricked *garlic* oil cap in the mouth. Nature's Path ionized SILVER-LYTE, or Allergy Research PROLIVE (*Olive leaf extract*) is effective.

WEAK SYSTEM: see Optimal Whole Foods Diet For Children in this chapter. Give Crystal Star SYS-TEMS STRENGTH™ broth daily. Add Nature's Path TRACE-LYTE minerals. Add 1 teasp. nutritional yeast for B-complex vitamins and protein. Hyland's BIOPLASMA is a good general homeopathic remedy. Give apple or carrot juice daily. Include a daily chewable interferon boosting vitamin C wafer as a preventive.

WHOOPING COUGH: (cases are rising almost 85% over the last several years.) Give a liquid diet during acute stage with plenty of juices, broths and water. Crystal Star ANTI-SPZ™ or *valerian-wild lettuce* extract, ZINC SOURCE™ drops and ANTI-BIO™ capsules. Use B & T COUGH & BRONCHIAL syrup or *thyme* extract in water. Give vitamin C with bioflavonoids $1/4$ teasp. every hour until stool turns soupy. Give *marshmallow root, slippery elm bark* or *osha root* tea, or *lobelia* extract to soothe respiratory tract. Apply hot *ginger-garlic* compresses to chest; use a *eucalyptus* steam at night.

A brief medicine chest for kids:

1: TEA TREE OIL: for infections that need antiseptic or antifungal activity, including mouth, teeth, gums, throat, ringworm, fungus, etc. Effective on stings, bites, burns, sunburns, cuts, and scrapes.

2: RESCUE REMEDY by Nelson Bach: For respiratory problems, coughing, gas, stomach ache and constipation. A rebalancing calmative for emotional stress and anxiety.

3: KIDS KIT from Hylands Homeopathic: A first aid kit with gentle, all-purpose remedies.

4: FIRST AID TEA FOR KIDS™: Crystal Star's tea addresses many childhood problems — for infant jaundice and teething pain; for a fever to induce a cleansing sweat; for stomach aches, diarrhea and when a child is whiney and sickly.

5: To help prevent contagious disease after exposure, give 1 *cayenne* capsule 3x a day, 1 chewable vitamin C 500mg wafers 3x a day, and a cup of roasted *dandelion root* tea daily for 3 or 4 days.

Should you vaccinate your child?

It depends on the vaccination — some have serious side effects for sensitive individuals, like the flu vaccination; some can wear off and allow a more serious disease to develop as an adult, like the chicken pox vaccination (a childhood case of chicken pox confers lifetime immunity). Medical literature from the last 70 years shows a high incidence of vaccination-related injuries and death. In just a 39 month period (July 1990-Nov. 1993), over 54,000 adverse reports, including 471 deaths as a result of vaccinations were reported to the FDA. (The homeopathic remedy *Silicea* is a specific remedy for adverse reactions to vaccinations.) My own sense is that most vaccines unnaturally stimulate and imbalance the immune system, eventually allowing many more immunological disorders like M.S., lupus, chronic fatigue syndrome, candida and herpes infections.

When Should You Call A Doctor?

Herbs are wonderful for most childhood health problems, but sometimes your child may need strong medicine. Here are the signs that tell you to call a doctor:

—If your child has a chronic stuffy nose and thick discharge that doesn't go away.

—If a fever persists longer than 3 days or returns after 3 days, or is unusually high.

—If a cold doesn't clear up and a rash or honking cough develops after 7 days.

—If your child shows rapid breathing, gasping, wheezing, or pale or bluish skin.

—If your child breaks a bone, or gets a deep, blood-gushing gash.

—If your child is recovering from chicken pox or flu virus, and goes into prolonged, vomiting with a fever followed by severe fatigue and confusion, he or she may have Reyes Syndrome, linked to aspirin reaction in children. Symptoms include: agitation, delirium, seizures, double vision, speech impairment, hearing loss and coma. Brain damage and death can result if the child does not get emergency treatment of intravenous glucose and electrolytes within 12 to 24 hours after vomiting starts.

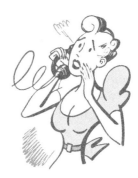

Special notes:

1: Do not use honey (linked to infant botulism) in teas for children less than one year old.

2: Do not use aspirin for children's viral infections. Aspirin given during a viral infection is linked to Reyes syndrome, a dangerous child's liver disease. Aspirin is also linked childhood allergies.

3: Antibiotic drugs can be tough on a small child's system, especially over a long period of time. Question your doctor if an antibiotic prescription seems automatic, especially if your child has a viral infection.

Can't find a recommended product? Call the 800 number in Product Resources for the store nearest you.

255

Slow Down Your Aging Clock

It's happening to everybody, most of the time faster than we'd like. Whenever the gold and silver years begin for you, it's when the fun begins, when hectic family life quiets down, financial strains and needs ease, business retirement is here or not far off, and we can do the things we've always wanted to do but never had time for — travel, art, music, a craft, gardening, writing, quiet walks, picnics, more social life...... doing what we want to do, not what we have to do. We all look forward to the treasure years of life, and picture ourselves on that tennis court, bicycle path or cruise ship, healthy and enjoying ourselves. But, there's a catch - our freedom comes in the latter half of life, and many of us don't age gracefully in today's world.

Anti-aging is the buzz word of the millennium. There are so many interesting things to do and see in the world..... without enough time to do them. We all want to extend our life spans with the best health possible.

Fortunately, youth is not a chronological age. It's good health and an optimistic spirit. Even if the hourglass tells us we're older, the passage of time isn't really what ages us. It's the process that reduces the number of healthy cells in our bodies.

Life expectancy lengthens as you age. It's a paradox of aging. The average American child born in 1993 has a life expectancy of 75.4 years. But average life expectancy for someone 85 years is *six more years*. The longer you live, the longer your total expected life span becomes. **Age is not the enemy.... illness is.**

Human life span is at least 20 to 30 years longer than most of us actually live today. It's astonishing to realize that we are living only two-thirds of the years our bodies are capable of!

Our cells don't age; they're sloughed off as their efficiency diminishes, to be replaced by new ones. With the right nutrients, cell restoration may continue for many years past current life expectancy. A long standing diet of chemical-laced foods, pollutants that cause nutrient deficiencies, overuse of prescription drugs and antibiotics, all prevent our seniority dreams from becoming a reality. Eighty percent of the population over 65 years old in industrialized nations today is chronically ill, usually with arthritis, heart disease, diabetes or high blood pressure. If stress is piled on top of poor health, our minds and spirits suffer, too. It's a prescription for aging.

Yet, human lifespan can be increased. **A balanced life is the key to long life.** You can strengthen your lean body mass, boost your metabolism and enhance your immune response. Your cell life is largely genetically controlled, but disease is more often the result of diet, lifestyle or environment. Natural anti-aging techniques are not hocus pocus or a magic potion. They are an integrated, hard-core approach to avoiding disease (the real enemy). In my opinion, they work far better than any of today's "superdrugs."

This chapter offers keys to slow down aging.... how to have a better memory with no senility, better skin tone with fewer wrinkles, a strong heart, bones and immune response, flexible joints and muscles, a youthful metabolic rate and a healthy sex life (good hormone activity keeps your whole body youthful).

Regular aerobic exercise, like a brisk daily walk, prolongs fitness at any age. Exercise helps maintain stamina, strength, circulation, joint mobility, and increases your lifespan! Stretch out every morning to limber up, oxygenate your tissues, and clear your body of last night's waste and metabolic eliminations. Stretch at night before you retire to insure muscle relaxation and a better night's rest.

Don't worry. Be happy. Think positive to stay young. Science is validating the mind-body connection in terms of the body's ability to heal. A well-rounded, optimistic life needs friends and family. It's important for you and for them. Doing for, and giving to others at the stage of your life when there is finally enough time to graciously do it, makes a world of difference to your spirit.

Can't find a recommended product? Call the 800 number in Product Resources for the store nearest you.

Are you aging faster than you want to? Don't be overly harsh, but an honest evaluation of the following widely accepted aging signs may identify areas where you can take action to slow down some of aging's effects.

Anti-Aging Check-Up:

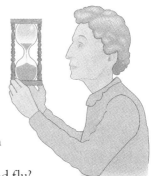

- Is your energy level at an all-time low?
- Have you noticed brown spots around your eyes, nose and hands?
- Has your hairline receded? Is your hair showing a lot of gray?
- Has constipation or irregular bowel movements become a problem for you?
- Do you have some hearing loss or annoying ringing in the ears?
- Do you have joint pain or joint crackling on one side? Do you have knobs on your index fingers? Are you stiff when you get up in the morning?
- Does it take longer for you to recover from respiratory infections like colds and flu? Do colds frequently become pneumonia for you?
- Is your eyesight worsening? Are you afraid you have macular degeneration, glaucoma or cataracts?
- Is it more difficult for you to lose weight? Have you put on 10-15 pounds that you just can't get rid of?
- Are your eyes noticeably dry? Do you have trouble tearing? Are your mouth and nasal passages always dry? If you are a woman, do you have chronic vaginal dryness?
- Is the skin on your hands, arms and neck crepe-y, thinner, bruising easily or getting strawberry marks?
- Are your teeth more brittle, with visible chip marks or discoloration? Have you lost teeth to gum disease? (Nothing makes you look older than poor teeth. See my "Dental Problems" program on pg. 363)
- Do you experience heartburn, indigestion or gas regularly after eating (a sign of low hydrochloric acid)?
- Have you lost some height? Look in the mirror. Is your neck starting to hunch over or at an angle?
- Have you had a recent bone fracture in a fall or accident that would never have meant a break in the past?
- Do you have poor circulation? Are your hands and feet cold even in mild weather?
- Do you have regular insomnia? (especially a sign of adrenal deficiency)
- Have you noticed a slight but constant trembling of your hands? Are you unsteady when you walk?
- Do you find yourself becoming seriously forgetful? Do you sometimes forget friends' names?
- Have your arms or legs become more flabby? Are your muscles noticeably weaker?
- Have you started to have heart palpitations? or small chest pains?

Start your anti-aging campaign with the lifestyle factors that affect aging the most.

—take a long hard look at the prescription drugs you use: Many drugs lead to serious body imbalancees by impairing your nutrient uptake, and they can spur a free radical assault that accelerates aging. They also tend to interact, especially drugs that affect hormones, like Viagra or Andro or Propecia.

—take another look at your diet: You've probably already cut the fat and fried food. But the chemicals in foods like lunch meats and pre-prepared meals are the culprits for early aging. They can create an over-acid condition in the blood, trigger many allergies, and like drugs, set up a free-radical cascade favorable to disease.

—if you eat a lot of sweets or have hard alcohol drinks regularly, your diet is probably high in sugar: sugar is also a hidden ingredient in most processed foods. A high sugar diet wipes out immunity and reduces tissue elasticity. Artificial sweeteners with aspartame are linked to degenerative nerve disorders.

—take a look at your teeth and gums: almost nothing shows age faster than discolored teeth, lost teeth or red, receding gums. Consider taking CoQ-10 right away for gum problems, about 200mg daily at least for the first month, and see a good holistic dentist to solve discoloration problems.

—take a look in the mirror: is your neck no longer straight, but at a slight angle, or if you shoulders are hunching, you may be losing bone density. Start a strengthening exercise program right away. Make sure it includes elongating, smooth muscle stretches and stick with it. Exercise can rapidly reverse this aging sign.

—if you've moved to a southern climate: 90% of skin cancers and wrinkles trace back to sun exposure. Use 40SPF for your face, up to 26SPF for your body and wear a hat.... or face those fine lines in the mirror.

Can't find a recommended product? Call the 800 number in Product Resources for the store nearest you.

257

Longevity begins with a good diet

A nutrition rich diet is the center piece of a vibrant long life. Most health experts agree that the food guide pyramid needs modification for better health as we age. Your diet must become *even more* nourishing and even higher in antioxidants as the years pass. A good diet improves health, provides a high level of energy, maintains harmonious system balance, keeps memory and thinking sharp, staves off disease, and contributes to a youthful appearance. The aging process slows down if you have a good internal environment.

Lower your daily calories to reduce the signs of aging. A low calorie diet protects DNA molecules from damage, preventing organ and tissue degeneration. Your body needs fewer calories and burns calories slower as you age; optimum body weight should be 10 to 15 pounds less than in your 20's and 30's. An easy way to control that annoying slow upward weight gain is to compose your diet of 50% fresh foods.

Focus on whole, fresh, organically grown foods to protect your skin from the signs of aging. Your skin is a window on your diet. The American diet was already saturated with chemicals from pesticides, preservatives and additives. Now over 70% of our foods are genetically altered. The brown age spots and rough texture we see on our skin are signs that our bodies are less able to process our foods correctly.

The Best Anti-Aging Foods:

—**Fresh fruits and vegetables!** Fresh produce gives you the most vitamins, minerals, fiber and enzymes. Plants have the widest array of nutrients and are the easiest for the body to use. Enzyme-rich fruits and vegetables are the essential link in stamina levels. Eat organically grown foods when possible to insure higher nutrient content and avoid toxic sprays. Have a green salad every day! New German research reveals the immune cells of vegetarians are twice as effective as meat eaters in killing cancer cells!

• **Fresh fruit and vegetable juices** offer quick absorption of high-quality nutrients, especially antioxidants, which protect the body against aging, heart disease, cancer, and degenerative conditions.

—**Sea greens are the ocean's superfoods.** They contain all the necessary elements of life and transmit the energies of the ocean to us as proteins, complex carbohydrates, vitamins, minerals, trace minerals, chlorophyll, enzymes and fiber. Sea greens and sea foods stand almost alone as potent sources of natural iodine. By regulating thyroid function, they promote higher energy levels and increased metabolism for faster weight loss after 40.

—**Whole grains, nuts, seeds and beans for protein, fiber, minerals and essential fatty acids.** Sprouted seeds, grains, and legumes are some of the healthiest foods you can eat. They are living nutrients that can go directly to your cells.

—**Cultured foods for friendly digestive flora.** Yogurt tops the list, but kefir and kefir cheese, miso, tamari, tofu, tempeh, even a glass of wine at the evening meal also promote better nutrient assimilation. Raw sauerkraut is especially good for boosting friendly bacteria. (Avoid sauerkraut processed with alum.)

—**Fish and fresh seafoods** two to three times a week enhance thyroid and metabolic balance.

—**Plenty of pure water every day** keeps your body hydrated and clean. See "Water" on pg.146 for more info.

—**Keep your system alkaline** with green drinks, green foods, miso, and grains like rice.

—**Healthy, unsaturated fats and oils,** 2 to 3 tablespoons a day are enough to keep your body at its best.

—**Poultry, other meats, butter, eggs, and dairy in moderation.** Avoid fried foods, excess caffeine, red meats, highly seasoned foods, refined and chemically processed foods altogether.

Plant Enzymes Are A Key To Anti-Aging

Enzymes are the cornerstone of anti-aging, because they support strong immune system health and provide the active food antioxidants which fight free-radicals. Replenishing your enzymes every day builds a body that resists disease, enables healing, and lengthens your life. In fact, Dr. Edward Howell, a founder of enzyme therapy said that "the actual length of life is tied to the increased use of food enzymes because they decrease the rate of body enzyme exhaustion."

Enzymes are the workhorses that power our bodies. Enzymes have been called our vital force, because without them we would be a pile of lifeless chemicals. At this very moment, millions of enzymes in your body are carrying out the vital functions that preserve your life.

Enzyme depletion and aging go hand in hand. Each of us is born with a battery charge of body enzyme energy. The faster you use up this enzyme supply - the shorter your life. Of course enzymes are used up in normal body functions like metabolism and healing. But enzymes are wasted haphazardly throughout life by alcohol, drugs and chemical-laced foods, and depleted by overcooked food and harmful environmental chemicals. Unless we do something to stop the one-way-flow out of the body of enzyme energy, our digestive and eliminative capacities weaken, obesity, and chronic illness set in, and lifespan shortens.

Enzyme rich foods assure us the main components of anti-aging, especially antioxidants. They bring into our bodies not only enzymes but the full array of plant nutrients that keep our immune systems strong. Enzymes are incredibly heat-sensitive; they're the first to be destroyed during cooking (above 118 degrees Fahrenheit), pasteurization, canning, microwaving, and fast food operations. Irradiated, highly processed and microwaved or overly cooked foods (even plant foods) are a poor choice, because their enzymes are dead.

Eating food devoid of enzymes means the pancreas and the liver have to use their enzyme stores for digestion. But even this substitute measure doesn't make up for the missing enzymes, because we need the food enzymes plants provide to break the food down correctly and deliver nutrients to the blood. We end up with undigested food in the blood. White blood cell immune defenses leave their jobs to take care of the undigested food, and immune response takes a dive.

I believe Nature intended us to eat a largely plant-based diet, rich in fresh foods, perhaps to ensure that a large percentage of the diet is enzyme rich. If you don't get enough fresh foods, or you need extra enzymes for healing, plant based, food enzyme supplements are the next best choice. Plant enzyme supplements are particularly useful for anti-aging, improving digestive and skin disorders (even age spots), inhibiting fibrosis related to atherosclerosis, and fighting free radicals that damage DNA.

Note: See ENZYMES AND ENZYME THERAPY, page 127 for more information.

The importance of vitamins, minerals and superfoods increases as you age.

Vitamins, minerals and superfoods optimize your healing potential. They offer potent armor to deal with the body-aging realities of today's environment. Mineral depleted soils mean we get less important minerals. Strong chemicals everywhere expose our bodies to unhealthy toxins. Pollutants decrease the available oxygen we receive from the air. Fortifying your diet with supplements and superfoods strengthens your ability to function in a world which makes it tough to be healthy.

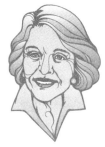

Note: In addition to the information offered here about vitamins, minerals and superfoods as they relate to aging, be sure to check THE ALTERNATIVE ARSENAL chapter (page 78) for broader data.

Can't find a recommended product? Call the 800 number in Product Resources for the store nearest you.

259

Antioxidants Are a Key To Anti-Aging

Important anti-aging antioxidants:

—**Alpha lipoic acid:** may slow or reverse the aging process by increasing metabolic activity and reducing oxidative damage; the only antioxidant known to significantly boost body glutathione, a key detoxifying antioxidant which begins to decline around age 60.

—**Bee pollen:** a food source, energy builder and health restorer since ancient times; a full-spectrum rejuvenative food that helps counteract the effects of aging and increases both mental and physical capability.

—**CoQ-10:** the body's ability to assimilate food source CoQ-10 declines with age. Supplements provide benefits for gum disease, cardiovascular health, and breast and prostate cancer protection.

—**Carotenes:** beta, alpha, lycopene, lutein, zeaxanthine and others are powerful anti-infectives and antioxidants for immune health, protection against environmental pollutants, slowing aging and allergy control.

　• **Lycopene:** with twice the antioxidant power of beta carotene, lycopene is an anti-cancer carotenoid reducing risk for prostate, cervical and pancreatic cancers.

—**Vitamin C:** a primary antioxidant for boosting immune strength. Protects against infections, cancer, heart disease, arthritis and allergies. Safeguards against radiation, heavy metal toxins and pollutants.

　• **Bioflavonoids:** part of the C-complex prevent artery hardening, enhance connective tissue, capillary and vein strength, and control bruising. They help lower cholesterol, and stimulate bile for digestion.

—**Vitamin E:** an anticoagulant and vasodilator against blood clots and heart disease. It retards cellular and mental aging, works as an anti-aging antioxidant with selenium to quench free radical fires and reduces infections in the elderly.

—**Germanium (organic):** a potent antioxidant mineral that detoxifies and boosts natural killer cells. Increases tissue oxygenation (poor oxygenation is one of the most common causes of cell injury and disease).

—**L-Glutathione:** an antioxidant amino acid that works to neutralize radiation toxicity and inhibit free radical formation. It also cleanses the blood from the effects of chemotherapy, X-rays and liver toxicity.

—**NAC (N-Acetyl-Cysteine):** an antioxidant amino acid and precursor of glutathione. Prevents age-related free radical damage to skin and arteries. Detoxifies the body from alcohol, heavy metals, smoke, x-rays and radiation. NAC is the acetylated form of cysteine, which provides better absorption.

—**NADH** (Co-enzyme Nicotinamide Adenine Dinucleotide): a powerful antioxidant coenzyme involved with the synthesis of ATP (chemical energy) in the body. Used sucessfully to treat Alzheimer's, Parkinson's, chronic fatigue syndrome and depression. Kal NADH tablets.

—**Oligomeric Proanthocyanidins (OPC's):** highy potent antioxidants that strengthen capillaries and connective tissue. OPC's reduce LDL cholesterol that accumulates on arteries causing atherosclerosis.

—**Selenium:** an antioxidant trace mineral that protects the body from heavy metal toxicity.

—**Royal Jelly:** an anti-aging superfood which stimulates the immune system, deep cellular health and longevity, boosts circulation to the skin and supplies key nutrients for energy and mental alertness.

—**Zinc:** limits the amount of free radicals the body naturally produces, like malondialdehyde (MDA).

Super green foods are widely popular antioxidants. They should be part of your anti-aging picture. Check out the sections in this book on sea greens, chlorella, spirulina, aloe vera, barley and wheat grass.

Nootropic brain nutrients are another anti-aging key.

—**Choline:** one of the lipotropic B vitamins, improves fat metabolism, and it's a memory "vitamin," easily converted to the brain neurotransmitter acetylcholine. Studies show lecithin, a rich source of choline, greatly improves memory. Just eating 2 TBS. a day for five weeks can do the job!

—**Phosphatidylserine:** a phospholipid nutrient that helps maintain cell membrane integrity and fluidity. Boosts brain health by increasing neurotransmitter activity and improving glucose metabolism. Now available in supplement form, PS is shown in 25 different human studies to improve or maintain cognition and concentration in older adults. Allergy Research Group PHOSSERINE.

Herbs Can Help Slow The Effects Of Aging

People have searched for the Fountain of Youth since ancient times. The answer may have been available all along in the youth-extending nutrients of herbs.

Herbs have wide ranging properties and far reaching possibilities as revitalizers. Herbs are at their best in this type of role... balancing, toning and normalizing our bodies. Herbs have antioxidant properties that guard against free radical destruction of tissue. Herbs are full of whole essence vitamins, minerals and phytochemicals — potent nutrients that can address aging concerns — better memory, strong gland and metabolic activity, smoother skin, energy, and good muscle tone. Herbs have powerful enzymes that make their nutrients easy to absorb.

The three main causes of aging are:
1: cell and tissue damage by free radicals that aren't neutralized because the body lacks antioxidants.
2: reduced immune response that puts the body at risk for disease.
3: enzyme depletion in the body due to lack of enzyme reinforcements from food & supplement choices.

Herbal therapy is one of the best defenders your body has for these aging actions.
   —**Anti-oxidant herbs** scavenge and neutralize free radicals, energize and tone.
   —**Adaptogen herbs** strengthen immunity, and equip your body to handle stress.

Free radicals play a key role in body aging. They are highly active compounds that spark with an oxidating fire when fat molecules react with oxygen. Although they occur in normal metabolic breakdown, our bodies experience excesses of these cell damagers from air and environmental pollutants. Your body takes 10,000 free radical hits a day just in normal, everyday living!

Free radicals that go unchecked by antioxidants are dangerous — they can actually reprogram your DNA, degrade collagen and cause premature aging, immune system breakdown and inflammatory reactions. Free radicals are the missing link to many diseases including cancer, atherosclerosis, Alzheimer's disease and immune compromised diseases like fibromyalgia and chronic fatigue syndrome.

Lowering the saturated fat in your diet is the single most beneficial step you can take to reduce free radical damage. Heavy, saturated fats depress the body's antioxidant enzyme response to free radical attacks.

Potent herbal antioxidants for anti-aging:
   —**Arjuna:** an Ayurvedic heart tonic effective for angina pain, arrhythmia and congestive heart failure. High antioxidants in the tannins amd flavones prevent oxidative damage linked to heart disease.
   —**Cat's Claw:** a Peruvian rainforest herb known for its benefits for arthritis, irritable bowel syndrome (IBS), immunity, and tumorous growths. Plentiful antioxidants, including proanthocyanidins for anti-aging.
   —**Pine bark, and grapeseed:** contain powerful proanthocyanidins (OPCs or PCOs), concentrated, highly active bioflavonoids. Fifty times stronger than vitamin E, 20 times stronger than vitamin C, they are one of the few dietary antioxidants that readily crosses the blood-brain barrier to protect brain cells and aid memory.
   —**Ginkgo biloba:** is used worldwide to combat the effects of aging. It protects the cells against damage from free radicals, reduces blood cell clumping which leads to congestive heart disease, improves memory and brain activity, restores circulation, helps improve hearing and vision and fights allergic reactions. Studies show ginkgo extracts stablize and, in some cases, improve cognition function and social behavior of severely demented Alzheimer's patients. New studies reveal that ginkgo actually reduces the "stress" hormone cortisol linked to immune suppression, atherosclerosis and brain cell toxicity.
   A biological super tree, ginkgo has survived almost unchanged for over 150 million years and is so hardy that a solitary ginkgo was the only tree to survive the atomic blast in Hiroshima! This tree is still alive today, standing near the epicenter of the blast, a testament to ginkgo's remarkable ability to survive.
   —**Shiitake mushrooms:** promote vitality and are especially valuable as a treatment for systemic conditions related to age-related sexual dysfunction.

Can't find a recommended product? Call the 800 number in Product Resources for the store nearest you.

261

—**Reishi mushrooms** (*ganoderma*): tonic herbs that increase vitality and enhance immunity. They lower cholesterol and high blood pressure, combat bacteria and viruses, may help prevent cancer and aid in the treatment of chronic fatigue syndrome, ulcers and heart disease.

—**Astragalus:** a strong immune enhancer, adrenal stimulant and gland tonic; a vasodilator that helps lower blood pressure, increases metabolism and improves circulation. It is a specific in liver dysfunction and respiratory problems that involve allergies.

—**Alfalfa:** is rich in chlorophyll, which helps heal damaged tissue and promotes growth of new tissue. It is one of the oldest fatigue remedies known.

—**Hawthorn:** bioflavonoid-rich, and adept at counteracting the damaging effects of free radicals on the cardiovascular system. Hawthorn helps make the heart a more efficient pump, increasing output of blood from the heart and decreasing resistance from the blood vessels.

—**Licorice:** offers immune-enhancing properties that increase the overall number of lymphocytes, and the activity of killer T-cells. It is antiviral and antibacterial, with powerful antioxidant properties. Tests indicate it may also have cancer-inhibiting properties.

—**Wheat germ oil:** 1 tablespoon provides the antioxidant equivalent of an oxygen tent for 30 minutes.

Herbal adaptogens have tonic, anti-stress action. They increase resistance to adverse influences by helping the body adapt or normalize. Herbs like *astragalus, shiitake and reishi mushrooms* already mentioned in the anti-oxidant section are also adaptogens.

Potent herbal adaptogens for anti-aging:

—**Panax Ginseng** (*red, white and American ginsengs*): are the most effective of all adaptogen herbs. Ginseng is capable of stimulating both long and short term energy, has measurable amounts of germanium, provides energy to all body systems, promotes regeneration from stress and fatigue, and rebuilds foundation strength. A central nervous system stimulant, ginseng also nourishes reproductive and circulatory systems. Red ginseng is particularly beneficial for men since it promotes testosterone production. White and American ginsengs stimulate brain and memory centers for women as well as men.

—**Siberian Ginseng** (*eleuthero*): a tonic that supports the adrenal glands, circulation and memory.

—**Schizandra:** synergistic with eleuthero for stress, weight loss and sports endurance formulas, schizandra supports sugar regulation and liver function, helps keep aging skin healthy through better use of fats.

—**Suma:** an ancient herb with modern results for overcoming fatigue and hormonal imbalance. Widely used to rebuild the body from the ravages of cancer and diabetes.

—**Gotu Kola:** a brain and nervous system restorative. Considered an elixir of life and a longevity herb in Chinese medicine, it's a primary nerve and deep body healer after trauma or illness. Gotu kola has therapeutic applications for the skin, cellulite, wound repair, burns, scars (helps inhibit formation), and varicose veins.

—**Fo-Ti** (*Ho-Shou-Wu*): a flavonoid-rich herb with special success in longevity formulas. It is a cardiovascular strengthener, increasing blood flow to the heart.

—**Cordyceps:** an adaptogenic, antioxidant mushroom used for centuries in TCM. Gained its fame in 1993 after several Chinese long distance runners won gold medals following a Cordyceps-containing diet. Cordyceps boosts libido in men and women, improves impotence and increases sperm count.

—**Horsetail:** a nutritive herb rich in silica, a premier anti-aging mineral, which prevents wrinkling by boosting collagen formation, restores flexibility to arthritic joints, strengthens tooth and bone structure and, overall, increases the health of the body, especially the skin, hair and nails.

—**Noni:** a traditional Hawaiin medicinal herb highly effective for degenerative disease like diabetes, high blood pressure and heart disease. Regenerates at the cellular level, improving cell function and health. A pain reliever for carpal tunnel syndrome, tennis elbow and sciatica. Matrix NONI caps or liquid.

—**Bilberry:** a bioflavonoid-rich herb that helps keep connective tissues healthy and strengthens small blood vessels and capillaries, factors that keep skin youthful. Bilberry also protects against macular degeneration.

Note: Consider Crystal Star AGELESS VITALITY™ with the best of anti-aging, antioxidant, adaptogen herbs.

Are You Considering Anti-Aging Drugs or Supplements?
Read this chapter before you make a decision.

Many hormones, like melatonin, DHEA, Human Growth Hormone (hGH) and Pregnenolone are widely publicized for anti-aging.

1: Human growth hormone is the latest craze, but is it really an anti-aging miracle for men and women over 50?

hGH is produced by the pituitary gland height. It is available only by prescription, and a year! hGH treatment has some benefits. It hormone deficiency to grow, and it reduces improves skin elasticity and reduces wrinkles. sity, decreases body fat, and stimulate a sense

But before you rush to your doctor to get hGH is linked to carpal tunnel syndrome and youth); hGH increases diabetes risk; some sue growth. One of the most frightening re- who took the hGH to improve his perfor- because his bones literally grew through his

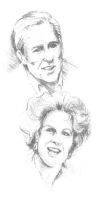

which promotes bone growth and regulates daily injections cost an astounding $8,000 helps very, very short children with growth tissue-wasting caused by advanced AIDS. It It even increases muscle mass and bone den- of well being in elderly men. your hGH prescription, know its cautions: aching joints (similar to "growing pains" in hGH users develop abnormal bone or tis- ports is the story of a professional athlete mance and had to have massive skin grafts skin!

You can boost growth hormone levels naturally! It's the best way to reap the benefits without the drawbacks. Weight training can boost hGH, as it increases the mass and strength of bones and muscle. The amino acids arginine and glutamine also affect the release of growth hormone. A 1995 study shows that oral glutamine supplements of 2000mg per day slightly increase hGH release. Arginine promotes an increase of hGH, especially when injected intravenously. A full spectrum amino acid complex like NutriCology FREE AMINOS in conjunction with weight training provides the best results.

Experts that I've spoken to at Allergy Research are developing a new, safer way to supplement the hGH superhormone. Growth hormone microdoses, monitored by a licensed health practitioner, appear to offer the same benefits with fewer health risks! Allergy Research Group BIOGEN PRO is a microdilution of growth hormone in a convenient spray delivery that is absorbed through the tissues of the mouth.

2: Pregenolone is popular today. Is it a good choice for anti-aging? Pregenenolone, (called PREG), is a steroid hormone made primarily in the adrenal glands from cholesterol. Considered by many the "grand-mother of all superhormones," PREG is the precursor to DHEA and progesterone in the body. PREG pro-duces a feeling of well being and increases energy levels; users also report heightened awareness and alertness (preliminary evidence suggests PREG stimulates brain receptors); in addition, it enhances visual and auditory perception (sometimes to hallucinatory levels at higher doses, especially in men). Like DHEA, pregenolone supplements can be synthesized in a lab from wild yam *diosgenin*.

There are cautions for using PREG: PREG induces central nervous system excitability and can cause in-somnia or shallow sleep; high doses (even 25mg a day) can cause irritability, anger, anxiety or headaches. Special groups of people like pregnant women, people with heart disease or people taking anti-depressant drugs or thyroid medication should avoid PREG. PREG is probably the most poorly researched of all the superhormones.

Are there natural alternatives to PREG? I recommend *gotu kola*, a ginseng-like adaptogen herb. Gotu kola boosts mental energy, promotes a feeling of well being, and heightens sensations without the safety risks of PREG. A good product choice with *gotu kola* and other ginseng-like herbs is Crystal Star's MENTAL INNER ENERGY™ formula. Meditation and deep breathing can also help you sharpen your awareness and help you live longer! A recent study finds that meditating just 20 minutes, twice a day, increases the average lifespan by 65%. Try it today!

3: Is melatonin really an anti-aging hormone?

We've all heard of the superhormone melatonin. Many people have used it as Nature's sleeping pill. Is it a safe choice for anti-aging? Melatonin, a hormone secreted by the pineal gland, sets our internal biological clock that governs our sleep/wake cycles or rhythms. One of the best benefits of melatonin is its ability to help with the effects of jet lag. Melatonin can even help the blind get better sleep, regulating sleep patterns for the sight-impaired by "telling" the person when it's time to sleep. I have met the medical doctor who discovered the hormone melatonin. Besides acknowledging that his melatonin work showed that our bodies sense night and day in a deeper way than by sight, he told me that if melatonin hadn't been labeled a hormone first, he would have called it an antioxidant!

Melatonin has some cautions. At high levels, it may temporarily shut down the reproductive system. A new contraceptive in Europe called B-Oval combines a very high dose of melatonin (75 mg) with progestin and is currently being used as birth control. Melatonin has become popular for other hormone effects as well. As an antioxidant, melatonin helps protect the body from free radical damage. Melatonin is also believed to reverse the shrinkage of the thymus a little, enabling it to produce more infection-fighting T-cells.

We know that every drug has side effects, and this is true of melatonin. Once melatonin supplementation begins, the body tends to shut down its own production of the hormone, perhaps putting an end to regular sleep for good. Melatonin can also cause nightmares, nausea and stomach cramps, decrease sex drive, and even shrink male gonads. In addition, there are many contraindications. Melatonin should not be taken with steroid medication, MAO inhibitors or sedative drugs. People with depression, SAD, mental illness, epilepsy, women trying to conceive or who are nursing should avoid melatonin.

4: DHEA, (*dehydro-epiandrosterone*), is being promoted for anti-aging for every adult over 45, but is there a downside?

DHEA is used by the body to manufacture other hormones, such as estrogen, testosterone, progesterone, and corticosterone. It has been touted as a substance that lowers serum cholesterol, reverses aging symptoms, and promotes energy and libido.

DHEA regulates the auto-immune mechanism, stimulating immune defenses to fight infections and monitoring over-reactions that might attack the body. It has thus proven helpful against lupus and rheumatoid arthritis. Research shows the importance of DHEA in preventing cancer, heart disease, and Alzheimer's disease.

DHEA supplements work for post-menopausal women with osteoporosis who are low in DHEA, much the same as estrogen replacement. Other symptoms of menopause are also relieved, and cancer risk associated with estrogen replacement is greatly reduced; it may even be prevented by DHEA's immune potential.

DHEA does have side effects. If you take too much, it suppresses your body's ability to make its own. Adult acne is a common side effect, as is excess perspiration, and facial and body hair. DHEA causes irritability, insomnia and mood swings in a significant number of people. It may also lead to confusion, headaches and liver damage, and should not be used by people with ovarian, thyroid or adrenal tumors. As a mild stimulant and blood thinner, it should not be used in combination with blood thinning drugs, aspirin or thyroid medication.

If DHEA is not right for you, you have other choices. Dioscorea (wild yam), contains *diosgenin* which some researchers think helps the body produce its own DHEA. In addition, breakthrough technology from Dr. C. Norman Shealy, M.D., Ph.D. , may increase your body's own production of DHEA. Shealy uses a subtle nerve stimulator and incorporates sythesized progesterone cream to stimulate 12 acupuncture points that boost your own DHEA production naturally. If you're interested, write to: Shealy Institute, 1328 East Evergreen, Springfield, MO 65803.

Note: For more information on these four super hormones, see THE ALTERNATIVE ARSENAL *section in this book.*

Exercise Is An Important Antioxidant Against Aging

Exercise doesn't have to be complicated. Simple mild stretches every morning oxygenate your tissues, limber your body, and help clear it of the previous night's waste. Stretches at night before bed help insure muscle relaxation and better rest. There are so many ways to bring exercise into your life: yoga, dance, sports like tennis or sailing, aerobic exercise, swimming, walking, jogging, bike riding or hiking.

There are two keys to maintaining regular exercise. Find something that you like, because that's something you'll do on a long term basis; and switch around your exercise activities so you don't get bored. Take an aerobics class one day, swim the next, play tennis on the weekend, etc.

Advantages of regular exercise for an anti-aging lifestyle:
—Exercise improves blood circulation and the body's ability to use oxygen for physical energy.
—Exercise helps reduce the risk for heart attacks and cancer.
—Exercise greatly contributes to weight control by fanning the metabolic fires.
—Exercise reduces stress and tension, and encourages relaxation.
—Exercise stimulates hormone production in men and women.
—Exercise contributes to strength and endurance. Inactivity contributes to fatigue.
—Weight bearing exercises trigger bone mineralization to help prevent osteoporosis.
—Exercise helps agility and joint mobility.

Amazingly, according to physical fitness experts, regular exercise makes the most difference in the oldest and *least* fit people. Take a walk every day, especially after your largest meal, for better circulation, energy, strength, stress reduction and enzyme function. Walking exercises both your body and your brain. Walking is an "antioxidant nutrient," that helps keep your immune system strong. Raising your heart rate just 20 beats per minute can markedly decrease your high blood pressure. Regular exercise also lowers your risk of falls as you age, one of the most serious health threats in our older years. Exercise becomes especially important to a man as he ages, because it helps maintain his sexual vigor and burns his excess fat. Don't leave exercise out of your anti-aging lifestyle program.

Deep breathing is a superb anti-aging technique

Deep breathing is a powerful way to decrease stress and increase calm energy. Low body oxygen can cause anxiety, depression, tight muscles, aches and pains and exacerbate chronic illness. Diaphragmatic breathing is the deepest kind of breathing. Deep diaphragm breathing lowers anxiety levels, relaxes and loosens muscles, and generates an inner feeling of peace and calm. Diaphragm breathing also strengthens heart and lungs, encourages more restful sleep and slows the aging process.

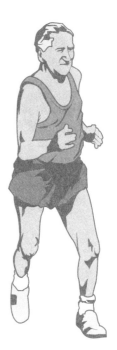

Here are some basic diaphragm breathing steps:
1) Inhale deeply through your nose. Try to fill your lungs.
2) Exhale slowly through your mouth.
3) Breathe deeply for 30 seconds. It takes less than a minute to calm and center yourself during anxious moments. Breathing deeply for just one minute prevents the short, quick breaths which negatively affect the oxygen-carbon dioxide content of your blood.
4) Now breathe deeply to fill the lower part of your lungs. Notice the pop-pop feeling in your chest as unused lung pockets open up. Your abdomen extends slightly as you fill it with air. Slowly exhale — your abdomen moves inward.
5) As you breathe in deeply, think of oxygen reaching and recharging all the cells of your body. As you exhale, imagine all the stress and tension leaving your body.

Can't find a recommended product? Call the 800 number in Product Resources for the store nearest you.

265

Anti-aging Techniques for Your Change of Life

The change of life comes to everyone. Both men and women experience body shape changes and hormonal fluctuations at mid-life. We all know menopause as the change of life for women. Mid-life change for men is much less discussed, even in the medical community. But "andropause" is a real phenomenon and, for some men, it can cause unusual fatigue, anxiety, even impotence!

Life changes are natural, but any change can be difficult. I find a change may be just what our bodies need at this phase of our lives. Most people I've talked to adjust, even embrace their changes, especially after they've taken steps in their diet and lifestyle to insure their health for the years to come.

Natural Therapies For Andropause

Eight in ten family physicians today recognize male andropause as a real change of life for men comparable to female menopause. Symptoms to watch for include: low energy; slow facial or head hair growth; decrease in muscle mass; lost height or early osteoporosis; enlarged prostate; depression; less strong or less frequent erections; lower than normal sex drive.

1: Reduce fried foods, red meats and fatty dairy foods (full of disrupting hormones), caffeine and sugar — all deplete the adrenals and drain male energy.

2: Don't go too far. An extremely low fat diet is disastrous for andropausal health. Penn State University studies find it may reduce testosterone levels... almost to preadolescent levels — definitely bad news for an older man! Include healthy fats from seafood and cold water fish, and lean meats such as hormone-free turkey and chicken regularly. Consider flax seed oil as a healthy oil to use in salad dressings. (Use about 1 TB.)

3: Increase your intake of zinc to renew sexual potency. Zinc, highly concentrated in semen, is the most important nutrient for male sexual function. Eat high zinc foods like liver, oysters, brewer's yeast, nuts and seeds regularly. Add zinc-rich spirulina to your superfood supplement list.

4: Check your alcohol intake. Heavy drinking can lead to prostate problems and impaired erections. DHT elevation, linked to testosterone decline and elevation of female hormones, is definitely undesirable for men.

5: Take care of your prostate. Research documented in the Quarterly Review of Natural Medicine finds *saw palmetto* reduces the symptoms of BPH by blocking DHT (di-hydro-testosterone), and inhibiting the enzyme 5-alpha reductase related to prostate enlargement. Consider Crystal Star PROX™ FOR MEN with *saw palmetto* and *pygeum* to help reduce prostate enlargement and dribbling urine. Morada Research Laboratories PROSTATE is a prostate tonic that reduces inflammation and enhances tissue repair.

6: For sexual virility, try the herb *tribulus terrestris.* An Ayurvedic herb, tribulus has been used since ancient times as a treatment for increasing libido and impotence in men. I recommend Nutritional Technologies T2 - TRIBULUS TERRESTIS. As an alternative, Crystal Star's MALE PERFORMANCE™ caps have a long history of success for strengthening the male system and enhancing the sexual experience.

7: Regular exercise is a vital component of male sexual health. It makes the body stronger, function more efficiently and have greater stamina. In one study, 78 healthy, but sedentary men were studied during nine months of regular exercise. The men exercised for 60 minutes a day, three days a week. Every man in the study reported significantly enhanced sexuality, including increased frequency, performance and satisfaction. Rising sexuality was even correlated with the degree of fitness improvement. The more physical fitness the men were able to attain, the better their sex life!

Renewing female balance during menopause is an area I've worked with for over 20 years. The best stories come from women who take menopause as an opportunity to become more in tune with the changing needs of their bodies. Gentle herbs are a good choice to regulate hormone fluctuations safely and naturally without the side effects and risks of harsh hormone drugs that overwhelm the body and disrupt delicate female balance.

Most women are highly sensitive to even small fluctuations in hormone levels. At menopause, this sensitivity tends to magnify as hormone shifts become even more pronounced. Symptoms to look for: great fatigue; hot flashes and night sweats; mood swings; nighttime panic attacks; weight gain; bone loss; vaginal dryness or atrophy (usually pain with intercourse); unusually dry skin; migraine headaches.

Natural Therapies For Menopause

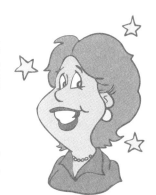

1: Reduce the bad fats in your diet. Fats are storage for excess estrogen that lead to many hormone-driven diseases (like breast cancer). Steam and bake foods — never fry. Especially avoid commercial red meats and fatty dairy products (regularly injected with hormones) that disrupt delicate female balance.

2: Add good fats, like those in seafood often for hormone balancing omega 3 essential fatty acids. Women I talk to report smoother skin, enhanced mental clarity and increased libido when they follow a high seafood diet. Salmon is particularly beneficial. I try to eat salmon at least once a week.

3: Eat soy foods like tofu, tempeh, miso or soy milk regularly. Recent Italian studies found women who took a soy protein isolate had a 45% reduction in hot flashes! An added perk: Several new studies find eating just 1.5 oz. of soy foods lowers total cholesterol 9%. LDL, bad cholesterol, drops as much as 13%!

4: Regulate your estrogen levels by increasing your fiber from whole grains and fresh vegetables. Add boron-containing foods like leafy greens, fruits, nuts and legumes to strengthen bones against menopausal bone loss.

5: Target menopausal symptoms with herbs. I've used Crystal Star EST-AID™ Caps with gentle, phytoestrogen herbs for years as a revitalizer that dramatically reduces hot flashes. The formula has been lab tested in over 200 tests by a third party, non-profit lab. It clearly inhibits breast cancer cell growth in test tubes! Transitions For Women HOT FLASH FORMULA is another good choice with bioflavonoids structurally similar to the body's own estrogen.

6: Herbs can come to your rescue if get panic attacks. I'm in the process of developing a complex herbal HEART STABILIZER formula for women with herbs like *hawthorn*, *arjuna*, and *passionflowers* to normalize heart palpitations and reduce stress-related panic attacks during menopause. Preliminary results look very good. Ask a knowledgable health professional if an herbal heart stabilizer is right for you.

7: Essential oils reduce menopausal depression. Add a few drops of clary sage, jasmine (also revs up libido), neroli, bergamot or geranium to a diffuser and inhale the aroma for 20 minutes.

8: During menopause, the vaginal lining may become thin and dry due to reduced circulating estrogen. Intercourse may become painful, and there's increased susceptibility to vaginal infection. I recommend Crystal Star WOMAN'S DRYNESS extract (works almost overnight); or apply pure aloe vera gel or natural vitamin E oil. Panax ginseng also helps your body produce more fluid.

Normalizing hormone balance with diet and herbs is a gentle and easy way to sail through menopausal and andropausal body changes. I know I'll keep my change!

Can't find a recommended product? Call the 800 number in Product Resources for the store nearest you.

267

Optimizing Exercise & Sports Performance
Getting The Most Out Of Your Exercise Choices

The latest statistics are shocking! We may all know exercise is critical to good health, that exercise speeds results in weight loss and strengthens our hearts, but new National Institute of Health studies reveal that as many as 58% of adult Americans get no or little exercise. A sedentary lifestyle has the same effect on heart disease risk as smoking a pack of cigarettes a day!

Regular exercise is also a significant part of a healing program. It strengthens your whole body — muscles, nerves, blood, glands, lungs, heart, brain, mind and mood. It increases your metabolic rate, muscle mass, oxygen uptake, circulation, and boosts the enzymes that help your body burn fat. Exercise is the key to stress control, low cholesterol and a sharper memory. It also stimulates antibody production, enhances immune response, and reduces fatigue. Exercise is the best mood elevator of all! By releasing pain-relieving endorphins, exercise reduces anxiety, relieves depression and extends your lifespan.

Exercise optimizes metabolism, especially brown fat activity. Brown fat is highly active metabolically, very different from yellow fat (the kind you see deposited around your body). Brown fat is bound to your skeleton and is filled with tiny, brown-colored, mitochondria and cytochromes, chemical powerhouses that produce energy in your cells. Brown fat is thermogenically responsive. When you take in excess calories, your body compensates in part by producing more heat to burn them off instead of storing them as yellow fat. Brown fat activity explains why some people can overeat and stay slim while other people gain weight easily.

For most of us, brown fat becomes less active and less thermogenically responsive as we age. Instead of calories being burned off, they get stored as yellow fat. Keeping your brown fat activated is a big key to weight control as you age. Brown fat activity goes down if your diet is poor and you don't get regular aerobic exercise to increase your lung capacity and elevate your heart rate. Putting on weight and not exercising causes lean muscle tissue to break down, leaving you flabby, with less energy, and ultimately, with even less brown fat activity to burn calories.

Exercise is easy and as available as your front door. A daily, thirty minute walk, breathing deeply, for even a mile a day ($\frac{1}{2}$ mile out, $\frac{1}{2}$ mile back) makes a big difference to brown fat activity. Deep exhalations release metabolic waste along with CO_2; deep inhalations flood your body with fresh oxygen. A walk cleans your circulatory system, and improves heart strength and muscle tone. It reduces heart attack risk, especially in women. Think of sunlight on your body as **heliotherapy** adding natural vitamin D for skin and bone health.

If you don't exercise, you'll not only lose muscle, you'll lose about 1% of your bone mass every year.... it can begin as early as age 35. Walking, jogging or cycling increases both muscle and bone mass.

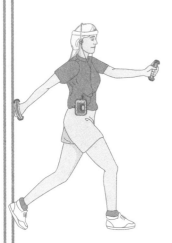

You don't need to overdo it to reap the rewards of exercise. Two different studies published in the Journal of the American Medical Association show moderate exercise is as beneficial for the cardiovascular system and overall fitness as high intensity workouts. Pick an exercise that you enjoy and stick to it!

Dancing is one of the best aerobic exercises I know. Legs and lungs both show rapid improvement, not to mention the fun you have. Any kind of dancing is a good workout, and the breathlessness you feel afterward is the best sign of aerobic benefits. **Swimming** works all parts of your body at once. Noticeable upper arm and thigh definition improvement comes quickly with regular swimming. Just fifteen to twenty steady laps, two or three times a week, and a more streamlined body is yours. (I use water weights when I swim to maximize my exercise.) **Cycling** gets you somewhere while you exercise. **Exercise classes** are easily available, everyday, everywhere at low prices.

Can't find a recommended product? Call the 800 number in Product Resources for the store nearest you.

If your schedule is so busy that you hardly have time to breathe, let alone exercise, but still want the benefits of bodywork, there is an all-in-one aerobic exercise. It has gotten resounding enthusiasm and response rates for aerobic activity and muscle tone - all in one minute. The exercise sounds very easy, but is actually very difficult, and that is why it works so well. You will be breathless (the sign of an effective aerobic workout) before you know it.

Simply lie flat on your back on a rug or carpet. Rise to a full standing position any way you can, and lie down flat on your back again. That's the whole exercise. Stand and lie down, stand and lie down — for one minute. Typical repetitions for most people with average body tone are six to ten times in 60 seconds. The record time for an athlete in top competitive condition is 20-24 times in a minute. Be very easy on yourself. Repeat only as many times as you feel comfortable and work up gradually. It is worth a try because it exercises muscles, lung capacity and circulatory system so well.... but don't overdo it.

Whatever exercise program you choose for yourself, make rest a part of it. Work out harder one day, go easy the next; or exercise for several days and take two days off. It's better for body balance, and will increase your energy levels when you exercise the next time. After a regular program is started, exercising four days a week will increase fitness level; exercising three days a week maintains fitness level; exercising two days a week will decrease a high fitness level. But any amount of exercise is better than nothing at all.

Choose those that work for you conveniently and easily. Vigorous physical exercise is the most efficient way to burn yellow fat, but every series of stretches and exercises you do tones, elasticizes, shapes and contours your skin, connective tissue and muscles.

Eating For Energy & Performance

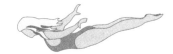

Body building is 85% nutrition. Nutrition is the most important factor for exercise or sports performance, at any level. Long-term, optimal nutrition is the basis for high performance. Protein or carbo-loading before an event can't make up for nutrient short-falls. No anabolic supplement of any kind can give you athletic excellence if you have an inferior diet. Good nutrition helps eliminate fluctuating energy levels, abnormal fatigue, and susceptibility to injury or illness. When you eat junk foods, you pay the penalty of poor performance.

Exercise is integral to good nutrition. Most of us notice that when we're exercising we're not hungry. We're thirsty after a workout as our bodies call for water and electrolyte replacement, but not hungry. One of the reasons rapid results are achieved in a body streamlining program is this phenomenon. Muscles become toned, heart and lungs become stronger, and fats are lost, but the body doesn't call for calorie replacement right away. Its own glycogens lift blood sugar levels for a feeling of well being. **Exercise becomes a nutrient in itself.**

The breakdown of a high performance diet: Sixty to seventy-five percent should be in clean-burning complex carbohydrates — from whole grains, pasta, vegetables, rice, beans and fruits. They improve performance, promote muscle fuel storage, and absorb easily without excess fats that slow down weight loss and sap energy.

Twenty to twenty-five percent should be in protein from whole grains, nuts, beans, low fat dairy products, soy foods, yogurt, kefir, eggs, and some poultry, fish, and seafood. Vegetable protein is best for mineral absorption and bone density. Strength and muscle mass decline if you get too little protein. But eating too much protein, especially from red meats (as is in the highly popular "Zone" and "Zone clone" diets) hampers performance. Excess amino acids from too much protein cause toxic ammonia to form in the body. Too much protein may overload your kidneys (you'll feel lower back pain) as your body struggles to eliminate waste by-products from inefficient metabolism. To learn more, see "Protein in a Healing Diet" on pg 133 of this book.

Can't find a recommended product? Call the 800 number in Product Resources for the store nearest you.

269

Ten to fifteen percent of an athletic diet should be in energy-producing fats and oils necessary for glycogen storage. The best fats are mono-or polyunsaturated oils, a little butter, nuts, low fat cheeses and whole grain snacks.

Other diet fuel should be liquid nutrients; fruit juices for natural sugars, mineral waters and electrolyte replacement drinks for potassium, magnesium and sodium, and "superfoods." Superfoods are highly concentrated, bio-available nutrients that can give an athlete the edge in strength and stamina. Green superfood blends contain concentrates of spirulina, alfalfa, chlorella, barley grass, blue-green algae and wheat grass. Bee pollen and royal jelly are rich in essential nutritional elements. Aged garlic has valuable properties for the athlete, providing anti-fatigue and anti-stress effects, and potent antioxidants for free radical protection.

Drink plenty of water. Without an ample fluids, waste and impurities don't get filtered or released, and the liver doesn't metabolize stored fats for energy. Six to eight glass of water a day are a must, even if you don't feel thirsty. Drink at least 16-oz. of water two hours before exercise to prepare for exercise-related water-mineral loss.

Three Proven Strength Diets

Strength nutrition enhances endurance, speed and focus. Strength nutrition helps prevent injury, reduces stress, lets you carry more oxygen, replaces ATP, removes lactic acid and improves electrolyte balance. For the serious athlete, strength nutrition can create the edge that makes the difference between winning and losing, especially in the last burst of energy for peak performance.

Three tried and true strength nutrition diets to choose from:

1: **HIGH ENERGY, ACTIVE LIFE STYLE DIET** - targeted for people who lack consistent daily energy and tire easily, and those who need more endurance and strength for hard physical jobs or long hours. It is also for weekend sports enthusiasts who wish to accomplish more than their present level of nutrition allows.

2: **MODERATE AEROBIC DIET** - for people who work out 3 to 4 times a week. It emphasizes complex carbohydrates for smooth muscle use, and moderate fat and protein amounts. Complex carbohydrates also produce glycogen for the body, resulting in better energy and endurance.

3: **HIGH PERFORMANCE-TRAINING DIET** - concentrates on energy for competitive sports action, and long range stamina. For the serious athlete, and for those who are consciously body building for high workout achievement, this diet is a good foundation for significantly improved performance. Sports tests show that adjusting the diet before competition can increase endurance 200% or more — well worth consideration.

Athletes' nutrition needs are considerably greater than those of the average person. Normal RDAs are far too low for high performance or competition needs. Consult a good sports nutritionist, or knowledgable person at a health food store or gym to determine your specific supplement requirements. The important consideration is not body weight, but body composition.

All three diets are useful for a serious, performing athlete. Competitive training and a training diet alone cannot insure success. Rest time and building energy reserves are also necessary to tune the body for maximum efficiency. When not in competition or pre-event training, extra high nutrient amounts are not needed, and can be hard for the body to handle. A reduced density diet is better for maintaining tone, and can be easily increased for competitive performance.

Note: See the following 2 pages for a FOOD EXCHANGE LIST and a FOOD AMOUNTS CHART by diet so you can adjust individual needs.

Food Exchange List

Any food in a category may be exchanged one-for-one with any other food in that category. Portion amounts are given for a man weighing 170 pounds, and a woman weighing 130 pounds.

Grains, Breads and Cereals: One serving is approximately one cup of cooked grains, such as brown rice, millet, barley, bulgur, kashi, couscous, corn, oats, and whole grain pasta;
> or one cup of dry cereals, such as bran flakes, Oatios, or Grapenuts;
> or three slices of wholegrain bread; or three six-inch corn tortillas; or two chapatis or whole wheat pita breads;
> or twelve small wholegrain crackers; or two rice cakes.

Vegetables:
Group A: One serving is as much as you want of lettuce (all kinds), Chinese greens and peas, raw spinach and carrots, celery, cucumbers, endive, sea greens, watercress, radishes, green onions and chives.
Group B: One serving is two cups cabbage or alfalfa sprouts; or $1\frac{1}{2}$ cups cooked bell peppers or mushrooms;
—or one cup cooked asparagus, cauliflower, chard, sauerkraut, eggplant, zucchini or summer squash;
—or $\frac{3}{4}$ cup cooked broccoli, green beans; onions or mung bean sprouts; or $\frac{1}{2}$ cup vegetable juice cocktail;
Group C: One serving is approximately $1\frac{1}{2}$ cups cooked carrots;
—or one cup cooked beets, potatoes, or leeks; or one cup fresh carrot or vegetable juice;
—or $\frac{1}{2}$ cup cooked peas, corn, artichokes, winter squash or yams.

Fruits: One serving is approximately one apple, nectarine, mango, pineapple, peach or orange;
—or 4 apricots, medjool dates or figs; or half a honeydew or cantaloupe;
—or 20 to 24 cherries or grapes; or one and a half cups strawberries or other berries.

Dairy: One serving is approximately one cup of whole milk, buttermilk or full fat yogurt, for 3mg of fat;
—or one cup of low-fat milk or yogurt, for 2gm. of fat;
—or one cup of skim milk or non-fat yogurt, for less than 1gm. of fat;
—or one ounce of low fat hard cheese, such as swiss or cheddar;
—or $\frac{1}{3}$ cup of non-fat dry milk powder.

Poultry, Fish and Seafood: One serving is approximately 4-oz. of white fish skinned, for 3gm of fat;
—or four ounces of chicken or turkey, white meat, no skin for 4gm of fat;
—or one cup of tuna or salmon, water packed for 3gm of fat;
—or one cup of shrimp, scallops, oysters, clams or crab for 3 to 4gm of fat.

Note: I recommend avoiding red meats – beef, veal, lamb, pork, sausage, ham, and bacon. They are high in saturated fats and cholesterol, and unsound as a use of planetary resources. Many are routinely injected with hormones and antibiotics.

High Protein Meat and Dairy Substitutes: One serving is approximately four ounces of tofu (one block);
—or $\frac{1}{2}$ cup low fat or dry cottage cheese; or $\frac{1}{3}$ cup ricotta, parmesan or mozzarella;
—or one egg; or $\frac{1}{2}$ cup cooked beans or brown rice.

Fats and Oils: One serving is approximately one teaspoon of butter, margarine or shortening for 5gm of fat;
—or one tablespoon of salad dressing or mayonnaise for 5gm. of fat;
—or 2 teaspoons of poly-unsaturated or mono-unsaturated vegetable oil for 5gm. of fat.

The following foods are high in fat; amounts are equivalent to 1 fat serving on the diet chart. Use sparingly.
—2 tablespoons of light cream, half and half, or sour cream; 1 tablespoon of heavy cream;
—$\frac{1}{6}$ slice of avocado; $\frac{1}{4}$ cup of sunflower, sesame, or pumpkin seeds;
—12 almonds, cashews or peanuts; 20 pistachios or Spanish peanuts; 4 walnut or pecan halves.

Food Amounts Chart By Diet

Scale servings up or down to fit your individual weight and type of active diet.

Daily Diet for Men Approx. 170 pounds			**Daily Diet for Women** Approx. 130 pounds		
High Energy, Active Life Diet Calories 2800 Protein 17% Carbos 70% Fat 13%	**Moderate Aerobic Diet** Calories 3250 Protein 20% Carbos 65% Fat 15%	**Training & Competition Diet** Calories 3950 Protein 23% Carbos 65% Fat 12%	**High Energy, Active Life Diet** Calories 2000 Protein 17% Carbos 70% Fat 13%	**Moderate Aerobic Diet** Calories 2200 Protein 20% Carbos 65% Fat 15%	**Training & Competition Diet** Calories 2750 Protein 23% Carbos 65% Fat 12%
6 whole grain servings	7 whole grain servings	8 whole grain servings	4 whole grain servings	4 whole grain servings	6 whole grain servings
Group A vegetables - all you want	Group A vegetables - all you want	Group A vegetables - all you want	Group A vegetables - all you want	Group A vegetables - all you want	Group A vegetables - all you want
Group B vegetables - 6 servings	Group B vegetables - 6 servings	Group B vegetables - 7 servings	Group B vegetables - 4 servings	Group B vegetables - 4 servings	Group B vegetables - 6 servings
Group C vegetables - 6 servings	Group C vegetables - 6 servings	Group C vegetables - 8 servings	Group C vegetables - 3 servings	Group C vegetables - 4 servings	Group C vegetables - 5 servings
5 fruit servings	5 fruit servings	6 fruit servings	3 fruit servings	`4 fruit servings	4 fruit servings
3 dairy servings	4 dairy servings	4 dairy servings	2 dairy servings	3 dairy servings	3 dairy servings
2 poultry or seafood servings	4 poultry or seafood servings	5 poultry or seafood servings	1 poultry or seafood servings	1 poultry or seafood servings	3 poultry or seafood servings
5 fat servings	5 fat servings	6 fat servings	3 fat servings	3 fat servings	3 fat servings

Can't find a recommended product? Call the 800 number in Product Resources for the store nearest you.

Supplements & Herbs For Bodybuilding & Sports Performance

Strength training supplements are good for both the serious and casual athlete. They help build muscle tissue, maintain low body fat, and improve endurance when the body is under the stress of a workout series. Supplements optimize recuperation time between workouts, are proven for muscle growth and speed healing from sports-related injuries. Antioxidant supplements are a byword for sports performance, because they help maintain the body's defenses against exercise-induced free radicals to combat injury and speed muscle recovery.

How you take training supplements is as important as what you take. Your program will be more productive if you balance supplements between workout days and rest days. Muscle growth occurs on rest days as your body uses the training you've been giving it. Increase enhancement by taking vitamins, minerals, and glandulars on your rest days. Take proteins, amino acids, anabolics and herbs on workout days, before the workout.

Herbal supplements are efficient partners in your exercise program. Herbs act as concentrated food nutrients for body building. They offer extra strength for energy and endurance, and they have been used since ancient times by athletes. Yarrow and other herbs were used by the gladiators to help heal wounds. Chinese and Japanese warriors and wrestlers used herbs to increase endurance and strength from pre-history to the present. In Russia, Germany, Japan and Korea, herbs are extremely popular with sports enthusiasts and athletes. American athletes are just beginning to see the value of herbs for a winning body.

Herbal supplements work better in combination, and they work best when taken on exercise days, either in the morning with a protein drink, or 30 minutes before exertion.

Herbs you can use for your exercise program:
—**Antioxidant Herbs For Aerobic Support:** *Siberian ginseng, ginkgo biloba, barley grass, spirulina, chlorella, American and Chinese panax ginseng, rosemary, white pine bark*; Crystal Star ANTI-OXIDANT™ extract.
—**Adaptogen Herbs For Body Stress:** *American and Chinese panax ginseng, Chinese astragalus, schizandra, ashwaganda, fo-ti, Siberian ginseng, damiana*; Crystal Star ACTIVE PHYSICAL ENERGY™ extract.
—**Anti-Inflammatory Herbs For Injuries:** *turmeric, St. John's wort, and arnica*; Crystal Star STRESSED OUT™ extract (usually results in 20 minutes). *Lavender* essential oil, mixed with almond oil, relieves inflammation.
—**Energy Stimulants:** *guarana, ginkgo biloba, damiana, kola nut, gotu kola*; Crystal Star HIGH PERFORMANCE™ caps, HIGH ENERGY™ tea, or RAINFOREST ENERGY™ caps. Nutritional Technologies T2-TRIBULUS TERRESTRIS.
—**Stamina and Endurance Herbs:** *Siberian ginseng, sarsaparilla, wild yam, schizandra, spirulina, American and Chinese panax ginseng, fo-ti*; Crystal Star HIGH PERFORMANCE™ caps.
—**Adrenal Tonics:** *licorice, ginseng*; Crystal Star ADRN-ACTIVE™ or GINSENG-LICORICE extracts.
—**Blood Tonic Herbs:** *chlorella, spirulina, barley grass, yellow dock root, sarsaparilla* and *goldenseal*; Crystal Star ENERGY GREEN™ drink, SYSTEMS STRENGTH™ drink or caps.
—**Circulation Activators:** *ginkgo biloba, cayenne, ginger*; Crystal Star HEARTSEASE CIRCU-CLEANSE™.
—**Metabolic Enhancers:** *sarsaparilla, licorice root, bee pollen, royal jelly, panax ginseng*, green tea; Crystal Star MALE PERFORMANCE™ caps and THERMO-CITRIN GINSENG™ caps and extract.
—**Anabolic Stimulants:** *suma*; Crystal Star GINSENG 6 SUPER CAPS™.
—**Muscle Relaxers for Soreness:** *valerian, passionflowers*; Crystal Star STRESSED OUT™ extract.
—**Workout Recovery and Nerve Strength:** *sarsaparilla, suma, carrot rt.*; Crystal Star BODY REBUILDER™.
—**Mineral-Rich Herbs:** *yellow dock root, barley grass, dandelion*; Crystal Star MINERAL SPECTRUM™ caps.

Note: Mineral balance is critical for an athlete at any level. Macro and trace minerals are built into every bio-chemical action of athletic movement... energy, digestion, use of vitamins and protein, nerve transmission, muscle contraction, metabolism, cholesterol levels and blood sugar. Athletes should replace electrolytes lost after workouts. Nature's Path TRACE-LYTE is a true electrolyte formula.

Do You Really Need Steroids For High Performance?

As standards of excellence rise in sports competition, steroid use, legal and illegal is increasing. Steroids lead to wholesale destruction of gland tissue, stunted growth from bone closure, male testicle shrinkage, low sperm counts with sterility (noticeable after only a few months of use), male breast enlargement, weakening of connective tissue, jaundice from liver malfunction, poor circulation, and hostile personality behavior and facial changes.

Superhormone steroids like ANDRO (*androstenedione*) are highly popular today. ANDRO, a by-product of DHEA is synthesized from the seeds of the Scotch Pine tree. Studies show ANDRO increases the body's testosterone supply up to three times the normal level. According to experts at Allergy Research, ANDRO is most effective for accelerating healing from sports injuries. However, ANDRO should be used cautiously, and under the supervision of a health professional. It can boost testosterone levels too much and too fast, causing aggressive behavior and acne. ANDRO may actually convert into estrogen in the body, possibly leading to breast growth or water retention in men. And, the conversion of androstenedione to estrogen accelerates aging in both men and women! Don't use ANDRO if you have any hormone-related problems like cancers of the breast, prostate or testes. People with acne, liver disorders, BPH, dysmenorrhea or Cushing's adrenal syndrome should also avoid ANDRO.

Creatine (*methyl guanidine-acetic acid*), a popular steroid-like supplement, is a booming $100 million business. It's found in large amounts in the muscles, formed when the amino acids arginine, methionine and glycine are combined in the body. Its food sources are meats and fish. Creatine helps provide the energy (ATP) muscles need to move. It is especially useful for the rapid, explosive movements required in many sports. But there are risk factors that you need to know about. Creatine forces muscles to retain too much water, leading to strains and dehydration. I spoke to Rod Fleming, respected member of the advisory board for my newsletter, Natural Healing Report, and registered physical therapist. Fleming say, "Dehydration is consistently a problem for people using creatine. I have also personally seen very unusual muscle tears (pectoral) in people taking this supplement. I advise against it." If you choose to try creatine, take it only as directed and drink plenty of fluids. (Don't mix it with fruit juice; creatine can react with fruit juice and transform into creatinine, a metabolic waste product.)

Ribose is a sports' supplement with some advantages over ANDRO and creatine. Ribose is a simple sugar our cells use to convert nutrients into ATP. As a supplement, ribose increases energy stores in the heart and muscle cells, especially useful for people with cardiac insufficiency (diminished blood flow to the heart) and athletes who want to increase muscle endurance and decrease recovery time from workouts. Natural Balance RIBOSE RIBOMAX — maintenance doses equal 3 to 5 grams per day.

Can herbal steroids do the strength enhancement job? There are no magic bullets for energy or endurance in sports, but plant-derived steroids called phytosterols do have growth activity similar to that of free form amino acids and anabolic steroids. Amino acids can act as steroid alternatives to help build the body to competitive levels without chemical steroid consequences. They also help release growth hormone, detox ammonia, promote fast recuperation, increase stamina, and support peak performance.

The most well-known of these herbs are:
—Damiana, a mild aphrodisiac and nerve stimulant.
—Sarsaparilla Root, *Smilax*, coaxes the body to produce more anabolic hormones, testosterone and cortisone.
—Saw Palmetto, a urethral toning herb that increases blood flow to the sexual organs; balances testosterone.
—Siberian and Panax Ginsengs, adaptogens for over-all body balance and energy.
—Wild Yam, an anti-spasmodic that prevents cramping. Contains diosgenin, a phyto progesterone.
—Yohimbe, a testosterone precursor for body building, and potent aphrodisiac for both men and women.
—Tribulus Terrestris,= an ancient treatment for low libido and impotence; increases strength and stamina.

Supplementing Your Individual Exercise Requirements

The following pages detail three separate supplement programs:
1) high energy active lifestyle, 2) moderate aerobic workout, 3) high performance and competitive training.

Supplements for a high energy active lifestyle:

Use superfoods to supercharge your diet for energy. Here are some to try:

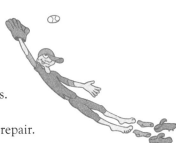

—**Crystal Star ENERGY GREEN DRINK™** - a concentrated, body-building, whole green drink with herbs.
—**NutriCology PRO-GREENS with EFA's** - green superfoods, herbs, sea greens.
—**Nature's Path TRACE-MIN-LYTE** - full spectrum minerals from sea greens.
—**Herbal Products Development POWER-PLUS** - food enzymes- healing and repair.
—**Esteem SUPER PRO** - an ultra-multi plus megaforce nutrients.
—**Natural Balance RIBOSE RIBO-MAX** to replenish ATP energy
—**Futurebiotics MAXATIVA** - for men; **Floradix HERBAL IRON** for women.
—**Jones Products SPORTS STAR HEALTH pak** - vitamin, mineral, antioxidant multi-pak.

Supplements for a moderate aerobics workout:

Superfoods: *For deep body strength and faster recovery.*
—**Green Foods MAGMA PLUS** - a phytonutrient-rich combination of organic barley grass powder plus 57 other natural ingredients including antioxidants, chlorophyll, digestive enzymes, prebiotics (FOS) and probiotics.
—**Pines MIGHTY GREENS SUPERFOOD BLEND** - a blend of premium organic cereal grasses and alfalfa, plus spirulina, chlorella, ginkgo biloba, royal jelly and 18 other superfoods and herbs.
—**Futurebiotics VITAL GREEN** - contains alfalfa leaf juice, barley grass juice, spirulina, and chlorella.

Minerals: *You need minerals to run - for bone density, speed and endurance; as anabolic enhancers.*
—**Potassium-magnesium-bromelain combo** - relieves muscle fatigue/lactic acid buildup.
—**Cal-mag-zinc combo with boron** - to prevent muscle cramping and maintain bone integrity.
—**Chromium picolinate**, 200mcg - for sugar regulation and glucose energy use.
—**Zinc picolinate**, 30-50mg daily for athletes - for immunity, healing of epithelial injuries.
—**Crystal Star MINERAL SPECTRUM™, IRON and CALCIUM SOURCE™** extract and capsules.
—**Nature's Path CAL-LYTE or HEMA-LYTE iron**, electrolytes for strong muscles.

Vitamins: *Metabolize blood and body fats, and enhance muscle growth.*
—**B-complex, 100mg or more** - for nerve health, muscle cramping, carbohydrate metabolism.
—**Lewis Labs BREWER'S YEAST** - chromium fortified to stimulate protein synthesis.
—**Unipro TRIMETABOLIC** and **PRO-OPTIMIZER.**
—**Jones Pro SPORTS STAR ATHLETIC PAK** - vitamins, minerals, amino acids, support nutrients.

Antioxidants: *To increase oxygen use, reduce free radical damage, and to protect against pollutants.*
—**CoQ-10** - a catalyst co-enzyme factor to produce and release energy.
—**Wakunaga KYOLIC SUPER FORMULA 105** - several potent antioxidants.
—**NutriCology ANTIOX FORMULA 11**- offers a potent mixed antioxidant formulation.

Sports Drinks/Electrolyte Replacements: *Use after exertion to replace body minerals.*
—**Champion Nutrition REVENGE**
—**Twin Lab ULTRA FUEL**
—**Anabol Naturals CARBO SURGE** and **Nature's Path TRACE-LYTE** liquid electrolytes
—**Unipro ENDURA**
—**Knudsens RECHARGE**

Can't find a recommended product? Call the 800 number in Product Resources for the store nearest you.

Testosterone Support: *As part of a natural anabolic program for increased male muscle hardness.*
—Crystal Star ACTIVE PHYSICAL ENERGY™ with panax ginseng
—Muira Pauma Bark (potency wood), saw palmetto and sarsaparilla (*smilax*) herbs
—Anabol Naturals DHEA REJUVAPLEX with L-Glutamine and crystalline vitamine B-12
—Unipro TRIBULUS SYNERGY

Stimulants: *for quick, temporary, energy.*
—Natural Balance RIBOSE RIBO-MAX to replenish ATP energy
—Crystal Star ACTIVE PHYSICAL ENERGY™ or HIGH PERFORMANCE™ caps

Free Form Amino Acids: *Activators to increase body structure and strength.*
—Arginine/Ornithine/Lysine combo, 750mg, to burn fats for energy - Anabol Naturals GH RELEASERS
—Anabol Naturals AMINO BALANCE - 23 crystalline free-form amino acids for tissue repair and energy.
—AmeriFit GOLD PAK, pre-digested amino acids - easily absorbed for better performance.
—Carnitine, 500mg - to strengthen heart and circulatory system during long exercise bouts.
—Anabol Naturals MUSCLE OCTANE or AMINO NITRO MAX, BCAAs for ATP energy conversion.
—Glutamine, strong growth hormone release.
—Unipro BCAA 1000

Protein/Amino Drinks: *Mainstays for muscle building, weight gain, energy, endurance.*
—Twin Lab AMINO FUEL liquid - effective twice daily for endurance energy.
—Twin Lab GAINERS FUEL 1000 - for maximum weight gain.
—Nature's Life SUPER-GREEN PRO-96 green protein.
—Champion LEAN GAINER - low-fat weight gainer.
—Unipro PERFECT PROTEIN
—Bee pollen - complete, natural full spectrum amino acids.

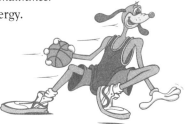

Fat Burners: *Metabolize blood and body fats, and enhance muscle growth.*
—Nature's Path SLIM-LYTE 1200 - chromium to burn fat, not muscle tissue.
—Anabol Naturals GH RELEASERS - metabolic fat burner
—Unipro TRIMETABOLIC

Sports Bars: *Rich sources of carbohydrates, protein and fiber.*
—EAS® MYOPLEX DELUXE™
—EAS® MYOPLEX LITE™
—Power Foods POWER BARS; SOURCE OF LIFE ENERGY BARS
—Unipro BURN BAR

Glandulars: *For gland and hormone stimulation.*
—Pituitary, 200mg - the master gland, for upper body development.
—Adrenal, 500mg - Country Life ADRENAL w. L-Tyrosine, Crystal Star ADR-ACTIVE™ phyto-glandular.
—Liver, 400mg - for fat metabolism, Enzymatic Therapy LIQUID LIVER EXTRACT with *Siberian Ginseng*.
—Unipro PRO-OPTIMIZER

Recovery Acceleration: *For muscles, joints, ligaments, tendons.*
—Proteolytic Enzymes - break down scar tissue build-up and shortens recovery time after injury.
—Bromelain-Papain 500mg - for muscle and ligament repair and strength.
—Natural Balance RIBOSE RIBO-MAX to replenish ATP energy

Can't find a recommended product? Call the 800 number in Product Resources for the store nearest you.

Supplements for the training needs of the serious athlete: *Before you work out:*

High Protein Drinks:
—Champion PRO-SCORE 100, PHOSPHAGAIN, MET MAX
—Unipro MYO SYSTEM XL
—Twin Lab AMINO FUEL liquid and CREATINE FUEL PLUS
 —Jones Products SPORTS STAR MILK & EGG PROTEIN

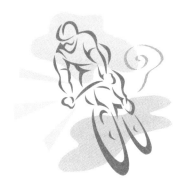

Oxygenators and Antioxidants:
—CoQ-10 75mg daily
—UniPro LIQUID DMG
—Real Life Research CoQ 20/20 liquid sublingual plus antioxidants,
—Nature's Path HEMA-LYTE w. electrolytes
—Nutricology GERMANIUM 150mg to protect the thymus.

Free form amino acids: *to increase workout performance.*
—Arginine-ornithine-lysine to metabolize fats, carnitine to strengthen muscle activity
—Anabol Naturals ANABOLIC AMINO BALANCE, AMINO GH RELEASERS, AMINO NITRO MAX
—Unipro AMINO 1000
—Champion MUSCLE-NITRO, (BCAAs) - for ATP energy conversion.

Non-steroidal Anabolic Agents:
—Radiant Life SUMAX 5 derived from suma, shown to be as effective as the illegal synthetic steroid, dianabol without the side effects. Highly recommended.
    —Anabol Naturals DIBENCOPLEX 10,000 - dibencozide (coenzyme B-12) activates protein biosynthesis.
—Natural Balance RIBOSE RIBO-MAX to replenish ATP energy

Testosterone Support: *To increase muscle hardness.*
—Unipro TRIBULUS SYNERGY
—Country Life LIQUID FARMACY SUPER STRENGTH YOHIMBE (Use with caution.)
—Crystal Star ACTIVE PHYSICAL ENERGY™ with panax ginseng; raw orchic extract, 6 to 10x strength.

Fat Burners:
—Anabol Naturals GH RELEASERS - metabolic fat burner; or **Unipro TRIMETABOLIC**
—Bricker Labs CUT-UP PLUS, Carnitine and Chromium fat-burner; **MAXIMAL BURNER** - with HCA.

Herbs:
—Crystal Star GINSENG ACTIVE PHYSICAL ENERGY™, HIGH PERFORMANCE™
—Futurebiotics MALE POWER - high-potency herbal plus glandular formula to rev-up your engine.

Vitamins and Minerals:
—Jones Products SPORTS STAR TRAINING PAK - a mega potent combination of vitamins, minerals, amino acids, and support nutrients for the serious athlete that demands the best.

Recovery Acceleration:
—EAS® BETAGEN™
—Champion CORTISTAT-PS to reduce cortisol levels and inflammation during a "burning" workout.
—Nature's Path TRACE-LYTE, Knudsen RECHARGE, Alacer MIRACLE WATER bring lost minerals.
—Unipro GLUTAGEN, Eidon SILICA, Now MSM caps help to rebuild and protect joints from injuries.
—NutriCology PHOS-SERINE - reduces muscle breakdown and soreness by lowering cortisol levels.
—Anabol Naturals ANABOLIC AMINO BALANCE, AMINO NITRO MAX.

Bodywork Watchwords for Body Building, Training & Competition:

Cross train. Besides your major sport or activity, supplement it with auxiliary exercise such as bicycling, jogging, walking, or swimming and aerobics. This balances muscle use and keeps heart and lungs strong.

Recuperate. Muscles don't grow during exercise. They grow during rest periods. Alternate muscle workouts with rest days. Exercise different muscle sets on different days, resting each set in between.

Breathe deep. Lung capacity is a prime training factor. Muscles and tissues must have enough oxygen for stamina. Breathe in during exertion, out as you relax for the next rep. Vigorous exhaling is as important as inhaling for the athlete, to expel all carbon dioxide and increase lung capacity for oxygen.

Stretch out. Muscle extensions before and after a workout keep cramping down and muscles loose. Get morning sunlight on the body every day possible for optimal absorption of nutrient fuel.

No pain does not mean no gain. Your exercise doesn't have to hurt to be good for you. Once you work up to a good aerobic level and routine, pushing yourself ever harder won't offer benefits.

Water. Good hydration is necessary for high performance, cardiovascular activity and overheating. Take an electrolyte replacement drink after a workout or anytime during the day.

Weight training. It's good for everybody, no matter what your sport, age or fitness goals. Forty-five minutes of weight bearing exercise three times a week boosts endurance, and strengthens the heart and bones. Women do not get a bulky, masculine physique from lifting weights. They have low levels of testosterone, which influences their type of muscle development. *Note: Vitamin E prevents muscle damage from weight training.*

How much fat are you burning?

Check your heart rate to see how many fat calories you're burning during your workout. If your heart rate is 70% of maximum, you are burning 20% fat of the total calories per hour/exercise time. If your heart rate is 45% of maximum, you are burning 40% fat of the total calories per hour/exercise time. More fat is burned in low intensity activities because you can take in the extra oxygen needed to burn fat - more than twice as much as carbohydrates per fat gram. (If you reduce maximal effort, you will need to exercise longer to burn the fat.)

Calorie burning choices:
—Aerobic dancing- 300-700 calories per hour
—Calisthenics- 360 calories per hour
—Cross Country Skiing- 350-1,400 calories per hour
—Cycling- 200-850 calories per hour
—Running- 400-1,300 calories per hour
—Stretching- 60-120 calories per hour
—Swimming- 380-850 calories per hour
—Walking- 240-430 calories per hour
—Water Aerobics- 180-880 calories per hour
—Weight training- 260-480

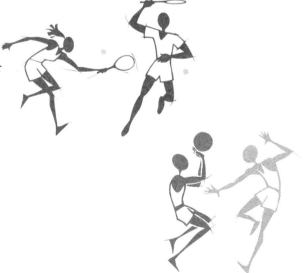

Alternative Healing Options For Pets

Americans are animal lovers. Over sixty percent of American families have at least one pet. In many ways we depend on them. They love us no matter what, lower our stress levels, ease our pain and add incredible joy to our lives. Over three-quarters of us feel guilty when we leave our pets at home alone. But of course they depend on us too, and somehow, pets have been left behind in good nutrition and health care!

Cats and dogs usually need better nutrition than they get today from today's animal foods. Commercial foods often contain low quality ingredients rejected for human consumption, even diseased animal meat laced with high levels of antibiotics. If these foods are the mainstay of your pet's diet they may destroy its health.

Most brands are saturated with the ingredients we fight against for ourselves...... chemical additives, artificial colors, dyes, preservatives like BHT and BHA — ingredients with known toxicity that are banned for human consumption. Further, much of the meat used in commercial pet food comes from dead, dying, disabled or diseased animals! Did you know that euthanized pets, trapped animals and roadkill are making their way into your pet's food? Almost all pet food is cooked, pasteurized, canned or microwaved, killing most of the enzymes critical to your pet's healthy body processes.

Our pets' diets are in a sad state. It's easy to see why so many pets are now victims of the same health problems we face: arthritis, heart disease, diabetes and hypoglycemia, allergies, and skin, eye and digestive disorders. Like us, animals need the live energy of fresh foods and quality, whole ingredients. Their bodies rely on enzymes even more than ours to protect them from degenerative diseases. It's the reason some animals, even some breeds, tend to eat waste excrement — for the enzymes.

It takes a little more time and effort to feed fresh foods to your pet. I use it as a communication-training time, often with a little by-hand feeding that we both love. Actually, a leftover salad is full of enzyme-rich fresh vegetables, and it makes a big difference to your pet's health. Start them on some veggies young if you can. I remember the day our cat (now 24 years old) turned up her nose at her own cat food and jumped on the kitchen table to eat our dinner salad!

Diet For Healthy Dogs & Cats

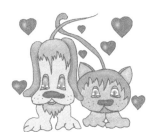

Cats and dogs thrive on the healthy foods that are good for people. A whole grain, additive-free kibble, a little meat and plenty of fresh water are basic staples. (*Note: Cats need more meat, and do better with fresh meat. If you have an indoor cat, you need to make up for their inability to catch fresh mice or birds, and offer them uncooked meat.*) Most pets need some fresh vegetables every day, too. We've all seen our pets chewing on grass. Mix greens with a little fish, raw liver and kidney, chicken, low-ash canned or dry food (use meat free of chemicals, and organic vegetables if possible). Most animals like salad greens, cucumbers, green peppers, carrots, green onions, parsley, celery and vegetable juice. Both dogs and cats like oatmeal, too.

I recommend the chemical-free pet foods found in health food stores. Several veterinarians that use natural healing methods on pets who advise us for this book, feel that many of today's pet ailments are a result of chemical-laced foods and environmental pollutants....just like people.

Note: Animals like people, can become addicted to particular foods if they have been given them for long periods of time. Some pets make quick adjustments to diet improvements; for others, you may need to introduce new foods gradually. Try a short all-water fast (no more than 24 hours) for an especially finicky pet until it's hungry enough to try the new diet.

Diet watchwords for pets:

1: Try high quality natural pet food instead of commercial brands. Halo-Purely For Pets manufacturers the first 100% human grade wet food (SPOT'S STEW) with all natural ingredients for dogs and cats. Flint River Ranch makes one of the best dry dog and cat food and it can be mixed with some water.

2: Give your pets occasional fish (especially salmon) and game meats like canned rabbit or venison for protein-amino acid energy building blocks, and essential fatty acids for a healthy, shiny coat. These meats, at least, haven't been treated with hormones or antibiotics.

3: Offer them some dairy foods. Most animals like yogurt, kefir and cottage cheese and goat's milk.

4: A little fruit is OK occasionally to loosen up a clogged system, but give sparingly. Dogs and cats like raisins, coconut, cantaloupe and apples.

5: Give dogs and cats plenty of omega-3 oils from sea greens, spinach, asparagus and corn. My pets like sea greens so much they eat them dry right from my hand. Add sea veggies (in granular form for ease of use) to your pets food daily to help insure adequate minerals and EFA's in their diet. Sea greens also boost metabolism for overweight pets

6: Have fresh water available all day long. Animals need plenty of liquids.

7: Feeding time is "together" time for people and animals. Your attention is focused on your pet; they know it and love it. But if you're pressed for time, make a meal up all at once and divide it between feedings.

For three to four servings: mix lightly, 1 small can quality fish or poultry (fresh fish or meat is even better), 4 TBS whole grain kibble, 3 teasp. nutritional yeast, 1 teasp. of a green superfood powder like spirulina or barley grass, 1 raw egg, 1 cup chopped vegetables, a little broth or water to moisten.

Instead of commercial dry kibble, mix in a spoonful of brown rice, oatmeal or other whole grains for strength and energy. I mix sea greens like nutrient-rich kelp, dulse or nori in with brown rice.

Cats and dogs need slightly different diets. Be aware of these tips:

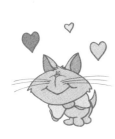

—**Key foods for cats:** include liver, bone meal, sea vegetables, whole grains, brown rice and vegetables to provide sustained energy with the correct proportions of proteins and carbohydrates. Add some wheat bran, corn germ or oatmeal, vegetable oil and leafy greens three times a week. The amino-acid taurine, found in meat and fish is critical to cats. Without taurine, a cat may develop heart problems and possibly go blind. If liver is used, be aware that if it is more than 10% of a cat's diet (too much vitamin A), it may lead to distorted bones, gingivitis, and stiff joints. Raw fish and raw egg whites contain an enzyme, thiaminase which inactivates vitamin B_1, a nutrient animals need to repel fleas and mosquitos.

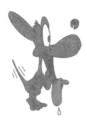

—**Key foods for dogs:** include high quality proteins and whole grains for easier digestibility. Dog foods should be low in saturated fat. Contrary to popular advertising, dogs do not need meat as an essential part of their diet. Their quality protein can come from eggs, low fat dairy products, as well as occasional fish or poultry. Dogs tolerate a vegetable diet better than cats because dogs are able to synthesize enough taurine. Make sure your dog's diet doesn't consist of your leftover table scraps (especially spicy foods like cold pizza or anything with onions). Don't feed chocolate of any kind to dogs.

Remember:
• Both puppies and kittens need twice the nutrients and calories as adult animals.
• Pregnant and nursing females need more protein, vitamins and minerals.
• Older animals need very digestible foods, less fat and less vitamins, minerals, proteins and sodium.
• Enzymes are essential to health; add in grated veggies to their food.

Can't find a recommended product? Call the 800 number in Product Resources for the store nearest you.

Herbs and Supplements For Your Healthy Pet

Food source supplements are good for animals. Wheat germ oil, spirulina, kelp, brewer's yeast, bran and lecithin all help keep pets in tip top condition. Homeopathic remedies are good for animals, too. They are effective, gentle, non-toxic, and free of side effects. They heal without harming.

Other supplement tips:

• Just like us, virtually all pet chronic diseases are directly linked to free radical damage. Consider BioVet International PET ANTIOXIDANT WAFERS for protection against free radicals. PET-LYTE by Nature's Path is a water-based solution of trace minerals for energy and balance.

• Supplement with oils high in omega-3's like *flax* oil or *borage* oil to balance the effects of omega-6 overload, common in pet commercial foods. Noah's Ark ROYAL COAT is a good choice.

• Many of today's foods are enzyme deficient, I highly recommend an enzyme supplement for pets. Consider Transformation CAREZYME. Green Foods BARLEY DOG and BARLEY CAT are powdered barley grass supplements with garlic, brown rice and nutritional yeast for all the chlorophyll and enzymes these foods give to us.

• I keep Bach Flower RESCUE REMEDY on hand as a first aid remedy for pet emergencies. RESCUE REMEDY works well for animals that are nervous, scratch compulsively, are depressed or have behavior disorders. It can also help calm an injured animal.

• **Crystal Star Herbal Nutrition has three highly beneficial food supplements for pets.**

—HEALTHY LIFE ANIMAL MIX™ gives dogs and cats the benefits of chlorophyll-rich greens to keep their blood strong, their bodies regular and their breath sweet. Rich in carotenes for natural immune strength, high in antioxidants like vitamin E and life-giving enzymes. HEALTHY LIFE ANIMAL MIX™ helps control arthritis and dysplasia symptoms, and protects against damage from rancid fats or poor quality foods. All kinds of animals love it, from hamsters to horses. Some, including our own, won't eat without it!

—AR-EASE FOR ANIMALS™ eases stiff joints and boosts mobility in older animals, especially larger dogs.

—SYSTEMS STRENGTH™ drink is an advanced healing combination for pets as well as people. I find this mix to be rapidly restorative for animal systems. Even sick or injured animals seem to know instinctively that it is good for them, and will eagerly take it as a broth from an eye dropper.

Bodywork For A Healthy Pet

• Give your pet plenty of fresh air, exercise and water. Brush and comb your animals often. It keeps their coats shiny, circulation stimulated, and they love the attention. (Brush cats gently; their skin is very sensitive.)

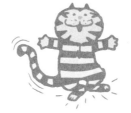

• Avoid chemical-impregnated flea collars. They often have DDT or a nerve gas in them — potentially toxic to your children, your pet, and the environment. Use a mild shampoo with herbal oils like *eucalyptus* and *rosemary* instead. The oils interfere with an insect's ability to sense the moisture, heat and breath of the animal.

• Sprinkle cedar shavings around your animal's bed to keep insects away and to make the area smell nice.

• Halo-Purely For Pets, DERMA-AIDE are natural healing skin salves for DREAM and Nature's Path PET-HEAL-mange, skin sores and insect bites.

• Consider massage therapy for older pets who have dysplasia or arthritis.

• Finally, Pet your pet. Love is always the best medicine. They need it as much as you do.

Can't find a recommended product? Call the 800 number in Product Resources for the store nearest you.

281

Nutritional Healing For Animals

Except in emergency situations, an optimal diet should be your key concern for natural animal healing. Concerned vets tell me that many animal health problems are actually caused by poor diets. A wholesome diet with a greens supplement (see previous pages) needs to be at the base of every healing program. Health problems are much harder to turn around when highly processed foods are used as the major part of your pet's diet. If possible, use meats without hormones or nitrates and also organically grown veggies.

AMYLOIDOSIS:
—Amyloid, a protein-polysaccharide complex is produced and deposited in tissues during certain pathological states. The liver, spleen and kidney can be affected, as well as any other body tissues.
—Protease product: Transformation PUREZYME or Enzymedica PURIFY - use as directed , 2 to 4 times daily between meals to break down amyloid (glycoprotein).

ANEMIA:
—Give a diet high in protein, iron, and vitamin B-12. Add land and sea greens ($^1/_2$ teasp. snipped) for iron, minerals and enzymes. Add some beef or chicken liver occasionally for protein, B complex, extra B-12 and iron.
—Give 500 to 2,000mg vitamin C, depending on size of animal.
—Sprinkle nutritional yeast flakes on food; or Nature's Path TOTAL-LYTE, an electrolyte yeast mix.
—Monas CHLORELLA - high chlorophyll content helps stimulate production of healthy blood.

ARTHRITIS:
—Avoid giving refined foods, especially white flour and sugar. Reduce red meat, canned foods and preserved meats like bologna. Add fresh green foods, particularly grated carrots, beets and celery.
—Make a barley grass or alfalfa tea, and add to animal's drinking water, or use Green Foods BARLEY CAT or BARLEY DOG in food.
—Give a dilute *devil's claw* herb solution daily.
—Give 2 teasp. cod liver oil or flaxseed oil (1 tsp. for cats, 1 TB. for dogs), 100IU vitamin E daily, 2 to 8 alfalfa tablets (most dogs eat these from your hand).
—Give $^1/_4$ teasp. <u>sodium</u> ascorbate or Ester C powder daily. Or open vitamin C capsules, depending on the size and age of animal, give 250 to 2,000mg a day (a puppy - 250mg, a great dane - 2,000mg). Natural Animal ESTER-C (dog formula and cat formula).
—Crystal Star AR-EASE FOR ANIMALS™; or SYSTEMS STRENGTH™ broth mix, $^1/_2$ teasp. daily.
—Give shark cartilage (dose by weight); give continually until no evidence of the problem.
—Open 1 capsule MICROHYDRIN, available from Healthy House, dissolve in water; feed one daily.
—Dancing Paws HI-POTENCY JOINT RECOVERY (therapeutic formula) and JOINT MAINTENANCE (preventive formula).
—Nature's Path PET-BONE-AIDE (shark cartilage with electrolytes) to aid movement and functions of animals suffering from osteoarthritis.
—Homeopathic *Rhus tox* 12c, one dose per month.

BAD BREATH:
—Feed more fresh foods, less canned processed foods. Snip fresh parsley into food at each meal.
—Sprinkle a little spirulina powder or Green Foods BARLEY DOG or BARLEY CAT on food.
—Monas CHLORELLA; add $^1/_4$ to $^1/_2$ teasp. to food - high chlorophyll content deodorizes bad breath and other body odors

282

BLADDER INFECTION and FELINE UROLOGICAL SYNDROME (FUS) - INCONTINENCE:

—Put animal on a liquid diet for 24 hours of veggie juices and broths - no solid foods, plenty of water.

—Avoid dried food entirely during healing. Focus on fresh foods. To make your own healthy cat food: mix together a handful of raw hormone-free meat (cut in small pieces), some grated vegetables (like carrot, zucchini, greens).

—Add $1/2$ tsp. Transformation CAREZYME, $1/2$ tsp. sea greens flakes, $1/2$ teasp. Monas CHLORELLA, 1 TB flax oil, $1/2$ to 1 cap probiotic (friendly bacteria), and 1 TB nutritional yeast. Add in enough water to make a juicy meal. Add 1 TB of brown rice occasionally.

—Enzyme supplements are important. Add a digestive formula like Transformation CAREZYME to all meals. Give a protease product like Enzymedica PURIFY or Transformation PUREZYME, 2 caps, between meals 2 times per day.

—Open 1 capsule MICROHYDRIN, available from Healthy House, dissolve in water; feed one daily.

—Extra vitamin C daily. Natural Animal ESTER-C for cats - use as directed.

—Vitamin E 100IU daily for a month, then decrease to 400IU once a week.

—Use Wysong URETIC cat food for cat bladder infections and blockage.

—For acute attacks, acidify the urine. Different types of crystal formations can occur in FUS. For struvite crystals only (diagnoses needed by veterinarian), Orthomolecular Specialties CARPON (treats and prevents FUS by acidifying urine and breaking up struvite crystals).

—Nature's Path PET-LYTE - use as directed.

—Designing Health THE MISSING LINK - use as directed.

—To reduce stress, Natural Labs DEVA FLOWER STRESS/TENSION.

—Avoid "clumping" type kitty litter brands which can contribute to blockage problems. Natural Animal LITTER PLUS - made from 100% organic plant material (peanut shell meal). Many feed stores have a corn cob mixture that works great as a healthy kitty litter.

—For kidney, liver or bladder disease, protease and digestive enzymes help detoxify fibrosis of affected organs. Use Transformation CAREZYME, (excellent results), mix into meals as directed.

CANCERS - LEUKEMIA - MALIGNANT TUMORS:

—Avoid commercial foods; use as much fresh, unprocessed foods as the animal will accept.

—Animal cancers have shown dramatic improvement with enzyme therapy from plant proteases against tumor growth. Protease enzymes may be used with or without conventional therapy. Use Enzymedica PURIFY or Transformation PUREZYME 3 to 6 times daily (on empty stomach with water, or mixed into a small amount of food if necessary). Add digestive aid Transformation CAREZYME (good results) into meals

—Open 1 capsule MICROHYDRIN, available from Healthy House, dissolve in water; feed one daily.

—Natural Energy Plus CAISSE'S tea - 6 to 15 lb animal, use $1/2$ to 1 teasp. dilute tea daily. 16 to 30 lbs- 1 to 2 teasp. dilute tea. Call 888-633-9233 for more info.

—Give vitamin C as sodium ascorbate powder, $1/4$ teasp. twice daily for larger animals and cats with leukemia or Alacer EMERGEN-C in water. As tumor shrinks, decrease to a small daily pinch.

—Give Crystal Star SYSTEM STRENGTH™ broth 2x daily, $1/4$ cup or as much as animal will take.

—Shark cartilage, give continually until no evidence of the problem.

—Apply Crystal Star ANTI-BIO™ gel to tumorous areas.

—The herb *chaparral* shows success (check carefully with your holistic vet as to dosage for your pet).

—Dilute a *goldenseal-echinacea* extract to $1/2$ strength. Give $1/4$ teasp. daily (dogs only).

—Herbal Answers HERBAL ALOE FORCE JUICE, 2 to 3 teasp. daily; apply HERBAL ALOE FORCE GEL if tumor is visible.

Can't find a recommended product? Call the 800 number in Product Resources for the store nearest you.

283

COAT and SKIN HEALTH:
—Crystal Star HEALTHY LIFE MIX™ in food daily.
—Add 1-2 TB lecithin granules or Nature's Path LECI-LYTE daily to meals.
—Give vitamin E 100IU daily. Apply E oil or jojoba oil to affected skin areas.
—Add 1 teasp. spirulina or kelp powder to food daily. Use PET-SKIN-AIDE by Nature's Path.
—EFA's are a key. Squeeze 1 black currant oil capsule onto food daily. Add 1 TB flax oil or meal to food.
—Halo-Purely For Pets DREAM COAT (EFA formula).
—Dancing Paws BREWER'S YEAST PLUS (Edible Skin and Coat Conditioner).
—For allergy-related skin/coat problems, try an oatstraw soak (add 4 oz dried oatstraw tops to a hot bath).

CONSTIPATION:
—Add greens and veggies to the diet; mix $\frac{1}{2}$ teasp. to 1 TB bran to each meal; decrease canned food.
—Add Crystal Star HEALTHY LIFE MIX™ or fresh dandelion greens for soluble food fiber.
—Mix a little garlic powder with 1 TB. olive oil and add to food.
—Natural Animal GENTLE DRAGON INTESTINAL CLEANSER (cat and dog formulas).
—Monas CHLORELLA - $\frac{1}{2}$ teasp. daily in food - chlorella's unique cell walls stimulate the intestine's linings and increase the number of friendly bacteria.
—Exercise the animal more often. Let it outside more often for relief.
—Give *aloe vera* juice, 2 to 3 teasp. daily.

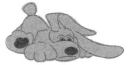

CUTS, SORES and WOUNDS:
—Apply a goldenseal/myrrh solution, or comfrey salve.
—Apply vitamin E oil. Give vitamin E 100IU daily. Give RESCUE REMEDY for trauma.
—Apply aloe vera gel and give desiccated liver tabs or powder in food daily.
—Give vitamin C crystals $\frac{1}{4}$ to $\frac{1}{2}$ teasp. in water. Apply on sore and give internally during the day.
—Nelson Bach RESCUE REMEDY CREAM.
—Nature's Path PET-HEAL-AIDE.

DEHYDRATION: *A major emergency for cats. Check for dehydration by pulling up the scruff of the neck. If skin is slow to return, the animal is dehydrated. Take to a vet as soon as possible.*
—Use comfrey tea, or Crystal Star SYSTEMS STRENGTH™ broth immediately. Force feed if necessary about 2-oz. an hour. Mix bran, tomato juice and sesame oil. Feed each hour until improvement.
—Try to feed green veggies; especially celery, lettuce and carrots for electrolyte replacement. Once the crisis has passed, add kelp, spirulina or a green drink to the diet.
—PET-LYTE by Nature's Path is liquid minerals in electrolyte solution.
—Check for worms, often a cause of dehydration.
—Give the animal lots of love and attention. Dehydration may be caused by depression. The animal simply curls up and will not eat or drink anything. Bach Flower RESCUE REMEDY is excellent in this case, or Natural Labs DEVA FLOWER STRESS/TENSION drops.

DIABETES:
—Strictly avoid sugary foods, especially soft moist animal foods that come in cellophane bags - (very high in sugar, preservatives and artificial colors).
—Lower fat intake. (Use omega-3 oils like flax, $\frac{1}{2}$ teasp. cod liver oil; alternate with a vegetable oil.)
—Beneficial foods for diabetes: Grains - millet, rice, oats, cornmeal, and rye bread. Vegetables - green beans (pods contain hormonal substances closely related to insulin), dandelion greens, alfalfa sprouts, corn, parsley, onion (not for dogs) and garlic reduce blood sugar. Alkalizing foods - grated vegetables, fermented foods like yogurt help counter overacidity due to the disordered metabolism of diabetes.
—Sprinkle nutritional yeast on food; add $\frac{1}{2}$ teasp. to 1 TB. lecithin in granular or liquid form.
—Add vitamin C - 500mg to 2000mg daily depending on pet size - divide into 2 or more doses.

Can't find a recommended product? Call the 800 number in Product Resources for the store nearest you.

DIARRHEA:
—Diarrhea is caused by spoiled food, non-food items, worms of harmful bacteria. Put the animal on a 24 hour liquid diet with aloe vera juice, 2 to 3 TBS daily, vegetable juices, broths and lots of water.
—Give plain yogurt, acidophilus liquid and brewer's yeast at every feeding until diarrhea ends.
—Sprinkle crushed activated charcoal tablets on food.
—Use Dr. Goodpet DIAR-RELIEF homeopathic remedy.
—Use Transformation PLANTADOPHILUS powder, about $1/4$ teasp sprinkled omn food.

DISTEMPER:
—If the problem is acute, put the animal on a short liquid diet with vegetable juices and broths.
—Give vitamin C crystals (sodium ascorbate if possible), $1/4$ teasp. in water, divided through the day, in an eye dropper if necessary. If vomiting and loss of fluids, give some vitamin C liquid every hour.
—Give Dr. Goodpet CALM STRESS homeopathic remedy to calm vomiting.
—Add $1/2$ dropperful B complex liquid and 1 teasp. bonemeal to food daily.
—Give a dilute (1 drop extract in 2 teasp. water) *goldenseal-myrrh*, or *echinacea* solution.
—Give yogurt or acidophilus liquid to rebuild friendly flora; add Green Foods BARLEY DOG to diet.
—Give fresh garlic, or a garlic-honey mixture daily. Give raw liver or liver tablets several times a week.
—Add brown rice and bran to daily food for B vitamins and system tone.

ECZEMA:
—Give zinc 25mg internally, and apply zinc ointment to infected areas.
—Mix cottage cheese, corn or cod liver oil, vitamin E oil, garlic powder brewer's yeast. Give 1 TB. daily.
—Give Green Foods BARLEY DOG daily. Apply solution locally to sores.
—Reduce meat and canned foods. Add fresh veggies and sea greens to the diet.
—Use Nature's Path PET-SKIN-AIDE for healing and rebuilding the skin.
—Add 1 TB. flax oil or meal to food daily.

EAR MITES:
—Use NATURAL HERBAL EAR WASH by Purely For Pets. Prevents infection, heals abrasions, promotes healthy cell formation and eliminates ear wax and odors.
—Apply Crystal Star ANTI-BIO GEL™; or make a homemade oil treatment:
    #1 Combine $1/2$ oz. olive oil and 400IU vitamin E from a capsule in a $1/2$ oz dropper bottle. Put a dropperful in each ear, massage ear canal, let animal shake its head. Gently clean out ear (not deep into ear) with cotton swab. Repeat for 3 days. Let ear rest for 3 days to smother the mites.
    #2 Grind 1-oz dried or 2-oz fresh *thyme* and *rosemary* and combine with $1/2$ cup olive oil - let sit in a sunny windowsill or on top of a water heater to rest for 3 days. Shake daily to help extract essential oils. Strain mixture into a 1-oz dropper bottle and add 400IU vitamin E. Once a day for 3 days put warmed mixture in each ear as above. Let ear rest for 10 days. Repeat oil treatment for 3 days to catch egg mites. Note: Do not use *Tea Tree oil* on cats - it is toxic to them.

EYE and EAR INFECTION:
—1 teasp. cod liver oil and vitamin E 100IU to the diet. Apply cod liver oil and E oil locally.
—Give goat's milk daily in food, and apply with cotton balls to the eye.
—ANITRA'S HERBAL EYEWASH kit by Halo for eye infections.
—For ear infection, try a "apple cider vinegar flush" (2 TBS. to 1 cup of water) twice a week.
—Give homeopathic *Nat. Mur*, early stages; *Silicea*, later stages to arrest cataract development. Or Hepar *sulphuris calcareum* 12c. - one dose every 3 days. Three doses total.
—Apply an *eyebright* herb tea or Crystal Star EYEBRIGHT HERBAL™ tea to infected area.

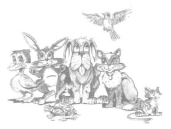

FLEAS - TICKS - MITES: Give floppy-eared pets a weekly ear inspection for mites and ticks.
   —Give nutritional yeast and garlic powder for B vitamins and protection against infestation.
      Dust $1/4$ teasp. nutritional yeast and $1/2$ teasp. garlic powder on pets' food at least 3 times a week.
   —Use CLOUD-NINE HERBAL DIP by Halo-Purely For Pets.
   —Dancing Paws NATURAL FLEA EZE (cat and dog formulas).
   —Natural Animal HERBAL FLEA POWDER for dogs and cats with *pyrenthrum* kills fleas on contact.
   —String *eucalyptus* buds around animal's neck and sleeping area. Stuff a pillow with *rosemary, pennyroyal,*
      eucalyptus and mint leaves, and place on animal's bed. Rub *rosemary oil* on coat between shampoos.
   —Give $1/2$ of a 100mg vitamin B_1 tablet daily to ward off insects.
   —Apply *tea tree* oil directly on insect to kill it. Add a few *tea tree* oil drops to pet's regular shampoo.
      Leave on 3 to 5 minutes before rinsing. Note: Do not use *Tea Tree* oil with cats - it is toxic to them.
   —Apply *jojoba* oil on the bitten place to heal it faster.

House treatments for fleas, tick and mites:
   —Vacuum carpets and bare floors. For carpet infestation, use inorganic salts (sodium borate).
      Use only 100% pure, non-toxic borates such as TERMINATOR by Canine Care.
   —Use carpet and bedding sprays containing citronella, eucalyptus, tea tree oil, and lemon grass oils.

FOOD ALLERGIES:
   —Give Enzymedica DIGEST or Transformation CAREZYME.
   —Give Enzymedica PURIFY or Transformation PUREZYME as directed.

GAS and FLATULENCE:
   —Give alfalfa tabs, spirulina, or Green Foods BARLEY DOG or CAT at
      each feeding.
   —Sprinkle a pinch of ginger powder on food at each feeding.
   —Give *comfrey, chamomile, cinnamon, fenugreek* (not for pregnant animals),
      or *peppermint* tea daily.

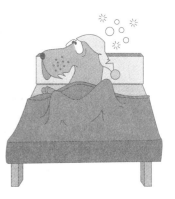

GUM and TOOTH PROBLEMS:
   —Apply a dilute goldenseal/myrrh or propolis solution to gums.
   —Bee balm to help reduce gum inflammation and to fight gingivitis.
   —Give a natural fresh foods diet, adding crunchy raw veggies and whole grains.
   —Apply vitamin E oil, or calendula oil to gums.
   —Rub vitamin C - a weak solution of ascorbate crystals in water on the gums.
   —Open 1 capsule MICROHYDRIN, available from Healthy House, dissolve in water; feed one daily.
   —Hepar *sulphuris calcareum* 12 c. - one dose every 3 days - 3 doses total.

HIP DYSPLASIA and LAMENESS *(See also ARTHRITIS):*
   —Add more whole grains like brown rice and oatmeal, and lean meats like turkey and chicken to the diet.
   —Mix 1 teasp. sodium ascorbate, or Ester C crystals in water and give throughout the day, every day.
   —Natural Animal ESTER-C (dog formula and cat formula), as directed.
   —Mix 1 teasp. bonemeal powder in 1 c. tomato juice, with 1 tsp. bran and $1/2$ tsp. sesame oil; give daily.
   —Give Crystal Star AR-EASE FOR ANIMALS™ daily, or NU-PET PLUS for pets from Biogenetics.
   —Give shark cartilage as directed, continually until no evidence of problem.
   —Dancing Paws HI-POTENCY JOINT RECOVERY (therapeutic formula) and
      JOINT MAINTENANCE (preventive formula).
   —Protease enzymes, like Transformation PUREZYME or Enzymedica PURIFY as directed 3 times daily.
   —Nature's Path CAL-LYTE and PET-LYTE.

Can't find a recommended product? Call the 800 number in Product Resources for the store nearest you.

HORMONE IMBALANCE: *Neutered pets really benefit from herbs that support hormonal systems.*
—Herbs for spayed female pets: *wild yam, dong quai, oats, Siberian ginseng.*
—Herbs for neutered male pets: *saw palmetto, damiana and Asian ginseng.*

INTESTINAL, DIGESTIVE DISORDER: *often caused by spoiled food, non-food items or worms.*
—Put the animal on a short 24 hour liquid diet with vegetable juices, broths, and plenty of water.
—Give yogurt, acidophilus liquid or brewer's yeast at every feeding until diarrhea ends.
—Sprinkle crushed activated charcoal tablets on food; use Dr. Goodpet DIAR-RELIEF remedy.
—Give aloe vera juice, 2 to 3 teasp. daily.
—Give Crystal Star HEALTHY LIFE MIX™ with $1/2$ teasp. extra garlic powder daily.
—Give *garlic, mullein-myrrh* extract, or *echinacea* or *black walnut* extract diluted in water, or *mugwort* tea.
—Give *comfrey* or dilute *cinnamon* tea in the water bowl.
—Use enzyme therapy for inflammatory bowel disease or intestinal disorders: Transformation CAREZYME or Enzymedica DIGEST, mix in meals as directed. Protease - Transformation PUREZYME or Enzymedica PURIFY protease, as directed mixed into a treat like cottage cheese.
—Diarrhea: *podophyllum peltatum* 12c. - 1 to 2 doses as needed.

MANGE & FUNGAL INFECTION:
—Put drops of *tea tree* oil in the animal's shampoo; use every 2 or 3 days. Use *tea tree* oil directly on infected areas by itself or diluted with olive oil. Do not use *Tea Tree* oil with cats - it is toxic to them.
—Apply *pau d' arco* salve, *mahonia* ointment or zinc ointment and fresh lemon juice to relieve area.
—Apply dilute *echinacea* tincture, or *goldenseal-echinacea-myrrh* water solution to affected areas daily.
—Apply Nature's Path PET-SKIN-AIDE for skin healing-rebuilding, or Crystal Star FUNGEX GEL™.
—Give 1 teasp. lecithin granules daily. Mix 2 teasp. cod liver oil with 1 TB. nutritional yeast and 2 teasp. desiccated liver powder. Give daily.

OVERWEIGHT:
—Reduce canned and saturated fat foods. Increase fresh foods, whole grains and organ meats.
—Crystal Star HEALTHY LIFE™ for fiber without calories. Lecithin 750mg daily (dogs and cats).
—Sea greens daily to boost metabolism (1 teasp. of snipped sea veggies for dogs and just a pinch for cats.)
—Apple cider vinegar 1 teasp. (dogs) $1/8$ to $1/4$ teasp. (cats) in water 2x daily.
—Add more exercise to the animal's life.

PANCREATIC INSUFFICIENCY:
—Digestive aid product: Enzymedica DIGEST or Transformation CAREZYME - mix into all meals according to directions.
—Protease helps clean up and prevent fibrosis- Enzymedica PURIFY or Transformation PUREZYME, mixed into a small treat 3 times daily between meals.

PREGNANCY and BIRTH:
—Give red raspberry tea daily during the last half of gestation for easier birth.
—Give daily spirulina tabs or powder for extra protein.
—Give desiccated liver tabs (dogs), extra bonemeal, and cod liver oil daily.
—Give extra vitamin C 100mg chewable, and vitamin E 100IU daily.

Can't find a recommended product? Call the 800 number in Product Resources for the store nearest you.

RESPIRATORY INFECTIONS and IMMUNE STRENGTH:
—Put animal on a liquid diet for 24 hours to cleanse the system, with vegetable juices, broths and water. Offer *comfrey* tea to flush toxins faster. (Nibbling on growing comfrey plants is a pet natural therapy.)
—Give Crystal Star HEALTHY LIFE MIX™ for immune strength. COFEX TEA™ for hacking cough.
—Give Crystal Star SYSTEMS STRENGTH™ broth 2 times daily, about $\frac{1}{4}$ cup. Add *astragalus* herb (well tolerated by both dogs and cats) to the broth.
—Add 1 teasp. bee pollen, vitamin E 100IU, and $\frac{1}{4}$ teasp. vitamin C (as sodium ascorbate if possible), dissolved in a cup of water to diet.
—Add 2 to 4 garlic tablets and 6 alfalfa tablets to the daily diet.
—East Park OLIVE LEAF EXTRACT - (works, but difficult to get cats to take this bitter antibiotic.)

WORMS and PARASITES:
For most parasitic diseases, treatment must also include medicinal measures.
—Build up parasite immunity with Crystal Star HEALTHY LIFE ANIMAL MIX™, as directed daily.
—Put the animal on a short 24 hour liquid fast with water to weaken the parasites. Then give Crystal Star VERMEX CAPS™ as directed with charcoal tabs in water or an electuary for 3 to 7 days. Repeat process in a week to kill newly hatched eggs.
—Mix $\frac{1}{2}$ teasp. garlic powder and a pinch cloves; sprinkle on food daily until worms are gone. Give spirulina or Green Foods BARLEY DOG or BARLEY CAT for a month after worming.
—Garlic, *mullein/myrrh* blend; *echinacea* or *black walnut* extract diluted in water; or *mugwort* tea.
—Protease - Transformation PUREZYME or Enzymedica PURIFY, as directed 2x daily between meals.
—Digestion - Transformation CAREZYME or Enzymedica DIGEST - mix into all meals.

Note: Acupuncture has been a very successful alternative treatment for animals - especially in cases of arthritis, hip dysplasia, asthma, epilepsy, cervical-disk displacements and chronic infections. To find a certified veterinary acupuncturist, contact the International Veterinary Acupuncture Society (IVAS) at 303-682-1167 or visit them on the web: www.ivas.org.

Special contributions to Animal Healing section come from esteemed experts in holistic animal care.
1) Dr. Jim R. Smith, DVM, AAVD who does extensive research on enzymes for dietary, theraputic use with animals. He owns the Animal Allergy Clinics and is a board member of Transformation Enzyme Corporation.
2) Linda A. Mower, D.Hom, is a homeopathic educator, writer and consultant for humans and animals.
3) Howard Peiper is a nationally recognized expert in the holistic counseling field. He has coauthored 12 books including "Super Nutrition for Animals."

About Animals & Toxic Substances

There is a wide range of substances that are harmful or lethal to animals. They include pesticides from lawn and garden products, rat poison, commercial flea killers, herbicides like Round-Up, and others. House cleaning products and disinfectants, building and decorating hazards (like paint and outgassing from synthetic carpets) are hazardous when you're only 12 inches off the ground and have to live so close to them. Use products that are environmentally safe as a general rule.

Many people are unaware of plant poisoning. Laurel, commonly used in dried flower arrangements, Christmas mistletoe, poinsettias, jimson weed, and oleander can cause death in a pet. Dogs who love to dig and chew the bulbs of the hyacinth can experience convulsions.

I recommend the medicine-chest information from The ASPCA's National Animal Poison Control Center, 1717 S. Philo Road, Suite #36, Urbana, IL., 61802. It's a good idea to call them before you have an emergency at 217-337-5030. This organization is the first animal-oriented poison center in the United States. The phones are answered by licensed veterinarians and board-certified veterinary toxicologists.

Emergency calls go to 1-888-426-4435 (credit cards, no charge).

Dear reader, let me tell you a true story about healthy healing...

I embrace things very enthusiastically. When I first heard about a cleansing diet in the 70's I thought it sounded like just the thing for me. I had fought my weight all my life. I was tired all the time (probably from all the crazy diets I went on to lose weight), and I felt "toxic," constantly getting fever blisters, urinary tract and yeast infections. I had dull hair, poor skin texture, peeling feet and breaking nails. Oh, I remember those days well.

Detoxification seemed like it would solve of lot of health problems. I thought I would be on a cleansing diet all my life.

The trouble was, I had almost no idea how to go about it. The 60's and 70's were the decades that the FDA had what amounted to a "gag order" on all books and information about alternative health methods, healing techniques and products. (You would not be reading this book now if the owner and employees of a very brave health food store in California had not finally challenged this regulation in the early 1980s in the courts and won, after many years and enormous expense.)

But I had a little knowledge and some enthusiastic friends who were detoxing, too, so I started on what was essentially a 5 food diet — cabbage, lettuce with a little salad dressing, apples, oranges, peanut butter (for protein), and a few whole wheat crackers occasionally. I was delighted with my weight loss (I averaged about 90 pounds for my 5 foot frame). I rarely ate other things; this went on for several years. I didn't realize it, but my body was going into major malnutrition decline.

Today, with all the information we have about nutrition, most people know this type of diet is not a cleansing diet. It's a prescription for terrible health. All I saw was that I was finally thin.

One week, in the winter of 1981, my energy had dropped so low that I couldn't make it to my job. I had just started working at the town's small health food store, and I loved my work, so this was very unusual.

I didn't realize it but I had already slipped into shock — the hours and days were slipping by like a dream. I lived alone with my dogs and cats, but my colleagues from work wondered why I wasn't there. Thankfully, one of them came to check up on me. He saved my life.

I had already collapsed, and was lying by my front screen door. He scooped me up and got me to the nearest emergency room. It was eight-thirty in the morning, at a very small Seventh Day Adventist hospital in a small California town. There were 12 people in the building. Everyone worked feverishly to save me, but my blood pressure dropped rapidly. The staff saw me slip into a coma — they thought they had lost me.

All I knew was that I was floating, above my body, the operating table and the doctors who were working on me. It was all very interesting. I saw all the frantic emergency room procedures — like a TV show.
And then... I can see as clearly as when it happened, I floated to a top corner of the room. A million colors were swirling around me. I saw a dark tunnel with a white pinpoint of light miles away at the end. I turned to go to it... then everything went black, and I don't remember any more.

I was in a coma, and even though I didn't know it, I had made it.

Eventually I regained consciousness, and woke up full of tubes and needles on a breathing machine. My blood was so toxic, the hospital had to have plasma flown in every 5 hours to give me a slow but complete transfusion. It kept me alive, but I wasn't regaining health. I was slipping back and forth into unconsciousness. The doctors wanted to MED-Evac me to Stanford for specialized treatment, but I knew that I would just become a number, so I wouldn't go.

One of the wonderful things about a Seventh Day Adventist hospital (especially in those days) was that they listened to the patient. I couldn't speak, of course, but I could write. So, I asked for green drinks from the health food store and the hospital staff allowed a small refrigerator in. It was like a miracle. Within hours I felt stronger; within days, they removed the respirator; within a few more, they removed all the tubes and needles. In a total of twelve days after I regained consciousness, I left the hospital, very very weak, weighing 69 pounds, and unable to walk because my legs would not support my weight.

I knew I had been given another chance at life and a tremendous challenge to regain my health. My hair had either fallen out or turned white; some of my veins has collapsed from the needles. I had pulled retinal tissue in one eye; my skin was peeling off at my fingertips. The hospital thought they might have to amputate my toes unless I regained circulation in my feet fast.

I started reading everything I could get my hands on about natural healing and herbal remedies. I started formulating herbal formulas to bring each part of my body back to health. It began to happen. I could see a new me emerging, with curly hair, and a better skin tone and texture (no wrinkles) than I had before the illness. My circulation came back (no toe amputations); my energy returned and was stronger than it had been in many years.

The experience and the healing changed my life. I saw that herbs are far more than remedies for colds and flu. They can bring your health back from serious illness... literally from death's door. I was enormously impressed. I decided to devote my life to reaching out to others — to talk about the power of herbs, to write about their healing abilities, to return some of the essential universal knowledge that we've lost. I gained my degrees from Clayton College of Natural Health.

That early attempt at cleansing was almost fatally misguided. One of the reasons I wanted to write this book was to pass along all I've learned about healthy healing. Hundreds of thousands of people have been helped by this information. I hope you will be too. Pass it along!

To your best health,

Linda Page

PS: Please read what others have said....

"I have used your book, Healthy Healing, *as a reference, actually almost a bible, for the past few years after my yoga instructor suggested it for infertility advice. Your book, and some of your products have made a profound difference in the quality of my life!" -Kathleen D.*

"Thank you for your book, Healthy Healing. *With it I have succeeded in improving my general health dramatically -- despite the diagnosis of Chronic Lymphocytic Leukemia. I have passed on tons of information to others." -Margie M.*

"I purchased a copy of your book, Healthy Healing *while on a recent trip to Washington State. I am very impressed by the completeness and practicality of the information!" -Ron G.*

An Important Message to Interested Readers

The **Ailment Healing Section** of this book recommends many fine natural health products that I and my staff have used and reviewed for effectiveness and safety under label dosage and conditions.

There are special recommendations for Crystal Star Herbal Nutrition products in the Herb and Supplement heading. I formulated these products and have been involved in healing experiences with them for almost 25 years. The suggested uses for them in this book are for conditions I have either witnessed or heard directly from the first hand knowledge of people who used the products successfully for their health problems.

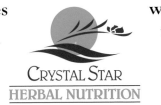

Although I no longer own Crystal Star Herbal Nutrition, my goal is to pass on to you all the information I have gained in the health field with products I have used and worked with. You can have every confidence that the products suggested under the health conditions in this book have had success for their recommendation.

This book is all about furthering real knowledge about what really works for human health — not just laboratory results, or even animal studies — but what works for us. I consider first person knowledge to be incredibly valuable in this effort.

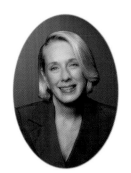

Linda Page, ND, PhD.

Access is important.

If you are interested in knowing more about the Crystal Star herbal formulas,
call Crystal Star Herbal Nutrition directly 1-800-736-6015.
Crystal Star is carried nationwide. If you know the product you want go to your natural food store. If they don't have it, they can easily order it for you.

If you prefer the convenience of ordering via the internet or by mail order, contact
The Healthy House - Home of The Natural Health Shopping Service, a service which automatically delivers products to you so you'll never run out of your favorite product.
Go online to: www.healthyhealing.com
or call 1-888-447-2939 to place an order or to receive a catalog.

How to Use the Ailment charts...

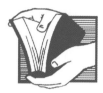

Each ailment chart includes three remedy categories:
—Diet and Superfood Therapy
—Herb and Supplement Therapy
—Lifestyle Support Therapy (bodywork and relaxation techniques)

There are many effective recommendations to choose from in each category. You can easily put together the best healing program for yourself. **Choosing one recommendation from each healing target under the interceptive therapy plan, for example, then using your choices together, may be considered a complete healing program**. All given doses are daily amounts unless otherwise specified. Dosage listed is for the major time of healing, and is not to be considered as maintenance or long term. The rule of thumb for natural healing is one month for every year you have had the problem.

Where a remedy is especially effective for women, a female symbol ♀ appears by the recommendation.
Where a remedy is especially effective for men, a male symbol ♂ appears by the recommendation.
Where a remedy is proven effective for children, a small child's face 😊 appears by the recommendation.

No matter what your health problem is, consider your diet as your primary healing tool. The diets I recommend are "real people" diets. People with specific health conditions have used them and have related their experiences to me. Over the years, diseases change — through mutation, environment, or treatment, for instance — and a person's immune response to them changes. HEALTHY HEALING's diet programs are continually modified to meet new, changing health needs.

The "foot" and "hand" diagrams in the ailment programs show the reflexology pressure points for each body area. You can use reflexology therapy when it is indicated. In some cases, the points are very tiny, particularly for the glands. It takes practice to pinpoint. The best sign that you have reached the right spot is that it will be very tender, denoting crystalline deposits or congestion in the corresponding body part. There is often a feeling of immediate relief in the area as the waste deposit breaks up for removal by your body.

Every edition of HEALTHY HEALING offers you the latest knowledge from a wide network of natural healing professionals — nutritional consultants, holistic practitioners, naturopaths, nurses, world health studies and traditional physicians in America and around the world.

You can have every confidence that the recommended remedies have been used and found to be effective, in some cases by thousands of people. I've developed and worked with the healing programs over the years; they are constantly updated with new information.

The most significant information is the evidence of people who have tried the natural healing methods for themselves, experienced real improvement in their health, and wish to share their success with others. Pick the suggestions that you instinctively feel strongly about. They are invariably the best for you, and will be the easiest to incorporate into your lifestyle. Refer to the ALTERNATIVE HEALTH CARE ARSENAL — "Look It Up," on page 78 for more information about any recommended healing agent.

No prescription is as valuable as knowledge.

Ailments: Table of Contents

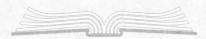

290

An Important Message About Your Health Care Responsibility

The material on the following pages is intended as an educational tool to offer information about alternative healing and health maintenance options available to the health care consumer today.

I believe we must be respectful of all ways of healing. The crisis intervention measures of drug therapy are sometimes needed to stabilize an emergency or life-threatening situation, but for long term well-being, disease prevention, and many common, self-limiting problems, diet improvement, exercise, and natural medicine choices make good sense. They are gentle, non-invasive, and in almost every case, free of any side effects.

The optional recommendations in this section are not intended as a substitute for the advice and treatment of a physician or other licensed health care professionals. In many cases, they may be used as adjuncts to professional care, to help shorten the time you may have to use drug treatment, and to help overcome any side effects.

Are there interactions between drugs and herbs? It is important to remember that herbs are foods, remarkably safe in their naturally-occurring state, and especially in combinations. They do not normally interact with drugs any more than a food would interact. However, be fair to your doctor and yourself. Discuss your alternative choices with your physician, and always inform your doctor or pharmacist of any other medication you are taking. Pregnant women are especially urged to consult with their health care provider before using any therapy.

I feel that education is the key to making wise health decisions. Part of the job of taking more command of your own health care is using your common sense, intelligence, and adult judgement based on the knowledge of your own body experiences. Ultimately, you must take the full responsibility for your choices and how you use the information presented here.

Abscesses

Boils, Carbuncles, Furuncles, Dental Abscesses

Pus accumulation that forms due to infection anywhere in the body - both externally and internally. Boils and furuncles are usually staph infections of sebaceous glands, especially around hair follicles (often caused by a rough or contaminated razor blade). Carbuncles are groups of adjacent boils where the staph infection extends out into the subcutaneous layers of the skin. Recurrent attacks of boils and abscesses indicate a depressed immune system.

Diet & Superfood Therapy

—**Nutritional therapy plan:**

1—Start with a short cleanse: 1 to 3 days of fresh juices (pg. 191), followed by a diet of fresh foods for 1 to 2 weeks to rebalance body chemistry pH.

2—Eat cultured foods - yogurt, kefir, etc. for friendly intestinal flora. Add acidophilus to your diet, either sprinkled over food or as a supplement, if taking high dose courses of antibiotics for abscess infections.

3—Drink 6 to 8 glasses of pure water daily.

—**Medicinal food applications:**

• Simmer flax and fenugreek seeds together until soft. Mash pulp. Apply as a compress.

• Mix fresh grated garlic or onion with lemon juice and apply directly to abscess.

—**Superfood therapy:** (Choose one or two)
• Crystal Star ENERGY GREEN™ for EFA's.
• Nutricology PROGREENS with EFA's.
• Liquid chlorophyll - apply to abscess. Take internally, 3 teasp. daily as a blood purifier.
• Propolis tincture - apply directly and take internally, twice daily.
• AloeLife FIBERMATE drink daily to cleanse intestinal tract.
• ALOE VERA JUICE each morning.

Herb & Supplement Therapy

—**Interceptive therapy plan:** (**Choose 2 to 3 recommendations**)

1—**For the infection:** • Crystal Star ANTI-BIO™ caps, 6 daily for 3 days, then 4 daily for a week; with • CLEANSING & PURIFYING™ tea for one week, or • Aloe vera juice, 2 TBS in juice morning and evening; or • Myrrh tincture.

2—**For swelling and pain:** • Crystal Star ANTI-FLAM™ caps as needed. Apply Crystal Star • ANTI-BIO™ gel, or • Echinacea extract 3x daily directly on abscess.

3—**Apply:** • Nutribiotic GRAPEFRUIT SEED SKIN SPRAY to abscess. Take • Nutribiotic GRAPEFRUIT SEED EXTRACT capsules if desired.

4—**For healing:** • Dr. Diamond HERPANACINE capsules, 6 daily.

—**Herbal healing resources:** (choose one)
• Garlic or nettles extract caps, 2 caps 3x daily to purify the blood.
• Cleavers tea, several times daily to take down inflammation.
• Burdock root tea 2 c. daily, a blood purifier to restore sebaceous gland function.

—**Effective skin healing applications:**
• AloeLife ALOE SKIN GEL, or Herbal Answers HERBAL ALOE FORCE gel.
• Tea tree oil or Thursday Plantation *tea tree* ANTISEPTIC CREAM.

—**For dental abscesses:**
• Colloidal silver - take internally as directed; apply directly.
• Use sage tea mouthwash twice daily, especially for dry socket abscesses.
• Apply *myrrh* extract 2x daily directly on abscess.

—**Preventive measures:** (choose one or more)
• Beta carotene 100,000IU daily, vitamin E 800IU daily, zinc 50mg daily, vitamin C with bioflavs. 3 to 5 grams daily for 1 month (may also apply a C solution).
• Prof. Nutrition DR. DOPHILUS + FOS caps or other probiotics 3x daily.
• Biotec CELL GUARD with SOD for 1 month to rebalance body chemistry.

Lifestyle Support Therapy

Warning: Squeezing a boil or abscess can force infectious bacteria into the bloodstream. Use hot compresses to bring boil to a head instead – 3 compresses, 3x daily. Dab with *tea tree oil.*

—**Bodywork:**

1—A *catnip, aloe vera juice,* or *wheat grass juice* enema at least once to clean out toxins.

2—Expose abscess area to early morning sunlight for 15 minutes a day.

—**Herbal healing; applications:** (choose 1)
• Hot epsom salts compress - 2 TBS salts to 1 cup hot water to bring to a head.
• Fenugreek seed compress to soften boil.
• Earth's Bounty O₂ spray, skin biocleanser
• A green or white clay compress 3 times daily to bring to a head.

—**For dental abscesses:** (choose one)
Homeopathic remedies are very successful. See a homeopathic professional.
• *Belladonna* for throbbing pain.
• *Bryonia* for acute inflammation.
• *Silicea* to increase pus drainage.
• *Mercurius* for foul breath.
    and
• Dissolve 1 tsp. acidophilus in water and rinse your mouth out 3x daily.

Common Symptoms: Boils are often part of your body's self-cleansing mechanism. Inflammation and infection of the skin layers, along with swelling of the nearest lymph glands; weeping, white, rather than clear drainage; pus-filled sores, often accompanied by chills and fever. Most common sites are buttocks, the back of neck and armpits.

Common Causes: Toxic system, especially the colon and blood, usually from an acid-forming diet high in chocolate, trans fats and sweets; lack of vegetable protein and essential fatty acids; a low resistance condition following a staph infection, viral or bacterial infection; an infection of a hair follicle, especially under the arms.

Can't find a recommended product? Call the 800 number listed in Product Resources for the store nearest you.

Acidity, Acidosis
Restoring Body Chemistry Balance

Balanced body chemistry pH is vital to immune health and disease correction. Your body has alkaline parts (like the blood) and acid parts (like the inside of the stomach), but when your over-all body chemistry is over-acid you open yourself up for arthritis type diseases. Duodenal ulcers are almost always in the wings if the body is continually over acidic. A healthy body keeps large alkaline reserves to meet the demands of too many acid-producing foods. When these are depleted beyond a 3:1 ratio, health can be seriously threatened. Take the Acid/Alkaline Test on page 542 to check your body chemistry balance and progress.

Diet & Superfood Therapy

–Nutritional therapy plan:

1–Go on a short 24 hour (pg. 192) liquid diet to cleanse excess acid wastes.

Drink an alkalizing juice: 8-oz. tomato juice, 1 tsp. each wheat germ, brewer's yeast and lecithin daily. ♀

Drink 1 to 2 glasses of cranberry juice daily, or Knudsen JUST CRANBERRY juice. ♀

2–For the next 3 days, eat only fresh, raw foods to complete the body: alkalizing process. (Cooked foods tend to increase acidity.)

3–Eat a diet of 75% alkalizing foods, including fresh and steamed vegetables, sprouts, fruits and fruit juices, miso soups, brown rice, green drinks, ume plums, honey, etc.

4–Acid-forming foods should be no more than 25% for 2 to 3 weeks. Avoid foods like coffee and caffeine-containing foods, meats, dairy foods (except yogurt or kefir), poultry, eggs, lentils, peanuts and legumes, cheeses, yeasted breads, most pre-prepared foods and most condiments.

5–Have a glass of wine at dinner to relax.

–Superfood therapy: (Choose one)
• AloeLife ALOE GOLD concentrate.
• Green Foods CARROT ESSENCE blend.
• Nutricology PRO GREENS with EFAs. ♀
• Crystal Star SYSTEMS STRENGTH™.
• Solgar WHEY TO GO.

Herb & Supplement Therapy

–Interceptive therapy plan: (Choose 1 or 2 recommendations)

1–For biochemistry balance: • Crystal Star FIBER & HERBS CLEANSE™ caps, or • Planetary Formulas TRIPHALA for 1 month; with • Crystal Star IODINE-POTASSIUM™ caps or 2 TBS snipped dry sea greens daily. And take • one teasp. cider vinegar in a glass of water each morning for a month.

2–To increase elimination of toxins: • Ginger compresses on the kidneys, and take • two ginger caps with each meal; or • Crystal Star AFTER-MEAL ENZ™ extract, or • HCL Pepsin tabs after meals.

–Other effective herbal healing resources: (choose one)
• Chamomile tea ♀
• Fennel seed tea
• Wisdom of the Ancients YERBA MATÉ tea

–Preventive measures: (choose one or more)
• High potency alkalizing enzymes, like Prevail FIBER ENZYME formula.
• B-complex 100mg with extra pantothenic acid 500mg, 2 daily.
• Ascorbate vitamin C crystals with bioflavonoids - 3000mg daily for 4 weeks.
• Future Biotics VITAL K PLUS, 2 tsp. daily.
• Arise and Shine FLORA GROW (friendly bacteria) for better pH.

–Supplements for kids: (choose one or two)
• Prevail VITASE for kids.
• Green Foods BARLEY ESSENCE (berry flavor).
• Catnip tea
• Probiotics: Natren LIFE START or Professional Nutrition DR. DOPHILUS powder in the morning.

Lifestyle Support Therapy

–Bodywork:
• Get some mild exercise every day for body oxygen. A daily walk is a good choice, with deep breathing exercises. Take another walk before you go to bed to relax and settle your system for the night.

–Herbal healing application:
• Crystal Star ALKALIZING ENZYME BODY WRAP™ for almost immediate change in body pH.

–Reflexology point:

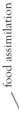

food assimilation

Common Symptoms: *Frequent skin eruptions that don't go away; sunken eyes with darkness around the eyes; rheumatoid arthritis; burning, foul-smelling stools and anal itching; chronic poor digestion; latent ulcers or ulcer flare-ups; bad breath and body odor; alternating constipation and diarrhea; insomnia; water retention; excessively low blood pressure; frequent migraine headaches.*

Common Causes: *Mental stress and tension; kidney, liver or adrenal malfunction; poor diet with excess acid-forming foods, such as caffeine, fried foods, tobacco, or sweets. Acidosis is often related to or caused by arthritis, diabetes or borderline diabetes. (Refer to those pages in this book.)*

Can't find a recommended product? Call the 800 number listed in Product Resources for the store nearest you.

Acne

Pimples, Blemishes

Acne is a hormone-related problem involved with the action of male testosterone on the sebaceous skin glands. Although teenage acne is common (4 out of 5 teenagers develop it) adult acne is also prevalent - clear signs of chronic stress and a poor diet. Whiteheads (comedones) are plugs of oil and dead skin cells under the surface of the skin that block oil from flowing to the skin surface. They may turn into blackheads (open comedones) when they reach the skin surface, or spread under the skin, rupture and inflame. Mega-doses of vitamins may aggravate acne because too much iodine and vitamin E can stimulate sebaceous glands to produce too much oil.

Diet & Superfood Therapy

—Nutritional therapy plan:

1—Go on a short 3 day liquid cleanse (pg. 191) to clean out acid wastes. Use apple, carrot, pineapple, papaya juices, and 6 glasses of water daily.

2—Add more fiber - especially from fresh foods. Have a salad every day. Add often to the diet: whole grains, green veggies, brown rice, sprouts, low-fat dairy and apples.

3—Choose turkey, chicken and vegetable protein (beans, tofu, sprouts) instead of red meat.

4—Limit acne triggers: wheat germ, shellfish, kelp, cheese, citrus, eggs, salt and foods with high iodine.

5—Drink Japanese green tea each morning or Crystal Star GREEN TEA CLEANSER™.

6—Eliminate acne trigger foods: white flour foods, sugary and fried foods, soft drinks, caffeine, chocolate, fatty dairy, hard cheeses, nightshade plants - eggplant, peppers, tobacco, tomatoes, peanut butter, additive-laden foods.

7—Add acidophilus and vitamin C if taking antibiotics for acne. Mix 1/4 teasp. vitamin C crystals with 1 TB acidophilus liquid, take 4x daily.

—Superfood therapy: (Choose one or two)

• Crystal Star ZINC SOURCE™ extract.
• AloeLife FIBER-MATE drink, 1/2 teasp.
• Y.S. ROYAL JELLY with GINSENG 2 teasp. daily.
• Green Foods CARROT ESSENCE blend.
• Wakunaga KYO-GREEN.

Herb & Supplement Therapy

—Interceptive therapy plan: (Choose 1 or 2 recommendations)

1—**Relieve inflammation and infection first:** • Crystal Star ANTI-BIO™ caps, 4x daily for 1 week. Use • Dr. Diamond HERPANACINE caps.♀

2—**Rapid improvement:** • Crystal Star BEAUTIFUL SKIN™ tea. Drink and apply with cotton balls, or dab on • Crystal Star HEALTHY SKIN GEL™.

3—**Tissue healing:** • Anabol Naturals AMINO BALANCE; homeopathic • *Ledum palustre* for adult acne, • *Hepar sulphuris* for youth acne.

4—**Add EFA's:** • *Evening primrose oil* 4-6 daily, or • *lemon grass*, or • *ginger* tea daily.

—For adult acne: (choose 2 or more remedies)

• Dr. Diamond HERPANACINE capsules 3 to 6 daily depending on severity.
• Honey facials: Use a tablespoon of honey; pat onto face for 5 minutes to remove dead skin cells. Rinse with water. Pat dry with cloth.
• *Burdock* tincture under the tongue 3x daily til clear. Add *yarrow* tea 2 c. daily.
• *Stevia* extract drops - apply directly.
• B-complex 100mg daily for stress-caused acne (appearing around chin). Add 100mg zinc daily with beta carotene 100,000IU.♂

—Acne skin healing applications: (choose one to pat on)

• *Goldenseal-myrrh* tea. • Jason NEW CELL ACNE THERAPY 5 1/2 roll-on.
• Propolis tincture, or • Beehive Botanicals PROPOLIS tincture.
• Acne soothing essential oils: *chamomile, tea tree, rosemary, lavender or geranium.*
• **For acne scars:** • Place fresh pineapple on the scars for enzyme therapy, and take bromelain 1500mg daily. • Take extra omega-3 oils for EFA's. • Use AHA's, like Noni of Beverly Hills AHA's regularly, or • Beta hydroxy acids if your skin is delicate. • Apply Camocare CAMOCARE GOLD clear solution.♀

—Preventive measures: (choose one or more)

• Pancreatin to digest oils. Vitamin E with selenium to normalize glutathione levels.♀
• **Liver detox:** especially with milk thistle seed extract for 2 to 3 months.

Lifestyle Support Therapy

—Bodywork:

• Apply Earth's Bounty O₂ SPRAY to affected areas. Do not squeeze. Whiteheads will come to the surface for elimination.
• Apply Nutribiotic FIRST AID skin spray to stop infected eruptions.
• Wash areas with *tea tree* or *calendula* soap. Then use Nonie of Beverly Hills NEW CONDITION for OILY PROBLEM SKIN.
• Herbal Answers ALOE FORCE gel.
• Apply cider vinegar. Dab on sores at night for 2 to 3 weeks. Sometimes amazing results.

—Lifestyle measures:

• **Sleep more.** Hormone levels and sebum levels increase when sleep is disrupted. Go to bed one hour earlier than usual.
• **Ice it.** As soon as you feel a pimple coming on, wrap an ice cube in saran wrap and hold it on the pimple for a few minutes. (Doesn't work for existing zits, though.)
• **Get sunshine.** Early morning sun on the face is best. Get fresh air and exercise daily.

—Herbal healing applications:

• Steam face with Swiss Kriss Herbs, or an aromatherapy *red clover-elder-eucalyptus* steam.
• Zia Cosmetics: ALOE CITRUS WASH, or ACNE TREATMENT MASK (adult acne).

See also ACNE ROSACEA page 502.

Common Symptoms: Inflamed and infected pustules on the face, chest and back. Often itching and scarring from Cystic Acne where fluid-filled cysts develop.

Common Causes: Gland (particularly pituitary), and hormone (particularly male) imbalance during teenage years, and before menstruation. Both teenage and adult acne are aggravated by a diet with lots of fatty foods, poor digestion of fats and essential fatty acid deficiency. Sugar-saturated skin is susceptible to acne, because a rise in blood sugar is multiplied by 5 when it gets to the skin. Poor liver function, poor elimination/constipation, heredity, some oral contraceptives, high oil cosmetics, emotional stress, and lack of green veggies are also related to acne's development.

Can't find a recommended product? Call the 800 number listed in Product Resources for the store nearest you.

Addictions

Alcohol Abuse, Rehabilitation

One-third of Americans are heavy drinkers, consuming more than 15 drinks a week, /accounting for 95% of the alcohol sold in the U.S. It's a disease, not a character flaw, and it leads to other problems. (For example, you may not be aware that all over-the-counter pain relievers now carry a liver damage warning for anyone who drinks 3 or more drinks a day.) As with other addictive practices, alcohol abuse is both brought on and marked by stress, depression, a no-confidence vote about one's self, as well as nutritional deficiencies. It also runs in families; over 76% of alcoholics have a genetic disorder metabolizing alcohol. As fatuous as it seems, purposely making a major life style improvement is sometimes the best medicine for changing body chemistry. This step works at the cause of the problem to curb the craving for alcohol's effects.

Diet & Superfood Therapy

—Nutritional therapy plan:

1—No alcohol detox program will work without liver regeneration. Go on a short liver cleanse (pg. 204) to clean out alcohol residues.

2—Follow the HYPOGLYCEMIA DIET in this book for 3 months. Take a daily protein drink, like Solgar WHEY TO GO to balance body chemistry and replace electrolytes quickly. Add 1 TB. lecithin granules or flax oil to control fatty liver.

3—Think B-vitamins, EFA's, protein and minerals for a solid nutrition base, especially magnesium-rich foods like wheat germ, sea greens, brewer's yeast, whole grains, brown rice, green leafy veggies, potatoes, low-fat dairy, eggs and fish.

4—Avoid fried foods, sugary or heavily spiced foods and caffeine. They aggravate alcohol craving. Sodas speed up alcohol release in the blood.

5—Sovex nutritional yeast broth or miso soup every night for B vitamins and to curb craving.

6—Dehydration is a hallmark of alcohol abuse. Drink 6 glasses of water every day.

—Superfood therapy: (Choose one or two)
• Crystal Star ENERGY GREEN™.
• Unipro PERFECT PROTEIN drink.
• **Nutricology PRO GREENS with EFA's.**
• Pines MIGHTY GREENS SUPERFOOD.
• Rainbow Light HAWAIIAN SPIRULINA drink.
• YS GINSENG-ROYAL JELLY tea for EFA's.

Herb & Supplement Therapy

—Interceptive therapy plan: (Choose 1 or 2 recommendations)

1—**Start your detox:** Crystal Star •WITHDRAWAL SUPPORT™ caps 3 months, with •REISHI-GINSENG extract, or •Country Life SHIITAKE/REISHI COMPLEX.

2—**Improve brain communication:** •Crystal Star CALCIUM SOURCE™ extract in water, a rapid calmer; or •5-HTP 50-100mg. Add •spirulina 500mg daily.

3—**Liver detox shortens withdrawal significantly:** •Crystal Star LIV-ALIVE™, •ADR-ACTIVE™ caps and •MENTAL INNER ENERGY™ caps for energy, or •Prevail DETOX ENZYME formula. Add •Milk Thistle Seed extract for 6 months.

4—**To curb alcohol craving:** take supplements below daily with meals for a month: •Glutamine, 2000mg daily to reduce cravings; •Carnitine 1000mg daily to reduce liver damage; •Time Release Niacin 500mg 2x daily; •Tyrosine 1000mg.

—Other effective herbal healing resources: (choose one)
• *Kava kava* calms nerves, (but also magnifies intoxification levels.)
• *Angelica-scullcap* tea to ease withdrawal and control craving, 3 cups daily.
• *Passionflower-hops* tea to control craving and regulate blood sugar.
• *Scullcap-black cohosh* tea calms nerves and overcomes depression.
• Evening primrose oil 500mg 2x daily for EFA's.

—Supplements can make up for critical deficiencies: (choose one or more)
—Vitamin C, up to 10,000mg daily (or until stool turns soupy).
—B-complex, 100mg 2x daily (B-vitamin deficiency increases desire for alcohol).
—Critical enzymes for alcohol detox are zinc dependent - Zinc 50mg 2x daily.

—Preventive measures: (choose one or more)
• DLPA 750mg with magnesium 500mg daily to help calm and curb cravings.
• Lithium orotate 5mg for 6 weeks especially if their is bipolar disorder, too.
• For nerve and withdrawal effects: •Solaray CHROMIACIN to regulate blood sugar, •Country Life B-15, 125mg for energy; •Taurine 500mg for nerve health.

Lifestyle Support Therapy

MEN: The liver controls hormone balance. Excessive drinking especially affects men and their estrogen levels through liver damage; abuse often means enlarged breasts, reduced sex drive and beard growth, and shrunken testes.

—Although it states the obvious, avoid the places, people and circumstances that sharpen your desire to escape through alcohol. This usually means a major life change and may seem impossible. But it almost always starts the road to lasting success and is often the only way.

—Bodywork:
• Acupuncture and massage therapy realignment help curb craving for alcohol.
• Improved fitness and system oxygen are important. Aerobic exercise like a daily walk reinforces your supplement therapy.
• Foot reflexology points:

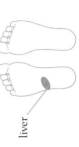

liver

See the LIVER DETOX program in this book for more information.

Common Symptoms: Alcohol dependence, and using alcohol for daily calories instead of food; short term memory loss; liver degeneration and disease; nervousness and poor coordination; high LDL cholesterol and blood sugar (there is a stress/sugar connection for both conditions); immune depression; poor enzyme production leading to poor fat and protein metabolism, and especially to mineral deficiency; anger, lack of emotional control, aggressive/compulsive behavior towards friends and family members.

Common Causes: Excessive intake of alcohol influenced by socio-psychological factors, genetic disorder, hypoglycemia from too much sugary food and too little fresh food; unrelieved daily stress.

Can't find a recommended product? Call the 800 number listed in Product Resources for the store nearest you.

Addictions

Alcohol Poisoning and Toxicity Reactions, Hangover

A high-stress, fast-paced, jet-lag lifestyle overloads your biochemical detox systems so that you get a steamroller effect the "morning after." A hangover should be gone by five o'clock the next day. If it isn't, you probably have alcohol poisoning. This severe type of hangover is alcohol poisoning with dehydration thrown in. Your body can't work adequately unless you give yourself a break. There are effective natural means of reducing alcohol's damage to your body and brain, but the real idea is to reduce alcohol consumption below the toxicity level.

Diet & Superfood Therapy

—Nutritional therapy plan:

1—Restabilize your body with vitamin B-rich, high fiber foods like brown rice and vegetables to soak up alcohol. Add antioxidant foods like cruciferous veggies and soy foods to help detoxify.

2—Drink cranberry juice to protect your liver.

3—NO "hair of the dog" drinks; they drag out a hangover. Eat crackers and honey at bedtime instead to burn up and soak up alcohol.

4—Drink several glasses of water at bedtime and in the morning to stave off a killer headache.

—Antioxidant hangover chasers:

• **Drink plenty of O.J. and tomato juice. Fructose helps your body burn alcohol.**

• Mix tomato juice, green and yellow onions, celery, parsley, hot pepper sauce, rosemary leaves, fennel seeds, basil, water, and Bragg's LIQUID AMINOS. Drink straight down.

• Knudsen's VERY VEGGIE SPICY juice.

—Superfood therapy: (Choose one or two)

• Crystal Star BIOFLAV., FIBER & C SUPPORT™ drink. Rapid results within a half hour.

• Knudsen's RECHARGE electrolyte replacement.

• Herbal Answers HERBAL ALOE FORCE juice.

• Red Star NUTRITIONAL YEAST $1/4$ teasp. in water to alleviate nausea.

Herb & Supplement Therapy

—Interceptive therapy plan:

1—**Before drinking, to minimize toxicity to the brain: (choose 1 or 2)** Take • Cysteine 500mg (or NAC) with • 2 Evening Primrose oil 500mg caps and • B-complex 100mg before drinking and before retiring to boost glutathione. • Kudzu caps, 2 to 6, or • Planetary KUDZU HERBAL 750mg to suppress ethanol.

—**Liver support:** • Milk Thistle Seed 120mg extract.

—**Curb cravings-boost energy:** *Siberian ginseng extract drops in angelica root tea.*

2—**After you drink to minimize toxicity to the brain: (choose 1 or 2)** Take Crystal Star ASPIR-SOURCE™ caps, with 2 MENTAL INNER ENERGY™ caps.

—**For withdrawal:** • Alacer EMERGEN-C with bioflavonoids $1/2$ teasp. in water, with a • B-complex 100mg capsule, zinc 30mg, and • 5-HTP - 50mg.

—**For energy:** • Crystal Star GINSENG 6 SUPER™ tea, or • Dragon Eggs SAGES GINSENG tablets.

—Nervines and enzyme therapy if you have a hangover:

• *Kava kava* calms nerves, (but also magnifies intoxication levels).

• *Cayenne-ginger* capsules settle the stomach and relieve headaches.

• *Dandelion-burdock-ginger* tea with honey to quell nausea.

• *Scullcap* tea soothes nerves and oxygenates the brain.

• BILBERRY extract protects the liver; MILK THISTLE extract supports the liver.

—Antioxidants end the misery and heal a hangover:

Take 1 each - EVENING PRIMROSE oil 1000mg, Source Naturals CO-ENZYMATE-B, (or 4 bee pollen tablets), Country Life B-12 sublingual, 2500mcg; Country Life DMG, 125mg tablet, Glutamine 1000mg.

—A quick liver tonic if you have alcohol poisoning: Steep for 20 minutes - hibiscus, cloves, allspice, and juice of 2 lemons in grape or orange juice. Drink slowly.

Lifestyle Support Therapy

If you take kava kava for depression or tension, don't drink alcohol for at least 6 hours after taking it. You'll get highly intoxicated. Both are sedatives-depressants.

Get outside in the fresh air - the more oxygen in the lungs and tissues, the better.

If the case is severe, you may need a stomach pump at an urgent care center.

—Bodywork:

• If your hangover doesn't go away, you may have alcohol poisoning. Take a catnip, chlorophyll or coffee enema, and the liver tonic on this page.

• Apply cold compresses to the head before and after a long hot shower to wash off toxins coming out through the skin. (You won't believe what a difference this makes.) Or, take alternating hot and cool showers to stimulate circulation and eliminate blood alcohol.

• **Take a sauna for 20 minutes. Scrub skin with a dry skin brush.**

—Hand reflexology:

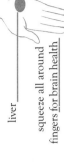

liver

squeeze all around
fingers for brain health

Common Symptoms: Sensitivity to light, headache, eyeache, bad taste in the mouth, weakness and debility, shakiness, dull mind and senses, stomach queasiness, lethargy. Initial withdrawal symptoms include high anxiety, rapid pulse with tremors, hot flashes and drenching perspiration, dehydration, insomnia and sometimes hallucinations.

Common Causes: Alcohol poisoning from too much alcohol; liver exhaustion and consequent malfunction.

A cleanse can start your program right. Call the 800 number listed in Product Resources for the store nearest you.

Can't find a recommended product? See page 208 for more information and my book DETOXIFICATION for a complete cleanse.

Addictions

Drug Abuse, Rehabilitation

Most people begin taking drugs to alleviate boredom and fatigue, or to relieve physical or psychological pain. In almost every case, nutritional health is severely compromised regardless of whether the drug being abused is a prescription or pleasure substance. Multiple depletions of critical nutrients like vitamins, minerals, essential fatty acids and enzymes set off addictive chain reactions. It takes a year or more to detoxify the blood of drugs. No program is successful against drug abuse without consistent therapy and awareness. Lifestyle therapy helps treat addictions successfully by minimizing the discomfort and maximizing the healing process as you go about your life. Don't be fooled.... all street drugs, whether chemical or so-called herbal are strong, usually adulterated and can cause brain damage.

Diet & Superfood Therapy

—Nutritional therapy plan:

1—Most addictive drugs create malnutrition. A good diet is essential for overcoming nutrient deficiencies caused by substance abuse. Include plenty of slow-burning complex carbohydrates from whole grains and fresh vegetables, and vegetable protein from soy, grains and sprouts.

2—The brain is dependent on glucose as an energy source. Drug withdrawals often mean blood glucose levels drop with the consequent results of sweating, tremor, palpitations, anxiety and cravings. Eliminate sugars, alcohol and caffeine from the diet. They aggravate the craving for drugs. Follow the Hypoglycemia Diet, page 427.

3—Enzymes are important: include plenty of fresh foods for plant enzymes (or take Enzymedica DIGEST) to restabilize your body chemistry.

Note: A cleanse can help get rid of drug residues quickly. See page 186 for more information and my book DETOXIFICATION for a complete cleanse.

—Superfood therapy: (Choose one or two)
• YS ROYAL JELLY-GINSENG tea blend.
• Body Ecology VITALITY SUPER GREEN with royal jelly and evening primrose oil.
• Crystal Star SYSTEMS STRENGTH™ (especially for prescription drugs).♂
• Nutricology PRO GREENS with EFA's.

Herb & Supplement Therapy

—Interceptive therapy 7-step plan:

1—**Normalize body chemistry:** • Crystal Star GINSENG 6 SUPER TEA™, • WITHDRAWAL SUPPORT™ caps, or • GINSENG/REISHI extract.

2—**Clean out drug residues:** • Crystal Star HEAVY METAL™ or • DETOX™ capsules 4 daily; • Sun CHLORELLA tabs; • M.D. Labs DAILY DETOX tea.

3—**Detoxify the liver:** • Crystal Star LIV-ALIVE™ tea, or • GREEN TEA CLEANSER™ with • milk thistle seed extract for 2 months, and • B-complex 150mg daily.

4—**Reduce anxiety and relax nerves:** • Crystal Star RELAX™ caps; gotu kola caps.

5—**Curb cravings and boost circulation:** • licorice tea or • ginkgo biloba extract; • Crystal Star GINSENG-REISHI extract, • Glutamine 1000mg 2x daily.

6—**Increase energy:** • Crystal Star GINSENG 6 SUPER ENERGY™ caps, or • MENTAL INNER ENERGY™ extract; • Siberian ginseng; • astragalus extract.

7—**Replenish neurotransmitters:** • Enzymatic Therapy THYROID/TYROSINE caps, • 5-HTP, 50mg 2x daily, • Country Life RELAXER (GABA with taurine).

—Minimize withdrawal discomfort: (choose 2 or 3)
• Rosemary tea, or glutamine 1000mg; DLPA 750mg for cravings and depression.
• Oatstraw tea or valerian-wild lettuce extract in water for sleeplessness and anxiety.
• Chamomile for stress, scullcap for nerves, ginkgo biloba for memory loss.
• Amino Acids for stabilizing protein - full spectrum 1000mg daily.

—Withdrawal help for specific drugs: Methionine for heroine; Tyrosine and Siberian ginseng for cocaine; CoQ-10 up to 300mg for prescription drugs; LITHIUM orotate 5mg for uppers and depressants; B-complex 150mg for LSD.

—Preventive measures:
• Vitamin C crystals - up to 10,000mg daily, with niacin 1000mg 3x daily.
• Acidophilus - to replace friendly G.I. flora; chromium to rebalance sugar levels.
• Enzymes- Enzymedia DIGEST; Rainbow Light ADVANCED ENZYME SYSTEM.

Lifestyle Support Therapy

Note: Strong drugs, from LSD to hard alcohol to nicotine to heroin, can put you at higher risk for Alzheimer's disease due to microvascular blockage and cerebral dementia.

Nicotine increases craving for drugs by stripping the body of stabilizing nutrients.

—Bodywork:
• Biofeedback, chiropractic, massage therapy, yoga and acupuncture techniques have a high success rate in overcoming drug addictions.

• Apply tea tree oil, or B&T CALI-FLORA GEL to heal ulcers in the nose.

• Lobelia extract drops every half hour can sometimes help normalize from an overdose situation.

• Reflexology point:

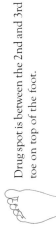

Drug spot is between the 2nd and 3rd toe on top of the foot.

See the HYPOGLYCEMIA DIET, pg. 427 for more information.

Can't find a recommended product? Call the 800 number listed in Product Resources for the store nearest you.

Common Symptoms: Metabolic disorders like low blood sugar, hypothyroidism, poor adrenal function, liver malfunction and depression; general irritability, fatigue, unusual drowsiness, shakiness, nervousness, disorientation, memory loss, wired feeling, anxiety and paranoia; headaches, sweating and cramps; palpitations; poor food absorption even when meals are good.
Common Causes: Addictive origins cover a broad spectrum of factors, ranging from inherited genetics, childhood social behavior patterns, poor nutrition, along with allergies to certain foods, and metabolic physiology.

Caffeine Addiction

Caffeine is one of the most widely used stimulant drugs in the world. It is found in coffee, tea, cocoa, chocolate and herbs such as cola nuts and yerba mate tea. It is a constituent of prescription medicines like Excedrin, Anacin, Vanquish and Bromo-seltzer. It is an ingredient of almost every appetite suppressant and many soft drinks. More than 80% of American adults use coffee, and almost everybody else gets caffeine in one of its other forms. There is good news and bad news about caffeine. Clearly it is a quick energy pick-me-up, and a memory stimulant, but just as clearly, excessive use of caffeine (over 5 cups of coffee a day) can lead to anxiety, sleeplessness, increased blood sugar levels, rapid heartbeat, exhausted adrenals and increased tolerance to its effects - all signs of addiction.

Good ideas for successfully cutting down on caffeine without the agony of withdrawal:
1: Drink a cup of energizing herbal tea instead of coffee, such as •Crystal Star HIGH ENERGY™ tea (energy rise is rapid), or •GINSENG SIX SUPER™ tea (slower, longer energy).
2: Strengthen your adrenal glands with herbal formulas like •Crystal Star FEM SUPPORT™ extract for women, or •ADR-ACTIVE™ extract for men.
3: Normalize your body chemistry with a ginseng adaptogen compound, containing herbs like •Siberian ginseng, panax ginseng, ashwagandha, gotu kola and reishi mushroom.
4: Take •Natra-Bio homeopathic CAFFEINE WITHDRAWAL RELIEF, zinc 30mg daily (caffeine leaches out body zinc stores), and add a B-Complex 100mg daily.

Prescription Drug Dependence

One of the most serious addictions today is the widespread dependence on prescription drugs - especially mood altering drugs like tranquilizers, anti-depressants and anti-psychotics. Others, like amphetamines, create an addictive high through a metabolic process similar to the effect of the body's endorphins. A 1998 study showed that 17% of Americans over 60 are addicted, and that many of seniors mix alcohol with their prescription drugs for additional risk.

Signs that addiction is occurring: 1) The body builds up a tolerance to the drug, so that the user increases the dosage regularly. 2) There is a decreased desire to work, with inattentiveness, mood swings, restlessness, temper tantrums, crying spells, or all of the above. 3) There is unusual susceptibility to illness because the immune system has been weakened by the drug. 4) Withdrawal symptoms of headaches, insomnia, light sensitivity, hot flashes, diarrhea and disorientation occur when the individual stops the drug.

Some tranquilizers and anti-depressants can be replaced with herbal remedies to avoid dependence, but specific prescription information is necessary to make the withdrawal process straightforward and safe. A good holistic doctor or naturopath should be able to help you.

Three types of herbs are needed to wean yourself from addictive prescription drugs.
—Nervines, such as scullcap and passionflower, to relax and rebuild the nervous system. Try •Crystal Star RELAX caps as needed.
—Tonic adaptogens, such as ginseng, astragalus, or chlorella strengthen and normalize the body.
—Liver detoxification herbs, such as milk thistle seed extract, or turmeric (curcumin), help rebalance your entire system.

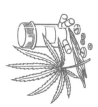

About Marijuana Use

The use of marijuana is rising again in the U.S., this time with new propagation techniques that make THC content over 200% greater than 20 or 30 years ago. We should be clear about what marijuana is and what it isn't. Marijuana is no longer the mildly euphoric 3 or 4 hour high of the 60's and 70's. It is addictive. Those who are dependent on it are either constantly thinking about it, under intoxication, or recovering from its influence. Both mental and physical health are clearly affected, especially in terms of blood sugar balance, muscle coordination, reaction time and emotional deterioration. Work habits suffer from lack of ambition and direction, family life and relationships suffer because of apathy and non-communication.

However, many casual marijuana users are not aware of new research about this drug. Its newly increased strength means many more people are experiencing exaggerated effects, such as acute anxiety, paranoia, incoherent speech, extreme disorientation and hallucinations lasting up to 12 hours. Marijuana also impairs the reproductive system, especially in terms of reduced male sperm count, both short term and long term memory, and depressed immune response (by as much as 40%). Marijuana smoke today contains the same health-damaging carcinogens as tobacco smoke, only now in much higher concentrations. Because its smoke is inhaled more deeply and held in the lungs longer than tobacco, it leads to severe lung damage. All the attendant diseases of nicotine smokers are now besetting marijuana smokers - especially chronic bronchitis, emphysema and lung cancer.

Marijuana withdrawal is characterized by anxiety, sleeplessness, tremors and chills. Simple nutrition and lifestyle changes can go a long way toward minimizing the discomfort and mental craving.
•Marijuana leaches B vitamins; make brown rice and broccoli mainstays of your diet during the withdrawal period. Follow the diet for HYPOGLYCEMIA (pg. 427) to control sugar cravings.
•Take a protein drink every morning, like •ALL ONE MULTIPLE grren plant base, •Unipro PERFECT PROTEIN, or •Crystal Star SYSTEMS STRENGTH™ drink with sea greens.
•Take antioxidants like tyrosine, plenty of •vitamin C with bioflavonoids, •B-complex, and herbal nerve relaxers such as rosemary aromatherapy, or •Crystal Star RELAX CAPS™.
•Exercise - it re-oxygenates your tissues to help you kick the craving. Marijuana makes for flabby bodies.

See my book DETOXIFICATION for a complete drug rehabilitation program.

Can't find a recommended product? Call the 800 number listed in Product Resources for the store nearest you.

Does your body need to clean out drug or alcohol toxins?

Americans have an expensive river of chemicals coursing through our national veins. We take almost $20 billion worth of prescription drugs each year. Ten million Americans are officially classified as addicted to alcohol. At a cost to taxpayers of nearly $300 billion dollars a year, some believe that it's the nation's number one health problem. The use of "hard" or "pleasure" drugs in today's society is also prevalent. Still, experts believe that the most serious addictions are those to prescription drugs. More than one million people a year (3 to 5 percent of admissions) end up in hospitals as a result of negative reactions to prescription drugs.

Clearly, modern drugs play lifesaving roles in emergency situations and they can help numerous health problems, especially short term, but most people begin taking drugs to alleviate boredom and fatigue, or to relieve physical or psychological pain. A detox program helps enormously to release drugs and alcohol from your system, but withdrawing after long time use can produce harsh effects. I highly recommend the supervision of a qualified health professional for an addictions cleanse, especially if the dependency has been long term and highly addictive. Sometimes, the best way is to wean yourself gradually from the addictive substance while you do your addiction cleanse.

The dis-ease feelings that drugs or excessive alcohol alleviates are merely warning signs of deeper internal imbalances. Alcohol abuse especially may be brought on and marked by stress and depression. Drugs and alcohol can even aggravate an original health problem and add to the poisons in your body. Drug detoxification is a process of releasing the stored residues, at the same time changing lifestyle habits so that you are no longer dependent on them. It is critical to fortify your body enough to give it the power to resist returning to the addictive substance. I have found that only a well-nourished body can offer both your body and mind enough of a sense of well being and strength to melt the relapse urges and desires.

Do you think you might be addicted?

—Do you only feel happy and relaxed after having a drink or taking an antidepressant or mood elevating drug?
—Do you find that you can't relieve daily stress without a drink or a drug? Do you get frequent headaches that feel like a continual hangover?
—Do you have liver problems? Does your stomach protrude but you are thin everywhere else? It's a sign of liver enlargement and inflammation.
—Do you have esophagus impairment, reflux after eating, high blood pressure, or pancreatitis? Are your stools pale?
—Are the whites of your eyes dingy? Is the eye lower lid yellow? Is your skin slightly jaundiced? Do you sweat a lot? Signs of liver exhaustion.
—Have you lost your appetite? Have you gotten noticeably, or unusually thin? Do you have a marked intolerance for fatty foods?
—Is your digestion always bad? Do you have a metallic taste in your mouth? Are you drowsy after meals? Are you often foggy mentally? Have you become intolerant to certain foods? Are you overly sensitive to chemicals? Do you crave sweets? Is your blood sugar usually low? Do you ever get dizzy or black out? These signs indicate rampant hypoglycemia from alcohol or drug overload.
—Do you feel shaky and sweaty? Do you often get a "wired," nervous feeling, sometimes with heart palpitations? Central nervous system overload is a sign of addiction.
—Do you have frequent memory loss? Short term memory loss is one of the first signs of alcohol abuse; damage to the brain is another.
—Are you unusually anxious, even paranoid? Do you lose your temper or get in a bad mood easily? Do you feel depressed and cry a lot? Typically late symptoms of alcohol abuse.
—Is there pain on your right side or under your right shoulder blade? Do you get stomach or muscle cramps frequently?
—Are you continually tired? Extreme fatigue usually results from poor liver health, adrenal exhaustion or thyroid malfunction
—Is your immune response low? Do you seem to have a cold or flu all the time? All drugs weaken the immune system over time.

In the overwhelming number of cases, habitual drug and alcohol users suffer from chronic subclinical malnutrition, and from multiple depletions of critical nutrients. Vitamins, minerals, amino acids, fatty acids and enzymes are all depleted, some by 50 to 60 percent.

What does it feel like to withdraw from drugs or alcohol?

Withdrawal symptoms are the same as addiction symptoms, only worse and more frequent. Breaking destructive habits is hard. Your body reacts when a substance it thinks it depends on is removed. The initial withdrawal phase is usually the most difficult part of an addiction detox and can last from a day or two to a week or more. You'll get chronic headaches, usually with diarrhea as your body tries to release toxins faster, and a lot of irritability. Some people experience hallucinations, disorientation or irrational thinking. Some go into depression. You'll probably sleep poorly, and your sleep will be interrupted during the night. Most people in withdrawal are sensitive to light and noise, hot and cold flashes, and sweating.

But every day gets easier. I encourage people to look at each episode of discomfort as a little victory on the road to recovery. One of the laws of the universe is that we don't have to fight the same battle twice. As your body dislodges and removes more toxins day by day, you have the satisfaction of knowing they can be gone for good. Natural mood enhancers, like St. John's Wort and Kava Kava, that our bodies are equipped to handle, help in the weaning process from addictive substances. Ginkgo biloba extract for a month speeds up your brain processes.

See my book DETOXIFICATION for a complete drug rehabilitation program.

Can't find a recommended product? Call the 800 number listed in Product Resources for the store nearest you.

Adrenal Gland Health

Adrenal Exhaustion

Small glands resting on top of the kidneys, the adrenals are comprised of two parts: the medulla, which secretes adrenaline, and norepinephrine to help the body cope with stress by increasing metabolism; and the cortex, responsible for maintaining body balance, regulating sugar metabolism, and a complex array of steroid hormones, including cortisone, DHEA, aldosterone, progesterone, estrogen, and testosterone. Adrenal function is impaired by long term cortico-steroid drug use, because these drugs cause the adrenals to shrink in size.

Diet & Superfood Therapy

—Nutritional therapy plan:

1—Eat small, instead of large meals, low in sugar and fats. Eat lots of fresh foods, cold water fish, brown rice, legumes and whole grains.

2—Put sea greens at the top of your list of adrenal enhancing foods. Add more potassium-rich foods like potatoes, salmon, seafood and avocados to your diet. Intake should be about 3 to 5 grams daily. Cut down on high sodium foods.

3—Avoid stimulants like hard liquor, tobacco and excess caffeine during healing.

4—Avoid fats, fried foods, red meats and highly processed foods for long term adrenal health.

5—Make a fresh mix daily: flax seed, bran, miso broth and honey. Take some each morning to feed adrenals. Or, take 2 teasp. each Red Star Nutritional yeast and wheat germ daily in fruit juice.

—Superfood therapy: (Choose one or two)

• Crystal Star SYSTEMS STRENGTH™ drink, or BIOFLAV., FIBER & C SUPPORT™ drink.
• Y.S. ROYAL JELLY with GINSENG 2 tsp. daily.
• Wakunaga KYO-GREEN drink.
• Green Kamut JUST BARLEY drink.
• Nutricology PRO-GREENS with EFA's.

Herb & Supplement Therapy

—Interceptive therapy plan: (Choose 1 or 2 recommendations)

1—**Stimulate hormone and adrenal rebalance:** • Crystal Star ADR-ACTIVE™ capsules or ADRN™ extract, 2x daily with BODY REBUILDER™ caps; • CC Pollen HIGH DESERT ROYAL JELLY with ginseng, 2 teasp. daily; • Nutricology GERMANIUM 150mg daily.

  —For women: Add • Morada Research Labs ADRENAL GLANDS or • Crystal Star IODINE SOURCE™ extract as a potassium-rich source. ♀

  —For men: Add • Crystal Star GINSENG-LICORICE ELIXIR™ extract 2x daily, • Panax ginseng root, or Siberian ginseng-astragalus capsules, 4 daily. ♂

—Long term adrenal support from herbs: (choose one or more)

• Evening primrose oil 4-6 daily.
• Siberian ginseng **and** panax ginsengs directly support the medulla.
• Licorice root tea (deglyrrhizinated capsules if you have high blood pressure).
• Hawthorn leaf, berry and flower extract.
• Gotu kola extract caps 6 daily.
• Milk thistle seed extract.

—Preventive measures:

Adrenal nutrients include essential fatty acids, amino acids, pantothenic acid, vitamins E, A, C, fat soluble vitamins D and K, bioflavonoids, and the minerals zinc, selenium, potassium, manganese, chromium and magnesium.
• Adrenal complex glandular, such as Country Life ADRENAL with TYROSINE.
• Enzymatic Therapy LIQUID LIVER with Siberian Ginseng.♂
• Pantothenic acid 1000mg daily, with B-complex 100mg and Tyrosine 500mg daily. ♀
• Ascorbate vitamin C 3000mg or Ester C 1500mg daily.
• Enzymes: CoQ-10 60mg 2x daily as an enzyme antioxidant; Enzymedica DIGEST or Prevail VITASE to stimulate adrenal cortex.

Lifestyle Support Therapy

—Warning signs of adrenal exhaustion:

1: poor memory and low energy; 2: nervous moistness of hands and soles of feet; 3: brittle, peeling nails and extremely dry skin; 4: heart palpitations and panic attacks; 5: chronic low back pain; 6: hypoglycemia and cravings for salt or sweets; 7: severe reactions to odors or certain foods; 8: and a high incidence of yeast and fungal infections.

—Bodywork:

• Massage therapy is effective in improving adrenal function. Therapists use muscle testing to determine the degree of dysfunction and then work to clear the adrenal pathways.
• Take a Crystal Star HOT SEAWEED bath for a noticeable adrenal energy boost.
• Take an arm-swinging walk every day for adrenal health.

• Reflexology point:

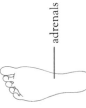

adrenals

Common Symptoms: *Lack of energy and alertness; a sense of being "driven" and anxious, followed by great fatigue, weakness and lethargy; poor memory, low blood pressure and poor circulation; moodiness and irritability; sugar dysfunctions (hypoglycemia and diabetes); low immunity; brittle nails, dry skin; food cravings (especially for sugar).*
Common Causes: *Continuing stress; extensive use of corticosteroid drugs for arthritis, asthma, allergies, etc.; pituitary disease or T.B.; poor diet with too much sugar and refined carbohydrates; over use of alcohol, nicotine, or recreational drugs; too much caffeine; vitamin B and C deficiencies, especially during menopause years.*

See DIET FOR HYPOGLYCEMIA in this book for more specifics.

Can't find a recommended product? Call the 800 number listed in Product Resources for the store nearest you.

Adrenal Exhaustion

Adrenal exhaustion is an epidemic in this country. No other gland is more affected by stress, emotional strain or anger than the adrenals. Your adrenal glands are responsible for a myriad of body functions including the production of steroid hormones like cortisone, DHEA, aldosterone, progesterone, estrogen and testosterone, maintaining body balance and regulating sugar metabolism. When you're under pressure, the adrenal medulla secretes adrenaline and norepinephrine to accelerate metabolism, heart rate, respiration and perspiration. It's a response vital to our survival, strengthening the body and increasing its resistance to stress. But when the adrenals release too few or too many hormones, exhaustion or overstimulation can result. Corticosteroid drugs, temperature changes, excessive exercise, too much caffeine or sugar, chronic stress and infections all exhaust the adrenal glands. Chronic, unexplained fatigue, low blood sugar attacks and increased allergies are often the result of exhausted adrenals.

A good diet and plenty of rest is essential to adrenal health. Potassium is the principal mineral lost when adrenal health is compromised. Eating more potassium rich foods like sea vegetables, bananas, kiwis, potatoes and fish can help recharge your adrenals so you'll have more energy. Other key nutrients for recovery from adrenal exhaustion: B vitamins (royal jelly as a rich food source of pantothenic acid shows excellent results); vitamin C (important in maintaining adrenal integrity and in helping convert cholesterol to adrenal hormones); zinc foods, like brown rice, grains, sunflower seeds, pumpkin seeds, brewer's yeast, bran, eggs, oysters, etc.; magnesium foods like dark green leafy vegetables, almonds, dried apricots, avocado, raw carrots, citrus fruits, lentils, salmon, flounder, etc.; and the amino acid tyrosine. Recommended herbs to include: Korean ginseng, sarsaparilla, kelp and garlic.

Important note for menopausal women: Adrenal health is critical for women after menopause as these glands begin to shore up the work of hormone production to keep a woman healthy, active, and beautiful after estrogen production is reduced by the ovaries. Certain herbs like licorice, sarsaparilla and Siberian ginseng work specifically to stimulate the adrenal glands to regulate body energy after menopause.

Do you have Addison's Disease?

In Addison's disease, adrenal exhaustion is so severe that the adrenal glands are completely unable to secrete their steroid hormones. Immune response decreases, energy levels fall rapidly, even small stresses lead to serious collapse of health. Addison's disease may be lifelong and life threatening. Warning signs to watch for include: unexplained weight loss; chronic fatigue (especially muscular weakness); severe nausea and/or vomiting; changes in pigmentation (skin darkening); unusual irritability and depression; light-headedness and dizziness upon standing from low blood pressure; and cravings for salty foods (loss of body salt from electrolyte imbalance is common in Addison's disease).

—A good diet is critical for overcoming Addison's disease. Alcohol, caffeine, tobacco, and highly processed foods must be avoided.
—Take Enzymatic Therapy ADRENAL CORTEX concentrate, with PITUITARY concentrate to stimulate and balance ACTH output.
—Take Lewis Labs BREWERS YEAST, 2 TBS daily, or brewer's yeast tablets, with extra B Complex 100mg and pantothenic acid 1000mg.
—Take royal jelly, 60,000 to 100,000mg or more, 2x daily; YS ORGANIC ROYAL JELLY with GINSENG TEA is an excellent choice.
—Take licorice extract or Crystal Star GINSENG/LICORICE ELIXIR™, under the tongue or in water, 2x daily.

Cushing's Syndrome

A rare, dysfunctional disease caused by an overactive adrenal cortex, Cushing's syndrome is an opportunistic condition, allowed by immune suppression, and sometimes brought on by overdose of cortico-steroid drugs, (particularly those used for rheumatoid arthritis). It is also a metabolic disease that causes the formation of kidney stones. It is characterized by obesity in the stomach, face and buttocks, but severe thinness in the limbs. There is muscle wasting and weakness, poor wound healing, thinning of the skin leading to stretch marks and bruising. Peptic ulcers, high blood pressure, mental instability, and diabetes also accompany Cushing's. The face may get acne-like sores and the eyelids are often swollen. Cushing's appears in women five times more than men; there is scalp balding, excess body and facial hair (hirsutism), brittle bones, along with a wide variety of menstrual disorders.

Because of its rarity, our experience has been limited with this disease. The following protocols have been found helpful:
•Follow a vegetarian diet, low in fat, sodium and sugar. Add high potassium foods daily - bananas, broccoli, sea greens, etc.
•Add green drinks, like Nutricology PRO-GREENS with EFA's, chlorella, germanium and protein for healing, or Crystal Star ENERGY GREEN™ drink regularly.
•Take potassium in large doses - daily sea greens, herbal potassium drinks, like Future Biotics VITAL K, 2 teasp. daily, or Crystal Star IODINE/POTASSIUM SOURCE™ capsules.

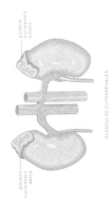

glandula
suprarenalis
sinistra

glandula
suprarenalis
dextra

GLANDULAE SUPRARENALES

Can't find a recommended product? Call the 800 number listed in Product Resources for the store nearest you.

AIDS and HIV Infection

AIDS and its cousin diseases are the result of immune system breakdown. The body becomes unable to defend itself. Long believed to be caused by the HIV (human immunodeficiency virus), a retro-virus that affects DNA and T-cells, there is a growing body of evidence that severe AIDS is influenced by nutritional factors. AIDS occurs in stages: an asymptomatic state (when the disease is most often passed), a mononucleosis-like stage with one or more AIDS-related complexes, and "full blown" AIDS. The protocols here are for those who are diagnosed with HIV, but are asymptomatic, for those who decide to reject orthodox AIDS treatment for alternative methods, and for those who have tried orthodox treatment, but showed no improvement and have decided to use alternative techniques (evidence shows that even new highly acclaimed drugs are failing, and may increase diabetes risk). If you decide to use a combination of orthodox and alternative treatments, seek out advice from a knowledgeable naturopath. Mixing natural products with the powerful drugs used for AIDS can be dangerous.

Diet & Superfood Therapy

—**Nutritional therapy plan:**

Compromised nutrition is clearly tied to low immune response. Diet improvement is the key to keeping HIV infection from becoming AIDS. Intestinal chemistry and pH environment must be changed to optimize disease protection.

1—The extreme toxicity, fatigue and malabsorption of AIDS forestalls a liquid detox plan - it is too harsh for an already weakened system. **Three glasses of fresh carrot juice and a potassium broth (pg. 215) daily keep a good detox ongoing. A good juicer is really necessary.**

2—Your diet plan should have the highest possible nutrition. A modified macrobiotic diet is ideal for high resistance and immune strength. All produce should be fresh and organically grown when possible. See diet recommendations on page 306.

3—No fried, fatty foods (they aggravate diarrhea). Avoid concentrated sweeteners, and highly processed, chemicalized foods of all kinds.

4—Eat plenty of foods with anti-parasitic enzymes: cranberries, pineapple, papaya.

5—Flush your body with 6 to 8 glasses of mild herb teas and bottled water daily. Add $\frac{1}{2}$ teasp. ascorbate vitamin C and $\frac{1}{4}$ teasp Natren bifidobacteria to each daily drink for optimum results.

—**Superfood therapy: (Choose one or two)**
• Monas CHLORELLA drink.
• Crystal Star GREEN TEA CLEANSER™.
• Imperial Elixir GINSENG/ROYAL JELLY drink.
• Solgar WHEY TO GO to deter HIV.
• Nutricology PRO-GREENS with EFA's.

Herb & Supplement Therapy

—**Interceptive therapy plan: (Choose 2 or more recommendations)**

Plant anti-virals have been among the most effective treatments against HIV.
• Transformation enzyme PUREZYME 360m, see directions for HIV infection.
• East Park OLIVE LEAF EXTRACT helps drop viral loads.
• Licorice root, Nettles, Calophyllum lanegirum and Hyssop inhibit HIV replication.
• Milk thistle seed boosts immune response and protects the liver.
• Turmeric (curcumin) inhibits TNF, a cytokine that increases HIV in T-cells.
• Garlic inhibits TNF, and is a measureable selenium source.
• Una da gato and St. John's wort extract, proven effective against retro-viruses.
• Siberian ginseng extract or Imperial Elixir SIBERIAN GINSENG, T-cell helpers.
• Chinese herbal antivirals - immunomodulators effective against HIV: Astragalus, Reishi and Shiitake mushrooms, Grifon PRO MAITAKE D-FRACTION extract, Atractylodes, Schizandra, Ligustrum.
• Chinese bitter melon and wheat grass juice are selectively anti-tumor.
• Evening primrose oil, infected cells crack up and die when bombarded with GLA.

—**Detoxification and purifying supplements: (choose one or more)**
• Egg yolk lecithin. Active lipids help make cell walls virally resistant.
• American Biologics DIOXYCHLOR or Crystal Star DETOX™ caps.
• Enzymatic Therapy LIVA-TOX caps, or Jarrow LIPOIC ACID 150mg 3x daily.
• Herbal Answers ALOE FORCE JUICE, 2 to 4 TBS daily to curb virus spread with echinacea extract to stimulate interleukin, and turmeric to inhibit TNF.
• Nutricology CAR-T-CELL shark cartilage vials, 15ml under the tongue daily.

—**Body normalizing measures: (choose one or more)**
• Vitamin C powder with bioflavonoids, 10-30g daily, injection or orally.
• 300,000IU mixed carotenes to stimulate T-cell activity.
• NAC (N-acetyl-cysteine), high potency as directed.
• Nutricology GERMANIUM 150-200mg daily for interferon production.
• CoQ₁₀ 300mg daily, with GLUTATHIONE 100mg 2 daily.
• Quercetin (blocks HIV same way as AZT) with BROMELAIN 1500mg daily.
• Enzyme therapy: Bromelain 1500mg daily; and Biotec Foods CELL GUARD.
• OPC's from grape seed and white pine 100mg 4 daily.
• Prof. Nutrition DOCTOR DOPHILUS with FOS powder, (7 potent cultures).

Lifestyle Support Therapy

—**Detoxification bodywork:**
• It is absolutely necessary to detoxify the liver for holistic healing to be effective. See LIVER CLEANSING in this book.
• Remove infected feces from the intestinal tract. Take both a colonic and an enema implant with aloe vera, wheat grass or spirulina once a week until recovery is well underway.

—**Bodywork:**
• Acupuncture, meditation, massage therapy and visualization help in normalizing from AIDS symptoms.
• Get fresh air and sunlight on the body every day. Get mild exercise daily, and plenty of rest. Do deep breathing exercises morning and evening.
• Overheating therapy helps kill the virus. See pg. 225 in this book.

—**Reflexology point:**

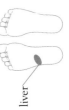

liver

—**Lifestyle practices to avoid HIV:**
• Practice safe sex.
• Avoid anal intercourse.
• Avoid needle-injected pleasure drugs.
• Make sure any blood transfusion plasma has been tested for HIV virus.

Can't find a recommended product? Call the 800 number listed in Product Resources for the store nearest you.

A 302

Is there hope if you are HIV positive?

Testing "anti-body positive" does not mean that you have AIDS, only that you has been exposed to the HIV virus. Being HIV positive does not even mean that you will develop AIDS. **It is a warning, not a sentence.** Some research attests that only 60% of people diagnosed as HIV positive develop full-blown AIDS. Even more encouraging, the face of AIDS has changed dramatically just within the last two years (1999). Protease inhibitor "cocktails" and genetic modifying drugs, coupled with a healthy diet, elimination of recreational drugs and responsible sexual behavior are showing promise in HIV status. Even though HIV infection has gone way beyond the gay community, to heterosexuals, and to babies from infected parents, HIV positive people are recognizing that the destructive lifestyle factors leading to their diagnosis can be changed to prevent further re-infection, and that they can greatly improve their health condition with lifestyle therapies that can help keep them symptom free.

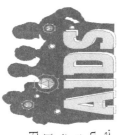

What does it take to survive AIDS?

New drugs may offer new hope, but researchers find that even when 99% of the virus seems to be destroyed, resistant strains can appear within days. Most infected people today find they can co-exist with HIV and lead a normal life. There are thousands of long term AIDS survivors who are free of HIV symptoms. In every case that I know of, the survivor consciously decided to take charge of his or her own life and healing. All energies were channeled into the therapies that the survivors thought were correct for themselves. They faced reality, acknowledged that there was no silver bullet, realized that the process would be long and hard, and that the battle would take a great deal of courage. Almost universally, AIDS survivors believe that they grew a great deal in their humanity, compassion and maturity by taking responsibility for such an enormous task. They also felt that they gained great strength, confidence and control of their lives - and indeed, have become the kind of person they always wanted to be.

A phenomenon of AIDS survival is the intense desire to reach out to other sufferers to share the experience through encouragement and hope. Here are their survival watchwords:

1: You cannot think or behave like a victim - you must fight for your life. There is no invariably fatal diagnosis - no mortal can decide when or if someone will die. Expect favorable results for courageous lifestyle steps. 2: You must take charge of your own healing. Educate yourself about alternative approaches and treatment - lifestyle therapy must be part of recovery. Destructive life patterns must be stopped. 3: Seek life re-inforcing, healing modalities. Avoid stress, learn to laugh, engage in some form of physical exercise, eliminate harmful drugs and alcohol, reduce red meat and sugar. 4: Seek the healing power of God and of Love. You are not alone - seek people and relationships that support your great effort. Have no fear of death - look forward to your life.

AIDS risks and symptoms you may not know

—It is relatively easy to transfer HIV virus through anal intercourse, more difficult through vaginal or oral sex. Powerful proteins in tears, saliva and pregnant women's urine, friendly flora in the intestinal tract, and HCl in the stomach produce a hostile environment that destroys HIV. There is no such protection in the colon. Suppression of the immune system is believed to occur when the HIV virus slips through the intestinal wall and into the bloodstream. Normal immune response is to attack the virus with macrophages that then die and are removed through the lymphatic system. These toxic wastes are finally dumped into the colon on its last leg of clearance from the body, but in an unprotected colon without friendly bacteria or good defensive pH environment, new HIV viruses hatch from the dead macrophages and multiply in the feces all over again, repeating the same cycle. The immune system cannot detect the virus in the colon and does not marshal its forces until the infection is in the bloodstream; often too late if immune defenses are exhausted.

—Parasites are a co-factor in the development of AIDS. Amoebic parasites rupture immune defense cells that have engulfed the HIV virus in an effort to destroy it allowing the virus to spread.

—HIV never stands alone as the only culprit in the AIDS connection. Immuno-suppression comes before HIV. Syphilis is usually present in AIDS victims, as are parasites and other viruses that set the stage for AIDS and related conditions. Parasites are also, many times, a co-factor in HIV development. If you are frequently diagnosed with a bacterial infection and treated with antibiotics that don't help, have your stool tested for parasites. If your lifestyle is immuno-suppressing, parasites can easily take hold, and they are becoming an epidemic in the U.S.

—You can continually re-infect yourself! The most destructive immune-suppressing lifestyle elements are continual exposure to HIV and other STD's through sexual excess and multiple sex partners, and excessive use of chemicals, drugs and alcohol.

—Hepatitis predisposes you to AIDS, because the liver is so weakened it cannot play its part in resisting infection. HIV also predisposes you to hepatitis by grinding down liver defenses.

—Environmental factors, such as water, air and soil, are now full of chemical pollutants that affect delicate immune balance. You must consciously make healthy choices for yourself.

—Symptoms can appear anywhere from 6 months to 3 years after infection. If you feel you are at risk, here are the early symptoms: swollen glands and lymph nodes in the neck area, armpits and groin; inability to heal even minor ailments like a small cut, bruise or cold; unusual fatigue; white patches in the mouth and trouble swallowing (thrush), nail ringworm fungus.

—Continuing symptoms mean that AIDS is undeniable: purplish blotches that look like hard bruises occurring on or under the skin, inside the mouth, nose, eyelids or rectum that do not go away (Kaposi's Sarcoma); swollen glands that never go away; persistent dry, hacking cough (unrelated to smoking) that doesn't go away; fevers and night sweats that last for days or weeks; severe, unexplained fatigue; persistent diarrhea; unexplained, rapid weight loss; visual disturbances; personality changes; memory loss, confusion and depression.

Can't find a recommended product? Call the 800 number listed in Product Resources for the store nearest you.

Addressing AIDS Related Syndromes

The following are "opportunistic" diseases that accompany AIDS and play a major role in the body's susceptibility to it. Studies show many of these side-effect syndromes can be addressed with natural, lifestyle therapies.

—PNEUMOCYSTIS CARINII (PCP): a rare form of pneumonia that develops with AIDS, and the leading cause of AIDS-related death, affecting over 70% of all AIDS cases. It is thought to be caused by a parasite. Alternative healing protocols for PCP: •*Black Carrot* extract, (an anti-viral, anti-fungal and anti-bacterial immune stimulant, 30 drops 4x daily, available from naturopaths that treat HIV), and/or •Colloidal silver as directed; •Earth's Bounty O$_2$ caps as directed, and O$_2$ skin spray rubbed on the feet morning and evening; •Nutricology GERMANIUM 150mg daily for interferon production; •Crystal Star ALRG-HST™ extract to ventilate the lungs and stimulate the liver to produce anti-histamines; •Enzymatic Therapy MEGA-ZYME and LIVA-TOX to stimulate the pancreas to attack foreign protein in the blood; *milk thistle seed* extract to strengthen the liver; •a potassium broth (page 215) to increase cell metabolism; •Ester C with minerals and bioflavonoids 5000mg for collagen production and healing of infected tissue; •Natren BIFIDO FACTORS powder (rinse mouth 3x daily); •Solaray quercetin with bromelain (QBC PLEX) 4x daily; •CC Pollen HIGH DESERT ROYAL JELLY drink as a prime source of pantothenic acid; •Aloe Answers ALOE FORCE or •Aloe Life ALOE GOLD drink to rebuild immunity. Note: vegetables in your diet should be lightly steamed rather than eaten raw, because the protozoan parasite thought to cause pneumocystis lives in the soil and is destroyed by heat. Do deep breathing exercises morning and evening, especially when recovering from pneumocystis.

—KAPOSI'S SARCOMA (KS):usually benign skin tumors, but when they accompany AIDS drugs, KS lesions become a serious connective tissue cancer. (When the drugs are stopped, the lesions often regress.) Alternative healing protocols for KS: •Curcumin (*turmeric*) extract 8-10 capsules daily (or more) to inhibit tumor necrosis factor; •Crystal Star ANTI-BIO™ gel with *una da gato* and ginseng; •Nutricology CAR-T-CELL shark cartilage liquid vials, 15ml daily; astragalus extract; •CoQ$_{10}$ 300mg daily; •PCOs from *white pine* or *grape seed* oil to restore interleukin 100mg 3x daily; •*Dfraction Maitake* mushroom extract or *Maitake* mushrooms in food or •Grifon MAITAKE MUSHROOM extract to boost macrophages and T-cell production; •Herbal Answers HERBAL ALOE FORCE gel applied directly to lesions; •*Black Carrot* extract (see a clinical naturopath); •Nutribiotic GRAPEFRUIT SEED EXTRACT and SKIN SPRAY as a healing antibiotic. A daily potassium broth (page 215) and •Green Foods CARROT ESSENCE are important for healing, along with the macrobiotic diet on page 306.

—EPSTEIN-BARR VIRUS (EBV): a chronic fatigue disease of the herpes family, and a cause of mononucleosis. EBV lives and hides in the B-cells of your immune system, producing anti-bodies that react against your tissue cells to affect immune response. Symptoms are swollen lymph nodes, fever, chills, severe fatigue, chronic sore throat, usually pneumonia. Alternative healing protocols for HIV-related Epstein Barr: •garlic suppositories and/or •Crystal Star ANTI-VI™ extract to kill the virus; •American Biologics DIOXYCHLOR or •Earth's Bounty OXY CAPS; •Prof. Nutrition Dr. DOPHILUS +FOS for all-important micro-flora; •AloeLife ALOE GOLD juice every morning; •*Ashwagandha* extract and •Crystal Star ZINC SOURCE™ extract to strengthen immune response; •Crystal Star *echinacea* or *maitake* mushroom extract to stimulate interferon, and •GINSENG/LICORICE ELIXIR™ to mobilize anti-bodies; •Earth's Bounty O$_2$ CAPS as directed or O$_2$ SPRAY rubbed on the feet twice daily; •Crystal Star ENERGY GREEN™ drink to rebuild immune strength; •Enzymatic LIQUID LIVER, or Crystal Star LIV-ALIVE™ caps with MILK THISTLE SEED extract and •Crystal Star GINSENG-REISHI extract for 3 to 6 months; •Enzymatic Therapy LYMPHO-CLEAR for lymph node swelling.

—WASTING SYNDROME: malabsorption characterized by severe, unhealthy weight loss which can be addressed with superfoods. Normalizing body fluid levels, calories and protein is critical to fighting infections and inflammation. In addition, many drugs for AIDS leach valuable nutrients from already weak bodies, making superfoods such as •Mona's CHLORELLA, •Crystal Star SYSTEMS STRENGTH™ drink, or •Solgar WHEY TO GO protein drink even more important. Alternative healing protocols for HIV-related wasting syndrome: •Nature's Path CAL-LYTE, take with food for malabsorption, food allergies, healing of gastric membranes and leaky gut, and detoxifying lymph glands; •Chinese bitter melon to inhibit the virus and treat gastrointestinal infection; •Crystal Star GINSENG/LICORICE ELIXIR™ for digestion, sugar balance, and to inhibit virus replication; •CoQ-10 300mg daily for stronger blood; •Arginine 2000mg and •Glutamine 2000mg to defeat muscle loss of wasting disease. Diet should concentrate on metabolic care, with large amounts of vegetable juices (especially potassium broth (page 215) and •Pines MIGHTY GREENS drink, yogurt, kefir and kefir cheese, and high sulphur foods like garlic and onions. Eat complex carbohydrate foods first, protein foods last, and plenty of high fiber foods. Avoid absolutely: caffeine, (drink herbal teas), all pork and other fatty meats, enzyme-inhibiting foods like soy products and peanuts, table salt and sugary foods.

—CYTOMEGALOVIRUS (CMV): a salivary, herpes-type virus, associated with Epstein Barr infection, CMV produces fever, low white blood cell count and fungal infections of the gastrointestinal tract. Alternative healing protocols for HIV-related Cytomegalovirus: •*nettles* extract; •*tea tree* oil mouthwash; •Earth's Bounty OXY CAPS as directed or O$_2$ SPRAY rubbed on the feet twice daily; •Enzymatic Therapy MEGA-ZYME to digest foreign proteins and •PHYTO-BIOTIC 816 formula for parasitic infestation; •acupuncture treatments with accompanying *shiitake* and *maitake* mushroom and *astragalus* extracts (or ASTRA-8 Chinese herb compound) to strengthen the body's major organs; •Crystal Star MIGR-EASE™ extract with feverfew to reduce severe headaches; •Enzymatic Therapy ADRENAL CORTEX COMPLEX; •black carrot extract (from a clinical naturopath) or •Crystal Star ANTI-VI™ extract with •MILK THISTLE SEED extract.

—HERPES SIMPLEX VIRUS: AIDS-related herpes is activated and aggravated by UV sunlight; antioxidants have been shown to protect against this. See HERPES SIMPLEX pg. 355 in this book.

The Holistic Approach to Overcoming HIV Infection and AIDS

Holistic therapies show more promise than ever for AIDS, and its related immune syndromes. Alternative treatments have been enormous factors in showing that HIV infection and AIDS are no longer inevitably fatal as they once were. In fact, holistic programs are the key to abating symptoms. The advance of the virus itself has been slowed and the quality of life has improved. More alternative expertise is coming into the field via holistic physicians, homeopaths, naturopaths, chiropractors, therapists, nutritional counselors and others. The following protocol is a well-received holistic therapy program that has achieved measureable success with AIDS and its attendant conditions. Doses are generally quite high in the beginning. They may be reduced as improvement is observed. Treatments may be used together or separately as desired by each individual, along with the recommendations of a competent professional who has personal case knowledge. Note: Address allergies and malabsorption before beginning alternative HIV treatment.

—DETOXIFY: These products and protocols work during the detox phase, especially to cleanse the lymph and liver tissue, HIV targets: (choose 2 or 3)
• Lymph and liver cleansing is the key: American Biologics DIOXYCHLOR, Enzymatic Therapy LIVA-TOX; or Crystal Star LIV-ALIVE™ with GREEN TEA CLEANSER™.
• Use calcium ascorbate vitamin C crystals, or a mixed mineral ascorbate with bioflavonoids to flush and detoxify the tissues. Take orally 10-20 teasp. daily for 2 to 3 weeks, then reduce to 10 grams daily for maintenance.) Intravenous dose, 100-150 grams daily for 2-3 weeks, reducing to 30 grams every week for maintenance.)
• If not too weak, detoxify with a weekly wheat grass colonic to clean out toxic wastes, and to stimulate and normalize organs, gland function and mental balance.
• Use thermo-therapy - both a sauna and an overheating bath (pages 225) severely attenuate virus and tumor cells by the sudden raising of body temperature. In vitro tests show an amazing reduction of infected cels by as much as 40%." Karl Kroyer, France 1998. (patents pending).

—DIET: These products and protocols work to normalze your body chemistry: (choose 2 or 3)
• Rebalance body pH with micro-flora - an acidophilus complex with bifidus, like Natren BIFIDO FACTORS, 3 teasp. daily. Sprinkle acidophilus on food, too for an extra probiotics boost.
• Take carrot juice and other fresh vegetable juices daily - a good juicer is critical to potency. Take a potassium juice (page 215) twice daily with garlic extract and flax oil added for omega-3 EFA's.
• Chew DGL tablets to neutralize acids. Add egg lipids from egg yolk lecithin - highest potency, Jarrow Corp., or Source Naturals EGGS ACT liquid. Drink plenty of distilled water every day.
• Whey protein to inhibit HIV as part of every meal or as Solgar WHEY TO GO drink.

—PHYTOBIOTIC HERBAL THERAPY: (choose 2 or 3)
• St. John's wort extract or Crystal Star ANTI-VI™ EXTRACT (50% St. John's Wort/50% Lomatium) and ANTI-BIO™ caps with echinacea, goldenseal and myrrh; and evening primrose oil 1000mg 2x daily work as immunomodulators and to block HIV replication. Echinacea stimulates interferon against HIV virus that hides in memory T-cells.
• Aged aloe vera juice, 2-3 glasses daily, blocks the virus spread, and reduces herpes lesions. Take with black carrot extract 30 drops 4x daily to fight infection.
• Essiac tea 3x daily, Flora FLOR-ESSENCE extract, or Crystal Star CAN-SSIAC™ extract solution with panax ginseng enhance the body's own immune forces.
• Drink 4-6 cups daily of the following immune restorative tea: prince ginseng roots, dry shiitake mushrooms and soaking water, echinacea angustifolia root, schizandra berries, astragalus, ma huang, pau d' arco bark, St. John's wort. Steep 30 minutes. (See also Crystal Star GINSENG SUPER SIX™ TEA.)

—SUPERFOOD THERAPY: (choose 1 or 2)
• Propolis extract with Wakunaga KYO-Green garlic extract, or YS ROYAL JELLY with GINSENG drink.
• Sun CHLORELLA - 15-20 tablets or 2 pkts granules daily, Green Foods GREEN ESSENCE or CARROT ESSENCE; Crystal Star ENERGY GREEN™ or SYSTEMS STRENGTH™ drinks.
• Solgar WHEY TO GO protein drink, or Wakunaga KYO-GREEN, or Nutricology PRO-GREENS with EFA's for better brain performance.

—ANTIOXIDANT & ENZYME THERAPY: (choose 2 or 3)
• American Biologics SHARKILAGE 740mg - 1 cap for every 12 pounds of body weight for 3 weeks before meals then 4-6 caps daily - increases leukocytes and white blood cell activity.
• Carnitine - 500mg daily for 3 days. Rest for 7 days, then 1000mg for 3 days. Rest for 7 days. Take with high omega 3 flax oils, 3 to 6x daily, or evening primrose oil 500mg 3 x daily.
• Germanium, highest potency 200mg 6x daily, or 150mg sublingually, 4x daily, with astragalus capsules, 4 daily, with digestive enzymes, like Enzymatic Therapy MEGA-ZYME with pancreatin
• CoQ10 300mg daily, Pycnogenol or grape seed PCO's, 50mg 4x daily,. Solaray QUERCETIN PLUS 500mg 3x daily for respiratory improvement.
• Glutathione 50mg 2x daily to overcome the side effects and nerve damage from AZT, and to strengthen white blood cell and T-cell activity.
• NAC - a stable form of L-cysteine that helps deactivate HIV, with glutathione 50mg 2x daily.
• MICROHYDRIN a superior antioxidant, available at Healthy House, 2 daily.
• The body produces H_2O_2 naturally as part of its immune defenses. Change the cell environment with Bio-oxidation therapy (catalytic H_2O_2 with shark cartilage) by injection, (with a qualified practitioner only), or rub Earth's Bounty O_2 SPRAY on the feet morning and evening. Alternate H_2O_2 use, 4 days on and one week off for best results.

—BODYWORK THERAPY: These lifestyle measures magnify the results of your supplement and diet programs.
• Thermo-therapy is effective for inhibiting growth of the invading virus. Hydrotherapy is effective in re-stimulating circulation. Take a sauna or overheating bath. (see page 225.)
• Use implant-enemas with either supergreen foods such as chlorella or spirulina, or micro-flora, or Enzymatic Therapy PHYTO-BIOTIC HERBAL FORMULA.

For additional protocols and information, visit the Bastyr AIDS Research Center website: http://www.bastyr.edu/research/buarc/

Can't find a recommended product? Call the 800 number listed in Product Resources for the store nearest you.

Diet Defense Against HIV and AIDS

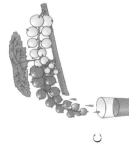

Malnutrition is the number one reason for low immune response. HIV itself isn't deadly. It simply weakens the immune system to the point where it can't fight. A high resistance, immune-building diet is the key to success. Your intestinal environment must be changed to create a hostile site for the pathogenic bacteria. AIDS victims need about 4000 calories a day, double the usual amount, to sustain body weight. The following liquid and fresh foods diet represents the first "crash course" stage of the change from cooked to living foods. It is for the ill person who needs dramatic measures - a great deal of concentrated defense strength in a short time. It has been extremely helpful in keeping an HIV positive person free of symptoms, and in symptom recession during full-blown AIDS. This program also helps prevent other attendant diseases associated with immune deficiency. The space in this book only allows for a "jump start" form of this diet. The complete program with supporting recipes, may be found in my book "COOKING FOR HEALTHY HEALING."

The suggested step-by-step program below is a modified, enhanced macrobiotic diet, emphasizing more fresh than cooked foods, and mixing in acidophilus powder with foods that are cooked to convert them to living nourishment with friendly flora. As with other immune-depressing viral diseases, HIV lives on dead and waste matter. For several months at least, the diet should be vegetarian, low in dairy, yeasted breads and saturated fats. Meats, fried foods, dairy products except yogurt and kefir, coffee, alcohol, salty, sugary foods, and all refined foods must be eliminated. Of course, all recreational drugs should be eliminated, as well as unnecessary prescription drugs. The ultra purity of this diet controls the multiple allergies and sensitivities that occur in the auto-immune state, yet still supplies the needs of a body that is suffering primary nutrient deprivation. For most people, this way of eating is a radical change, with major limitations, but the health improvement against HIV is excellent.

The goal for overcoming HIV infection is staying strong. System strength greatly reduces the chances of succumbing to full-blown AIDS or to another infection. It allows you to survive while research for answers against the HIV virus goes on. In some cases, a strong person can develop resistance to the virus effects for many years.

On rising: take 3 TBS cranberry concentrate in 8-oz. of water with ¹/₂ teasp. ascorbate vitamin C crystals with bioflavonoids and ¹/₂ teasp. Natren BIFIDO FACTORS; or a Solgar WHEY TO GO protein drink.
Take a brisk walk for exercise and morning sunlight.

Breakfast: have a glass of fresh carrot juice with 1 teasp. Bragg's LIQUID AMINOS, and whole grain muffins or rice cakes with kefir cheese; or a cup of plain yogurt blended with a cup of fresh fruit, sesame seeds, walnuts, or oatmeal, amaranth or buckwheat pancakes with yogurt and fresh fruit; and ¹/₂ teasp. Prof. Nutrition DOCTOR DOPHILUS with FOS, or Enzymedica PURIFY powder mixed in 8-oz. of aloe vera juice or AloeLife ALOE GOLD.

Midmorning: take a weekly colonic. On non-colonic days, take potassium essence (page 215), with 1 teasp Bragg's LIQUID AMINOS and ¹/₂ tsp. ascorbate vitamin C crystals with bioflavonoids; and have another fresh carrot juice, or *pau d'arco* tea, with ¹/₂ teasp. Natren BIFIDO FACTORS added.

Lunch: have a fresh green salad with lemon-flax oil dressing, with plenty of avocado, nuts, seeds and alfalfa or broccoli sprouts; or an open-faced sandwich on rice cakes, or a chapati with fresh veggies and kefir cheese; or a cup of miso soup with rice noodles or brown rice, and some steamed veggies and tofu with millet or brown rice; and take a cup of *pau d'arco* tea or aloe vera juice with ¹/₂ teasp. ascorbate vit. C, and ¹/₂ teasp. Natren BIFIDO FACTORS added.

Midafternoon: have another carrot juice with Bragg's LIQUID AMINOS and ¹/₂ teasp. Natren BIFIDO FACTORS added; and a green drink such as Mona's CHLORELLA, Green Foods GREEN ESSENCE, or Crystal Star ENERGY GREEN™, with ¹/₂ teasp. ascorbate vitamin C crystals and bioflavs added.

Dinner: have a baked potato with Bragg's LIQUID AMINOS, low-fat cheese or kefir cheese and a green salad, and black bean or lentil soup with ¹/₂ teasp. Natren BIFIDO FACTORS added; or a fresh spinach or artichoke pasta with steamed veggies and lemon/flax oil dressing; or a Chinese steam stir-fry with shiitake mushrooms, brown rice and vegetables. Sprinkle ¹/₂ teasp. Natren BIFIDO FACTORS or Alta Health CANGEST powder over any cooked food at this meal.

Before Bed: take a glass of aloe vera juice with ¹/₂ teasp. ascorbate vit. C crystals and ¹/₂ teasp. Natren BIFIDO FACTORS; and a fresh carrot or papaya juice, or body chemistry balancing drink such as Crystal Star SYSTEMS STRENGTH™.

Note 1: Unsweetened mild herb teas and bottled water are recommended throughout the day for additional toxin cleansing and system alkalizing.
Note 2: For optimum results, add ¹/₂ teasp. ascorbate vitamin C powder with bioflavonoids to any drink throughout the day until the stool turns soupy.

Can't find a recommended product? Call the 800 number listed in Product Resources for the store nearest you.

Allergies

Multiple Chemical Sensitivities (MCS), Environmental Illness, Drug and Contaminant Reactions

Multiple chemical sensitivities are multiplying. We're exposed to more chemicals every day than any generation in history; 30% of Americans have sensitivities to chemicals! Over 2¹/₂ billion pounds of pesticides are used in America every year! (300 million pounds in the home.) Benzene, formaldehyde, and carcinogens from carpeting and dry cleaning affect our brains. Repeated chemical exposures set off rampant free radical reactions, and allergic response. Those making the news today, environmental illness, sick buildings, Gulf War syndrome, breast cancer, nerve damage, attention deficit disorder in children, latex and insecticide allergies, are just the latest in a growing list. Worse, our bodies use up enormous amounts of nutrients trying to detoxify us from these chemicals, nutrients that could have been used to keep us happy and healthy.

Diet & Superfood Therapy

—Nutritional therapy plan:

1—Go on a short blood purifying cleanse (pg. 208) to begin toxin release. Have one each daily:
• a glass of fresh carrot juice
• a carrot-beet-cucumber juice
• a cup of miso soup with sea greens.
• a bowl of high fiber cereal to bind / eliminate toxins in the G.I. tract. Sprinkle on brewer's yeast, toasted wheat germ and lecithin granules.

2—Eat organically grown foods as much as possible. Avoid caffeine, which inhibits liver filtering function, and foods sprayed with colorants, waxes or ripening agents.

3—Eat legumes and sea greens to excrete lead. Have an apple a day if you work in a polluted area. Apple pectin removes metal toxins.

4—Lower bad saturated and trans fats; add good omega-3 fats with essential fatty acids: sea greens, flax, canola and olive oils for resistance.

—Superfood therapy: chemical exposure sets off rampant free radicals. (Choose one or two)
• Crystal Star ENERGY GREEN™; Sun Wellness CHLORELLA; or Green Foods GREEN MAGMA for blood detoxification
• AloeLife ALOE GOLD juice.
• Green Foods BETA CARROT blend.
• Pines MIGHTY GREENS drink.

Herb & Supplement Therapy

—Interceptive therapy plan: (Choose 2 or 3 recommendations)

1—Detoxify your blood: •Crystal Star DETOX™ caps with GREEN TEA CLEANSER™ or CLEANSING & PURIFYING™ TEA for 6 weeks; Glutathione 50mg 3 daily; Tyrosine 500mg daily; magnesium 800mg if there are TIA episodes.

2—Support your liver: •Crystal Star LIV-ALIVE™ tea or caps for 1 month to restore the liver. Then •FIBER & HERBS COLON CLEANSE™ caps with milk thistle seed extract; •B-complex 100mg daily with extra B₆ and pantothenic acid.

3—Neutralize histamine reactions: •Crystal Star ANTI-HIST™ caps and BITTERS & LEMON™ extract for enzyme therapy. •Bilberry extract with natural quercetin, or Quercetin1000mg caps with bromelain 500mg to take down swelling. •CELL GUARD by Biotec Foods with SOD, 6 daily offers key protection.

4—Neutralize allergen response: • MSM 400mg 2x daily, or Astragalus extract caps; Evening primrose 500mg daily, or • Nature's Secret ULTIMATE OIL capsules, Kelp 10 tabs daily, or •Crystal Star IODINE THERAPY caps 4 daily.

—Other effective herbal healing resources: (choose one)
• Garlic oil caps, 2-4 daily.
• Dandelion-nettles caps, 6 daily.
• Pau d'arco tea every 4 hours.
• GRAPEFRUIT SEED EXTRACT caps.

Reinforce your body against chemical assault and boost immune response:
• Key antioxidants: 1) Vitamin C with bioflavonoids, 3-5000mg daily boosts immunity against MCS. 2) Vitamin E 400IU w/selenium 200mcg daily. 3) CoQ-10, 60mg 2x daily. Grapeseed PCO's 100mg 2x daily. 4) Quercetin 1000mg daily. 5) Vitamin B-12 2000mcg daily. 6) Beta/marine carotene 150,000IU.

—Glandulars reinforce the body at its deepest level:
• Enzymatic Therapy ADRENAL CORTEX COMPLEX, THYMU-PLEX caps.

Lifestyle Support Therapy

—Bodywork:
• Use Coca's Pulse Test or muscle testing to identify allergens. (See page 538.)
• Acupuncture, chiropractic, massage therapy are most effective for chemical allergies.

—Lifestyle measures: avoid contaminants.
• Seek out trees to live around. Trees produce oxygen and remove many air pollutants.
• Avoid antacids; they interfere with enzymes, and your body's ability to carry off chemical residues.
• Invest in an air filter.
• Pay attention to unhealthy air alerts; stay indoors if you have chemical sensitivities. Don't exercise near freeways.
• Avoid as much as possible: smoking and secondary smoke, pesticides and herbicides, phosphorus fertilizers, fluorescent lights, aluminum cookware and deodorants, electric blankets; microwave ovens.

—Hand reflexology:

liver   also press webbing between thumb and index finger

A 307

Common Symptoms: Always feeling "under the weather" regardless of how much sleep you get; brain fog mental sluggishness; abnormal metabolism; learning and behavior disabilities; skin rashes; chronic respiratory infection; ringing in the ears; nausea; diarrhea; headaches; low immune response. Drug reactions mimic many allergy reactions but usually don't involve the immune system (IgE antibodies).
Common Causes: Repeated exposure and sensitivity to toxic chemicals, like chlorine, dry cleaning chemicals, latex, plastic food containers, synthetic perfumes, solvents, mercury dental fillings, aspirin; and environmental pollutants like auto exhaust, pesticide sprays and smoke; inherited tendency (affecting more women and children than men).

See also CHEMICAL AND CONTAMINANT POISONING page 480.

Can't find a recommended product? Call the 800 number listed in Product Resources for the store nearest you.

Allergies

Seasonal Hayfever, Allergic Rhinitis, Respiratory Allergies

Allergies are an epidemic at the turn of the millenium. Over 60 million Americans suffer from allergies - that's 20% of the population! Respiratory allergies (35 million people) include environmental pollutants, like asbestos and smoke fumes, and seasonal conditions, like dust, pollen or spores. This type of allergic reaction often occurs when the body has an excess accumulation of mucous which harbors environmental irritants. Common drugstore medications generally mask symptoms and also have a rebound effect - the more you use them, the more you need them. The newest ones are strong medicine.... and have strong side effects like rapid heartbeat, even possible tumors. Steroid drugs for hayfever allergies, if taken for long periods, do not cure and often make the situation worse by depressing immune defenses, and impeding allergen elimination.

Diet & Superfood Therapy

—Nutritional therapy plan:

1—Diet change and cleansing your internal environment is the most beneficial thing you can do to control allergic rhinitis reactions.

2—Begin with a 3 to 7 day cleanse (pg. 195) to get rid of mucous build-up, and release allergens. Drink plenty of water during your cleanse.

3—**Have a cup of green tea each morning.** Take hot miso or chicken soup to release mucous.

4—Eat non-mucous-forming foods: fresh vegetables and fruits, whole grains, cultured foods like yogurt, high vitamin C foods like citrus and berries, seafoods, and fundamental sulphur from cabbage, onions and garlic. Get plenty of essential fatty acids from omega-3 oils like flax, sea greens and spinach.

5—Avoid preserved and canned foods, sugary foods, caffeine, and fatty, mucous-forming foods during healing. This means dairy products.

—Superfood therapy: (Choose one or two)
• Nutri-Cology PRO GREENS with EFA's.
• CC Pollen ALLER BEE-GONE.
• Herbal Magic ALLERGY SEASON herbal.
• Crystal Star BIOFLAV., FIBER and C SUPPORT™ for absorbable vitamin C benefits.
• Beehive Botanicals 24-HOUR ROYAL JELLY, or Y.S. ROYAL JELLY-GINSENG drink for pantothenic acid.

Herb & Supplement Therapy

—Interceptive therapy plan: (Choose 2 or more recommendations)

Natural therapies build rsistance and offer symptom relief without side effects.

1—**Herbal antihistamines:** • Crystal Star ALRG™ or ANTI-HST™ caps, or
• Futurebiotics MSM 400mg 2x daily to counter IgE antibody response; • Ascorbate Vitamin C or Ester C with bioflavonoids 5000mg daily. Grapeseed PCO's 100mg or • Country Life ALLER-MAX w. pycnogenol are natural antihistamines.

2—**Liver support:** Dandelion-nettles teas, 2 cups daily.

3—**Flush mucous congestion:** • Crystal Star ANTI-BIO™ caps or • Zand DE-CONGEST HERBAL to control congestion. • AloeLife FIBER-MATE as directed.

4—**Feed your adrenals:** • B-complex with extra pantothenic acid 500mg; • Crystal Star ADR-ACTIVE™ extract or caps; raw thymus and adrenal 3x daily.

5—**Stabilize your body's reaction to hayfever allergens:** • Crystal Star GINSENG-REISHI extract with RESPIR-TEA™, 2 cups daily. • Quercetin 2000mg daily with bromelain 500mg • CC Pollen ALLER-BEE-GONE; Herbs, Etc. ALLER-TONIC.

—Homeopathic remedies can help even even acute attacks without side effects:
• Euphrasia tabs or drops.
• BioForce POLLINOSAN tabs
• BioForce SINUSAN tabs
• Bio-Allers POLLEN-HAYFEVER, 3x daily.
• Similasan EYE DROPS #1 and NASAL SPRAY.

—Reinforce your body's defenses against allergens:
• Evening primrose oil 4-6 daily for several months as a preventive.
• CoQ-10 30mg 3x daily to reinforce defenses.
• Nutricology GERMANIUM 150mg with Country Life B₁₂ SL 2500mcg daily.
• CC Pollen PROPOLIS caps.
• Freeze-dried nettles caps for allergic rhinitis.
• Tyrosine 500mg 2x daily.

Lifestyle Support Therapy

—Bodywork:
• Use Coca's Pulse Test or muscle testing to identify allergens. (See page 538)
• Take 1 teasp. fresh grated horseradish in a spoon with lemon juice. Hang over a sink to release great quantities of excess mucous fast.
• Apply MSM gel topically to skin rashes.
• Apply BREATHE RIGHT post nasal strips.
• Apply cayenne-ginger chest compresses.
• Exercise is important to increase oxygen uptake. Take a daily walk with deep breathing.
• Use relaxation techniques. Stress depresses immunity and aggravates allergies.
• Acupuncture and chiropractic have both proven effective for allergies.

—Lifestyle measures: avoid allergens.
• Stay indoors, esp. in the a.m. and exercise indoors on dry, windy days.
• Invest in an air filter.
• Stop smoking and avoid secondary smoke. It magnifies allergies reactions.

—Acupressure points:
1—During an attack, press tip of nose hard as needed for relief.
2—Press hollow above the center of upper lip as needed.
3—Press underneath cheekbones beside nose, angling pressure upwards.

A 308

Common Symptoms: Runny, watery, itchy nose and eyes; sneezing and coughing attacks; dark circles under the eyes that don't go away with sleep; sore, irritated throat; chronic lung, bronchial and sinus infections; skin itching and rashes; asthma; frontal headaches; insomnia; menstrual disorders; hypoglycemia; learning disabilities.

Common Causes: Sensitivity to pollen, spore, mold and other airborne allergens reacting with excess mucous and waste accumulation in the body; adrenal exhaustion; free radical damage lowering antihistamine levels and liver function; stress; hypoglycemia; candida albicans yeast overgrowth; EFA deficiency. If you are taking loratadine (Claritin) for allergies, it has been shown to cause liver tumors, including cancers.

For a complete diet to overcome allergies, see my book COOKING FOR HEALTHY HEALING.

Can't find a recommended product? Call the 800 number listed in Product Resources for the store nearest you.

Allergies

Food Sensitivities and Intolerances, Celiac Disease

Food allergy: an immune system antibody response to a certain food. Food intolerance: a non-immune reaction, usually an enzyme deficiency to digest a certain food. Celiac disease: a sensitivity to gluten, a wheat protein (some estimate celiac disease affects 20% of Americans). Ninety percent of food reactions are caused by certain proteins in cow's milk, peanuts, egg whites, wheat and soybeans. Food sensitivities are growing fast as people are more exposed to chemically altered, enzyme-depleted, processed foods. Without enzyme active foods, total food assimilation does not occur, and large amounts of undigested fats and proteins are left that the immune system treats as potentially toxic. It releases prostaglandins, leukotrienes, and histamines into the bloodstream and allergy reactions occur.

Diet & Superfood Therapy

—Nutritional therapy plan:

1—Go on a short cleansing diet (page 191) to clear the system of allergens. Then follow a diet emphasizing enzyme-rich fresh foods and grains.

2—A food rotation diet can eliminate suspected allergen foods, especially if you are overweight, have candida, sluggish thyroid or hypoglycemia.

3—Take 2 TBS apple cider vinegar with honey at each meal to acidify saliva.

4—Eat cultured foods, like yogurt to add friendly flora to the G.I. tract.

5—Common allergy foods: wheat, dairy products, fruits, sugar, yeast, mushrooms, peanuts, eggs, soy, coffee, corn, beer and greens. Some of these foods are healthy in themselves, but are often heavily sprayed, and in the case of animal products affected by antibiotics and hormones.

6—Safer food choices: rice milk, goat's milk, almond milk, flat breads, quick breads, brown or wild rice, millet, buckwheat, amaranth, quinoa, date sugar, maple syrup, almond butter, sesame butter, egg replacer made from flax or arrowroot.

—Superfood therapy: (Choose one or two)

• Crystal Star BIOFLAVONOID, FIBER & C SUPPORT™ drink to guard against leaky-gut.
• New Moon GINGER WONDER syrup to help block inflammation.
• Aloe Falls ALOE GINGER JUICE.

Herb & Supplement Therapy

—Interceptive therapy plan: (Choose 2 or 3 recommendations)

1—**Produce antihistamines:** • Crystal Star ANTI-HST™ or ALRG-HST™ caps; • CoQ-10 60mg 3x daily

2—**Reduce allergic reactions:** • MSM 400-1000mg 2x daily; • Crystal Star GINSENG-REISHI extract; • Omega-3 flax oil with meals for essential fatty acids (EFA's); • Liquid chlorophyll 1 teasp. in water 3x daily before meals.

3—**Cleanse the G.I. tract:** • Crystal Star BITTERS & LEMON CLEANSE™, or green tea; or aloe vera juice each morning.

4—**Add proteolytic enzymes:** • Quercetin 500mg daily between meals with bromelain 500mg 3x daily for antioxidant activity plus enzymes. A full spectrum enzyme like Herbal Products POWER PLUS ENZYMES ♂, or Enzymedica DI-GEST. ♀; • Enzymedica PURIFY • Transformation PUREZYME caps (protease); • Source Naturals CO-ENZYMATE B with meals, • Alta Health CANGEST, .

5—**Add probiotics:** • Prof. Nutr. Dr. DOPHILUS 1/4 tsp. in liquid before meals;

6—**Support the adrenals:** • Crystal Star GINSENG-LICORICE ELIXIR™; • Ester C up to 5000mg daily with bioflavonoids.

—Herbal enzymes boost immunity and normalize digestion: (choose one)

• Milk thistle seed extract; • Dandelion root-nettles tea; • Echinacea-goldenseal root caps; • Gaia SWEETISH BITTERS or • Crystal Star AFTER MEAL ENZ™ caps.

—For gluten intolerance: See also CANDIDA ALBICANS page 341.
• Crystal Star CAND-EX™ caps especially if there is unexplained weight gain.
• Bio-Allers FOOD ALLERGY GRAIN.

—For lactose intolerance: (choose one) • Lactaid drops or tablets; • Nature's Plus SAY YES TO DAIRY; • Country Life DAIRY-ZYME; • Prevail DAIRY ENZYME FORMULA 3x daily; • Prevail DAIRY ENZYMES.

Lifestyle Support Therapy

Food allergies are common in children; many result from feeding babies meats and commercial dairy foods before 10-12 months. Babies do not have the right enzymes to digest these foods. Feed mother's milk, soy milk or goat's milk for 10 months to avoid food allergies.

—Bodywork:

• Use Coca's Pulse Test or muscle testing to identify allergens. (See page 538) Both skin-prick and RAST tests used by many allergists often misdiagnose food allergies unless a rotation-reintroduction diet is also used.
• Use a garlic-catnip enema to cleanse the digestive tract and balance colon pH.

—Hand reflexology:

food assimilation

One of the most insidious effects of food allergy is weight gain. Eliminate wheat from your diet to stop allergy-related weight gain.

Common Symptoms: Itchy, watery eyes, blurred vision; I.B.S., or diarrhea; headaches; hypothyroidism; osteoarthritis; hypoglycemia; hyperactivity, irritability and flushing in children; excessively swollen stomach; gas and constipation; nausea or mental fuzziness after eating; heart palpitations, sweating, hives; ringing in the ears, chronic ear infections; chronic congestion; unexplained obesity.

Common Causes: Eating chemically altered, sprayed, or injected foods that the body cannot handle; inherited food sensitivities; food additives such as nitrites, aspartame, MSG and sulfites; stress; fast-food diet; alkalosis with low gastric pH and enzyme deficiency; insufficient sleep; emotional trauma; chronic infections; a particular allergen food like gluten foods.

See FOOD POISONING page 481, and my book COOKING FOR HEALTHY HEALING for a complete diet.

Can't find a recommended product? Call the 800 number listed in Product Resources for the store nearest you.

Does your body need to clean out toxins that are causing allergies or asthma?

Allergies used to be defined as inappropriate immune responses to substances (like cat hair, dust or wheat) that weren't normally harmful. Today, the dramatic rise in allergies is due to substances that *are* harmful. Not only does the toxic overload from chemicals in our food and environment cause allergic reactions, it also impairs the body's immune response to them. A strong immune system is critical to preventing or overcoming opportunistic diseases like herpes, candida albicans or chronic fatigue syndrome that have allergic reaction symptomology. Immune system studies show that allergy-prone people produce an overabundance of complex proteins known as antibodies—which trigger special cells known as mast cells—which release inflammation-causing chemicals called histamines and leukotrienes throughout the body. A "histamine reaction" occurs when your body tries to neutralize the chemicals by a severe allergic reaction. Conventional medical treatment for most allergies consists of antihistamines, steroids and desensitization shots. Laser surgery can now vaporize mucous-forming nasal tissue. People with allergies know that these treatments seldom work because they don't get to the cause of the problem. At best they provide temporary relief of symptoms; at worst, they create side effects which may be worse than the allergy itself.

The substances that cause allergies are called allergens.

—**Allergies to environmental allergens like air pollutants, asbestos or heavy metals, and seasonal allergens like dust, pollen, spores and mold, are called Type 1 allergies.** Excess mucous accumulations harbor Type 1 allergen irritants. Drugstore medications for environmental allergies only mask symptoms, often cause drowsiness and have a rebound effect. The more you use them, the more you need them. Steroid drugs for Type 1 allergies, especially if taken over a long period of time, depress immune response and impede allergen elimination. Allergens may interact in the bodies of allergy sufferers, activating and aggravating other offending irritants. When this is the case, even the most powerful drugs do not relieve symptoms.

—**Allergies to chemicals and contaminant allergens are called Type 2 allergies.** Reactions to chemicals are frequently a defense mechanism, the body's attempt to isolate an offending substance by storing it in fatty tissue. An allergic reaction of this type only occurs after the second exposure to the irritant as the body's inflammatory histamine response is alerted. Repeated exposures to the irritant set off massive free radical reactions as the body's contaminant toleration levels are reached, toxic overload results and a severe allergic reaction sets in. Chemical sensitivity also initiates other allergy reactions, so that the sufferer becomes allergic to nearly everything else. Common chemical/contaminant irritants vary, from a wide range of petrochemicals and estrogenic chemicals to combustion residues from household appliances and heating systems, to various kinds of sprays, paints and exhaust fumes. Other culprits include chlorine bleach, moth balls and insect repellents, dry cleaning chemicals, and clothes that have been chemically treated.

—**Allergies, intolerances and sensitivities to foods or food additives are also called Type 2 allergies.** They're extremely widespread, the fastest growing allergic reactions in the U.S. today, as we become exposed to chemically altered foods. Food intolerances are often confused with food allergies. A **food allergy** is an IgE antibody immune response to a food it views as a pathogen or parasite. Food allergies may be hereditary, with a child being twice as likely to develop allergies if one parent has them, or four times as likely if both parents have them. A **food intolerance** is an enzyme deficiency for digesting a certain food. For example, people with a lactose intolerance experience the bloating, cramping and diarrhea of an allergy reaction. But the symptoms are really due to a deficiency of the enzyme lactase, which helps digest milk sugar. Common food intolerances include those to wheat, dairy foods, fruits, sugar, yeast, mushrooms, eggs, corn and greens. Although these foods may be healthy in themselves, they are often heavily sprayed or treated; in the case of animal products, also affected by antibiotics and hormones. **Food sensitivities** are similar to allergy reactions, but differ in that no antigen-specific antibodies are present. In general, they are not a permanent condition.

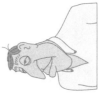

Signs you might need an allergy or asthma cleanse:

—**You may have a Type 1 seasonal allergy, or asthma, the most serious Type 1 allergy reaction if:** 1) you have chronic sinus congestion with itchy, watery nose and eyes. 2) you get headaches with sneezing, coughing and scratchy throat. 3) your face swells up, with itchy, rashy skin. (all the first three symptom listings are signs of excess mucous that forms as a shield around the offending allergens.) 4) you are unusually tired and have trouble sleeping at night.

—**You may have a Type 2 allergy to chemicals and contaminants if:** 1) you get unexplained migraine headache. 2) you are frequently moody and depressed for no reason 3) your friends and family tell you that your personality changes, that you are often spacey or that your memory is getting unusually bad. 4) you have a child that's chronically hyperactive.

—**You may have a Type 2 food allergy if:** 1) you get cyclical headaches with mental fuzziness after eating. 2) you get heart palpitations, with sweating, rashes or puffiness around the eyes after eating. 3) your abdomen becomes excessively swollen after eating with heartburn or stomach cramps. 4) you've gained significant weight even though your diet hasn't changed. 5) you have a child that's irritable, flushed and hyperactive after eating. (Regardless of the food, most food allergy symptoms are similar. Inflammation is generated by a release of histamines into tissue mast cells, walling off the affected body area until immune response agents can restore health. But this process takes time. If the body is re-exposed before health is renewed, inflammation and symptoms, especially mucous congestion become chronic.)

Can't find a recommended product? Call the 800 number listed in Product Resources for the store nearest you.

Alzheimer's Disease

Senility, Cerebral Atherosclerosis, Loss of Memory, Senile Dementia

The number one fear of older Americans isn't heart disease or cancer.... it's Alzheimer's. As more people live into their 80's and 90's, cases of Alzheimer's and dementia are rising fast. Alzheimer's disease now affects 4 million Americans at a cost of over $100 billion in nursing care and lost wages of family members. By 2050, 14 million more Americans will fall victim to the disease. Alzheimer's disease progresses slowly. Memory loss and disorientation are the first symptoms, but eventually there is almost complete loss of physical function and reversion to childhood in terms of care. Many of those diagnosed are really victims of too many drugs, or have nutritional deficiencies that can be reversed. Although orthodox medicine has been unable to make a difference in this relentless disease, natural therapies have been successful in slowing brain deterioration.

Diet & Superfood Therapy

—Nutritional therapy plan:

1—Good nutrition clearly deters Alzheimer's onset. Red meats and sugar appear to be the biggest culprits. Add high fiber foods and good fats like omega-3 oils from sea greens, flax, ginger, nuts, eggs and soy for brain-nourishing EFA's.

Make a brain mix: lecithin granules, brewer's yeast, wheat germ, oat bran, flax oil and molasses. Take 2 TBS each morning with cereal or juice.

2—Eat a largely vegetarian diet. Especially reduce red meats. Excess meat protein and fat accelerate amyloid neurofiber tangle build-up. Alzheimer's has been linked to synthetic estrogens injected into some red meats. Eat organic foods to avoid estrogens from pesticides.

3—Eat B vitamin foods - brown rice, whole grains, brewer's yeast, molasses, liver, fish and wheat germ. (They block aluminum toxicity.)

5—Eat tryptophan-rich foods - poultry, low-fat dairy, avocados. Low tryptophan is linked to Alzheimer's. Use pain killers or sleeping pills sparingly; they can leach acetylcholine from brain tissue.

6—Drink unfluoridated water. Fluoridated water increases aluminum absorption!

—Superfood therapy: (Choose one or two)

- Crystal Star SYSTEMS STRENGTH™ drink.
- Nutricology PRO-GREENS with EFA's.
- Pines MIGHTY GREENS superfood blend.

Herb & Supplement Therapy

—Interceptive therapy plan: (Choose 2 or more recommendations)

1—**Reduce glyco-protein amyloid strings and overcome brain damage:** • Enzymedica PURIFY, powerful protease, 3 to 5 capsules; • Ethical Nutrients MAGNESIUM-MALIC ACID. • Country Life Phosphatidyl Choline 5000-10,000mg.

2—**Normalize body chemistry:** Crystal Star GINSENG-REISHI extract; • Siberian ginseng extract; • ginseng-gotu kola caps 4 daily; • MICROHYDRIN from Healthy House. Transformation EXCELLZYME; Nutricology ANTI-OX II.

3—**Enhance memory retention:** • Huperzine-A, 50mcg, 2 daily. Phyto-hormones from herbal sources like panax ginseng and royal jelly; • Crystal Star MENTAL INNER ENERGY™ caps, or CREATIVI-TEA™ 2x daily; • Y.S. ROYAL JELLY-GINSENG drink. • Ginkgo biloba extract caps, 60mg 3x daily stabilizes symptoms.

4—**Nourish the brain:** • Crystal Star BRAIN DEFENSE™ caps and • SILICA SOURCE™ or • Flora VEGE-SIL to prevent aluminum build-up; • Biotec CELL GUARD w. SOD; • Herbal Magic GINSENG-GOTU KOLA; • Brain oils - Evening primrose 500mg 4 daily, vitamin E 800IU daily, omega-3 flax oil for EFA's. • Chelation therapy cleans up arterial pathways - Golden Pride FORMULA ONE.

5—**Preserve brain cells with amino acid therapy:** • NADH - 10mg in the morning before eating. • Phosphatidyl serine 100mg 3x daily or choline 650mg, for 3 months, or DHA for 3 months (nature's calcium channel blocker); • Lysine 1000mg daily; • Carnitine 500mg 2 daily, or Acetyl-L-Carnitine; • CoQ-10, 60mg 4x daily.

—Herbal brain boosting resources: (choose one)

- Rosemary tea daily; add extra • cat's claw extract drops.
- Crystal Star IRON SOURCE drops daily often improve conversation ability.
- Moderate wine drinking appears to boost brain activity AND deter Alzheimer's.

—B-complex for mental power and to lower homocysteine levels:

- Extra pantothenic acid 1000mg and B-6 100mg and folic acid 400mcg.
- Extra B-1 (thiamine) 100mg and B-12 2500mcg.

Lifestyle Support Therapy

—Lifestyle measures:

• Alzheimer's is aluminum related. Beware of fluoridated water. It increases absorption of aluminum from deodorants, pots and pans, etc. by over 600%. Avoid aluminum and alum containing products: cookware, deodorants, dandruff shampoos, anti-diarrhea compounds, canned foods, salt, buffered aspirin and analgesics, antacids, refined and fast foods, relishes, pickles, tobacco, etc. Read labels!

• Consider removing silver amalgam dental fillings. Mercury toxicity releases into the brain and affects brain health.

• Decrease prescription diuretics if possible. They leach potassium and nutrients needed by the brain.

• Daily exercise is medicine against Alzheimer's. Take hot and cold hydrotherapy showers for brain and circulation stimulation.

—Reflexology brain pressure points:

—Squeeze all around the hand and fingers.
—Pinch end of each toe. Hold 5 seconds.

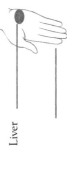

Liver

A 311

See Diagnostics, Tests and Procedures pages 529 for more information.

Can't find a recommended product? Call the 800 number listed in Product Resources for the store nearest you.

Common Symptoms: Loss of ability to remember past or present facts, names or places; inability to learn new information; loss of touch with reality; confusion; difficulty in completing thoughts or following directions; getting lost; constantly repeating oneself; personality and behaioral changes. In final stages, almost a return to infancy, communication is almost non-existent, feeding and elimination functions uncontrolled.

Common Causes: Acetylcholine deficiency; poor or obstructed circulation; arteriosclerosis; anemia; estrogen disrupters like those in pesticides; lack of exercise, and body-brain oxygen; a brown fluid (lipofuscin) forms on brain neurons; thyroid malfunction; aluminum toxicity; possible mercury toxicity; reaction to drugs like oxybutynin chloride for incontinence or some antihistamines.

Anemia

Hemolytic, Iron-Deficiency, Folic Acid, Aplastic, Pernicious, Thalassemia, Sickle Cell

Iron-Deficiency: *a chronic state of diminished hemoglobin caused by a lack of iron, or poor absorption of iron. Twenty percent of American women suffer from iron-deficiency anemia.* **Hemolytic:** *vitamin B-12 and/or folic acid deficiency causing red blood cells to be destroyed more quickly than they are replaced.* **Thalassemia:** *an inherited defect, usually affecting people of Mediterranean origin.* **Sickle Cell:** *an inherited hemoglobin defect among blacks.* **Pernicious:** *a heredity prone, auto-immune disease caused by failure of the digestive tract to absorb vitamin B-12, affecting nerve and digestive systems; common among elderly people;* **Folic acid:** *lack of folic acid interferes with red blood cells.* **Aplastic:** *progressive bone marrow failure, generally caused by exposure to a chemical toxin.*

Diet & Superfood Therapy

—Nutritional therapy plan:

1—Good nutrition is a good remedy. Eating patterns show that vegetarians consume more iron than meat eaters. Eat vegetable and herbal iron sources are best for absorbability.

2—Eat some iron-rich foods every day: liver, organ meats, figs, seafood, molasses, beets, brown rice, spinach and dark greens, whole grains, poultry, eggs, grapes, raisins, yams, almonds, beans.

3—Eat manganese and vitamin C foods for iron uptake: whole grains, greens, legumes, nuts, pineapples and eggs, citrus fruits, cruciferous vegetables, tomatoes and green pepper.

4—Eat cultured foods for friendly flora and vit. B-12: yogurt, kefir, miso. sauerfraut, soyfoods.

5—Eat potassium rich foods until red blood count improves: broccoli, bananas, sunflower seeds, vegetables, whole grains, kiwi, dried fruits; or a potassium broth (pg. 215).

6—Avoid iron-depleting foods: sodas, caffeine, chocolate, red meat, cow's milk.

7—Mix brewer's yeast, molasses, wheat germ, sesame seeds, dry snipped sea greens; sprinkle 2 TBS daily over food.

—Superfood therapy: (Choose one or two)

• Nutricology PRO-GREENS with EFA's.
• Nature Care CHAWAN PRASH.
• Beehive ROYAL JELLY/GINSENG.

Herb & Supplement Therapy

—Interceptive therapy plan: (Choose 2 to 3 recommendations)

1—**Improve red blood cell count:** • Crystal Star IRON SOURCE™ caps or extract daily ○ or • Monas CHLORELLA or Floradix LIQUID IRON 2x daily. ⚥

2—**Improve iron absorption:** • Crystal Star ENERGY GREEN™ drink daily for both extra iron, and zinc needed for iron absorption; • Planetary Formulas TRIPHALA COMPLEX; • Solaray ALFA-JUICE caps to help stimulate bone marrow production and help digestion of protein. Iron-enhancing herbs include: *yellow dock root, red raspberry, dandelion, kelp* (especially during pregnancy).

3—**Add B vitamins and B-12:** • Morada Reasearch BLOOD formula; Transformation SUPER-CELLZYME formula; • *Spirulina*-bee pollen caps 6 daily, a source of plant B-12; • B-complex 100mg with extra B_6 100mg, folic acid 800mcg daily, and biotin; • Country Life sublingual B-12, 2500mcg or • Solaray 2000mcg B-12.

—Other iron-enhancing resources:

• Crystal Star POTASSIUM-IODINE™ caps, 2 daily. ⚥
• Siberian ginseng, or Enzymatic Therapy LIQUID LIVER w. *Siberian Ginseng.*
• Nature's Secret ULTIMATE IRON, Betaine HCl or manganese at meals.
• *Dong quai/damiana* extract as a blood tonic.
• Zinc 50mg daily with your iron source, or • Source Naturals OPTI-ZINC caps.

—Folic acid anemia:

Folic acid with B-12 and zinc 50mg (regains menstrual periods); and Sun Wellness CHLORELLA tabs, 15 daily. ⚥

—Sickle-cell anemia:

Folic acid 800mcg, vitamin B-6 100mg 2x daily, zinc 50mg daily, and vitamin E 400IU 2x daily. ○

—Thalassemia:

vitamin E 800IU with CoQ₁₀ 30mg 3x daily.

—Pernicious anemia:

Folic acid 800mcg daily.

Lifestyle Support Therapy

—Watchwords:

• If your baby is pale, lacks energy and drinks cow's milk instead of breast milk, he or she may be anemic. Cow's milk may promote loss of iron in stools.

• Methotrexate drugs used during chemotherapy may cause anemia by interfering with folic acid activity.

—Bodywork:

• Get some mild exercise daily to enhance oxygen uptake. Get morning sunlight every day possible for vitamin D.

—Lifestyle measures:

• Avoid pesticides, sprays and fluorescent lighting that cause mineral leaching from your body.

• Poor food combining accounts for an amazing amount of iron deficiency. See the FOOD COMBINING CHART on page 555.

Common Symptoms: *Overall weakness; dizziness and fainting; heart palpitations; shortness of breath; lack of libido; gastro-intestinal bleeding; ulcers; slow healing; fatigue; skin pallor; violent mood swings; irritability; spots before the eyes. Secondary signs: vision problems; apathy, brittle nails, poor appetite, hair loss, yellowish skin, headaches, dark urine, poor memory.*
Common Causes: *Recurring infections and diseases indicating low immunity and mineral deficiency; vitamin B-12 and folic acid deficiency; pregnancy effect; rapid growth in childhood; poor diet or poor food assimilation; candida albicans, lupus, or other auto-immune condition; blood loss from an ulcer; parasites; excessive menstruation; lack of green vegetables; alcoholism.*

Can't find a recommended product? Call the 800 number listed in Product Resources for the store nearest you.

Anxiety

Panic Attacks, Phobias, Obsessive-Compulsive Disorder

Over 30 million Americans have been diagnosed with clinical anxiety and panic disorders, and phobias (fear taken to extremes). Another 35 million suffer mild to moderate symptoms. A Harvard study shows that people who react to stress this way are 4 times more likely to become ill than those who don't. For some, the overall feeling is that they are going to die. Anxiety and phobias are more than just frightening. They are closely tied to high blood pressure, heart spasms and heart disease. During a panic attack, terror is so great that a person loses all reason and reality. Continued economic insecurity can generate this kind of fear.

Diet & Superfood Therapy

—Nutritional therapy plan:

1—If you get panic attacks, avoid alcohol, caffeine and smoking. They deplete B vitamins, your body's natural tranquilizers.

2—Avoid trigger foods: sugar, aspartame loaded foods, nitrate-preserved meats, MSG, fast, salty, fried foods, cola drinks.

3—Eat simple, calming, comfort foods during the day to prevent a panic attack at night..brown rice, mashed potatoes, creamy yogurt, oatmeal, steamed vegetables, etc. Consider goat's milk instead of cow's milk.

—Nutrients to be aware of for your diet:

• Foods rich in calcium for both stress and immune response: sesame seeds, almonds, soy foods, low fat dairy products, and leafy greens.

• Foods rich in magnesium to protect nerves: kelp, wheat germ, bran, most nuts, soy foods.

• Foods rich in B vitamins to support the adrenals and fuel the nerves: nutritional yeast, whole grains and brans, nuts, beans.

• Foods rich in vitamin C for stress response: peppers, greens, broccoli, kiwi, acerola cherries.

—Superfood therapy: (Choose one or two)

• Crystal Star SYSTEM STRENGTH™ w. EFA's.
• Nutritional yeast or miso broth before bed.
• Green Foods CARROT ESSENCE.

Herb & Supplement Therapy

—Interceptive therapy plan: (Choose 2 to 3 recommendations)

1—**Herbal calmers help, often within 20 minutes:** • Nelson Bach RESCUE REMEDY; • *Kava kava,* • *ashwagandha* or • *Siberian ginseng* extracts under the tongue; • Crystal Star RELAX CAPS™, 2-4 as needed; • Enzymatic Therapy KAVA-TROL.

2—**Rebuild nerves-relieve anxiety:** • *Gotu kola, scullcap* or *passionflower* extracts, • St. John's *wort* extract, or • Crystal Star VALERIAN/WILD LETTUCE extract; • B-complex 100mg with extra B$_6$ 50mg, niacinimide 500mg, thiamine 500mg and taurine 500mg, 3x daily. • Phosphatidyl choline 1000mg 3x daily.

3—**Adrenal boost:** • Crystal Star STRESSED OUT™ extract and • ADR-ACTIVE™ caps; • *Evening Primrose oil* 3000mg daily, boosts adrenals and adds EFA's.

4—**Aromatherapy can often help right away:** • *Lavender* or *ylang-ylang* oil on the temples, • *chamomile* or *rose* oil; • *aromas of apples and cinnamon.*

—Tonic adaptogens to rebalance body chemistry:

• Crystal Star GINSENG-LICORICE ELIXIR™. ♂
• Crystal Star FEM-SUPPORT or *Dong Quai-Damiana* extracts. ♀
• Crystal Star MENTAL INNER ENERGY™ with *kava kava* and *panax ginseng.*
• *Hawthorn* extract as needed for heart palpitations.

—Anti-stress amino acids and minerals are calmers and balancers:

• GABA 750-1000mg daily and as needed during an attack, to mimic valium effects without sedation.
• 5-HTP 50-100mg especially at night before bed; or Cal-Mag-Zinc, 4 at night.
• Magnesium is critical support for heart stability and calcium balance.
• Tyrosine 500mg a.m-/p.m., between meals.

—Homeopathic remedies for anxiety are effective:

• Enzymatic Therapy ANTI-ANXIETY.
• *Ignatia*

Lifestyle Support Therapy

—Bodywork:

• **Hypnotherapy** has been extremely successful for panic attacks and anxiety.
• **Relax.** Take a quiet bath, get a massage therapy treatment, do yoga or meditate.
• **Deep breathing** is a natural tranquilizer: 1) exhale with a whoosh. 2) inhale through your nose slowly. 3) hold your breath for a count of six. 4) exhale with a whoosh. Repeat four more times.

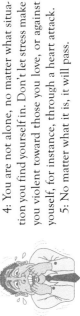

—Lifestyle measures:

• Most panic attacks take place in the early hours of the morning. Next time, put the 5 a.m. willys into perspective:

1: Get out of bed, turn on a TV show, take a shower; see the sun rising and life going on. Get dressed and walk outside.

2: Stretch, exercise a little, or walk your dog. There is a body chemical basis for fear, released in hormone secretions. Exercise oxygenates the body, replacing that function.

3: Think positive. Review a recent success, remind yourself of your talents and abilities.

4: You are not alone, no matter what situation you find yourself in. Don't let stress make you violent toward those you love, or against youself, for instance, through a heart attack.

5: No matter what it is, it will pass.

See DEPRESSION page 366 for more information.

A 313

Common Symptoms: "nerves" type attacks; trembling, rapid heartbeat, indigestion, ulcer or colitis attacks; irritability; insomnia; high blood pressure; head and neck aches; loss of appetite; dizziness.

Common Causes: Fear, sometimes fear of fear, is at the heart of all panic disorders. Anxiety is the result of emotional and physical stress encountered in daily life - relationship difficulties, severe, long term financial problems, job demands, food allergies and nutrient deficiencies of B-vitamins, and magnesium; traffic jams and our increasingly crowded and noisy environment. Anti-depression drugs like Prozac, besides their side effects, change your body chemistry, making you more at risk for a panic attack, and abnormal behavior.

Can't find a recommended product? Call the 800 number listed in Product Resources for the store nearest you.

Appendicitis
Chronic Appendix Inflammation

Appendicitis is an inflammation of the appendix, a small 2 inch tube opening into the beginning of the large intestine. It is usually caused by blockage from a small, hard lump of fecal matter, which itself results from a fiber-deficient diet. The blockage stops the natural flow of fluids, unfriendly bacteria swarm in and inflammation and infection result. The suggestions on this page are for chronic, recurring appendicitis. Perforation and rupture of the organ is a major medical emergency, and you need emergency treatment. DON'T DELAY!

Diet & Superfood Therapy

—Nutritional therapy plan:

1—Go on a short spring cleanse (pg. 191) to gently clear and clean the intestine. Take one potassium drink (pg. 215) daily during your cleanse.

2—Eat sweet fruits for a day to encourage healing. Then, resume a simply cooked, mild foods diet. Include a glass of carrot juice daily for 2 weeks.

3—Reduce the risk of developing appendicitis by making sure your diet is high in fiber.

4—Avoid chemicalized and fried foods on a continuing basis.

—Warning: Take no solid food or laxatives during an appendicitis flare-up.

—Superfood therapy: (Choose one or two)
• Crystal Star SYSTEMS STRENGTH™ drink for alkalinity and better food absorption.
• Crystal Star CHO-LO FIBER TONE™ drink or AloeLife FIBERMATE to provide fiber.
• Nutricology PROGREENS with EFA's.
• Green Foods CARROT ESSENCE.

Herb & Supplement Therapy

Chronic or grumbling appendicitis can be treated herbally with some success. Any hint of complications or deterioration of your condition must be taken seriously. **Get to an emergency room!**

—Interceptive therapy plan: (Choose 2 to 3 recommendations) Take liquid supplements as much as possible to make it easier on your system.

1—**Reduce infection:** • Crystal Star ANTI-BIO™ extract in water every 2 hours.

2—**Reduce inflammation:** • Crystal Star ANTI-FLAM™ extract.

3—**Reduce spasms:** • Crystal Star CRAMP BARK COMBO HERBS™ extract.

4—**Flush lymph toxins:** • Echinacea extract 4x daily under the tongue for a month after an attack to keep the lymph glands flushed.

—Appendix specific teas: (choose one)
• 2 TBS *agrimony*, 2 TBS *echinacea root*, 1 TB *chamomile*, 1 TB *wild yam root*.
• 2 TBS *agrimony and calendula flowers*.

—After an attack has subsided, clean the colon of infection: (choose one)
• Solaray TETRA CLEANSE or • Planetary TRIPHALA caps.
• Yerba Prima COLON CARE SYSTEM.
• Crystal Star FIBER & HERBS CLEANSE™ caps.

—Preventive measures: (choose one or more)
• **Vitamins:** • Beta carotene 25,000IU 4x daily; • vitamin E 400IU 2x daily; • zinc picolinate 30mg daily; • Ester C or vitamin C crystals ¹/₄ teasp. in water 4x daily; • Transformation SUPERCELL-ZYME capsules daily.
• **Plant enzymes:** • Liquid chlorophyll in water 3x daily; • Rainbow Light ADVANCED ENZYME SYSTEM tablets at meals.
• **Probiotics:** • Prof. Nutrition Dr. DOPHILUS lactobacillus powder ¹/₄ tsp. in water 3x daily; or • Natren LIFE START powder - for friendly flora, better peristalsis.

Lifestyle Support Therapy

—Lifestyle measures:
• Do not take high colonics or enemas *during an attack.*
• But keep the colon clean. Constipation is usually at the heart of an attack. Use a mild catnip enema if necessary.

—Bodywork:
• Use alternating hot and cold cayenne/ginger compresses on affected region and along spinal area.

—Reflexology point:

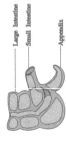

appendix

—Position of appendix:

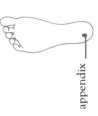

The **Appendix**

Large Intestine
Small Intestine
Appendix

Common Symptoms: Early symptoms: colicky, central abdominal pain followed by nausea and vomiting; then pain shifting to the right lower abdomen as the inflammation spreads; intense, recurring sharp pain on the lower right side at the waist.

Common Causes: Poor diet, lacking in fiber and roughage; too many laxatives resulting in lack of peristalsis and friendly bowel flora; toxic build-up causing depressed immunity.

Can't find a recommended product? Call the 800 number listed in Product Resources for the store nearest you.

Arteriosclerosis - Atherosclerosis
Clogging and Hardening of the Arteries

Both arteriosclerosis and atherosclerosis block the flow of blood from the arteries to the heart, and damage the circulatory system. Atherosclerotic plaque is largely composed of cholesterol. It begins under the inner wall of the artery suggesting that a vitamin B_6 deficiency and a diet high in animal fats is the cause rather than cholesterol as previously thought. Arteriosclerosic plaque is the build-up of calcium on the inside of the artery walls. Both conditions are not only preventable, but reversable. Love and affection, both given and taken, really reduces heart and arterial problems.

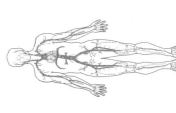

Diet & Superfood Therapy

—Nutritional therapy plan:

1—Reduce coffee to 1 cup daily. Drink green tea every morning instead.

2—Reduce dietary cholesterol. Avoid saturated fat-containing foods, like red meats, fatty dairy products, fried foods and low fiber foods.

3—Reduce high phosphorus foods: soft drinks, beef, pork, and poultry. They promote negative calcium balance.

4—Eat antioxidant-rich vegetables. In tests, vegetarians have healthier hearts and arteries. The risk of stroke from clogged arteries decreases by over 35% for each increase of 3 fruit or vegetable servings per day.

5—Eat plenty of high fiber whole grains, in the form of cereals, rather than bread or pasta, and lots of fresh greens.

6—Take a healthy artery drink twice a week: in a cup fenugreek tea, add 2 tsp. wheat germ, 2 tsp. honey, 1 TB lecithin granules.

7—Have a little wine at dinner; wine has an enzyme that breaks up blood clots. Eat smaller meals, especially at night.

—Superfood therapy: (Choose one or two)
• Nature's Secret ULTIMATE FIBER.
• Crystal Star CHO-LO FIBER TONE™, low cholesterol means clearer arteries.
• Aloe Falls ALOE VERA GINGER JUICE, 1 8-oz. glass daily.

Herb & Supplement Therapy

—Interceptive therapy plan: (Choose 2 to 3 recommendations)

1—**Normalize blood circulation:** • Crystal Star HEARTSEASE-HAWTHORN™ capsules, or •HEARTSEASE CIRCU-CLEANSE™ tea with *butcher's broom*; *astragalus tea* or *ginseng-cayenne* caps daily. Silica helps good circulation return: • Flora VEGESIL or •Eidon SILICA as directed.

2—**Oral chelation shows good results:** • Golden Pride FORMULA 1 oral chelation therapy with EDTA; • Enzymatic Therapy ORAL NUTRIENT CHELATES.

3—**Inhibit development of atherosclerosis:** •Ginkgo biloba extract also relieves claudication; chromium picolinate 200mcg daily.

4—**Lower cholesterol and triglycerides:** • Ester C 3-5000mg daily with bioflavonoids keeps LDL cholesterol from being oxidized; • Vitamin E 400IU w. selenium daily also lowers intermittent claudication. • Add magnesium, at least 400mg daily to raise HDL (good cholesterol).

5—**Liver support for fat metabolism:** • Milk thistle seed extract for 3 to 6 months; •Crystal Star GREEN TEA CLEANSER; • Enzymatic Therapy CO-ENZYMATE B-complex; Carnitine 1000mg; •Niacin 500mg 2x daily with pancreatin 1400mg.

6—**Good fats help your liver:** •High omega-3 flax oil, 3x daily, or *evening primrose oil caps*, 4-6 daily for 1 month, then 3-4 daily.

—Lower homocysteine levels: (see complete program on page 535).
1) B Complex, 100mg daily. Add 50mg extra of B_6 and 400mcg extra of folic acid; 2) Four garlic capsules (about 1200mg a day) maintain aortic elasticity; 3) Daily ginger prevents blood "stickiness"; 4) Red wine, one glass with dinner.

—Antioxidants are front line defense: Their negatively charged electrons help prevent and remove positively charged plaque build-up. MICROHYDRIN 2 to 3 daily, available at Healthy House; •PCO's from grape seed or white pine 100mg daily; •CoQ-10, 30mg 3x daily, or •Sun Force CoQ$_{10}$ in flax oil; •Phosphatidyl choline 1000mg daily; •Zinc picolinate, 30mg daily.

Lifestyle Support Therapy

—Lifestyle measures:
•Stop smoking. Keep your weight down. Relax. Meditation has proven to be good for your arteries.
•For arteriosclerotic retinopathy: reduce fats, especially saturated fats from meats in your diet. Reduce sugar intake to help normalize blood sugar balance. Take garlic capsules daily to help normalize blood pressure levels.

—Bodywork:
•Take a brisk walk daily. Aerobic exercise helps raise HDL levels. Then, use a dry skin brush over the body to stimulate circulation.
•Take an alternating hot and cold shower to increase blood circulation.

Common Symptoms: Intermittent claudication (pain upon exertion); poor circulation with cold hands and feet, and leg cramps; mild heart attacks; mental and respiratory deterioration; blurred vision; high blood pressure; sometimes impotence.

Common Causes: High risk factors include smoking, high cholesterol, high blood pressure, diabetes, too much saturated fat and refined food in the diet; vitamin B_6 deficiency; being overweight; stress; lack of aerobic exercise; too much caffeine and alcohol; excess salt.

See HEALTHY HEART DIET pg. 410.

Can't find a recommended product? Call the 800 number listed in Product Resources for the store nearest you.

Arthritis

Joint and Connective Tissue Diseases

The term arthritis, meaning joint inflammation, refers to over 100 diseases that attack joints and connective tissue. Up to 50 million Americans are afflicted by one or more of these crippling conditions. Other degenerative joint diseases include gout, lupus erythematosus, ankylosing spondylitis (arthritic spine), psoriatic arthritis (skin and nail arthritis), infective arthritis (bacterial joint infection) and rheumatism. Arthritis is not a simple disease in any form, affecting not only the bones and joints, but also the blood vessels, kidneys, skin, eyes, brain and immune response. Conventional medicine has not been able to address arthritis successfully. Natural therapies, based on lifestyle changes, however, do work extremely well, addressing the causes of arthritis while reducing pain and discomfort.

Diet & Superfood Therapy

—Nutritional therapy plan:

1–Change to a low-fat, mostly vegetarian diet - the single most beneficial thing you can do to control any kind of arthritis, even in long-standing cases. See following page for an arthritis cleansing diet.

2–Avoid arthritis trigger foods: corn, wheat, rye breads, bacon and pork, beef, eggs, coffee, oranges, oats and milk. Nightshade foods like peppers, eggplant, tomatoes and potatoes; mustard, colas, chocolate.

3–Cut down on: alcohol, fried foods, dairy foods, black tea, salty, highly spiced foods.

4–Add body balancing foods: green tea, artichokes, cherries, cabbages, brown rice, oats, shiitake mushrooms, cold water fish, sea greens, fresh fruits, vegetables, leafy greens, garlic, onions, olive oil, sweet potatoes, squashes, ginger and parsley.

5–Arthritis V-8 Special: add to a bottle of Knudsen's VERY VEGGIE JUICE, 4 TBS each: wheat germ, lecithin granules and brewer's yeast flakes. Take 8-oz. twice daily.

—Superfood therapy: (Choose one or two)

• Crystal Star ENERGY GREEN™ drink and ZINC SOURCE™ drops. (If you take cortisone for arthritis, you are probably deficient in zinc.)
• Green Foods MAGMA PLUS barley grass.
• Wakunaga KYO-GREEN - take with glucosamine sulfate for 1 month. When symptoms abate, continue with KYO-GREEN for 3 months.
• Aloe Life ALOE GOLD drink.
• Nutricology PRO-GREENS with EFA's.

Herb & Supplement Therapy

—Interceptive therapy plan: (Choose 2 to 3 recommendations)

1–Repair joints, reduce pain: • Metabolic Response Modifiers or Solgar GLU-COSAMINE-CHONDROITIN 4 daily; (Shark cartilage has natural chondroitin sulfates.). Use with • CMO (cetyl-myristoleate), 500mg, like Jarrow TRUE CMO for EFA's.
• Omega-3 flax or fish oil 3x daily. Expect pain diminishment in 2 to 4 months.

2–Reduce inflammation: • Enzymedica PURIFY; • MSM, 750 to 1000mg.
• Quercetin 1000mg w/Bromelain 750mg, 2 daily; • DLPA 1000mg for pain.
• **Herbal anti-inflammatories:** • Crystal Star AR EASE™ caps; • nettles extract; • cat's claw caps; • Earth's Bounty NONI liquid or caps. **Ocean anti-inflammatories:**
• Green-lipped mussel cap and sea cucumber caps 1500-2000mg for 2 months.

3–Antioxidants help regenerate cartilage and immune response: • SAMe protects cushioning synovial fluid and blocks enzymes that degrade cartilage. • CoQ$_{10}$ 60mg 3x daily; • Carnitine 1000mg 2x daily; • Grapeseed or white pine PCO's 300mg daily; • Vitamin E 800IU daily.

4–Boost new collagen synthesis: • American Biologics SHARKILAGE or bovine tracheal cartilage 1000mg; • Ester C 500mg with bioflavonoids, up to 10 daily;
• Country Life LIGA-TEND as needed.

5–Enzymes help normalize body chemistry: • Rainbow Light ADVANCED ENZYME SYSTEM; • Crystal Star ALKALIZING ENZYME™ herbal wrap.

6–Enhance adrenal activity: • Y.S. royal jelly/ginseng 2 tsp. daily; • Enzymatic Therapy ADRENAL CORTEX COMPLEX; • Crystal Star ADR-ACTIVE™ caps daily with Evening Primrose Oil 3000mg daily.

7–Stimulate natural cortisone production: • Alfalfa tabs 10 daily; • Solaray ALFA-JUICE caps; • Sun Wellness, or Mona's CHLORELLA 1 teasp. daily.

—Ayurvedic arthritis medicines: Boswellin creme, turmeric caps 4 daily; ashwagandha extract, ♀ cayenne-ginger caps 2 daily; apply cayenne-ginger compresses.

—Desert healers are some of the best: Yucca extract, Jojoba oil to apply, Aloe vera gel and juice, devil's claw root.

—Homeopathic remedies for arthritis: Rhus tox for aching joints; Arnica and arnica cream for soreness; Bryonia for swollen joints and pain.

Lifestyle Support Therapy

—Lifestyle measures:

• High doses of aspirin, NSAIDS and cortisone for arthritic pain can hamper your body's ability to maintain bone strength.
• Nightshade plants may trigger arthritis: Tobacco is a nightshade plant. MOTRIN is also a nightshade derivative, and should not be used by nightshade-sensitive people.

—Bodywork:

• **An arthritis sweat can help right away.** See page 540 for details.
• To relieve pain, press the highest spot of the muscle between the two fingers, closer in the webbing between thumb and index finger. Press toward the bone that attaches to the index finger. Press into the web muscle, angling the pressure toward the bone of the index finger. Press for 10 seconds at a time.
• Massage therapy, acupuncture, hot and cold hydrotherapy (page 228), epsom salts baths, chiropractic treatments and overheating therapy (page 225) are all effective.
• Get some sun on your body for vitamin D.

—Local healing applications: (choose 1)

• Transitions PRO-GEST wild yam cream.
• Wakunaga FREEDOM ARTHRITIS RELIEF CREAM.
• Biochemics PAIN RELIEF lotion.
• capsaicin creme, or Nature's Way CAYENNE PAIN RELIEVING OINTMENT.
• Emu oil (with omega-3, omega-6 EFA's.)

A 316

See my book COOKING FOR HEALTHY HEALING for a complete diet with recipes.

Can't find a recommended product? Call the 800 number listed in Product Resources for the store nearest you.

The Different Faces Of Arthritis

Arthritis is not a single disease. It is many diseases with the common result of connective tissue breakdown. The causes of arthritic diseases also vary widely - from lifestyle wear and tear to emotional resentments, to viruses and bacterial origins. Specific natural therapies for the most common types are offered on this page.

—OSTEOARTHRITIS: degenerative joint disease, is the most common form of arthritis. OA most often appears in the weight-bearing joints like the knees, hips and spine, and in the hands, where there is much cartilage destruction followed by hardening and the formation of large bone spurs on the joints. The first signs of osteoarthritis show up as morning stiffness especially in damp weather, then pain in motion that worsens with prolonged activity. Osteoarthritis is a condition of age, (we see it in the creaking and cracking of joints on movement), because decades of use lead to degenerative changes in joints, and the body has less ability to repair itself. Although osteoarthritis affects more women than men, a man who is more than 20 pounds overweight doubles his risk of knee and hip arthritis. Repair ability can be greatly increased with body chemistry improvement. Food allergies almost always contribute to osteoarthritis symptoms, so a good body detox followed by a diet with plenty of fresh vegetables is the first place to start. Standard drug therapy with aspirin or NSAIDS drugs like MOTRIN suppress pain and inflammation, but may actually promote the progression of the disease by damaging cartilage and inhibiting the ability of the body to maintain normal collagen structures. Osteoarthritis is repairable. Numerous studies show that glucosamine sulfate (NAG), a natural body substance that stimulates the production of cartilage components works even better than NSAIDS drugs. The dose is 500mg 3x daily.

—In addition to the general recommendations, previous page, natural therapies for osteoarthritis: cherries and cherry juice take the bumps out of the knuckles by helping eliminate acids; take with a mild diuretic like •Crystal Star TINKLE CAPS™ to flush. •Crystal Star PRO-EST OSTEO-PLUS™ roll-on gel with wild yam, and •ADRN-ACTIVE caps for women for adrenal exhaustion; •Ayurvedic BOSWELLIA with zinc 50mg for men. Bitters herbs stimulate bile and better digestion: •Crystal Star BITTERS & LEMON CLEANSE™ extract. •Vitamin B-12 2500mcg daily. New pain relievers: •Biochemics PAIN RELEAF; •W.F.Young ABSORBINE CHRONIC arthritis strength formula. Daily outdoor exercise for extra vitamin D helps osteoarthritis.

—RHEUMATOID ARTHRITIS: affects more than 6 million Americans, the vast majority of them women. RA is a chronic, auto-immune, inflammatory disease in which rogue immune cells attack the synovial membrane that cushions joints. When this connective membrane becomes inflamed, it invades and damages nearby bone and cartilage, resulting in pain, stiffness, loss of movement, and eventually destruction of joints. Damage goes even further, because RA also causes inflammation of the blood vessels and the outer lining of the heart and lungs. Most RA sufferers also have food allergies, amoeba infestation, anemia, ulcerative colitis, chronic lung and bronchial congestion and liver malfunction. Common causes include calcium depletion, adrenal exhaustion, prolonged use of aspirin or cortico-steroid drugs, that eventually impair the body's own healing powers; poor diet, lacking in fresh vegetables, and high in acid and mucous-forming foods; auto-toxemia from constipation; inability to relax; resentments and a negative attitude toward life that locks up the body's healing ability.

—In addition to the general recommendations, previous page, specific natural therapies for rheumatoid arthritis: Add fresh salmon or tuna to your diet twice a week. Take •Vita Carte BOVINE TRACHEAL CARTILAGE (natural chondroitin sulfates), •Evening Primrose Oil 4000mg daily, •Nutricology PRO-GREENS drink with EFA's; •vitamin E 800IU along with ginger caps daily; •PCO's from grape seed oil, up to 300mg daily significantly reduce joint inflammation; •CAPSAICIN and Tiger Balm rub-on cremes, hot sulphur and mud baths at your favorite spa. Enzyme therapy alleviates pain and swelling: •Transformation PUREZYME 6 caps 3x daily, •bromelain 1500mg; •Rainbow Light ADVANCED ENZYME SYSTEM full-strength pancreatic enzymes. •B-complex 100mg with extra pantothenic acid 500mg and folic acid 400mcg significantly reduce morning stiffness and pain. •Thymus extracts boost critical immune deficiencies.

—RHEUMATISM, rheumatism myalgia: characterized by pain, muscle stiffness, and tenderness in soft-tissue structures, where excess acid settles in the joints causing pain and inflammation, and inhibits the production of natural cortisone in the body. (Cortisone feeds your adrenals and helps your body metabolize proteins.) Improve your body chemistry to relieve rheumatism.

Start with a sage cleansing tea, such as •Crystal Star CLEANSING & PURIFYING™ tea. Add a glass of cider vinegar and water each morning. Then build your diet around low acid foods and foods that help to absorb acid, such as potatoes, turnips, green beans and root vegetables like carrots. Low acid fruits like white grape juice and apples can help to stimulate digestion. Alfalfa has a long tradition of success for rheumatism - eat alfalfa sprouts often, take alfalfa tablets or •Solaray ALFA-JUICE caps, or •Crystal Star ENERGY GREEN™ drink with alfalfa daily. Anti-rheumatics - •Enzymatic Therapy AR-MAX or •Crystal Star AR-EASE™; anti-inflammatories, like a glucosamine-chondroitan complex supplement, or ginger, both as compress and a supplement 2-4 capsules daily, work for rheumatism. A long term musculo-skeletal support herbal formula might be •Crystal Star SYSTEMS STRENGTH™, along with circulatory stimulants, like cayenne/ginger capsules and Capsaicin rub on cream. A mild diuretic like •Crystal Star TINKLE CAPS™ helps release congestive sediments. Since muscle tension is often at the core of rheumatic aches, •Crystal Star RELAX CAPS™ is also recommended. Topical rub-on creams for pain relief include •wintergreen oil and •Wakunaga FREEDOM ARTHRITIS RELIEF cream.

—PSORIATIC ARTHRITIS: an easily aggravated rheumatoid-like condition, associated with psoriasis. Burdock tea, 2 cups daily and daily applications of wild yam cream are two specifics for this type of arthritis. Immune support is essential. I recommend Biotec Foods ANTI-STRESS ENZYMES, 6 daily for several months. Crystal Star 4 each daily LIV-ALIVE™ and BLDR-K caps support liver function and kidney elimination of toxins.

—GOUT: a metabolic disorder that results in pain in the hands, knees and toe joints, sometimes produces arthritis as its primary symptom. Barley grass juice, like •Green Kamut JUST BARLEY is a specific for gout. See GOUT PAGE 398 in this book for more information.

Note: Dr. Dombach's spa and clinic for arthritis comes highly recommended. You can investigate further. Call 1-800-359-6547.

Can't find a recommended product? Call the 800 number listed in Product Resources for the store nearest you.

Does your body need an arthritis detox for better joints, connective tissue and immune response?

Arthritis is already the country's number one crippling disease, affecting up to 80% of people over 50. When you add to that number, people suffering from arthritis-like diseases - gout, bursitis, tendonitis and lupus, and the figure becomes staggering. Arthritis isn't a simple disease in any form, affecting not only the bones and joints, but also the blood vessels (Reynaud's disease), kidneys, skin (psoriasis), eyes and brain. The confusing array of new products in both the conventional and the alternative healing worlds for arthritis is rising at an almost exponential rate as the baby boomer generation creeps into the "age of arthritis." NSAIDS drugs, cortisone drugs, even the newest biogenetic drugs for arthritis have side effects and unknowns in terms of immune response. Natural therapies, based in lifestyle and diet changes, however, work extremely well because they address the causes of arthritis. In fact, diet improvement to normalize body chemistry is the single most beneficial thing you can do to control an arthritic condition. I have personally seen notable reduction of swelling, and deformity even in long-standing cases. Arthritis is unique in its close ties to emotional health. Emotional stress frequently brings onset of the disease. Acid-causing, emotional resentments and negative obsessive-compulsive actions aggravate arthritis. Most arthritis sufferers have a marked inability to relax (relaxation techniques are essential to arthritis healing). Many have a negative attitude toward life that locks up the body's healing ability.

Is your body showing signs that it needs an arthritis detox?

–Are you unusually stiff when you get up in the morning? Do you notice marked redness and swelling in your fingers, shoulders or neck when the weather turns cold and damp?
–Have you started to notice bony bumps on your index fingers? Or bony spurs on any other joints?
–Are your joints starting to crack and pop? Do you experience back or joint pain when you move? Does it get worse with prolonged activity?
–Are you anemic? Is your complexion unusually pale? Have you recently lost weight but weren't on a diet?
–Is your digestion poor? Do you have food allergies or intolerances?
–Are you more than 20 pounds overweight and starting to feel the effects of the extra weight in your knees and hips?
–Do you have a lot of long-standing lung and bronchial congestion?
–Are you usually constipated? Do you suffer from ulcerative colitis?
–Do you regularly take more than 6 aspirin a day? Are you on a long-term prescription of corticosteroid drugs? Either of these may eventually impair the body's own healing powers.

Start with this 3 day nutritional arthritis cleanse:

–**On Rising:** take a glass of lemon juice and water; or a glass of fresh grapefruit juice. (Acidic citrus fruits help enzymes alkalize the body); or Crystal Star GREEN TEA CLEANSER™.
–**Breakfast:** take a potassium broth or essence (pg. 215); or a glass of carrot/beet/cucumber juice.
–**Mid-morning:** have apple or black cherry juice; or a green drink, like Green Foods GREEN ESSENCE, Personal Best V-8 (pg. 218) or Crystal Star ENERGY GREEN™ drink.
–**Lunch:** have a cup of miso soup with sea greens snipped on top, and a glass of fresh carrot juice with 1 teasp. Bragg's LIQUID AMINOS.
–**Mid-afternoon:** have another green drink, or alfalfa/mint tea, or Crystal Star CLEANSING & PURIFYING™ tea.
–**Dinner:** have a glass of cranberry/apple, or papaya juice, or another glass of black cherry juice.
–**Before Bed:** take a glass of celery juice, or a cup of miso soup with 1 TB of nutritional yeast.

Follow your detox with a fresh foods diet for 1 month. 1) Fresh fruits and vegetables, with lots of green leafy greens, rich in enzymes. 2) There is a link between a sulfur deficiency and arthritis. Eat sulfur-containing foods like broccoli, onions, cabbage and garlic. 3) Fiber keeps crystalline wastes flushed. Eat whole grains like rice and oats. 4) Bioflavonoids strengthen connective tissue. Eat (and drink) cranberries, grapes, papayas and citrus fruits, or Crystal Star BIOFLAVONOID, FIBER & C SUPPORT™ drink. 5) Have cold water fish like salmon for high omega-3 oils twice a week.

Lack of water is linked to arthritis pain and stiffness. Chondroitin sulfate, a specific nutrient for arthritis, is the molecule in cartilage that attracts and holds water. Healthy joints are 85 to 90% water, but since cartilage doesn't have its own blood supply, chondroitin sulfate aids the chondroitin "molecular sponge" in providing joint nourishment, waste removal and lubrication. Water often helps restore healthy cartilage as it relieves osteoarthritis symptoms. Include eight 8-oz. glasses of water daily in your arthritis healing diet. Limit your alcoholic beverages since they are especially dehydrating.

A 318

Can't find a recommended product? Call the 800 number listed in Product Resources for the store nearest you.

Asthma

Allergic Breathing Disorder

Asthma, inflammation of the bronchial tubes, is a severe respiratory allergy reaction and it's experienced almost a 50% rise in the last decade, mainly because of increased environmental pollutants. It now affects 3 percent of the U.S. population, about 15 million people, 2 million of whom have needed emergency treatment. It is the leading serious, chronic illness among children under the age of ten, (a 2:1 ratio of boys to girls), and a death rate of about 5,000 kids yearly. In asthma, the lung airways become red, swollen and full of thick mucous. Bronchial spasms constrict airways. The inflamed, constricted airways react, often progressively, to asthma triggers: allergens like certain foods, food additives, animal dander or molds, irritants like smoke, chemical toxins and factory emissions, infections like a cold or flu, even emotional stress.

Diet & Superfood Therapy

Nutritional therapy plan:

1—Food sensitivities play a major role in asthma attacks. During an attack - eat only fresh foods. Include fresh apple or carrot juice daily. Add plenty of water to thin mucous secretions.

2—To control asthma nutritionally: Go on a short mucous cleansing liquid diet (see page 195).

3—Avoid dairy products: they generate the most mucous. Avoid foods with sulfites, preservatives or MSG, high gluten breads, oily and fried foods and sugary foods. Avoid soft drinks and caffeine.

4—Add green leafy veggies (their magnesium relaxes bronchial muscles). Fresh fish offer EFA's.

5—**A largely vegetarian diet offers significant improvement.** Leukotrienes that contribute ro asthma reactions are derived from arachidonic acid found only in animal products.

6—Reduce salt and starchy foods. Asthma is common when salt intake is high.

• Make a syrup of pressed garlic juice, cayenne, olive oil and honey. Take 1 teasp. daily as a liver cleansing bile stimulant for fatty-acid metabolism.

—Superfood therapy: (Choose one or two)

• AloeLife FIBERMATE drink.
• Crystal Star BIOFLAV. FIBER & C drink.
• Klamath BLUE GREEN SUPREME.

Herb & Supplement Therapy

—Interceptive therapy plan: (Choose 2 to 3 recommendations)

1—**Clear the chest of mucous and control spasms:** • Crystal Star ASTH-AID™ tea or capsules clear the chest; • ANTI-HST™ caps or ALRG-HST™ for antihistamines. • Crystal Star ANTI-SPZ™ caps or • Ginkgo biloba extract eases breathing.

—**For acute attacks:** • Lobelia extract under the tongue as needed relaxes chest constriction; or sniff an anti-spasmodic oil like *lavender, rosemary,* or *anise.*
—Effective Ayurvedic bronchodilators: • *Coleus Forskholi* and • *Sida condifolia.*

2—**Minimize allergic reactions:** • Futurebiotics MSM 400mg 2x daily, with • MICROHYDRIN available from Healthy House. • Ease stress with • *Reishi* mushroom extract drops in water. • **Multiple reactions**- *una da gato* extract.

3—**Ease coughing, release mucous:** • Herbs Etc. LUNG TONIC; • Crystal Star X-PECT™ tea; • *wild cherry syrup;* • *Echinacea-goldenseal* extract thins mucous.

4—**Correct prostaglandin imbalance with EFA's:** • *Evening Primrose oil* 500mg (kids), 2000mg (adults). • Omega Nutrition ESSENTIAL BALANCE, 2 daily.

5—**Normalize adrenal activity:** • Crystal Star ADR-ACTIVE™ capsules; • raw adrenal complex and • raw thymus glandular 2x daily.

6—**Strengthen the immune system:** • Astragalus-echinacea extract drops in water; • Enzymedica PURIFY protease.

—Magnesium-B₁₂ therapy for kids:
• Calcium 500mg. • Magnesium 250mg, • B-12 2000mcg every other day, • Vitamin C 1000mg and • B-complex 50mg.

—Antioxidants for asthmatics: (Choose one or more)
• Quercetin 1000-2000mg daily, with • Bromelain 500mg; • Vitamin C 3000mg with bioflavs. and rutin; • Vitamin E 400IU with selenium 200mcg; • CoQ₁₀ 60mg 2x daily.; • Green tea or • Crystal Star GREEN TEA CLEANSER™ every morning.

—Pantothenic acid therapy:
Royal jelly 2 teasp. daily (unless allergic to bee products); B-complex 150mg daily with extra pantothenic acid 1000mg, extra B₆ 100mg.

Lifestyle Support Therapy

Try to stay away from cortisone compounds that eventually weaken the immune system, and over-the-counter drugs that often drive congestion deeper.

—Bodywork:

• Use eucalyptus oil in a vaporizer at night for relief and tissue oxygen.
• Oshadi FRANKINCENSE aromatherapy.
• A twenty minute oxygen bath helps right away. See page 229 for instructions.
• Take a catnip-garlic enema once a week.
• Apply a hot ginger compress to the chest.
• Acupuncture, biofeedback, guided imagery and massage therapy are effective.
• Gently scratch the lung meridian from top of shoulder to end of thumb to clear chest of mucous. Massage between the shoulder blades.

—Home and lifestyle measures:

• Avoid tobacco smoke, wood and gas stoves.
• Keep house temperature less than 70 degrees, humidity less than 55%. Launder with perfume/dye-free detergents. Vacuum often.
• Keep indoor plants in your home as natural air filters.
• Deep breathing exercises bring asthmatic breathing under control. Expel toxins by taking a walk, a day at the beach, (helps 85% of asthmatics), or bicycle ride.

Common Symptoms: *Difficult breathing (actually a failure to exhale, not inhale); choking, wheezing, coughing, often with heart palpitations. Colds are often accompanied by ear infections, and a croupy cough. Accompanying hyperactivity in kids, high blood pressure in adults.*
Common Causes: *Food allergies especially to sugar, dairy products and wheat, sensitivity to food additives and sprayed produce; Beware of aspirin if you are at asthma risk. In kids, a chronic fungal or parasite infection; in adults, adrenal exhaustion and imbalance; hypoglycemia; constipation; an increased toxic load from chemical environmental pollutants; emotional stress or excessively cold air; low thyroid.*

See page 310 for more info and my book COOKING FOR HEALTHY HEALING for a complete Asthma Control diet.

Can't find a recommended product? Call the 800 number listed in Product Resources for the store nearest you.

Attention Deficit Hyperactivity Disorder
Learning Disabilities, Autism, Tourette's Syndrome

Hyperactive behavior and Attention Deficit Disorder are serious problems affecting up to 10% of children today. Hyperactivity may be the expression of either hypoglycemia or food allergies or both. Attention Deficit Disorder is slow learning caused by any or all of the learning disorders. Autism is almost a "mind-blind" condition, characterized by withdrawn behavior, lack of emotion and speech, extreme sensitivity to sound and touch. Autistic children have a brain malfunction that creates a barrier between them and the rest of the world. Children at greatest risk are male, with a history of family diabetes or alcoholism. Tourette's Syndrome is an involuntary movement and vocal disorder, often socially disabling. Nutritional improvement and stress-calming herbs are the cornerstones of successful treatment in overcoming hyperactivity disorders.

Diet & Superfood Therapy

Nutritional therapy plan:

1—Diet improvement is the key to changing ADD behavior. Results are almost immediately evident, generally within 1 to 3 weeks. When behavior normalizes, maintain the improved diet to prevent reversion.

2—Food sensitivities play a major part in attention disorders. **Reduce sugar intake** (almost always involved in ADHD reactions). Make sure any sugary foods are part of a well-balanced meal. Reduce carbonated drinks (Excess phosphorus). Eliminate red meats (nitrates).

3—Use applied kinesiology to determine allergens, or test foods like milk, wheat, corn, chocolate, and citrus with an elimination diet.

4—The ongoing diet should be high in vegetable proteins and whole grains, with plenty of fresh fruits and vegetables, and no junk or fast foods. Use organically grown foods when possible. **Have a green salad every day.**

5—Include calming tryptophan-rich foods like turkey, tuna, wheat germ, yogurt and eggs.

6—Add EFA-rich foods: sea greens, spinach and other leafy greens, soy foods, fish and seafoods.

—**Superfood therapy: (Choose one or two)**
• Lewis Labs high phosphatide lecithin and-or Red Star NUTRITIONAL YEAST.
• Miso soup before bed.

Herb & Supplement Therapy

—**Interceptive therapy plan: (Choose 2 to 3 recommendations)**

1—**Improve behavior problems:** • DMAE, 100 to 500mg daily in divided doses; • Crystal Star RELAX CAPS™, • Herbs Etc. KIDALIN, or • Planetary Formulas CALM CHILD drops as needed. • Homeopathic *Camomilla* (very young kids).

2—**Focus attention:** • **NADH 2.5mg daily.** • Rosemary tea or aromatherapy oil.

3—**Calming herbs:** • Crystal Star CALCIUM SOURCE™ extract in water is a rapid calmative. • Crystal Star *valerian-wild lettuce* extract or *catnip* tea for extra calming; • *gotu kola* or *hawthorn* drops for nerve stress or • Taurine 500mg daily.

4—**Enhance neurotransmitters - brain serotonin:** • Stress B Complex with extra pantothenic acid 100mg and B₆ 100mg; • *Gotu kola, kava kava* or *St. John's wort* extract drops in water. • Ginkgo biloba drops (older kids) 60mg 3x daily also helps inner ear balance. • GABA, 100mg and-or • Phos. Serine 100mg daily.

5—**Add electrolyte minerals:** • Nature's Path TRACE-LYTE minerals. • Add magnesium 400mg and • Premier Lithium .5mg. Check you child's iron- a deficiency often results in a learning disability.

6—**Minimize allergic reactions:** • Chromium 150mcg 3x daily with • Vanadium 150mcg to regulate blood sugar metabolism.

7—**Correct prostaglandin imbalance with EFA's:** • Sea-Lutions TUNA OIL (Omega-3's with DHA fatty acids for kids); • Black currant or borage oil • *Evening Primrose oil*, 500mg; • Omega-3 flax oil; • or Source Naturals FOCUS DHA 100mg.

—**Homeopathic remedies for ADD: (choose one)**
• Hylands CALMS and CALMS FORTE
• Nature's Way RESTLESS CHILD

—**Natural Autism therapy:** Magnesium 400mg, B-complex with extra B₆ 100mg (Natren HEALTHY TRINITY for synthesis of B vitamins), • *Black walnut* as an anti-fungal medicine. Ask a qualified practitioner for dosage. • Vitamin C with bioflavonoids, up to 2000mg daily - best in powder, ¹/₄ teasp. every 2 hours in juice.

Lifestyle Support Therapy

Avoid aspirin and amphetamines of all kinds if your child has any of these disorders.

Prescriptions for Ritalin, Cylertor, and Atarax, short-term sedative drugs for hyperactive disorders, often make the condition worse. Some researchers say Ritalin is almost identical to cocaine! Side effects include nervousness, insomnia, unhealthy weight loss, stunted growth, stomach aches, skin rashes, headaches and hallucinations. Avoid them if you can. Try diet improvement first.

Read food labels carefully. Avoid all food products with preservatives, BHT, MSG, BHA, additives and colors.

—**Bodywork:**
• Massage therapy, acupressure and biofeedback have shown some success.
• Take warm baking soda and sea salt baths.

—**Reflexology points:**

adrenals
diaphragm
pituitary
brain

Common Symptoms: *Behavior:* extreme emotional instability, compulsive-aggressive destructive behavior, short attention span, not sitting still; self-mutilation, chronic liar, doesn't follow directions or listen, impatient, defiant. Poor motor coordination and muscle harmony, speech problems; dyslexia; accident proneness. *Cognitive/perceptual:* slow learning-reasoning, chronic thirst, chronic cold symptoms, sneezing, coughing.

Common Causes: Mineral and EFA deficiencies from too many refined, junk foods; food allergies to corn, wheat and additives; prostaglandin imbalance; hypoglycemia; heavy metal (esp. lead) poisoning causing excess ammonia waste in the brain; prescription drugs that block EFA conversion in the brain. Autism almost certainly has allergy, parasite, yeast infection or fungal links.

Thanks to Dr. Howard Peiper and Rachel Bell for their work and book The A.D.D. and A.D.H.D. Diet.

Can't find a recommended product? Call the 800 number listed in Product Resources for the store nearest you.

Back Pain

Lumbago, Herniated Disc, Scoliosis, Sciatica

Friend and fellow author Art Brownstein (Healing Back Pain Naturally) says that "back pain....can drive a person to thoughts of suicide." The spine is the seat of human nerve structure, so it manifests much of your body's stress. 80% of Americans suffer back pain at some point in their lives and almost 40% wind up with crippling back pain. Lumbago is any pain in the lower back. Sciatica is pain radiating along the sciatic nerve, buttocks and back of the leg. Scoliosis is a particular curvature of the spine. A herniated disc occurs when the outer covering of the disc ruptures and the soft filling bulges into the spot. Major back surgery, like removing discs may do more harm than good. Diet improvement, supplements, a chiropractor or massage therapist who treats more than just the physical problem is often the best answer.

Diet & Superfood Therapy

—**Nutritional therapy plan:**

1—Your diet should be high in minerals and vegetable proteins. Vegetarians have stronger bone density.

2—It is critical to drink at least 6 glasses of water daily. Much back and rheumatoid pain is due to chronic dehydration. You need to keep acid particles flushed to keep kidneys functioning well.

3—Uric acid aggravates back pain. Avoid red meats, pasteurized dairy and caffeine.

3—Reduce the fat in your diet. The greater the deposits of fatty plaque, the greater the degeneration of spinal discs.

—**Superfood therapy: (Choose one or two)**
• Crystal Star ENERGY GREEN™ drink, or SYSTEMS STRENGTH™ for absorbable minerals, esp. potassium, and chlorophyll strength.
• A protein drink, like Unipro PERFECT PROTEIN, or Solgar WHEY TO GO.
• Nutricology PRO-GREENS with EFA'S
• Take a potassium drink (pg. 215) once a week for kidney cleansing.
• AloeLife ALOE GOLD concentrate, 2 TBS in water as an anti-inflammatory.

Herb & Supplement Therapy

—**Interceptive therapy plan: (Choose 2 to 3 recommendations)**

1—**Relieve pain:** • Crystal Star STRESSED OUT™ extract under the tongue usually helps within 20 minutes. • Apply cayenne-ginger heat packs - work wonders (page 233). • Crystal Star BACK TO RELIEF™ caps, an analgesic, or • ANTI-SPZ™ caps 4 at a time, for spasm control. • DLPA 1000mg. • MSM, 750 to 1000mg for chronic pain.

2—**Build stronger cartilage:** • Morada Research BONES/CALCIUM (silica calcium); • Crystal Star SILICA SOURCE™ extract; • Country Life LIGATEND 6 daily.
• Bovine tracheal cartilage 750-1000mg daily; • Rainforest Remedies BACK SUPPORT.

3—**Reduce swelling and inflammation:** • Quercetin 1000mg with Bromelain 1500mg daily or • Nature's Life BROMELAIN/PAPAIN; • Glucosamine-chondroitin, 1500/1200mg daily with vitamin C 3-5000mg and boron 3mg daily for better uptake.
• Crystal Star ANTI-FLAM™ caps for longer term pain control. • Homeopathic *Horse Chestnut* - results in about 3 to 6 days. • Apply ice packs if pain lasts more than 48 hours.

—**Effective herbal compresses and topical remedies for your back:**
• *Hops-comfrey-lobelia* compress; *lavender* or *chamomile* essential oils to control spasms.
• Home Health CASTOR OIL PACKS.
• B &T TRIFLORA GEL, or Chinese WHITE FLOWER oil.
• Biochemics PAIN RELIEF lotion.
• DMSO with ALOE GEL.
• New Chapter *Arnica-Ginger* gel.

—**For scoliosis — arthritis-like back pain:** • Glucosamine-chondroitin complex, 1500/1200mg daily; • Vitamin B-12, 5000mcg daily for spine cell development; • Vitamin D 400IU; • Evening primrose oil 2000mg daily for EFA's; • Calcium 1500mg-magnesium 750mg-zinc 25mg compound; • *devil's claw* herbal compound. Avoid sugar; eat a high protein diet from the sea - seafoods, cold water fresh fish, sea greens.

—**For sciatica:** Look to potassium drinks (page 218) and green drinks (page 218). Add extra potassium, up to 500mg daily for 1 to 2 weeks and CoQ-10, 60mg 3x daily.

Lifestyle Support Therapy

If you have fallen or bruised your spine or tailbone, and have persistent pain after 5 days, see a massage therapist or chiropractor.

Acupuncture, chiropractic and massage therapy are all successful for all types of back pain or injury. Ozone pools work for backs. (See pg. 229), and your favorite spa.

—**Bodywork:**
• Spring Life POLARIZERS.
• Exercise regularly to build back strength.
• Seventy-five percent of all lower back problems can be prevented by strengthening abdominal muscles. Aim for 12 to 15 crunches each morning.
• Be sure to watch for my American Holistic Healer Directory available spring 2000 for complete information on recommended back pain experts.
• More than 2 days bed rest with a bad back weakens muscles. Sleep on a firm mattress.

—**Reflexology points:**

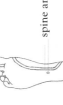

spine and kidney

Common Symptoms: *Spinal stress and pain; inability to do even small bending or pushing actions; sometimes inability to move at all. Sciatic nerve pain can be excruciating.*
Common Causes: *Causes for back conditions can be as wide-ranging as a herniated disc, artery blockage or family financial problems. Poor posture; improper lifting, sitting or standing; arthritis or osteoarthritis; deep-seated emotional stress; kidney malfunction, usually from dehydration; high heels; being overweight; protein, calcium and other nutrient deficiency; low green vegetable intake; osteoporosis; sleeping on a mattress that is too soft; congenitally poor spinal alignment. Scoliosis curvature is thought to be an inherited tendency.*

Can't find a recommended product? Call the 800 number listed in Product Resources for the store nearest you.

Bad Breath & Body Odor

Halitosis, Bromidrosis

Both of these conditions are manifestations of the same problem - poor diet, poor food digestion, causing rotting food and bacteria formation that the body throws off through the skin and breath. There are many very effective natural mouth fresheners and deodorizers. Make sure you don't have a more serious problem than just poor food assimilation. Rule out cavities, gum disease and sinus infections for bad breath first.

Diet & Superfood Therapy

—Nutritional therapy plan:

1—Diet change to keep your internal environment clean is the single most beneficial thing you can do to get rid of bad breath and body odor.

2—Start with a 24 hour liquid diet (pg.192) with apple juice and 1 TB psyllium husks, or Crystal Star CHO-LO FIBER TONE™ to cleanse the bowel.

3—For one week, add liquid chlorophyll to apple or carrot juice to neutralize stomach acids and cleanse the digestive tract.

4—Then make sure your diet has crunchy, cleansing, fiber-rich foods like fresh fruits and vegetables. Eat high chlorophyll foods like parsley, leafy greens and sprouts.

5—Eat plenty of cultured foods such as yogurt or kefir for intestinal flora activity.

6—Drink 6 glasses of water daily to flush your GI tract. When your body is dehydrated, mouth secretions become concentrated and odorous.

7—Eat light, less concentrated foods - especially reduce or avoid red meats and heavy animal protein, caffeine, fried foods, and heavy sweets.

8—Eat smaller meals, and chew well for best enzyme activity. Drink green tea after each meal.

—Superfood therapy: (Choose one or two)

• Crystal Star ENERGY GREEN™ drink.
• GreenFoods CARROT ESSENCE.
• Mona's CHLORELLA, 1 tsp. in juice.

Herb & Supplement Therapy

—Interceptive therapy plan: (Choose 2 to 3 recommendations)

1—**Bitters compounds stimulate complete digestion:** •Crystal Star BITTERS & LEMON CLEANSE™ extract each morning, •PRE-MEAL ENZ™ extract before meals, or •AFTER MEAL ENZ™ extract after meals; •BioForce GOLDEN-ROD extract. (Bitters don't work unless you can taste them in the mouth.)

2—**Deodorize your digestive tract with chlorophyll-rich compounds:** •Alfalfa-Mint tea; •Liquid chlorophyll, 1 teasp. in water after meals.

3—**Spices break up gas and act as natural antacids:** Put pinches of *cloves*, *ginger*, *cinnamon*, *nutmeg* or *anise* in a cup of water and drink down.

4—**Intestinal and bowel cleansers:** •Crystal Star GREEN TEA CLEANSER™ every morning; •HERBAL-TONE gentle laxative tabs at night; •Crystal Star LAXA-TEA™, or •AloeLife FIBER-MATE. ♀

5—**Breath and body fresheners:** •BioForce DENTAFORCE breath spray; •Desert Essence TEA TREE mouthwash; •TIBS essential oil breath drops. •Chew a few aromatic seeds like *anise*, *cardamom* or *fennel*. Drink *peppermint* or *spearmint* tea.

6—**Control low-grade mouth and gum infections:** •*propolis* lozenges daily, or •*tea tree* oil rubbed on gums; ♂ •Home Health PERI-DENT gum massage. •Use *myrrh, myrrh gum powder,* or Toms toothpaste with *myrrh*.

7—**Aid digestion with probiotics and enzymes:** •Acidophilus caps 4-6x daily; •1 TB cider vinegar in water before each meal; •Betaine HCl with papain before each meal (especially before meat protein); •Schiff ENZYMALL tabs with ox bile. ♀

—Expressly for body odor: •**Think zinc. Take 15-50mg daily;** •*Fenugreek-sage* tea; •Dilute essential oils of *lavender, thyme, juniper, rosemary* or *myrrh* - put a few drops on a cotton pad and apply to your underarms.

—Expressly for morning breath: Just before bedtime, floss well. Then brush the back of your tongue and teeth with baking soda rather than toothpaste. Don't use mouthwash. Morning breath should be eliminated or greatly reduced.

Lifestyle Support Therapy

Give your body a chance to digest your food. Don't eat for 2 hours before bed.

—Bodywork:

•Exercise to cleanse metabolic wastes being improperly expelled through skin and lungs.

•Use mineral salts: Take a mineral salts bath like Para Labs BATH THERAPY once a week.

•Natural mineral crystals are deodorants.

•Use a dry skin brush, loofah, or exfoliating skin cloth all over the body daily to remove toxins coming out through the skin. Then shower with an oatmeal/honey scrub soap.

•Wear natural fiber clothing so the skin can breathe. Wear sandals when possible.

—Natural body deodorants:

• Dab underarms/feet with vinegar.
• Earth Science LiKEN deodorant.
• Tom's deodorants (all kinds).
• Apply aloe vera gel under arms.
• Essential oils: Wyndemere Peppermint; Oshadhi LAVENDER. ♀

—Reflexology point:

food assimilation

♂

B 322

Common Symptoms: Bad taste in the mouth and mouth odor; foul smelling perspiration.
Common Causes: Poor diet with a green vegetable deficiency; poor digestion; enzyme deficiency; inadequate protein digestion, leading to indigestion; bacteria on and around the back of the tongue; sluggish intestinal system and chronic constipation; stress and anxiety; gum disease and tooth decay; food intolerances; HCl deficiency; low grade chronic throat infection; candida yeast infection; smoking; liver malfunction; post-nasal drip from a chronic sinus infection; candida yeast infection.

Can't find a recommended product? Call the 800 number listed in Product Resources for the store nearest you.

Bedwetting

Child and Adult Enuresis

Bedwetting, after the normal age of 3 to 7 years old, affects about 5 million children, (10%) mostly male. It also affects over 150,000 adults. Most experts agree that barring any physical/mechanical obstruction or infection, bedwetting is probably psychologically based. However, nutritional therapies have had such notable success in this area that I cannot help but believe that nutritional deficiencies are also a part of the problem.

Diet & Superfood Therapy

—**Nutritional therapy plan:**

1–Avoid oxalic acid-forming foods, such as cooked spinach, rhubarb, caffeine, cocoa, chocolate, etc.

2–No junk foods. Avoid refined sugars, salty or extra spicy foods as irritants.

3–Avoid food colorings, preservatives and pasteurized cow's milk as possible allergens.

4–Take a small glass of cranberry/apple juice each morning to clean the kidneys.

5–No liquids before bed. Eat a little celery instead to balance organic salts.

6–A spoonful of honey before bed.

—**Superfood therapy: (Choose one)**

•Twin Lab LIQUID K PLUS to strengthen tissues.

•AloeLife FIBER-MATE drink, $^1/_2$ teasp.

•Country Life CAL SNACK, milk-free chewable calcium.

•Green Foods CARROT ESSENCE blend drink or BERRY BARLEY ESSENCE.

Herb & Supplement Therapy

—**Interceptive therapy plan: (Choose 1 or 2 recommendations)**

1–Crystal Star BLDR-K™ extract drops in water before dinner. Use half strength for children. •Give the child *cinnamon* sticks to chew on before bed, or make a *cinnamon* tea from *cinnamon* extract drops in water. •*Cornsilk* or *plantain* extract drops in water. •*Ginkgo biloba* extract drops in water, mixed with a little honey before bed for better circulation, are a key.

2–**Relax stress before bed:** •Crystal Star RELAX CAPS™ or •*valerian/wild lettuce* extract in water; •*scullcap* extract drops in water.

3–**Minerals to strengthen tissues:** •Crystal Star CALCIUM SOURCE™ capsules, or extract drops in water; •*Parsley-oatstraw-juniperava ursi* tea daily (not at bedtime). •Twin Lab Chondroitan sulfate A 250mg 1 daily; •Mezotrace SEA MINERAL COMPLEX chewable; •Flora FLORADIX children's multivitamin daily; •Magnesium 100mg daily; •*Horsetail* herb extract drops in water at dinner; rub on abdomen, Body Essentials SILICA GEL.

—**Highly effective homeopathic remedies:**

•Hylands *BEDWETTING* tablets before bed.

•BSI *Equisetum* for bedwetting during dreams or nightmares.

•Standard Homeopathics *Enuraid* (adults).

Lifestyle Support Therapy

—**Bodywork:**

•See a good chiropractor or massage therapist if a compressed nerve or an obstruction is the suspected cause.

•Muscle testing (applied kinesiology) is effective here in determining what allergies may be the cause.

•Guided imagery techniques have had some success. Within the first few hours of sleep, give the child reassuring messages without waking him.

•Good circulation is a key. Good daily exercise is an answer; especially bicycle riding.

—**Lifestyle TLC:**

•Leave a night light on so the child will feel free to get up at night.

•Give a relaxing massage before bed to ease muscles and fears. Try lavender oil.

•Decrease your child's stress about bedwetting by giving encouragement rather than punishment. Praise him for not wetting the bed. Sometimes a reward system helps.

•Make sure home emotional environment is supportive.

•Make sure bedtime is regular and stress-free. Consider a happy bedtime story.

Common Symptoms: *Involuntary urination during the night beyond toilet training age.*

Common Causes: *Unusually deep sleep patterns with decreased REM sleep; inherited organ weakness; allergies - especially food allergies; excess sugar, salt, spices or dairy in the diet; bladder infection; stress, emotional anxiety and behavioral disturbances; bad dreams; hypoglycemia or diabetes; compressed nerve or congenital obstruction in the bladder area.*

Can't find a recommended product? Call the 800 number listed in Product Resources for the store nearest you.

Bladder, Urinary Tract Infections

Bacterial Cystitis, Incontinence

Recurrent bladder infections are common in women; less common in men (infection for them is largely tied to prostate problems). Bladder infections are the most frequent reason a woman seeks medical attention; pain can be all-consuming during the acute stage. Over 75% of American women have at least one urinary tract infection in a ten year period, almost 30% have one once a year. Staph and strep infections, and diabetes may also affect the kidneys, making the problem more serious - an alarming number of cases result in kidney failure. Note: The active chemical in many spermicidal creams and foams, nonoxynol-9, causes recurring cystitis and yeast infections. Some oral contraceptives are also implicated. Treatment should begin at the very first sign of infection. Consult a holistic clinic if there is no improvement within 5 days.

Diet & Superfood Therapy

—Nutritional therapy plan:

1—Changing body pH is important. Eat a yeast-free diet, with no baked breads during healing.

2—Flush the bladder: Most UTI's are not a problem of bacteria getting into the bladder but of bacteria getting out. Dilute cranberry juice (unsweetened), 6 to 8 glasses daily (cranberries contain substantial D-Mannose against E. coli infection).

3—Purify the bladder and urethra with watermelon seed tea or a carrot/beet/cucumber juice every other day to reduce infection.

4—Increase urine flow: Drink 10 glasses of distilled water, diluted, unsweetened fruit juices and herbal teas daily to keep acid wastes flushed.

5—During acute stage: take 2 TBS cider vinegar and honey in water each a.m., yogurt at noon, a glass of white wine at night.

6—Avoid acid-forming foods - caffeine, tomatoes, cooked spinach, chocolate. Avoid sugary foods, carbonated drinks, fried, salty and fatty foods, pasteurized dairy foods. Reduce meat protein.

8—Add alkalizing foods: celery, watermelon, ume plum balls, blueberries, green drinks, potassium broth (pg. 215), garlic and onions.

—Superfood therapy: (Choose one or two)
• Green Foods GREEN MAGMA.
• Crystal Star BIOFLAV. FIBER & C SUP-PORT™ with cranberry.

Herb & Supplement Therapy

—Interceptive therapy plan: (Choose 2 to 3 recommendations)

1—**Control infection and bacterial adhesion:** •Crystal Star BLDR-K™ caps, 2 every 3 hours at the first hint of a bladder infection, and/or BLDR-K™ tea (with two •ANTI-BIO™ capsules each time if problem is severe). •D-Mannose by Biotech Pharmacal, Ark., inhibits E. coli infection (powder- 1 tsp. in water every 3 hours); • or take •cranberry caps every 3 hours. •Nutribiotic GRAPEFRUIT EXTRACT caps 2 daily, and a glass of water with 1 tsp. baking soda in it. •Homeopathic cantharis can sometimes stop a UTI immediately.

•If infections develop regularly after intercourse, rinse the vagina with •golden-seal-echinacea tea. Urinate as soon as possible after intercourse.

2—**Curb pain and inflammation:** •Goldenseal-echinacea extract; •or take Future Biotics VITAL K and •uva ursi caps for 14 days to disinfect. On the tenth day, begin Solaray CRAN-ACTIN caps or •Natural Balance CRAN-MAX caps, 2 daily. •Solaray CORNSILK BLEND caps, or uva ursi tea daily for 10 days, then •cat's claw extract for 10 days especially for chronic infections.

3—**Reduce muscle spasms:** •to a shallow sitz bath, add 3 drops tea tree oil, 2 drops bergamot oil, 2 drops juniper oil, 2 drops thyme oil, 1 drop eucalyptus oil. Take 2x daily for ¹/₂ hour. •Or massage your abdomen with a blend of 1-oz. almond oil, 3 drops sandalwood oil, 2 drops cedarwood oil, 2 drops cypress oil, 1 drop lavender, 1 drop frankincense oil.

4—**Re-establish vaginal flora to reduce recurrence rate:** •use a lactobacillus suppository, or 1 TB acidophilus powder in warm water as a douche for 4 days after treating a UTI with antibiotics; take •Dr. DOPHILUS 6 daily with garlic caps 6 daily; •take ascorbate vitamin C 1000mg and Lysine 1000mg every 2 to 3 hours.

—For incontinence: (add vitamin C to each suggestion for stronger tissue.)
• Crystal Star BLDR-K CONTROL™.
• Crystal Star PROX FOR MEN™ caps. (For BPH, results within 48 hours.)
• Standard Homeopathics Enuraid.

Lifestyle Support Therapy

—Bodywork:

• Acupuncture can sometimes relieve pain almost immediately.

• Apply wet heat, or hot comfrey compresses across lower back and kidneys or take hot sitz baths to relieve pain and ease urination.

• For accompanying hemorrhage, take 1 oz. marshmallow rt., steep in 1 pt. hot milk. Take every ¹/₂ hr. to staunch bleeding.

• Take a mild catnip or chlorophyll enema to clear acid wastes.

• Dyes in colored toilet paper may contribute to bladder infections.

• Do not use a diaphragm if you are prone to bladder infections.

—Reflexology point:

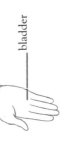

—— bladder

—For incontinence:

• Biofeedback and acupuncture have been successful for incontinence in both women and men, regardless of cause.

• Do toning Kegel exercises.

See also INTERSTITIAL CYSTITIS program next page.

Common Symptoms: Frequent, urgent, burning, painful urination, especially at night; pain in lower back and abdomen below the navel; often chills and fever as the body tries to throw off infection; strong, turbid, foul-smelling urine; cloudy or bloody urine. If you have pain above the waist, it may be a kidney infection or kidney stones instead of a bladder infection.
Common Causes: A staph, strep or colibacillus or even a rhinitis cold infection, aggravated by overuse of antibiotics; chlamydia infection; fecal bacteria, usually E.coli that migrate up the urethra; stress; spermicide and contraceptives; kidney malfunction; food allergens; lack of adequate fluids; aluminum cookware; poor elimination; tampons or diaphragms pinching the neck of the bladder, hampering waste elimination.

Can't find a recommended product? Call the 800 number listed in Product Resources for the store nearest you.

B 324

Bladder, Urinary Tract Infections

Interstitial Cystitis, Chronic Urethritis

Chronic UTI's may not be due to infection. Interstitial cystitis, a non-bacterial form affecting one in 20 women (usually menopausal) with bladder infections, has been called "migraine of the bladder," because many of the same things that either trigger or benefit migraine headaches affect interstitial cystitis the same way. It seems to be an auto-immune disease, resulting from low immune strength. Attend to healing immediately, because of the great pain, and because the bladder can shrink to a size where it will only hold 1 or 2 ounces. A natural approach is best. This type of infection is normally antibiotic-resistant and may be aggravated by drug treatment. Some can actually attack the bladder lining when there is no infection to attack. The active chemical in many spermicidal creams and foams, nonoxynol-9, increases the risk of all types of cystitis.

Diet & Superfood Therapy

—Nutritional therapy plan:

1—Cranberry juice is not beneficial for interstitial cystitis. Take veggie drinks (pg. 218) and carrot juice instead during acute stages, and as a preventive.

2—Begin drinking water immediately all during the day when you feel an infection coming.

3—Cleanse the bladder and kidneys with watermelon juice, or watermelon seed tea. Strengthen them with well-cooked beans and sea greens.

4—Avoid triggers: Aged protein foods such as yogurt, pickled herring, preserved or smoked meats, cheeses, yeasted breads, sauerkraut, citrus fruits, citrus juices and red wine until condition normalizes.

Avoid acid-forming foods - like coffee, black tea, colas, chocolate, citrus fruits, tomatoes, spicy foods, soy sauce, and foods with additives like NutraSweet.

3—Increase leafy greens and high fiber foods.

—Superfood therapy: (Choose one or two)

• Crystal Star ENERGY GREEN™ provides critical minerals for the urinary system.
• Nutricology PRO-GREENS with EFA's.
• Solaray ALFAJUICE as a potent anti-oxidant.
• Sun CHLORELLA 1 pkt. daily for 1 month.
• Herbal Aloe ALOE FORCE juice.

Herb & Supplement Therapy

—Interceptive therapy plans: (choose 2 or 3 recommendations)

1—Control swelling and pain: • Crystal Star BLDR-K™ extract and/or BLDR-K™ tea, or • cat's claw tea 3 cups daily. If necessary, add • 6 extra goldenseal-echinacea compound capsules, or • Crystal Star ANTI-BIO™ caps, 6 a day during acute periods. • Solaray CORNSILK BLEND caps, or • uva ursi tea daily for 10 days, then • cat's claw extract for 10 days for chronic infections. • Crystal Star ANTI-SPZ caps, 4 at a time, or • scullcap tea every few hours for pain.

2—Control inflammation: • At the first signs of an impending infection, take a teasp. of baking soda in 8-oz. of water to alkalize the urine before it reaches the bladder. • Then, take a calcium carbonate capsule every 12 hours for a time-release effect. • Or, Enzymatic Therapy ACID-A-CAL caps until pain is reduced, then • Nutribiotic GRAPEFRUIT SEED extract drops in water as directed for 1 month.

3—Combat auto-immune reaction: • Licorice root extract; • a full course of Echinacea-Goldenseal extract; • Astragalus extract. • Vitamin C therapy: ascorbate or Ester C powder, ¼ teasp. every 2 hours during acute stages, then • Lysine 1000mg with bromelain 1500mg daily, or • Enzymedica PURIFY to help restore immunity.

4—Reduce interstitial scarring: • Solaray Centella Asiatica extract caps to heal the ulcers. • CoQ10 30mg 3x daily; • mycelized vitamin A & E, or • Nature's Plus vitamin E 800IU and zinc 30mg daily to combat re-infection.

—Bladder infection teas: may also be used on a hot or cold cloth as a compress.

• Cornsilk tea, Dandelion-nettles tea, Horsetail tea.
• Make a tea blend: 1 handful uva ursi or buchu leaves, 1 handful echinacea root, cut, 1 handful nettle leaves. Take for 6 days.

For chronic urethritis:

• Cat's claw tea 3 cups daily for 2 weeks (results usually within 3 days).
• Ginkgo Biloba extract (proven more effective than tetracycline).
• Bilberry extract as an anti-inflammatory and tissue strengthener.

Lifestyle Support Therapy

Do not wear tampons if you have recurring cystitis.

—Bodywork:

• Acupuncture works well for symptom relief and pain reduction.
• Press alternating hot and cold compresses against the pubic bone and clitoris. Press hard.
• Hot sitz baths during an infection help bring cleansing circulation to the infected area. See aromatherapy sitz baths on the previous page.
• Apply compresses - both hot and cold have been effective. Put the compress between your legs, and press against your pubic bone and clitoris.

—Reflexology point:

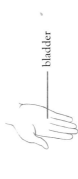

bladder

Common Symptoms: Small sores and cracks scarring the bladder lining; tough, atrophied bladder, so that normal urination is impossible; pain goes away during urination, then immediately returns; breakdown of bladder tissue, even when infection is not present; cloudy urine with foul odor; systemic fever and aching.
Common Causes: Leaks in the bladder wall that allow urine to irritate bladder tissue, even to destroy bladder lining; sometimes accompanies endometriosis; environmental and food allergies; lowered immunity; dietary "triggers" causing acidity in the system; pelvic congestion from chronic constipation, lowered libido, or heavy, painful menstrual periods; dehydration.

See also BACTERIAL CYSTITIS program previous page.

Can't find a recommended product? Call the 800 number listed in Product Resources for the store nearest you.

Bone Health

Healing Bone Breaks, Preventing Brittle Bones, Regrowing Strong Cartilage

Your bones are alive! Bone is far more complex than we ever thought.... and it needs far more nutrition than we ever think about giving it. We tend to think about our bones as we age, but nearly 87% of teenage girls and 64% of teenage boys aren't getting enough calcium, let alone other bone-building nutrients. Extending those nutrient deficiency numbers through life means over half of America's future women and one in eight men will develop osteoporosis fractures. Pay extra attention to your bone health. New French research shows a significant correlation with increased hip fractures and fluoride in drinking water. Most of America's tap water (64%) is already fluoridated, with pending legislation on the books for the rest of our cities. If you have prematurely gray hair, it may be a sign you have decreased mineral bone mass.

Diet & Superfood Therapy

—Nutritional therapy plan:

1—Feed your bones for total body health. Vegetarians have denser, better formed bones, and stronger immune systems.

2—Focus on mineral-rich vegetable proteins (sesame seeds, almonds, nutritional yeast, sea greens for vitamin K, too, etc.). Love your liver. It is vital to forming bone marrow.

3—Your diet should be alkalizing: **For calcium and silicon:** green vegetables, fish and seafood, sea vegetables, whole grains, soy protein, yogurt. **For boron:** dried fruits, nuts and seeds, honey, a little wine. **For vitamin C:** papayas, kiwi, strawberries, bell peppers, broccoli, cantaloupe.

4—Avoid bone leaching foods: red meats, refined foods, and acid-forming foods like fried and fast foods, and sodas.

—Sugar inhibits calcium absorption.
—Caffeine causes a loss of calcium.
—Excess salt decreases bone density.

5—Red Star NUTRITIONAL YEAST extract drink or MISO broth before bed.

—Superfood therapy: (Choose one or two)

• Crystal Star SYSTEMS STRENGTH™.
• Lewis Labs BREWER'S YEAST.
• Green Foods CARROT ESSENCE.
• Solaray ALFAJUICE for active vitamin K.
• AloeLife ALOE GOLD for HCl.

Herb & Supplement Therapy

—Interceptive therapy plans: (choose 2 or 3 recommendations)

1—Add more bone nutrients to build bones: There is much more to strong bones than just calcium. Without the proper amounts of other minerals as well as vitamin D - you won't absorb the calcium. Herbs are one of the best ways to get bone-builders. • Add silica: Crystal Star SILICA SOURCE™ extract, • Body Essentials SILICA GEL. or • Flora VEGE-SIL for collagen formation. • Add balanced herbal calcium - Crystal Star CALCIUM SOURCE™ caps or extract; or • Ethical Nutrients BONE BUILDER.

2—Improve assimilation of bone nutrients: • Magnesium, 400mg daily; • Vitamin D 400IU daily; • B-complex 100mg daily with extra B-6 100mg and folic acid, 400mcg. • Manganese, 5mg; • Morada Research BONES/CALCIUM (silica-calcium); • Enzymedica DIGEST; or • Transformation Enzyme DIGESTZYME.

3—Keep your glands healthy for good bones: Phytohormone herbs can be an important part of continuing bone health and formation. Effective estrogen/progesterone balancing herbs: • Crystal Star FEM-SUPPORT™ ♀ or • *damiana-dong quai* compound; • YS ROYAL JELLY-GINSENG drink or *royal jelly-ginseng* capsules; ♂ • Crystal Star PRO-EST OSTEOPLUS, a plant progesterone roll-on; • DHEA 25mg daily; • Transitions PROGEST CREAM; • Enzymatic Therapy OSTEO PRIME.

4—Help your body remodel your bones: • Calcium ascorbate C 3000mg. • Vitamin A & D 25,000IU/1000IU daily. • Nature's Path TRACE-MIN-LYTE; Vitamin E 400IU; • CoQ₁₀ 60mg 2x daily; • Jarrow HYDROXYAPATITE caps; • Bilberry extract (herbal bioflavonoids also have estrogen-like activity.)

—Effective bone knitters and healers:

• Homeopathic Arnica Montana; apply Arnica gel for swelling.
• Country Life sublingual B-12, 2500mcg every 3 days.
• Apply a Comfrey poultice. Take Nettles caps or Horsetail extract.
• Chondroitin sulfate A capsules 1000mg daily, or shark cartilage 1400mg daily.
• Suspected bone cancer - yarrow tea, or • Natural Energy Plus CAISSE'S TEA.

Lifestyle Support Therapy

—Bodywork:

• Aerobic exercise and light weight training are primary bones builders and strengtheners.
• Get some sunlight on the body every day possible for natural vitamin D.
• Don't smoke. It increases bone brittleness and inhibits bone growth.
• Swim or walk in the ocean when possible.
• Avoid aluminum pots and pans, deodorants and fluorescent lighting. Both leach calcium from the body.

• Common medicines put bone health at risk: *L-thyroxine*, a thyroid stimulant; *corticosteroid* drugs like hydrocortisome, cortisone and prednisone - prescribed for rheumatic conditions and respiratory diseases; *phenytoin and phenobarbital (anti-seizure drugs); heparin,* a blood thinner; *furosemide*, a diuretic; and *No-DOZ*, a stimulant.

• The following drugs can hamper your body's ability to maintain and repair bone: *Ibuprofen*, *NSAIDS* drugs like *Naproxen, Fenclofenac, Indomethacin, Sulindac, Kato-profen, Diclofenac, Aspirin, Piroxicam, Flurbiprofen, Asopro-pazone.* (British LANCET.)

See also OSTEOPOROSIS, pg. 468 for more information.

Common Symptoms: Brittle bones with easy bone breaks; poor bone healing; weak muscles, shifting teeth, gum disease, lots of plaque on the teeth; brittle nails that break too easily; joint and tendon soreness; chronic lower back pain; very thin skin and prematurely gray hair (before 40), is sometimes a sign of decreased bone mineral mass.

Common Causes: Mineral deficiency or poor assimilation; poor diet with too many refined foods, and too much meat protein, causing phosphorus imbalance; enzyme deficiency; heavy metal or drug toxicity; steroids or too many cortico-steroid drugs; stress; too much alcohol, caffeine or tobacco; fluoridated water supply.

Can't find a recommended product? Call the 800 number listed in Product Resources for the store nearest you.

Brain Health

Better Memory, More Mental Activity, Less Mental Exhaustion

The brain controls the entire body. It is our primary health maintenance organ and the seat of energy production. Although it makes up only 2 1/2% of our body weight, it uses almost 25% of our available oxygen, more than 25% of available glucose and 20% of our blood supply! The brain is an incredibly sensitive organ, responding quickly but only temporarily to drugs and short term stimulants. The best way to get good, long term, brain enhancement is to feed it and use it. Brain nutrients have a rapidly noticeable effect on increased brain performance. Good, consistent brain nourishment can straighten out even grave mental, emotional and coordination problems. One expert calls the brain, with its tens of billions of neurons, a million times more powerful than a computer!

Diet & Superfood Therapy

—Nutritional therapy plan:

1—Your brain needs constant, rich nutrition sources of vitamins, minerals, amino acids and antioxidants to function optimally. Avoid sugary foods. They decrease the blood sugar available to nourish the brain.

2—Brain cells are about 60% EFA's. Keep your brain well oiled with omega-3 oils for EFA's: Sea greens, spinach and other leafy greens, cold water fish, and shellfish have plenty of DHA and EPA oils; also have sprouts, fertile eggs, wheat germ, olive, canola, flax oils, brown rice, tofu, apples, oranges, grapefruit, cantaloupe, wheat germ and beans.

2—Add glutathione foods for neurotransmitter energy: eggs, spinach, parsley.

2—Make a brain food: mix 2TBS. each: lecithin for phosphatides and memory lapses., brewer's yeast for myelin formation. Take 1-2TBS. daily.

2—A glass or two of wine at dinner appears to boost brain activity.

—Superfood therapy: (Choose one or two)

• Nutricology PRO-GREENS with EFA's.
• Solgar EARTH SOURCE GREENS & MORE w. EFA's.
• Crystal Star SYSTEMS STRENGTH for brain minerals and EFA's.
• Y.S. ROYAL JELLY with GINSENG 2 tsp. daily. ♀
• Future Biotics VITAL K drink. ♀

Herb & Supplement Therapy

—Interceptive therapy plan: (Choose 2 to 4 recommendations)

1—**Boost neurotransmission for good brain connections:** • Phosphatidyl Serine (PS) 1000mg, GABA or Choline 600mg. (If your choline levels are low, try Huperzine A 50mg to allow levels to rise.) • Evening primrose oil 2-4 daily; • Enzymedica PURIFY. • For bad moods, add 5-HTP 50mg at night for serotonin connection.

2—**Enhance blood flow to the brain:** • Ginkgo Biloba extract 3x daily; • cayenne caps, or ginger-cayenne caps; • Rosemary aromatherapy applied on the temples. • Take 1/4 teasp. each: Glutamine powder and Glycine powder; • Magnesium 800mg.

3—**Nourish your brain with EFA's:** Ginseng brain nutrients: • Crystal Star SUPER GINSENG 6™ caps or tea, or MENTAL INNER ENERGY™ extract; EYE-Q, DHA available at Healthy House. • Royal jelly caps or YS royal jelly-ginseng drink; • Omega-3 flax oils. Ginseng-Gotu Kola, Ashwagandha and Fo-Ti root are brain tonics.

4—**Sharpen your memory:** • ACL (Acetyl-L-Carnitine), up to 2500mg daily; • Crystal Star MENTAL CLARITY™ capsules, CREATIVI-TEA™, ♀ or MEDITATION™ tea; • Dr. Diamond DIAMOND MIND caps; • Source Naturals HIGHER MIND; • Super Nutrition EINSTEIN'S FORMULA; Klamath POWER 3 caps. ♂
• DHEA, esp. with pregnenolone boosts long and short term memory. ♂

—Antioxidants for more brain energy:

• Glutathione 50 mg 2x daily.
• Alpha Lipoic Acid neutralizes toxins and recycles glutathione for better use.
• CoQ$_{10}$, 60mg 2x daily. Take with vitamin E 400IU for best results.
• NADH 5 to 15mg daily, or NADA by Kal as directed.

—B's are for brain power: B-complex 150mg - extra niacin 500mg and B-6 250mg. Country Life sublingual active B-12, 2500mg.

Brain tumor defense: MICROHYDRIIN available at Healthy House; Premier GERMANIUM with DMG daily or Nutricology GERMANIUM 150mg daily. ♂

Lifestyle Support Therapy

Note: Alcohol, tobacco and marijuana inhibit brain release of vasopressin, impairing memory, attention and concentration and increase the need for neurotransmitter replenishment through brain nutrients.

—Bodywork:

• More oxygen and better circulation are the bodywork goals for better brain function. Build more brain circuits by reading and playing mental games. (Do a Sunday crossword puzzle.)
• Breathe for your brain. Deep brain breathing works wonders. (See also Dr. Bragg's book on BRAIN BREATHING.)
• Try TM for TLC. Transcendental meditation been proven to help you reach a state of restful alertness to reduce stress and enhance your ability to think at your best.
• Takes a daily, arm-swinging 1/2 hour walk.
• Cheerfulness, optimism and relaxation assure better brain function. (New studies show classical music is especially good.)

—Reflexology point:

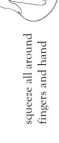

squeeze all around fingers and hand

See MENTAL HEALTH PAGE 485 for more specifics.

Can't find a recommended product? Call the 800 number listed in Product Resources for the store nearest you.

Common Symptoms: Spaciness and lack of concentration; unexplained depression, gloominess and frequent bad moods; inability to remember well or for a reasonable length of time; constant stress and overwork with no rejuvenating "down time"; stress; sometimes viral activity; poor diet.
Common Causes: Lack of protein, potassium or other minerals that causes mental burnout; constant stress and overwork with no rejuvenating "down time"; stress; sometimes viral activity; poor diet.

Bronchitis

Acute and Chronic

Chronic bronchitis is an infectious inflammation of the bronchi. It appears to be a direct result of prolonged exposure to irritants like cigarette smoke and environmental chemicals. The typical victim is forty or older, with lowered immunity from prolonged stress, fatigue or smoking. The disease usually develops slowly over a course of years, but will not go away on its own. Bronchial walls thicken and the number of mucous glands increases. The person becomes increasingly susceptible to respiratory infections. The recent type of viral bronchitis, which affects women, is very hard to treat, and lasts from 3 weeks to 5 months. Chronic bronchitis can be incapacitating, and lead to serious, even potentially fatal lung disease. Acute bronchitis, inflammation of the bronchial tree, is generally self-limiting, like a bad chest cold, with eventual complete healing.

Diet & Superfood Therapy

—Nutritional therapy plan:

1—Go on a short mucous cleansing liquid diet (pg. 195) to get rid of the thick mucous. Then follow a largely vegetarian, cleansing diet for 3 weeks. Reduce fats, dairy, salt and clogging heavy foods.

2—Take cleansing soups broths, hot tonics, high vitamin C juices, vegetable juices and green drinks (pg. 218).

3—Take lemon juice in water each morning and flax seed tea each night during acute stages to alkalize the blood and cleanse the colon.

4—Avoid sugars, dairy, and starchy and fatty foods during healing to reduce congestion. Keep the bowels clean so that your body can eliminate excess mucous.

5—Make a traditional onion-honey syrup: Put 5 to 6 chopped onions and 1/2 cup honey in a pot and cook over very low heat for two hours. Strain and take 1 TB every two hours.

—Superfood therapy: (Choose one or two)

• Crystal Star SYSTEMS STRENGTH™ drink mix daily for 1 month.
• AloeLife ALOE GOLD 2 TBS daily.
• Liquid chlorophyll 1 tsp. in water before each meal.

• Transitions for Health EASY GREENS.

Herb & Supplement Therapy

—Interceptive therapy plan: (Choose 2 to 4 recommendations)

1—Reduce inflammation and infection: • Oregano oil, or Oshadi OREGANO oil as directed. • Crystal Star BRNX™ extract with ANTI-BIO™ capsules 6x daily; • usnea extract or Crystal Star BIO-VI™ extract for direct effect. • Add reishi mushroom extract, or • Crystal Star GINSENG-REISHI extract, for T-cell defenses. • Flora VEGE-SIL or • Crystal Star SILICA SOURCE™ for bio-available silica.

2—Expectorants get rid of thick, irritating mucous: • Lobelia extract drops in water as needed; • cayenne-ginger capsules; Also apply cayenne-ginger compresses to the chest. • Bayberry tea, or hyssop-horehound tea. • NAC (N-acetyl-cysteine), or Nutricology NAC 2 daily; • Crystal Star X-PECT TEA™ expectorant, or • GINSENG/LICORICE ELIXIR™, a tonic expectorant.

3—Soothe the hacking cough: • Han HONEY LOQUAT syrup; • marshmallow root tea - gargle twice daily and at night; • Zinc lozenges as needed every two hours, or Crystal Star ZINC SOURCE™ drops as needed. ♂ Note: Avoid commercial cough suppressants. Coughing helps get rid of mucous.

4—Use antioxidants to re-establish lung capacity: • Crystal Star FIRST AID™ caps, 4 to 6 daily, a powerful antioxidant to relieve acute conditions. • Vitamin A 10,000IU with vitamin C with bioflavonoids up to 5000mg and magnesium 800mg daily. • Twin Lab LYCOPENE for the lungs.

—For chronic bronchitis: CoQ10 100mg 2x daily; mullein tea 2 cups daily; cayenne-garlic or elecampane caps 6 daily; Cordyceps extract, or Metabolic Response Modifiers CORDYCEPS 750mg; or echinacea extract drops for 2 months.

—Acute bronchitis tonic tea: Make a tonic bronchitis herbal tea: Steep 1TB each in 4 cups hot water for 25 minutes - licorice rt., horehound, lemon grass, osha, coltsfoot, lobelia, pleurisy rt., mullein. ☺ Or use homeopathic B&T Bronchitis/Asthma Aid.

—Restabilize immunity: raw thymus or Enzymatic Therapy THYMU-PLEX caps.

Lifestyle Support Therapy

Air pollutants are probably responsible for more chronic bronchitis than any other one cause. Avoid smoking, secondary smoke and smog-plagued areas. Get fresh air and sunshine every day.

—Bodywork:

• Take a hot sauna; follow with a brisk rub-down, and chest-back percussion with a cupped hand to loosen mucous.

• Apply alternating hot and cold witch hazel compresses to the chest. Use eucalyptus oil in a vaporizer.

• Do deep breathing exercises daily, morning and before bed to clear lungs.

• Avoid inhaling cold air. Cover mouth and nose with a scarf or mask so that infectious micro-organisms are not sucked into the lungs.

• Rub tea tree oil on the chest, or apply Earth's Bounty O₂ OXY-SPRAY on the chest.

—Reflexology point:

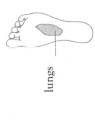

lungs

B 328

See pg. 196 for a non-mucous-forming diet.

Common Symptoms: Acute Bronchitis: symptoms like a deep chest cold; slight fever; inflammation; headache, nausea, lung and body aches; hacking, mucous-producing cough. **Chronic Bronchitis:** bronchial tissue becomes inflamed, and mucous becomes thicker and more profuse; difficult breathing and shortness of breath from clogged airways; repeated attacks of acute bronchitis; chest congestion; mucous-producing cough and wheezing that lasts for 3 months or more; fatigue, weakness and weight loss; low grade lung infection.
Common Causes: High mucous and acid-forming diet; suppressive "cold preparations"; lack of exercise and poor circulation; smoking, air pollutants; low immunity, stress and fatigue.

Can't find a recommended product? Call the 800 number listed in Product Resources for the store nearest you.

Bruises, Cuts, Abrasions
Easy Bruising, Blisters, Black Eyes, Hard To Heal Wounds

Easy bruising usually means you have weak capillaries; it's the response of your skin to a minor trauma. It can also be a signal of anemia or even a bleeding disorder, such as the inability of your blood to coagulate. But its root cause is almost always a flavonoid deficiency (the nutrients that strengthen your vein and capillary walls). As we age the layer of skin below the dermis becomes weaker and thinner, collagen fibers become coarse and random, and there's less support for capillaries. If there is continued, excessive and frequent bruising see a physician for a clotting time blood test. Do not take aspirin if you bruise easily. It allows blood seepage that leads to discoloration.

Diet & Superfood Therapy

—Nutritional therapy plan for bruises:

1—Your diet should be light, low fat, and mineral-rich to lay a solid foundation for strong capillaries and skin.

2—Eat plenty of fresh greens every day.

3—Eat enzyme rich foods like papayas and pineapple to encourage enzyme therapy healing.

4—Eat vitamin K rich foods - alfalfa sprouts, sea greens, leafy greens, peppers, citrus fruits. Eat vitamin C and bioflavonoid-rich foods like citrus, strawberries and other berries, grapes, peppers and broccoli.

5—Apply pineapple slices directly to a bruise; orange to a black eye; milk to a blister.

6—Avoid clogging dairy foods during healing.

—Nutritional therapy plan for cuts:

1—Take a green veggie drink once a week, especially for hard-to-heal wounds (page 218).

2—Apply wheat germ oil-honey mix directly.

—Superfood therapy: (Choose one or two) Give yourself more protein to heal.

• Crystal Star ENERGY GREEN™ drink.
• Crystal Star BIOFLAV. FIBER & C SUPPORT™ drink.
• Unipro PERFECT PROTEIN drink.
• Solaray ALFAJUICE with high vitamin K.
• Y. S. ROYAL JELLY/GINSENG drink.

Herb & Supplement Therapy

—Interceptive therapy plan for bruises: (Choose 2 or 3 recommendations)

1—Reduce bruises: • Homeopathic Arnica or B & T ARNIFLORA gel; *Ledum* for severe bruises. ♀ • *Horse Chestnut Seed* extract can take down a bruise as you watch or • Enzymatic Theray VARI-CARE tabs. • Rosemary essential oil disperses bruising by raising circulation. • Other essential oils to apply: *tea tree oil, fennel oil* or *lavender oil* (also for pain); • apply *marigold* tincture or salve; • Solaray TUR-MERIC capsules, or *cayenne-ginger* capsules disperse bruise. • *Ginkgo biloba* extract 4 x daily brings up circulation quickly to relieve a bruise.

2—Rebuild healthy skin and capillary strength: • *bilberry* extract or • Crystal Star SILICA SOURCE™ or Eidon SILICA minerals for collagen; • *gotu kola* capsules 6 daily. Apply • *wheat germ oil* directly. • Ascorbate vitamin C with bioflavs and rutin 1000mg every 2 hrs. during healing.

3—Enzyme therapy: • Take papaya tabs, • Enzymedica DIGEST or • Biotec BIO-GESTIN; • Bromelain 750mg daily, or • Nature's Plus ULTRA BRO-MELAIN 1500mg; or • make and apply a paste of bromelain/papain powders.

—Interceptive therapy plan for cuts: (Choose 2 or 3 recommendations)

1—Reduce risk of infection: • Apply *cayenne* tincture to stop bleeding; take drops on back of tongue as needed for shock (or • Nelson Bach RESCUE REMEDY). • Apply Crystal Star ANTI-BIO™ gel (with *una da gato*), or • °GINSENG SKIN CARE™ gel (with *germanium*); or a • *goldenseal-myrrh* salve. • Take Crystal Star ANTI-BIO™ caps or extract for a week. • Apply Nutribiotic GRAPEFRUIT SEED extract SKIN SPRAY. • Apply *echinacea* or *yarrow* extract; • Vitamin K 100mcg daily.

2—Encourage healing: *Evening Primrose* oil with bromelain 1500mg for hard to heal wounds. Take zinc picolinate 50mg 2x daily; • *gotu kola* capsules 6 daily. • Apply *St. John's wort* oil or • °Nature's Pharmacy MYR-E-CAL. • Take Ester C with bioflavonoids and rutin, 5 grams daily. Apply a weak C solution directly to cut.

3—Rebuild connective tissue: • B-complex with extra pantothenic acid 500mg for collagen. • Nutricology GERMANIUM 150mg for a month if healing is slow.

Lifestyle Support Therapy

—Applications for bruising:

• Apply ice cubes wrapped in a cloth for at least 15 minutes after a bruise occurs. Remove for 10 minutes, then repeat ice pack. The next day repeat the procedure with a hot and cold washcloths on the bruise for 10 minutes each.

• A Springlife POLARIZER with seaweed crystals can avoid a bruise if used immediately.

• Take a bruise bath: make strong *rosemary-thyme* tea. Strain; add to a hot bath. Soak.

• Apply a *comfrey* or *comfrey cream* compress.
• Aloelife ALOE VERA SKIN gel compress.
• Apply DMSO a.m. and p.m. for 3 days.

—For a cut or abrasion:

• Place ice packs on the area immediately. Apply a thick honey (or sugar) coat -natural antibiotics- to the cut and wrap.

• Apply alternating hot and cold witch hazel compresses, or clean with H_2O_2 and apply tea tree oil drops every 2 to 3 hours.

• Apply B & T CALIFLORA, or a good *calendula* gel. Note: For a deep cut do not apply calendula gel right away. It heals so fast that the outside closes up before the inside is healed. Apply after the inside begins to heal.

• Essential *thyme* oil - white blood cells.
• Apply *aloe vera* gel as needed.

See also CHEMICAL AND CONTAMINANT POISONING page 480.

Can't find a recommended product? Call the 800 number listed in Product Resources for the store nearest you.

Common Symptoms: For bruises: Black and blue skin discoloration; sometimes vein damage.

Common Causes: Bruises: Vitamin K deficiency; thin capillary and vein walls; poor collagen formation; mineral-poor diet. Easy bruising is usually found in people who are overweight, or who take anti-clotting drugs. Unusual easy bruising is also an early warning sign of cancer. Hard to heal wounds: occur because bioflavonoids are deficient.

Burns

1st, 2nd and 3rd Degree Burns, Sunstroke, Heatstroke

Burns are classified as first, second, or third degree by the severity of the tissue damage and by how many tissue layers are affected. First degree burns only affect the epidermis, or top layer of the skin; second degree burns damage the dermis, the next lower layer, causing swelling and blistering; third degree burns injure all skin layers, and often damage muscles and other tissue as well. Get medical help fast for anything other than a first degree or small second degree burn. Don't use over-the-counter-burn medications over large body areas or for serious burns. They are for minor burns only. If there is severe itching, redness or swelling, or if fever, chills or great fatigue appear, get to a medical clinic. The recommendations on this page are for first degree or small second-degree burns only. If the burn is 3rd degree, treat for shock until help arrives.

Diet & Superfood Therapy

—Nutritional therapy plan:

1—Apply ice water immediately, then vinegar soaked compresses.

2—Drink plenty of fluids, especially potassium broth (pg. 215) and veggie drinks (pg. 218). Get plenty of protein and mineral-rich foods for fast tissue repair.

3—For immediate relief with no blistering or irritation, dip cotton balls in strong fresh ginger juice or strong black tea or green tea and apply.

4—Electrolyte replacements for heatstroke-sunstroke: Alacer EMERGEN-C, 2 pkts. in water. Lemonade, limeade, mineral water.

—Effective kitchen compresses:

• Honey
• Inside of a banana peel
• Egg whites or raw potato for scalds
• Baking soda or cider vinegar in warm water for acid/chemical burns

—Superfood therapy: (Choose one or two)

• Nutribiotic PRO GREENS with EFA's.
• Crystal Star ENERGY GREEN™ drink.
• Crystal Star BIOFLAVONOID, FIBER & C SUPPORT™ drink.
• Future Biotics VITAL K several times daily for fluid loss.
• Sun Wellness CHLORELLA 1 pkt. daily.

Herb & Supplement Therapy

—Interceptive therapy plan: (Choose 2 or more recommendations)

1—Reduce pain and swelling: •Apply Aloe Life ALOE SKIN GEL to stop burning, or •mix and apply aloe vera gel with a few drops of *lavender* or *chamomile* essential oil; then apply •Crystal Star ANTI-BIO™ GEL, or •*St. John's wort* oil, or •*Tea tree* oil. 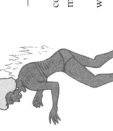 Use •Crystal Star ANTI-FLAM™ caps or extract or •*fresh ginger* juice to take down swelling. •Make a strong burn tea and apply: *Elder blossoms, red clover, yarrow* and *goldenseal.* •Nutribiotic grapefruit seed extract SKIN SPRAY or colloidal silver to counter infection. •Take vitamin C 3-5000mg daily. Make a water solution of ascorbate crystals and apply.

2—Reduce risk of shock: •Nelson Bach RESCUE REMEDY. •For fluid loss: B-complex 100mg a calcium-magnesium tablet with vitamin D and potassium for fluid/potassium loss.

3—Accelerate healing: •Apply *Calendula* gel or •*Thyme* oil. •Make a skin healing tea and apply several times daily: *Comfrey, nettles, marshmallow, scullcap, red clover.* •Take Flora VEGE-SIL caps, •Crystal Star SILICA SOURCE™ extract, or •*horsetail* tea to help new collagen formation. •*Green* tea or *gotu kola* caps and tea, 2 cups daily for nerve and tissue healing. •Take Nutricology GERMANIUM 150mg.

4—Normalize your skin and tissue: •Proteolytic enzymes for healing, especially bromelain 750mg and papain. •American Biologics SUB-ADRENE for skin cortex formation 3 drops, 3x daily. •Take vitamin E w. selenium.

—Homeopathic burn remedies:

Use Arnica for bad burns, followed by:
• *Hypericum* tincture
• *Apis* for a stinging burn
• *Phosphorus* for electrical burns
• *Urtica Urens* for 2nd degree burns that itch and sting

Lifestyle Support Therapy

—Immediate procedures:

•Flush with cold water; then apply ice packs until pain is relieved. Cut away loose clothing that has not adhered to the skin.

•Apply ice water if skin is not charred. If charred, apply cloths dipped in *aloe vera* gel or juice, or a fresh *comfrey leaf* poultice.

•Use a Springlife POLARIZER immediately after the burn for very rapid healing.

•*Cayenne:* $1/4$ teasp. tincture, or 2 opened capsules in 1 tsp. warm water for shock.

—Soothing applications: (choose 2 to 3)

• Matrix Genesis OXY-SPRAY.
• Body Essentials SILICA GEL.
• New Chapter ARNICA-GINGER GEL.
• *Peppermint* oil drops mixed with wheat germ oil and honey. *(Rosemary Gladstar)*
• *White oak bark* compress
• *Flax* oil and *mullein leaf* compress
• Fresh *plantain* herb leaves

—For sunstroke or heatstroke:

•Apply ice packs and wrap the person in a cold wet sheet. Get medical help for shock immediately. See SHOCK THERAPY, page 495.

•Give an electrolyte drink or a little salty water. No alcoholic drinks; they dehydrate.

Common Symptoms: *1st degree - sunburn or heat exposure, minor blistering and pain. 2nd degree - blistering, scarring; gland structure damage; hair follicles burned off. 3rd degree - extensive tissue damage; oozing, charring, severe loss of body fluids; electrolyte loss and shock. Heat and sunstroke are an overreaction to heat and sun exposure, characterized by rapid pulse, and a "shocky" condition which can even lead to brain damage.*

See also SUNBURN AND SKIN *page 501.*

Can't find a recommended product? Call the 800 number listed in Product Resources for the store nearest you.

Bursitis

Acute or Chronic Tendonitis, Tennis Elbow

Bursitis is acute or chronic inflammation of a bursa, the sac-like membrane of connective tissue that contains joint protecting fluids. Tendonitis is an inflammatory condition of the lining of the tendon sheath and its enclosed tendon, especially where tendons pass near bones. Both conditions usually develop calcified deposits in the shoulder, elbow, hip or knee. Both can result from strain, a blow to the affected body part, or in the case of bursitis, as a secondary symptom of arthritis or rheumatism.

Diet & Superfood Therapy

—Nutritional therapy plan:

1—Avoid acid-forming foods, such as caffeine, salts, refined foods, red meats, and nightshade plants like tomatoes, potatoes and eggplant.

2—Keep the body vegetarian and alkaline with foods like celery, avocados, potatoes, wheat germ, sweet fruits, sprouts, greens, brewer's yeast, oats and sea greens.

3—Eat high magnesium fods like leafy greens, green and yellow veggies, and sea greens.

4—Take 2 TBS cider vinegar and 2 TBS honey in water each morning for 2 weeks.

5—Have a carrot-beet-cucumber juice twice a week to "scour" out sediment residues.

6—Take high Omega-3 flax oil 1 tsp. 3x daily. Improvement usually in 2- 6 weeks.

—For organic calcium-magnesium uptake:
• Salmon and sea foods
• Dark leafy greens, broccoli and cauliflower
• Cultured foods

—Superfood therapy: (Choose one or two)
• Crystal Star BIOFLAVONOID, FIBER & C SUPPORT™ drink.
• Solaray ALFAJUICE.
• New Chapter GINGER WONDER syrup or Aloe Falls ALOE-GINGER JUICE to block inflammation.

Herb & Supplement Therapy

—Interceptive therapy plan: (Choose 2 or 3 recommendations)

1—**Reduce inflammation:** • Nature's Bounty B₁₂ nasal gel on a daily basis for 2 weeks, then every other day for two weeks. (Injections for a week also highly recommended.) • Country Life LIGA-TEND as needed, or 4 daily; • Crystal Star ANTI-FLAM™ caps or extract; • Solaray TURMERIC capsules- 500mg; • Enzymatic Therapy ACID-A-CAL capsules to dissolve sediment.

2—**Neutralize arthritis-like symptoms:** • Biotec EXTRA ENERGY ENZYMES with SOD 6-10 daily; • Quercetin 1000mg3 daily with extra bromelain 1500mg; • Alive Energy MAXIMUM MOBILITY; • Prevail MOBIL-EASE.

3—**Reduce spasms and pain:** • Crystal Star STRESSED OUT extract or RELAX™ capsules for relief. • Take DLPA 1000mg as needed. • Nutricology GERMANIUM 150mg and apply. Apply • Chinese WHITE FLOWER oil, or • B&T TRI-FLORA analgesic gel; • lobelia-mullein or crampbark tincture as an antispasmodic rub; • burdock-lobela tea applied as a poultice; • hot comfrey-olive oil compresses; • Nature's Way CAYENNE HERBAL PAIN RELIEVING ointment;

4—**Rebuild connective tissue:** • Crystal Star ADR-ACTIVE™ capsules, or • American Biologic SUB-ADRENE extract for essential cortex formation. Apply • Body Essentials SILICA GEL to joints, take internally as directed, or • Eidon SILICA MINERAL supplement. • Ascorbate vitamin C or Ester C with bioflavonoids and rutin 3000mg daily for collagen formation.

—Improve body pH for long term help:
• Crystal Star ALKALIZING/ENZYME BODY WRAP™ (almost immediate).
• Cornsilk tea to flush kidneys.
• Crystal Star CLEANSING & PURIFYING TEA™.
• Prof. Nutrition DOCTOR DOPHILUS + FOS caps or Natren BIFIDO FACTORS between meals.
• Solaray BIO-ZINC or zinc picolinate daily.
• Niacinamide 500mg 2x daily for 1 week, then once daily with DMG 125mg.

Lifestyle Support Therapy

Smoking and tobacco produce excess acid.

—Bodywork:
• Apply ice packs to inflamed area during acute stages. Apply wet warm compresses in later stages for fast healing.
• Hot castor oil packs on affected areas.
• Take an epsom salts bath once a week with several drops of rosemary essential oil.
• Apply Earth's Bounty O₂ OXY-SPRAY to affected areas every 24 hours.
• Apply DMSO roll-on as needed.
• Biochemics PAIN RELEAF.
• Acupuncture and reflexology treatments have proven excellent for bursitis.
• Magnet therapy has now been proven effective for bursitis.
• Regular mild aerobic and stretching exercises keep your joint system flexible. Use affected area gently. Intense athletic activity is inadvisable until trauma is relieved.

—Reflexology points:

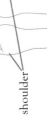

shoulder

See Arthritis page 316 for more information.

B 331

Common Symptoms: Both tendonitis and bursitis involve inflammation and tenderness where tendons affix to bones, causing limited motion in the affected body part. The pains are usually severe and shooting with swelling and redness, especially in the morning and in damp weather. Intense pain usually occurs when lifting or backward rotating the arm.
Common Causes: An acid-forming diet opens the door, causing metabolic imbalance; stress; toxemia; a direct blow or repetitive pressure to a bursa area.

Can't find a recommended product? Call the 800 number listed in Product Resources for the store nearest you.

Cancer

Whole Body Recommendations

More than 3 million Americans are being treated for cancer. 1.3 million are newly diagnosed each year. Cancer used to be extremely rare. Is our late twentieth century lifestyle really that bad? The dramatic increase is only minimally due to new diagnostic tests, or to calling old diseases, like consumption, cancers. The devastating disease we know as cancer today emerged gradually and then started rising at extraordinary rates as industrial societies became more dependent on technology instead of nature. Over 200 different diseases are now classified as cancer. Chasing every cancer classification with a drug for the different requirements and ramifications of each one is futile. Evidence from a rising group of cancer survivors shows us that using every part of our lifestyle to normalize cells that are out of control offers the best chance for success.

Diet & Superfood Therapy

Research links diet to the prevention of 70% of all cancers. 1/3 of cancer deaths are related to nutrition. Dramatic diet changes can mean dramatic results.

Consider the macrobiotic diet on the next page to begin healing.

—Nutritional therapy plan for prevention:
1—Boost your intake of veggie juices, citrus juice and green tea. Add a glass of red wine a day.
2—Have miso, shiitake mushrooms, sea veggies and brewer's yeast several times a week.
3—Reduce meat proteins and fat.

—The best cancer-fighting foods:
• carotene-rich foods: all red, orange and yellow fruits and veggies; tomatoes; green vegetables.
• antioxidant foods soak up free radicals: garlic, onions, broccoli, wheat germ, sea greens, leafy veggies, chile peppers, grapes, berries, carrots.
• steamed cruciferous vegetables: broccoli and broccoli sprouts, cabbage, cauliflower, kale.
• protease inhibitors: beans (esp. soy), potatoes, corn, hibiscus tea, brown rice.
• high fiber foods: whole grains, especially brown rice, apples, fruits and vegetables.
• lignan foods: fish, flax oil, walnuts, berries.

—Superfood therapy: (Choose one or two)
• AloeLife ALOE GOLD juice.
• Green Foods GREEN ESSENCE drink.
• Y.S. ROYAL JELLY-GINSENG drink.
• Sun Wellness CHLORELLA 2 pkts. daily.
• Green Kamut JUST BARLEY.

Herb & Supplement Therapy

—Interceptive therapy plan: (Choose 2 to 3 recommendations)
1—**Detoxification support:** • Crystal Star DETOX™ capsules extract as directed, and • GREEN TEA CLEANSER™ every morning. Give yourself a weekly • vitamin C flush (also relieves pain for men) - up to 10g daily (or until stool turns soupy). • *Una da gato*, especially if liver fluke parasites are involved (many cancers).
2—**Discourage tumor growth:** • *Gotu kola* caps; • *Ginger* extract; • *Ginkgo Biloba* extract; • European mistletoe helps repair damaged DNA; • Nutricology MODIFIED CITRUS PECTIN as directed for metastasis; • *Maitake* mushroom extract; • Crystal Star SYSTEMS STRENGTH™ drink daily for iodine therapy. • Full spectrum probiotics, like Prof. Nutrition DOCTOR DOPHILUS retard cancer cell growth.
3—**Ginseng therapy reinforces tumor immunity:** • Imperial Elixir Siberian Ginseng-Royal Jelly, or • *Siberian ginseng* extract; • Crystal Star CAN-SSIAC caps™ 6 daily; • Flora FLOR-ESSENCE tea; • GINSENG-REISHI extract.
4—**Protect against free radical damage:** • Glutathione 150mg daily; • Lipoic acid, or Jarrow ALPHA LIPOIC ACID 600mg daily; • *Rosemary* essential oil.
5—**Boost anti-angiogenesis to block tumor nourishment:** • Shark cartilage - Lane Labs BENE-FIN caps, • Nutricology CAR-T-CELL emulsion; or • VitaCarte BOVINE TRACHEAL cartilage. • *Garlic* 10 tabs daily; • *Pau d'arco* tea, 4 cups daily.
6—**Add polyphenol compounds:** • red wine, • green tea, • aloe vera juice, • *Maitake* mushroom extract, or • Grifon PRO MAITAKE D-FRACTION extract.
7—**Natural anti-neoplastic substances reduce tumors:** • Green tea; • folic acid 800mcg. • EFA's and Omega-3 oils: • *Evening Primrose* oil 1000mg 3x daily; fish or flaxseed oil, 1-oz daily for cancer; • selenium 400mg daily with vitamin E 800IU.
8—**Use enzyme therapy:** • Quercetin 1000mg with Bromelain 1500mg daily; • CoQ$_{10}$ 200mg 3x daily; • Transformation Enzyme PURE-ZYME, protease therapy, 3 to 5 daily - empty stomach; • Enzymedica PURIFY as directed.
9—**Anti-oxidants are anti-carcinogenic:** • Nutricology GERMANIUM 150mg; • grape seed PCO's 100mg 3x daily. • Beta carotene 100,000IU 2x daily; • Ester C with bioflavs 3000mg daily; • MICROHYDRIN available at Healthy House; • Biotec CELL GUARD w. SOD, 8 daily.

—Reduce the effects of chemotherapy and radiation: • *Reishi* mushroom extract; • *Astragalus* extract; • *Nettles* tea to dissolve adhesions. • Apply *kukui nut* oil for chemotherapy or radiation burning.

Lifestyle Support Therapy

—Bodywork:
• Get aerobic exercise regularly. It is an antioxidant nutrient in itself. No healing program will make it without some exercise.
• Get some sunlight on the body every day possible (esp. for organ cancers).
• Guided imagery has been effective in helping the immune system work better, and the hormone system to stop producing abnormal cells.
• Enemas can clean out putrefaction fast: Take a coffee enema once a week for a month (1 cup strong brewed in a qt. of water) or chlorella implants, or a wheat grass retention enema.

—Poultices for external growths:
• AloeLife ALOE SKIN GEL.
• Garlic/onion poultice.
• Comfrey leaf poultice.
• Green clay poultice.
• Crystal Star GINSENG SKIN REPAIR™ GEL or ANTI-BIO™ gel with *una da gato*.

—Lifestyle measures:
• Avoid tobacco in all forms, synthetic hormones, particularly estrogen, X-Rays, excessive alcohol (especially beer) and caffeine.
• Experts have finally linked alternating electromagnetic fields (not static as appear in nature) and some types of cancer.
• Watch your barbecue - blackened meat has carcinogenic hydrocarbons.

See the following pages for signs, early symptoms and recommendations for specific cancer sites.

Can't find a recommended product? Call the 800 number listed in Product Resources for the store nearest you.

A Macrobiotic Cleansing and Balancing Diet for Cancer

A macrobiotic diet is effective against cancer, helping to rebuild healthy blood and cells, and preventing diseased tissue from continued growth. This way of eating is non-mucous forming, low in fat foods that can alter body chemistry and enhance cancer potential in the cells, and high in vegetable fiber and protein. It is stimulating to the heart and circulatory system through its emphasis on oriental foods such as miso, bancha green tea, and shiitake mushrooms. It is alkalizing with umeboshi plums, sea greens and soy food. It is high in potassium, natural iodine and other minerals. Its greatest benefit is that it is cleansing and strengthening at the same time, and offers a truly balanced way of eating that is easily individualized for one's environment, the seasons, and the constitution of the person using it. The strict form recommended here for an intensive healing program should be followed for three to six months.

Before each meal, and before bed: take 2 to 4 TBS. aloe juice concentrate in water (detoxifies and eases nausea if you are undergoing chemotherapy or radiation).

On rising: take a potassium broth or essence (page 215); or carrot-beet-cucumber juice to clean liver and kidneys; or cranberry concentrate (2 teasp. in water) or red grape juice; or a ginseng restorative tea like Crystal Star GINSENG SIX™, or Crystal Star SYSTEMS STRENGTH™; or a vegetable superfood drink like Green Foods CARROT ESSENCE.

Breakfast: have Pulsating Parsley Juice: 6 carrots, 1 beet, 8 spinach leaves and 1/4 cup fresh parsley; a mix of 2 TBS. each: brewer's yeast, wheat germ, lecithin, bee pollen granules. Sprinkle some on a whole grain cereal, granola or muesli, or mix with yogurt and dried fruit; use on fresh fruit, such as strawberries or apples with kefir or kefir cheese; add a whole grain breakfast pilaf such as Kashi, bulgur or millet, with apple juice or kefir cheese topping.

Mid-morning: take a cup of Crystal Star CLEANSING & PURIFYING™ TEA; or a veggie drink (pg. 218); Mona's CHLORELLA, Green Foods GREEN MAGMA; Crystal Star ENERGY GREEN™ or fresh wheat grass juice. Or take an herb tea, like pau d'arco, Essiac tea, or Crystal Star CAN-SSIAC™ drops in water as a tea; or a glass of fresh carrot juice; or a cup of miso soup with fresh ginger and sea greens snipped on top. (Have 2 TBS dry sea greens daily.)

Lunch: have a Super V-7 veggie juice: 2 carrots, 2 tomatoes, handful each of spinach and parsley, 2 celery ribs, 1/2 cucumber, 1/2 green bell pepper. Add 1 TB of a green superfood: Crystal Star ENERGY GREEN™; NutriCology PRO-GREENS; Ethical Nutrients FUNCTIONAL GREENS; Vibrant Health VITALITY SUPERGREEN. Or, have some steamed broccoli or cauliflower with brown rice, or an oriental stir fry with brown rice and miso sauce; or a fresh green salad with whole grain pitas; or a black bean, onion or lentil soup, or a 3 bean salad.

Mid-afternoon: a cup of green tea, Crystal Star GREEN TEA CLEANSER™, and some whole grain crackers with kefir cheese or a soy spread; or raw veggies dipped in gomashio.

Dinner: have brown rice and steamed vegetables with maitake or shiitake mushrooms. Snip on dry sea vegetables, 1 TB flax or olive oil, and nutritional yeast; or have a brown rice, millet, bulgur, or kasha casserole with tofu, or tempeh and some steamed vegetables, or a hearty dinner salad with sea greens, nuts and seeds, and whole grain bread or chapatis, or baked, broiled or steamed fish or seafood with rice and peas or other veggies, or stuffed cabbage rolls with rice, and baked carrots with tamari and a little honey.

Before bed: have a cup of shiitake mushroom or ginger broth, or green tea - exhibits anticancer and cancer chemoprotective effects; or a glass of organic apple juice.

Note: In order for the macrobiotic balance to work correctly with your body, several foods and food types must be avoided:

—Red meat, poultry, preserved, smoked or cured meats of all kinds, and dairy products.
—Coffee, black teas and carbonated drinks. All refined, frozen, canned and processed foods; hot spices, white vinegar, and table salt.
—Nightshade plants - tomatoes, potatoes, peppers and eggplant.
—Sugars, corn syrup and artificial sweeteners; and tropical and sweet fruits.

Supplements and herbal aids for an intensive macrobiotic cleanse:

Cleansing support: DAILY DETOX by M.D.; Arise & Shine CLEANSE THYSELF PROGRAM - a specific for cancer patients, with many reports of success.

Enzyme support: Transformation Enzyme PUREZYME between meals dissolves the fibrin coating on cancer cells allowing immune defenses to work. Purifies the blood by breaking down protein invaders. Source Naturals COENZYME Q10 ULTRA POTENCY; Herbal Answers HERBAL ALOE FORCE - proteolytic enzymes.

Immune supoport: Herbs: *panax ginseng, echinacea, ashwaganda, Siberian ginseng, goldenseal, licorice, astragalus, ligustrum, suma, dandelion and cayenne.* Supplements: Allergy Research THIODOX (lipoic glutathione); NutriCology LAKTOFERRIN with colostrum and TOTAL IMMUNE SUPPLEMENT.

Green superfood support: Crystal Star ENERGY GREEN™; NutriCology PRO-GREENS with EFA'S; Vibrant Health GREEN VIBRANCE; Country Life SHIITAKE/REISHI COMPLEX with *Chlorella*.

Antioxidant support: Biotec CELL GUARD; NutriCology ANTIOX FORMULA II; Country Life SUPER 10 ANTIOXIDANT; MICROHYDRIN available at Healthy House.

Cancer Fighters: NutriCology GERMANIUM and MODIFIED CITRUS PECTIN inhibit tumor metastasis; NutriCology CAR-T-CELL.

Note: Get morning sunlight and mild exercise every day possible to accelerate the passage of toxins.

See my book COOKING FOR HEALTHY HEALING for a complete diet program for cancer control.

Can't find a recommended product? Call the 800 number listed in Product Resources for the store nearest you.

An Objective Look At Cancer

Our knowledge about cancer has changed. Here's what we know today that can help you make more choices to help yourself.

Cancer cells are normal cells that have been altered by a chemical or other enabler that allows the cell to survive, but without the controls of normal cells. Cancer-filled cells can no longer do their assigned job for your body. Cancer cells have only one job....to survive. To reduce your risk for cancer (and to treat cancer successfully), you must boost your immune response first. Cancers are opportunistic, attacking when immune defenses and bloodstream health are low. Promote an environment where cancer and degenerative disease can't live - where inherent immunity can remain effective. These diseases do not seem to grow or take hold where oxygen and minerals (particularly potassium) are high in the vital fluids. Love your liver! It is a powerful chemical plant that keeps the immune system going. Love your thymus! It is the seat of the immune system.

Many cancers respond well to diet improvement because most cancers are related to poor nutrition. Nutritional deficiencies accumulate over a long period of time - too much refined food, fats and red meats, and too little fiber and fresh foods all lead to natural vitamin and mineral imbalances. These deficiencies eventually change body chemistry. The immune system cannot defend the body properly when biochemistry is altered. It can't tell its own cells from invading toxic cells, and sometimes attacks everything or nothing in confusion. Cancerous cells seem to crave dead de-mineralized foods. They find it easy to live and grow in the unreleased waste and mucous deposits in the body. Avoid red meats, pork, fried foods, refined carbohydrates, sugars, caffeine, preserved or artificially colored foods, heavy pesticides and sprayed foods. All of these clog the system so that the vital organs cannot clean out enough of the waste to maintain health. If you like junk foods, starving cancer cells out is difficult, but as healthy cells rebuild, your cravings for these chemical-laced foods will subside.

Enzyme therapy is effective against cancer. It improves immune response, chemically alters tumor by-products to lessen cancer's side effects, and changes the tumor's surface to make it vulnerable to immune system response. Avoid antacids. They interfere with enzyme production, and the body's ability to carry off heavy metal toxins.

Regular exercise is almost a "cancer defense" in itself. Exercise at least 3 times a week. While one out of three Americans falls victim to cancer, only one out of seven active Americans does. Exercise acts as an antioxidant to enhance body oxygen use; it alters body chemistry to control fat retention, and also accelerates passage of waste out of the body.

Knowing The Early Detection Signs

You can bring on your risk reducers early if you're alerted by early tell-tale signs: 1) a change in bowel or bladder habits, especially blood in the stool. **2)** chronic indigestion, bloating and heartburn, especially difficulty swallowing. **3)** unusual bleeding or discharge from the vagina. **4)** lumps or thickening of the breasts or testicles. **5)** a chronic cough or constant voice hoarseness; bloody sputum. **6)** growth or changes in warts or moles, or scaly skin patches that never go away, especially if they become inflamed or ulcerate. **7)** unusual weight loss.

Cutting Your Risk

How can we take more control of our health and our lives to prevent cancer? Cancer is not a single disease with a single cause, but a multi-dimensional disease with many factors. Ninety percent of all types of cancer relate to diet, lifestyle habits and environmental pollutants and chemicals. At least 20,000 of the 70,000 chemicals people come in contact with regularly are toxic. Hereditary factors account for 5% of cancer cases, but even these are largely influenced by diet and environment. It seems like we're assaulted from all sides by cancer activators that we can't control. It's easy to get the idea that anything and everything can cause cancer. Yet, most cancer is preventable. Lifestyle causes mean that we can positively affect many cancer source factors ourselves - both to prevent cancer from occurring and helping ourselves when it has.

Six watchwords for cutting your risk:

•Improve your diet in 3 ways: **#1) Reduce your intake of fat.** Environmental toxins become lodged in the fatty tissue of the animals in our food chain, and in tissue of humans who eat them. Fat from cancer tissue regularly tests almost double the safe amount of chlorinated pesticides. **#2) Reduce your intake of red meats.** Cancer is closely related to the protein and fat in red meats, fast foods and fried foods. **#3) Eat vegetables every day.** The best chance for cancer isn't drugs or surgery - it's diet and lifestyle choices you can make yourself. Fresh foods, superfoods and herbs (and the phyto-chemicals they contain), are powerful cancer fighters. The more fruits and vegetables you eat, the less your cancer risk, regardless of the type of cancer. People who eat plenty of fruits and vegetables have half the risk of people who eat few fruits and vegetables. Even small to moderate amounts of fruits and vegetables make a big difference. Two fruits and three vegetable servings a day show amazing anti-cancer results. Eating fruit twice a day, instead of twice a week, can cut the risk of lung cancer by 75%, even in smokers.

•Keep your immune system strong. U.S. industries alone generate 88 billion pounds of toxic waste per year. The EPA estimates 90% of them are improperly disposed of. Environmental toxins can damage cell DNA, which leads to cell mutation and tumor development.

•Use enzyme therapy in 2 ways: #1) Have a fresh green salad every day as a source of hydrolytic enzymes to stimulate immune response. #2) Take CoQ$_{10}$ 30mg daily to boost immunity.

•Detoxify and cleanse your body at least twice a year. Certain superfoods and juices accelerate natural body detox activity and prevent the genetic ruin of cells, a prelude to cancer.

Experimental Anti-Neoplaston Therapy. Ask your alternative health care provider.

Can't find a recommended product? Call the 800 number listed in Product Resources for the store nearest you.

Recommendations For Specific Cancer Sites

Cancer is not one disease, but many. There are four types of cancerous growths: 1) carcinomas- affecting the skin, glands, organs and mucous membranes; 2) leukemias- blood cancers; 3) sarcomas- affecting connective tissue, bones and muscles; 4) lymphomas- affecting the lymph system. There can be more than one type of cancer in a location. The link between all cancers is that certain cells have been de-sensitized to normal growth constraints. The damaged cells grow uncontrolled and may move (metastasize) to other sites in the body. Obviously, cancer is complex. There is no simple solution. Vigorous treatment is necessary on all fronts. But, more people are overcoming this devastating disease every day. Use the specific site recommendations along with the general cancer healing recommendations on page 331.

Breast Cancer

Over 185,000 women fall victim to breast cancer every year (up 60% from a generation ago). Over 50,000 die of it annually. Post-menopausal, overweight women have the highest risk, with 75% of all cases occurring in women over 40. If you're more than 25% above your recommended weight your risk increases because fat cells store environmental estrogens, pesticides, organo-chlorine residues and other chemical toxins that cause cancer. Weight gain around age 30 increases the long-term risk of breast cancer, too. A 10-pound increase raises the risk by 23%, a 15-pound increase by 37%, and a 20-pound increase by 52%. Also at risk are women who have overly high, or imbalanced estrogen secretions, e.g., those who had their first period before age 12, those who did not go through menopause until after age 55, those who did not have a child before age 30, and those who did not carry a pregnancy full-term. Women who eat a diet high in meats and dairy products have a higher risk. Many food animals are injected with hormones that add to the environmental estrogens circulating in a woman's body. Women who eat soy foods have lower levels of circulating estrogen. Vegetarians have fewer instances of breast cancer because they process estrogen differently....and they are less exposed to hormone-injected animals like beef and pork. Long term synthetic estrogen and/or oral contraceptive use, and estrogen-containing pesticides are also a risk factor for breast cancer. Indeed, there is a veritable assault on female hormone balance from man-made estrogens. Regular exercise is a key to fighting breast cancer, because it favorably alters body chemistry to control fat retention which stores excess estrogen, and increases fat metabolism, which helps flush out excess and environmental estrogens. Try to limit your exposure to environmental estrogens.

The largest breast cancer increase is in women who were born in the years after World War II, an era that ushered in massive amounts of new chemicals and drugs, like super-strong antibiotics, hormone therapy, and processed foods into American life. Most were developed during the press of wartime, without the normal years of testing for long term health effects. After the war, a great many of these substances found their way into agriculture and household products. Most pesticides, household chemicals and common plastics (the major estrogen imitators) did not exist before World War II. Man-made and environmental estrogens alone can stack the deck against women by increasing their estrogen levels hundreds of times. Only in the last five years has anyone realized how common synthetic estrogens are in today's world. Smoking and long smoke exposure increase risk; women who work around electromagnetic fields have a 38% greater risk. Breast or prostate cancer in a woman's father's family doubles her risk. Chemotherapy does not seem to improve a woman's chances for survival, especially if the cancer has spread to the lymph nodes.

About mammograms: Radiation from X-Rays can severely harm breast tissue and cell balance. Although mammograms have improved in the last 20 years, I still hear enough horror stories about swift fibroid onset to feel that mammograms should not be done routinely or without suspected cause. Because a younger women's breasts are dense, a mammogram screening of her breasts only detects dangerous lesions about 50% of the time. No study has shown that death rates from breast cancer are reduced by mammogram screening in women under 50. Since even low-dose radiation can cause breast fibroids, mammograms in this age group should only be necessary if there are abnormal lumps or nipple infections. Even in women over 50, where the effect of radiation is less, if there is no suspected reason for alarm, mammograms should be undertaken with care. False positive diagnoses cause unbelievable emotional trauma for a woman and her family. Check out your chosen facility thoroughly. By the time a tumor has reached the size that can be detected, it has probably been growing for 10 years or more and has likely spread to other body areas. While early detection can mean less radical medical intervention, early detection is not prevention. A healthy lifestyle should be the primary goal.

Signs and symptoms: discharge from, or scaly skin patches around, the nipple, breast lumps or thickening; change in breast texture or color; persistent enlargement of lymph nodes in the armpit; breast changes not related to your regular menstrual cycle; chronic swelling or sores around the mouth, gums or jaw; severe unusual morning nausea; hypothyroidism linked to low iodine.

Alternative healing protocols: Reduce your saturated fats. Especially avoid fats from sugary foods, dairy products and high sugar alcohol. Increase your fiber and antioxidants from fruits, vegetables, whole grains and soy. Add vegetables like broccoli, cabbage, and cauliflower which have estrogen-reducing effects. Add tomatoes - lycopene from tomatoes protects against tumors. Reduce all meats in your diet, even chicken and turkey, unless you can find an organic supply that has no hormone injections. Fish is fine. Salmon is especially beneficial. Certain minerals, like copper, zinc, chromium, manganese and magnesium are critical to detoxification pathways in the body, protecting us from the cancer-promoting effects of chemical overload. Sea greens are a highly absorbable source of protective plant minerals. •Hypothyroidism is regularly involved in breast cancer. Sea greens are a naturally-occurring iodine source that balances thyroid activity. Two TBS. daily of dried sea greens are a therapeutic dose; or take Crystal Star POTASSIUM-IODINE caps. •Add vitamin E 400IU, selenium, 200mcg. daily and folic acid 400mcg for protection.

•Take Crystal Star EST-AID™ extract or use •PRO-EST WOMEN'S DEFENSE™ roll-on, lab-tested, proven cancer inhibiting formulas. Take Crystal Star REISHI-GINSENG extract for 6 months. •Take royal jelly, 1/4 teasp. daily in panax ginseng tea to boost adrenal activity. •Take Evening Primrose Oil, 3000mg daily. Use fresh rosemary in your cooking; drink rosemary tea frequently. •Add vitamin C, up to 10,000mg with bioflavonoids, (or quercetin 1000mg), and •CoQ-10, 300mg daily. Add •shark or bovine tracheal cartilage (or Nutricology CART-CELL), to inhibit angiogenesis that feeds tumor growth. Cartilage show remarkable activity, even when standard therapy fails. •Take PCOs, 100mg 3x daily (from white pine bark or grape seeds) - some of the most potent antioxidants and free radical scavengers known... 50% more potent than vitamins E or C. Consider •New Life hormone-free COLOSTRUM and Nutricology MCP stimulate glutathiobe - new therapies with great promise for breast cancer. Low body levels of the antioxidant hormone melatonin may raise breast cancer risk. •melatonin, .1 to .3mg at night.

Prostate Cancer

Prostate cancer is the most common cancer in males in the U.S., striking one in nine men over age seventy. Striking at an ever earlier age, over 200,000 new cases of prostate cancer are detected each year, (up 100% over the last 30 years), with the annual death rate approaching 50,000 men. Prostate cancer is clearly associated with the conversion of normal testosterone to di-hydro-testosterone by the enzyme 5-alpha reductase, which is itself a consequence of a high fat, high sugar, low fiber diet and high cholesterol foods like red meats. A low-fat, vegetarian diet is a proven weapon against prostate cancer, since high fiber, low-fat foods excrete hormones linked to its onset. Since sperm counts have dropped by 50% and prostate cancer has doubled in the last 50 years, new research focuses on environmental estrogens, androgens and pollutants that appear to put men at risk. A monthly self-exam should be a part of your prevention plan, especially if you are over fifty. Consider with caution, supplemental melatonin .1 to .3mg. at night as a prostate cancer deterrent.

About the PSA test: The medical world has gotten better at diagnosing prostate cancer, largely because of super-sensitive blood tests like the Prostate Specific Antigen (PSA) test. In fact, the PSA test is producing an epidemic of prostate radiation and surgery, the treatment of choice for prostate cancer in America. Radiation and surgery procedures are escalating even though they can be as devastating as the disease. Studies indicate that surgery only extends life a few months at best. Almost 2% of men die within 90 days of prostate cancer surgery, and 8% experience severe heart and lung complications. Because surgery and radiation damage nerves that lead to the penis and rectum, both treatments regularly cause incontinence and impotence. Over 10% of men become impotent after surgery for prostate cancer, and more than 12% become incontinent. Radiation treatments also frequently initiate a free radical cascade that reduces immune response. Always get a second opinion if you are diagnosed with prostate cancer. It may all be a waste of time, pain and money since two out of three men with border-line high PSA levels don't have prostate cancer. While most elderly men have some prostate cancer cells, most do not die of prostate cancer. It is such a localized, non-invasive form of cancer, that life expectancy with surgery and radiation is practically the same as with no treatment. The European way of "watchful waiting" may be a better choice for avoiding the enormous pain and disability if surgery is not absolutely necessary. There is, however, growing concern worldwide about invasive prostate cancer, which rapidly engulfs the organ and spreads throughout the body. The incidence of this deadly form of prostate cancer is noticeably increasing among men in their 40's and 50's in all industrialized countries.

Signs and symptoms: lumps in prostate and/or testicles; thickening and fluid retention in the scrotum; persistent, unexplained back pain; frequency of urination; difficulty in starting and stopping urination; urgency or straining at urination; and other symptoms similar to prostatitis. As the cancer outgrows the small prostate gland, it often eats its way into the bladder or rectum, even the pelvis and back, causing severe damage. *Note: if you're considering the new testosterone therapy for better sex drive, consider that testosterone therapy can stimulate prostate cancer.*

Alternative healing protocols: improve your diet immediately: Reduce saturated animal fats to 15% or less of calorie intake. No caffeine or sodas. Add 4 to 6 grams of fiber to your daily diet from complex carbohydrates such as those in whole grains, vegetables and fresh or dried fruits. •Add green tea to your daily diet. Especially add cruciferous vegetables like broccoli and cauliflower, and other green and orange vegetables. Include carotene-rich, antioxidant, lycopene-rich foods like tomatoes, (or take a 10mg lycopene supplement) and/or beta-carotene 100,000IU daily. •Add soy foods to your diet. The soybean has at least five proven anti-cancer agents, with anti-estrogenic activity that can retard the development of hormone related prostate cancer.

•Ginseng-royal jelly therapy has been successful. Take Y.S. or Beehive Botanical products with these two ingredients daily. •Take *una da gato* and Crystal Star GINSENG-LICORICE ELIXIR™. Both the ginsenosides of panax ginseng and the triterpenoids of licorice root have been tested for their ability to stifle quick-growing cancer cells and in some cases, cause pre-cancerous cells to return to normal. Add a phyto-hormone-rich herbal compound to balance hormone levels. •Crystal Star PROX™ and PRO-EST PROX™ roll-on with *saw palmetto, pygeum,* and *potency wood* have been lab tested for inhibiting the DHT form of testosterone. Take •EVENING PRIMROSE oil as an EFA, 1000mg 4 daily to suppress the growth of prostate cancer cells, and •zinc 50mg daily. Take a three month course of •*milk thistle seed extract* or *nettle extract* to help your liver metabolize unwanted fats from your system. •Include a glycine, alanine, and glutamic acid amino acid combination to normalize sugar use in the body; antioxidants like •CoQ₁₀, 300mg daily; shark or bovine tracheal cartilage capsules (or Nutricology CAR-T-CELL); and garlic capsules 8 daily to retard cancer cell growth. •Take vitamin C 10,000mg daily (best as an ascorbic acid flush - page 234). Add rich antioxidants like •glutathione 50mg 2x daily, • vitamin E 400IU with selenium 200mcg daily, and •cysteine 500mg daily. •Add PCO's from grapeseed or white pine, 100mg 2x daily, especially for invasive prostate cancer. Take •MCP (modified citrus pectin) Nutricology MCP, recommended to prevent cancer metastasis. Exercise is a must for men dealing with prostate cancer, as well as early morning sunlight on the body for vitamin D, at least 15 minutes every day possible. (African American men have a 40% higher rate of prostate cancer than white men because they synthesize less vitamin D. Black men should consider supplementing with 400IU vitamin D daily.) •Note: if you have prostate cancer, avoid DHEA supplements. DHEA can be converted to testosterone which may stimulate the cancer.

Testicular Cancer

About 7,000 men a year are diagnosed with testicular cancer. Unlike prostate cancer, it's a younger man's disease, usually striking men under 35. It's much more common among sedentary men than active men (over 70% higher for men who sit more than 10 hours a day than those who sit less than 2 hours a day).

Signs and symptoms: Unlike other hormone driven cancers, testicular cancer spreads quickly - even in a few months it can spread to lymph nodes. Early detection can mean much better virility, less impotence, even higher survival rates. Roll each testicle between your thumb and forefinger to check for any bumps, tenderness or swelling.

Alternative healing protocols: most recommendations for prostate cancer apply to testicular cancer. (See above.) Add green tea to your morning diet. Especially add EFA's from *Evening primrose oil* and sea greens to your diet. Vitamin C should be a target nutrient, along with selenium 200mcg and beta-carotene 100,000IU daily.

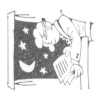

C 336

Can't find a recommended product? Call the 800 number listed in Product Resources for the store nearest you.

Cervical, Uterine (Endometrial) Cancer

Overweight women, especially those who smoke, are at significant risk for cancer of the cervix and/or uterine lining. Post menopausal women, between the ages of 55 and 75, especially those who have never been pregnant, (or conversely, have had more than five births), are vulnerable. Women who take estrogen replacement therapy for menopausal symptoms are especially at risk (symptoms are clearly aggravated by excess estrogen). Using oral contraceptives for 5 or more years at a time, having a history of frequent abortions or sexually transmitted diseases, especially cervical dysplasia, and having benign uterine fibroids are all linked to cervical and uterine cancer. If localized cervical cancer is not treated, it usually spreads to underlying connective tissue, nearby lymph glands, the uterus, and the genito-urinary tract. Serious vaginal infections like trichomonas, and exposure to carcinogenic substances, such as heavy metals, asbestos and herbicides, should be warning signs. Avoid tobacco - it secretes toxins into cervical mucous, significantly increasing the risk of cervical and endometrial cancer. The drug tamoxifen may also increase the risk of endometrial cancer.

Signs and symptoms: Symptoms advance steadily - unusual bleeding or discharge between menstrual periods, painful, heavy periods, vaginal discharge or bleeding during intercourse indicating the presence of polyps. Infertility or difficulty getting pregnant should alert you to question. A class 4 PAP smear is a definite pre-cancerous sign.

Alternative healing protocols: Even after displaysia surgery, recurrence is common if lifestyle changes aren't made. • Reduce fatty meats and dairy foods in your diet immediately. These animal crops receive hormone and antibiotic injections. The excess estrogen correlation between these foods and uterine cancer is undeniable. Fresh fruits and vegetables (especially cruciferous vegetables, oranges, carrots and artichokes) are protective anti-carcinogens. Include • soy foods in your diet 3 times a week; add 2 TBS bee pollen daily (tested effective). • Add sea greens for broad spectrum carotenes or take a carotene supplement 100,000IU daily. Take • Crystal Star CALCIUM SOURCE™ or other herbal calcium with nettles to prevent pre-cancerous lesions from becoming cancerous. • Take Evening Primrose Oil, or high Omega-3 flax oil daily. • Ester C 5 to 10,000mg daily and vitamin E 800IU daily with selenium 200mcg. Take • high potency royal jelly 2 teasp. daily. • Use • Transitions PROGEST CREAM for natural progesterone protection.
• Take green superfoods - Green Foods GREEN MAGMA, or Crystal Star ENERGY GREEN™ drink. Use • Crystal Star WOMAN'S BEST FRIEND™ capsules for 3 to 6 months. • Lane Labs BENE-FIN shark cartilage 6 daily, and • folic acid 800mcg daily.

Note: the American Cancer Society has quietly dropped its recommendation that women have a PAP test every year - advocating it only if the woman is at high risk. If you have a Type II PAP smear, take • green drinks daily, use • Crystal Star ENERGY GREEN MAGMA, or Crystal Star ENERGY GREEN™ drink. Use • Transitions PROGEST CREAM for natural progesterone protection.

Ovarian Cancer

Women at risk seem to be those who have never had children, didn't breastfeed, who are past menopause or are overweight from a high fat diet. Long term estrogen replacement therapy increases ovarian cancer risk. Excess ovulation is a high risk factor. Fertility drugs add to the risk. NutraSweet is implicated in ovarian cancer. Avoid it, especially in hot drinks. Check the dates on products that contain NutraSweet. Old NutraSweet breaks down into DKP, a tumor-causing product. Talcum powder is linked to ovarian cancer. The mineral particles get trapped in the ovarian (and fallopian) tissue. Use a talc-free condom during intercourse; do not dust your perineum with talcum. Asbestos exposure is also implicated, as well as some anti-inflammatory drugs (salicylates, non-steroidals, and cortico-steroids). Some reports show that the risk of developing leukemia from chemotherapy for ovarian cancer is high enough to outweigh the benefits.

Signs and symptoms: In early stages, ovarian cancer is asymptomatic, except for some bloating and abdominal discomfort. There are often no symptoms until the cancer has metastasized.

Alternative healing protocols: Add omega-3 rich flax oil to your diet, or take • Evening Primrose Oil 1000mg daily. Enrich your diet with fresh fruits and vegetables, especially cruciferous vegetables. Keep fats low, and include soy foods for protein instead of meats or dairy products, especially if you have a lactose intolerance. Add sea greens, 2 TBS daily as a source of iodine therapy and carotenes, especially if a thyroid disorder is involved. Avoid fried foods and eggs. • Take shark cartilage or bovine tracheal cartilage as directed to arrest angiogenesis of tumors. Take high potency • royal jelly 2 teasp. daily with ginseng. Take • Crystal Star GINSENG/LICORICE ELIXIR™. • Add anti-oxidant supplements: beta-carotene 150,000IU daily, especially from marine sources; Ester C, up to 10,000mg with bioflavonoids daily, vitamin E 800IU daily with selenium 200mcg. Take • garlic 8 - 10 capsules daily. Take • milk thistle seed extract for 3 months. Take green superfoods such as • Green Foods GREEN MAGMA, or • Crystal Star ENERGY GREEN™ drink. Use • Transitions PROGEST CREAM for natural progesterone protection. Early morning sunlight protects the ovaries with vitamin D. Get 15 minutes of sunlight on the body daily.

Bladder / Kidney Cancer (Renal Cell Carcinoma)

Bladder and kidney cancers are rising in America, (more than 50,000 new cases every year) especially in women who smoke. Smoking has been implicated as the main cause in both bladder and kidney cancers. A history of cystitis and polycystic kidney disease add to the risk. High use of diuretic drugs increases risk of renal cell cancer.

Signs and symptoms: Blood in the urine; urinary difficulty; sometimes side or loin pain. (These can also be signs of problems other than cancer.)

Alternative healing protocols: Increase your intake of fresh vegetables, especially carrots, or • Green Foods CARROT ESSENCE. Drink up to ten 8-oz glasses of water a day to dilute potential carcinogens. Have fruit in the morning and at night before retiring. Have cold water fish twice a week. Take • garlic 10 tablets daily. Take • una da gato extract twice daily. Probiotics, like high potency lactobacillus, or • Prof. Nutrition DOCTOR DOPHILUS with FOS along with antioxidants vitamin A 40,000IU, B-6 250mg, vitamin C 3000mg, vitamin E 400IU with selenium 200mcg and zinc 50mg help prevent bladder cancer recurrence. Take • Nutricology MODIFIED CITRUS PECTIN (MCP) to inhibit growth into other sites. Add • sea greens to your diet for further antioxidants and iodine therapy, 2 TBS daily.

Can't find a recommended product? Call the 800 number listed in Product Resources for the store nearest you.

Colon & Colo-rectal Cancer

Because America's diet is still loaded with fat and low in fiber, colon cancer has become the number two cause of cancer death in the United States, 150,000 people die every year from colon cancer. Overweight men are particularly at risk. A low fat, high fiber diet can dramatically reduce the development of benign polyps that usually lead to colon cancer. Experts estimate that 90% of colon cancer is avoidable through diet improvement! Other risk factors include a family history of colon cancer (mostly from family diet habits), diabetes, severe ulcerative colitis or Crohn's disease. Smoking is linked to colon cancer. I find a seasonal colon cleanse (see page 200) may be your best defense against colon cancer.

Signs and symptoms: persistent diarrhea, changing to persistent constipation for no apparent reason, blood in the bowel movement, and a change in shape of the stool to a thin, flattened appearance. There may be pain and gas in the lower right abdomen. There is also unusual weight loss and fatigue. Colon cancer begins as polyps on the colon walls. For precancerous polyps, •take vitamin C with bioflavonoids 5000mg daily and Green Foods GREEN MAGMA drink. You can test for colon cancer yourself. See self test on page 542.

Alternative healing protocols: high food fiber, (especially an apple or banana a day) and low fat food are still the dietary key for colon cancer. Reduce the meat in your diet. It moves through the colon too slowly. Add whole grain cereals (particularly wheat bran), fresh vegetables (especially cruciferous vegetables), soy foods as protease inhibitors and for genistein estrogen balance, legumes and other high fiber (but low roughage) foods, like dried fruits, to the diet. Include carotene-rich, antioxidant foods like tomatoes, fresh greens and cruciferous vegetables. Have a green salad every day. Add calcium rich foods like dark greens and broccoli. Numerous studies show that daily exercise, active leisure activities and sunshine lower the risk of colon cancer.

Inhibitory antioxidant vitamins: vitamin C 5000mg daily with bioflavonoids; beta carotene 100,000IU; **MSM, 750 to 1000mg** is a chemo-preventive for colon cancer. Omega-3 rich flax oil (effective in reversing pre-cancerous changes in the rectum) and folic acid 800mcg daily. Drink a cup of green tea or Crystal Star GREEN TEA CLEANSER™ each morning as a preventive; take *flax seed tea* for fiber. Take •Nutricology MODIFIED CITRUS PECTIN with flavonoids that help prevent spread of tumors. Take •B-complex 100mg daily; CoQ₁₀ 60mg 5x times daily; L-Carnitine 2000mg daily and acidophilus 3x daily with meals to normalize the colon environment.

•Garlic is a proven colon cancer inhibitor; 6 to 10 capsules daily (may reduce tumors by 75%). •*Cat's claw* extract (una da gato) reduces tumor development. •Take shark cartilage, to inhibit tumors from forming new blood vessels. Tumors even shrink from lack of nutrients as the blood vessels shrivel. Shark cartilage is also rich in calcium, a specific preventive for colon cancer. Bovine tracheal cartilage helps the immune system resist abnormal growth of cancer cells, by activating lymphocytes that slow down cell multiplication. Take a •GLA source such as EVENING PRIMROSE oil, 6 daily or flax seed oil. •Ginseng-based adaptogen combinations speed healing and normalize cell structure. Ginseng enhances antibody response, strengthens the immune properties of cellular connective substances, normalizes blood cells according to need, normalizes cell structure and has a distinct activity against radiation. •Crystal Star GINSENG/REISHI extract has shown clinical results against colon cancer cells. People who have had polyps surgically removed recover faster and build more healthy new cells when they drink a ginseng tea such as •Crystal Star GINSENG 6 SUPER TEA™ during healing.
•GINKGO BILOBA and *astragalus* extracts support body defenses against tumor development. •*Shiitake* mushrooms contain the polysaccharide, lentinan, an anti-cancer agent and immune cell stimulant. •Green drinks like Mona's CHLORELLA with easily absorbd calcium, help prevent recurrent colorectal tumors.

Note: The herbal formula •ESSIAC appears to be effective for colon cancer. But in my experience, it does not go far enough toward immune enhancement, nor is it complex enough to address cancer as it exists today. •Crystal Star CAN-SSIAC™ formula with pau d'arco for immune response, and panax ginseng for reverse transformation activity on malignant cells may be more effective.

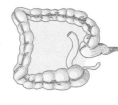

Stomach & Esophageal Cancer

A high fat, low fiber diet is always linked to stomach cancer and stomach polyps. The elderly are particularly at risk, because of decreasing HCl production and lack of dietary fiber. Stomach cancer takes a long time to develop, sometimes as much as fifteen years. Smoking is a high risk factor. Dietary habits contribute to onset - a high intake of meat proteins and nitrates, and low intake of fresh fruits, vegetables and olive oil (especially vitamins C and E in them). Vitamin C significantly inhibits the formation of nitrosamines. The common gastric pathogen *H. pylori* is strongly linked to stomach cancer (possibly another rsult of nitrite metabolism. Heavy metals from industry are also implicated.

Early signs and symptoms: Pernicious anemia; chronic indigestion and gastritis; pain after eating.

Alternative healing protocols: A diet with plenty of fresh vegetables, like broccoli and cabbage. I recommend at least 3 servings per meal for antioxidants and vitamin C. •Add soy foods to your diet, at least three times a week for protease inhibitors. Add whole wheat and wheat bran. Eat garlic and onions in some form every day, and add garlic 8 caps daily or Enzymatic Therapy GARLINASE. •Add glutathione-rich foods like avocados, asparagus, grapefruit, oranges and tomatoes, or take glutathione 50mg 2x daily. Limit alcohol to a small drink a day. Limit salt to less than 2500mg a day. Limit cured meats and smoked foods like bacon, ham or hot dogs, and eat them with a source of vitamin C like broccoli or green peppers. Reduce caffeine intake. •Drink green tea, or •Crystal Star GREEN TEA CLEANSER™ as therapy and a preventive. •Take green superfoods, like •Pines MIGHTY GREENS or Crystal Star ENERGY GREEN. •Take CoQ₁₀ 100mg 3x daily. Take proteolytic enzymes, like •bromelain 1500mg daily or Solaray HCL with PEPSIN and pancreatin 1400mg for protein digestion. Add soy foods and •Transformation Enzyme PURE-ZYME as directed, as protease inhibitors. Take •Crystal Star GINSENG/LICORICE ELIXIR™ daily. Eat small frequent meals - no large meals. Inhibitory vitamins are beta-carotene, C and E 800IU with selenium 200mcg. •*Cat's claw* extract (una da gato) reduces tumor development. •Take •shark cartilage caps, 8-14 daily before meals to inhibit angiogenesis. Strong probiotic like •Prof. Nutrition DOCTOR DOPHILUS with FOS.

Can't find a recommended product? Call the 800 number listed in Product Resources for the store nearest you.

Lung Cancer

Lung cancer is still the leading cause of cancer deaths worldwide. Smoking and second-hand smoke exposure hurts everybody and puts everyone more at risk for cancer, even unborn fetuses. Even with all the media and medical attention on the hazards of smoking, lung cancer is still rising in the U.S. up 262% in the last 30 years, at the astounding rate of 153,000 deaths per year, and 175,000 new cases annually. Eighty-five percent of lung cancer cases are attributable to cigarette smoke, (including the new, potentized marijuana strains, which are 100 times more likely to cause lung cancer than cigarettes!). The remaining 15% is attributed to heavy metal, toxic chemicals (pesticides and herbicides), radioactive exposure, chronic bronchitis and T.B. Excessive intake of cow's milk products may also be a factor in lung cancer.

Signs and symptoms: a persistent cough and chest pain, hoarseness, a sore throat, and increasingly, blood in the sputum. The cough changes and worsens, and chest pain increases as the cancer grows. There is unusual sweating, feverishness and unhealthy weight loss as the disease progresses.

Alternative healing protocols: Carotenes hold the key. There are over 600 carotenes in fresh orange, red and yellow fruits and vegetables. Add beta-carotene, particularly from marine sources like sea greens. Regard broccoli and lycopene-rich tomatoes as a healing gift for lung cancer. I recommend at least 3 servings of fresh vegetables 3 times a day. Lung cancer has been reduced by 75% with this nutritional therapy! •Reduce all dairy foods in your diet. Your increased vegetable intake can supply more absorbable calcium sources. Add sulphur-rich garlic and onions to your daily diet, and soy foods 3 times a week. Reduce saturated fat calories to no more than 20% of your diet. •Drink green tea daily or take Crystal Star GREEN TEA CLEANSER™. Take •Crystal Star MINERAL SPECTRUM™ capsules, rich in watercress, a proven lung cancer deterrent. •Add shiitake mushrooms to your recipes. Their lentinan is a specific proven against lung cancer. Add soyfoods. They're one of Nature's best protease inhibitors to block lung cancer. •Vitamin C is a critical protective nutrient against lung cancer. Take 5000mg or more daily if you are at high risk. •Take vitamin E 1000IU with selenium 200mcg, B complex 150mg, vitamin B₁₂ w/ folic acid, •Nutricology GERMANIUM 200mg, and •Nutricology LACTOFERRIN with colostrum; •garlic tabs 6 - 10 daily, •Y.S. ROYAL JELLY with *Siberian ginseng* drink 4x daily, and *reishi mushroom* tea or capsules for interferon. Apply •Earth's Bounty O₂ SPRAY to the chest regularly for more tissue oxygen. •Chinese herbal medicine has been a vanguard in bronchopulmonary cancers. Seek out a knowledgeable Traditional Chinese Medicine specialist.

Liver & Pancreatic Cancers

Organ cancers are some of the most difficult to deal with, because they are so deep in the body, because their influence on other parts of the system is so widespread, and because they metastasize quickly. Beware of the drug loratadine (brand name Claritin), an antihistamine. It causes liver tumors in animal testing.

Signs and symptoms: Extreme, unusual tiredness is usually the first sign.

Alternative healing protocols: Guided imagery is successful as a method of reaching liver and pancreatic cancers. Use magnetic therapy, especially to reduce abdominal bloating. Avoid alcohol consumption. Reduce fats and add soy foods to your diet at least three times a week as a protease inhibitor. A diet with plenty of fresh vegetables is the key, especially cruciferous vegetables, like broccoli and cabbage, and lycopene-rich foods like tomatoes. Liver cancer specifics are watercress and arugula with almost 500 different carotenes. I recommend at least 3 servings per meal for antioxidants and vitamin C. Six out of seven studies show that high vitamin C intake reduces the risk of pancreatic cancer. •Take up to 10,000mg with bioflavonoids daily. Green drinks are essential: Crystal Star ENERGY GREEN™. •Green Foods GREEN ESSENCE or AloeLife ALOE GOLD drink, or •Sun Wellness Chlorella WAKASA GOLD. Add high omega-3 flax oil 2 teasp. and Enzymatic Therapy LIQUID LIVER to any drink. Use •Nutricology CAR-T-CELL shark emulsion. or •Allergy Research Group LACTOFERRIN with colostrum. Herbal medicines have a proven record. Mega-doses are important at first. Include in your therapy: *schizandra, MILK THISTLE SEED, shiitake mushrooms, dandelion, GINKGO BILOBA, pau d'arco, ECHINACEA, goldenseal, saw palmetto*, and Crystal Star GINSENG/LICORICE ELIXIR™. •Enzyme therapy is critical in organ cancers, like Enzymedica PURIFY, pancreatin 1400mg, and proteolytic enzymes like bromelain 1500mg daily; I consider •CoQ-10 300mg daily, L-Carnitine 3000mg daily, Chromium picolinate 250mcg daily, Glutathione 100mg daily critical in your program.

Brain Cancer

Most brain tumors grow very slowly, for years, but when they become large, progressive problems develop quite rapidly. The use of pesticides in pest strips have been linked to brain cancer, especially in children. Excessive intake of Nutrasweet in sodas and pre-prepared foods has produced a high incidence link with brain tumors. The brain is also often a site for the metastasis of other tumors, usually from the lungs and breast. Question closely the call for a brain biopsy; it could set the cancer cells free to roam the rest of the body.

Signs and symptoms: recent onset of cluster headaches; weakness, lethargy; nausea for no reason; personality change; double vision; poor motor coordination; swollen spleen; unusual weight loss; night sweats; mental decline.

Alternative healing protocols: Find an acupuncturist with a track record in treating brain tumors. Add prayer and meditation to your life. Keep your immune system strong with plenty of •fresh vegetable juices and Herbal Answers ALOE FORCE juice (ALOE MASTERS for children). •Use superfoods like Green Foods GREEN ESSENCE, or WHEAT GERM extract. •Use a fresh grape juice poultice on the nape of the neck. Leave on until dry; continue treatment until tumor regresses. Take •Premier GERMANIUM w. DMG 3x daily. Take vitamin E with selenium 200mcg. •Take GINKGO BILOBA extract to increase brain circulation. •Use Nutricology VITA-CARTE bovine tracheal cartilage for glioblastoma multiform tumors.

Can't find a recommended product? Call the 800 number listed in Product Resources for the store nearest you.

Lymphoma

Lymphomas are cancers of the lymphatic system, including Hodgkin's and non-Hodgkin's lymphomas, and lymphatic leukemia. Lymphomas are related to mercury fillings in the mouth. Check them first to see if you should have them removed. Exposure to herbicides, solvents and vinyl chloride petro-chemicals have been implicated in both Hodgkin's and non-Hodgkin's diseases, especially when immunity was already compromised because of long term conditions like hypoglycemia or prescription drug addiction.

Early signs: swollen lymph nodes, especially in the neck. If the lymph nodes stay swollen for more than 3 weeks, you should get a medical diagnosis. Frequent and often painful, burning urination; blood in the urine; extreme lethargy; unexplained weight loss; night sweats; a fever that comes and goes; itchy skin.

Alternative healing protocols: Start with a liver cleansing diet, (page 205 in this book.) Green superfoods have shown the most promise for detoxification, especially • Sun Wellness Chlorella WAKASA GOLD, and • AloeLife ALOE GOLD drinks. Use • American Biologics DIOXYCHLOR as directed, *reishi* or *maitake* mushroom extracts, or • Crystal Star REISHI-CHLO-RELLA extract; • Nutricology GERMANIUM 200mg daily, • high potency royal jelly, $\frac{1}{2}$ teasp. 4x daily, and • Crystal Star ANTI-BIO™ extract 6 daily to clear the lymph nodes of poisons. Add carotenes, especially lycopene from tomatoes and watermelon to your diet. Add soy foods and cruciferous veggies like cabbage to block tumor nourishment.

Skin Cancer

Skin cancer is an undeclared epidemic of our time. It is the most common (one in every three cancers is skin cancer), and the fastest rising (800,000 new cases each year) of all cancers, claiming about 10,000 deaths a year. Over 90% of skin cancers are caused by over-exposure to the sun's harmful ultra-violet rays, radiation that is increasing in toxicity as the earth's protective ozone layer is steadily depleted. There is also evidence that a genetic predisposition to certain reactions with the sun's UV rays is involved. Exposure to coal tar, creosote, and radium all show up in skin cancers. Age (usually 55 or over) and gender (50% more males gets skin cancer) are factors. One in 75 people will be diagnosed with melanoma in their lifetime. Take great care of your skin.

There are 3 kinds of skin cancer: 1) squamous cell carcinoma, fast growing, characterized by a red papule or a psoriasis-looking patch with scaly crusted surface, appearing on sun-exposed areas of the body. Later, it becomes hard and nodular; may become a lesion on the face, lips or ears. Generally curable with appropriate treatment; 2) basal cell carcinoma, least dangerous, but most common. They do not metastasize, are characterized by small, shiny, firm nodules, or ulcerated crusted lesions that look like local dermatitis. A shiny, pearly border develops after 3 or 4 months with a central ulcer; 3) malignant melanoma, a deeply rooted cancer that arises from the same type of cells found in moles. It is serious, and can be fatal, because it can metastasize to other organs of the body, especially lymph nodes. Early signs of melanoma look just like a freckle or mole. Warning signs include itchiness, tenderness, hardening, or any visible change in size or color in the mole. Early stage melanomas are 95 to 100% curable.

Alternative healing protocols: Reduce the fat in your diet immediately. Stop smoking; it's linked to recurrence of skin cancers. Eliminate hard alcoholic drinks; reduce wine intake to 2 small drinks a day or less. Add soyfoods to your diet. Soy saponins slow the growth of some skin cancer cells. Eat leafy greens daily for carotenes like lutein. Eat orange and yellow vegetables 3 times a week for more carotenes. Eat cold water fish like salmon twice a week. Take 1 teasp. each, wheat germ oil and brewer's yeast in • AloeLife ALOE GOLD juice 2x daily: Avoid sugary foods and caffeine.
• Drink green tea, or take Crystal Star GREEN TEA CLEANSER™ tea and apply GINSENG SKIN REPAIR GEL™. • Take highest potency Beehive Botanicals ROYAL JELLY with propolis and ginseng to normalize skin cells. Alpha hydroxy acids help normalize the epidermis, like Noni of Beverly Hills AHA blends. • Take CoQ$_{10}$ 300mg daily, and EVENING PRIMROSE OIL caps 1000mg daily for better cell oxygenation. Take • Flora VEGE-SIL for connective tissue growth. Take proteolytic enzymes like • Enzymedica PURIFY, 10 daily between meals; and • bromelain 1500mg to reduce swelling. Take *turmeric* capsules with 2 cups of *burdock* tea daily to reduce skin cancer swelling. Take Nutricology GERMANIUM 150mg as an immuno-stimulant.

For basal cell carcinomas: Use • American Biologics DIOXYCHLOR, • Aloe Life ALOE SKIN GEL, • ascorbate or Ester C powder, $\frac{1}{2}$ teasp. hourly to bowel tolerance during healing, for collagen production and connective tissue growth; add shark cartilage capsules, up to 1400mg. • Also open a shark cartilage capsule and mix with $\frac{1}{4}$ teasp. vitamin C crystals and DMSO as a skin transporter and apply and take MSM 1000mg daily. Results usually in 3 to 4 weeks. Or, massage sandlewood essential oil into skin papillomas.

For squamous cell carcinoma: • Apply an escharotic salve through which tumor cells can exit: equal parts *garlic* powder, *goldenseal* powder, zinc powder - mix into calendula ointment. Apply daily until tumor is destroyed, usually 4 weeks. The commercial product is called • HERBAL VEIL 8 by Lenex Labs. Take • PHYCOTENE MICROCLUSTERS available at Healthy House, or • beta carotene 150,000IU; drink carrot juice daily, add • *garlic* capsules 6 to 8 daily. • Apply a combination of vitamin A and vitamin E oil to reverse skin cancers in early stages and prevent recurrence. • Add vitamin E 400IU and selenium 200mcg to your daily diet. Apply • *tea tree* oil, • BioForce ECHINACEA CREAM, or a germanium solution in water.

For malignant melanomas: • Add histidine to your supplements - 1000mg 3x daily. Take • *Milk Thistle Seed* extract drops 3x daily in a cup of *red clover* tea. Take • pycnogenol 100mg 3x daily, and apply Earth's Bounty O$_2$ SPRAY. Take • PHYCOTENE MICROCLUSTERS available at Healthy House; • apply Crystal Star ANTI-BIO™ gel, *calendula* gel, • *birch bark* extract or a • *goldenseal/myrrh* solution. Apply a • vitamin C/*garlic* paste solution, or a *turmeric* paste; open a • shark cartilage capsule, mix with $\frac{1}{4}$ teasp. vitamin C crystals and DMSO as a skin transporter and apply.
Wear protective clothing in the sun. Always use water-proof sun screen, and let it soak in before going out in the sun. Apply sunscreen before insect repellent or the sunscreen won't work. Avoid tanning salons and sunlamps if you are fair skinned. Get early morning sunlight on the skin every day for 15 minutes. Early sun can help heal ulcerations. Midday sun aggravates them. • Skin cancer healing applications include • hot *comfrey* compresses, • dry mustard plasters, • *tea tree* oil, • propolis tincture, • green clay poultices, • B & T CALIFLORA gel, or Earth's Bounty O$_2$ spray on affected area, and on to soles of feet. (Usually a noticeable change in 3 weeks.)

For more information on Lenex Labs incredible safe herbal escharotic skin cancer ointment, FAX 809.324.3434.

Can't find a recommended product? Call the 800 number listed in Product Resources for the store nearest you.

Candida

Candidiasis, Thrush, Leaky Gut Syndrome

Candidiasis is a state of inner imbalance, not a disease. It is a stress-related condition marked by a seriously compromised immune response. Candida albicans yeast is common, normally living harmlessly in the gastrointestinal tract and genito-urinary areas of the body. But when immune response is reduced from repeated rounds of antibiotics, birth control pills or steroid drugs, a high sugar or carbohydrate rich diet, and a lifestyle short on rest, the body loses its intestinal balance and candida yeasts multiply too rapidly, voraciously feeding on the excess sugars and carbohydrates in the digestive tract. As an immune-compromised condition, candida is extremely hard to overcome. Give your body's weakened defenses assistance or candida colonies will flourish throughout the body and keep releasing toxins into the bloodstream.

Diet & Superfood Therapy

—Nutritional therapy plan:

1—The food recommendations for the initial diet are critical for reducing candida yeast proliferation to normal levels. Candida yeasts grow on carbohydrates, preserved, over-processed and refined foods, molds and gluten breads.

2—**Do not eat the following foods for the first month to 6 weeks:** Sugar or sweeteners of any kind, gluten bread and yeasted baked goods, dairy products (except plain kefir or kefir cheese, yogurt or yogurt cheese), smoked, dried, pickled or cured foods, mushrooms, nuts or nut butters (except almonds or almond butter), fruits, fruit juices, dried or candied fruits, coffee, black tea, carbonated drinks (phosphoric acid binds up calcium and magnesium), alcohol or foods containing vinegar. Avoid antibiotics, steroid and corticosteroid drugs, and tobacco.

This is a long, restrictive list, but for the first critical weeks, when energy-sapping yeasts must be deprived of nutrients and killed off, it is the only way.

3—**Acceptable foods during the first stage:** Fresh and steamed veggies (especially onions, garlic, ginger, cabbage, and broccoli), raw cultured sauerkraut, poultry, seafoods and sea greens, olive oil, eggs, mayonnaise, brown rice, amaranth, buckwheat, barley, millet, miso soup and tofu, vegetable pastas, plain or vanilla yogurt, rice cakes-crackers, some citrus fruit and herb teas. Have a green drink, green tea and miso soup every day.

This is a short list, but diet restriction is the most important way to stop candida yeast overgrowth.

Herb & Supplement Therapy

—Interceptive therapy plan: (Choose a recommendation in each category)

Rotate anti-yeast and anti-fungal products, so that yeast strains do not build up resistance to any one formula. Use herbs to restore body homeostasis.

1—Kill the yeasts: • *Pau d' Arco* tea 4 cups daily (also soak nails for nail fungus, or use as a douche for vaginal fungus); • *Echinacea* extract or *echinacea-barberry* extract (if diarrhea), 15 drops 4x daily. Add • *Black Walnut* extract and *garlic* 10 capsules daily; • Crystal Star CAND-EX™ caps, 6 daily with CRAN-PLUS™ tea. • Nutribiotic GRAPEFRUIT SEED extract; • *Olive leaf* extract eats candida -East Park Olive Leaf extract or Nutricology PROLIVE, up to 1500mg daily; • Nature's Secret CANDISTROY or • Herbal Magic IMMUNE SYSTEM programs.

2—Clean out the dead yeasts and wastes: • AloeLife FIBER-MATE drink; • Crystal Star BWL-TONE IBS™ caps. • Gaia CANDIDA SUPREME VITAL CLEANSE.

3—Detoxify the liver: • Crystal Star LIV-ALIVE™ caps; • Vibrant Health RED MARINE ALGAE or 2 TBS snipped sea greens daily; • Milk Thistle Seed extract; • Oceanic carotenes 200,000IU; or • Planetary TRIPHALA caps as directed.

4—Enhance adrenal and thyroid activity: • Crystal Star SYSTEMS STRENGTH™ drink; • Crystal Star ADR-ACTIVE™ caps or Enzymatic Therapy ADRENAL complex; • Biotin 1000mcg with Nature's Secret ULTIMATE B tabs, and taurine 500mg.

5—Fight fungal activity and inhibit yeast overgrowth with EFA's: • Evening Primrose Oil caps, 1000mg 4 daily; • Solaray CAPRYL, or Solgar caprylic acid tabs up to 1200mg; • Allergy Research Group *oregano* oil caps, or Oshadi *oregano* oil, 1 drop 2x daily in 1 teasp. flax oil; • Coconut oil is a rich source of caprylic acid with 50% lauric acid, a disease-fighting fatty acid - • Body Ecology COCONUT OIL.

6—Probiotics re-establish your internal balance: • Natren BIFIDO-FACTORS; • Professional Nutr. DR. DOPHILUS +FOS; • Rejuvenative Foods VEGI-DELITE.

7—Boost your antioxidants and minerals to prevent further infection: • Nutricology *Germanium* 150mg; • rub Earth's Bounty O₂ SPRAY on abdomen. • Grapeseed PCO's 100mg 3x daily; • Nature's Path TRACE-MIN-LYTE.

8—Enzyme therapy for hidden allergies: • Bromelain 750mg daily; • Pancreatin 1400mg w. HCL; • Transformation Enzyme PUREZYME or • Enzymedica PURIFY.

9—Shift internal ecology from unhealthy to healthy: • Crystal Star GINSENG-LICORICE ELIXIR™; • Planetary Formulas TRIPHALA; • Glutamine to increase IgA levels, with NAG (N-acetyl-glucosamine) to deter adherence of candida.

Lifestyle Support Therapy

—Lifestyle measures:

• Use applied kinesiology to test for food and product sensitivities.

• Avoid antibiotics, birth control pills and steroids unless absolutely necessary.

—Detoxification bodywork:

• **Enema:** Take an enema the night before or the morning of your cleanse. Flushing the colon is one of the best ways to jump start a cleanse; it allows a more expedient release of dead yeast cells and toxins from the body.

• **Irrigate:** Have at least one colonic during your cleanse for best results.

• **Exercise:** Take a brisk walk for more body oxygen, and a positive mind and outlook. They are essential to overcome candida body stress. Try a good hearty laugh every day.

• **Rest:** Candida infection often means interrupted sleep patterns. Adequate rest is primary for the body to overcome debilitating, yeast-induced fatigue.

• **Flower remedies:** Natural Labs Deva Flower CLEANSING REMEDY or FEARFULNESS (dread is a primary emotion described by candida and chronic fatigue syndrome victims); Nelson Bach RESCUE REMEDY (for stress).

—Reflexology point:

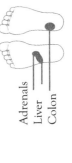

Adrenals
Liver
Colon

C 341

See also FOOD ALLERGIES, NAIL FUNGUS and SKIN FUNGAL INFECTIONS.

Can't find a recommended product? Call the 800 number listed in Product Resources for the store nearest you.

Do you have a Candida infection?

Most of the orthodox medical community still chooses not to recognize, diagnose or treat Candidiasis seriously. It's no wonder since three out of the four main contributors - overuse of antibiotics, excess consumption of sugar, mercury dental fillings and birth control pills come from conventional medical practice. Instead the alternative professions of Naturopathy, Homeopathy, Chiropractor and massage therapy have seen and dealt with most cases. Their energy and dedication have dramatically advanced the knowledge of the symptoms and etiology of Candidiasis to better pin-point symptoms and treatment, to investigate its far-reaching companion diseases, to shorten healing time, to lessen overkill, and to understand the large, overriding psychological aspect of the disease.

Watch out for these lifestyle factors that promote Candida infection: 1) Poor diet - especially excessive intake of sugar, starchy foods, yeasted breads and chemicalized foods. 2) Repeated use of antibiotics—long term use of antibiotics kill protective bacteria (that keep candida under control) as well as harmful bacteria. 3) Hormone medications like corticosteroid drugs and birth control pills. 4) A high stress life, too much alcohol, little rest.

Signs and symptoms that you may have a candida infection:

- Do you have recurrent digestive problems, gas, bloating or flatulence?
- Do you have rectal itching, or chronic constipation alternating to diarrhea?
- Do you have a white coating on your tongue (thrush)? Do you crave sugar, bread, or alcoholic beverages?
- Have you been unusually irritable or depressed? Do you catch frequent colds that take many weeks to go away?
- Are you bothered by unexplained frequent headaches, muscle aches and joint pain?
- Do you feel sick, yet the cause cannot be found? Do your symptoms worsen on muggy days?
- Has your memory been noticeably poor lately? Do you find it hard to concentrate or focus your thoughts? Do you have a spacey feeling?
- If you are a woman, do you have serious PMS, menstrual problems or endometriosis? or chronic vaginal yeast infections or frequent bladder infections?
- If you are a man, do you have abdominal pains, prostatitis, or loss of sexual interest?
- Do you have chronic fungal infections like ringworm, jock itch, nail fungus or athlete's foot?
- Do you have hives, psoriasis, eczema or chronic dermatitis?
- Are you bothered by erratic vision or spots before the eyes?
- Are you oversensitive to chemicals, tobacco, perfume or insecticides?
- Have you recently taken repeated rounds for 1 month or longer, of antibiotics or corticosteroid drugs, like Symycin, Panmycin, Decadron or Prednisone, or acne drugs?

Symptoms for candida albicans overgrowth occur in fairly defined stages:

1st symptoms: Bowel and bladder problems; heartburn; chronic indigestion with gas and bloating; recurring cystitis or vaginitis; chronic fungal skin rashes and nail infections.
2nd symptoms: Allergy-immune reactions- chronic bronchitis; hives, sinusitis, eczema, hayfever, acne; chronic headaches or migraines; muscle pain; earaches; sensitivity to odors.
3rd symptoms: Central nervous system reactions- extreme irritability; confusion, a "spacey" feeling and night time panic attacks; memory lapses and the inability to concentrate; chronic fatigue and lethargy, often followed by acute depression.
4th symptoms: Gland and organ dysfunctions: hypothyroidism, adrenal failure, and hypoglycemia; ovarian problems, frigidity and infertilty; male impotence; lack of sex drive.

Note: Not everyone can detect if they have Candida overgrowth.Candida albicans can mimic the symptoms of over 140 different disorders. For instance, chronic fatigue syndrome, salmonella, intestinal parasite infestation and mononucleosis exhibit similar symptoms, but are treated very differently. Have a test for candida before starting a healing program to save time, expense, and for more rapid improvement. Call ANTIBODY ASSAY LABS, 1-800-522-2611, for a blood test that includes both candida immune complexes and candida antibodies. Accuracy rate is 88%.

A comprehensive, successful protocol for overcoming candida includes the following stages:

Stage 1: Kill the yeasts through diet change and supplement therapy. Avoid antibiotics, cortico-steroid drugs and birth control pills, unless there is absolute medical need.
Stage 2: Cleanse the dead yeasts and waste cells from the body with a soluble fiber cleanser or bentonite. Colonic irrigation and herbal implants are effective here.
Stage 3: Strengthen the digestive system by enhancing its ability to assimilate nutrients. Strengthen the afflicted organs and glands, especially the liver. Restore normal metabolism, and promote friendly bacteria in the gastro-intestinal tract.
Stage 4: Rebuild the immune system. Stimulating immune well-being throughout the healing process supports faster results.

Can't find a recommended product? Call the 800 number listed in Product Resources for the store nearest you.

Addressing Candida Related Syndromes

Candida may infect virtually any part of the body. A wide range of opportunistic syndromes can be caused by a candida infection. The most common sites include nail beds, skin folds, feet, mouth, sinuses, ear canal, navel, esophagus, intestine, vaginal tract and urethra. Candida also infects deep internal organs, which sometimes results in serious disease. Likely sites of infection include the thyroid and adrenal glands, kidneys, bladder, bowel, esophagus, uterus, lungs and bone marrow.

—LEAKY GUT SYNDROME: a set of symptoms connected to disorders like the allergy-immune compromised response of candida, bowel diseases like Crohn's disease and chronic infections. Breaches in the gut wall and too much gut permeability allows foreign food and toxin molecules into the bloodstream where they are attacked by the immune system. Wide nutrient deficiencies occur because the inflamed gut can't absorb them. Fatigue and bloating set in. New food allergies usually appear. Natural treatment recommendations (use several): Reestablish normal permeability of the gut with vitamin C with bioflavonoids (an ascorbic acid flush once a week, page 234, and up to 5000mg daily); Omega-3 fatty acids from flax oil and sea greens inhibit inflammatory chemicals; L-Glutamine 500mg 3x daily to normalize gut barrier; probiotics – Professional Nutrition DOCTOR DOPHILUS + FOS to reseed colonic flora; NAG (N-acetyl-glucosamine) rich in mucopolysaccharides to restabilize connective tissue. Daily ginger tea helps take down inflammation; Crystal Star GINSENG-LICORICE ELIXIR™ also reduces inflammation and helps normalize gut mucous membranes. Zinc 50mg daily for a month and bromelain 1500mg daily for enzyme therapy should be added.

—THRUSH (oral candidiasis): Frequently a childhood candida condition, thrush usually appears as creamy white patches or sores on the tongue or mucous membranes of the mouth. The corners of the mouth may also be red and cracked. The primary cause of thrush is widespread antibiotic use. Natural treatment recommendations (use several): • Probiotics are a key - Nature's Path FLORA-LYTE or Natren LIFESTART by mouth, and use as a rectal suppository. • Add vitamin C 100mg or Ester C chewable. • Give garlic extract drops in water, or squirt a pricked garlic oil cap in the mouth or give KYOLIC by Wakunaga. • COLLOIDAL SILVER drops or Nature's Path SILVER-LYTE are effective. Use • tea tree oil; • homeopathic Thuja. • Nature's Pharmacy MYR-E-CAL, and • Black Walnut extract. • Disinfect toothbrush with 3% hydrogen peroxide frequently.

—VAGINAL CANDIDA (Vulvovaginitis): a thick, white, leukorrhea vaginal discharge with itching and redness all around the genitalia. Natural treatment recommendations (use one or more): • Natren GY-NA-TREN caps and inserts; • Prof. Nutr. DR. DOPHILUS as a vaginal application (apply powder to a tampon and insert or open a capsule and apply); garlic capsules 6 daily; • Pau d' Arco tea as a douche 2x daily; • Pro-Seed GRAPEFRUIT SEED EXTRACT liquid or capsules - May also be used as a vaginal douche or enema. • Beta-carotene 100,000IU daily, or 2 TBS dry snipped sea greens daily (a key diet source of mixed carotenes). • Soak infected areas in a dilute tea tree oil solution. Use in water as a vaginal douche. • Thursday Plantation TEA TREE OIL may be used as a douche to inhibit candida growth. Follow directions carefully. Or douche with • Nature's Phrmacy Golden MYR-E-CAL (see directions with product). Or make your own highly effective herbal douche for candida: • brew a strong tea of garlic cloves, echinacea root, myrrh, calendula flowers and thyme. Fill a squirt bottle - wash perenium after defecating to keep from re-infecting; may also douche the vagina. • Or insert a peeled garlic clove and leave in overnight. Note: Be sure to follow the treatment recommendations for intestinal candida on page 341. Vaginal candida is dependent on intestinal candida. Cure is not likely if you only address the vaginal infection.

—CANDIDA PENIS INFECTION: Infects the tip (glans penis); almost always a result of the ping-pong effect, where a man has a sexual partner who has candida vaginitis, and the infection bounces back and forth between them. Men most at risk are those who have diabetes. In most cases, the same treatment protocols effective for vaginitis are also effective for penile candidiasis. (See above.)

—PARASITE INFESTATION: parasites encourage candida growth by reducing normal immune response. Some naturopaths say that up to 2/3 of people suffering from candida also have a parasite infestation. Natural treatment recommendations: High dosage of probiotics is effective. Choose a broad spectrum, multi flora suplement like • Professional Nutrition DOCTOR DOPHILUS + FOS or Nature's Path FLORA-LYTE. Use for 12 weeks. • Garlic is a natural antiparasitic; use a garlic enema 2x a week. • COLLOIDAL SILVER or Nature's Path SILVER-LYTE are effective.

—NAIL FUNGUS: usually begins as painful swelling of the finger or toe tips, which later develops into a pus around the nails. If the infection occurs under the nails, it may cause loss of the nail. Natural treatment recommendations (use one or more): • apply tea tree oil on affected areas several times daily. • Soak nails in Pau d' Arco tea.

—CANDIDA SKIN INFECTION: characterized by itchy, scaly skin patches, candida fungus lesions are usually red-looking pustules that appear in moist places like the groin, under-arms, navel, anus, buttocks or webbing of fingers and toes. Crusts that form on the scalp usually cause hair loss. Natural treatment recommendations: Apply • Nature's Phrmacy Golden MYRECAL lotion several times daily.

Can't find a recommended product? Call the 800 number listed in Product Resources for the store nearest you.

Candida Cleansing Diet for the First Two Months of Healing

Diet change is the most effective way to rebuild strength and immunity from candida overgrowth. The initial cleansing diet on this page concentrates on releasing dead and diseased yeast cells from the body. This phase may require 2-3 months for complete cleansing. It may also be used as the basis for a "rotation diet," in which you slowly add back individual foods during healing that caused an allergic reaction to candida. As you start to see improvement, and symptoms decrease (usually after two months), start to add back some whole grains, fruits, juices, a little white wine, some fresh cheeses, nuts and beans. Go slowly, add gradually. Test for food sensitivity all along the way until it is gone. Don't forget that sugars and refined foods will allow candida to grow again.

I have been working successfully with candidiasis since 1984 and have found repeatedly that a too-rigid diet does not work over the long term, because the sufferer cannot stick to it (except in a very restricted, isolated environment), and the body becomes imbalanced in other ways. In fact, the disease itself, and the immune response to it are changing. The recommended diets in this book, and my book "COOKING FOR HEALTHY HEALING" are real people diets, used by people suffering from candida who have shared their experience with us. The diets are continually modified to meet changing needs and to take advantage of an ever-widening network of information.

—Superfood therapy: (Choose one or two and add any time) - Crystal Star ENERGY GREEN™ drink; Unipro PERFECT PROTEIN, whey protein; Nutricology PROGREENS with EFA's; Future-biotics VITAL K; Aloe Falls ALOE GINGER juice; AloeLife ALOE GOLD.

On rising: take 2 tsp. cranberry concentrate, or 2 tsp. lemon juice in water, or a fiber cleanser like AloeLife FIBERMATE or Crystal Star FIBER & HERBS COLON CLEANSE™ to clean the colon; or a cup of Crystal Star GREEN TEA CLEANSER™, or 1 teasp. raw unfiltered apple cider vinegar with 1 teasp. honey, if you have gas.

Breakfast: take NutriTech ALL 1 vitamin/mineral drink in water; then take 1 or 2 poached or hard boiled eggs on rice cakes with a little butter or flax oil; or almond butter on rice cakes or wheat free bread; or oatmeal with 1 TB Bragg's LIQUID AMINOS; or amaranth or buckwheat pancakes with a little butter and vanilla; or a vegetable omelette with broccoli; or scrambled eggs with onion, shiitake mushrooms and red pepper; or brown rice with onions and carrots; or oatmeal or cream of buckwheat.

Mid-morning: take a vegetable drink (page 218) or Sun Wellness CHLORELLA or Green Foods GREEN MAGMA, or Crystal Star SYSTEMS STRENGTH™ in water; or a cup of miso soup with sea greens snipped on top; or a cup of *pau d' arco* tea, *echinacea* or *chamomile* tea, or a small bottle of mineral water.

Lunch: have a fresh green salad with lemon/coconut, olive or flax oil dressing, some seafood, chicken or turkey; or a vegetable or miso soup with sea veggies snipped on top with butter and cornbread; Rejuvenative Foods VEGI DELITE cultured veggies; or steamed veggies with brown rice. or open face rice cake or wheat free bread sandwiches, with a little mayonnaise or butter, some veggies, seafood, chicken or turkey; or chicken, tuna or wheat-free pasta salad, with mayonnaise or lemon/oil dressing.

Mid-afternoon: have some rice crackers, or baked corn chips, with a little kefir cheese or butter; or some raw veggies dipped in lemon/oil dressing or spiced mayonnaise; or a small mineral water and hard boiled or deviled egg with sesame salt or sea vegetable seasoning.

Dinner: baked, broiled or poached fish or chicken with steamed brown rice or millet with flax oil and veggies; or a tofu and veggie casserole with sea greens; or a baked potato with Bragg's LIQUID AMINOS, Rejuvenative Foods VEGI DELITE cultured veggies; or a little kefir cheese, or lemon/oil dressing; or a vegetable stir fry with brown rice, sea veggies and a miso or light broth soup; or a vegetarian pizza with snipped sea veggies on top, on a chapati or pita crust; or a hot or cold wheat-free, vegetable pasta salad.

Before bed: have a cup of herb tea such as chamomile, peppermint, or Crystal Star AFTER MEAL ENZ™ extract drops in water, or a cup of miso soup.

Note: Brewer's yeast does not cause or aggravate candida albicans yeast overgrowth. It is one of the best immune-enhancing foods available. Candida yeasts need minerals to thrive, and they deplete the minerals from our bodies. Supplement minerals to shore up mineral deficiencies caused by the yeast - • Restricting sugar in your permanent diet is essential.

Golden Rules for controlling candida overgrowth:

The candida albicans yeast strain takes advantage of lowered immunity to overrun the body. A healthy liver and a strong immune system are the keys to lasting control of candida. The whole healing/rebuilding process may take 6 months or more, and is not easy. The changes in diet, habits and lifestyle are often radical. Some people feel better right away; others go through a rough "healing crisis." (Yeasts are living organisms - a part of the body. Killing them off is traumatic.) But most people with candida are feeling so bad anyway that the knowledge that they are getting better pulls them through the hard times. Be as gentle with your body as you can. Give yourself all the time you need, at least 3 to 6 months. I know you want to get better quickly, but multiple therapies all at once can be self-defeating, psychologically upsetting, and too traumatic on your system. Just stick to it and go at your own pace.

Can't find a recommended product? Call the 800 number listed in Product Resources for the store nearest you.

Carpal Tunnel Syndrome
Repetitive Strain Wrist Injury

Long a problem for knitters and needle-workers, and those doing repetitive task jobs like carpenters, musicians and assembly-line workers, carpal tunnel syndrome is the most common ailment of the computer age. Far more widely spread than originally thought, people with the wrist pain and tell-tale tingling are estimated to be one in five workers today. Research shows that other diseases like arthritis, diabetes, even thyroid disease, also cause the same type of pain and numbness in the wrist, arm and shoulder. Standard medical treatment is usually cortisone shots to control swelling, or in severe cases, surgery to enlarge the carpal tunnel opening. Natural therapies can both relieve pain and act as a preventive to the development of CTS.

Diet & Superfood Therapy

—Nutritional therapy plan:

1–Viatmin B_6 helps CTS. Make sure your diet is rich in vitamin B_6 foods, such as whole grains, liver, green leafy vegetables, beans and legumes.

2–Eat plenty of fresh foods with at least one green salad every day. Add sea greens or miso soup to alkalize.

3–Add fluid-balancing foods to keep from retaining excess fluid - hormone-free chicken and turkey, fish, beans, wheat germ and whole grains. Add celery for good cell salt activity.

4–Avoid acid-forming foods like caffeine, hard liquor and soft drinks. They bind magnesium.

5–Take a glass of lemon juice and water each morning. Make a mix with 2 teasp. each: lecithin granules, brewer's yeast, molasses, toasted wheat germ; add 1 TB to your daily diet.

—Superfood therapy: (Choose one or two)
• Green veggie drinks (pg. 218).
• Fresh carrot juice or Green Foods CARROT ESSENCE drink.
• Crystal Star BIOFLAV., FIBER & C SUPPORT DRINK™ for collagen support and tissue integrity.

Herb & Supplement Therapy

—Interceptive therapy plan: (Choose 2 or more recommendations)

1–Relax tingling nerves: • Crystal Star STRESSED OUT™ extract (relief usually felt within 25 minutes). • Country Life LIGA-TEND caps. Extracts of • *scullcap, passionflowers* or *lobelia* are good nerve relaxers. • Massage area with Earth's Bounty O_2 SPRAY.

2–Control pain and inflammation: Vitamin B_6 250mg daily, with B-complex 100mg and Bromelain 1500mg for 3 months. • Crystal Star ANTI-FLAM™ caps or extract, 4x daily, or • Solaray QBC-PLEX or TURMERIC capsules. • Metabolic Response Modifiers GLUCOSAMINE-CHONDROITIN 2-4 daily. • DLPA 500mg as needed. Massage affected areas frequently with • *cajeput* oil or • Chinese WHITE FLOWER oil. ♀

3–Restore nerve health: • Crystal Star RELAX CAPS™ as needed (usually relief felt within 30 minutes); Anabol Naturals AMINO BALANCE; ♂ • *Evening Primrose Oil* 500mg, 4 daily. • Homeopathic: Hylands NERVE TONIC or *Arsenicum* as needed.

4–Strengthen wrist tissue: • Crystal Star CALCIUM SOURCE™ or • Nutrapathic CALCIUM/COLLAGEN capsules. • Crystal Star SILICA SOURCE™ extract or • Flora VEGE-SIL 2 to 3x daily for rebuilding collagen and connective tissue. • Ascorbate vitamin C with bioflavonoids 3-5000mg daily for connective tissue formation. • Country Life GABA with Taurine.

5–Increase circulation to the painful area: • *Ginkgo Biloba* extract 2-3x daily; niacin (flush-free if desired) 500mg 2x daily.

Lifestyle Support Therapy

• **Self Test for CTS:** Hold out your right hand, bend your left index finger and tap the middle of your right wrist where the wrist joins your hand. If you get a tingling sensation or shooting pains down your fingers, you probably have carpal tunnel problems.

• Both chiropractic and hypnosis are effective for a variety of repetitive strain injuries. Surgery is usually unnecessary.

—Bodywork exercises for relief:
1) Stand with arms at your side.
2) Lift arm in front to shoulder level, palm up. Spread fingers and point them to the floor.
3) Bring fingers up into a fist and flex wrist toward you. Pull fist to your face.... slowly.
4) Move your arm and fist to the side to make a muscle. Turn your head toward the fist.
5) Straighten out your arm, open your fist. Spread fingers again and point them to the floor. Turn your head to your other shoulder and repeat the exercise.

—Reflexology point:

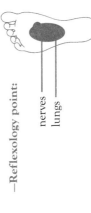

nerves
lungs

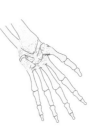

Common Symptoms: Poor grip; intense numbness, tingling, pain and swelling in the wrist and hand, often involving shoulder nerves as well; fluid retention; chronic muscular weakness and atrophy; nerve inflammation. Left untreated, muscle atrophy of the wrist and hand is likely to develop.

Common Causes: Continued stress on the wrist, hand and arm nerves from repetitive tasks; vitamin B_6 deficiency, and/or birth control pills creating a B_6 deficiency, leading to the disorder; underactive thyroid; too much protein; lack of magnesium; glandular imbalance during pregnancy; body electrical system "shorts" from prostaglandin imbalance; other diseases like arthritis or diabetes.

Can't find a recommended product? Call the 800 number listed in Product Resources for the store nearest you.

Cataracts & Macular Degeneration

Lens Opacity

Cataracts, when the lens of the eye becomes hardened and cloudy, affects over 4 million people. Cataracts are linked to smoking, diabetes, steroids drugs (and steroid inhalers for asthma), radiation and excessive exposure to UV light. Cataracts are ultimately related to free radical damage. Cataract surgery is the most common operation for people over 65, performed over 1 million times a year. Most operations have to be repeated in 2 to 5 years. Natural therapies can arrest and even reverse early cataracts. **Age-related macular degeneration (AMD),** a disease of the central part of the eye, is characterized by accumulation of oxidized fat (lipofuscin) and thinning of the macular pigment. It affects 13 million Americans and is the leading cause of blindness in people over 60. AMD can be greatly aided or reversed with nutritional therapy.

Diet & Superfood Therapy

—Nutritional therapy plan:

1—Reduce saturated fat foods and salt. Add magnesium foods: seafoods, whole grains, green veggies, molasses, nuts, eggs (full of zeaxanthin).

2—Avoid sugary foods, red meats, and caffeine.

3—Add berries of all kinds for anthocyanins.

4—Load up on vitamin A and C foods to reduce your risk of these eye diseases by up to 40%.

"See" foods to prevent cataracts:

•Stabilize blood sugar levels: green tea each morning, green leafy veggies (especially spinach), sea greens (2 TBS daily, seafood, celery, citrus fruits, brewer's yeast, sprouts, apples, apple juice.

•Take a daily carrot juice for three months.

"See" foods for macular degeneration:

•Leafy greens can cut your risk by 50%. Eat lutein-rich foods, especially kale, collard greens and spinach. (Good for cataracts, too.)

•Eat natural zinc-rich foods: fish and seafoods, sea greens, whole grains, beans, pumpkin seeds.

•New tests show just 2 to 4 glasses of wine a month can cut risk for AMD by 20%!

—Superfood therapy: (Choose one or two)

•Green Foods CARROT ESSENCE.

•Ethical Nutrients FUNCTIONAL GREENS ♀ high in carotenoids for macular degeneration.

Herb & Supplement Therapy

—Interceptive therapy plan: (Choose 2 or more recommendations)

1—Strengthen eye tissue and nerves: •Allergy Research Group OCUDYNE with Lutein; •Homeopathic *Silicea* tabs; •Solaray VIZION capsules; •Nature's Life I-SIGHT; •High potency royal jelly 2 teasp. daily, with spirulina tabs 8 daily; ♀ •Quercetin 1000mg daily with bromelain 1500mg daily. •Green Foods GREEN MAGMA drink; Futurebiotics BRIGHT EYES.

2—Boost eye strength with super bioflavonoids like PCO's: •Take BILBERRY extract for PCO activity as soon as cataracts or macular degeneration become known; or PCO's 100mg 3x daily from grapeseed or white pine. •*Ginkgo Biloba* extract. •Take Crystal Star EYEBRIGHT COMPLEX caps and use EYEBRIGHT HERBS™ tea as an eyewash. •Aloe vera juice as an eyewash or Quantum AQUALOGICS EYE LOTION. ♂

3—Boost antioxidants against free radical damage: especially de-activating heavy metals and pollutants: •Biotec CELL GUARD with SOD 6 daily; MICRO-HYDRIN available at Healthy House; •Cysteine 1000mg 2x daily or NAC (N-acetyl-cysteine) to boost glutathione; •Vitamin C with bioflavonoids 5000mg daily (use rosehips tea as a natural vitamin C eyewash); •Nutricology GERMANIUM 150mg; •CoQ-10 100mg 3x daily; •Glutathione 50mg 2x daily.

4—Carotene therapy and "eye" vitamins: *the higher the intake of carotenes, the lower the risk of macular degeneration.* •Beta carotene 150,000IU daily, or •PHYCO-TENE MICROCLUSTERS, mixed carotenes from sea greens available at Healthy House; or Ethical Nutrients CAROTENE PLUS. •B-complex 100mg daily with extra B-2, 25mg and B-3, 50mg daily; •Vitamin E 800IU with selenium 200mcg daily; •Taurine, up to 2000mg daily; •Zinc 50mg 2x daily. ♂

5—Bring more circulation to your eyes: •*Ginkgo Biloba* extract.

6—Balance your blood sugar to see better: •Crystal Star SUGAR STRATEGY HIGH™ capsules; •Bilberry extract decreases sorbitol accumulation, and helps remove chemicals from the eyes. •Enzymatic Therapy ACID-A-CAL caps, with chromium picolinate 200mcg. ♂

Lifestyle Support Therapy

—Bodywork:

•Do long slow neck rolls and other good eye exercises (see Bates Method book).

•Acupressure and massage therapy stimulate energy flow to your eyes. They are important techniques.

•Avoid long exposure to the sun. Get your exercise early in the day. Wear wrap around sunglasses for protection.

•Stop smoking and avoid secondary smoke. Smokers are 63% more likely to develop cataracts.

•Avoid aspirin, commercial antihistamines and cortisone as detrimental to eye health.

•Wear amber or blue-blocking sunglasses, especially when driving.

—Reflexology point:

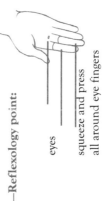

squeeze and press
all around eye fingers

eyes

—Cataract and AMD area:

C 346

Common Symptoms: Cataracts: appear as cloudy or opaque areas on the crystalline lens of the eye which focuses light, (they block light entering the eye). **Macular degeneration:** blurry, distorted vision; decreased reading ability, even with large type; faded colors. Glasses do not help. Driving is very difficult because of blind spots. People with light colored eyes are more at risk.

Common Causes: Cataracts: Free radical damage from heavy metal or environmental pollutants or UV rays; too much dietary fat (may boost risk as much as 80%), sugar, salt; diabetes, poor circulation and constipation; liver malfunction; protein deficiency with poor enzyme activity. **Macular degeneration:** poor digestion; linked to UV sunlight. Thinning of the ozone layer.

See the Diabetes Diet page 368 for more information.

Can't find a recommended product? Call the 800 number listed in Product Resources for the store nearest you.

Cerebral Palsy
Muscle-Nerve Dysfunction

Cerebral palsy is a crippling childhood disorder, almost always occurring as a birth defect in premature, very low birth weight babies. Cerebral palsy is a broad term for brain-centered motor disorders which usually occur before or during birth, or in the first few months after birth. Damage to the cerebrum causes a paralysis (palsy) in one or more parts of the body. The damage is sustained throughout adulthood. Premature infants with very low birth weight (less than 3½ pounds) are at high risk for developing cerebral palsy, especially if the mother has been addicted to drugs. Some experts now argue for intravenous magnesium during pregnancy for pregnant women to prevent cerebral palsy in premature births.

Diet & Superfood Therapy

–Nutritional therapy plan:

1–A modified macrobiotic diet is effective. See pg. 138 in this book, and "COOKING FOR HEALTHY HEALING" by Linda Rector-Page for a complete daily diet.

2–Eat organically grown foods as much as possible. Include plenty of leafy greens and a fresh salad every day.

3–Go on a gentle juice cleanse one day a week until symptoms improve (usually 3 to 4 months). Take a potassium broth (pg. 215) every other day during the cleanse.

4–Avoid chemicalized foods, saturated fats, red meats, fried foods, caffeine and canned foods.

5–Boost magnesium intake during pregnancy: dark green vegetables, seafood and sea greens, whole grains, cultured foods like yogurt, cottage cheese and kefir, beans and almonds.

6–Boost B vitamins and choline: Make a mix with 2 TBS each: brewer's yeast, lecithin, toasted wheat germ. Take some daily over cereal or in juice.

–Effective superfoods: (choose 1 or 2)
• Crystal Star SYSTEMS STRENGTH™.
• Red Star NUTRITIONAL YEAST broth or MISO extract, 2 TBS in water before bed.
• Beehive Botanicals ROYAL JELLY with Siberian Ginseng drink or capsules.

Herb & Supplement Therapy

–Interceptive therapy plan: (Choose 2 or 3 recommendations)

1–**Relax and repair nerves:** Crystal Star RELAX CAPS™ 2-4 daily as needed for tension, with Evening Primrose Oil caps 6 daily. • Centella asiatica, • Ginkgo Biloba extract for brain and nerve stability. • Make an effective nerve strengthening tea: one part each of gotu kola, bilberry, ginger, butcher's broom and scullcap. • Hawthorn extract 4x daily for circulation and a feeling of calm well-being. • Country Life RELAXER caps (GABA with Taurine); • Metabolic Response Modifiers Glucosamine-Chondroitin complex 3 to 4 caps daily for spinal and nerve pain; • Tyrosine 500mg daily for L-Dopa formation.

2–**Tone and strengthen muscles to help control spasms:** • Crystal Star ANTI-SPZ™ capsules, ♀ or • CRAMP BARK COMPLEX™ extract. ♀ • Crystal Star BLDR-K CONTROL™ extract drops in water for urinary incontinence.

3–**Boost mineral, especially magnesium intake for better muscle coordination:** • Magnesium 800mg; • Crystal Star MINERAL SPECTRUM™ caps for stability and alkalinity. • Pregnant women at risk for premature births and toxemia, especially from drugs, should take magnesium 400mg during prenatal months to reduce risk of brain injury associated with birth asphyxia.

4–**Choline therapy:** • Twin Lab CHOLINE/INOSITOL caps; • Country Life PHOSPHATIDYL CHOLINE 1200mg; • Jarrow Egg Yolk Lecithin 6 daily. ♀

5–**Boost your B's for calm and tension relief:** • B-complex 150mg daily; • REAL LIFE TOTAL B, liquid sublingual (contains 250% of B-12 RDA) to reduce muscle atrophy. ♀

–Effective antioxidants:
• Rosemary tea.
• Octacosanol 1000mg 4 daily.
• Natural vitamin E 400IU 3x daily.
• CoQ-10 60mg 2x daily.
• Earth's Bounty O₂ SPRAY applied to affected muscle areas.

Lifestyle Support Therapy

–Lifestyle measures:
• Stay away from all pesticides and agricultural sprays. Many affect the nervous system for a sensitive, fragile system.

–Bodywork:
• Use hot and cold hydrotherapy to stimulate nerve circulation.
• Continuing massage of the muscles is a key deterrent to atrophy.

–Reflexology pressure points:

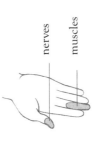

nerves

muscles

Common Symptoms: Characterized by a loss of control over voluntary muscles and abrupt, jerking, muscle contractions; spastic, convulsive seizures; often atrophy of the muscles; usually drooling and speech impairment. Typically, children with CP have above average intelligence.

Common Causes: Hereditary through drug abuse or over-use in the mother, especially when it causes inadequate oxygen supply to the brain; clogged motor control centers in different locations in the brain, malnutrition as an infant; infant diseases, such as encephalitis, meningitis, or herpes simplex; heavy metal poisoning; nerve malfunction through deficient prostaglandin formation.

See MULTIPLE SCLEROSIS page 458 for more information.

Can't find a recommended product? Call the 800 number listed in Product Resources for the store nearest you.

Chicken Pox
Varicella Zoster Virus

Chicken pox is a herpes-type viral disease, usually a childhood ailment, lasting from seven to ten days. One bout of chicken pox provides immunity against recurrence for the rest of your life. Adults are vulnerable if they did not have chicken pox as children. It can be life-threatening with a death toll of about 100 a year) if the child has a compromised immune system (such as a cancer patient undergoing chemotherapy treatment). Complications commonly include ear infections and secondary skin infections.

Diet & Superfood Therapy

—**Nutritional therapy plan:**

1—Take 2 lemons in water with a little honey every 4 hours to flush the system of toxins and clean the kidneys.

2—Stay on a liquid diet with plenty of fruit and vegetable juices for the first 3 days of infection. Then have a raw foods diet, with apples, bananas, yogurt, avocados and a fresh salad daily for the rest of the week.

3—Avoid all dairy products except a little yogurt or kefir cheese. Make a morning blender drink for kids: 8 strawberries, $1/2$ cup vanilla yogurt, 1 TB toasted wheat germ.

4—Dab honey or wheat germ oil on scabs to heal and prevent infection.

5—Get plenty of vitamin C in your diet: best sources are strawberries, pineapple, papaya, kiwi, cruciferous veggies like broccoli.

—**Effective superfoods: (choose 1 or 2)**

• Crystal Star SYSTEMS STRENGTH for minerals and body balance.
• Mona's CHLORELLA drink as an antiviral.
• Beehive Botanicals fresh royal jelly in honey. Take internally and apply to sores.
• Green Foods BERRY BARLEY.
• Knudsen's organic VERY VEGGIE JUICE.
• Aloe Falls ALOE-GINGER JUICE as a swishing mouth wash.

Herb & Supplement Therapy

—**Interceptive therapy plan: (Choose 2 to 3 recommendations)**

1—**Mineral-rich herbs provide key bio-chemical ingredients for effective neurotransmission:** •*cayenne-lobelia* caps every 3 to 4 hours; Herbs Etc. ECHINACEA TRIPLE SOURCE with *olive leaf, elder berry and spilanthes*; Klamath POWER 3 caps 4 daily.

2—**Antihistamine herbs help reduce itching and redness:** •Crystal Star ANTI-HST™ caps, or •Crystal Star ANTI-FLAM™ to reduce inflammation; •pat on licorice root tea; •Nutribiotic GRAPEFRUIT SEED skin spray for infection.

3—**Nervine herbs to help calm and relax:** •Crystal Star WILD LETTUCE-VALERIAN extract drops in water.

4—**Help heal sores:** •Apply Crystal Star LYSINE/LICORICE GEL to sores. •Apply Crystal Star ANTI-BIO™ gel frequently, or a *goldenseal-myrrh* solution if sores are infected. •Crystal Star THERA-DERM™ tea and wash. Take internally, apply with cotton balls to lesions; or •strong tea of *yellow dock, burdock roots and goldenseal root* every 4 hours. Apply •Home Health SCAR-GO to heal scars.

5—**Vitamins for chicken pox:** •Extra vitamin C is essential. Begin taking vitamin C when diagnosis is made: Vitamin C or Ester C crystals, $1/4$ teasp. every 3 hours to bowel tolerance, to relieve itching and neutralize viral activity. Also important: •Vitamin A 10,000IU or Beta carotene 25,000IU; natural vitamin E 400IU daily. •Apply vitamin A and E oil to scabs; zinc 30mg 2x daily for a month to reestablish immunity. •Raw thymus glandular for production of T-lymphocytes.

—**Effective topical applications:**

•Make a *rosemary-calendula* wash: 1 handful of each dried herb to 1 qt. water. Dab on sores every 2 to 3 hours.
• Comfrey salve, or fresh comfrey leaf compresses.
• St. John's wort oil or salve.

—**Effective homeopathic remedies:** • *Rhus Tox*; • *Pulsatilla*

Lifestyle Support Therapy

—**Watchwords:**

• Do not give aspirin to your child. It has been linked to Reye's syndrome, a rare but deadly disease that can afflict children after bouts of chicken pox or some types of flu. It also tends to aggravate sores.

—**Bodywork:**

• Use a catnip enema during acute stage to clean out toxins.

• **Apply:**
—Thursday Plantation ANTISEPTIC CREAM.
—Aloe vera gel, or AloeLife SKIN GEL.
—Witch Hazel
—B & T CALIFLORA gel.
— *Lemon Balm* cream to prevent scarring.
— *Pleurisy root* skin washes.
—Apply Earth's Bounty O₂ SPRAY to reduce scarring.

—**Baths for skin itching and skin healing:**

• Peppermint/ginger
• Cider vinegar/ sea salt
• Oatmeal
• Ginger root

Note: Wet compresses of any of the above baths may be applied often to control itching.

Common Symptoms: Mild fever and headache, with small, flat, pink, blister-type lesions all over the body that erupt, crust and leave a small scar. The blisters and scabs are highly infective and extremely itchy. Keep the child isolated from other children, frail elderly people, or those who have never had chicken pox.

Common Causes: An airborne viral infection, usually allowed to become virulent by reduced immunity from a poor diet - too many sugars, sweets, refined carbohydrates, and mucous-forming foods; lack of green vegetables.

See Childhood Diseases page 245 for more information.

Can't find a recommended product? Call the 800 number listed in Product Resources for the store nearest you.

Cholesterol

Hyperlipidemias, High Serum LDL or VLDL, High Triglycerides

Cholesterol is a fat-related substance essential to every body function. Poor metabolism and over-indulgence in artery clogging foods leads to serious deposits in arterial linings, and to gallstones. There are two kinds of cholesterol. HDL (high density lipo-protein, or good) cholesterol, LDL/VLDL (low density and very low density lipo-proteins, or bad) cholesterol. Triglycerides are a sugar-related blood fat that travels with cholesterol. Heart attack rate is twice as high if your triglyceride level is above 250. High triglycerides cause blood cells to stick together, impairing circulation and leading to heart attack.

Diet & Superfood Therapy

—Nutritional therapy plan:

1—Cholesterol in foods like eggs isn't the culprit. Eggs are a whole food, with phosphatides to balance the cholesterol. The big contributor to high blood cholesterol levels is saturated fat and over-eating. Focus instead on plant foods like red yeast rice. Vegetarians who occasionally eat eggs and small amounts of low fat dairy are at the lowest risk for arterial or heart disease.

2—A low fat, high fiber diet is still the key to reducing cholesterol. Reducing sugar is the key to lowering triglycerides.

3—Foods that lower bad cholesterol: soy foods (with isoflavones), olive oil, whole grains like oats, high fiber foods like fresh fruits and vegetables, beans, yogurt and cultured foods, and yams.

4—Substantially reduce or avoid animal fats, red meats, fried foods, fatty dairy foods, salty/sugary foods, refined foods.

5—Eat smaller meals, especially at night. A little wine with dinner reduces stress and raises HDL's.

—Effective superfoods: (choose 1 or 2)

• Crystal Star CHO-LO FIBER TONE™ drink daily for 1 to 2 months.
• Red Star NUTRITIONAL YEAST.
• Y.S. ROYAL JELLY-GINSENG drink.
• Green Foods BERRY BARLEY ESSENCE.
• Crystal Star GREEN TEA CLEANSER™ daily.

Herb & Supplement Therapy

—Interceptive therapy plan: (Choose 2 to 3 recommendations)

1—**Balance your LDL to HDL levels (the real secret):** • Crystal Star CHOL-EX™ caps, 3 daily for 2 months; • Crystal Star GINSENG-REISHI extract. • Red yeast rice.

2—**Support your cardiovascular health:** • Crystal Star HEARTSEASE-CIRCU-CLEANSE™ tea; • Hawthorn extract 3x daily. • Golden Pride FORMULA ONE oral chelation with EDTA. • Source Naturals TOCOTRIENOLS 34mg.

3—**Boost your antioxidant intake:** • CoQ$_{10}$ 60mg daily (especially if taking cholesterol-lowering drugs). • Grapeseed PCO's 100mg daily; or • BILBERRY extract 2x daily for PCO's; • Carlson E-ELITE soft gels; • Carnitine 1000mg. daily. ♂

4—**Good fats help your body balance out bad fats:** • Source Naturals MEGA-GLA or • Evening Primrose Oil 4 daily; • Omega-3 rich flax oil capsules daily.

5—**Raise your HDL's:** • Panax ginseng (also protects the liver); Suma root; • Solaray ALFA JUICE caps; ♀ Herbs Etc. CHOLESTERO-TONIC.

6—**Lower your LDL, VLDL and triglyceride levels:** • Grifon MAITAKE mushroom caplets; • Cayenne-Ginger capsules 2 daily; • Garlic, or Garlic-Fenugreek seed caps 6 daily (decrease bad cholesterol about 10%). • Nutricology NAC (N-acetyl-cysteine) 500mg 2x daily, or • Enzymatic Therapy GUGGUL-PLUS guggulipid 3x daily or to lower blood fats over all. • Chromium 200mcg for triglycerides.

7—**Help your liver metabolize cholesterol properly:** • Drink green tea or take Crystal Star GREEN TEA CLEANSER™ each morning; • Milk Thistle Seed extract for 3 months; • Dandelion root tea; • Herbal Magic GOLDENSEAL-MYRRH capsules. • Nature's Herbs CHOLESTEROL POWER; ♂ Solaray LIPOTROPIC 1000. • Planetary TRIPHALA caps as directed.

If dietary changes haven't helpd you, use niacin therapy to reduce harmful blood fats and benefit nerves. (Do not use if glucose intolerant, have liver disease or a peptic ulcer.) Flush free niacin is OK. Some common effective doses: 1500mg daily; ♀ 1000mg daily; ♂ • Bio-Resource LO-NIACIN with glycine 500mg if sugar sensitive. • Futurebiotics CHOLESTA-LO with garlic and niacin.

Lifestyle Support Therapy

—Bodywork:

• Ideal cholesterol levels should be from 140 to 165 mg/dl, with LDL cholesterol from 30 to 50 mg/dl, and HDL cholesterol from 80 to 90 mg/dl. (Over 244 is an ideal heart attack victim; 210 is the average American level.)

—Ideal triglyceride levels should be around 170 to 200mg/dl. Ideal is below 140. Every 1% increase in blood cholesterol translates into a 2% increase in heart disease risk. *See "What Level Should Your Cholesterol Be?" page 546.*

• Reduce your body weight. Many overweight people have abnormal metabolism. If you are 10 pounds overweight, your body produces an extra 100mg of cholesterol every day.

• Exercise is preventive medicine for cholesterol. Even if you cut your fat, you need to exercise to lower your LDL's. Take a brisk daily walk or other regular aerobic exercise of your choice to enhance circulation and boost HDL.

• Eliminate tobacco use of all kinds. Nicotine raises cholesterol levels.

• Practice a favorite stress reduction technique at least once a day. There is a correlation between high cholesterol and aggression. Men who are the most emotionally repressive have the highest cholesterol levels.

Common Symptoms: Plaque formation on the artery walls; poor circulation; leg cramps and pain; high blood pressure; difficult breathing; cold hands and feet; dry skin and hair; palpitations; lethargy; dizziness; allergies and kidney trouble. Note: High cholesterol levels do not seem to increase heart disease risk in people 70 and older; and some cholesterol-lowering drugs are actually harmful. Ask about yours.

Common Causes: Stress; diet high in saturated fats and sugars, low in soluble fiber; EFA deficiency. Oxidized LDL-cholesterol poses a particular health hazard to the heart, as it significantly contributes to the accumulation of arterial plaque. An English study shows that not only is this progression inhibited, but the process may be prevented from even occurring by taking PCO's.

See my book "COOKING FOR HEALTHY HEALING" for a complete daily diet.

Can't find a recommended product? Call the 800 number listed in Product Resources for the store nearest you.

Chronic Fatigue Syndrome

Epstein Barr Virus, Hypoadrenalism

Chronic fatigue syndrome (CFS) is sometimes referred to as a condition without a cause. In reality, the opposite is true. There are a wealth of causative factors. Most researchers accept that wide group of viruses are involved. Epstein-Barr virus (EBV), herpes simplex viruses (genital and oral), and cytomegalovirus (CMV) are clearly implicated. Candida albicans yeast and parasite infestations are also highly suspect. CFS association with hypoglycemia is well-known. Incredibly, new research shows that the polio virus, long considered conquered, may be resurfacing 20 to 30 years after childhood vaccinations against it, as Post-Polio Syndrome, now seen as Chronic Fatigue. Environmental contaminants contribute by lowering immune response and allowing CFS a path to develop through exhausted adrenal glands.

Diet & Superfood Therapy

—Nutritional therapy plan:

1— See the Diet for Hypoglycemia on page 427.
2—Keep the diet at least 50% fresh foods during intensive healing time. Emphasize foods that build immunity.

Include often: defense foods: cruciferous vegetables; antibody forming foods: onions and garlic; oxygenating foods: sea greens, brown rice; high fiber complex foods: prunes and bran; cultured foods: yogurt and miso; protein foods: sea foods and whole grains.

3—Avoid allergen-prone, body-stressing foods: junk and fast foods; caffeine, refined sugars, alcohol, dairy, gluten and chemicals.

—Lower your homocysteine levels:

— 4 garlic capsules (1200mg a day) to maintain aortic elasticity.
— B_6, 50mg and folic 800mg to help break down homocysteine.
— red wine, 1 glass with dinner.

—Effective superfoods: (choose 1 or 2)
Immune defense cells are created in bone marrow. Keep new cell development strong with protein. Take a protein drink every morning:
• Solgar WHEY TO GO (lactose-free).
• Crystal Star SYSTEMS STRENGTH™ (also combats hypothyroidism), and GREEN TEA CLEANSER™ to detox.
• Nutricology PRO-GREENS with EFA's, or Pines MIGHTY GREENS with EFA's.
• Beehive Botanicals Royal Jelly, Pollen, Propolis and Siberian Ginseng drink.

Herb & Supplement Therapy

—Interceptive therapy plan: (Choose several recommendations)

1—Fight the viral infection: • St. John's wort (also as an antidepressant); • Crystal Star ANTI-VI™ tea or extract (with St. John's wort); • Nutricology OLIVE LEAF extract caps; • Usnea extract 30 drops 2x daily or Crystal Star BIO-VI extract; • Garlic capsules 8 daily; • Nutribiotic GRAPEFRUIT SEED EXTRACT capsules. • Vitamin C or Ester C crystals with bioflavonoids, $1/4$ teasp. every half hour to bowel tolerance - to flush the tissues and act as an anti-viral agent, for 10 days. Then reduce to 3 - 5000mg daily.

2—Take non-depleting energizers: • Carnitine 2000mg daily (sometimes dramatic improvement); • Country Life sublingual B-12, 2500mcg; • Ethical Nutrients MALIC-MAGNESIUM caps; • Imperial Elixir SIBERIAN GINSENG; • Crystal Star FEM-SUPPORT™ extract (with ashwagandha); • Crystal Star ADRN-ACTIVE™ caps or extract, with BODY REBUILDER™ 4 daily.

3—Enzyme therapy is important for cellular energy, digestion and inflammation: • NADH 10mg or Kal NADA each morning; • CoQ-10 60mg 4 daily; Nature's Plus Bromelain 1500mg daily; • Future Biotics VITAL K; • Natren BIFIDO FACTORS; Prof. Nutrition DOCTOR DOPHILUS +FOS.

4—Relieve muscle pain and increase healing blood supply to affected organs: • L-lysine 500mg 4x daily; • Magnesium 1000mg daily; • chamomile tea, 2 cups daily.

5—Balance your body chemistry: take 15 to 30 drops in water of any of the following extracts: • Suma extract; • Ginseng-Reishi mushroom extract, • Hawthorn extract; • Siberian ginseng extract, or • Rainbow Light ADAPTO-GEM. • Crystal Star PRO-EST BALANCE™ roll-on, with • maitake mushroom caps for 3 months.

6—Detoxify and repair your liver: • Milk thistle seed extract; • Crystal Star LIV-ALIVE™ caps; • Biotec CELL GUARD tablets 6 daily; • B-complex 100mg daily with extra biotin 1000mcg.

7—Strengthen your nervous system: • SAMe (S-adenosyl methionine) to boost serotonin, dopamine and phos. serine levels, 800mg daily. • Ginkgo Biloba extract as needed; • Herbal Magic GINKGO-GINSENG caps; • Evening Primrose oil 4 daily. • Crystal Star GINSENG-LICORICE ELIXIR™;

8—Rebuild immune strength: • Crystal Star GINSENG-CHLORELLA™ extract; • Pau d'arco tea; • Vitamin E 400IU with selenium 200mc; • PCOs - pine or grapeseed, 50mg 3x daily. • Enzymatic Therapy THYMU-PLEX tablets; • Tyrosine 500mg daily.

Lifestyle Support Therapy

—Lifestyle measures:

• Note: High doses of aspirin, NSAIDS and cortisone for arthritic pain can hamper your body's ability to maintain bone strength and adrenal health.

—Bodywork:

• Take a daily deep-breathing walk for tissue oxygen uptake. Walk for a half hour to stimulate lymphatic system and cerebral circulation.
• Get some early morning sunlight on your body every day possible for vitamin D.
• Apply Matrix Health GENESIS OXY-SPRAY onto soles of the feet for body oxygen. Alternate use, one week on and one week off. Too much reactivates symptoms. A little is great; a lot is not.
• Relax. An optimistic mental attitude and frame of mind play a major role in releasing body stress, a big factor in lowered immunity. Remember that immune stimulation itself has an anti-viral effect.
• Stretching exercises and massage will cleanse the lymph system and enhance oxygenation. Use hot and cold alternating hydrotherapy to stimulate circulation.
• Take a wheat grass enema, once a week, to help detoxification.
• Avoid tobacco in all forms. Nicotine destroys immunity. It takes 3 months to rebuild immune response even after you quit.
• Overheating therapy helps control retroviruses. See page 225 for at-home technique.

Call the CFS Hotline (800) 442-3437, and see MONONUCLEOSS, page 456 for more information.

Can't find a recommended product? Call the 800 number listed in Product Resources for the store nearest you.

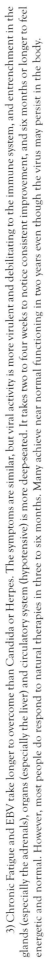

Do You Have Chronic Fatigue Syndrome?

Most researchers believe CFS is a result of mixed infections, with several pathogens involved. Susceptibility to chronic viral infections has become more and more prevalent in the last decades. Environmental pollutants and contaminants contribute to CFS by reducing immune response and allowing CFS a path to develop. In addition, growing evidence points to exhausted adrenal glands from high stress lifestyles and an imbalance in the hypothalamic-pituitary-adrenal (HPA) axis. CFS is a response (or lack of immune response) to the ever-increasing mental, emotional and physical stresses in our environment. As our immunity drops lower and lower, almost anything can be the final trigger for CFS. Onset is abrupt in almost 90% of cases.

Natural healers and therapists have now been working with fatigue syndromes since the early eighties. They are illnesses that represent a degenerative imbalance in the endocrine/metabolic systems of the entire body, so are quite difficult to diagnose and treat. Over 85% of CFS victims are women, usually between 30 and 50, who are outgoing, productive, independent, active, overachievers. It affects close to 2 million people in America today. The number of people suffering from medically incurable viral conditions is increasing at an alarming rate. No conventional medical treatment or drug on the market today can help fatigue syndromes; most hinder immune response and recovery.

Knowledge is part of the cure for CFS. Here are some things to recognize:

1) CFS develops from opportunistic retro-viruses that attack a weakened immune system. But it is maintained through other agents: a history of mononucleosis and/or yeast related problems, food allergies are either a related cause or a result; environmental pollutants that cause chemical sensitivities; smoking; widespread use of antibiotic or cortico-steroid drugs; a low nutrition diet; or low levels of cortisol (an immune-stimulating hormone that is secreted in response to stress). I suggest a test for candida albicans yeast, mononucleosis, herpes virus or other conditions with similar symptoms, so they can be ruled out first.

2) Chronic fatigue syndromes act like recurring systemic viral infections, viruses that often go undetected because their symptoms mimic simple illnesses like colds, flu, or acute, but less debilitating, mononucleosis. Following the acute stages these retro-viruses penetrate the nuclei of immune system T-cells where they are able to survive and replicate indefinitely. Multiplication of the virus and recurring symptoms appear with a rupturing of the organism and its release into the bloodstream. This can occur at any time, but almost always arises when a person is under stress or has reduced immune response due to a simpler illness such as a cold or cough.

3) Chronic Fatigue and EBV take longer to overcome than Candida or Herpes. The symptoms are similar, but viral activity is more virulent and debilitating to the immune system, and entrenchment in the glands (especially the adrenals), organs (especially the liver) and circulatory system (hypotensive) is more deep-seated. It takes two to four weeks to notice consistent improvement, and six months or longer to feel energetic and normal. However, most people do respond to natural therapies in three to six months. Many achieve near normal functioning in two years even though the virus may persist in the body.

4) CFS symptoms are greatly reduced by aerobic exercise. Even light stretching, shiatzu exercises, or short walks are noticeably effective when they are done regularly every day.

5) Good diet and lifestyle habits are paramount in keeping the body clear of toxic wastes and balancing the lymphatic system. Drink plenty of fresh liquids, and clear the bowels daily.

6) Mind and attitude play a critical role in the status of the immune system and energy levels for overcoming CFS. Be gentle with yourself. Don't get so wound up in the strictness of your program that it further depresses you and takes over your life. The people who learn to identify and manage mental, emotional and physical stress in their lives recover fastest. Laughter is still the best medicine.

Symptomology For Chronic Fatigue Syndrome - A CFS Profile

The outward symptoms for chronic fatigue conditions are similar to mononucleosis, HIV infection, candidiasis, cytomegalovirus, M.S., lupus, Lyme disease and fibrocystic myalgia. There are many AIDS-like reactions, but CFS does not kill, is not sexually transmitted as once thought, and tends to go into remission. Get tested for viral titers that measure your body's reaction to the virus, or elevated levels of EBV anti-bodies so that your treatment will be correct.

—First symptoms include persistent, debilitating fatigue where there has been no previous history of fatigue that does not resolve with bed rest, and that is severe enough to reduce average daily activity below 50% percent of normal for that person for at least 6 months. The person experiences classic flu or mononucleosis symptoms - chronic low grade fever, throat infections without pus, unexplained muscle weakness, lethargy, gastro-intestinal disturbance, and sore lymph nodes in the armpit and neck.

—Second symptoms include ringing in the ears, exhaustion, chronic depression and self-doubt, moodiness and irritability, fogginess, disorientation and muddled thinking, continued low grade infection and fever, worsening allergies, diarrhea, sharper muscle aches and weakness, numbness and tingling in the limbs, and vertigo.

—Third symptoms include extreme fatigue, isolation, herpes infections, aching ears and eyes, night sweats, blackouts, extremely low immune response resulting in frequent infections, paranoia, chronic exhaustion, weight loss and loss of appetite, MS-like nerve disorder with heart palpitations.

CFS Support Groups are a good idea. CFS Infoline: (800) 442-3437.

Can't find a recommended product? Call the 800 number listed in Product Resources for the store nearest you.

Circulation Problems

Sluggish Blood Flow, Intermittent Claudication, Chillblains, Raynaud's Disease

It isn't hard to see why our circulatory health is so important. It delivers our river of life throughout the body. It keeps us alert (15% of our blood supply goes to the brain). It transports heat from the inner body to the skin. It carries antibodies to areas of infection. It helps move waste products to channels of elimination. Sluggish circulation is one of the first signs of serious disorders. High blood pressure, arteriosclerosis, varicose veins, phlebitis, and heart disease are all connected with circulatory system health. Investigate further if your condition does not improve. Claudication is a peripheral artery disease, characterized by pain in the legs due to obstructed blood flow. Raynaud's disease is characterized by numbness and cold hands and feet even in warm weather. Chillblains are painful, itchy patches on the hands and feet.

Diet & Superfood Therapy

—**Nutritional therapy plan:**

1—Keep the colon clear and your cholesterol down with a high fiber diet; at least 60% fresh foods.

2—Eat citrus fruits, juices and dried fruits; they have good bioflavonoid content to strengthen vein and tissue walls.

3—Avoid red meats, fried and fatty foods, excess caffeine, salts, refined foods, sugar.

4—Drink plenty of healthy fluids, especially for Raynaud's disease. Have soy milk instead of dairy.

5—Eat smaller meals more often. Avoid large or heavy meals.

6—**Make a circulation drink:** take daily for almost immediate improvement: Mix $1/2$ cup tomato juice, $1/2$ cup lemon juice, 6 teasp. wheat germ oil, 1 teasp. brewer's yeast.

—**Effective superfoods: (choose 1 or 2)**

• Crystal Star BIOFLAV. FIBER & C SUPPORT™ drink, and on alternating days, CHOLO-FIBER TONE™ drink.

• Rainbow Light GARLIC & GREENS.

• Green tea daily or Crystal Star GREEN TEA CLEANSER™.

• New Moon GINSENG GINGER WONDER syrup as desired.

Herb & Supplement Therapy

—**Interceptive therapy plan: (Choose 2 to 3 recommendations)**

1—**Boost your circulation nutrients:** • Crystal Star *Heartsease-Hawthorn*™ capsules; • *Hawthorn* or *Ginkgo Biloba* extract; • Country Life sublingual B-12, 2500mcg.

2—**Stimulate a sluggish circulation:** • Crystal Star HEARTSEASE CIRCU-CLEANSE™ tea daily; ♂ • *Ginger* tea or extract daily. • Ginseng Company CY-CLONE CIDER; • Niacin therapy: 250mg 3x daily. • *Butcher's broom* caps or tea are a natural blood thinner. (Use only temporarily.) ♂

3—**Strengthen-elasticize veins and capillaries:** • Carnitine 500mg 2x daily; • Solaray CENTELLA ASIATICA caps; • Vitamin E 400IU with selenium 200mcg daily; • vitamin C or Ester C with bioflavonoids 500mg 4x daily; • Golden Pride HEART HEALTH PAK as directed.♂ • *Garlic* to keep blood pressure normal and HDL levels down, 6 daily; • *Horse chestnut* extract drops.♀

4—**Flavonoids tone your circulatory system:** • *Bilberry* extract 2-3x daily; SIBERIAN GINSENG extract; • Quercetin 1000mg with bromelain 1000mg.

5—**Balance your prostaglandins to smooth out circulation:** • Omega-3 flax oil 3x daily; • *Evening Primrose* oil 2000mg daily; Nature's Secret ULTIMATE OIL

6—**Antioxidants for long-term circulatory health:** • *Panax ginseng* 2x daily; • CoQ-10, 30mg 2x daily; • PCO's from pine or grapeseed, 100mg daily; ♀ • Crystal Star GINSENG-CHLORELLA extract.

—**For chillblains:** Nature's Way CAYENNE PAIN RELIEVING ointment or *cayenne-ginger* capsules, 2 daily.

—**For claudication:** rub • CAPSAICIN cream on legs; • take GINKGO BILOBA extract, 120mg daily; • apply hot sea salt compresses to the legs. Solaray CENTELLA VEIN caps; • Enzymedica PURIFY - a protease enzyme.

—**For Raynaud's Disease:** • *Cayenne/ginger* caps 4 daily, • Follow a hypoglycemic diet, take • Crystal Star IODINE-POTASSIUM caps, ♀ • New Moon GINGER WONDER syrup and • Magnesium 400mg 2x daily.

Lifestyle Support Therapy

—**Lifestyle measures:**

• Biofeedback has been notably successful for cold hands and feet.

• Avoid things that restrict blood flow, like smoking and alcohol.

—**Bodywork:**

• Apply alternating hot and cold *cayenne-ginger* compresses to areas in need of stimulation. Or wrap feet in towels soaked in *cayenne-ginger* solution.

• Use a dry skin brush before your daily shower.

• See a chiropractor or massage therapist for a structure work-out to clear any obstructions and open energy pathways.

• Take a brisk walk every day to get your blood moving.

• **Effective massage aromatherapy oils:** *Juniper* oil; *Rosemary* oil; *Sage* oil

—**For claudication:** sit with legs elevated when possible. Don't wear knee high hosiery. Massage your legs each morning.

• Take a daily morning walk.

Common Symptoms: Cold hands and feet; poor memory; migraine headaches; numbness; ringing in the ears and hearing loss; dizziness when standing quickly; shortness of breath; high triglyceride and cholesterol levels; varicose veins; irregular heartbeat; leg cramps; swelling ankles; nosebleeds. In Raynaud's disease, fingers turn white due to lack of blood because small arteries contract and cut off blood flow. Raynaud's disease is usually the result of an underlying circulatory cause like atherosclerosis or using a jackhammer or chain saw on the job over many years.

See HIGH BLOOD PRESSURE page 417 and HEART DISEASE page: 407

Can't find a recommended product? Call the 800 number listed in Product Resources for the store nearest you.

Colds

Upper Respiratory Infections

The common cold is quite common... Americans catch about 66 million colds a year. In any two week period during high risk seasons, almost one-third of the U.S. suffers from a cold. Your body is talking to you when you get a cold. A cold is usually your body's attempt to cleanse itself of wastes, toxins and bacterial overgrowth that build up to a point where natural immunity can't overcome them. The glands are always affected, and as the endocrine system is on a 6 day cycle, a normal cold usually runs for about a week as the body works through all its detoxification processes. Work with your body, not against it, to get over a cold. Natural remedies are effective in speeding recovery and reducing discomfort. In my experience, most drug store cold remedies halt the body cleansing/balancing processes, and generally make the cold last longer.

Diet & Superfood Therapy

—Nutritional therapy plan:

1–**When you have a cold:** Go on a liquid diet during acute stage, with green or potassium drinks (pg. 215) to clean out infection and mucous.

2–Take 2 TBS cider vinegar, and 2 teasp. honey in water, or garlic/ginger tea each morning, and garlic/miso soup each night.

Or 2 TBS each lemon juice and honey, and 1 teasp. fresh grated ginger at night.

3–When fever and acute stage has passed, eat light meals - fresh and steamed vegetables, fresh fruits and juices, and cultured foods for friendly intestinal flora.

4–Avoid dairy products of all kinds, red meats, sugary, fried or fatty foods during a cold.

5–Chicken soup increases mucous release.

6–Drink eight glasses of liquids daily, especially green tea, peppermint tea and orange juice.

7–To release quantities of mucous all at once if you have a streaming cold: take fresh grated horse-radish in a spoon with lemon juice, and hang over the sink; or use onion-garlic syrup for gentler mucous release.

8–Boost immunity with glutathione foods: avo-cado, asparagus, watermelon, oranges, peaches and green superfooods like chlorella and barley grass.

—Effective superfoods: (choose 1 or 2)

•Crystal Star BIOFLAV., FIBER & C SUP-PORT™ drink for nasal congestion - clears in 15 to 20 minutes; GREEN TEA CLEANSER™ to combat infection.

•Balance your intestinal structure with Solgar WHEY TO GO protein drink.

Herb & Supplement Therapy

—Interceptive therapy plan: (Choose 2 to 3 recommendations)

1–**During initial stage:** •Vitamin C crystals, $^1/_4$ teasp. every half hour to bowel tolerance to flush and neutralize toxins; COLLOIDAL SILVER drops every 3 hours.

2–**During acute phase:** •Crystal Star FIRST AID CAPS™ every hour during acute stages to promote sweating and eliminate toxins. (Use as a preventive in initial stage.) •Zand HERBAL LOZENGES, Crystal Star ZINC SOURCE™ throat spray or •Beehive Botanical PROPOLIS THROAT SPRAY every 2 hours. ☺

Relieve the infection with •Crystal Star ANTI-BIO™ caps or extract to flush lymph glands for 6 days. Use throat coats like • Crystal Star COFEX™ TEA, ☺ •*elderberry-mint-yarrow* tea as needed; •apply hot ginger compresses to the chest.

• A "cold" cocktail works great! Mix in a glass of aloe vera juice: $^1/_4$ teasp. vitamin C crystals, 2 tsp. SAMBUCOL elderberry syrup, $^1/_2$ teasp. *turmeric* powder (or open a *curcumin capsule*), 1 opened capsule *echinacea*, $^1/_2$ teasp. propolis extract.

Congestion cleansers: •*Cayenne-ginger* caps; •*Echinacea-goldenseal* caps; •*Cay-enne-garlic* capsules; •Crystal Star X-PECT-T™ tea; •Zand DECONGEST extract; •Nutribiotic GRAPEFRUIT SEED extract spray, or gargle (3 drops in 5-oz. water) to release mucous and phlegm. ♂

—Effective homeopathic remedies: •Boiron OSCILLOCOCCINUM; •B&T ALPHA CF tabs; •Aconite for fever, sneezing; •*Eupatorium Perfoliatum* for sweat-ing; •Hylands C-PLUS. ☺

3–**During recovery phase:** •*Usnea* extract or Crystal Star BIO-VI™ extract; glutamine 500mg 2x daily; •Nutribiotic NASAL SPRAY & EAR DROPS; •Zinc lozenges to kill throat bacteria; •Planetary formulas OLD INDIAN COUGH SYRUP; •Olbas COUGH SYRUP and pastilles. ♂

4–**Re-establish immune health:** •Vitamin C, up to 5000mg daily to decrease severity of colds; •Nutricology NAC (N-acetyl-cysteine) to boost glutathione; •*panax ginseng, astragalus* extract or Siberian ginseng extract to boost lymphocytes and inter-feron; •Crystal Star COLD SEASON DEFENSE™; •CoQ-10, 30mg 3x daily; •Nutricology LACTOFERRIN with colostrum caps. ◔ •Enzyme therapy: Prevail DEFENSE FORMULA; the "king of bitters," •Ayurvedic Concepts HEMO-CARE with *andrographis* or Flora FLORADIX HERBAL BITTERS.

5–**High risk season preventives:** •Crystal Star HERBAL DEFENSE TEAM™; •Zinc 30mg daily; •Acidophilus liquid 3 tsp. daily; ☺ •Garlic caps 6 daily; •Beta carotene 25,000IU 4x daily. •Enzymatic Therapy THYMU-PLEX tablets.

Lifestyle Support Therapy

—Bodywork:

•Open all channels of elimination with hot baths or showers, hot broths and tonics, brandy and lemon, and catnip enemas.

• A massage therapy treatment can open up blocked body meridians.

• For prevention, take daily alternating hot and cold showers at the beginning of cold sea-son to stimulate immune response. Repeat any time you feel the first signs of discomfort.

• Rest is important. Light exercise is better than vigorous exercise during a cold.

•Aromatherapy steams, with or without a vaporizer are effective:

—*Eucalyptus* opens sinus passages.

—*Wintergreen* relieves nasal congestion.

—*Mint or chamomile* relieve headaches.

—*Tea tree oil* combats infection.

• A nasal salt irrigation helps remove patho-gens from mucous membranes and clears breathing quickly: add $^1/_2$ teasp. sea salt to a cup of warm water. Fill a dropper with liquid, tilt your head and fill each nostril; then blow your nose.

—Acupressure press points:

—For a scratchy, hoarse throat: press be-tween the nail and the first joint of the thumb, just behind the nail, on the outside.

—To unclog a stuffy nose: press on the cheek, at the flare of the nostrils where they join the cheek.

See FLU page 387 for what to do for flu.

Can't find a recommended product? Call the 800 number listed in Product Resources for the store nearest you.

C 353

Do You Have Chronic Colds?

Although rhino-viruses are involved in the misery we know as a cold, we are constantly exposed to these organisms without them causing a cold. Your immune system health is the deciding factor in whether you "catch" a cold or not. There seem to be almost as many drugstore cold remedies as there are colds, most of them symptom-suppressing with side effects. Since a cold is usually a cleansing condition, I feel it may be better to just let it happen so your body can start fresh, with a stronger immune system. Yet, without a doubt, it is hard to work, sleep, and be around other people with miserable cold symptoms. Traditional wisdom is effective for minimizing misery while your body gets on with its job of cleaning house.

1) A daily walk revs up immune response and gives you some fresh air. A walk puts cleansing oxygen into your lungs, and stops you from feeling sorry for yourself. It works wonders!
2) Take ascorbate vitamin C or Ester C, 1000mg every hour, preferably in powder form with juice, throughout the day. Take zinc lozenges as needed, or propolis throat spray.
3) No smoking or alcohol (other than a little brandy and lemon). They suppress immunity. Avoid refined foods, sugar, and dairy foods. They increase production of thick mucous.
4) Eat lightly but with good nutrition. Nutrient absorption is less efficient during a cold. A vegetarian diet is best at this time so the body won't have to work so hard at digestion.
5) Drink plenty of liquids; 6-8 glasses daily of fresh fruit and vegetable juices, herb teas and water to help flush toxins through and out of your system.
6) Keep warm. Don't worry about a fever unless it is prolonged or very high. (See fevers as cleansers and healers, page 384).
7) Take a long hot bath, spa or sauna. Lots of toxins pass out though the skin. Increase room humidity so your mucous membranes will remain active against the virus or bacteria.
8) Stay relaxed. Let your body concentrate energy on cleaning out infection. Go to bed early, and get plenty of sleep. Most regeneration of cells occurs between midnight and 4 a.m.
9) Think positively about becoming well. Optimism is often a selffulfilling prophecy.

Do You Have a Cold or The Flu? Here's How to Tell.

Colds and flu are distinct and separate upper respiratory infections, triggered by different viruses. (Outdoor environment - drafts, wetness, temperature changes, etc. do not cause either of these illnesses.) The flu is more serious, because it can spread to the lungs, and cause severe bronchitis or pneumonia. In the beginning stages, the symptoms of colds and flu can be similar. Both conditions begin when one or more of the over 200 hundred viruses that cause a cold or flu penetrate the body's protective barriers. Viruses don't breathe, digest food or eliminate, but they replicate themselves with a vengeance. Nose, eyes and mouth are usually the sites of invasion from cold viruses. The most likely target for the flu virus is the respiratory tract. Colds and flu respond to different treatments. The following symptomatic chart can help identify your particular condition and allow you to deal with it better.

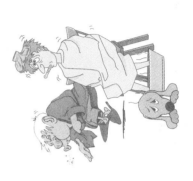

A Cold Profile Looks Like This:
   —Slow onset. No prostration.
   —Body aches - largely due to the release of interferon (an immune stimulator).
   —Rarely accompanied by fever and headache.
   —Localized symptoms such as sore throat, sinus congestion, listlessness, runny nose and sneezing.
   —Mild fatigue and weakness as a result of body cleansing.
   —Mild to moderate chest discomfort, usually with a hacking cough.
   —Sore or burning throat common.

A Flu Profile Looks Like This:
   —Swift and severe onset.
   —Early and prominent prostration with flushed, hot, moist skin.
   —Usually accompanied by high (102° -104°) fever, headache and sore eyes.
   —General symptoms like chills, depression and body aches.
   —Extreme fatigue, sometimes lasting 2-3 weeks.
   —Acute chest discomfort, with severe hacking cough.
   —Sore throat occasionally.

Can't find a recommended product? Call the 800 number listed in Product Resources for the store nearest you.

Cold Sores, Canker Sores, Fever Blisters
Mouth Herpes (Simplex 1)

Mouth sores caused by the Herpes Simple 1 virus are quite common. They're highly contagious - you can get them from kissing, or sharing eating utensils, drinking glasses, even a towel. Sores crop up about 20 days after exposure. They ususally indicate recurrent body chemistry imbalance, occurring after a fever, illness, body stress, and resulting reduced immunity, sometimes coupled with a hypothyroid condition or triggered by a food allergy. They can occur on the lips, tongue, inside the cheeks or on the gums. They can also be caused by nutrient deficiencies, or hormone imbalance. Mouth sores occur most often in women, generally because of hormone imbalances during the menstrual cycle. They are more prevalent in winter than warm months, unless the lips get sunburned.

Diet & Superfood Therapy

Nutritional therapy plan:

1—Body pH balance is important: Add more cultured foods to your diet for prevention: yogurt, kefir, raw sauerkraut, etc. Add sea greens (2 TBS snipped, dried) to your daily diet for a month.

2—Eat a mineral-rich diet: plenty of salads, lots of raw and cooked vegetables, whole grains; baked potatoes and steamed broccoli are especially good.

3—Avoid high arginine foods, such as coffee, peanut butter, nuts, seeds, corn, etc. Avoid nightshade plants like eggplant and peppers.

4—Avoid red meats, caffeine, refined and fried foods, especially sugary foods and sweet fruits.

5—Drink a fresh carrot juice once a week.

—Tannins and bioflavonoids help. Apply:
• Red wine residues
• Black and green tea - apply cold tea bags
• Grapes and grape juice
• Apples and apple juice
• Strawberries

—Effective superfoods: (choose 1 or 2)
• Crystal Star SYSTEMS STRENGTH™ drink to alkalize the body. Take BIOFLAV., FIBER & C SUPPORT drink for flavonoids.
• Red Star NUTRITIONAL YEAST, take 2 TBS daily.

Herb & Supplement Therapy

—Interceptive therapy plan: (Choose 2 to 3 recommendations)

1—**Reduce pain and inflammation:** Apply myrrh tincture; • take Crystal Star HRPS™ capsules 6 daily; • Crystal Star ANTI-FLAM™ to reduce pain and inflammation. Take daily and apply • *Echinacea-goldenseal* extract. Take • Ester C or ascorbate vitamin C crystals with bioflavonoids - ¼ teasp. every 2-3 hours in juice. Also make a strong solution in water and apply directly to sores every half hour until they subside. • Or apply CAT'S CLAW drops.♂

2—**Fight the virus:** • Take St. John's wort capsules or • Crystal Star ANTI-VI™ extract. • Apply St. John's wort salve. • Source Naturals RED ALGAE. • Take L-lysine 500mg 4x daily, to arrest virus replication; apply • Crystal Star LYSINE-LICORICE GEL™ or apply SUPER LYSINE PLUS cream on blisters.; Propolis lozenges - apply propolis extract directly, and take under the tongue to boost immune response, or use • Beehive Botanicals PROPOLIS THROAT SPRAY.

3—**Rebalance your body:** • Crystal Star RELAX CAPS™ as needed to calm the tension; • Burdock tea 2 cups daily to balance hormones. ♀ • Licorice extract, or Crystal Star GINSENG-LICORICE ELIXIR™, or a mouthwash made from • deglycyrrhizinated licorice chewable tablets - apply directly, take internally. • B Complex 100mg. daily with extra B₆ 250mg, and pantothenic acid 100mg 3x daily. • Prof. Nutrition DR. DOPHILUS, or Natren LIFE BIFIDO-FACTORS, ¼ teasp. 4x daily in water to rinse mouth 3x daily.

Proteolytic enzyme therapy for better body pH: • Bromelain 1500mg for 7 days; • Enzymatic Therapy DGL tabs 3 or 4 times daily.

4—**Heal your skin:** • Diamond HERPANACINE tablets as directed. • Enzymatic Therapy HERPILYN cream. • Apply geranium essential oil. ♀

—Effective herbal mouthwashes: swish around in mouth several times daily.
• White oak extract, an astringent; • Chamomile flowers tea; • Lemon balm tea.

—Homeopathic remedies: Hylands Hylavir; Natrum Muriaticum; Rhus Tox.

Lifestyle Support Therapy

—Bodywork:
• During the acute stage: Apply Nutribiotic GRAPEFRUIT SEED SKIN SPRAY as needed.

—Effective rinses to normalize mouth pH: Swish in mouth every half hour.
• Echinacea tea.
• Goldenseal tea, or *goldenseal-myrrh* tea.
• Aloe vera juice (also apply *aloe vera* gel).
• Salty water

—Effective topical applications:
• *Calendula* ointment
• Witch hazel
• Black walnut hulls tincture
• Tea tree oil as needed.
• Comfrey-aloe salve
• Lemon balm cream
• B & T homeopathic SSSTING STOP

• Apply ice packs frequently to stop movement of virus from nerves to the skin. Follow with vitamin E oil.

• Relax more. Get plenty of sleep and rest. Use sunblock more often.

See IMMUNITY page in this book for extra help.

Common Symptoms: Highly contagious herpes simplex virus sores on the face and mouth. (Don't kiss if you have a cold sore.) They begin with a small, sore bump, and turning into a very sore, often pussy blister. Lips and inside of the mouth are usually also sore. Accompanying flu like symptoms or a fever aren't unusual.

Common Causes: Herpes simplex virus 1; B Complex, iron or folic acid deficiency; high arginine foods diet; reduced immunity; Sodium-lauryl-sulfate toothpaste; premenstrual tension and consequent hormone imbalance; Crohn's disease; gluten sensitivity; over-acid diet; recurring virus infection; emotional stress. Check your toothpaste. It should be sodium-lauryl-sulfate free.

Can't find a recommended product? Call the 800 number listed in Product Resources for the store nearest you.

Colitis, Irritable Bowel Syndrome
Ulcerative Colitis, Spastic Colon, Ilietis

A chronically inflamed, painful colon is often a result of food allergies (65%), usually a gluten reaction to wheat, or cheese, corn or egg or other sensitivity. Lactose intolerance symptoms mimic those of IBS and colitis. Most victims are women between 20 and 40 with stressful jobs or lifestyles. Colon membranes become irritated, and the body forms pouchy pockets in reaction. In severe cases, ulcerous lesions line the sides of the colon (ulcerative colitis). Natural therapies are effective and reduce the need for drugs. Many sufferers see dramatic results. Diet changes are a must. Healing herbs and supplements will not work without diet changes. If there is appendicitis-like sharp pain, seek medical help immediately.

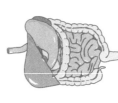

C 356

Diet & Superfood Therapy

Nutritional therapy plan:

1–**During the acute stage:** Go on a mono diet for 2 days with apples and apple juice.

2–Then eat a low fat diet with plenty of fiber, but low roughage. Foods should be lightly cooked, never fried, with few salts.

3–Include fresh fruits, fruit fiber from prunes, apples and raisins, green salads with olive oil and lemon dressing, whole grain cereals like oatmeal or brown rice (not wheat), and steamed veggies.

4–Have a glass of mixed vegetable juice (page 218) daily for the first two weeks. Have fresh carrot juice at least 3x a week. Keep your body well-hydrated - 6 to 8 glasses of water a day.

5–Eat cultured foods, such as yogurt and kefir for friendly intestinal flora.

6–Eat smaller, frequent meals. No large meals.

7–Clean up your diet: Avoid coffee and caffeine foods: nuts, seeds, dairy and citrus while healing. Cut back on saturated fat as much as possible. Eliminate refined sugars, sorbitol and wheat foods (the most irritating) of all kinds. Spicy foods are an irritant.

—**Effective superfoods: (choose 1 or 2)**
• Crystal Star CHO-LO FIBER TONE™ drink at bedtime for 2 weeks.
• Wakunaga KYO-GREEN.
• AloeLife FIBER MATE drink.

Herb & Supplement Therapy

Liquid and chewable supplements are best for colitis irritation.

—**Interceptive therapy plan: (Choose 2 to 3 recommendations)**

1–**Relieve the pain and inflammation:** • Take una da gato extract, 3 capsules or 3 droppers daily (cat's claw- usual results occur in 5 days); • peppermint oil or Now PEPEPERMINT oil is a specific for colitis and IBS, 2 capsules 3x daily, or 5 drops in tea. I like • Crystal Star GREEN TEA CLEANSER™ 2 cups daily with up to 5 peppermint oil drops added, 2x daily. • Glutamine 500mg 4x daily. • Take Planetary Formulas TRIPHALA caps or • Crystal Star BWL-TONE IBS™ (results within 2 to 3 days). • Curcumin caps twice daily; • High Omega-3 flax oil 3 capsules daily.

Effective anti-spasmodics: • Crystal Star RELAX CAPS™, • ANTI-SPZ caps or • CRAMP BARK COMPLEX™ extract. • Apply warm ginger compresses to spine and stomach.

2–**Neutralize or remove the allergen:** • Crystal Sar BITTERS & LEMON CLEANSE™ drops, or • Milk Thistle Seed drops in water each morning.

3–**Soothe the intestines:** Take • chamomile tea 4 cups daily; • slippery elm or pau d'arco tea as needed; • Take an electrolyte replacement drink if there is diarrhea.

4–**Calm tension:** • Crystal Star VALERIAN-WILD LETTUCE extract drops in water or scullcap tea.

5–**Enzyme therapy rebalances the entire digestive system:** • Bromelain 750mg 2x daily; • American Health papaya enzyme chewables; • Biotec BIO-GESTIN; • pancreatin 1400mg before meals. • Alta Health CANGEST powder (especially for wheat allergies); • Enzymatic Therapy chewable DGL tabs before meals, PEPPERMINT PLUS (enteric-coated peppermint oil) between meals and GUGGUL-PLUS each morning. • Natren TRINITY powder in water to rebalance bowel flora.

6–**Immune system support is crucial:** • Allergy Research Group NAG 500mg or Source Naturals Glucosamine sulfate 500mg for mucous membrane health. • Royal Jelly with ginseng 2 teasp. daily in water. • Sun Wellness chlorella powder in water or • chlorophyll liquid 3 teasp. daily in water before meals; • Bee pollen 2 teasp. daily.

Lifestyle Support Therapy

—**Watchwords:**
• Do not take aspirin. Use an herbal analgesic, or non-aspirin pain killer.
• Avoid antacids. They often do more harm than good by neutralizing body HCl.
• Consciously practice relaxation techniques like meditation to reduce stress.

—**Bodywork:**
• Effective gentle enemas to rid the colon of fermenting wastes and relieve pain:
  –Peppermint tea
  –White oak bark
  –Slippery elm
  –Chamomile
  –Lobelia
• Reduce stress: Biofeedback is especially helpful for IBS.
• Acupressure helps: Stroke abdomen up, across and down.

Common Symptoms: First symptoms include weakness, lethargy and fatigue; then abdominal cramps, distention and pain (relieved by bowel movements); recurrent constipation, usually alternating with bloody diarrhea; rectal hemorrhoids, fistulas and abscesses; mucous in the stool; urgency to defecate; dehydration and mineral loss; unhealthy weight loss with abdominal distention.

Common Causes: Excess refined foods and sweets; lack of dietary fiber; food allergies; yeast disease like candida albicans; heavy smoking and/ or caffeine use; vitamin K deficiency; anemia and electrolyte imbalance; emotional stress, depression and anxiety; too many antibiotics, causing reduced immunity; a small number of cases are genetically prone.

See also CROHN'S DISEASE page 360 for more information.

Can't find a recommended product? Call the 800 number listed in Product Resources for the store nearest you.

Constipation & Waste Management
Colon and Bowel Health

The colon and bowel are the depository for all waste material after food nutrients are extracted and processed into the bloodstream. Decaying food ferments, forms gases as well as 2nd, even 3rd generation toxins, and the colon becomes a breeding ground for putrefactive bacteria, viruses, parasites, yeasts and more. Most naturopaths believe that this old, infected material in bowel pockets (diverticulosis), which often reabsorbs into the body and nearby organs, is a cause for up to 90% of all disease. Ideally, one should eliminate after each meal, but some experts say the average American is 50,000 bowel movements short over a lifetime because our bowels are so sluggish. Bowel transit time should be about 12 hours. Healthy intestines are your body's second immune system. Take in plenty of fiber and liquids, exercise regularly and have a regular daily time for elimination.

Diet & Superfood Therapy

Nutritional therapy plan:

1—Start with a short colon cleansing juice diet (pg. 200). A glass of lemon juice and water starts your cleanse right.

2—Fiber foods, like prunes are the diet key - most experts recommend 40-45 grams daily: fiber isn't digested; it simply moves through your system, helping other foods move along with it.

Make an easy fiber drink: mix equal parts of flax seed and oat bran in water. Let sit overnight. Take 2 TBS in the morning in juice.

3—Follow a low fat, largely vegetarian diet, with plenty of intestinal brooms - fruits, whole grains, greens, veggies and cultured foods like yogurt.

4—Avoid high fat, sugary, fried foods and dairy foods; they don't allow your body to get rid of waste easily.

5—Drink 6-8 glasses of healthy liquids every day; avoid cow's milk and dairy drinks.

6—Chew food well, and eat smaller meals.

—Effective superfoods: (choose 1 or 2)

•Crystal Star BIOFLAV., FIBER & C SUP-PORT™ drink for 3 gms. fiber per serving, or CHO-LO-FIBER TONE™ drink.
•Aloe Falls ALOE JUICE with GINGER.
•Nutricology PRO GREENS with flax.
•Solgar WHEY TO GO protein drink.
•Green Kamut Corp. GREEN KAMUT.

Herb & Supplement Therapy

—Interceptive therapy plan: (Choose 2 to 3 recommendations)

1—Cleanse the body of old wastes: •Crystal Star FIBER & HERBS COLON CLEANSE™ capsules 2, 3x daily (one to three months for a complete cleanse). •Nature's Secret A.M./P.M. ULTIMATE CLEANSE. •Earth's Bounty OXY-CLEANSE removes old hardened wastes.

For a quick occasional cleanse- •take 3000 to 5000mg vitamin C with bioflavonoids over a two hour period; or •Crystal Star LAXA-TEA™ to flush wastes gently over a 24-hour period; or •Zand QUICK CLEANSE.

2—Prevent constipation: Omega-3 flax seed oil caps; magnesium 400mg daily; •Probiotics prevent constipation and overcome antibiotic residues: •Professional Nutrition Dr. DOPHILUS with FOS; •Solaray MULTI-DOPHILUS; •Transformation PLANTADOPHILUS powder (also helps liver function); •Prevail INNER ECOLOGY. Note: Think twice about taking drugstore antibiotics, antacids and milk of magnesia. They kill friendly intestinal flora.

3—Normalize digestion and intestinal functions: •Solaray TETRA CLEANSE or •Nature's Way 5 SYSTEM CLEANSE; •Fennel-ginger caps 4 daily; •Garlic caps, 4 daily; •Turmeric or •goldenseal-myrrh extract drops in water enhance bile flow.

4—Promote a healthy, odor-free stool: •Planetary Formulas TRIPHALA as directed; •Milk thistle seed, or dandelion extract enhance bile output and soften stool.

5—Natural laxatives and regulators: •Bee pollen 2 tsp. daily; •Senna leaf/pods (sparingly, a little goes a long way); una da gato caps 6 daily; •Cascara caps increase peristalsis.

6—Enzyme therapy re-establishes acid-alkaline balance: •Prevail FIBER-ZYME 2x daily; •Papaya enzymes 1000mg daily, to digest milk proteins and sugars. •Peppermint or ginger tea provide plant enzymes that specifically balance digestion.

7—Add food-source fiber: (Take a food source multi-vitamin to control initial gas and stomach rumbling as the additional dietary fiber combines with the minerals in the G.I. tract.) •AloeLife FIBER-MATE drink; •Apple pectin tabs; •Maitake mushroom holds moisture in bowel-increases peristalsis.

Lifestyle Support Therapy

—Bodywork:

•Fiber is your body's best friend. A protective level of fiber in your diet can be measured:
1) the stool should be light enough to float.
2) bowel movements should be regular, daily and effortless.
3) the stool should be almost odorless, signalling less transit time in the bowel.
4) there should be no gas or flatulence.

•Take a colonic irrigation to start your program. A grapefruit seed extract colonic is extremely effective; a wheat grass retention enema is effective if there is colon toxicity along with constipation. (Dilute to 15 to 20 drops per gallon of water.)

•Consider a catnip enema once a week to keep cleansing going. (See page 539) Note: Enemas may be given to children. Use small amounts according to size and age. Allow water to enter very slowly; let them to expel when they wish.

•Take a daily walk to stimulate regularity.
•Stroke and press each reflexology point for 5 minutes:

colon points

Common Symptoms: Infrequent bowel movements; flatulence and gas; fatigue, nausea and depression; nervous irritability; coated tongue; headaches; bad breath and body odor; mental dullness; sallow skin.
Common Causes: Poor diet with too little fiber, and too much fast, fried, sugary, low-residue foods; often food allergies to cheese and cow's milk, especially in kids; drugs, travel and stress all affect bowel regularity; too much red meat, pasteurized dairy, caffeine and alcohol; overeating and eating late at night; overuse of drugs and laxatives; hypothyroidism; lack of exercise.

Can't find a recommended product? Call the 800 number listed in Product Resources for the store nearest you.

Step-By-Step Diet Change For Colon Health

Most poor health conditions stem from poor elimination in some way. Elements causing constipation and colon toxicity come from three basic areas:

1) **Chemical-laced foods, and pollutants in the environment, ranging from relatively harmless to very dangerous.** The body can tolerate a certain level of contamination. When that individual level is reached, and immune defenses are low, toxic overload causes illness. A strong system can metabolize and excrete many of these toxins, but when the body is weak or constipated, they are stored as unusable substances. As more and different chemicals enter and build up in the body they tend to interreact with those that are already there, forming mutant, second generation chemicals far more harmful than the originals. Evidence in recent years has shown that much bowel cancer is caused by environmental agents.

2) **Over-accumulation of body wastes and metabolic byproducts that are not excreted properly.** Unreleased wastes can also become a breeding ground for parasite infestation. A nationwide survey reveals that one in every six people studied has one or more parasites living somewhere in their bodies! An astounding figure.

3) **Slowed elimination time, allowing waste materials to ferment, become rancid, and then recirculate** through the body tissues as toxic substances, usually resulting in sluggish organ and glandular functions, poor digestion and assimilation, lowered immunity, faulty circulation, and tissue degeneration.

The key to avoiding bowel problems is almost always nutritional. A high fiber, low fat diet, with lots of fresh foods is important to both cure and prevent waste elimination problems. Diet improvement can also correct the diseases waste elimination problems cause. Even a gentle and gradual change is often better than a sudden, drastic about-face, especially when the colon, bowel or bladder are painful and inflamed. Constipation is normally a chronic problem, and while body cleansing progress can be felt fairly quickly with a diet change, it takes from three to six months to rebuild bowel and colon elasticity with good systolic/diastolic action. There is no easy route, but the rewards of a regular, energetic life are worth it. See also THE BODY SMART SYSTEM by Helene Silver for more information.

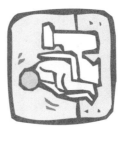

After the initial cleansing juice diet, (see page 200), the second part of a good colon health program is rebuilding healthy tissue and body energy. This stage may be used for 1 to 2 months. It emphasizes high fiber through fresh vegetables and fruits, cultured foods for increased assimilation and enzyme production, and alkalizing foods to prevent irritation while healing. During this diet avoid refined foods, saturated fats or oils, fried foods, meats, caffeine or other acid or mucous forming foods, such as pasteurized dairy products.

On rising: take a glass of Herbal Answers HERBAL ALOE FORCE JUICE with herbs, with 1 teasp. liquid acidophilus added; or Crystal Star CHO-LO FIBER TONE™ capsules or drink in apple or orange juice.

Breakfast: soak a mix of dried prunes, figs and raisins the night before; take 2 to 4 TBS with 1 TB blackstrap molasses, or mix with yogurt; or make a mix of flax seed, oat bran, raisins, and pumpkin seeds, and mix with yogurt or apple juice, or a light veggie broth. Add 2 teasp. brewer's yeast or Lewis Labs FIBER YEAST; and have some oatmeal or a whole grain cereal, granola or muesli with yogurt or apple juice; or have a bowl of mixed fresh fruits with apple juice or yogurt.

Mid-morning: take a veggie drink (page 218), Sun Wellness CHLORELLA, Green Foods GREEN ESSENCE, or Crystal Star ENERGY GREEN™ drink; or pau d'arco, green tea or Crystal Star GREEN TEA CLEANSER™ to alkalize the system; or a fresh carrot juice.

Lunch: have a fresh green salad every day with lemon/olive oil dressing, or yogurt cheese or kefir cheese; or steamed veggies and a baked potato with soy or kefir cheese; or a fresh fruit salad with a little yogurt or raw cottage cheese topping.

Mid-afternoon: have another fresh carrot juice, or Crystal Star SYSTEMS STRENGTH™ drink; and/or green tea or slippery elm tea; and-or some raw crunchy veggies with a vegetable or kefir cheese dip, or soy spread.

Dinner: have a large dinner salad with black bean or lentil soup; or an oriental stir fry and miso soup with sea vegetables snipped on top; or a steamed or baked vegetable casserole with a yogurt or soy cheese sauce; or a vegetable or whole grain pasta with a light lemon or yogurt sauce.

Before bed: have some apple or papaya juice; or another glass of aloe vera juice with herbs; or Crystal Star CHOL-LO FIBER TONE™ drink or capsules, or BIOFLAV, FIBER & C SUPPORT™ drink.

Can't find a recommended product? Call the 800 number listed in Product Resources for the store nearest you.

C 358

Cough

Chronic Cough, Dry, Hacking Cough, Smoker's Cough

Coughs are one of the main signs of an inflammatory respiratory tract infection. It's a body defense mechanism, a protective reflex for cleansing the trachea and bronchial tree of excess mucous and toxic material. A continuing cough, however (one that lasts more than 2 or 3 weeks), is not usually the result of infection per se, but evidence of continuing throat irritation from smoking, environmental pollens, or chemical pollutants. It should be regarded as a sign of reduced immune response and treated both topically, and as part of an immune-stimulating program.

Diet & Superfood Therapy

Nutritional therapy plan:

1—Start with a short colon cleansing juice diet (pg. 200) to rid the bowel of current wastes. Avoid all dairy products during acute stages.

2—Take 2 TBS honey and 2 TBS lemon juice in water or cider vinegar to stop the tickle; or take a cup of hot black tea with the juice of 1 lemon and 1 teasp. honey.

3—Take a cup of hot water with 2 TBS brandy and 2 TBS lemon juice to help stop a cough at night.

4—Drink cleansing fruit juices. Eat high vitamin C foods, such as sprouts, green peppers, broccoli, citrus and cherries.

5—Help your body expel mucous if your cough is from a cold: eat hot, pungent foods like chilies and garlic to bring up phlegm.

—Make your own honey/onion cough syrup: Slice a large onion into rings and place in a bowl. Cover with honey and let stand 24 hours. Strain off liquid mixture and you have an anti-microbial cough elixir.

—**Effective superfoods: (choose 1 or 2)**
• Crystal Star BIOFLAV., FIBER & C SUPPORT™ drink.
• Aloe vera juice with herbs.
• Y.S. ROYAL JELLY with ginseng drink.

Herb & Supplement Therapy

—**Interceptive therapy plan: (Choose 2 to 3 recommendations)**

1—**Soothe and control the cough:** • Crystal Star COFEX TEA™, especially at night. Usually works in 24 hours. • Herbs, Etc. OSHA ROOT COMPLEX syrup.

2—**Get rid of excess mucous:** • Crystal Star X-PECT™ TEA as an expectorant; • Herbs, Etc. RESPIRATONIC and • Echinacea to release mucous.

3—**Reduce throat inflammation:** • Crystal Star ANTI-SPZ™ capsules, 4 at a time for spasmodic coughing, or • Nature's Way SORE THROAT (homeopathic).

4—**Overcome the infection:** • Propolis extract under the tongue or lozenges as desired, or • Beehive Botanicals PROPOLIS THROAT SPRAY; • Garlic capsules 6 daily; • Nature's Path THROAT-LYTE.

6—**Strengthen immune response:** • Beta-carotene 25,000IU 2x daily. • Ascorbate vitamin C or Ester C powder: $\frac{1}{4}$ teasp. every half hour to bowel tolerance.

—**Use these topicals directly on the throat (choose 1):** • Crystal Star GINSENG-LICORICE ELIXIR™ drops; • slippery elm lozenges; • Zinc gluconate lozenges, or • Zand HERBAL lozenges; • horehound, licorice or wild cherry drops or syrups; • Olbas Cough Syrup and pastilles.

• Make the popular thyme-honey cough syrup: put 3 TBS thyme leaves in a quart jar. Add 2 cups boiling water. Close lid and let steep til cool. Strain off liquid; add 1 cup honey, a 1" piece ginger or a piece of orange peel. Refrigerate. Take 1 teasp. every hour as needed.

—**Cough teas or head steams (choose 1):** • Wild cherry to suppress a cough; • Clove tea for spasmodic coughing; • Marshmallow for a dry cough; • Coltsfoot for a cough with mucous (small amounts only); • Sage-rosehips tea with lemon juice, honey, and ginger root.

—**Effective homeopathic remedies (choose 1):** • BioForce Biotussin drops and tabs; • Hylands Cough Syrup; • B&T Cough Syrup; • Standard Hylavir tablets.

Lifestyle Support Therapy

—**Bodywork:**
• Eliminate smoking and secondary smoke from your environment.

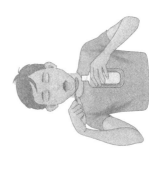

• Effective gargles:
   Tea tree oil drops in water
   Slippery elm tea
   Aloe vera juice
   Echinacea-goldenseal solution

• Steam eucalyptus, peppermint or tincture of benzoin in a vaporizer at night to clear respiratory passages.

• Avoid commercial cough syrups, and drugstore over-the-counter medicines. They often make the problem worse by suppression, which forces the infection deeper into the tissues.

Common Symptoms: Hacking, dry or chronic coughing with no phlegm or mucous eliminated; a reflex reaction to an obstruction of the airways; chronic, rough smoker's-throat cough from constant irritation.
Common Causes: Low grade chronic infection of throat and sinuses (often the hanging-on result of a cold or flu); mucous-forming diet; allergies; environmental irritants; cigarette smoking or secondary smoking irritation.

See SORE THROAT, COLDS AND FLU pages in this book for more information.

Can't find a recommended product? Call the 800 number listed in Product Resources for the store nearest you.

Crohn's Disease
Regional Enteritis

More than 30,000 Americans are diagnosed each year with Crohn's disease, chronic inflammation of the digestive tract. It affects about 2 million Americans today and its incidence is rising. It is characterized by painful ulcers that form in one or more sections, or all along the length of the gastrointestinal lining. When the ulcers heal they leave thick scar tissue that narrows and hardens the tract and adversely affects elimination. Poor assimilation of nutrients is always involved; accompanying ulcerous bleeding often causes anemia. A strictly followed, highly nutritious, mild foods diet is an effective, non-toxic alternative to cortico-steroid drugs. Crohn's disease sufferers can react to almost anything, no matter how mild or soothing. Start slowly, noting your reactions carefully.

Diet & Superfood Therapy

—Nutritional therapy plan:

1—Nutrition spells relief for Crohn's: Start with an alkalizing liquid diet for 3 days: carrot and apple juice, grape juice, pineapple and green vegetable drinks.

2—Add mild fruits and vegetables for a week: carrots, lettuce, potatoes, yams, apples, papayas, bananas and sea greens. Add steamed and raw vegetables, brans, cultured foods for 2 weeks: yogurt, kefir, miso, etc., and especially fresh salads.

3—Add rice, whole grains, wheat germ, tofu, fish and seafood for healing protein and EFA's.

4—Your continuing diet should be high in fiber and fresh vegetables, and low in fats. (Avoid too much fiber during flare-ups.)

5—Most people experience relief with a disaccharide-free diet - mainly avoid table sugar and milk sugars.

6—Avoid foods like popcorn, nuts, seeds, and citrus while healing. Eliminate red and fatty meats, saturated fats (especially from dairy and fried foods) and chemicalized foods.

7—Drink only bottled water. Over-treated tap water can wreak havoc on an inflamed bowel.

—Effective superfoods: (choose 1 or 2) ☿

• Lewis Labs FIBER YEAST each A.M. ☿
• AloeLife ALOE GOLD JUICE.
• Solgar WHEY TO GO protein drink.

Herb & Supplement Therapy

Use liquid or powdered supplements whenever possible for the least irritation.

—Interceptive therapy plan: (Choose 2 to 3 recommendations)

1—Ease the pain: •Crystal Star ANTI-FLAM™ extract in water to ease pain without aspirin salicylates. •Una da gato caps 4 to 6 daily; •Enzymatic Therapy IBS capsules and with chewable DGL tablets as needed. ♀

2—Reduce inflammation with essential fatty acids (EFA's): •Evening primrose oil caps 200mg daily; •Omega-3 flax oil 2 TBS daily, or Barleans FLAX caps 3 daily.

3—Normalize your bowel functions: •Crystal Star BWL TONE™ caps with GREEN TEA CLEANSER™ for 3 months. •ALOE VERA JUICE 4 glasses daily; •Mix 1 teasp. bee pollen in a cup of chamomile tea - take 2x daily. •Garlic capsules 4-6 daily. •Enzymatic Therapy LIQUID LIVER with Siberian ginseng. **Plant enzyme therapy normalizes quickly:** •Quercetin with bromelain 750mg; or •chewable bromelain 40mg or papaya enzymes after meals ♂ or •Solaray QBC complex; •Planetary TRIPHALA caps as directed.

4—Heal injured, damaged tissues: •Crystal Star ZINC SOURCE™ herbal drops; •Emulsified vitamin A and E drops 2x daily; •Pau d' Arco tea; •Bilberry or Hawthorn extract several times daily in rose hips tea.

5—Antioxidants scavenge free radicals to re-establish immune response: •Glutamine 500mg - as effective as prednisone in controlling Crohn's and GI integrity. •Ascorbate vitamin C with bioflavonoids powder, 1/4 teasp. 4 to 6x daily. •OPC's from grapeseed, 50mg 3x daily. •Y.S. ROYAL JELLY with ginseng drink.

5—Reculture your friendly flora: •Professional Nutr. DOCTOR-DOPHILUS + FOS; •Wakunaga KYO-DOPHILUS; •Natren TRINITY powder 1/4 teasp. 3x daily, before meals. •Flora ESSENCE liquid, 2-oz. daily in a cup of fenugreek tea. ♀

6—Replace depleted nutrients: •Flora FLORADIX MULTI-VITAMIN; •Real Life Research sublingual TOTAL B; •Country Life sublingual B-12, 2500mcg; •Zinc picolinate 15-30mg daily; ♂ •Magnesium 200mg 3x daily.

Lifestyle Support Therapy

—Lifestyle measures:

• Avoid commercial antacids. They eventually make the inflammation worse by causing the stomach to produce more acids.

• Consciously work to reduce stress in your life. Acupuncture, yoga and meditation have all been successful with Crohn's.

—Bodywork:

• Eat smaller meals, more frequently.
• Use peppermint tea enemas once a week for the first month of healing.
• Apply hot, wet ginger compresses to stomach and lower back.

—Reflexology points:

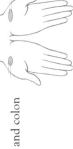

stomach and colon

—Crohn's disease region:

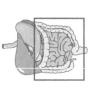

Common Symptoms: Inflammation and soreness along the entire G.I. tract (early signs are diarrhea and abdominal pain below the navel); bouts of diarrhea with a low grade fever; raised white blood cell counts; abdominal distention, tenderness and pain from food residue and gas; abnormal weight loss and depression; anemia. Intolerance to wheat foods (celiac disease is common in Crohn's sufferers).
Common Causes: A diet with low fiber, excess refined sugar and acid-forming foods, leading to a severely inflamed colon which forms deep ulcers along the entire length of the digestive tract from rectum to mouth. Smoking is a risk factor. Malnutrition is common in Crohn's disease. Multiple food intolerances - as in candida yeast overgrowths - are common; emotional stress; zinc deficiency.

For a Crohn's friendly practitioner, call the California Naturopathic Assn. (530) 676-4842. See also DIVERTICULITIS page 371 and COLITIS page 356.

Can't find a recommended product? Call the 800 number listed in Product Resources for the store nearest you.

Cysts & Polyps
Benign Tumors, Lipomas, Wens

Benign growths of varying size · found both internally on the intestinal, urethral, genital passage linings, and externally anywhere on the skin. They often arise from an excessive growth of fat cells. They are responsive to the body's growth-regulating mechanisms and quite receptive to natural therapies. They can be annoying, unsightly, and in some cases lead to cancer.

Diet & Superfood Therapy

—**Nutritional therapy plan:**

1—Go on a short 1 to 3 day liquid diet (page 191) to set up a healing environment, stimulate the liver and clean the blood. Then follow with a fresh foods diet for the rest of the week.

2—Avoid red meats, caffeine, pasteurized dairy products and acid-forming foods.

3—Eliminate saturated fats (mostly animal fats), fried foods, chocolate, margarine, shortening and other refined fats.

4—Add red peppers with plenty of capsaicin to your diet.

5—Add more fish, seafoods, sea vegetables and unsaturated oils, such as flax and sunflower oil to the diet.

—**Effective superfoods: (choose 1 or 2)**
• Crystal Star SYSTEMS STRENGTH™ drink.
• Monas CHLORELLA- anti-tumor properties.
• Herbal Answers HERBAL ALOE FORCE JUICE, and apply ALOE FORCE SKIN gel.
• Add 1 TB wheat bran to any can of BE WELL JUICE daily for 3 months to prevent colon polyps. Take in the morning. ♂

Herb & Supplement Therapy

—**Interceptive therapy plan: (Choose 2 to 3 recommendations)**

1—**If the growth is increasing in size:** • Crystal Star ANTI-BIO™ extract as an anti-infective, and apply ANTI-BIO™ gel directly. • Apply Nutribiotic GRAPE-FRUIT SEED EXTRACT directly, 2x daily, especially if the growth is increasing in size. • *Una da gato* caps 4 to 6 daily for 3 months; • *Pau d' arco* tea, 3 cups daily for a month. Take • *turmeric* caps 6 daily, (*curcumin*) extract 4x daily for 2 months. Add • Solaray CENTELLA ASIATICA caps 4 daily for cytotoxic effects.

•Make and apply an escharotic salve through which tumor cells can exit: equal parts *garlic powder, goldenseal powder, comfrey* or *cayenne* powder - mix into *calendula* ointment. Apply daily until tumor is destroyed, usually 4 weeks.

2—**Clear the lymph system and regulate your liver metabolism:** • *Echinacea* extract 2x daily; • *Chaparral* caps 6 daily for one month; • *Milk Thistle Seed* extract 4x daily; Diamond HERPANACINE caps 4 daily for 2 months. ♂

3—**Balance fat metabolism:** • *Evening primrose* oil 500mg 6 daily; • Omega-3 rich flax oil 2 TBS daily.

4—**Shield your immune warriors from toxins that aggravate tumor cells:** • Beta carotene 25,000IU 4x daily for a month; • Ascorbate vitamin C crystals with bioflavonoids ¼ teasp. 4x daily for a month; • CoQ-10 60mg 4x daily for a month; • Zinc picolinate 50mg 2x daily for a month, then 30mg daily for a month.

—**For lipomas and wens:** • Lane Labs BENE-FIN shark cartilage caps, 9 daily for 3 to 4 months; • Carnitine 500mg 2x daily; • high omega 3 flax oil 3x daily.
• I have used a version Michael Tierra's capsule formula several times with success for lipomas: Combine *pau d' arco, echinacea root, chaparral, red clover, poria mushroom, gotu kola, kelp and panax ginseng.* Take 4 daily for 2 months. ♂

—**For colon polyps:** • 1500mg daily calcium with Nature's Secret ULTIMATE A.M./P.M. CLEANSE; • Nutricology GERMANIUM 150mg daily; • Folic acid 400mcg; • Vitamin E 800IU with selenium 200mcg daily until condition clears. ♂

Lifestyle Support Therapy

—**Bodywork:**
• Homeopathic remedies work to reduce cysts and polyps. See a good homeopath who can recommend the correct treatment for your type of growth.

• Apply Crystal Star GINSENG SKIN RE-PAIR GEL™ (with germanium and vitamin C) for several weeks.

• Apply propolis extract directly. ♂
• Apply liquid garlic directly with a cotton swab.

• Apply *tea tree* oil for 4 to 6 weeks. ⚹
• Apply fresh *comfrey* compresses until cysts shrinks. ♂

• Scrub skin with a loofah or dry skin brush regularly to keep sebaceous glands unclogged.
• Massage into affected area daily, Earth's Bounty O₂ SPRAY for 3 weeks, for noticeable reduction without pain.
• Don't smoke. Nicotine aggravates gland imbalances that allow deposits to form.

Common Symptoms: A lump or bulge seen or felt under the skin (usually movable); in the case of vaginal cysts, there is often bleeding during intercourse; where there are colon, bladder or cervical polyps there is often rectal, urinal or vaginal bleeding; wens usually form over nerve ganglia.

Common Causes: Internal toxicity and infection; diet containing excess acid or mucous forming foods; poor assimilation/digestion of fats; for sebaceous cysts, gland outflow blocked with sebum deposits; accumulation of dead skin cells; local cosmetic irritants.

See FIBROIDS page 385 and TUMORS page 513 for more information.

Can't find a recommended product? Call the 800 number listed in Product Resources for the store nearest you.

Dandruff

Seborrheic Dermatitis, Pityriasis

Pityriasis (simple dandruff) is a dry skin problem, and can usually be controlled with a better diet, cleansing and brushing. Seborrheic dandruff appears as dry, flaky particles of skin in the hair. While it looks like a dry skin condition, it is actually the opposite - too much oil is produced, clogging the highly active sebaceous glands. Seborrhea appears when skin cells turn over at a faster rate than normal and break away in large flakes into the hair. Commercial dandruff preparations have become suspect because some contain coal tar, and some contain selenium sulfide a chemical that reduces the production of skin tissue and has been linked to hair loss (because it dries your hair out even more) and nerve damage. Diet improvement is the key to long term dandruff control for either kind of dandruff.

Diet & Superfood Therapy

—Nutritional therapy plan:

1—Eat vegetable proteins like soy, brewer's yeast and wheat germ, with plenty of fresh fruits and vegetables to keep your metabolically active scalp cells working right.

2—Reduce sugars, starchy foods and animal fats. Sugar depletes the body of B vitamins.

3—Eliminate fried foods. They clog the body so it can't eliminate wastes properly.

4—Avoid allergenic foods like dairy products, refined flours, chocolate, nuts and shellfish. These are sometimes involved with dandruff.

5—Add sulphur-rich foods: Lettuce, oats, green pepper, onions, cucumber, eggs, fish, cabbage, wheat germ.

6—Eat cultured products like yogurt and kefir to encourage healthy intestinal flora and better digestion.

—Superfood therapy: (Choose one or two)

• Crystal Star SYSTEMS STRENGTH™ for absorbable minerals.

• Crystal Star GREEN TEA CLEANSER™ to keep the system metabolically active.

• Nature's Life SUPER GREEN PRO-96, or Green Foods VEGGIE MAGMA, for extra vegetable protein.

• Nutricology PRO-GREENS with EFA's.

• Y.S. ROYAL JELLY 3-4 teasp. daily.

Herb & Supplement Therapy

—Interceptive therapy plan: (Choose 2 to 3 recommendations)

1—Control the flaking: Add a few drops • Nutribiotic GRAPEFRUIT SEED EXTRACT to shampoo and use daily; or use • Crystal Star ANTI-BIO™ extract or capsules with MINERAL SPECTRUM™ capsules. • Jason NATURAL JOJOBA SHAMPOO; • Rinse hair with cider vinegar after every wash to keep sebum deposits from clogging pores. • Use Rosemary/yarrow tea hair rinse.

2—Restore your scalp's natural oil balance with EFA's: • *Evening Primrose Oil* capsules for EFA's. • Ecco Bella NEEM SHAMPOO; • Omega-3 flax oils 3x daily.

Oil balancing herbal conditioning treatments 1) Mix the juice from fresh grated *ginger* with an equal amount of sesame oil. Rub on scalp at night. Rinse in the morning. Use for 1 week. 2) Steep *bay leaves* in olive oil until fragrant. Rub on scalp before shampoo. Leave on 30 minutes and shampoo out. 3) Massage *jojoba* or *rosemary* oil into scalp. Leave on 1 hour. Shampoo out. 4) Steep cider vinegar and *peppermint* oil drops in 1 cup water. Rinse hair.

3—Lubricate and balance with oil-based vitamins: • Take vitamin E 400IU with selenium 200mcg daily; • Schiff EMULSIFIED A & D; • Lecithin caps or choline/inositol caps, 2 daily; • Rainbow Light MULTI-CAROTENE COMPLEX; • Nature's Secret ULTIMATE OIL.

4—Nourish your skin-scalp with minerals: • Futurebiotics HAIR, SKIN, and NAILS tabs 2 daily; • Crystal Star SILICA SOURCE™ extract, or Flora VEGE-SIL for healthy hair growth. • Zinc picolinate 50mg 2x daily; • B Complex 100mg daily with extra B-6 100mg, folic acid 400mcg, PABA 1000mg and niacin 500mg for increased circulation; • Biotin 600mcg daily. • Mineral rich herbs like nettles and *chaparral* (also controls infection).

Lifestyle Support Therapy

—Bodywork:

• Avoid over-the-counter commercial ointments that often do more harm than good by clogging sebaceous glands.

• Get some regular circulation-stimulating exercise daily.

• Make your own disinfecting dandruff treatment: Add to a glass bowl, 1 small handfull each *nettles leaves, witch hazel* and *rosemary leaves.* Add enough boiling water to cover and let steep one hour. Strain. Add ¹⁄₂ teasp. tea tree oil. Pour mixture into a mild, unscented shampoo and use twice weekly.

• Use *jojoba, aloe vera,* biotin based or *tea tree* oil shampoo. Or *Oregon grape* hair rinse.

• Add drops of *tea tree* oil or *burdock* oil to any hair rinse; massage in - use daily.

• For oily scalp: apply about 1 cup white vinegar. Leave on 15 minutes. Rinse.

• For dry scalp: Mix 2 drops *vanilla* extract with 2 TBS mayonnaise. Massage into scalp. Put on a shower cap. Leave on 20 minutes. Rinse out.

• Massage head with both hands and all the fingers at once, for 5 minutes every day to stimulate scalp circulation and slough dead skin cells.

Common Symptoms: Scaling flakes on scalp, eyebrows and sometimes the face; redness, weeping and itching, burning scalp; sometimes a crust formation.
Common Causes: Sebaceous gland malfunction; an allergic reaction to a hair care product; too much alcohol, saturated fat, sugar and starch in the diet; a scalp imbalance caused by an essential fatty acid deficiency; lack of green vegetables; excessively strong or harsh hair dyes.

See also EczEMA-PsORIASIS page 375 for more information.

Can't find a recommended product? Call the 800 number listed in Product Resources for the store nearest you.

Dental Problems

Tooth Tartar and Plaque, Tooth Decay, Bruxism, Salivary Stones

Plaque is the film in which harmful mouth bacteria live, and it can begin to damage teeth and gums within 12 hours after a meal. It is important to brush at least twice a day and to floss or water-pick just before going to bed. Relax more. Stress reduces salivary flow allowing bacteria to flourish; although not all people with these fillings are sensitive to the mercury release, there seems to be no doubt that there are definite immuno-toxic effects for people who are. Mercury is a heavy metal that kills beneficial bacteria and allows resistant strains, which are also antibiotic-resistant, to flourish. The best choice is still to have the fillings gradually removed and replaced. After removal, go on a 2 to 3 month detox program to release the mercury from your bloodstream.

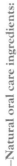

Diet & Superfood Therapy

—Nutritional therapy plan:

1—Eat crunchy teeth-cleaning foods: fresh vegetables, celery, carrots, broccoli, cauliflower, apples, etc. Chew well.

2—Eat high mineral foods for strong teeth - lots of green leafy vegetables and high fiber whole grains. Have a large fresh salad every day.

3—Focus on cranberries, cashews, cardamom seeds and especially green tea. All have anti-adhesion properties to arrest production of plaque acid and keep plaque from adhering to teeth. Strawberries are a good tooth cleanser. Rub strawberry halves on the teeth.

4—Reduce fats and sugars. A high fat diet results in high lipid levels in the saliva and a higher risk of tooth decay. Sugars significantly increase plaque accumulation. (Nibbling low fat cheese after eating sugar neutralizes cavity-causing acids.)

5—Avoid soft, gooey foods and dairy products like ice cream that leave a film on the teeth.

6—Add hot chili peppers that make your mouth water (also good sources of C). Add yogurt as a viable source of calcium for your teeth.

—Superfood therapy: (Choose one or two)

• Crystal Star GREEN TEA CLEANSER™ and BIOFLAV., FIBER & C SUPPORT™ drinks. ♀
• Sun Wellness CHLORELLA, 1 packet daily.

Herb & Supplement Therapy

Take care of your teeth. Studies show that the more natural teeth you are missing, the quicker you will age. If you're pregnant, breast-fed babies develop straighter teeth.

—Interceptive therapy plan: (Choose 2 to 3 recommendations)

1—**Boost antibacterial mouth activity:** • Crystal Star GINSENG-LICORICE ELIXIR™ extract drops in water as a mouthwash to inhibit bacteria and harmful sugars. • MICROBRITE, whitening powder available at Healthy House to remove and prevent tarter build-up; • Beehive Botanical PROPOLIS & HERBS THROAT SPRAY as needed. • *Eucalyptus* extract to prevent cavities; • *Neem* toothpaste helps remove tarter; • Bloodroot (*sanguinaria*) helps remove plaque.

2—**Rebuild tooth enamel:** • Crystal Star SILICA SOURCE™ extract drops in water as a mouthwash; or take • Flora VEGE-SIL caps 2 daily. • Apply baking soda mixed with water drops in a paste to teeth. Leave on 5 minutes to remineralize.

3—**Strengthen teeth and gums:** • Ester C crystals with bioflavs. and rutin, ¼ teasp. 3x daily in water. Swish and hold in mouth before swallowing for best results. Or, use Ester C chewables as needed. • *Spirulina* tabs 6 daily; or • Klamath POWER 3 capsules. Massage gums with • vitamin E oil; take internally 400IU daily.

4—**Control mouth infections:** • CoQ-10, 60mg 3x daily, or use Real Life Research SUBLINGUAL CoQ-10; • Myrrh drops as needed; • B complex 100mg daily; • Beehive Botanicals PROPOLIS TINCTURE, hold as long as possible. • Pain chewables; 🐝 • Omega-3 fatty acids like flax oil help control inflammation.

—For salivary duct stones: • Rinse mouth with equal parts *goldenseal root* and *white oak bark* tea to reduce swelling and bleeding. • Rinse mouth with *ginger root* tea; apply *ginger* compresses to area. • Rinse mouth with Crystal Star IODINE SOURCE™ extract in water or take *kelp* tabs 6 daily. • Alacer EMERGEN-C daily.

—For bruxism: take a calcium-magnesium-zinc combination daily to reduce stress. ♂

Lifestyle Support Therapy

Fluoride build-up is linked to health problems from skin eruptions to thyroid problems and immune weakening. (See Water page 146.)

—Bodywork:

• To remove tarter: Mix equal parts cream of tartar and sea salt, or baking soda and sea salt and scrub teeth.

• Floss daily. Nothing makes you look older than bad teeth.

—Natural oral care ingredients:

• Xylitol toothpaste (or sweetener) does not cause plaque formation.

• Papain powder helps kill harmful bacteria, is less abrasive than commercial toothpastes.

• *Tea tree oil* is anti-bacterial and anti-fungal for almost every mouth problem.

• Peelu has natural chlorine that whitens, removes tarter and controls plaque; it also has natural vitamin C.

• Propolis, a bee-collected product, is a natural immune booster and antibiotic.

—Make your own natural mouthwashes:

• Nutribiotic GRAPEFRUIT SEED EXTRACT in water as a mouthwash.

• Add 3 drops *tea tree oil* to water.

Common Symptoms: *Bad breath; noticeable sticky film on the teeth; bad mouth taste. Salivary stones cause swelling and pain in the jaw just in front of the ear, and a stone-like growth that blocks saliva.*
Common Causes: *Too many refined carbohydrates and sugars; excess red meat, caffeine and soft drinks that cause constipation and acid in the system; vitamin and fresh food deficiency; mercury poisoning from silver amalgam fillings; stress.*

See next two pages for more information.

Can't find a recommended product? Call the 800 number listed in Product Resources for the store nearest you.

Dental Problems

Toothaches, Wisdom Tooth Inflammation, TMJ (Temperomandibular Joint Syndrome)

An astonishing 90% of Americans have some form of gum disease or tooth decay. Almost 15 million Americans have lost all their teeth. Ignore them and you'll lose them. Many dentists now realize that you need to see a nutritionist along with a dentist if you have chronic toothaches and infections. The number one way to keep your mouth clean is to eat a natural diet. Natural healing wisdom about wisdom teeth - check to see that they're growing in straight; eat right so they don't decay; clean them well to keep them. They help the immune system of the mouth to work. TMJ is a painful syndrome that links various dental and other health problems to jaw misalignment. Approximately 10 million people suffer from TMJ, three times as many women as men.

Diet & Superfood Therapy

—Nutritional therapy plan:

1—Eat primarily fresh foods during acute stages to speed healing, with plenty of leafy greens and vegetable drinks (pg. 218).

2—To prevent recurring tooth problems, eat lots of crunchy, crisp foods, such as celery, and other raw vegetables, nuts and seeds, and whole grain crackers.

3—Eat calcium-rich foods: greens and shellfish.

4—Reduce acid citrus juices if you have weak teeth. They are great for your insides, but not for your teeth. Avoid soft, gooey foods. No sweets, or sodas (they especially damage weak teeth).

—For pain:

1) Ice the jaw; take a little wine or brandy and hold on the aching area as long as possible.

2) Mix 20 drops of clove oil with 1-oz. brandy. Apply with a cotton swab to toothache area.

3) Chew food very well.

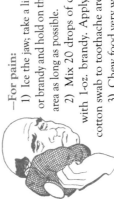

—Superfood therapy: (Choose one or two)
• Wakunaga KYO-GREEN - excellent for jaw arthritis.
• Nutricology PRO-GREENS with flax.
• Crystal Star ENERGY GREEN™ drink.
• Rainbow Light HAWAIIAN SPIRULINA.

Herb & Supplement Therapy

—Interceptive therapy plan: (Choose 2 to 3 recommendations)

1—**Control the infection:** • Crystal Star ANTI-BIO™ caps, or apply ANTI-BIO™ extract with a cotton swab directly on infected area as an effective disinfectant after a root canal. • Black walnut extract; • Echinacea-myrrh extract drops. • Twin Labs PROPO-LIS extract. ♂ • MICROBRITE, available at Healthy House, reduces plaque that causes gum infection.

2—**Reduce inflammation and swelling:** • Apply clove oil directly to painful tooth as needed. • Apply lobelia tincture; ⊛ • Solaray TURMERIC caps, or • Crystal Star ANTI-FLAM™ CAPS, 4 as needed for pain; or • Nature's Plus BROMELAIN 1500mg, or • Apply Bilberry or Hawthorn extract drops for on-the-spot bioflavonoids.

3—**Rebuild strong teeth:** • Nature's Life LIQUID CALCIUM PHOS. FREE with vitamin D. • Crystal Star CALCIUM SOURCE™ and SILICA SOURCE™ extract drops; or • Flora VEGE-SIL silica caps 4 daily. • Solgar CAL-MAG-ZINC, 4 daily, with boron 3mg for better tooth growth.

4—**Rebalance mouth pH:** • Reculture your mouth with Bio Energy Systems BIO-CULTURE 2000, especially after wisdom tooth problems. • Swish and hold De Souza liquid chlorophyll (in a small amount of water) for one month.

—For TMJ: Take
• B-complex 100mg with extra B₆ 100mg, niacin 100mg. • Take DLPA 1000mg as needed for pain. • Take CoQ₁₀ 100mg daily on a regular basis as a preventive. • Take nerve relaxing herbs like Kava Kava caps, Valerian-Wild Lettuce extract to calm from pain. • Crystal Star ASPIR-SOURCE™ capsules for nerve pain. • Cayenne-ginger caps take down inflammation. • Homeopathic remedies for TMJ - Cal. Phos., Mag. Phos., and Rhus Tox.

—Effective homeopathic remedies: • NatraBio TEETH & GUMS tincture;
• Chamomilla - neuralgic aches; • Belladonna - wisdom tooth pain and ache with pressure; • Hypericum - pain after extraction.

Lifestyle Support Therapy

—Bodywork:
• Relaxation techniques such as massage therapy, biofeedback and chiropractic adjustments are effective for TMJ.
• Acupressure technique: Squeeze the sides of each index finger at the end. Hold hard for 30 seconds.
• Rinse mouth with a solution of equal parts goldenseal and white oak bark tea to take down pain and swelling.

—Effective jaw compresses:
• Hot comfrey root
• Ginger root

—Apply directly to area with cotton swab:
• Chinese WHITE FLOWER oil
• Propolis tincture (Beehive Botanicals)
• Eucalyptus oil

—Reflexology point:

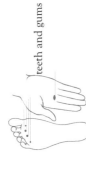

teeth and gums

See previous page for more information

Common Symptoms: Sore jaw and/or gums; dull or shooting pains; tooth or root nerve pain from a cavity; tooth and jaw crowding from wisdom teeth coming in too big, misaligned, etc.; pain from bruxism (tooth grinding at night); periodontal disease, and/or bleeding gums. TMJ symptoms, usually felt only on one side, include painful jaw movement; headaches, ringing in the ears, sinus pain, hearing loss, depression, dizziness and facial neuralgia.

Common Causes: TMJ - poor bite with frequent clenching of the teeth and grinding of the teeth at night (bruxism); neck injury that doesn't heal; stress.

Can't find a recommended product? Call the 800 number listed in Product Resources for the store nearest you.

Dental Problems

Periodontal (Gum) Disease, Pyorrhea, Gingivitis

Periodontal (surrounding the teeth) disease is a progressive disorder affecting not only the gums but also the bone structure around the teeth. Almost half the U.S. population over 35 years of age has some form of periodontal disease and it's a clear sign of accelerated aging. Unfortunately today, many children show signs of gingivitis. New findings show that risk of gum and mouth cancers are related to highly fluoridated water. Gum disease is a sign of body chemistry out of balance. New research indicates that there is a high correspondence between gum disease and other biochemical imbalance disorders like arthritis, diabetes and cadiovascular diseases. In many cases, holistic therapies are successful alternatives to surgery, involving body chemistry change through diet improvement, supplements and irrigation techniques.

Diet & Superfood Therapy

—Nutritional therapy plan:

1—Focus on cranberries, cashews, cardamom seeds and green tea. All have anti-adhesion properties to arrest production of plaque acid and keep plaque from adhering to teeth - a major cause of gum disease.

2—Eat raw, crunchy, fiber foods to stimulate the gums; apples, celery, Grape Nuts cereal, seeds, whole, chewy grains. Have a green salad every day. Chew well.

3—Eat high vitamin C foods, such as broccoli, green peppers, sea greens, kiwi, papaya, cantaloupe, and citrus fruits.

4—Eat vitamin A and carotene-rich foods, such as dark green leafy vegetables, yellow and orange vegetables and fruits, fish and sea vegetables.

5—Clean, soothe and rebalance gums with fresh strawberry halves, baking soda, honey, or lemon juice.

6—Eat cultured foods for digestive bacteria.

7—Avoid acid-forming foods, such as caffeine, sugars, refined foods and carbonated drinks.

—Superfood therapy: (Choose one or two)
• Crystal Star BIOFLAV., FIBER & C SUPPORT™ drink (no sugars).
• Sun Wellness CHLORELLA drink daily.
• AloeLife ALOE GOLD drink with myrrh extract drops added.

Herb & Supplement Therapy

—Interceptive therapy plan: (Choose 2 to 3 recommendations)

1—**Control the infection:** • Crystal Star ANTI-BIO™ caps or rub ANTI-BIO™ extract or myrrh extract drops directly on gums. • CoQ$_{10}$ 60mg 2x daily or • Real Life Research CoQ 20/20 for almost immediate relief. Continue for prevention. • Rub *Tea Tree Oil* directly on gums. Make up a C solution with water and ascorbate vitamin C powder with bioflavonoids - rub directly onto gums. Take vitamin C 5000mg daily. • MICROBRITE, available at Healthy House, reduces plaque that causes gum infection. • *Licorice Root* extract is anti-bacterial; *Lobelia* extract. 📶

2—**Reduce inflammation, stop bleeding, relieve pain:** • *Calendula* tincture directly on gums to relieve pain; • *Myrrh-goldenseal* mouthwash (a few drops in water) to stop bleeding; or *red raspberry* tea mouthwash; • Take three anti-inflammatories 2x daily - Quercetin 1000mg, bromelain 1500mg, Lysine 500mg. • Crystal Star ANTI-FLAM™ caps for gingivitis and abscesses. • *Echinacea* extract drops 2-3x daily.
• Take Body Essentials SILICA GEL, 1 TB in 3-oz. water 3x daily - or rub directly on gums as an anti-inflammatory. • Rub American Biologics DIOXYCHLOR gel directly on gums. • Enzymatic Therapy ORA BASICS with WILLOCIN caps for pain.

3—**Heal and strengthen gums:** • *Gotu Kola* extract or St. John's wort tea promotes healing; • *Ginkgo Biloba* extract for healing circulation and flavonoids; • Crystal Star MINERAL SPECTRUM™ caps strengthen gums (takes about 3 weeks). • Quantum GUM THERAPY; ♂ • vitamin A & E emulsion caps, 25000IU. Take internally, or prick caps to rub oil directly on gums. • Nature's Life liquid CALCIUM PHOS. FREE with vitamin D; ♂ or • Cal/Mag/Zinc to reduce alveolar bone loss.

4—**Add EFA's to rebalance body chemistry:** • Evening Primrose Oil caps 1000mg daily; • omega-3 flax oil 2 TBS daily; • a good multivitamin like Country Life MAX ♂ or MAXINE ♀ to prevent gum disease. • Chlorophyll liquid 3 teasp. daily before meals; or dilute with water and apply directly to gums.

—Effective homeopathic remedies: *Arsenicum Album, Ferrum Phos., Hypericum.*

Lifestyle Support Therapy

—Bodywork:
• Chew propolis lozenges. Use propolis toothpaste. Rub on propolis tincture.
• Beehive Botanical toothpaste, or Thursday Plantation TEA TREE toothpaste.
• Rinse with a salt water solution whenever you feel the first signs of gum infection.
• Put 4-5 drops tea tree oil, or Nutribiotic GRAPEFRUIT SEED extract or Rainbow Light HERBA-DENT extract in a water pik and use daily for recurring gum infections.
• Effective gum massages control pain:
  Clove oil - dilute ♂
  Eucalyptus oil - dilute ♀
  Witch hazel
  Make a *Goldenseal-Myrrh* powder poultice and place directly on gums.

• Daily watchwords for gum health:
  Brush teeth well twice a day.
  Floss, floss, floss - at least once a day.
  Rinse your mouth immediately after eating.

—Reflexology point:

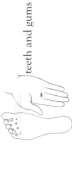

teeth and gums

Common Symptoms: Red, swollen, tender gums that bleed when you brush, chronic bad breath that no amount of mouthwash will help, loose or shifting teeth, pus between the teeth and gums, receding gums that leave the root surface of teeth exposed, the loss of even cavity-free teeth; changes in the bite; hot and cold sensitivity in the mouth. Don't smoke - smoking sabotages gum health.

Common Causes: Plaque formation on the gums that hardens into tarter, forming deep pockets between gums and teeth roots leading to loosened teeth and eventual bone damage; nutritional deficiencies, especially vitamins A, C, D and calcium; allergies; lack of fresh foods; too much red meat, refined foods, sugar, alcohol and soft drinks; stress; diabetes. Mood elevating medicines can cause saliva reduction and thus gum disease.

Can't find a recommended product? Call the 800 number listed in Product Resources for the store nearest you.

Depression

Bi-Polar Disorder, Paranoia, Mood Affective Disorder

Depression is the most common adult psychiatric disorder, and it's on the rise worldwide. Mood disorders affect 19 million Americans and we spend over $20 billion on treatment. Depression is both a mental and emotional state and affects women more than men. It's closely tied to disease. (Over 80% of terminal cancer patients have a history of chronic depression.) A common expression of depression I hear is the feeling of being in a box that you can't escape. Underlying origins for depression: 1) Great loss, as of a spouse or child, and the inability to express grief; 2) Bottled-up anger and aggression turned inward; 3) Negative emotional behavior, often learned as a child to control relationships; 4) Biochemical imbalance involved with amino acid and other nutrient deficiencies; 5) Drug-induced depression. Many prescription drugs create nutrient deficiencies.

Diet & Superfood Therapy

—Nutritional therapy plan:

1—If you are taking MAO inhibitor drugs, you must control your diet with care: avoid alcohol, cheese, red meat, yeast extract and broad beans - foods rich in tyrosine. Eliminate all preserved, refined and junk foods. Avoid sugary foods and caffeine - they wreak havoc on blood sugar levels.

2—Nutrition is a key to your brain's behavior. Make vegetable protein about 15% of total calorie intake. Include fatty acid foods like fish, sea foods, sea greens, spinach and legumes. Eat tryptophan foods like turkey, potatoes and bananas.

3—Eat foods rich in calcium, magnesium and B vitamins. Have a glass of carrot juice 2 to 3x a week with a pinch of sage and 1 teasp. Bragg's LIQUID AMINOS for adrenal stress.

4—Drink bottled water. Treated water can cause neurotransmitter imbalances.

5—Make a brain mix of lecithin granules, brewer's yeast, wheat germ, pumpkin seeds; take 2 TBS daily.

—Superfood therapy: (Choose one or two)

• Crystal Star SYSTEMS STRENGTH™.
• GreenFoods WHEAT GERM extract.
• Rainbow Light HAWAIIAN SPIRULINA. ♂
• Beehive Botanicals ROYAL JELLY with GINSENG and bee pollen. ♀

Herb & Supplement Therapy

Be aware that the two major classes of antidepressant drugs seem to block the effect of herbal nervines. St. John's wort is contra-indicated if you are taking PROZAC.

—Interceptive therapy plan: (Choose 2 to 3 recommendations)

1—**Relieve depression, improve your mood:** • Crystal Star DEPRESS-EX™ extract or caps for mental calm; • NADH 10mg daily with St. John's Wort, a natural MAO inhibitor. • *Kava-Kava* caps 2 daily or Enzymatic Therapy KAVA TONE. • *Ginkgo Biloba* or *Hawthorn* extract for a feeling of well-being. • Magnesium 500mg 2x daily. *Rhodiola Rosea* is an herbal serotonin booster effective against depression.

2—**Fight depression with essential fatty acids:** • *Evening Primrose* oil 1000mg 2x daily; omega-3 flax oil 2 TBS daily; or • Omega Nutrition OMEGA PLUS caps.

3—**Amino acids boost your brain energy:** • SAMe 400mg daily (important in synthesizing brain chemicals); • Glutamine 1000mg daily; • Country Life Maxi-B with taurine or MOOD FACTORS capsules as needed; • Tyrosine 500mg or • DLPA 1000mg as needed; • GABA 1000mg to mimic valium without sedation.

4—**Nerve tonics and relaxers:** • Crystal Star RELAX™ caps for nerve repair; • *Gotu Kola* for nerve support; • Flora NERVE GUARD drops; Country Life sublingual B-12, 2500mcg every other day for 2 months; • 5-HTP 50-100mg daily for 2 months. • Vitamin C with bioflavonoids, 3000mg daily helps withdrawal from chemical dependencies. • B-complex 150mg with extra B-6 250mg daily. • Take *Black cohosh*, Natrol SAF capsules, or melatonin 3mg at bedtime for 3 months if depression is hormone related. ♀ Allergy Research PROZA-PLEX caps. ♂

Drink • Crystal Star INCREDIBLE DREAMS™ tea before retiring; or make an • anti-depression pillow with fresh-dried *mugwort leaves, rosemary, California poppies, lemon balm and mint.* Stuff a pillow for sweet sleep. ♀

5—**Adaptogen herbs help normalize your body chemistry:** • High potency *panax ginseng* or *suma* • Crystal Star MENTAL INNER ENERGY™ formula with *kava kava;* • *Siberian ginseng* extract, or • Rainbow Light ADAPTOGEM caps; • Nelson Bach RESCUE REMEDY. ♀

Lifestyle Support Therapy

—Lifestyle thoughts:

• 67% of people with no apparent cause for their depression benefit from sleep deprivation. A single sleepless night can wash away depressive symptoms.

• Before you try PROZAC, (it has had more side effect complaints than any other drug) ask your doctor about hypnotherapy, biofeedback or acupuncture. These relaxation techniques have success in overcoming chronic depression.

—Bodywork:

• Exercise worry and anxiety away. Give yourself plenty of body oxygen. Exercise is an anti-depressant nutrient in itself.

• Prolonged depression increases risk of osteoporosis. Sunlight therapy - get some on the body every day possible for vitamin D. ♀

• Do deep brain breathing exercises. (See Paul Bragg's BRAIN BREATHING book).

• Yoga stretches or a regular massage can clear the mind and refresh the body.

• Stop smoking. It constricts capillaries and arteries, and slows circulation to the brain.

• Aromatherapy helps: Essential oils of jasmine, geranium, rosemary and basil.

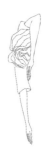

D 366

Common Symptoms: Manic episodes alternating with deep depression; excessive self-reproach and guilt; fatigue; inability to think and disorientation; memory loss; wired feeling; paranoia attacks; headaches; sweating; palpitations; loss of interest in pleasure; poor food absorption and significant weight loss even if meals are good; recurrent thoughts of death or suicide.
Common Causes: Hypoglycemia or other sugar imbalance; sugar or alcohol dependency; chemical or food allergies; glandular imbalance with high copper levels; drug abuse; hypothyroidism; prescription drug addiction or intolerance; negative emotions; the inability to cope with prolonged and intense stress.

See also ANXIETY and CHRONIC FATIGUE SYNDROME pages for more information.

Can't find a recommended product? Call the 800 number listed in Product Resources for the store nearest you.

Diabetes

High Blood Sugar, Type 1 (Juvenile Diabetes), Type 2 (Adult-Onset Diabetes)

Type 2, adult-onset, non-insulin dependent diabetes, affects about 85% of diabetics, striking one in 20 (more than 15 million) Americans. With its complications, it is the third leading cause of death in the U. S. It's a chronic degenerative disease in which disturbances in normal insulin mechanisms impair the body's ability to use carbohydrates. Type 2 diabetics produce insulin, the hormone that helps convert food into energy, but it isn't used properly (insulin resistance), causing glucose to build up in the bloodstream, depriving cells of the nutrients they need. Type 1 diabetes, a juvenile condition, is more severe and almost entirely dependent on insulin to sustain life. Both types benefit from diet improvement, exercise and natural supplements. Diet improvement is absolutely necessary to overcoming diabetes. High blood sugar is also an indication of high triglycerides.

Diet & Superfood Therapy

—Nutritional therapy plan:

1—Eliminate sugars, alcohol, fried, fatty, refined and high cholesterol foods. Avoid cow's milk especially and all fatty dairy foods.

2—Slow-burning complex carbohydrate, like whole grains and vegetables reduce insulin requirements.

3—High fiber foods are a key, and, in some mild cases, can lead to discontinuation of insulin therapy. Fiber improves control of glycemia and glucose metabolism, lowers cholesterol and triglyceride levels, and promotes weight loss.

4—Chromium-rich foods are a key: whole grains, brewer's yeast, string beans, eggs, cucumbers, soy foods, liver, onions and garlic, fruits, cheese, shiitake mushrooms, wheat germ, etc.

5—Have a daily green salad with Omega-3 flax oil dressing for EFA's. Eat salmon twice a week.

6—Your ongoing diet should be low in fats and total calories, largely vegetarian, rich in good fats like olive oil and proteins mostly from sea foods, sea greens and vegetable sources.

—Superfood therapy: (Choose one or two)
• Herbal Answers ALOE FORCE JUICE.
• Futurebiotics VITAL K.
• Sun Wellness CHLORELLA 20 tabs daily.
• Green Kamut JUST BARLEY.
• Green Foods BARLEY ESSENCE.

Herb & Supplement Therapy

—Interceptive therapy plan: (Choose 1 or 2 recommendations)

1—Stabilize blood sugar: •Crystal Star SUGAR STRATEGY HIGH™ capsules to encourage insulin balance; •GTF Chromium or chromium picolinate 100mcg 2x daily; •Siberian ginseng extract or •Imperial Elixir SIBERIAN GINSENG or •Grifon MAITAKE MUSHROOM caps to stabilize blood sugar. ♀ •Crystal Star GINSENG-LICORICE ELIXIR™ or *dandelion-licorice* tea; •vitamin E, 800IU daily; •Fenugreek seed, bitter melon or *rosemary* tea balance blood sugar. •Neem and turmeric powders (¼ teasp each in 1 teasp. honey before a meal).

2—Lower blood sugar levels: •Alpha Lipoic acid 600mg daily (lowers glucose levels up to 30%); •Crystal Star GINSENG 6 SUPER TEA™ or •Bilberry extract or •Olive Leaf extract as directed; •high dose biotin treatments - 3000mcg daily. ♂ •Vitamin C 3000mg daily with •magnesium 400mg daily combat insulin resistance.

3—Normalize pancreas activity and insulin function: •Take *gymnema sylvestre* extract before meals to help repair the pancreas, and damage to the liver and kidneys. •Ester C 3000mg daily increases insulin tolerance, normalizes pancreatic activity. •Glutamine 1000mg with carnitine 1000mg; ♀ •Nutricology PRO-LIVE olive leaf extract as directed; •DHEA 25mg daily increases cell sensitivity to insulin. •*Burdock*, *Pau d'arco* or *Astragalus* tea, 2 cups daily for 3 months; or •garlic capsules 6 daily; •raw pancreas glandular or •Premier VANADIUM 25mcg daily.

4—Help prevent nerve damage with EFA's: •Evening *Primrose* Oil capsules 1000mg daily, •Omega-3 flax or fish oil (for DHA) 3000mg daily.

5—Raise your antioxidant defenses: •Pycnogenol or grape seed PCO's 200mg daily; •Crystal Star ADR-ACTIVE™ caps for cortex support with BODY REBUILDER™ for stable energy. •*Spirulina* tablets 6 daily to elevate mood.♂

6—Boost energy: •Crystal Star ADR-ACTIVE™ caps for cortex support with BODY REBUILDER™ for stable energy.

—A vitamin regimen maintains many aspects of diabetic needs: Solaray B-12 2500mcg, B-complex 100mg, with pantothenic acid 500mg daily for adrenal activity, niacin 250mg to stimulate circulation, and zinc 50mg for more immune strength. Magnesium/ potassium/bromelain 3 daily to control blood pressure. ♂

Lifestyle Support Therapy

Don't smoke. Nicotine increases the desire for sugar and sugary foods. Don't stop or reduce insulin without monitoring by your physician.

—Bodywork:
•Walking is good exercise for diabetics to increase metabolic processes and reduce need for insulin.

•Alternating hot and cold hydrotherapy to stimulate circulation.

•A regular deep therapy massage is effective in regulating sugar use.

•Avoid phenylalanine. No Nutra-Sweet or Aspartame products. (Check labels on colas, diet drinks, etc.) They may trigger diabetes.

•If you're overweight, loose the excess. Poor bio-chemistry often results from being over-weight. A fiber weight loss drink, like Crystal Star CHO-LO FIBER TONE™ or AloeLife FIBER-MATE are effective.

—Reflexology points:

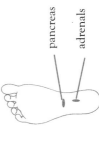

pancreas

adrenals

D 367

Common Symptoms: High blood sugar; constant hunger with rapid weight change; blurred vision; a tendency to infections; leg cramps, tingling in the extremeties; impotence; dry, itching skin; insatiable thirst; lack of energy; kidney malfunction leading to bladder and prostate problems, and excessive urination with high sugar in the urine; obesity; hypertension; accelerated aging.

Common Causes: Strongly linked to a modern fast food diet - too many refined foods, fats and carbohydrates; glucose and fat metabolism malfunction leading to obesity (the leading cause); chromium, HCL deficiency; possibly a virus; pancreas and liver malfunction from excess caffeine, alcohol and stress overloads; inherited proneness usually accompanied by several allergies; hypothyroidism.

See the Diabetes Control Diet on the following page.

Can't find a recommended product? Call the 800 number listed in Product Resources for the store nearest you.

Do You Think You or Your Child Might Have Diabetes? Here Are The Signs.

Type II - Adult-Onset Diabetes

—Are you always thirsty? Do you urinate too often?
—Do cuts and bruises heal slowly?
—Have you lost weight but weren't on a diet?
—Are you constantly tired? or drowsy?
—Do you get frequent infections?
—Do you get leg cramps, or prickling in your fingers or toes?
—Have you experienced episodes of impotence?
—Is your vision blurry from time to time?

Juvenile Diabetes

—Is your child unusually thirsty?
—Does he or she urinate too often?
—Is your child extremely hungry?
—Is your child unusually irritable?
—Is he or she unusually tired? or drowsy?
—Has your child lost weight lately?

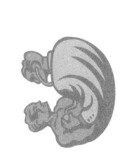

Blood Sugar Balancing Diet For Diabetes Control

Although many Type 2 diabetics must take insulin to regulate blood sugar levels, others can balance their blood sugar without drugs by following a controlled diet along with regular exercise.

Diabetes makes a person want to eat more, so it can be brought on by eating too much fat, too many sugary foods and excess refined foods. Exposure to this type of diet overworks, then damages the pancreas and other organs, your body loses the ability to produce or use insulin correctly, and high blood sugar results. As less and less simple carbohydrates and sugars are metabolized, they keep accumulating in the body and are stored as fat. Excess body fat and lack of exercise bring on insulin resistance, so less energy is moved into the cells. The following diet, in addition to reducing insulin requirements and balancing blood sugar use, has the nice "side effect" of healthy weight loss.

This is a low-glycemic diet, supplying slow-burning complex carbohydrate fuel, primarily from vegetables that don't need much insulin for metabolism, preventing rapid blood sugar spikes. Some people can even reduce or stop their prescription medications. (Check with your doctor.) Good diabetic meals are small, frequent, largely vegetarian, and low in saturated fats. Proteins come from soy foods and whole grains that are rich in lecithin and chromium. Fifty to sixty percent of the diet consists of fresh and simply cooked vegetables for low calories. All sugars, fried and fatty foods are excluded. Use *stevia* herb instead of sugar for sweetening. It does not have sugar's insulin requirements.

—**On Rising:** take the juice of two lemons in a glass of water with 2 teasp. Mona's CHLORELLA granules.

—**Breakfast:** take a glass of aloe vera juice, or NutriTech ALL ONE drink mix in apple juice or water to regulate and balance sugar curve; or make a mix of 2 TBS each: brewer's yeast, wheat germ, lecithin granules and rice or oat bran. Sprinkle some daily on your choice of breakfast foods, or simply mix into yogurt with fresh fruit and some grated almonds on top; or have 1) poached egg on whole grain toast; 2) muesli, whole grain or granola cereal with apple juice or vanilla soy milk; 3) buckwheat or whole grain pancakes with apple juice or molasses.

—**Mid-morning:** have a green drink such as Crystal Star ENERGY GREEN™ or Green Foods GREEN MAGMA; and some whole grain crackers or muffins with a little soy spread or kefir cheese; and a refreshing, sugar balancing herb tea, such as *licorice, dandelion, or pau d'arco* tea.

—**Lunch:** have a green salad, with celery, sprouts, green pepper, marinated tofu, and mushroom soup; or baked tofu, tofu burgers or turkey with some steamed veggies and rice or cornbread; or a baked potato with a little yogurt or kefir cheese, or soy cheese and some miso soup with sea vegetables; or a whole grain sandwich, with avocado, low fat or soy cheese, a low fat sandwich spread and watercress leaves.

—**Mid-afternoon:** have a glass of carrot juice, diluted with water; and/or fruit juice sweetened cookies with a bottle of mineral water or herb tea; or some watercress/cucumber sandwiches with a kefir cheese sandwich spread; or a hard boiled egg with sesame salt, or a veggie dip, and a bottle of mineral water.

—**Dinner:** Keep it light - have a baked or broiled seafood dish with brown rice and peas; or a Chinese stir-fry with rice, veggies and miso soup; or a Spanish beans and rice dish with onions and peppers; or a light northern Italian polenta with a hearty vegetable soup, or whole grain or veggie pasta salad; or a mushroom quiche with whole grain crust and yogurt/wine sauce, and a small green salad. A little white wine is fine with dinner for relaxation and has surprisingly high chromium content. Beware of overconsumption of alcohol, it can cause blood sugar to soar.

—**Before bed:** take another heaping teasp. CHOL-LO FIBER TONE™ mix in apple juice; and/or Red Star NUTRITIONAL YEAST or MISO, 1 teasp. in warm water.
Avoid caffeine and caffeine foods, hard liquor, food coloring and sodas. Even "diet" sodas have phenylalanine that can affect blood sugar levels.

D 368

Can't find a recommended product? Call the 800 number listed in Product Resources for the store nearest you.

Controlling Complications Associated With Diabetes

Diabetes frequently leads to other health problems. Use the recommendations as needed for specific diabetic complications along with your diabetes healing program.

—**DIABETIC CATARACTS, GLAUCOMA, DIABETIC RETINOPATHY (DAMAGED RETINA), RETINITIS AND IMPAIRED VISION:** the leading cause of new blindness in the U.S., a disorder of the light sensitive retina caused by diabetes. **Alternative healing protocols:** • Bilberry extract 2x daily for effective flavonoids; • Ginkgo biloba extract 3x daily for blood vessel circulation to the eyes; • PCO's from grapeseed or white pine bark, 100mg 3 to 4 times daily to reduce vascular fragility; • Quercetin 1000mg with bromelain 750mg 2x daily; • Lane Labs BENE-FIN shark cartilage caps 1200mg for blood vessel and capillary support; • magnesium 400mg 3x daily; • Vitamin C or Ester C powder with bioflavonoids, $1/4$ teasp. at a time, 4 to 6x daily; • vitamin E 400IU 3x daily, especially for retinitis; • Planetary TRIPHALA caps as directed; or • Solaray CENTELLA ASIATICA for optic nerve support; • B-complex 100mg daily with taurine 500mg.

—**DIABETIC CARDIOVASCULAR COMPLICATIONS:** People with diabetes are twice as likely to suffer from coronary heart disease and stroke; they are five times as likely to suffer from arterial disease as non-diabetics. **Alternative healing protocols:** • Ginkgo biloba 3x daily; • PCO's from grapeseed or white pine bark, 100mg 3 to 4 times daily; • *gymnema sylvestre* extract to lower blood lipids; taurine to reverse blood clotting; • CoQ-10 100mg daily with vitamin E 400IU daily to increase blood flow and decrease platelet aggregation; or • Golden Pride HEART HEALTH PAK daily. • Omega-3 flax oil 3x daily helps keep arteries and circulatory system free of fats. Take • Country Life vitamin B-12 sublingual 2500mcg with carnitine 1000mg and • Bilberry extract. To help lower cholesterol: • MICROHYDRIN available from Healthy House (rapid results); • niacinamide 500mg 2x daily, and • chromium picolinate 200mcg daily, or • Solaray CHROMIACIN.

—**DIABETIC OBESITY:** Weight control problems and heart disease are in a vicious circle. Obesity is a risk factor for heart disease; obesity is a risk factor for diabetes. Therefore diabetes is a risk factor for heart disease. Excess body fat plays a key role in Type II diabetes by contributing to insulin resistance - the inability of the body to deliver glucose to the cells for energy. **Alternative healing protocols:** You must lower your sugar and saturated fat food intake. Get help with this from • *stevia herb*, or • *gymnema sylvestre* herb before each meal for pancreatic normalization and increase in insulin output; • Lewis Labs FIBER YEAST daily in the morning, or • Lewis Labs WEIGH DOWN DIET DRINK with chromium picolinate; or take • chromium picolinate 200mcg daily; • L-carnitine 1000mg daily; • Magnesium 800mg daily and •vitamin E 400IU daily to overcome insulin resistance. Take in more "good" fats. Most diabetics suffer from EFA deficiency. My favorite sources for diabetic related obesity are • Evening Primrose oil 1000mg 4x daily, flax seed oil, 2 tablespoons daily on soup, salad or rice. A weekly dry sauna helps regulate sugar use and control cravings. Smaller, more frequent meals helps, too.

—**DIABETIC NEPHROPATHY:** Kidney disease resulting from diabetic small blood vessel malfunction. **Alternative healing protocols:** Avoid red meats - eat fish or chicken instead - especially salmon; take • *gymnema sylvestre* water soluble extract before meals; • alpha lipoic acid 600mg daily; • Lane Labs BENE-FIN shark cartilage capsules for blood vessel and capillary support.

—**DIABETIC CIRCULATORY PROBLEMS AND ULCERS: Alternative healing protocols:** consider chelation therapy. Today, it is an easy clinic procedure... and it works. • Golden Pride FORMULA ONE as directed. Take • American Biologics emulsified vitamin A & D 25,000/1,000 IU (beta-carotene is not effective for diabetics, who cannot convert it to A in the liver). Drink aloe vera juice every morning. Take • zinc/methionine 30mg 2x daily to improve zinc status without affecting copper levels. Clean diabetic ulcers of necrotic tissue and apply a comfrey poultice, • B & T CALIFLORA gel, • AloeLife SKIN GEL, tea tree oil/olive oil compresses, or • Country Comfort GOLDENSEAL/MYRRH salve.

—**FOOD ALLERGIES:** When being tested for glucose tolerance, be sure to take food tolerance tests to determine food allergies. There is a definite link between cow's milk and Type 1 Juvenile Diabetes. Aspartame (especially in sweeteners like NutraSweet, Sweet 'N' Low and Equal) deplete insulin reserves. **Alternative healing protocols:** • HCL with meals, digestive enzymes after meals, such as • Solaray DIGEST-AWAY or • Enzymedica PURIFY, or • Prevail DAIRY ENZYME FORMULA for lactose intolerance. Keep the diet high in fresh raw fruits and vegetables, with lots of soluble vegetable and grain fiber. Avoid acid-forming foods like red meats and hard cheeses, refined carbohydrates, and preserved foods.

—**DIABETIC NEUROPATHY:** Damage to the peripheral nerves characterized by numbness, tingling, pain and cramping in hands and feet. **Alternative healing protocols:** Follow a vegetarian diet; take • Quercetin with Bromelain 2x daily (or Solaray QBC COMPLEX); take • alpha lipoic acid 600mg daily to help lower blood sugar; • PCO's from *grapeseed* or *white pine bark*, 100mg 3x daily to reduce vascular fragility; *gotu kola* capsules 6 daily for nerve support. Take • Ginkgo Biloba, Hawthorn or Bilberry extract 3x daily; • Evening Primrose Oil capsules 1000mg 4 daily or • choline 600mg for nerve damage; • biotin 1000mcg 6x daily; • Apply capsaicin cream or Nature's Way CAYENNE PAIN RELIEVING OINTMENT to affected areas for pain relief; • Country Life vitamin B-12 sublingual 2500mcg, every other day for a month; vitamin C 3000mg daily; • Magnesium 400mg 2x daily; • L-carnitine 2000mg daily.

—**DIABETIC RELATED ACCELERATED AGING (ESPECIALLY ARTERIOSCLEROSIS):** **Alternative healing protocols:** antioxidants are the key: • chromium picolinate 200mcg 3x daily. Caution note: Diabetics progressively lose the ability to heal from cuts and wounds as they age (particularly cut toenails straight across or have a professional do it). Antioxidants help prevent all the other complications for diabetes by quenching free radical production.

Can't find a recommended product? Call the 800 number listed in Product Resources for the store nearest you.

Diarrhea

Chronic Diarrhea, Traveler's Diarrhea, Poor Nutrient Absorption

Uncomfortably frequent, fluid and excessive bowel movements, diarrhea is your body's way of ridding itself of something disagreeable or harmful. Diarrhea is one of the body's best methods of rapidly throwing off toxins. Unless diarrhea is chronic, or continues for more than two to three days, it is best to let it run its cleansing course. Note: No drugstore remedy I have found is as effective as diet correction with herbs or natural supplements.

Diet & Superfood Therapy

—**Nutritional therapy plan:**

1—**For chronic diarrhea:** Go on a juice fast for 24 hours (pg. 192) to clean out harmful bacteria. Then take daily for 3 days: Miso soup with sea greens, papaya juice, a green salad, toast, and brown rice with steamed vegetables. Add pectin foods like apples or bananas to absorb water.

2—Add fiber to your continuing diet with whole grain brans, amaranth cereal (an astringent), brown rice and fresh vegetables. Add yogurt, kefir and cultured foods for friendly flora. Drink plenty of liquids to keep from getting dehydrated and losing minerals.

3—Avoid dairy products, and fatty and fried foods during healing.

4—Eat small meals and chew food well.

1—**For travel diarrhea and irregularity:** Eat only very ripe bananas for 24 hours - esp. if in a 3rd world country to help your body retain water and absorb salt. Eat high fiber foods during your trip, especially brown rice, salads and vegetables. Add yogurt to your travel diet.

2—Drink black *orange pekoe* tea with a lemon and a pinch of cloves.

3—Have a glass of wine with meals - 6 times more effective killing bacteria than Pepto Bismol.

Herb & Supplement Therapy

—**Interceptive therapy plans:** (choose 2 or 3 recommendations)

1—**Control the infection:** •Crystal Star ANTI-BIO™ caps or extract to counter gastrointestinal infections. •Nutribiotics GRAPEFRUIT SEED extract caps.

2—**Soothe discomfort and cramping:** •*Peppermint-Slippery Elm tea; Blackberry-elderberry-cinnamon tea;* •New Chapter GINGER WONDER syrup as needed. ☜

3—**Astringent herbs help dry up diarrhea:** •Carob powder drink with honey or applesauce; ☜ •*Catnip, nettles, sage or thyme tea.* Activated charcoal tabs on a temporary basis with Cal/Mag/Zinc caps at night. ♂

4—**Rebalance your bowel functions:** •BWL TONE-IBS™ capsules for gentle rebalance. •Prof. Nutrition DR. DOPHILUS, or •Natren TRINITY, or •Transformation Enzyme PLANTADOPHILUS pwd. ½ teasp. 3x daily in water or juice. •Sun Wellness CHLORELLA 20 tabs daily. •Vitamin A 10,000IU daily; •*Garlic* capsules 6 daily; •*Bayberry-barberry* tea; •Pancreatin 1200mg daily. •Quercetin 1000 with bromelain 750mg if you have food allergies. •Niacin therapy 250mg daily.

5—**Rebuild strong bowel tissue:** •Crystal Star SILICA SOURCE™ extract; •*Red Raspberry* tea, rich in needed minerals; ♀•Planetary TRIPHALA caps as directed.

—**All-in-one diarrhea aid:** Crystal Star GREEN TEA CLEANSER™ with ¼ teasp. ginger powder, 15 drops *myrrh* extract and 1 teasp. Bragg's LIQUID AMINOS added.

—**For traveler's diarrhea:** Crystal Star TRAVELERS COMFORT™ (with *ginger*); •Bee pollen, 2 tsp. daily, or Beehive Botanical POLLEN PLUS; kelp tabs 6 daily.

—**Homeopathic diarrhea remedies:** *Nux Vomica,* Hylands *Diarrex,* ☜ *Chamomilla.*

—**Superfood therapy:** (Choose one or two)
•Crystal Star SYSTEMS STRENGTH™ to replace lost electrolytes - stimulate enzymes.
•Salute ALOE VERA JUICE with HERBS morning and evening.
•Lewis Labs FIBER YEAST daily, B vitamins and fiber, or brewer's yeast tabs.

Lifestyle Support Therapy

—**Bodywork:**
•Mix 1 TB each: *psyllium husk, flax seed, chia seed,* and *slippery elm* in water. Let the mix soak for 30 minutes. Take 2 TBS at night for 2 days before bed.
•If no inflammation is present, use mild catnip enemas to rid the body of toxic matter.
•Take *fenugreek* seed tea enemas to soothe inflamed tissues.
•Apply ice packs to the middle and lower back to stimulate nerve force.

—**To curb symptoms:**
•Two teasp. roasted carob powder in water with 1 teasp. of cinnamon 2x daily. ☜
•Two TBS cider vinegar in hot water with honey 2 to 3x daily.
•BLACK WALNUT HULLS extract.
•Apple pectin capsules 3 daily.
•For babies: give finely grated apples followed by oatmeal. ☜
•For older children: give oat flakes; let them chew and wet them with saliva; don't give any other food for at least 2 hours. ☜

See PARASITE INFECTIONS page 476 for more information.

Can't find a recommended product? Call the 800 number listed in Product Resources for the store nearest you.

Common Symptoms: *Loose, watery, frequent stools, often with abdominal pain and dehydration; sometimes vomiting and fever; general fatigue.*
Common Causes: *Poor food absorption, and lack of fiber in the diet; enzyme and chronic vitamin A deficiency; intestinal parasites; colitis; food poisoning; reaction to rancid or unripe foods; food allergy- particularly lactose intolerance; stress; reactions to chemicals in foods or drugs (antibiotics); reaction to water and/or foods in foreign countries; flu infection. Note: hemorrhoids are linked to diarrhea and obesity conditions - not constipation as one might think.*

Diverticulosis

Diverticulitis, Inflamed Bowel Disease

*Diverticular disease is common today, affecting almost 40% of Americans over 50. It mimics many of the symptoms of Irritable Bowel Syndrome. **Diverticulosis** is characterized by small hernias that protrude through the wall of the sigmoid colon. **Diverticulitis** occurs when these small sacs become infected and inflamed. A highly refined diet lacking enough fiber and bulk leads to fermented, uneliminated food residues. A constipated colon is most at risk for the pouch-like hernias which essentially trap toxic waste to protect the body from main-canal infection. However, if constipation continues, and the diet is not improved, the pouches (diverticula) themselves become painfully infected, and may perforate leading to contamination in the abdominal, vaginal or contiguous area.*

Diet & Superfood Therapy

—Nutritional therapy plan:

1—Diet improvement is the main solution: Start with a short juice diet for 3 days (pg. 191). Use carrot, apple, grape or carrot/spinach juice.

2—Fiber is the diet key: to prevent constipation: Add oat or rice bran and take 2 TBS molasses with a banana and plain yogurt daily. Eat prunes for occasional constipation.

3—Then add mild fruits and vegetables, such as carrots, bananas, potatoes, yams, papayas, broccoli, well-cooked beans (especially black beans).

4—As inflammation subsides and healing begins, add brown rice, millet, cous cous, tofu, baked fish or seafood as lean protein sources.

5—Eat plenty of cultured foods for healthy G.I. flora; yogurt, kefir, miso, sea greens for EFA's.

6—Eliminate dairy products, fatty and sugary foods, red meats and fried foods during healing. Reduce wheat and dense grains, nuts and seeds during healing.

7—Drink 6 to 8 glasses of water and plenty of apple juice, cranberry juice or ginger ale (add New Moon GINGER WONDER syrup to any drink).

—Superfood therapy: (Choose one or two)
• Crystal Star CHO-LO-FIBER TONE™.♂
• Green Foods BARLEY ESSENCE.
• AloeLife ALOE GOLD juice drink to soothe pain and gently aid bowel action. ♀

Herb & Supplement Therapy

Liquid and chewable supplements are preferable for ease and gentleness.

—Interceptive therapy plan: (Choose 2 to 4 recommendations)

1—**Heal and tone bowel tissue:** • Crystal Star BWL TONE IBS™ caps with *wild yam* (wild yam is a specific for diverticular disease) 2-3x daily for 3 months. • Evening Primrose Oil for EFAs to normalize bowel function. *Pau d'arco or una da gato* tea 3 cups daily for a month. • Planetary TRIPHALA caps as directed.

2—**Ease gas and flatulence:** • B-complex vitamins, like Nature's Secret ULTIMATE B, • Source Naturals Co-ENZYMATE B complex, or • Real Life Research TOTAL B liquid sublingual (highly recommended), to curb stomach gas and rumbling as fiber combines with minerals.

3—**Reduce inflammation and pain:** • Crystal Star ANTI-FLAM™ drops in water or other white willow combination. ♂ • Crystal Star ANTI-SPZ™ capsules 4 at a time, or other cramp bark combination. ♀ • *Alfalfa*-mint tea or Solaray ALFA-JUICE caps 6 daily; *Slippery elm* tea; *Comfrey-fenugreek* tea.

4—**Control infection:** • Crystal Star ANTI-BIO™ drops in water, or other • *echinacea-goldenseal* combination; • *garlic* extract caps 6 daily.

5—**Soothe stress and tension leading to diverticular spasms:** • Crystal Star STRESS OUT extract drops in water. (usually results in 20 minutes or less.) • Enzymatic Therapy THYMU-PLEX to help immune response.

—Enzyme therapy is very important: • Dr. DOPHILUS or Transformation Enzymes PLANTADOHILUS powder ½ teasp. 3x daily with meals; • Nature's Plus chewable BROMELAIN 40mg or chewable PAPAYA ENZYMES at each meal; • Enzymatic Therapy DGL chewables; • Chlorophyll liquid, 1 teasp. in water before meals; • Whey complex powder after meals for bowel rebalance; • Rainbow Light ADVANCED ENZYME SYSTEM capsules.

Lifestyle Support Therapy

—Bodywork:
• Avoid drugstore antacids. They eventually make the problems worse by causing the stomach to produce more acids.

• Take *peppermint, fenugreek*, or *catnip* enemas once or twice a week for bowel cleansing and rebalancing.

• Massage therapy treatments often help.

• Active people are less prone to diverticular disease. Take a brisk walk every day possible. Walk outdoors to get a vitamin D boost.

• Apply wet hot ginger compresses to abdomen and lower back to stimulate systolic/diastolic action.

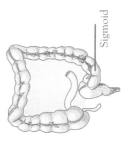

Sigmoid

—Diverticulitis area:

D 371

Common Symptoms: *Usually no symptoms of diverticulosis unless the small protruding sacs become infected. Diverticulitis is characterized by abdominal pain, cramping and distention caused by inflammation in the colon mucous membranes from unpassed food residues and gas; chronic constipation or alternating constipation and diarrhea; sometimes severe bleeding from the rectum especially in the elderly.*
Common Causes: *Fiber deficiency from too many refined foods, leading to weakening of the colon wall, and formation of pockets that look like worn out tire bulges; chronic constipation; thyroid deficiency; emotional stress causing colon spasms; obesity; causing compressed or prolapsed colon structure.*

See also COLITIS-IBS page 356 and the CONSTIPATION CLEANSING DIET page 357 for more information.

Can't find a recommended product? Call the 800 number listed in Product Resources for the store nearest you.

Down Syndrome

Genetic Mental Retardation, Mongolism

Down syndrome, a genetic condition caused by an extra 21st chromosome, is characterized by both physical and mental retardation. Untreatable by conventional medicine, innovative vanguard work is being done with nutritional therapies. Studies show that some retarded dysfunction and behavior is learned, not inherited, and that Down syndrome victims have immune deficiencies, particularly greatly accelerated free radical damage, that are thought to be largely responsible for the accelerated aging progress of the condition. Because of this, most Down victims do not live very long lives. Those that do almost always fall prey to Alzheimer's disease.

Diet & Superfood Therapy

—Nutritional therapy plan:
Better nutrition can improve IQ and physical health in Down syndrome, which is both a glycogen storage and protein metabolism problem.

1—Eat only fresh foods for 3 or 4 days to clear the body of toxic waste, and provide a clean working ground for nutritional therapy.

2—Then, insist on a highly nutritious diet of fresh and whole foods, rich in vegetable proteins, magnesium and EFA rich foods like leafy greens, sea foods and sea greens.

3—Eliminate all refined foods, sugars, pasteurized dairy and alcohol. Reduce high gluten foods.

4—Take Alacer MIRACLE WATER for brain potassium. ♂

5—Make a mix of brewer's yeast, lecithin and wheat germ; take 2 TBS daily over cereal.

—Superfood therapy: (Choose one or two)
Down Syndrome may be a metabolism disease today rather than an inherited disease. Enzyme therapy from superfoods is critical.
• Nutricology PRO-GREENS with flax EFA's.
• New Moon GINGER WONDER syrup. ☺
• Crystal Star SYSTEMS STRENGTH™.
• Green Kamut JUST BARLEY.
• Unipro PERFECT PROTEIN.
• Long Life IMPERIAL TONIC w. EPO.
• Knudsen organic VERY VEGGIE juice.

Herb & Supplement Therapy

—Interceptive therapy plan: (Choose 2 to 4 recommendations)

1—**Thyroid balance is a key:** •Crystal Star IODINE/POTASSIUM caps, or 4 kelp tablets daily, or •2 TBS of sea greens daily sprinkled on soup, rice or a salad.

2—**Strengthen nerves and thinking centers:** •Crystal Star CREATIVI-TEA™ daily as needed. • Gotu kola or Solaray CENTELLA ASIASTICA caps for nerves. •Chamomile tea to relax spasms. •Choline 600mg 4 daily, or phosphatidyl choline (PC 55), or phosphatidyl serine (PS) as directed. • Country Life MAXI-B with taurine, and extra B_6 100mg for nerve strength.

3—**Lower homocysteine levels:** 1: B vitamins to the rescue. Take B-complex, 100mg daily. Add 50mg extra B_6 and 400mcg extra folic acid to help break down homocysteine. Or, use Y.S. high potency royal jelly, ginseng and honey tea, 1 cup daily, or use the royal jelly paste, 2 teasp. daily and Real Life Research TOTAL B (has B-12) daily. 2: Garlic caps, 4 daily to maintain aortic elasticity; Ginkgo biloba extract 3x daily; 3: Take daily ginger - it inhibits an enzyme that makes blood prone to stickiness. Crystal Star TINKLE TEA™ helps gently reduce fluid retention.

4—**Supply abundant antioxidants to counteract free radical damage:** •CoQ_{10} 30mg 3x daily, •Vitamin E 400IU with selenium 200mcg •Ester C 550mg with bioflavonoids 4 to 6 daily all help Down Syndrome. Add •DMG sublingual 1 daily or Premier GERMANIUM with DMG (half dose for children).

5—**Nourish the brain with EFA's and produce better collagen:** •Evening Primrose Oil caps 4-6 daily for 3-4 months. •Crystal Star SILICA SOURCE™ drops or •Flora VEGE-SIL caps help the body produce collagen.

6—**Stimulate better immune response:** •Crystal Star GINSENG-REISHI extract, •Crystal Star CHLORELLA-GINSENG extract or • Siberian ginseng extract drops in water daily. • Marine carotene 25,000IU 3x daily. • Solaray pancreatin 1300mg with • Enzymatic Therapy THYMUPLEX for immune strength.

7—**Amino acid therapy:** •Country Life RELAXER capsules with Taurine 500mg; •Acetyl-carnitine (20mg for every 20lbs, of body weight); •GABA 100mg daily and •L-glutamine are the cutting edge of Down's treatment. Ask your naturopath.

Lifestyle Support Therapy

—Lifestyle measures:
•Music bypasses the brain to touch our emotional core. Play soothing classical or new age music in the home. I have seen it work wonders to calm behavioral stress problems.
•Avoid pesticides, heavy metals, (cadmium, lead and mercury), and aluminum.

—Bodywork:
•More oxygen and increased circulation are the bodywork goals for better brain function. Build more brain circuits by reading and playing mental games. Do deep breathing exercises every morning to oxygenate the brain.
•Expose the body to early morning sunshine daily if possible for vitamin D.
•Massage therapy helps circulation and tissue strength.
•Stay interactive with other people and especially animals.

—Reflexology points:
•Pinch the end of each toe. Hold 5 seconds.
•Squeeze all around the hand and fingers.

D 372

Common Symptoms: *Slow reactions and motor dysfunction; poor collagen and connective tissue causing weakness, poor muscle tone and joints; learning disability; social withdrawal and poor behavior with people; thyroid disease; gland and hormone deficiencies giving the person a "retarded," mongoloid appearance.*
Common Causes: *Drugs, either given to the child or taken by the mother when pregnant; immune system dysfunction from free radical damage from excessive SOD production; excess water fluoridation; too much sugar and refined foods; heavy metal poisoning altering brain chemistry; hypoglycemia and glycogen storage deficiency; allergies; birth trauma.*

See the HYPOGLYCEMIA DIET *page* 427 *and* ALZHEIMER'S DISEASE *page* 311 *for more.*

Can't find a recommended product? Call the 800 number listed in Product Resources for the store nearest you.

Earaches

Excessive Earwax, Otitis Media, Otitis Externa (Swimmer's Ear)

The most common type of infection in adults is swimmer's ear - inflammation of the outer ear canal. Middle ear infections are common in children (accounting for a third of all childhood doctor visits) whose eustachian tubes have not fully formed. Lavish use of antibiotics for ear infections is almost never justified, because common use often results in thrush in children and candidiasis in adults. Breast feed your baby; breast fed kids have far less ear infections as they grow up. Nursing mothers should avoid dairy products if their babies are prone to ear infections. Enhancing immune defenses is a primary factor in controlling chronic earaches in both adults and children. Question having medical drainage tubes placed in children's ears. They may damage hearing.

Diet & Superfood Therapy

—Nutritional therapy plan:

1—Many ear infections are the result of food reactions. Eliminate MSG, and check for food additives and preservatives, the biggest offenders. If earaches are chronic, keep the diet low in fats and reduce mucous-forming foods like dairy products.

2—During healing, eliminate all milk and dairy products, sugars and protein-concentrated foods, such as peanut butter. Do not take sweet fruit juices in full strength. The high natural sugars may feed bacteria.

3—Reduce all sugary, fried and refined foods.

4—Drink lots of water and diluted juices to keep mucous secretions thinned.

—For pain: Use ice packs instead of heat on the ear to relieve pain.

• Press out and strain onion juice onto a small cotton plug. Place in the ear for fast, effective relief and infection fighting,

• Mix warm vegetable glycerine and witch hazel. Soak a piece of cotton and insert in the ear to draw out infection. ☺

—Superfood therapy: (Choose one or two)

• Crystal Star BIOFLAVONOID, FIBER & C SUPPORT™ drink as needed.

• Liquid chlorophyll in water 3x daily.

Herb & Supplement Therapy

—Interceptive therapy plan: (Choose 2 to 3 recommendations)

1—Control the infection: •Crystal Star ANTI-BIO™ capsules 4 to 6 daily, or extract 4x daily to clear infection. (Extract may also be used as ear drops morning and evening.) •Nutribiotic GRAPEFRUIT SEED extract to clear infection. Warm •Lobelia extract in the ear. ☺ •Use •Echinacea extract, or BD Herbs organic Echinacea in water internally. •Mix 1-oz. white vinegar and 1-oz. 70% isopropyl alcohol; drop in the ear for 30 seconds. Rinse out. Three times daily.

2—Reduce swelling and inflammation: •Crystal Star ANTI-HST™ capsules to shrink swollen membranes. (Also use before an airplane flight to relieve ear congestion.) Chewing •Xylitol gum can sometimes open swollen ear canal. ☺ •Enzymatic Therapy LYMPHO-CLEAR to flush lymph glands.

3—Relieve pain and throbbing: •Crystal Star ASPIR-SOURCE™ capsules 4 at a time (open in juice for kids); ☺ or •Crystal Star ANTI-FLAM™ 4 at a time for for inflammation in adults. •Chamomile tea.

4—Enhance immune defenses: •Crystal Star ZINC SOURCE spray or drops or •Zand ZINC HERBAL lozenges. •Vitamin C 500mg for each year of child's age daily; •Acidophilus pwdr. $\frac{1}{4}$ teasp. in juice 4x daily; beta carotene 25,000IU daily.

5—Effective homeopathic remedies: •NatraBio EARACHE; •Pulsatilla; •Chamomilla for irritability; •Belladonna for throbbing pain.

—Effective ear drops: (use a dropper and flush ear gently) •Mullein oil drops; ☺ or •Herbs Etc. MULLEIN-GARLIC ear drops; •Turtle Island warm EAR OIL drops; •Calendula oil ear drops; warm •garlic oil or •Gaia GARLIC oil ear drops; •take garlic tabs 4x daily, too. •Castor oil drops; or food grade dilute solution, 3% H₂O₂ to cleanse infection.

—Make an aromatherapy ear massage: 6 drops chamomile oil, 3 drops tea tree oil and 3 drops lavender or calendula oil. Add to 1-oz. vitamin E oil. Rub around the ear and massage down the neck.

Lifestyle Support Therapy

—Bodywork:

• Massage ear, neck and temples. Pull ear lobe 10 times on each ear. Fold ear shell over and back repeatedly until blood suffuses area. Big yawn several times.

• Ear candles are effective used as directed.

• Most childhood earaches can be treated at home. Get medical help if you see these signs:
—if acute pain and loss of hearing does not respond within 48 hours.
—if fever does not abate within 3 days.
—if dizziness, difficult breathing or vomiting, bloody discharge, or redness around the ear.

—For excess earwax: Have the ear flushed for infection at a clinic.

• Then press firmly but gently behind, then in front of the ear. Pull lobe up and down to work wax out. Fold ear shell in half. Open and fold repeatedly for circulation.

• Put 3 drops of warm olive oil in each ear to soften wax; flush with warm water.

—Reflexology point:

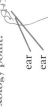

ear
ear

Common Symptoms: *Acute, stabbing pain in the mastoid, eustachian and ear area; swelling, inflammation, thickness and temporary loss of hearing in the ear; slight fever and general fussiness in a child - nausea and vomiting in a baby; bleeding or pusy discharge from the ear; extreme tenderness when the earlobe is pulled; ear congestion.*

Common Causes: *Residue of a cold, flu or bronchial infection settling in the ear; too many mucous-forming foods like dairy products; food allergies esp. to sulfires; high altitude, cold and decompression in air travel; in children, eustachian tubes become easy breeding areas for bacterial infection. A ruptured eardrum can result from diving, a hard slap on the ear, a loud explosion or a serious middle ear infection.*

See also COLD page 353 and FLU page 387 for more information.

Can't find a recommended product? Call the 800 number listed in Product Resources for the store nearest you.

Eating Disorders

Anorexia Nervosa, Bulimia

Almost 15% of Americans have some type of eating disorder. For 35% of women, and over 75% of American teen-age girls, looking good means being bone thin. Fashion models are seen as the aesthetic standard and **the health standard.** Striving to meet this abnormal standard means thinness at any cost, leading to eating disorders that are extremely hard to overcome, and may be fatal. Within 20 years of diagnosis, there is a mortality rate of almost 40%! Men are not completely exempt. Bodybuilders, male models, etc. compete with ever-thinner rivals, and can suffer reduced testicular function from starving. Bulimia is a binge-purge cycle - consumption of huge amounts of food in a very short time and then vomiting to purge it from the system. Anorexia is self-starvation, distorted body image, extreme preoccupation with food, sometimes binge eating.

Diet & Superfood Therapy

—**Nutritional therapy plan:**

1—Emphasize optimal nutrient foods for body regeneration. Eat a high vegetable protein, high complex carbohydrate diet. Don't skip breakfast - with whole grain cereals, fruit and yogurt.

2—Carrot juice (page 219) or Green Foods CARROT ESSENCE daily.

3—NO junk foods, heavy starches or sugars. They disrupt normalization of body chemistry.

4—Eat slowly; chew well; have small meals often for best absorption.

5—Boost B vitamins: Make a mix of Red Star NUTRITIONAL YEAST, bee pollen granules, toasted wheat germ, molasses; take 2 TBS daily.

—**Superfoods are lifesavers (choose 2 or 3):**
- Crystal Star SYSTEMS STRENGTH™.
- Future Biotics VITAL K - liquid poassium.
- Protein drinks: Unipro PERFECT PROTEIN, or Solgar WHEY TO GO.
- Green drinks for blood-building: (pg. 218) or Crystal Star ENERGY GREEN™.
- Rainbow Light HAWAIIAN SPIRULINA.
- Crystal Star BIOFLAV., FIBER & C SUPPORT™ drink daily for 1 month.
- Y.S. ROYAL JELLY-GINSENG drink daily.
- Crystal Star nutrient-rich drink, LIGHT WEIGHT™ meal replacement is well-accepted by people struggling with eating disorders.

Herb & Supplement Therapy

—**Interceptive therapy plan: (Choose 2 to 3 recommendations)**

1—**Normalize appetite and metabolism:** • Zinc is a key. Severely zinc-deficient people can't manufacture a key protein that allows them to taste. Chewable zinc lozenges help, or • Crystal Star ZINC SOURCE™ extract or capsules with POTASSIUM-IODINE SOURCE™ caps; (Add extra tyrosine 500mg if desired.)
• Crystal Star BODY REBUILDER™ caps with ADR-ACTIVE™ caps, 2 each daily.

2—**Herbal serotonin boosters help regulate mood-appetite brain chemicals:**
• Natural Balance 5-HTP CALM, 100mg daily. • Crystal Star RELAX CAPS™ 4 daily (especially for bulimics) to rebuild nerve structure.

3—**Control stress reactions:** • B-complex like Nature's Secret ULTIMATE B or Country Life SUBLINGUAL B-12 3000mcg with folic acid 200mcg for healthy cell growth and energy. GABA compounds relieve stress relief - • Natrol SAF or Country Life RELAXER tabs.

4—**Stimulate appetite, digestion and nutrient assimilation:** • Enzymedica DIGEST speeds digestion, takes stress off enzyme reserves; • Ginseng-Gotu Kola caps, 4 daily; • Rainforest Remedies BELLY BE GOOD herbs; • Rainbow Light ADVANCED ENZYME SYSTEM; • Acidophilus complex powder ¹/₄ tsp. 3x daily.

—**Ginseng is a key for energy and balance without calories:** • Root To Health POWER PIECES (panax ginseng in honey); • Beehive Botanical GINSENG/ROYAL JELLY caps; • Crystal Star GINSENG SUPER 6™ 2 daily, or • Crystal Star FEEL GREAT™ capsules 2x daily for a feeling of well-being and strength.

—**Mineral therapy is effective:** The minerals people with eating disorders lose through vomiting are the ones that help control their weight - potassium and iodine stimulate the thyroid to keep metabolism and calorie-burning strong. (Minerals also help restore normal menstrual periods.) • Crystal Star MINERAL SPECTRUM caps; • Nature's Path TRACE-MIN-LYTE (with sea greens); • Flora VEGE-SIL caps, or • Crystal Star SILICA SOURCE™ extract for new collagen growth.

Lifestyle Support Therapy

See Eating Disorder Test on page 524.

—**Bodywork:**
• Since there is a high correlation between sexual abuse and eating disorders, psychological counseling is often helpful. It can help in understanding the universal problem of low self-esteem that triggers this behavior. Therapy during healing reinforces the idea that destructive thinking and behavior can change, and the self-confidence of the sufferer reestablished. However, from experience I know it is almost impossible for an anorectic or bulimic person to seek help until they are almost beyond help.
• To improve self-esteem, cultivate relationships with positive people. Keep company with those in whose company you feel good about yourself.
• Get some mild exercise every day for lung, heart and muscle rebuilding.
• Get regular massage therapy treatments.

—**Reflexology point:**

food assimilation

Common Symptoms: Extreme malnutrition from vomiting/laxatives (bulimia) that discharges most nutrients; or refusing to eat (anorexia); belligerent, impolite, aggressive behavior; low blood pressure, slow heartbeat; hard fecal stools; fluid retention; reduced metabolism; cold hands and feet; dry skin, brittle, dull hair; tooth decay and yellow teeth; cessation of menses. Bulimia sufferers have a swollen neck and eroded tooth enamel from excessive vomiting, broken blood vessels on the face, low pulse rate and blood pressure, and extreme weakness.

Common Causes: Eating disorders are usually caused by complex cultural or emotional problems that end up turning into a form of compulsive psychosis. Sometimes yeasts or celiac disease are involved.

For more information contact the National Eating Disorder Organization (800) 322-5173 x5600.

E 374

Can't find a recommended product? Call the 800 number listed in Product Resources for the store nearest you.

Eczema and Psoriasis

Atopic Dermatitis

Eczema is an intense, itchy, inflammatory skin disease found on the tender areas of elbows, knees, wrists and neck. It is most common in infants and children. **Psoriasis** is a common adult skin disorder, marked by plaques and silvery scales on the skin, caused by a too-rapid replication and pile up of skin cells. It usually affects the scalp, and the outsides of the elbows, wrists, knees, etc. Drugs can produce dramatic short-term results, but the problem reappears after they are discontinued. Natural therapies have had notable achievement in both skin conditions because they get to the root of the problem. Natural methods take several months to produce consistent improvement, but they offer lasting results.

Diet & Superfood Therapy

—Nutritional therapy plan:

1–A healthy, low fat diet is a key factor. Most severe psoriasis sufferers are overweight.

2–A high fiber, high mineral diet with lots of vegetable protein is the key to clearing and preventing eczema.

3–Go on a short 3 day cleansing diet (pg. 191) to release acid wastes. Take 1 TB psyllium husk, Sonné bentonite or Crystal Star CHOL-LO-FIBER TONE™ in water morning and evening.

4–Take three cranberry or apple juices daily.

5–Eliminate refined fatty or fried foods, alcohol and red meats. Then follow a sugar-free, milk-free, low-fat and alkalizing diet with 60-70% fresh foods, whole grains, seafood and sea vegetables for iodine therapy.

6–Make a skin health mix of lecithin granules, brewer's yeast, and unsulphured molasses and take 2 TBS daily.

—Superfood therapy:
Take a green drink daily.
• Crystal Star BIOFLAV, FIBER & C SUPPORT™ to help tissue integrity.
• Nutricology PROGREENS with EFA's.
• AloeLife ALOE JUICE drink with herbs.
• Green Foods GREEN MAGMA.
• Crystal Star ENERGY GREEN™ with sea greens for EFA's.

Herb & Supplement Therapy

—Interceptive therapy plan: (Choose 2 to 3 recommendations)

1—Control the infection: • Take Crystal Star ANTI-BIO™ caps, and apply • ANTI-BIO™ extract or ANTI-BIO™ gel; • Una da gato caps 6 daily; • Myrrh-Goldenseal root extract; • Echinacea extract or Pau d' arco tea for 3 months as a lymphatic cleanser.

2—Reduce the inflammation and scaliness: • MSM, 750 to 1000mg • Turmeric therapy: take equivalent of 1-oz. (twelve "00" capsules) turmeric daily for 6 weeks. Often dramatic results in new skin without recurrence. Apply • Mahonia bark ointment to heal psoriasis plaques. • Chamomile tea reduces inflammation. For excellent results with eczema: • Licorice root or burdock tea; apply • witch hazel or chickweed tea relieves eczema itching. • Diamond HERPANACINE capsules as directed.

3—Heal the skin with minerals: Spray • Crystal Star ZINC SOURCE™ on sore areas; take • Crystal Star BEAUTIFUL SKIN™ tea internally 2 cups daily, and apply to lesions with soaked cotton balls. • Zinc picolinate 50mg daily; with • vitamin E 400IU and selenium 200mcg (or mix zinc oxide with pricked vitamin E oil capsules and apply to sores). • Add copper 2mg 3x daily for 2 months; • Nutricology GERMANIUM 150mg daily. For psoriasis, • Alta Health SILICA with bioflavs.; apply • Body Essentials SILICA GEL • Aloe vera gel or • Nettles extract.

4—Boost omega-3 oils for more EFA's: Use for at least 3 to 6 months • Evening primrose oil 4000mg daily; • Barleans's lignan-rich flax oil 3x daily; • Nature's Secret ULTIMATE OIL; • Lane Labs BENE-FIN shark cartilage caps 3 daily for 3 months.

5—Reduce stress to help psoriasis: • Crystal Star ADRN™ extract drops help form adrenal cortex; • Crystal Star RELAX CAPS™ ease stress.

6—Nourish the skin to prevent recurrence: • Crystal Star BEAUTIFUL SKIN™ gel daily; • Abkit CAMO-CARE cream; • Ester C with bioflavonoids 3000mg daily for tissue regrowth and less histamine reactions. • Beta carotene 100,000IU daily, or • PHYCOTENE MICROCLUSTERS mixed carotenes and sea greens, available at Healthy House; and vitamin A & D 1000/400IU 4 daily. • B-complex 100mg with extra pantothenic acid 500mg, PABA 1000mg. Keep the liver healthy- • yellow dock root tea 2 cups daily. • MILK THISTLE SEED extract drops 2x daily; • yellow dock root tea 2 cups daily.

Lifestyle Support Therapy

—Bodywork:

• Exercise keeps circulation healthy and body wastes released.

• Expose affected areas to early morning sunlight daily for healing vitamin D.

• Swim or wade in the ocean, or take kelp foot baths for iodine therapy.

• Take a catnip or chlorophyll enema once a week to release acid toxins that come out on the skin.

• For childhood eczema: bathe areas with strong chamomile tea, then apply an oatmeal paste and let dry. Repeat for 4 days until clear.

—Effective skin applications:

• Tea tree oil for psoriasis.
• Aloe vera gel.
• Jojoba oil (for scalp psoriasis).
• Capsaicin cream reduces psoriasis itching.
• Hot ginger, goldenseal or fresh comfrey leaf compresses.

—Stress management is a key:
Depression and emotional stress can cause and aggravate psoriasis flare-ups. Meditation seems to relieve psoriasis outbreaks.

• Overheating therapy (pg. 225) is effective for psoriasis.

Common Symptoms: Chronic silvery red, scaly, skin rash or patches on knees, elbows, buttocks, scalp or chest that flare up irregularly; skin is continually dry and thickened even when not in the weeping, blistered stages; "oil drop" stippling of the nails; sometimes accompanying arthritis. Great susceptibility to staph infections and herpes outbreaks.

Common Causes: Overuse of drugs/antibiotics; chronic stress or depression; eczema is associated with diabetes, asthma, candida yeast; psoriasis with arthritis; hypothyroidism; EFA deficiency; liver malfunction; thin bowel walls allowing wastes elimination through the skin; excess fatty foods in the diet and poor protein digestion; food allergies also play a role, especially to wheat, dairy, soy and nuts; heavy smoking.

See also SKIN HEALING page 497 for more information.

Can't find a recommended product? Call the 800 number listed in Product Resources for the store nearest you.

E 375

Emphysema

Smoker's Pulmonary Disease

Emphysema is a wasting pulmonary disease that affects smokers almost exclusively. It is characterized by loss of elasticity and dilation ability, then scarring and thickening of delicate lung tissue. Breathing becomes ever more difficult as the lungs progressively scar. The lung exchange of oxygen and carbon-dioxide is seriously affected to the point of extreme breathlessness and the inability to take a deep breath at all. The person feels asphyxiated and struggles for every breath. Severe pneumonia bouts almost always occur. Natural therapies can help, but if an emphysema sufferer continues to smoke, emphysema is usually fatal (for 50,000 men alone each year). See STOP SMOKING, page 553 in this book.

Diet & Superfood Therapy

—Nutritional therapy plan:

1—Eliminate food and inhalant allergens, especially mucous-forming foods that provide storage for the allergens, like pasteurized dairy, (mucous), red meats (saturated fat). Go on a short mucous cleansing juice diet for 3-5 days (pg. 196).

2—Make sure your diet is low in sugars and fats to reduce your breathlessness. Eat largely fresh foods. Increase your vegetable protein from whole grains, tofu, nuts, seeds and sprouts. Have a green salad every day, and add vitamin B rich foods such as brown rice and eggs frequently.

3—Add extra protein to your diet from sea foods like salmon and sea greens for more B$_{12}$

4—Have a glass of fresh carrot juice every day for a month (pg. 219), then every other day for a month.

—Superfood therapy: (Choose one or more)

• Wakunaga KYO-GREEN drink.
• Crystal Star SYSTEMS STRENGTH™ drink.
• Solgar EARTH SOURCE GREEN & MORE drink.♂
• Beehive Botanical ROYAL JELLY with Siberian ginseng 2 teasp. daily, or Long Life IMPERIAL TONIC with royal jelly and EPO.♀
• AloeLife ALOE GOLD juice 2x daily.
• Mona's CHLORELLA drink or tabs.

Herb & Supplement Therapy

—Interceptive therapy plan: (Choose 2 to 3 recommendations)

1—Control the infection: •Crystal Star ANTI-BIO™ caps 6 daily followed by •Propolis extract, or Beehive Botanicals PROPOLIS TINCTURE 65%, 3x daily, or •Crystal Star BIO-VI™ extract with propolis. •Crystal Star GINSENG-LICO-RICE ELIXIR™ reduces lung inflammation.

2—Thin, loosen, expel phlegmy bronchial mucous: •Crystal Star X-PECT™ tea expels mucous congestion. •Rainbow Light GARLIC & GREENS caps, 6x daily, or •Crystal Star IODINE THERAPY extract with 1 tsp. olive oil in juice dissolves mucous. •NAC (N-acetyl-cysteine) 1000mg, or Nutricology NAC 500mg daily.

3—Help your lungs detoxify from pollutants: •Vitamin C crystals with bioflavonoids $\frac{1}{4}$ teasp. every hour to bowel tolerance daily for a month (an ascorbic acid flush to neutralize lung poisons and encourage tissue elasticity); then reduce to 5000mg daily for 3 months. •Crystal Star HEAVY METAL CLEANZ™ caps if pollutants are the cause. •Crystal Star WITHDRAWAL SUPPORT™ capsules if marijuana smoking is the cause. •Nutricology Germanium 150mg, or •Crystal Star IODINE-POTASSIUM SOURCE™ caps 3x daily for tobacco smoke.

4—Enhance breathing muscles: •Carnitine 500mg 2x daily; •magnesium citrate, 400mg daily; •Crystal Star RSPR™ caps 2x daily for tissue oxygen uptake.

5—Nourish the lungs and bronchial tubes: •High B-complex 150mg daily with pantothenic acid 500mg, and extra folic acid 800mcg. •Mullein-lobelia caps or extract drops in water daily; •Comfrey-fenugreek or Pleurisy root tea; •Lycopene caps, 4 daily, a carotene specific for the lungs. •Transformation Enzymes PUREZYME protease enzymes (excellent results for scarring). •Enzymatic Therapy LUNG COMPLEX and THYMUPLEX COMPLEX. •PCOs from grapeseed or white pine, 100mg 3x daily strengthen collagen and elastin tissue and reduce inflammation.

6—Antioxidants are critical for lung tissue oxygen: •Beta carotene 150,000IU or mixed carotenes like •PHYCOTENE MICROCLUSTERS from Healthy House, with copper 2mg daily for lung tissue elasticity; •Vitamin E 1000IU with selenium 400mcg daily; •CoQ-10 100mg 2x daily; •Premier GERMANIUM w. DMG.

Lifestyle Support Therapy

—Bodywork:

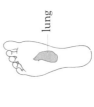

• Avoid smoking and secondary smoke, including smog and other air pollution. (Use Enzymatic Therapy NICO-STOP formula to help stop smoking.)

• Do deep breathing exercises for 3 minutes every morning when rising to clean out the lungs.

• Take a brisk deep breathing daily walk to increase oxygen.

• Get some early sunlight on the body every day possible.

• Steam head and nasal passages with *eucalyptus* and *wintergreen* herbs.

• Use 1 teasp. food grade 3% solution H$_2$O$_2$ in 8-oz. water in a vaporizer at night.

—Reflexology point:

lung

E 376

Common Symptoms: Chronic bronchitis with shortness of breath, continuing post-nasal drip and congestion; frequent colds; coated tongue; bad breath; frequent hacking cough, especially during exhalation and speaking; lack of energy and general vitality because of lack of oxygen.

Common Causes: Smoking and secondary smoke; air and environmental pollution; excess refined foods and dairy products; allergies (both foods and chemicals) are usually involved; heavy metal pollution from industry; poor circulation; poor elimination of poisons by the lungs.

See also the HYPOGLYCEMIA DIET in this book, or COOKING FOR HEALTHY HEALING by Linda Rector-Page.

Can't find a recommended product? Call the 800 number listed in Product Resources for the store nearest you.

Endometriosis

Pelvic Inflammatory Disease (PID), Polycystic Ovarian Syndrome

Endometriosis is a condition caused by endometrial tissue that is not shed during menstruation. The tissue escapes the uterus and spreads attaching to other areas of the body (ovaries, lymph nodes, fallopian tubes, bladder, rectum, even the lungs). There it grows as normal tissue in abnormal places, bleeding, usually severely during the menstrual cycle from the vagina or the rectum or bladder or back through the fallopian tubes instead of through the vagina normally. Endometriosis increases risk for uterine and breast fibroids. It is credited with up to 50% of infertility cases in American women. It is often followed by CFS or Fibromyalgia. An immune-enhancing program that addresses liver therapy, improves emotional stress, body trauma, and relieves pain is effective. Question corticosteroid drugs commonly given for endometriosis - esp. prednisone.

Diet & Superfood Therapy

—Nutritional therapy plan:

1—Go on a short 24 hour juice diet (pg. 192) to clear out acid wastes. (This helps you to work on the integrity of the liver and digestive system first. Repeat the cleanse for 24 hours before menses.)

2—Decrease estrogen production with a low fat diet (20 grams daily). Especially avoid dairy foods.

3—Then follow a vegan diet with the addition of cold water fish. Eat cultured foods, fresh fruits and green salads, whole grains and cereals until condition clears. Especially add soy foods and sea greens (2 TBS daily) for estrogen balancing power.

4—**Eat an immune power diet:** Eliminate alcohol and caffeine during healing. Restrict refined sugars, red meats and dairy products during healing. Keep all animal fats and high cholesterol foods low, to prevent excess estrogen production, a clear cause of endometriosis. Particularly avoid chocolate, tropical oils, fried and fast food of all kinds.

5—See the Hypoglycemia Diet, page 427 for long term eating habits.

—Superfood therapy: (Choose one or more)
• Body Ecology VITALITY SUPERGREEN.
• Crystal Star ENERGY GREEN™ drinks.
• Crystal Star SYSTEMS STRENGTH™ for iodine and potassium therapy.
• Nature's Secret ULTIMATE GREEN - EFA's.

Herb & Supplement Therapy

—Interceptive therapy plan: (Choose 2 to 3 recommendations)

1—**Relieve pain and clear our wastes:** • Crystal Star WOMAN'S BEST FRIEND™ caps 6 daily, and burdock tea 2 cups daily for 3 months or • Transitions PRO-GEST cream or oil rubbed on the abdomen. • Black cohosh extract or • Transformation Enzyme PURE-ZYME tablets to dissolve adhesions of abnormally placed tissue; • Crystal Star PRO-EST BALANCE™ roll-on, controls pain and stimulates progesterone balance. • Enzymatic Therapy NUCLEO-PRO F for pain relief. Chew tablets for faster results. • Ascorbic acid flush: ascorbate vitamin C powder with bioflavonoids - $\frac{1}{4}$ teasp. in juice every hour until stool turns soupy.

2—**Reduce inflammation and spasms:** • Crystal Star ANTI-FLAM™ caps or ANTI-SPZ caps 4 at a time each; • Enzymatic Therapy LYMPHO-CLEAR 3x daily.
• American Biologics SHARKILAGE 750mg as an anti-infective.

3—**EFA's are important for metabolizing and balancing excess estrogen:** • Evening Primrose Oil caps 1000mg 4 daily; • Omega-rich flax or fish oil; • Solaray LIPOTROPIC PLUS complex; • Barlean's ESSENTIAL WOMAN oils; • Dandelion leaf tea.

4—**Energy-building liver therapy:** • Echinacea and Milk Thistle Seed extracts; • NatureWorks SWEDISH BITTERS or Crystal Star BITTERS & LEMON CLEANSE™. (Note: Bitters herbs can be excellent cleansers of pelvic congestion, but should be avoided during painful flare-ups.) • Nature's Secret ULTIMATE B, and extra folic acid 400mcg; • Floradix HERBAL IRON 3x daily; Enzymedica PURIFY protease.

5—**Balance hormones for long term relief:** • Crystal Star WOMEN'S STRENGTH ENDO™ tea -a gland and hormone balancer for 3 months. • Choline 1000mg with inositol 500mg; • Crystal Star ADRN™ extract for adrenal cortex balance; • VITEX extract for pituitary support; • Bernard Jensen LIQUI-DULS for thyroid balance.

6—**For emotional stress and tension:** • Crystal Star RELAX CAPS™ for stress reduction - 2 at a time as needed.

7—**Enhance immune response:** • CoQ-10, 60mg 3x daily. • Solgar OCEANIC CAROTENE 100,000IU daily; • Ester C with bioflavonoids 3000mg; • Future Biotics VITAL K liquid potassium 3 teasp. daily; • Vitamin E 400IU daily.

Lifestyle Support Therapy

Before you jump into surgery or any drastic treatment decision, endometriosis fibroids often go away when glands and hormones rebalance, such as after pregnancy and birth, or menopause.

—Bodywork:
• Use stress reduction techniques like massage therapy and acupuncture.
• Avoid all chloro-fluorocarbon products and any other known toxic chemical or environmental pollutants.
• Avoid all IUD's. They are a major contributor to endometriosis.
• Get mild exercise and early morning sunlight on the body every day.

—Effective cleansing douches:
• Garlic
• Mineral water

—Reflexology point:
• Press both sides of the foot just below the ankle bone, 2x daily for 10 seconds each.
• Boluses and vaginal packs are effective in drawing out internal infection. Use castor oil packs or see the formula in HOME PROTOCOLS in this book. Make sure there are long rest times between pack or bolus use - 1 week of use to 3 weeks rest.

Common Symptoms: *Severe cramping and abdominal-rectal pain, swelling and bleeding just before menses, during ovulation and sex; fluid retention; enlarged ovaries; irritable bowel and gas; pinched nerve-type pain; unusual insomnia; excessive menstruation and prolonged cycles; irregular bowel movements or diarrhea during menses.*

Common Causes: *Excess levels of estrogen, deficient progesterone, hormone imbalance that causes abnormal behavior of the endometrium; sexually transmitted chlamydia, cervical dysplasia or vaginal warts; linked to yeast infections such as candida; magnesium deficiency; hypoglycemia; EFA deficiency and prostaglandin imbalance; X-Ray consequences; high fat diet with too much caffeine and alcohol.*

Call the ENDOMETRIOSIS hotline 1-800-992-ENDO: for updated information.

Can't find a recommended product? Call the 800 number listed in Product Resources for the store nearest you.

Energy

Increasing Stamina and Endurance, Overcoming Fatigue, Nerve Exhaustion and Mental Burn-Out

There's no doubt about it - stress and fatigue are becoming more a part of our lives - eight out of ten Americans say they feel tired most of the time. Almost all of us feel the need for a pick-me-up during a long day. Yet, turning to drugs or controlled substances for stimulation is asking for trouble. The result of overuse of stimulants is dependency, irritability and lethargy, further reducing energy in a downward spiral. Even traditional food energizers like caffeine, sodas or sugar can end up making us feel more nervous and restless. Natural energizers have great advantages over chemically processed stimulants. They don't exhaust the body, and are supporting rather than depleting. They can be strong or gentle as needed.

Diet & Superfood Therapy

—Nutritional therapy plan:

1—A balanced, high energy diet should consist of 65-70% complex carbohydrates, fresh fruits, vegetables, whole grains and legumes; 20-25% protein, from nuts, seeds, whole grains, legumes, soy, yogurt and kefir, sea foods and poultry; 10-15% fats from sources such as unrefined vegetable, nut and seed oils, eggs and low-fat dairy.

2—Foods that fight fatigue: potassium and magnesium-rich foods, complex carbohydrates, high vitamin B and C foods, and iron-rich foods.

3—Reduce sugar, caffeine, (drains adrenals) and dairy foods (produces clogging mucous).

4—Take a protein drink every morning (pg. 276). Add spirulina or bee pollen granules or Bragg's LIQUID AMINOS to any drink as a booster.

1—Drink plenty of healthy liquids. Dehydration's first sign is fatigue. Have a little wine at dinner for mental relaxation and good digestion.

—Superfoods are a key to rapid energy:

• Alacer EMERGEN-C granules in water.
• Nutri-Tech ALL 1 vit./mineral drink.
• Crystal Star ENERGY GREEN™.
• Unipro PERFECT PROTEIN.
• Nature's Life SUPER-PRO 96 drink.
• Beehive Botanicals ginseng/royal jelly.
• Nutrex HAWAIIAN SPIRULINA.
• Nature's Secret BEYOND ENDURANCE.

Herb & Supplement Therapy

—Interceptive therapy plan: (Choose 1 or 2 recommendations)

1—**Energizers for men:** • Crystal Star HIGH PERFORMANCE™ caps; SUPER MAN'S ENERGY™ tonic; MALE GINSIAC™, and ADRN™ extracts. • Chinese red ginseng; • Allergy Research BIOGEN PRO growth hormone. • Zinc picolinate 50-75mg.

2—**Energizers for women:** • Crystal Star BODY REBUILDER™ and ADR-ACTIVE™ caps; FEM-SUPPORT™ extract with ashwagandha, RAINFOREST ENERGY™ caps, FEEL GREAT tea. • Enzymatic Therapy THYROID-TYROSINE COMPLEX.
• Evening Primrose Oil for fatigue recovery; • Hawthorn extract for well-being.

3—**Ginseng is a natural energizer for both sexes:** • Crystal Star ACTIVE PHYSICAL ENERGY caps, FEEL GREAT™ caps, GINSENG SUPER 6 ENERGY™ capsules and tea; • Rainbow Light TEN GINSENGS; • Siberian ginseng extract;
• Suma caps; • Bioforce GINSAVENA.♂ Hsu's WILD AMERICAN GINSENG.

4—**Mental energizers:** • Crystal Star MENTAL INNER ENERGY™ caps and extract; • Ginkgo biloba extract or • Rainbow Light GINKGO SUPER COMPLEX;♀
• Enzymatic Therapy BRAIN NUTRITION caps; • NADH 10mg in the morning.

5—**Central Nervous System energizers:** • Crystal Star HIGH ENERGY™ tea and RAINFOREST ENERGY™ caps; • Futurebiotics LIVING ENERGY caps; • L-Glutamine 1000mg daily; • Nature's Secret ULTIMATE ENERGY.

6—**Metabolic energizers improve the performance of your body:** • Enzymedica PURIFY capsules on an empty stomach; • CoQ-10, 30mg 2x daily or Nutricology CoQ-10 with tocotrienols; • L-Carnitine 1000mg daily; • Alpha Lipoic acid 100mg 3x daily; • B-complex 100mg with extra pantothenic acid 500mg 2x daily.

7—**Nutrient boosters to overcome fatigue:** • Country Life sublingual B-12 2500mcg with folic acid 200mcg; take with tyrosine 500mg for best results. • Chromium picolinate 200mcg daily. • Source Naturals OPTI-ZINC.♂ • Nature's Path TRACE-LYTE minerals; ♀ Country Life INSTA-FIZZ energy enhancer.

8—**Antioxidant energizers:** • Vitamin C with bioflavonoids, 3000mg daily.
• Country Life DMG sublingual tabs or • Unipro LIQUID DMG. ♀ • A full spectrum, pre-digested amino acid compound, 1000mg. daily. ♂

Lifestyle Support Therapy

—Bodywork:

• If symptoms are chronic for more than 6 months, get a test for EBV, chronic fatigue syndrome, or Candida albicans.

• Take a brisk walk or other aerobic exercise every day for tissue oxygen. Aerobic exercise stimulates endorphins and replenishes oxygen in the entire body.

• Stretch out for 5 minutes both morning and before bed to release energy blocks.

• Get some early morning sunlight on the body every day possible.

• Have a full spinal massage for increased nerve force.

• Take alternating hot and cold hydrotherapy showers to increase circulation.

• Get good sleep. Feeling rested has everything to do with the amount of energy you have.

• Acupressure energizer: squeeze point between eyes where brows come together.

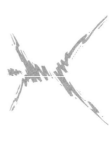

These two pages express just a tiny part of the natural energizers I've worked with. See my STRESS and ENERGY book for much more.

Can't find a recommended product? Call the 800 number listed in Product Resources for the store nearest you.

Common Symptoms: Lack of energy for even everyday tasks; mental depression; lethargy.
Common Causes: What's zapping our energy today? Why do some people drag through their daily lives, while others run marathons or juggle demanding career and family responsibilities without blinking an eye? Sickness, body imbalances, dietary deficiencies and prolonged stress, negativity and hopelessness all zap body energy. There are as many causes for fatigue as there are cures. Turn the page for a look at energy sappers and what you can do about them.

What's sapping your energy? Here are the 5 most common energy depleters.

—**LACK OF SLEEP:** 60 million Americans are sleep-deprived. Further, almost half of the U.S. population has sleep-related problems like insomnia. Lack of sleep may be one of the biggest health problems our society faces today. Americans sleep 20% less today than our ancestors did a century ago. A study from the National Center on Sleep Disorders Research reports that an astounding 25% of adults feel that they cannot be successful and still get adequate sleep. NEWSFLASH! We are not designed to stay awake deep into the night. This is why we become tired when it gets dark. We spend close to a third of our lives asleep. Lack of sleep zaps energy, reduces immunity, lowers libido, and raises blood pressure. When lack of sleep becomes absence of sleep, insanity results. Most people need 8 hours of sleep a night to recharge. Cutting into sleep time just by hour and a half reduces daytime alertness up to 33%!

Are you getting enough sleep? Signs that you may need more shuteye: 1) cuts, scrapes, blemishes or other injuries heal too slowly; 2) you have dark circles under your eyes; 3) you have difficulty getting up; 4) your are always tired; 5) your memory is poor and your thinking is fuzzy; 6) you sleep late regularly on the weekends; 7) you find yourself relying on stimulants like coffee, tea, nicotine or other drugs to get through the day.

—**STRESS:** No one is immune to all stress. The presence of stress depends on how you react to the changes and demands of your life. A little stress can even be good, motivating you towards meeting a goal. Too much stress can be disastrous to health. Chronic stress especially drains your energy, targeting organs like the adrenal glands and wiping out their stores. It shows up in how you look and how you feel. The more "stressed out" you become, the vulnerable you are to colds, flu, ulcers, allergies or even cardiovascular disease and high blood pressure.

Are you "stressed out"? Signs you may be on stress overload: 1) you get frequent tension headaches or migraines, chronic backaches or neck pain; 2) your brow is furrowed, you grimace a lot; 3) you have a tendency to "fly off the handle" easily; 4) you have fuzzy thinking or a poor memory; 5) you have chronic indigestion and unexplained weight loss; 6) you have chronic insomnia and daytime fatigue; 7) you have difficulty performing creative projects; 8) you get unusually frequent colds or flu.

—**ADRENAL EXHAUSTION:** Adrenal exhaustion is an epidemic in this country. No other gland is more affected by stress, emotional strain or anger than the adrenals. Your adrenal glands rest on top of kidneys and are responsible for a myriad of body functions including the production of steroid hormones like cortisone, DHEA, aldosterone, progesterone, estrogen and testosterone, maintaining body balance and regulating sugar metabolism. When you're under pressure, the adrenal medulla secretes adrenaline and norepinephrine which accelerates metabolism, heart rate, respiration and perspiration. This response is vital to our survival, strengthening the body and increasing its resistance to stress. But when the adrenals release too few or too many hormones, exhaustion can result. Corticosteroid drugs, temperature changes, excessive exercise, chronic stress and infections all exhaust your adrenal glands.

Are your adrenals exhausted? Body markers to watch out for: 1) constant fatigue or muscular weakness; 2) mood swings or spells of paranoia; 3) depression that is often relieved by eating; 4) chronic heartburn, indigestion or abdominal pain; 5) frequent heart palpitations, panic attacks or fainting spells; 6) unusually low blood pressure or excessively low cholesterol levels; 7) blood sugar disturbances or cravings for salt or sweets; 8) extreme sensitivity to odors and/or noises; 9) difficulty concentrating; 10) being easily frustrated with a tendency to cry or feel guilty; 11) chronic insomnia and headaches, particularly migraines; 12) clenching or grinding your teeth, especially at night; 13) frequent yeast or fungal infections.

—**THYROID MALFUNCTION:** Your thyroid is the gland which governs your metabolism, providing vital energy resources to all parts of the body. Since World War II, an above average number of people have thyroid problems. Thyroid disease affects 13 million people, most of whom are women. Today, hypothyroidism (low thyroid) is a common problem, largely because of all the chemicals and pollutants in our environment which put such a strain on our glandular health.

Is a sluggish thyroid slowing you down? Signs to watch out for: 1) lethargy or fatigue in the morning; 2) swollen ankles, hands and eyelids; 3) bloating, gas and indigestion after eating; 4) unusual depression; 5) unusual hair loss, especially in women; 6) unexplained obesity; 7) breast fibroid growths; 8) poor immune response.

—**OVER-USE OF STIMULANTS LIKE CAFFEINE, SUGAR OR DRUGS:** America is a quick fix society. We want something that works fast and we often end up paying the price in terms of our health. Overusing stimulants is one of the biggest energy zappers affecting Americans today. Nine out of ten Americans use caffeine in some form, averaging about 2 cups of coffee a day. The average person consumes 120 pounds of sugar a year, a whopping 1,000% increase from a century ago. We can get a quick lift from these substances, but they're one of the primary reasons we are so tired. Over-use of caffeine or sugar raises blood sugar. In the effort to clean up the excess sugar in the blood, insulin, the hormone which regulates blood sugar, removes too much sugar, causing low blood sugar reactions for more fatigue. Caffeine, a central nervous system stimulant, is also notorious for wiping out the adrenals, leading to low energy.

Are you hooked on caffeine and sugar? Here are a few clues: 1) easy agitation, frequent mood swings; 2) headaches and exhaustion when stimulants are eliminated; 3) increased tolerance to caffeine or sugar; 4) elevated blood sugar levels; 5) exhausted adrenals; 6) chronic insomnia; 7) dark circles under the eyes; 8) constipation when caffeine is eliminated.

Can't find a recommended product? Call the 800 number listed in Product Resources for the store nearest you.

E 379

Epilepsy
Petit Mal, Partial Seizures

Epilepsy is a neurological disorder very akin to an electrical short circuit in the brain, causing seizures. **1) Petit mal** *- a short seizure with a blank stare; most common in children;* **2) Grand mal** *- a long seizure with falling, muscle twitching, incontinence, gasping, and ashen skin.* **3) Partial seizures** *- muscle jerking, sensing things that do not exist. Most people have no memory of an attack. Many commonly used anti-convulsant drugs today are so strong and so habit forming that even non-epileptic people have bad reactions and seizures when cut off suddenly. Nutritional medicines can make drugs unnecessary. If you decide to use natural therapies, or try methods other than drugs, taper off gradually. If seizures recur, return to the anti-convulsants briefly to let the body adjust.*

Diet & Superfood Therapy

—Nutritional therapy plan:

1—There must be a diet and lifestyle change for there to be permanent control and improvement. Consider a rotation diet to check for food allergy reactions.

2—Start with a 3 day liquid diet (pg. 191) to release mucous from the system.

3—Then follow a diet with at least 70% fresh foods. Have a green salad every day.

4—Add cultured foods such as yogurt and kefir, tofu, brown rice and other whole grains.

5—After a month, add eggs, small amounts of low fat dairy, legumes, seafoods and sea greens.

6—Eat organically grown foods whenever possible to avoid seizure triggers in pesticides.

7—Eliminate foods with preservatives or colorings; refined foods, sugars, fried and canned foods, red meats, pork, alcohol, caffeine, and pasteurized dairy products.

—Superfood therapy: (Choose one or more)

• Crystal Star SYSTEMS STRENGTH™ for iodine, potassium, broad spectrum nutrients.
• Red Star NUTRITIONAL YEAST drink or MISO soup before bed.
• Amazake RICE DRINKS.
• AloeLife ALOE GOLD drink.
• Futurebiotics VITAL K.

Herb & Supplement Therapy

—Interceptive therapy plans: (choose 2 or 3 recommendations)

1—**Stabilize and nourish the nerves:** • Crystal Star RELAX CAPS™ and ANTI-SPZ™ caps as needed.; • Glutamine 500mg daily; • Country Life MAXI-B; • taurine 1500mg daily and • B-6 250mg as an anti-convulsant. • Country Life SUB-LINGUAL B-12 3000mcg with folic acid 200mcg; or • Alta Health SL MANGA-NESE with B-12.

2—**Natural sedatives help calm nerve convulsions:** • Lobelia extract drops in water daily; • Scullcap, or Catnip tea, 2 to 3 cups daily. • Nutremedix CALM as directed. • A calcium 1000mg/magnesium 500mg supplement daily to reduce excitability of the nerves. • Siberian ginseng or • Rainbow Light ADAPTO-GEM caps. • Country Life RELAXER caps with GABA and taurine 500mg 2x daily.

3—**Extra EFA's offer better brain balance:** • Evening Primrose Oil caps 4-6 daily for 2 months, then 3-4 daily for 1 month to balance body electrical activity.

4—**Protect your liver:** • Choline 600mg, or Choline-inositol or phosphatidyl choline for brain balance.; • Reishi mushroom extract 2x daily; • vitamin E 400IU; vitamin C, 500mg for each year of the child. • Crystal Star LIV-ALIVE™ caps and • Milk Thistle Seed extract especially if you are taking Dilantin or other anti-seizure drugs.

5—**Minerals help rebalance body chemistry:** • Atrium LITHIUM 5mg as directed; • Nature's Life TRACE MINERAL COMPLEX, or • Nature's Path TRACE-MIN LYTE; • Mezotrace SEA MINERAL caps; • American Biologics MANGA-NESE FORTE. Consider • oral chelation Golden Pride FORMULA 1 with EDTA.

—For young childhood epilepsy:

• Floradix liquid multiple vitamin-mineral complex for body balance.
• Nature's Way ANTSP tincture drops, or • lobelia tincture under the tongue as emergency measures.
• Carnitine 250mg with • folic acid 400mcg especially if taking Dilantin.
• Natren TRINITY for probiotic aid.

Lifestyle Support Therapy

—Bodywork:

• Take lemon juice or catnip enemas once a month keep the body pH balanced, toxin-free.
• Get some outdoor exercise every day for healthy circulation.
• New evidence shows that magnet therapy is effective in smoothing out the "electrical shorts" that accompany seizures.

• **Epileptic seizures are usually short,** with immediate recovery of consciousness.

—Do not attempt to restrain the person. Catch him if he falls. Loosen any constricting clothing.

—Let the person lie down and get plenty of fresh air. Clear away sharp or hard objects. Cushion the head.

—Squeeze the little finger very firmly during a seizure.

—Do not put anything in the person's mouth or throw water on the face. Turn head to let excess saliva drain out.

—Deep sleep usually follows a seizure.

• Biofeedback has been successful in shortening and limiting seizure attacks.

Common Symptoms: *Brief seizures, often with motor disability; loss of memory, sensory confusion, sometimes convulsions with jerking and foam at the mouth; sometimes there is falling down and loss of consciousness. Before a seizure there is often chest discomfort, nausea, or dizziness, heart palpitations or headaches, impaired speech, shortness of breath and numbness in the hands, lips and tongue.*
Common Causes: *Inability of the body to eliminate wastes properly with a resultant overload on the nervous system; heavy metal toxicity; allergies; EFA, magnesium and other mineral deficiency; hypoglycemia; sometimes drugs or alcohol; deficient metabolic function and prostaglandin formation; sometimes linked to allergies.*

See the HYPOGLYCEMIA DIET page 427 or my book COOKING FOR HEALTHY HEALING for more.

Can't find a recommended product? Call the 800 number listed in Product Resources for the store nearest you.

Eyesight

Weak Eyes, Blurred Vision, Bloodshot, Burning Eyes, Itchy, Watery Eyes

Ninety percent of what we learn during our lives we learn through sight. The eyes are not only the windows of the soul, but windows to body health as well. Eyes often reflect imbalances or poor health conditions elsewhere in the system. No other sense is so prone to poor health conditions. Your lifestyle profoundly affects your "eyestyle." Many drugs, prescription, recreational and over-the-counter, react with your eyes. The worst offenders are cocaine, excessive use of chemical diuretics, sulfa drugs or tetracycline, aspirin, nicotine, phenylalanine and hydrocortisone. As with so many other body systems, the liver is the key to healthy eyes. The most stressful eyesight situations are reading, using a computer for most of your workday, and a sedentary lifestyle. Most eye-improving supplements need 2 to 3 months for effectiveness.

Diet & Superfood Therapy

—Nutritional therapy plan:

1—Liver malfunction is a common cause of eye problems. Keep it clean and well-functioning.

2—Eat protein from the sea and soy foods (rich in omega-3 fatty acids), whole grains, low fat dairy foods, eggs (full of zeaxanthin), sprouts and seeds.

3—Increase vitamin A and high mineral foods: leafy greens (kale), sea greens are loaded with carotenoids and EFA's (2 dry TBS daily), orange and yellow veggies, broccoli, seafood and parsley.

4—Include vision foods like broccoli, sunflower and sesame seeds; leeks, onions, cabbage and cauliflower, corn, barley, blueberries, watercress.

5—A vision drink 2x a week: Mix 1 cup carrot juice, ½ cup eyebright tea, 1 egg, 1 TB wheat germ, 1 tsp. rose hips powder, 1 TB honey, 1 tsp. sesame seeds, 1 tsp. nutritional yeast, 1 tsp. kelp.

6—Reduce sugar intake. Avoid chemicalized foods, especially fried and saturated fat foods, pasteurized dairy and red meats. These foods cause the body to metabolize slowly, use sugars poorly, and form crystallized clogs.

—Superfood therapy:

• Solgar EARTH SOURCE GREENS & MORE w. EFA's.
• Green Foods CARROT ESSENCE.
• Ethical Nutrients FUNCTIONAL GREENS.
• Crystal Star SYSTEMS STRENGTH™ drink.

Herb & Supplement Therapy

—Interceptive therapy plan: (Choose 2 to 4 recommendations)

1—**Expand your eye power:** • Crystal Star EYEBRIGHT HERBAL™ capsules 4-6 daily; • Ginkgo biloba extract for healthy circulation to the eye area. • Chromium picolinate 200mcg regulate sugar use, with extra • vitamin B-2, 100mg daily.

2—**Bioflavonoids strengthen eye vessels:** • Bilberry extract; • Quercetin 1000mg with bromelain 1500mg daily; • PCO's (grape seed or white pine), 100mg 2x daily;
• Enzymatic Therapy I-TONE; • Source Naturals VISUAL EYES with zeaxanthin.

3—**Liver health means eye health:** • Crystal Star LIV-ALIVE™ capsules 4-6 daily;
• Milk Thistle Seed extract; • Dandelion root tea.

4—**Antioxidants boost eye health:** • Parsley root caps 4 daily; • eyebright tea; • beta carotene 150,000IU daily, or • PHYCO-TENE MICROCLUSTERS, mixed carotenes from sea greens available at Healthy House; • zinc 30 to 50mg daily;
• taurine 500mg daily; • vitamin E 400IU w. selenium 200mcg; vitamin D 400IU.

5—**For itchy red eyes:** • Aloe vera juice (apply and take internally); • B-complex 100mg; • Boiron OPTIQUE (allergy reactions); • Quorum AQUALOGICS drops.

6—**For strain and eye fatigue** (seeing sparks of light or color with your eyes closed indicates stress): • BILBERRY extract drops 4x daily. Apply cool black tea bags to eyes for 15 minutes. Works almost immediately to reduce puffy eyes. For clarity and brightness: bathe eyes in a rosemary solution. (better than Visine)

7—**For "computer" eyes:** • Press points under eyebrows; press points in inner corners of eyes; squeeze eyebrows; look up, down, right and left every half hour.
• Tape page one of a newpaper to a wall about 8 feet from your computer. Every 30 minutes, look at the newspaper, bring the headlines into focus, then look back at your monitor. (See yoga eye stretches on this page.) • Clean your screen.

—Clarifying natural eye treatments (use as an eyewash and take internally):

• Crystal Star EYEBRIGHT HERBAL™ tea; • Sea greens tea for blurry vision;
• Raspberry tea bags or green tea bags for bloodshot eyes; • Borage seed tea for sore eyes; • Calendula tea for scleroderma.

Lifestyle Support Therapy

—Yoga stretches for your eyes:

• Eye relaxation techniques are a key if your eyes are under strain. It takes two minutes out of every hour to strengthen your eyes. (See the Bates Method book for more information.)

—**Eye relaxation techniques:**

• Blink to cleanse, lubricate and destress.
• Look right; look up; look left; look down; look diagonally up down and to the sides. Rotate your gaze in a circle. (don't do these exercise if you wear contacts).
• For eyestrain: Massage temples, pinch skin between the brows; then palm your eyes for 10 seconds at a time.
• Bathe eyes in a cool saline solution, witch hazel, or chamomile tea; or bathe eyes in ice water - then squeeze them shut for a few seconds to increase blood flow to the area.
• For irritated eyes from smog or allergies: splash eyes with cool water. Then warm them with a hot washcloth over closed lids. Press eyes gently with your fingertips and repeat.

—Reflexology area:

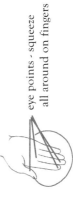

eye points - squeeze all around on fingers

Common Symptoms: *Poor, often degenerating vision; easily strained eyes, blurring more as the day goes on; frequent headaches over the eyes; spots and floaters before the eyes.*
Common Causes: *Liver malfunction; environmental pollutants; allergies; poor diet deficient in usable proteins and minerals, excessive in sugars and refined foods; thyroid problems; allergies; serious illness; prescription and other drug abuse.*

See the following pages for information on other vision problems.

Can't find a recommended product? Call the 800 number listed in Product Resources for the store nearest you.

Natural Therapy For Specific Vision Problems

The mind/body connection plays a big role in good vision. Emotional harmony has an impact on the willingness to see.

—**CATARACTS:** See page 346. Consider Enzymatic Therapy CATA-COMP.

—**CONJUNCTIVITIS INFECTION:** an inflammation of the eyelid, often caused by a viral infection; can be extremely contagious. **Alternative healing protocols:** • Take a pineapple carrot juice daily; use *goldenseal root, mullein, yarrow* or *eyebright* tea eyewashes and • *aloe vera* juice eyewashes; • BILBERRY extract; • Palm eyes to release infection and stimulate circulation. • Apply yogurt, grated potato or apple to inflammation; or a *calendula* compress to draw out infection - just make a warm tea; soak a washcloth in the tea and press on the eye. Or, simply use an egg white and spread it on a cloth or bandage; then apply to affected area. Use • colloidal silver eyedrops, or • Boiron OPTIQUE remedy or homeopathic *Belladonna* 30C. Take • PCO's from grapeseed to help new tissue grow back, 100mg 2x daily. • Add ascorbate vitamin C 2000mg daily.

—**DRY EYES, (Sjögren's syndrome)** a sudden onset problem, characterized by dry eyes, mouth, skin and all mucous membranes, and the inability to tear, often accompanies rheumatoid arthritis, scleroderma and systemic lupus. It is caused by a vitamin A deficiency and lowered immune response, and affects 9 times more women than men, usually after menopause. **Alternative healing protocols:** Reduce all refined sugars, red meats and saturated fats, milk and pasteurized dairy foods, corn, wheat, and nightshade plants (including tobacco and the drug Motrin, nightshade-based.) • Increase green vegetable, whole grain and fiber intake. • Increase cold water fish, sea foods and calcium foods like broccoli in your diet. Increase water and healthy fluid intake. • Bathe the eyes daily with *aloe vera* juice. • Take high omega-3 flax or *Evening Primrose Oil* capsules 4 daily. • Take 3000mg ascorbate vitamin C daily; • emulsified vitamin A and E 25,000IU/400IU, to clear and support tear pathways; • taurine 500mg 2x daily; • *butcher's broom* tea or • Crystal Star HEARTSEASE-CIRCU-CLEANSE™ tea to clear circulation; • BILBERRY and GINKGO BILOBA extracts act as natural antihistamines; • Ginseng caps 2 to 3 daily or • Crystal Star GINSENG 6™ caps for 3 months help your eyes to produce moisture. • B complex 100mg with extra B_2, and zinc 30-50mg daily. Take • Crystal Star CALCIUM SOURCE™ capsules for extra absorbable calcium.

—**DARK CIRCLES UNDER THE EYES :** usually caused by iron deficiency, but also an indication of liver or kidney malfunction or chronic allergies. **Alternative healing protocols:** • Take Floradix liquid iron; • Planetary TRIPHALA caps as directed for 3 months; • use *chamomile* or *green tea* teabags over the eyes for 15 minutes.

—**DYSLEXIA:** a signal-scrambling disorder affecting over 40 million Americans, both children and adults! It may have more to do with the inner ear than the eyes. **Alternative healing protocols:** Essential fatty acids are essential, especially • DHA and omega-3 rich fatty acids. Take • *ginkgo biloba* extract 3 to 4x daily; • *ginger* extract 3 to 4x daily; • lecithin caps 1400mg or choline 600mg; • Source Naturals DMAE 2 daily. Color therapy eyewear has had some success. Pick the color glasses that make your ability to read easier. Wear for 30 minutes at a time.

—**FLOATERS AND SPOTS BEFORE THE EYES:** extremely common in today's world, many are caused by drugs or a toxic overload from surgery or illness, candida yeast overgrowth or working in a polluted environment. A good liver detox can usually help floaters. Other floaters may be Bitot's spots, hard, elevated white spots on the whites of the eyes, bits of harmless debris that cast shadows over the retina, or scotoma, blind spots in the vision field because of retina trouble. To make debris floaters disappear, close your eyes and move your eyeballs up and down. **Alternative healing protocols:** Take • bioflavonoids 1000mg daily and • Planetary TRIPHALA caps as directed to cleanse the liver-3 months; • Vitamin K 100mcg 2 daily; • Vitamin A & D, 25,000IU/400IU, or • emulsified A & E 25,000IU/400IU to help remove lens particles, 4x daily; • pantothenic acid 500mg with B_6 250mg; • Vitamin C or Ester C; rub Earth's Bounty O_2 SPRAY on the feet at night for several months; • *dandelion* root tea and eyewash and a 2 month course of • MILK THISTLE SEED extract helps the liver.

—**GLAUCOMA:** caused by a build-up of pressure in the front compartment of the eye; may cause partial (or even full) blindness if not treated. See page 397.

—**MACULAR DEGENERATION:** AMD, age-related macular degeneration happens because oxidation to the macular blood vessels causes the tissues to break down. People with light-colored eyes seem to be more at risk. Macular degeneration is often reversible with nutritional therapy. A high fat diet, smoking and over-exposure to ultra-violet light all increase your risk. Don't smoke. Smoking increases your risk of macular degeneration up to three times over non smokers. **Alternative healing protocols:** Eat more dark green leafy veggies! Carotenoids, (specifically lutein and zeaxanthin) in foods like spinach and dark greens can cut your risk up to 50%. I recommend 2000mcg of mixed carotenoids. See page 346 for therapy information.

—**MYOPIA (Nearsightedness):** only 2% of second grade children are nearsighted; by the end of high school, the figure is 40%; by the end of college, more than 60% of students are nearsighted! **Alternative healing protocols:** In addition to the recommendations for better eyesight on the previous page, use • vitamin C up to 5000mg daily; • Vitamin D 1000IU; • Planetary TRIPHALA caps as directed; • BILBERRY extract or caps; • Enzymatic Therapy VISION ESSENTIALS capsules.

Can't find a recommended product? Call the 800 number listed in Product Resources for the store nearest you.

E 382

—NIGHT BLINDNESS: The inability of the eyes to adjust to changes in light intensity. **Alternative healing protocols:** • Add spinach and sea greens several times a week to your diet. Take • BILBERRY or • GINKGO BILOBA extract capsules or liquid; • CoQ-10 60mg 4x daily; • zinc 30 to 50mg daily; add • vitamin D 400IU daily. • Carotenoids, up to 200,000IU daily or • PHYCOTENE MICROCLUSTERS available from Healthy House, or • vitamin A 25,000IU (night blindness is usually a sign of a vitamin A deficiency). Take for 1 month, then 10,000IU for 2 months. May improve night vision up to 65%! • Take Enzymatic Therapy HERBAL FLAVONOIDS 4 daily. Blink as many times as you can for 5 seconds to help your eyes adjust. Use amber glasses when doing daytime driving. • **For color blindness:** Solgar oceanic carotene 25,000IU (from *Dunaliella Salina*).

—OVER-SENSITIVITY TO LIGHT (photophobia): **Alternative healing protocols:** • Ascorbate vitamin C 3000mg daily; • American Biologics A & E EMULSION as directed; or vitamin A & D 1000IU/400IU 4 daily; • Planetary TRIPHALA caps as directed for better balance; • BILBERRY extract. Natural sunlight nourishes eyes. Face the sun with eyes **CLOSED** for 5 seconds. Then cover eyes with palms for 5 seconds. Repeat 10 times to relax eyes and reduce light sensitivity.

—PRESBYOPIA (middle age far-sightedness): If you have to wear glasses, use an under-corrected prescription to encourage your eyes to work with the glasses, not passively depend on them. **Alternative healing protocols:** • Add B-complex vitamins like Nature's Secret ULTIMATE B daily; • taurine 600mg daily.

—PROTRUDING/BULGING EYES: generally denotes a thyroid problem. Iodine therapy has had some success in these cases. See page 178.

—RETINITUS PIGMENTOSA: the progressive degeneration of the rods and cones of the retina. Common signs are night blindness and a narrow vision field. **Alternative healing protocols:** Take • BILBERRY or • GINKGO BILOBA extract capsules or liquid. Take • CoQ-10, 60mg 4x daily (especially effective if the case is not severe); • PCO's from grapeseed or white pine 100mg 3x daily, taurine 500mg daily, • zinc picolinate 50mg daily. • Omega-3 fatty acids like flax or fish oils, or • Barleans' lignan-rich flax oil 3x daily; and • beta carotene 100,000IU or • vitamin A 15,000IU. Take • vitamin E 400IU 2x daily if retinitis is hemorrhagic.

—RETINAL DETERIORATION: occurs when the retinal epithelium, the thin layer of cells located behind the receptor cells does not function properly in providing nutrients to or removing wastes from the crucial light receptor cells. The photo-receptors die and vision loss is irreversible. **Alternative healing protocols:** • GINKGO BILOBA and • BILBERRY extracts and • PCO's from grapeseed 100mg 3x daily have proven effective. • *Gotu Kola* or • Solaray CENTELLA ASIATICA caps help strengthen optic and retinal nerves.

—SHINGLES NEAR THE EYES (herpes zoster): **Alternative healing protocols:** high dose • vitamin C crystals $1/4$ teasp. in water every hour until the stool turns soupy - about 8000-10,000mg daily; • vitamin E 400IU with selenium 200mcg daily. • Country Life SUBLINGUAL B-12 3000mcg with folic acid 200mcg (See also HERPES page in this book).

—STYES & EYE INFLAMMATION: painful, pimple-like infections of the eyelids. Natural therapies work well when treatment is early. Origins stem from allergic, viral, or herpes-type infections. **Alternative healing protocols:** use • buffered vitamin C eye drops (must be sterile solution), vitamin A, and zinc. If the cause is a bacterial infection, do not squeeze, use • Crystal Star ANTI-BIO™ extract drops in water (may also be used to bathe the affected area); or bathe eyes in • *aloe vera juice*, • *chamomile tea*, • *raspberry leaf tea*, • *eyebright tea*, • *yellow dock tea* or *goldenseal root tea*. • Mix one drop aged *garlic* extract in 4 drops distilled water and drop into infected eye. • Take vitamin A and D capsules 25,000IU/400IU, and • omega-3 flax oil. Use • Boiron OPTIQUE homeopathic eye irritation remedy. • Alternating hot and cold compresses on affected area to stimulate drainage of infection. Or use a • *calendula* flowers compress to draw out a stye infection - just make a warm tea; soak a washcloth in the tea and press on the eye. • Eye inflammation compress: 1 TB *eyebright* herb, $1/2$ TB powdered *comfrey* or *parsley root*, $1/2$ TB powdered *goldenseal* root, 1 pint boiling water. Add herbs and steep for 30 minutes, covered. Apply to cotton balls and then to affected areas. Or simply use • the white of an egg and spread it on a cloth or bandage; then apply to affected area. (If an eyelash is in the infected follicle, gently pull it out after drawing the pus to a head with the hot compress; the pus will be released.

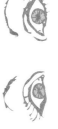

Can't find a recommended product? Call the 800 number listed in Product Resources for the store nearest you.

Fevers

Nature's Cleansers and Healers

A slight fever is often your body's way of clearing up an infection or toxic overload quickly. Body temperature is naturally raised to literally "burn out" harmful poisons, to throw them off through heat and then through sweating. The heat from a fever can also de-activate virus replication, so unless a fever is exceptionally high (over 103° for kids and 102° for adults) or long lasting (more than two full days), it is sometimes a wise choice to let it run its natural course. Often they will get better faster. Don't overmedicate. Fevers are usually a result of the problem and a part of the cure.

Administer plenty of liquids during a fever - juices, water, broths. Bathe morning and night during a feverish illness. Infection and wastes from the illness are largely thrown off through the skin. If not regularly washed off, these substances just lay on the skin and become partially reabsorbed into the body. There is usually substantial body odor during a cleansing fever as toxins are being eliminated, so frequent baths and showers help you feel better, too. A cup of hot bayberry or elderflower tea, or cayenne and ginger capsules, will speed up the cleansing process by encouraging sweating and by stimulating circulation.

Watchwords for fevers and kids: It's probably ok unless: 1) you have an infant with a temperature over 100°; 2) the fever has not abated after three days, and is accompanied by vomiting, a cough and trouble breathing; 3) your child displays extreme lethargy and looks severely ill, and looks severely ill and is making strange, twitching movements.

Diet & Superfood Therapy

Don't forget - use child dosage for kids. See page 250.

—Nutritional therapy plan:

1—Stay on a liquid diet during a fever to maximize the cleansing process: bottled water, fruit juices, broths and herb teas.

2—Carrot/beet/cucumber juice is a specific to clean the kidneys and help bring a fever down.

3—Sip on lemon juice with honey all during the morning; grapefruit juice during the evening.

4—Add plenty of healthy liquids to the daily diet all during the illness.

5—After a fever breaks, take enzyme therapy drinks (pg. 222).

—Superfood therapy: (Choose one or two)

• Crystal Star SYSTEMS STRENGTH™.
• Solgar WHEY TO GO - lactose-free with probiotics.
• New Moon GINGER WONDER syrup.
• AloeLife ALOE GOLD concentrate, 2 TBS in water as an anti-inflammatory.

Herb & Supplement Therapy

Don't forget - use child dosage for kids. See page 250.

—Interceptive therapy plan: (Choose 2 to 3 recommendations)

1—**Control the infection:** • Crystal Star ANTI-BIO™ caps or drops; • *Lobelia* tincture drops in water every few hours and Crystal Star FIRST AID TEA FOR KIDS™. • *Fenugreek* tea with lemon and honey. • Vitamin A 10,000IU or beta carotene 25,000IU every 6 hours.

2—**Use a fever to fight a cold or flu. Encourage sweating:** Take • Crystal Star FIRST AID CAPS™, or • *Calendula* tea, • *Elderflower-sage* tea or • *Boneset-white willow-yarrow* tea or • *thyme* tea until sweating occurs, usually within 24 hours.

3—**Help your body normalize from a fever and speed up healing:** • Vitamin C crystals ¼ teasp. every ½ hour in juice or water to bowel tolerance as an ascorbic acid flush. • Add garlic capsules 3x daily.

4—**If you decide to reduce the fever:** Do not give aspirin to children to reduce a fever. Give herb teas instead, • like peppermint or catnip.

5—**Rebuild immune strength:** • Crystal Star COLD SEASON DEFENSE™ caps.

—Effective homeopathic remedies: • Bioforce *Fiebresan* drops; • Natra-Bio Fever tincture; • Hylands *Hylavir* flu or cold tablets. **Homeopathic remedies for sudden fever onset:** • *Arsenicum album*, • *Belladonna*, • *Aconite*.

Lifestyle Support Therapy

—Bodywork:

• *Catnip* enemas cleanse the elimination channels.

• Use cool water sponges, or alcohol rub-downs to reduce a fever.

• Apply *peppermint* tea cooling compresses to the head.

• Take ECHINACEA extract to encourage the lymph glands to throw off toxins.

• Take a sauna to sweat toxins out.

• Then sponge off with cool water, and follow with a brisk towel rub.

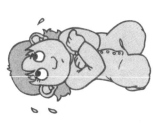

Common Symptoms: Hot, dry, flushed skin; then chill followed by fever; lethargy.
Common Causes: Bacterial or viral infection in the system that the body is trying to throw off; sometimes a sign of more serious problems, such as mononucleosis, Epstein-Barr virus, or diabetes.

See also INFECTIONS page 434 for more information.

Can't find a recommended product? Call the 800 number listed in Product Resources for the store nearest you.

Fibroids

Breast (Cystic Mastitis), Uterine (Myomas or Fibromas)

Up to 40 percent of American women 35 and older have fibroids. Uterine fibroids are more common than blue eyes! Hormone imbalances, primarily too much estrogen that isn't being processed smoothly by the liver and an under-active thyroid, are the normal cause for both breast and uterine fibroids. Fibroids are not cancer, and have little chance of becoming cancerous before menopause. Natural therapies have been consistently successful in helping a woman avoid fibroid surgery. Painful breast swelling and excessive uterine bleeding have disappeared within weeks after a change to a low fat, vegetarian diet. Care for your liver to prevent fibroids. The liver metabolizes and regulates body hormones (particularly estrogens). Avoid synthetic estrogen compounds if possible. They keep fibroids growing even after menopause.

Diet & Superfood Therapy

—Nutritional therapy plan:

1—Follow a low fat, fresh foods vegetarian diet (50-60% fresh foods) to rebalance gland functions and relieve symptoms. High fats mean imbalanced estrogen levels - a clear cause of fibroids. Obesity from a high fat diet also increases risk.

2—Coffee clearly aggravates fibroids. Avoid caffeine foods like chocolate and carbonated sodas. Avoid concentrated starches like pastries and fatty dairy foods. Avoid hormone-laden meats and refined sugars that can cause iodine deficiency.

3—During menses, avoid fried, sugary and salty foods, especially smoked or preserved meats.

4—Get high quality protein daily (about 60-70 grams) from largely-vegetable sources to avoid saturated fats: whole grains, sprouts, tofu and soy foods, sea foods, low fat dairy and poultry, etc.

5—Increase your intake of B vitamin-rich foods - brown rice, wheat germ and wheat germ oil (4 teasp. daily) and brewer's yeast.

6—Add miso, sea greens, and leafy greens to neutralize toxins. Eat diuretic foods - cucumber and watermelon to flush them out. Have fresh apple or carrot juice every day during healing.

—Superfood supplements:
• Crystal Star ENERGY GREEN™ drink.
• Y.S. ROYAL JELLY-GINSENG drink.
• Mona's CHLORELLA drink.

Herb & Supplement Therapy

—Interceptive therapy plan: (Choose 2 to 3 recommendations)

For breast fibroids:

1—**Normalize hormone levels:** • Crystal Star WOMEN'S BALANCE FIBRO™ caps for 3 months, then • Crystal Star FEMALE HARMONY™ caps or *Vitex* extract 2x daily with *burdock* tea 2 cups daily. • *Evening Primrose* 3000mg daily, or •vitamin E 800IU with folic acid 800mcg daily. • Enzymatic Therapy Raw Mammary.

2—**Help dissolve adhesions:** • Crystal Star CALCIUM SOURCE™ extract or •*nettles* extract. • Earth's Bounty O₂ SPRAY directly on fibroids; noticeable reduction in 3-6 weeks. Apply a •fresh *comfrey leaf* poultice to nodules. • Nutricology Germanium 150mg daily; •Vitamin C or Ester C powder w/ bioflavonoids 5000mg daily.

3—**Drain lymph tissue and excess fluids:** • Herbs, Etc. LYMPHATONIC.

For uterine fibroids:

1—**Normalize hormone levels:** • Crystal Star WOMAN'S BEST FRIEND™ 6 daily for 3 months; or Crystal Star PRO-EST BALANCE™ roll-on for fibrous areas. •*Evening Primrose* Oil 3000mg daily. • Crystal Star BITTERS & LEMON CLEANSE™ helps metabolize estrogens. Metabolic Response Modifiers CORDYCEPS 750mg.

2—**Liver support is important for balancing hormone levels:** • Crystal Star LIV-ALIVE™ caps, or • Milk Thistle Seed extract. • B-complex 150mg 3x daily; •beta carotene 300,000IU daily; •CoQ-10 60mg 4-6x daily

3—**Nervine relaxers and antispasmodics help with pain:** • Crystal Star CRAMP BARK extract. Beware of straight *dong quai* extract if you have uterine fibroids - it may increase bleeding. • Use *centella asiatica* instead.

4—**Help dissolve adhesions:** • Transformation Energy PURE-ZYME protease therapy, 3 to 5 daily on an empty stomach.

—Iodine therapy is significant in healing fibroids. Use for 3-4 months:
• Nature's Path TRACE-MIN-LYTE with sea greens; or • Crystal Star IODINE SOURCE™ extract, 2-3x daily; •Bernard Jensen's LIQUI-DULS. Take with •vitamin E 400IU for best results.

Lifestyle Support Therapy

• The medical answer for fibroids is early detection, surgical biopsies and then removal. But, the tests are often inaccurate (15% false negatives and 30% false positives), and the attendant invasive medical procedures cause anxiety, pain and expense. We have found that there is a very real risk in receiving regular doses of radiation through mammograms, even low dose radiation. Breast tissue is so sensitive that the time between a mammogram and fibroid growth is sometimes as little as three months.

• Try to avoid mammograms and chest X-rays. (See above.) X-rays also contribute to iodine deficiency.

—Bodywork:

• Get some outdoor exercise every day for tissue oxygen.
• No smoking. Avoid secondary smoke.
• External poultices: green clay and castor oil packs, applied directly.

—Reflexology points:

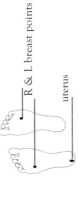

R & L breast points

uterus

F 385

Common Symptoms: *Breast fibroids: moveable, rubbery nodules near the surface of the breasts, causing painful breast swelling. Uterine fibroids: benign growths (between the size of a walnut and an orange) that appear on the uterine walls cause excessive menstrual bleeding; back and abdominal pain, and bladder infections; painful intercourse; infertility or the inability to sustain pregnancy.*
Common Causes: *Too much caffeine and too much fat in the diet; EFA deficiency; hormone imbalance with an abnormal response to estrogen and progesterone and an underactive thyroid; obesity; genetic factors; high-dose birth control pills; X-rays. Benign growths usually cease after menopause; new growths after menopause may mean breast or uterine cancer.*

Can't find a recommended product? Call the 800 number listed in Product Resources for the store nearest you.

Fibromyalgia

Immune Compromised Musculo-Skeletal Pain

Fibromyalgia is an arthritic muscle disease. Our parents and grandparents called it rheumatism. It's characterized by pain all over the body with identifiable tender spots that hurt significantly when pressed. There is considerable depression that often involves deep-seated resentment, and chronic headaches and fatigue with nerve and hormone imbalances that impair deep sleep. A stress-related immune disorder, the central cause seems to be a low level of serotonin in the brain and reduced growth hormone. Fibromyalgia shares many symptoms with Chronic Fatigue Syndrome (CFS), TMJ, and rheumatoid arthritis. Researchers estimate that up to ten million Americans (mostly midlife women) suffer from fibromyalgia. Although labeled untreatable largely because NSAIDS drugs do not help, FM may be vastly helped by natural therapies.

Diet & Superfood Therapy

—Nutritional therapy plan:

1—The HYPOGLYCEMIA diet page 427 is a good place to start diet improvement.

2—Go on a short 3 day cleansing diet (page 191).

3—Keep your diet at least 50% fresh foods during intensive healing time. A largely vegetarian diet can have very beneficial influence on blood toxins and fibrinogen that affects coagulation.

4—Add plenty of cruciferous veggies like broccoli for 3-indole carbinole to reduce pain.

5—Reduce processed foods, sugars, and saturated fats. Avoid red meats and caffeine. Watch out for common food allergens.

—Lower your homocysteine levels:

— 4 garlic capsules (1200mg a day) to maintain aortic elasticity.

— B_6, 50mg and folic acid 800mg to help break down homocysteine.

— red wine, 1 glass with dinner.

—Superfood therapy: (Choose one or two)

- Crystal Star GREEN TEA CLEANSER™.
- Mona's CHLORELLA packets or tabs.
- All One GREEN PHYTOBASE drink for pain.
- Green Kamut JUST BARLEY.
- Aloe Life ALOE GOLD drink.
- Solgar EARTH SOURCE GREENS.
- Y.S. ROYAL JELLY/GINSENG drink.

Herb & Supplement Therapy

—Interceptive therapy plan: (Choose 1 or 2 recommendations)

1—Reduce inflammation, manage pain: • Homeopathic Hormonegentics HGH 2c-30c; • MSM caps 800mg daily or • Futurebiotics MSM; • Crystal Star PRO-EST BALANCE™ roll-on; • Quercetin 1000mg and bromelain 1500mg daily. • Solaray TURMERIC (curcumin). Apply • Biochemics PAIN RELIEF lotion; • Transitions PRO-GEST wild yam cream; • Wakunaga FREEDOM ARTHRITIS RELIEF cream.

2—Balance brain chemistry and nerve transmission: • Ginkgo Biloba improves memory and circulation. • Crystal Star RELAX CAPS™, 6 daily as needed. • Gotu kola extract or • Solaray CENTELLA ASIATICA caps. • Crystal Star ADRN-ACTIVE™ capsules for adrenal deficiency.

3—Improve musculo-skeletal system: • Acetyl-L-Carnitine 1000mg daily. • Glucosamine-chondroitin combination, a cartilage nutrient -1500/1200mg 6 daily. • Crystal Star AR-EASE™ caps, joint rebuilder and collagen tonic; very relieving. • Burdock tea 2 cups daily as a blood cleanser for the musculo-skeletal system. Take with • Crystal Star FEM SUPPORT™ extract and una da gato caps for best results.

4—Enhance your natural energy sources: • Crystal Star MENTAL INNER ENERGY™ with kava kava and ginseng; • Country Life sublingual B-12 2500mcg.

5—Natural antidepressants raise serotonin levels: • SAMe (S-adenosyl methionine) 800mg daily boosts serotonin-dopamine levels. • St. John's wort, 300mg daily; • Enzymatic Therapy KAVA-TONE for headaches. • Rosemary tea, a memory booster.

6—Improve sleep quality: • 5-HTP 100mg; • St. John's wort extract or Crystal Star NIGHT CAPS™ for REM sleep. • Melatonin .1mg for better sleep patterns.

7—Add magnesium and B-vitamins: • Magnesium 400mg 2x daily or • Ethical Nutrients MALIC/MAGNESIUM to alleviate tender points; • B-complex 150mg 3x daily, or • Nature's Secret ULTIMATE B tabs.

8—Antioxidants boost immune response: • Nutricology LAKTOFERRIN with colostrum; • glutathione 100mg daily; • PCO's from grapeseed 100mg 3x daily; • Vitamin C up to 5000mg daily with extra bioflavonoids 500mg; • CoQ-10 60mg 3x daily; • Beta-carotene 100,000IU daily.

Lifestyle Support Therapy

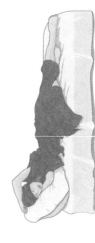

—Bodywork:

• Those with fibromyalgia are generally not physically fit. Build up a slow, low-impact aerobic exercise program - 20 minutes a day for body oxygen and muscle tone.

• Add light weight bearing exercise for 10 minutes a day to start.

—Relaxation techniques are crucial:

• Choose from meditation, guided imagery, yoga, biofeedback, and progressive muscle relaxation - all of which have had success with fibromyalgia in developing a positive mind/body stance to work with the disease.

• Regular monthly massage therapy treatments have had notable success.

• Local, gentle heat applications are effective, especially with a gentle massage.

Common Symptoms: Painful, tender, recurrent points aching all over the body; persistent, diffuse musculo-skeletal pain and stiffness; fatigue, weakness, headaches, confusion, migraine headaches, chronic diarrhea and irritable bowel, poor sleep patterns and nervous symptoms like anxiety and depression, and hypoglycemia - symptoms of mild cortisol deficiency; stomach and digestive problems; shortness of breath with high uric acid. Other symptoms include cardiovascular problems and unexplained allergies. Being overweight and a smoker compounds fibromyalgia. Aluminum toxicity may be linked to the magnesium deficiency; possible virus involvement; associated with mitral valve prolapse.

Common Causes: An immune compromised condition with no known real cause.

Access the FIBROMYALGIA/ CHRONIC FATIGUE SYNDROME Network for more information. (800) 853-2929.

Can't find a recommended product? Call the 800 number listed in Product Resources for the store nearest you.

F 386

Flu

Severe Viral Respiratory Infection

Like the common cold, the flu is an upper respiratory infection caused by a rhino-virus. Unlike a cold, flu infections are more severe, longer-lasting and highly contagious. Some twenty thousand people die each year from flu. Flu treatment programs work best in a series of stages. The ACUTE, or infective stage, includes aches, chills, prostration, fever, sore throat, etc., and usually lasts for 2 to 4 days. The RECUPERATION, or healing stage, replenishes the body's natural resistance. This phase should be followed for one to two weeks. The IMMUNE SUPPORT stage should be followed for two to three weeks, especially in high risk seasons. Recovery from flu is often slow with a good deal of weakness. Flu shots can affect immune response. Beware.

Diet & Superfood Therapy

—Nutritional therapy plan:

1—**During the acute stage:** take only liquid nutrients - plenty of hot, steamy chicken soup, hot tonics and broths to stimulate mucous release (pg. 215). Vegetable juices and green drinks (pg. 218) to rebuild the blood and immune system. Have ginger-garlic broth every day.

2—**During the recuperation stage:** follow a vegetarian, light "green" diet. Have a salad every day, cultured foods like yogurt and kefir for friendly flora replacement, and steamed vegetables with brown rice for strength.

3—**For immune support and all stages:** Avoid refined foods, sugars, and pasteurized dairy foods which increase mucous clogging and allow a place for the virus to live. Avoid alcohol and tobacco; they are immune suppressors. Avoid caffeine foods; they inhibit iron and zinc absorption.

4—**If you just can't seem to "get over it:"** make up 1 gallon of Crystal Star CLEANSING & PURIFYING™ tea, and take 5 to 6 cups daily with 15 FIBER & HERBS CLEANSE™ capsules daily until the virus is removed.

—Superfood therapy: (Choose one or two)

• Crystal Star SYSTEMS STRENGTH™ alkalizes, returns body vitality and rebuilds healthy blood.
• Wakunaga KYO-GREEN.
• Green Foods GREEN MAGMA.
• Mona's CHLORELLA.

Herb & Supplement Therapy

—Interceptive therapy plan: (Choose 2 to 4 recommendations)

1—**During the acute stage:** • Ester C or ascorbic acid crystals: $1/4$ teasp. every half hour to bowel tolerance to flush the body and neutralize toxins. • Crystal Star FIRST AID CAPS™ to raise body temperature and reduce virus replication, and CLEANSING & PURIFYING TEA™ sipped all during the day. • Nutribiotic GRAPE-FRUIT SEED extract drops. or • East Park FLU BAN olive leaf extract caps.

2—**During the infection fighting stage:** • Crystal Star ANTI-VI™ extract as needed several times daily, or • ANTI-BIO™ extract or capsules every 2 hours until improvement is noticed. • Nature's Path Silver-Lyte - ionized silver, a powerful infection fighter; • Ginseng Co. CYCLONE CIDER for achy, sore throat.♂ • *Garlic-ginger tea* 2 cups daily; • Boneset tea (or homeopathic *Eupatorium Perfoliatum*) to inhibit flu virus, relieve pain and induce sweating. Take • Nature's Way SAMBUCOL - *elderberry syrup* as needed ☺ or • Zinc lozenges to deactivate throat virus activity.

Effective congestion cleansers: • *Cayenne-ginger caps*; • *Echinacea-goldenseal caps*; • *Cayenne-garlic capsules.*

Effective anti-viral herbs: • *Usnea extract*, or • Crystal Star BIO-VI™ extract with propolis; • *Echinacea extract tea*; • *St. John's Wort*; • *Osha root tea.* ☺

3—**Speed up your recovery time:** • Glutamine 1000mg 2x daily; • *astragalus* or *reishi mushroom extract* 15 drops 4x daily; • *Cayenne-bayberry* capsules to normalize gland activity; • *chamomile tea* to relieve aches and pains (highly effective); • Wisdom of the Ancients SYMFRE tea. • Nutricology GERMANIUM 150mg; • Calendula tea 4 cups daily.

4—**Enhance and restablish immune response:** • Nutricology NAC a powerful immune booster, 1000mg daily; • *panax ginseng, astragalus extract* or *Siberian ginseng extract* to boost lymphocytes and interferon; • Sun Wellness CHLORELLA; • Nutricology LACTOFERRIN with colostrum as directed. • OPC's from white pine or grapeseed, 100mg 3x daily; • CoQ-10, 60mg 3x daily; • Beta-carotene 100,000IU. • Prof. Nutrition DR. DOPHILUS in papaya juice. ☺ • Raw thymus to build cell immunity, or • Enzymatic Therapy THYMUPLEX.

—Homeopathic remedies against flu: • Boiron OSCILLOCOCCINUM; • B&T Alpha CF; • BioForce FLU RELIEF; • Hylands remedies specific to individual symptoms of the flu.

Lifestyle Support Therapy

—Bodywork:

• **During the acute stage:** Sweating is effective at the first sign of infection.
1) Take 1 *cayenne cap* and 1 *ginger cap.*
2) Take a hot bath with *tea tree oil* drops. ☺
3) Go to bed for a long sleep, so the body can concentrate on healing.
4) During the next several days, take a hot sauna, spa, or bath to raise body temperature and increase circulation.

• A hyperthermia bath can helps deactivate viruses: See page 225 for How To Take An Overheating Bath in your home.

• Gargle with a few drops of *tea tree oil* or *ginger root tea* in water for sore throat; or use New Chapter GINGER WONDER SYRUP.

• Do several nasal irrigations to disinfect your mucous membranes and clear breathing quickly: add $1/2$ teasp. sea salt to a cup of warm water. Fill a dropper with liquid, tilt your head and fill each nostril; then blow your nose.

• Take a *catnip* enema to cleanse out flu virus from the intestinal tract.

• Get a complete massage therapy treatment to cleanse remaining pockets of toxins, and clear body meridians. Plus it makes you feel so good again!

See COLDS page 353 and IMMUNITY page 429 in this book for extra help.

Can't find a recommended product? Call the 800 number listed in Product Resources for the store nearest you.

Foot Problems

Bone Spurs, Plantar Warts, Calluses, Corns, Bunions

Bunions: thickened layers of skin on the sides of the big toe. **Calluses:** thick, dead skin pads your body builds up as protection on the site of continual pressure - usually on heels and balls of feet. **Corns:** painful hardened skin found mainly on the toe joints (hard corns) or between the toes (soft corns). May accompany rheumatoid arthritis, alkalosis or tendonitis because people with this disease are deficient in stomach acid and normal enzyme production. Note: If you decide to try magnets for relief of your foot problem (successful for 90% of diabetic DPN foot problems), most tests show that when the magnets are removed the problem reappears. **Bone spurs:** a calcium deposit out growth, usually on the foot sole. **Plantar warts:** painful, sometimes ingrowing, warts on the body.

Diet & Superfood Therapy

—Nutritional therapy plan:

1—Go on a 24 hour (pg. 192) vegetable juice diet to clear out acid wastes. Then eat plenty of fresh raw foods for a month. Have a green salad every day.

2—Drink black cherry juice daily. Take a green drink or carrot-beet-cucumber juice every 3 days to flush the kidneys and re-balance your body pH.

3—Eat two apples a day.

4—Make sure your diet is rich in whole foods, vegetables and fiber, low in sugars, meat, fried foods and saturated fats. Avoid acid-forming foods - red meats, caffeine, chocolate, carbonated sodas. Eliminate hard liquor and fried food.

5—Effective enzyme balancing foods: miso soup, lecithin 2 tsp. daily, fresh vegetables, brewer's yeast, cranberry juice.

—Superfood therapy: (Choose one or two)
• Crystal Star ENERGY GREEN™ drink.
• Sun Wellness CHLORELLA packets or tabs.
• Kyolic KYO-GREEN with EFA's.
• Aloe Life ALOE GOLD drink.
• Solaray ALFA-JUICE tabs.

Herb & Supplement Therapy

—Interceptive therapy plan: (Choose 2 to 3 recommendations)

1—**Dissolve crystalline deposits and flush them out:** • Crystal Star AR-EASE™ capsules with • BITTERS & LEMON CLEANSE™ extract each morning and evening. • Echinacea extract or apply BioForce ECHINACEA cream. • Country Life LIGA-TEND for at least 1 month; • Enzymatic Therapy ACID-A-CAL tabs. Apply Nutribiotic GRAPEFRUIT SEED skin spray or ointment and take the capsules 2x daily. • Flora VEGE-SIL, or apply • Eidon SILICA MOISTURIZING LOTION.

2—**Reduce pain and inflammation:** • Quercetin 2000mg daily with Bromelain 1500mg daily; • Crystal Star ANTI-FLAM™ caps to take down inflammation.

3—**For calluses:** • apply celandine tincture to dissolve hard skin. Use • vitamin A 25,000IU (not beta carotene) 3x daily for 3 months; apply • Calendula ointment.

4—**For bone spurs:** • Mix vitamin C crystals with water to a paste. Apply and take vitamin C up to 5000mg daily with extra bioflavonoids 500mg. • Take Cal/mag/zinc 4 daily with • B-complex 100mg 4 daily.

5—**For corns or bunions, apply:** • tea tree oil 2-3x daily; • a weak goldenseal root-aloe vera juice solution; • Bromelain 1500mg daily to reduce pain; • a mixture of wintergreen oil, witch hazel, and black walnut extract; • Apply CAPSAICIN cream.

6—**For foot odor:** Make a big pot of black tea. Pour into a basin; soak feet 15 minutes. The tannic acid eliminates odor.

7—**For cracked, occasionally bleeding heels:** For 3 months take • zinc picolinate 30mg 3x daily, • vitamin E 600IU, 2 TBS each flax oil and snipped dried sea greens daily in your salad dressing for essential fatty acids (EFA's). Add • B-complex 100mg or • Nature's Secret ULTIMATE B for EFA metabolism.

8—**For heel pain (often a low thyroid problem):** • Take Evening Primrose oil 2000mg, • omega-3 flax oil caps 3 daily, or Nature's Secret ULTIMATE OIL and 2 TBS dry sea greens daily. Add • Crystal Star POTASSIUM-IODINE caps and magnesium 800mg.

9—**Enzyme therapy controls inflammation, balances body pH:** • Magnesium-Potassium-Bromelain caps; • Prevail VITASE with meals; • Betaine HCl for better calcium uptake; • Gaia Herbs SWEETISH BITTERS.

Lifestyle Support Therapy

—Healing foot soaks:
• Add 2 handfuls comfrey root to 1 gallon warm water. Soak for 15 minutes.
• For ingrown nail, soak in Epsom salts bath.
• For blisters, add 2 TBS Aloe Vera gel to 1 gallon hot water. Soak for 15 minutes.

—For corns, calluses, bunions:
Soak feet in warm water first, then apply:
• Biochemics PAIN RELIEF.
• Body Essentials SILICA GEL.
• For corns, olive oil or lemon compresses; apply
• For bunions, aloe vera gel or castor oil or a Flaxseed-garlic paste poultices.
• Miracle of Aloe FOOT REPAIR.

—For plantar warts and bone spurs:
Soak feet in the hottest water you can stand for as long as you can; then apply:
• Earth's Bounty O₂ SPRAY directly on wart or bone spur 2x daily. Removal takes about 2 months.
• DMSO to dissolve crystalline deposits.
• Home Health CASTOR OIL PACKS.
• Mix vitamin C crystals and water to a paste. Apply to spur; secure with tape. Leave on all day for several weeks.

F 388

Common Symptoms: Pain and inflammation of nodules and growths on the feet. Note: Griseofulvin™ tabs for nail fungus can affect liver function.
Common Causes: Staph or strep type infection; kidney malfunction causing acid/alkaline imbalance; too many sweets, caffeine and saturated fats; excess sebaceous gland output causing poor skin elimination of wastes; poor circulation, (especially from diabetes); poor calcium elimination. Low acid diet aggravating liver congestion and poor or irregular kidney function; insufficient stomach acid; constipation and toxemia from excess fats and refined carbohydrates; too little vegetable protein.

See additional suggestions on NAIL FUNGUS page 462 and GOUT page 398.

Can't find a recommended product? Call the 800 number listed in Product Resources for the store nearest you.

Frostbite

Chillblains, Possibility of Gangrene

If untreated, severe frostbite of the extremities can turn into a gangrenous condition, in which blood flow stops, tissue becomes oxygen-deprived, numb and dies. The fluid between the cells freezes, causing them to rupture, and slough off into nearby blood vessels. Rubbing accelerates this skin damage. If treated right away, this type of dry, non-infected gangrene responds successfully to natural self-therapy. Wet gangrene is the result of an infected wound, which prevents drainage and deprives the affected tissues of cleansing blood supply and oxygen. See an emergency clinic if you have wet gangrene.

Diet & Superfood Therapy

—Nutritional therapy plan:

1—For frostbite: paint on, but do not rub in, warm olive oil. Massage in for gangrene.

2—Or paint on honey to arrest infective bacteria development and stabilize the skin balance.

3—Give the person warm drinks or green drinks, but no alcohol. It constricts blood flow.

4—Eat a high protein diet for the two weeks after exposure, with plenty of whole grains to speed recovery.

—Superfood therapy: (Choose one or two)

• Crystal Star ENERGY GREEN™ drink and capsules.

• Pines MIGHTY GREENS drink.

• Beehive Botanicals ROYAL JELLY-GINSENG and bee pollen drink.

• Sun Wellness CHLORELLA 1 pkt. daily.

• FutureBiotics VITAL K 3 teasp. daily.

Herb & Supplement Therapy

—Interceptive therapy plan: (Choose 2 or more recommendations)

1—**Enhance circulation:** • Nelson BACH RESCUE REMEDY every 5 minutes under the tongue as needed for shock. • *Ginkgo Biloba* extract; • Crystal Star HEARTSEASE-CIRCU-CLEANSE™ tea or • HEARTSEASE-HAWTHORN™ caps 4 daily. • CoQ-10 60mg 3x daily; • apply *Butcher's broom* extract mixed in water (also take internally, temporarily only). • *Sage* tea 2 cups daily.

2—**Help raise body temperature:** • Crystal Star FIRST AID CAPS™, or • Ginseng Co. CYCLONE CIDER. • Apply CAPSAICIN creme or a • *Ginger-Cayenne* powder compress mixed in olive oil.

3—**Control infection:** • *Myrrh* gum extract; • *Witch Hazel*; • *Black Walnut Hulls* extract; • Nutricology GERMANIUM for wound healing, 150mg for 2 months. • Earth's Bounty O₂ SPRAY, rub on affected area several times daily until healing begins. • *Calendula-comfrey* salve, or • *Slippery elm* or • *Comfrey/plantain* compresses mixed with olive oil.

4—**Repair damaged tissue:** • Vitamin C powder with bioflavs. and rutin, ¼ teasp. every half hour for 6 days for collagen and tissue rebuilding. • Vitamin E 400IU. Take internally and prick a capsule - apply oil to affected areas. • Apply AloeLife ALOE SKIN GEL often to affected areas. • Body Essentials SILICA GEL

5—**Enhance immune response:** • PCO's from grapeseed or pine, 100mg 3x daily; • Enzymatic Therapy ORAL NUTRIENT CHELATES. Then follow with a full-spectrum multi-vitamin complex for 1 month to help redevelop tissue.

Lifestyle Support Therapy

—Immediate procedures:

• Get the person to a heated room immediately. Cover warmly, so frostbitten areas will warm up gradually. Warm the entire body with hot drinks, dry clothing or human body heat.

• Gently stroke the kidneys toward the middle of the back.

• If case is severe, wrap in gauze so blisters don't break. Elevate legs. Do not rub blisters.

• Use alternating warm and cool hydrotherapy to stimulate circulation. No hot water bottles, hair dryers, or heating pads. Don't rub a frostbite. It makes it worse. Slow warming is the key.

• If case is very severe, immerse areas in warm water and massage very gently under water for 5 to 10 minutes.

—Stimulating and healing oils:

• *Cajeput* oil

• *Mullein* oil

• *Tea tree* oil, which sloughs off old and infected tissue, and leaves healthy tissue intact.

• Biochemics PAIN RELIEF.

See also SHOCK THERAPY page 495.

Common Symptoms: *Frostbite is the freezing of cold-exposed extremities, and its effects of redness, swelling, blistering, numbness, etc. Circulation slows, causing skin to become hard, blue-white and numb. Dry gangrene symptoms include dull, aching pain and coldness in the area. Pain and skin pallor are early signs of dry gangrene. As the flesh dies, pain can be intense; once it is dead, the flesh becomes numb and turns dark.*

Common Causes: *Prolonged exposure of the feet, hands, ears and face to severe cold; poor circulation; arteriosclerosis; an infected wound; a diabetic condition.*

Can't find a recommended product? Call the 800 number listed in Product Resources for the store nearest you.

Fungal Skin Infections
Athlete's Foot, Ringworm, Impetigo

Fungal infections are characterized by moist, weepy, red patches on the body. Although opportunities for risk seem to be everywhere, (new evidence even points to involvement with sinusitis), fungal infections do not take hold when there is healthy immune response. Stimulating and rebuilding immunity is the key to controlling recurring infections. Athlete's foot (ringworm of the feet) and other fungal infections thrive in dampness and warmth. Make sure that any concurrently occurring fungal infections (such as athlete's foot and "jock itch") are treated simultaneously, so that infection is not continually passed from one area to another. Avoid drug overuse, particularly long courses of antibiotics and cortisones.

Diet & Superfood Therapy

—Nutritional therapy plan:

1—Eat plenty of cultured foods like yogurt, tofu and kefir to promote healthy intestinal flora and allow full nutrient absorption.

2—Add lots of fresh fruits and vegetables to the diet during healing.

3—Keep dietary protein high for fastest healing: eat sea foods and sea greens, sprouts, eggs, soy foods, poultry and whole grains often.

4—Drink 6 glasses of water daily to keep elimination system free and flowing.

5—Avoid foods that promote a fungal growth environment: sugary foods are the biggest culprit, also red meats, pasteurized dairy food, cola drinks, caffeine, and fried foods.

6—Reduce most carbohydrates during healing pasta, pastries, breads, nuts and all sweet foods, (vegetable carbohydrates are fine).

—Superfood therapy: (Choose one or two)

• Apply AloeLife SKIN GEL; drink aloe vera juice daily.

• Balance your intestinal structure with Solgar WHEY TO GO protein drink.

Herb & Supplement Therapy

—Interceptive therapy plan: (Choose 2 or 3 recommendations)

1—**Control the infection and destroy fungal organisms:** • Apply Crystal Star FUNGEX™ gel or ANTI-BIO™ gel with *una da gato*. • East Park olive leaf extract caps; or • Allergy Research OREGANO OIL caps; • Apply Nutribiotic GRAPE-FRUIT SEED SKIN SPRAY or • American Biologics DIOXYCHLOR liquid. Take • Garlic extract or *turmeric* extract capsules 6 daily daily. Use • colloidal silver - Nature's Path SILVER-LYTE as directed internally, SILVER-SKIN-LYTE, an effective topical spray. • Apply *lomatium* extract to area, or Crystal Star ANTI-VI™ extract. Make a paste of an opened Crystal Star anti-fungal • WHITES OUT #2™ and water. Dab twice daily onto affected areas.♀

2—**Add EFA's to stop skin peeling and heal the skin:** • *Evening Primrose Oil* caps 4 daily for 2 weeks for fungal peeling. Apply • Miracle of Aloe FOOT REPAIR; East Park OLIVE LEAF gel; or • *Mahonia* ointment; or • *tea tree* oil as needed.☺

3—**Enzyme therapy and probiotics keep your body environment healthy so fungal infections can't take hold:** • Acidophilus is a key - 1) take acidophilus caps before meals, 2) dissolve acidophilus in water and apply to area directly. • Nature's Plus JR. DOPHILUS, ☺ • Natren TRINITY; ♀ • Prof. Nutrition Dr. DOPHILUS + FOS. • Schiff ENZYMALL; ♀ • Enzymedica PURIFY.

4—**Stimulating immune response is the key to preventing recurring infection:** • Beta carotene 50,000IU; • Zinc 50mg 2x daily; • Lysine 1000mg daily.

—For ringworm: Apply a *Basil* tea skin wash; use *Myrrh* extract - internally and applied; *Thuja* - externally and internally for both thrush and ringworm. ☺ Earth's Bounty O₂ SPRAY; *yellow dock root* tea, 2 cups daily

—For athlete's foot: • Make an antifungal paste: Crush or open and mix together in a bowl: B₂ 500mg, niacin 1000mg, pantothenic acid 500mg. Add 2 tsp. sesame oil and 2 tsp. brewer's yeast. Put on a sock to cover - leave on overnight. ♂

• Make an anti-fungal footbath with *tea tree oil* drops, *marshmallow root* and *black walnut hulls* extract. Soak feet for 20 minutes daily.

Lifestyle Support Therapy

—Bodywork:

• Expose affected areas to natural sunlight every day possible to inhibit fungal growth.

—For athlete's foot and toenail fungus:

• Keep feet well aired and dry. Keep shoes well-aired and change socks daily. Go barefoot as much as possible where appropriate.

• Soak in vinegar for athlete's foot. Dab vinegar between toes daily.

• Apply opened garlic capsules between the toes every morning and night.

• Apply *tea tree* oil; use *tea tree* oil soap.

• Apply baking soda daily and soak your feet in warm epsom salts water for 10 minutes; dry then apply *witch hazel* before you go to bed.

—For ringworm and impetigo:

• Take garlic oil capsules 6 daily. Apply a garlic poultice and cover for 3 days.

• Apply Earth's Bounty O₂ SPRAY.

• Pat on vinegar, or garlic vinegar.

• Dab on *goldenseal-myrrh* strong tea.

• Take epsom salts baths for 20 minutes.

—For thrush: rinse mouth with dilute tea tree oil solution. Keep bathroom cups/toothbrushes clean to prevent re-infection. Soak toothbrush in grapefruit seed extract solution.

Common Symptoms: Patchy, itching skin infection; area will be dry, scaly, cracked, bleeding and tender, with bacterial odor. Or, moist, weepy skin patches that do not dry out, such as ringworm, foot and toenail fungus, a non-healing cut, mouth or nail infections; excessive belching from gas; unexplained allergies; persistent headaches; acne; diaper rash in babies.
Common Causes: Broad spectrum antibiotic and prescription drug use that kills friendly digestive flora and lowers immune defenses allowing infection from fungus micro-organisms to grow; synthetic steroid use; birth control pills; poor hygiene. For athlete's foot or toenail fungus, tight or non-porous shoes.

Can't find a recommended product? Call the 800 number listed in Product Resources for the store nearest you.

F 390

Gallbladder Disease
Gallstones, Cholecystitis

The gallbladder helps digest fats by producing bile (a compound of cholesterol, bile pigments and salts). When the gallbladder bile fluids become saturated with cholesterol, the cholesterol precipitates into solid crystals and then accumulates into stones. As the stones enlarge, the gallbladder becomes inflamed, causing severe pain that feels like a heart attack, and, in some cases, can be life threatening if left untreated. Stones can also block the bile passage, causing pain and digestive harm. High risk factors include poor diet with high cholesterol and low bile acids, obesity, certain drugs, age, and Crohn's disease. About 20 million Americans have gallstones, and gallbladder cholecystitis, (acute gallbladder inflammation); three-fourths of them are women. Yo-yo dieting increases risk of gallstones. Gallstones are far easier to prevent than to reverse.

Diet & Superfood Therapy

—Nutritional therapy plan:

1—The primary gallstone culprit is a diet high in saturated fats, especially from red meats and dairy products. A vegetarian, high fiber diet is the best choice.

2—Go on a short juice and gallbladder flush fast for 3 days. (See next page.) In the acute pain stage, all food should be avoided. Only pure water should be taken until pain subsides.

3—After your gallbladder flush, take a glass of cider vinegar and honey in water each morning.

4—Add 1 TB lecithin grains before each meal, one TB brewer's yeast and 1 TB olive oil daily.

5—Avoid all dairy foods, (especially eggs and milk). Yogurt and kefir are OK. Add artichokes, pears and apples to your diet.

6—A new study shows coffee lowers the risk of gallstone disease - for some men 2 cups a day reduces risk by 30 to 40%.

7—Eat small meals more frequently. No large meals. Drink 6 glasses of water daily.

—Superfood therapy: (Choose one or two)

Note: Since a predisposing factor for gallstones is excessive sugar consumption, do not take highly sweetened protein powder drinks.

• Crystal Star CHO-LO FIBER TONE™ morning and evening.

• AloeLife FIBER MATE drink.

Herb & Supplement Therapy

—Interceptive therapy plan: (Choose 2 or 3 recommendations)

1—**Increase bile solubility to reduce cholesterol levels:** • Enzymatic Therapy coated peppermint oil caps • PEPPERMINT PLUS; • Crystal Star BITTERS & LEMON CLEANSE™ extract to help dissolve bile solids. • Herbal Answers ALOE VERA JUICE with herbs daily, with • MILK THISTLE SEED extract drops added to each glass.

—**Enzyme therapy:** • Alta Health CANGEST, • Rainbow Light ADVANCED ENZYME SYSTEM or • Transformation Enzyme LYPOZYME. • Two acidophilus caps like • Prof. Nutrition DOCTOR DOPHILUS + FOS before meals, and 1 HCL tablet after meals; • Vitamin C up to 3000mg daily with bioflavonoids.

2—**Bitters herbs increase bile flow and help the gallbladder expel small stones:**
• Artemisia extract drops; • dandelion root tea, 3 cups daily; • Wild yam root capsules 6 daily; • Crystal Star LIV-ALIVE™ tea; • NatureWorks SWEDISH BITTERS or • Gaia SWEETISH BITTERS extract; • Taurine 1000mg daily helps keep bile thinned.

3—**Reduce inflammation and pain:** • Turmeric extract (curcumin) 2x daily.

4—**Help dissolve stones:** • Chamomile tea, 5-7 cups daily for a month to dissolve stones; or • Gaia HYDRANGEA ROOT extract; • Crystal Star STN-EX™ capsules with lemon juice and water.

5—**Prevent stone formation:** • Ascorbate vitamin C or Ester C 550mg with bioflavonoids 6 daily; • Solaray ALFAJUICE caps. Fiber supplements reduce the risk of stones. • Futurebiotics COLON GREEN; • Rainbow Light EVERYDAY FIBER SYSTEM; • All One WHOLE FIBER COMPLEX.

6—**Balance excess blood sugar to keep stones from forming:** • Spirulina caps in between meals with • vitamin B complex 100mg helps stabilize blood sugar with Biotin 600mcg; • Glycine caps and • Chromium picolinate 200mcg daily regulate blood sugar; • Gymemma sylvestre capsules, 2 before meals.

7—**Lipotropics control and regulate cholesterol overload:** • Choline-Inositol 2 daily; • Phosphatidyl choline 500mg daily, or • Solgar PHOSPHATIDYL-CHOLINE triple strength; with • Omega-3 flax seed oil 3x daily; • Vitamin A 25,000IU & D 1000IU. • Methionine tablets before meals; • Solaray LIPOTROPIC 1000.

Lifestyle Support Therapy

—Bodywork:

• Take coffee, garlic or catnip enemas every 3 days until relief.

• Take olive oil flushes for 2-3 weeks until stones pass. (See next page.)

• Apply castor packs or cold milk compresses to the abdomen area.

• A sedentary lifestyle is a major high risk factor. Get mild regular exercise and reduce body fat to keep gallstones away. Tests show that for men 2 to 3 hours of light jogging per week can reduce gallstone formation by as much as 40%.

• Acupuncture and acupressure have been successful for gallbladder disease.

—Reflexology point: right foot only

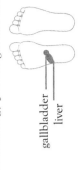
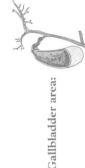

gallbladder
liver

—Gallbladder area:

See LIVER HEALING page 444 for more information.

Common Symptoms: Recurrent abdominal pain bloating and gas; intense pain in the upper right abdomen during an attack, sometimes accompanied by fever and nausea if there are gallstones; belching, pain, and bloating after a heavy meal; headache and bad temper; sluggishness, nervousness.

Common Causes: Too many fatty and fried foods, and lack of ability to digest them; chronic indigestion and gas from too much dairy and refined sugars; food allergies (eliminate the offending food to stop attacks); parasite infections can lead to calcium composition stones; high cholesterol sediment; birth control pills or ERT causing estrogen imbalance and increase of cholesterol by the liver; lack of regular exercise.

Can't find a recommended product? Call the 800 number listed in Product Resources for the store nearest you.

Do you need a gallstone cleanse?

In the United States, high bile cholesterol levels are the main cause of gallstones (bile cholesterol levels do not necessarily correlate with blood cholesterol levels). A stone may grow for 6 to 8 years before symptoms occur. Since continued formation of the gallstone is dependent on either an increased accumulation of cholesterol or reduced levels of bile acids or lecithin, it's easy to see that anywhere along the way, diet improvement will deter, even arrest, stone development.

What else causes gallstones? Other dietary factors like high blood sugar, and high calorie and saturated fat intake which leads to obesity are also involved. Gastrointestinal diseases, like Crohn's disease and diverticulitis are warning signs. Drugs like oral contraceptives and some estrogen replacement drugs have been implicated. Blood cholesterol lowering drugs that contain fibric acid derivatives like clofibrate and gemfibrozil increase the level of bile cholesterol. Gallstones are present in 95% of people suffering from cholecystitis (gallbladder inflammation). There may be no identifiable symptoms, except for periods of nausea and intense abdominal pain that radiates to the upper back. Ultrasound provides a definitive diagnosis.

Important note:

Although I have personally seen several gallstone sufferers use the 9 day program on this page pass gallstones without surgery, I recommend it only under the supervision of a qualified health professional. The liver and gallbladder are interconnecting, interworking organs. Problems with either affect both. Before undertaking a Gallstone Flush to pass gallstones, have an ultrasound test to determine the size of the stones. If they are too large to pass through the urethral ducts, other methods must be used.

The Nine-Day Gallstone Flush Plan

Gallbladder cleansing flushes have been very effective in passing and dissolving gallstones. Depending on the size of the stones and the length of time they have been forming, the flushing programs may last from 3 days to a month. Have a sonogram before embarking on a flush to determine the size of the stones. If they are too large to pass through the bile and urethral ducts, they must be dissolved first, using the STN-EX™ herbal program for 1 month, or other surgical methods must be used. Note: If olive oil is hard for you to take straight, sip it through a straw. See previous page and my book COOKING FOR HEALTHY HEALING for a complete diet program to prevent gallstones.

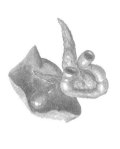

Three day Olive Oil and Lemon Juice Flush:

—**On rising:** take 2 TBS. olive oil and juice of 1 lemon in water. Sip through a straw if desired.
—**Breakfast:** have a glass of organic apple juice.
—**Mid-morning:** have 2 cups of *chamomile* or *cascara* tea.
—**Lunch:** take another glass of lemon juice and olive oil in water; and a glass of fresh apple juice.
—**Mid-afternoon:** have 2 cups of *chamomile* or *cascara* tea.
—**Dinner:** have a glass of carrot/beet/cucumber juice; or a potassium juice or broth (pages 215).
—**Before bed:** take another cup of *chamomile* tea.

Follow with a 5 day Alkalizing Diet:

—**On rising:** take 2 TBS. cider vinegar in water with 1 teasp. honey; or a glass of grapefruit juice.
—**Breakfast:** have a glass of carrot/beet/cucumber juice, or a potassium broth or juice.
—**Mid-morning:** have 2 cups of *chamomile* tea, and a glass of organic apple juice.
—**Lunch:** take a vegetable drink with Sun Wellness CHLORELLA, or Crystal Star ENERGY GREEN DRINK™, a small green salad with lemon-olive oil dressing and a cup of *dandelion* tea.
—**Mid-afternoon:** have 2 cups of *chamomile* tea, and another glass of apple juice.
—**Dinner:** have a small green salad with lemon-oil dressing; and another glass of apple juice.
—**Before bed:** 1 cup *chamomile* or *dandelion* tea.

End with a One Day Intensive Olive Oil Flush:

At 7 p.m. on the evening of the 5th day of the alkalizing diet, mix 1 pint olive oil and 10 juiced lemons; take ¹/₄ cup every 15 minutes until used. Lie on the right side for best assimilation.

Continuing diet notes: The key to prevention of gallstones is diet improvement. Increase your fresh fruit and vegetable intake for more fiber. Vegetable proteins from foods like soy, oat bran and sea greens help prevent gallstone formation. Reduce your intake of animal protein, especially dairy products (casein in dairy products increases formation of gallstones). Avoid fried foods and sugary foods altogether if you are at risk for gallstones.

Can't find a recommended product? Call the 800 number listed in Product Resources for the store nearest you.

Gastric Diseases

Chronic Gastritis, Gastroenteritis, Gastric Ulcers

Gastric diseases refer to ulcerative disorders of the upper gastro-intestinal tract. Stomach acids and some enzymes can damage the lining of the G.I. tract if natural protective factors are not functioning normally. Current medical treatment for these problems focuses on reducing stomach acidity - a symptom - rather than addressing the long term cause of the problem. Many of these treatments are extensive, with definite side effects, and a tendency to alter the normal structure of the digestive tract walls. The alternative approach focuses on rebuilding the integrity of the stomach lining and normalizing G.I. tract pH and function. Tagamet and Zantac, drugs prescribed regularly (one billion dollars in sales yearly) for ulcers and other gastric problems can be addictive. They also inhibit bone formation and proper liver function.

Diet & Superfood Therapy

—Nutritional therapy plan:

1—Emphasis should be on alkalizing foods. Include plenty of fiber foods, whole grains, brown rice, fresh fruits and vegetables. Eat cultured foods for friendly G.I. flora. Have a green salad daily.

2—Avoid alcohol, except a little wine at dinner. Eliminate caffeine, tobacco, aspirin and all fried foods. Chemicalized foods are irritants.

3—Avoid dairy products, except cultured foods; they contribute to stomach acidity.

4—Have a glass of non-carbonated mineral water every evening.

5—Eat small meals more frequently. No large meals. Chew everything well.

—Juices for stomach acid balance:
• Carrot for healing vitamin A.
• Carrot/cabbage, a stomach healer.
• Pineapple-papaya for extra enzymes.

—Superfood therapy: (Choose one or two)
• Crystal Star SYSTEMS STRENGTH™ drink.
• Solgar WHEY TO GO protein drink.
• Lewis Labs BREWER'S YEAST.
• Crystal Star ENERGY GREEN™.
• Herbal Answers ALOE FORCE JUICE.
• Green Foods CARROT ESSENCE.
• New Chapter GINGER WONDER syrup.
• Y.S. ROYAL JELLY 3 to 4 teasp. daily.

Herb & Supplement Therapy

—Interceptive therapy plan: (Choose 2 to 3 recommendations)

1—Reduce pain and inflammation: • MSM caps 800mg 2x daily or • Futurebiotics MSM caps 2 daily; • Enzymedica GASTRO as directed; • *Una da Gato* capsules 6 daily; • *Chamomile* tea or • *Ginger* tea tones intestinal walls; • *Goldenseal/myrrh* extract 3x daily curbs infection. • *Ginkgo Biloba* extract 3x daily; • Planetary TRIPHALA caps as directed; • Holistic PROPOLIS LOZENGES as needed.

2—Calm nerve and intestinal distress: • Crystal Star RELAX CAPS™ as needed, • *Pau D'arco* or Ginseng extract drops in water.

3—Soothe the stomach lining and lessen bleeding: • *Pau d'arco*-Peppermint tea combination; • *Calendula* tea; • *Plantain* tea; • *Slippery elm* tea; • *Turmeric* extract (curcumin) capsules; • *Celandine* extract tablets in water. • Magnesium to soothe membranes, or • Country Life magnesium-potassium-bromelain capsules 2 before meals. • Jarrow BIOSIL, 6 drops in warm water, or • Flora VEGE-SIL caps.

4—Balance stomach pH to help the body cleanse itself: • Aloe vera juice; • Crystal Star BITTERS & LEMON™ extract to balance gastrointestinal region; • gamma-oryzanol (GO) 300mg reduces abdominal distention.

5—Protease enzymes help curb leaky gut syndromes: • Enzymedica PURIFY as directed (results even in serious cases). • Glutamine 500mg 4x daily (or 1 teasp. glutamine powder in juice 3x a day) decreases permeability of small intestine to increase absorption.

6—Digestive enzymes and probiotics rebalance the gastric area: • Prevail ACID-EASE tablets; • Prof. Nutrition DR. DOPHILUS with FOS before meals or • Ethical Nutrients INTESTINAL CARE. • Betaine HCl for stomach acid; • Activated charcoal releases gas; • Pancreatin helps digest fats; Schiff ENZYMALL with ox bile. • Liquid chlorophyll 1 tsp. before meals; • Bromelain 750mg before meals, or • Enzymatic Therapy DGL chewable tablets after meals, and especially after taking antacid drugs.

Lifestyle Support Therapy

—Bodywork:
• Avoid cortico-steroid drugs. They often result in ulcers. Antacids offer minor symptomatic, or no relief. Excess use of aspirin increases gastric problem risk.
• Relaxation techniques like biofeedback are successful for many gastric problems.
• Take a "constitutional" walk after meals. Don't eat when upset, angry or anxious.

—Acupressure points:
Pull middle toe on each foot for 1 minute.

—Reflexology point:

solar plexus
diaphragm
stomach

—Upper gastro-intestinal region:

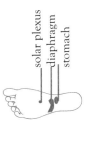

See next page DIVERTICULITIS, COLITIS AND CROHN'S DISEASE pages for more.

Common Symptoms: Chronic poor digestion, with sharp abdominal and chest pains; heartburn and tenderness; nausea and acid bile reflux in the throat; asthma-like symptoms, often irritable bowel symptoms; vomiting blood or a coffee groundlike material; loss of appetite; dark stools.

Common Causes: Too many fried, fatty foods, sugars, and refined foods; poor food combining; overeating - esp. excessively spiced foods; eating too fast, too much and too often; acidosis; intestinal parasites; food allergies or candida yeast overgrowth; too much caffeine and alcohol; steroid use; stress; drip from a chronic sinus infection; irritation from long use of NSAIDS drugs; H. pylori infection.

Can't find a recommended product? Call the 800 number listed in Product Resources for the store nearest you.

Gastric Diseases

GERD (Gastro-esophageal Reflux Disease), Hiatal Hernia

A hiatal hernia occurs when a part of the stomach protrudes through the diaphragm wall, causing difficulty swallowing, burning and reflux in the throat, and great nervous anxiety. Today's American diet habits mean that a hiatal condition is common. **GERD** (Esophageal reflux disease) is due to leaking of stomach acid back into the lower esophagus and acid coming up into the throat. This can also occur in severe cases of osteoporosis, when the rib cage and upper body have collapsed to the point where normal food transit is impeded. People who suffer from acid reflux are far more likely to develop cancer of the esophagus. Antacids do not reduce the cancer risk, only mask symptoms and often doing more harm than good. They don't prevent or cure the underlying condition and can upset stomach pH causing it to produce even more harmful acids.

Diet & Superfood Therapy

—Nutritional therapy plan:

1—Eat only raw or lightly steamed vegetable-source fiber foods during healing. Eat nothing within 3 hours of bedtime.

2—Drink 2 glasses of fresh carrot or apple juice every day.

3—Take 2 glasses of mineral water or aloe vera juice daily.

4—When digestion has normalized, follow a low fat, low salt, high fiber diet.

5—Eat smaller meals more frequently. No large meals. No liquids with meals. Eat slowly so that you are less likely to swallow air and belch.

6—Foods that aggravate a hiatal hernia are coffee, chocolate, red meats, hard alcohol drinks, and carbonated drinks.

7—Eliminate fried and spicy foods because they slow the rate at which your stomach empties, allowing food to travel backwards to the esophagus. Avoid nuts, seeds, acidic juices and gas-producing foods during healing.

—Superfood therapy: (Choose one or two)

• AloeLife or Saluté ALOE VERA juice.
• Crystal Star CHO-LO FIBER TONE™ drink for gentle cleansing fiber.
• Sun Wellness CHLORELLA 20 tabs daily for 1 month, or liquid chlorophyll 3 teasp. daily.
• Transitions EASY GREENS.

Herb & Supplement Therapy

—Interceptive therapy plan: (Choose 1 or 2 recommendations)

1—Lessen spasm and pain: •Glutamine 500mg 4x daily (or 1 teasp. glutamine powder in juice 3x a day) decreases permeability of small intestine to increase absorption. (Relief often within 30 minutes.) •Enzymedica GASTRO; •Crystal Star ANTI-FLAM™ caps 4 daily, and •ANTI-SPZ™ caps 2 with each meal, or •CRAMP BARK COMBO™ extract ½ dropperful at a time as needed for pain and spasms.
•Propolis extract ½ dropperful every 4 hours during an attack.

2—Soothe inflamed tissue of the stomach lining and esophagus: •Chamomile tea; •Pau d' arco tea; •Licorice root extract or •Crystal Star GINSENG-LICORICE ELIXIR™; •Slippery elm or marshmallow tea as needed. •Bromelain 1500mg as needed; or •Source Naturals ACTIVATED QUERCETIN or Quercetin 3 daily to reduce inflammation, with bromelain and vitamin C. •Enzymatic Therapy GASTRO-SOOTHE as directed. •Zinc gluconate lozenges under the tongue as needed. •Schiff EMULSIFIED A 25,000IU 2x daily to rebalance digestive tract.

3—After intial stages, bitters herbs stimulate the secretion of stomach acid, cleanse the stomach and balance its functions: •Crystal Star BITTERS & LEMON™ extract to balance gastrointestinal region; or •MILK THISTLE SEED extract for 1 to 3 months; •Planetary TRIPHALA caps as directed; or •Aloe vera juice daily.

4—Protease enzymes help curb leaky gut syndromes: •Enzymedica PURIFY as directed (results even in serious cases). •Glutamine 500mg 4x daily (or 1 teasp glutamine powder in juice 3x a day) decreases permeability of small intestine to increase absorption.

5—Digestive enzymes and area: •Herbal Products and DeFOOD ENZYMES; •Enzymatic needed; •Pancreatin 1400mg •Alta Health CANGEST caps

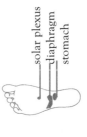

probiotics rebalance the gastric velopment POWER PLUS Therapy CHEWABLE DGL as with meals; •Prevail DIGEST; or powder 3x daily.

Lifestyle Support Therapy

—Bodywork:

• No smoking. Avoid all tobacco.
• Lose weight. Tone the abdomen with exercise. Watch posture to avoid slouching. Wear loose, comfortable, non-binding clothing.
• Apply a green clay pack to the upper abdominal area.
• Yellow color therapy eyewear - wear until hernia is gone, especially during meals.
• Have a chiropractic adjustment to the area or a massage therapy treatment at least once a month. (I have personally seen massage therapy work for many people.)
• To prevent night time reflux, elevate head of bed 6 to 8 inches. Don't eat within two hours of your bedtime.
• Don't lie down after eating.

—Reflexology point:

solar plexus
diaphragm
stomach

See previous page, Indigestion and Heartburn pages for more.

Common Symptoms: Chest pains and proneness to heartburn after eating; belching, excess gas and bloating; difficulty swallowing and a full feeling at the base of the throat; hiccups and regurgitation; pressure behind the breast-bone; raised blood pressure; diarrhea; inflammation and gastro-intestinal bleeding, usually with a stomach ulcer; mental confusion and nerves.
Common Causes: Food allergies; short esophagus; overeating; obesity; food allergies; enzyme deficiency; constipation from a low residue diet and too many refined and acid-forming foods; osteoporosis and bone collapse of upper body structure; tobacco; too tight jeans or underclothing.

Can't find a recommended product? Call the 800 number listed in Product Resources for the store nearest you.

Gastric Diseases - Ulcers
Stomach, Peptic, Duodenal

One in ten Americans now have, or have had, an ulcer. Our lifestyle habits of alcohol, smoking, rich, highly refined foods and too much aspirin (the latest figures show Americans take 85 million aspirin a day!) make us prime ulcer candidates. Every year, ten thousand people die of ulcer complications. A stomach or **gastric ulcer** occurs in the upper stomach lining. A **peptic ulcer**, the most common, is an erosion of the lining in the lower stomach, small intestine or esophagus. A **duodenal ulcer**, occurs in the duodenum (the first part of the small intestine). Most ulcers are caused by H. pylori, a common stomach bacterium which liberates copious amounts of damaging ammonia and carbon dioxide when the body's intestinal protective devices fail. Natural therapy focuses on gastric mucosal support and re-establishing intestinal balance.

Diet & Superfood Therapy

—Nutritional therapy plan:

1—Go on a short liquid diet (pg. 191) to cleanse the G.I. tract. Take 3 juices of your choice daily: 1) Potassium broth (pg. 215); 2) Veggie drinks (pg. 218) or see below; 3) Cabbage/celery/parsley juice; 4) Apple-alfalfa sprout juice with 1 teasp. spirulina powder added.

Drink 2-3 glasses mineral water daily.

2—Add easily digestible, fresh alkalizing foods, like leafy greens, steamed vegetables, whole grains and non-acidic fruits. Have a raw cabbage salad daily during healing.

3—Include cultured foods, such as yogurt, kefir and buttermilk for friendly G.I. flora.

4—Avoid sugars, fatty foods (interfere with buffer activity of protein and calcium), pasteurized dairy foods, red meat, heavy, spicy, refined foods. Reduce alcohol (a little wine is ok). Avoid cola drinks - provoke acid production.

5—Chew all food well. Eat small meals. No large, heavy meals. Avoid late night snacks.

—Superfoods are important against ulcers:
• New Moon GINGER WONDER syrup.
• Sun Wellness CHLORELLA tabs 15 daily, or liquid chlorophyll 3 teasp. daily with meals.
• Aloe Falls ALOE/GINGER juice, or Herbal Answers ALOE FORCE juice with herbs.
• Wakunaga KYO-GREEN with EFAs.

Herb & Supplement Therapy

—Interceptive therapy plan: (Choose 2 to 4 recommendations)

1—Reduce the pain and inflammation: • Crystal Star ULCR COMPLEX™ caps with meals; • ginger capsules before meals; • Jarrow Formulas CURCUMIN-97 capsules; • Goldenseal-cayenne caps; • Enzymedica GASTRO caps; • NAC (N-acetyl-cysteine) 600mg or Source Naturals N-ACETYL-CYSTEINE as directed.

For duodenal ulcers: • Crystal Star ANTI-SPZ™ caps to calm; a mild olive oil flush - 2 TBS oil through a straw before retiring for a week; and • Gamma Oryzanol (GO) as directed, - a rice bran extract; • Planetary TRIPHALA caps as directed.

2—Overcome H. pylori infection: • Crystal Star ANTI-BIO™ caps 6 daily or Nutricology PRO-LIVE (olive leaf extract caps) against H. pylori; • Una da gato tea, 3 cups daily; • Tea Tree oil mouth rinse as needed. ♂ • Quercetin 1000mg with bromelain 1500mg daily; • Propolis tincture as needed. ♀ • Evening Primrose Oil 2000mg daily or • Omega-3 flax oil, 2 teasp. daily retard H. pylori growth.

3—Herbal flavonoids have anti-ulcer properties and inhibit H. pylori bacteria: • Ginkgo Biloba extract; • Goldenseal-myrrh extract; • Garlic or garlic-parsley capsules 8 daily. • For duodenal ulcers: Bilberry extract 15 drops in calendula tea 3x daily. ♀

4—Soothe and heal the ulcerated areas: • Enzymatic Therapy DGL chewables as needed before meals; • Slippery elm tea heals mucous membranes and inflamed tissue; • Chamomile tea 3 cups daily; • Marshmallow root tea. • Stress B-complex 100mg with extra pantothenic acid 500mg and B-6, 50mg.

5—Restablish and improve the integrity of the gastrointestinal mucosa: • Glutamine 500mg 3x daily. • Crystal Star GINSENG-LICORICE ELIXIR™ inhibits H. pylori and balances G.I. tract. • Ascorbate vitamin C or Ester C, 3000mg daily for 3 months. • High potency Y.S. or Premier One ROYAL JELLY 2 teasp. daily. • Vitamin E 400IU 2x daily; • Schiff emulsified A 100,000IU for 6 days.

6—Rebuild immune response to prevent further ulcers: • Crystal Star CHLORELLA-GINSENG extract to normalize immune response and rebuild mucosa. • Zinc 30mg daily; • Chromium picolinate 200mcg daily; • Professional Nutrition DOCTOR DOPHILUS + FOS, 1/2 teasp. before meals.

Lifestyle Support Therapy

Note: Calcium carbonate antacids, like TUMS and ALKA-2 actually produce increased gastric acid secretions when medication is stopped, and may cause kidney stones. Sodium bi-carbonate antacids, like Alka-Seltzer and Rolaids elevate blood pH levels, interfering with metabolism, and they can increase blood pressure. Aluminum-magnesium antacids, like Maalox and Mylanta can cause calcium depletion and contribute to aluminum toxicity.

• Tagamet and Zantac drugs (over 1 billion dollars in sales yearly) suppress HCL formation in the stomach and may cause eventual liver damage. Both drugs interfere with the liver's ability to process and excrete toxic chemicals, making a person vulnerable to poisons from pesticides, herbicides, etc. Take DGL (deglycyrrhizinated licorice) to normalize after these drugs.

—Bodywork:
• Avoid smoking, caffeine, NSAIDS drugs and aspirin - key culprits in aggravating ulcers. Smoking particularly inhibits a natural bicarbonate secretion that neutralizes harmful acids.
• Take a catnip or garlic enema once a week during healing to detoxify the G.I. tract.

See previous two pages and the HYPOGLYCEMIA DIET, page 427 for more.

Common Symptoms: Open sores or lesions in the stomach/duodenum walls, causing burning, the urge to vomit and diarrhea; pain right after eating for a stomach ulcer - two or three hours later for a duodenal ulcer. If the vomit is bright red, and the feces are very dark, it is a duodenal ulcer.

Common Causes: Mental and emotional stress creating an acid system; gastrointestinal irritants like smoking, aspirin, NSAIDS drugs, coffee, alcohol; poor food combining and food irritants; eating too fast; excessive use of commercial antacids; food allergies; too many sugary foods; anemia; Candida albicans; hypoglycemia.

Can't find a recommended product? Call the 800 number listed in Product Resources for the store nearest you.

Gland Health
Deep Body Balance

Do you need a gland cleanse? Your glands and hormones work at your body's deepest levels. They are involved with almost every body function and biochemical reaction, so they're a key to good health, especially as you age. There are two types of glands: Exocrine glands, like salivary and mammary glands, regulated by the hypothalamus, secreting their fluids through ducts; and Endocrine glands, like the pituitary, pineal or ovaries, that emit their secretions (primarily hormones) directly into the bloodstream and lymph system. Hormones are chemical messengers exerting wide-ranging effects throughout our bodies. Hormones influence our moods, energy level, mental alertness, even metabolism. Hormone secretions like adrenaline, insulin, and thyroid hormone are extraordinarily affected by nutritional deficiencies, environmental pollutants, chemicalized foods and synthetic hormones. In fact, glands and hormones are affected first by harmful toxins and poor nutrition. A mineral deficiency, for instance, something that plagues most Americans, undermines the health of almost every gland and organ. The chronic stress loads most Americans live under have a direct effect on hormone balance, like the low levels of steroidal hormones produced by our "stressed out" adrenals.

Diet & Superfood Therapy

—Nutritional therapy plan:
1—Begin with a 3 day juice-liquid diet and follow with 1 to 4 days of a diet of all fresh foods.
2—The night before your gland cleanse.... take a gentle herbal laxative, like Crystal Star LAXA-TEA™, or M. D. Labs DAILY DETOX TEA.
3—The next day.... if in the season, go on a watermelon juice only cleanse. Drink throughout the day to rapidly flush and alkalize. If watermelon is not available, start with the following:
—On rising: take lemon juice in water with 1 tsp. honey. Add 2 tsp. brewer's yeast flakes.
—Breakfast: have a carrot juice with 1 TB any green superfood (next column).
—Mid-morning: take a carrot or mixed veggie drink. Add 1 tsp. sea greens (dulse or kelp).
—Lunch: have a bowl of miso soup. Sprinkle with dulse flakes and 1 tsp. brewer's yeast.
—Mid-afternoon: have a mixed vegetable-tomato base juice like Personal Best V-8 (page 218).
—Dinner: have a high mineral broth: Simmer 30 minutes: 3 carrots, 1 cup parsley, 1 onion, 2 potatoes, 2 stalks celery. Strain.
—Before Bed: have an apple or pineapple/papaya juice. If desired, blend in 1 fresh fig.

Herb & Supplement Therapy

—Interceptive therapy plan: (Choose 2 to 3 recommendations)
1—**Deep clean your glands:** • Gaia Herbs SUPREME CLEANSE.
2—**Enhance your gland functions:** Use herbal compounds that contain phyto-hormone-rich herbs, like ginseng, licorice root, sarsaparilla, dong quai, and black cohosh. • Crystal Star BIOFLAV., FIBER & C SUPPORT™ drink is a gland balancer. For gland homeostasis, • Crystal Star FEEL GREAT™ and ADRN™ formulas, or • Planetary Formulas SCHIZANDRA ADRENAL SUPPORT; use • Crystal Star HEAVY METAL CLEANZ™ caps if you are regularly exposed to toxic pollutants.
Raw gland extracts offer biochemical support for gland stress and fatigue: • Premier Labs RAW MULTIPLE GLANDULAR; • Enzymatic Therapy glandulars: THYMUPLEX, NUCLEO-PRO M, NUCLEO-PRO F and RAW MAMMARY.
3—**Essential fatty acids are essential:** • Barlean's Organic OMEGA TWIN FLAX/BORAGE COMBO. • Futurebiotics VITAL K LIQUID.
4—**Enzymes and probiotics assist detoxification and protect from toxins:** • Source Naturals LIFE FLORA; • Arise & Shine FLORA GROW; • Transformation Enzyme PUREZYME, or • Enzymedica DIGEST for adrenal exhaustion; • Rainbow Light DOUBLE-STRENGTH ALL-ZYME.
5—**Electrolytes expedite a gland cleanse:** • Nature's Path TRACE-LYTE LIQUID MINERALS; • Arise & Shine ALKALIZER.
6—**Your glands need greens! Chlorophyll rich superfoods:** • Body Ecology VITALITY SUPERGREEN; • Solgar EARTH SOURCE GREENS & MORE; • Crystal Star ENERGY GREEN™ or SYSTEMS STRENGTH drink; • Nutricology PRO GREENS with EFA's; • AloeLife ALOE GOLD JUICE; • Y.S. royal jelly with ginseng 4 teasp. daily.

Lifestyle Support Therapy

—Bodywork:
• Enema: Take an enema at least once during your gland cleanse to help release toxins.
• Exercise: Take a regular 20 minute "gland health" walk every day.
• Environmental: Avoid air and environmental pollutants as much as possible. Your glands are the first to feel the damaging effects.
• Acupressure points: Stroke the top of the foot on both feet for 5 minutes each to stimulate endocrine and hormone secretions.

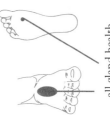

all gland health

• Massage therapy: Have a massage therapy treatment to stimulate circulation and re-establish clear meridian pathways in the body.
• Thump the thymus point briskly each morning 6 times for immune response.

Common Symptoms: **Is your body showing signs that it needs a gland cleanse?** Some of the first signs to look for might be unexplained weight gain and sluggish metabolism (indicating impaired thyroid activity), and blood sugar problems (indicating unbalanced insulin levels). Poor assimilation of nutrients may mean low enzyme output from a congested pancreas, chronic fatigue may indicate adrenal exhaustion.
Common Causes: Mineral deficiency; stress; hypothyroidism; environmental pollutants; too much sugar, alcohol, caffeine, tobacco and drugs.

See also KNOW YOUR GLANDS page 548 for more information.

Can't find a recommended product? Call the 800 number listed in Product Resources for the store nearest you.

Glaucoma
Eyeball Fluid Pressure and Hardening

Glaucoma affects over 3 million people over 65 in America. It is characterized by a build up of pressure in the eyeball but is often undetected because it is frequently asymptomatic in the early stages. If the pressure is not relieved, the eyeball may harden, harm the retina and progressively damage the eyes. Side vision becomes limited; if untreated, blindness can result. Collagen, as the most abundant and necessary protein in the eye, is responsible for eye tissue strength and integrity. Improved collagen metabolism can be a key to the relief of pressure on the eye. Glaucoma is also often the result of, and accompanied by, liver malfunction.

Diet & Superfood Therapy

—Nutritional therapy plan:

1—Go on a fresh foods diet for 2 weeks to clear the system of inorganic crystalline deposits. Take one of the following every day during these 2 weeks:

Carrot/beet/cucumber/parsley juice
Fresh carrot juice
Potassium broth (pg. 215)

2—Avoid all refined sugars, caffeine and foods containing caffeine. Avoid known food allergens.

•Vitamin A-rich foods for eyes: Endive and leafy greens, carrots, sea foods and sea vegetables, broccoli.

•Vitamin C sources for eyes: Citrus juice, green peppers, cucumbers, carrot juice, beets.

—Superfoods are important (the eyes require a great deal of nourishment.)
•Mona's CHLORELLA- 2 teasp. daily.
•Crystal Star ENERGY GREEN™ and BIOFLAV, FIBER & C SUPPORT™.
•Solgar EARTH SOURCE GREENS & MORE drink.
•Beehive Botanical ROYAL JELLY with Siberian ginseng 2 teasp. daily.
•AloeLife ALOE GOLD JUICE 2x daily, also dilute and use as an eyewash.

Herb & Supplement Therapy

—Interceptive therapy plan: (Choose 2 to 3 recommendations)

1—Vitamin C therapy reduces intra-ocular pressure of chronic glaucoma:
•Ascorbate Vitamin C with bioflavonoids and rutin, 10,000mg daily. As an ascorbic acid flush, take ¼ teasp. at a time in water every hour. Also bathe eyes daily with a dilute water ascorbate C/bioflavonoid solution. Add •Quercetin 1000mg with bromelain 750mg 6 daily. Add •Lane Labs BENE-FIN shark cartilage.

2—Lower intra-ocular pressure: •Crystal Star EYEBRIGHT COMPLEX™ capsules 4 daily; •Enzymatic Therapy Ayurvedic *coleus forskohlii* extract; •Enzymatic Therapy ORAL NUTRIENT CHELATES to help relieve pressure and crystallized particles in the eye. •Golden Pride FORMULA ONE with EDTA.

3—Improve and support the liver: •*Spirulina* 6 daily or •Solaray ALFAJUICE 2 daily as a liver cleanser. •Crystal Star BITTERS & LEMON CLEANSE™ extract.

4—Enhance eye circulation: •GINKGO BILOBA extract or •cayenne capsules, 2 daily to normalize circulation to the optical system. •Magnesium 400mg (Nature's calcium channel blocker) daily improves blood flow.

5—Improve collagen metabolism and tissue integrity: •BILBERRY extract several times daily; or •Solaray VIZION caps with *bilberry*; Source Naturals VISUAL EYES; •Herbal Magic GOTU KOLA-GINSENG caps 4 daily. •Vitamin E 400IU daily to help remove lens particles.

6—Antioxidants are critical to healing: •Alpha lipoic acid 300mg daily; •Nutricology OCUDYNE II with lutein; •OPCs from grapeseed or white pine, 100mg 3x daily; •Glutathione 50mg 2x daily; •Beta carotene 150,000IU daily or PHYCOTENE MICROCLUSTERS available from Healthy House.

7—Protect against glaucoma: •Carnitine 1000mg daily; •Crystal Star IODINE-POTASSIUM SOURCE™ for iodine imbalance; •Nature's Life I-SIGHT 2x daily.

—Glaucoma healing eye washes: •Crystal Star EYEBRIGHT™ tea; •Weak goldenseal solution; •Chamomile tea; •Fennel seed compresses.

Lifestyle Support Therapy

—Lifestyle measures:
•Relax more. Strive for a less stressful lifestyle.
•Stop smoking. It constricts eye blood vessels and increases pressure.
•Drugs to avoid for glaucoma: cortico-steroid drugs, tranquilizers, epinephrine-like or atropine drugs, aspirin and over-the-counter antihistamines. These drugs tend to inhibit or destroy collagen structures in the eye.
•Get a good spinal chiropractic adjustment or regular massage therapy treatments.

—Reflexology points: Important in breaking up crystalline deposits:

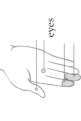

eyes

—Eyeball and muscles:

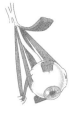

Common Symptoms: *Colored halos around lights or hazy vision; eye inflammation with reddened eyes; great pain in the eye area and headaches; tunnel vision, loss of peripheral vision; blurred vision; inability to tear; fixed and dilated pupils. Acute closed-angle glaucoma is extremely serious eye emergency with severe, throbbing eye pain, and loss of vision if pressure is not relieved within 36 hours.*
Common Causes: *Chronic glaucoma is more prevalent than acute glaucoma. Overuse of steroid and other drugs - see list above; diabetes; food allergies; poor collagen metabolism; too much dietary caffeine and sugar; prolonged emotional stress; allergies; adrenal exhaustion; liver malfunction; watching TV too long in the dark; thyroid imbalance; arteriosclerosis.*

See LIVER CLEANSING page 202 and EYESIGHT page 381 for more information.

Can't find a recommended product? Call the 800 number listed in Product Resources for the store nearest you.

Gout

Arthritis of the Toe and Peripheral Joints

Gout is a common type of arthritis, suffered primarily (90%) by overweight, middle-aged males. It is caused by poor metabolism that allows an accumulation of too much uric acid in the blood, tissues and urine. Although known as a toe problem, joints, tendons, fingers and kidneys are also gout sites. The natural healing approach is simple and successful. Improving gout involves diet change to eliminate high purine foods and heavy alcohol that causes sedimentary precipitates. It reduces dietary fat for weight loss and cholesterol reduction. It advocates cleansing of the kidneys to normalize uric acid levels in the blood and tissues.

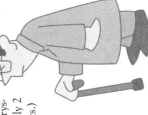

Diet & Superfood Therapy

—Nutritional therapy plan:

1—Gout is clearly caused by dietary factors. Reduce caffeine, white flour foods, fried foods, and all saturated fats, especially meat proteins. Avoid high levels of fructose in any food or drink.

2—Go on a bladder/kidney liquid cleansing diet (pg. 202) to rid the body of sediment wastes.

3—Follow with a diet of 75% fresh foods for a month to balance uric acid formation.

4—Drink 4 glasses of black cherry juice and 6 glasses of water daily to flush and neutralize uric acid. Eat plenty of cherries and other dark fruits.

5—Eat high potassium foods: fresh cherries of all kinds, bananas, strawberries, celery, broccoli, potatoes, and greens to put acid crystals in solution so they can be eliminated.

6—Avoid high purine foods: red meats, rich gravies, broths, sweetbreads, organ meats, mushrooms, asparagus, dry peas, legumes, spinach, rhubarb, sardines, anchovies, lobster, oysters, clams.

7—Eliminate alcohol during healing; it inhibits uric acid secretion from the kidneys.

—Superfood therapy: (Choose one or two)
• Potassium broth (page 215) or Crystal Star SYSTEMS STRENGTH™ for iodine - potassium.
• Crystal Star ENERGY GREEN™ drink.
• Nutricology PRO-GREENS with EFA's.
• Aloe vera juice each morning.

Herb & Supplement Therapy

—Interceptive therapy plan: (Choose 2 or more recommendations)

1—**Take down inflammation and pain:** •Crystal Star AR EASE™ or ANTI-FLAM™ capsules (with *white willow*), with ADRN™ extract 2x daily. •Enzymatic Therapy CHERRY JUICE extract. •Quercetin 1000mg with bromelain 1500mg 3x daily until relief. •Nutricology GERMANIUM 150mg reduces pain and swelling. •B-complex 100mg with extra B_6 250mg and folic acid 800mcg 3x daily inhibits xanthine oxidase.

Herbal diuretics are effective in reducing swelling without potassium loss:
•Crystal Star BLDR-K COMFORT™ caps or BLDR-K™ tea; or *Buchu* tea.

2—**Reduce uric acid accumulation:** •Vitamin C therapy is effective - take ascorbate Vitamin C with bioflavonoids and rutin, $\frac{1}{4}$ teasp. at a time in water every 4 hours for one week, then 5000mg daily for the rest of the month (almost immediate relief). Take with •lithium orotate, 5 to 10mg for best results. •Take Enzymatic Therapy ACID-A-CAL capsules as needed; •Enzymedica PURIFY, protease enzymes balance pH levels; or •BioForce DEVILS CLAW extract reduce both uric acid and cholesterol build-up. •*Celery* seed tea, 2 cups daily.

3—**Essential fatty acids inhibit inflammatory leukotriene production:** •Omega-3 rich *flax* oil 2 TBS daily; •*Evening Primrose* oil 3000mg daily.

4—**Enrich body flavonoids, a key to overcoming gout:** •*Hawthorn* or *Bilberry* extract 4x daily; •Crystal Star BIOFLAV, FIBER & C SUPPORT™ drink daily; •PCO's from grapeseed and white pine bark, 100mg 3x daily.

5—**Rebalance thyroid** (hypothyroidism is usually involved in gout): •Take sea greens 2 TBS daily, or •Crystal Star IODINE/POTASSIUM caps, or •Solaray ALFAJUICE tabs, or •FutureBiotics VITAL K 3 teasp. daily to normalize thyroid activity.

6—**Regulate blood sugar levels and increase circulation:** •Glycine 500mg daily. with chromium picolinate 200mcg; •Biotech CELL-GUARD with SOD, 6 daily; •vitamin E 400IU and •niacin 50mg to increase circulation.

Lifestyle Support Therapy

—Lifestyle measures:
•Weight reduction is a key factor to ease pressure on feet and legs. But lose it slowly. Rapid weight loss shocks your metabolism and may trigger a gout attack.
•Check your high blood pressure medicine. Several of them cause formation of inorganic crystal sediments.
•Avoid aspirin. It can raise uric acid levels.

—Bodywork:
•Apply *plantain*, *ginger*, or fresh *comfrey* compresses to inflamed area.
•Use Crystal Star ALKALIZING ENZYME HERBAL BODY WRAP™ to neutralize acids and balance body pH right away.
•Apply topical DMSO with aloe vera to painful area to help dissolve crystalline deposits (usually 2 to 4 days before results.)

See also ARTHRITIS THERAPY page 316.

Common Symptoms: *Extremely painful joints, usually in the foot and big toe; rapid onset of excruciating tenderness, redness, swelling - sometimes chills and fever; gradual joint destruction with longer and longer attacks.*

Common Causes: *Tiny, needle-like crystals of uric acid in blood and body fluids caused by overeating, too much red meat, refined food, alcohol, sugar, caffeine, etc. that an over-loaded kidney does not excrete properly; overuse of drugs, such as thiazide diuretics causing potassium deficiency; lead toxicity; obesity; hypoglycemia and hypothyroidism both appear to be factors.*

Can't find a recommended product? Call the 800 number listed in Product Resources for the store nearest you.

Grave's Disease

Hyperthyroidism, Hyper-parathyroidism

Grave's disease involves too much thyroid (thyroxine) secretion. Characterized by overactive metabolism, every body process seems to speed up - digestion, nervous energy, impatience, perspiration, tiredness (but the inability to rest adequately), hair loss, unhealthy weight loss, rapid heartbeat, climate sensitivity, even aging. Grave's disease affects women far more than men, and younger people far more than the elderly. The **parathyroid gland**, embedded in the thyroid, is responsible for blood levels of calcium. Hyperparathyroidism, too much PTH secretion, can lead to kidney stones and osteoporosis; it's a health problem for 65,000 women a year. Overactive thyroid conditions respond well to natural therapies. Some drugs, like over-the-counter diet pills, can both bring on and aggravate a thyroid problem.

Diet & Superfood Therapy

—Nutritional therapy plan:

1—For the first month of healing, follow a diet of about 75% fresh foods. Include plenty of vegetable proteins from sprouts, sea greens, soy foods and whole grains. Have a daily potassium drink (pg. 215) or green drink (pg. 218), and see below.

2—Add B vitamins and complex carbohydrates from brown rice and vegetables for stabilizing energy.

3—Eat plenty of cultured foods for friendly G.I. flora - yogurt, kefir, sauerkraut (cultured veggies).

4—Make a mix of brewer's yeast, wheat germ, lecithin; take 2 TBS daily.

5—Drink 8 glasses of water daily, and carrot juice 3x a week; take papaya juice for adrenal support. Avoid stimulants like caffeine and sodas.

—Thyroid-balancing foods: raw cruciferous vegetables, like cabbage, cauliflower, broccoli, kale and brussels sprouts, beets, spinach. (Cooking inactivates much of the thyroid lowering ability.)

—Superfood therapy: (Choose one or two)
• Crystal Star SYSTEMS STRENGTH™ drink for absorbable iodine and potassium.
• Nutri-Tech ALL ONE vitamin-mineral drink.
• Crystal Star ENERGY GREEN™ drink.
• CC Pollen POLLENENRGY.
• Future Biotics VITAL K, 2 teasp. daily.

Herb & Supplement Therapy

—Interceptive therapy plan: (Choose 2 or more recommendations)

1—**Help balance thyroid and metabolism:** •Crystal Star HEAVY METAL™ caps with *bugleweed* reduces the thyroid hormone T4 by inhibiting thyroid stimulating anibodies, (sometimes dramatic results); may be used with •Crystal Star IODINE-POTASSIUM™ capsules 2-4 daily or •Twin Lab LIQUID K, 2 teasp. daily. •*Ginkgo Biloba* extract; •*Mullein-Lobelia* extract; •Enzymatic Therapy THY-ROID/TYROSINE COMPLEX 4 daily. •*Astragalus* extract capsules 4 daily.

2—**Calm thyroid storms:** •Calcium citrate 4 daily; •EVENING PRIMROSE OIL or *borage* oil caps 500mg 4 to 6 daily; •Transformation Enzyme CALMZYME. •Lecithin 1900gr daily; or •Vitamin E 800IU daily; •Herbal Magic RELAXA HERBAL; •*Hawthorn leaf, berry and flower* extract.

3—**Support the liver:** •Crystal Star LIV-ALIVE™ tea for 1 month, then •Milk Thistle Seed extract for 2 months. •Enzymatic Therapy LIQUID LIVER with *Siberian* ginseng, or •*Siberian* ginseng extract capsules 2000mg.

4—**Ease stress and sleeplessness:** •Stress B-complex with extra B_2 100mg, and B_6 100mg. •Rainbow Light ADAPTOGEM caps; Morada Reasearch NERVOUS SYSTEM; •Country Life STRESS "M."

5—**Re-establish immune health:** •CoQ-10, 60 mg 3x daily; •Marine carotene, such as Solgar OCEANIC CAROTENE 100,000IU daily; •Ester C with bioflavs. 550mg 6 daily; •Zinc picolinate 50-75mg daily. •Rainbow Light MASTER NUTRIENT SYSTEM food-source multiple daily.

Lifestyle Support Therapy

—Bodywork:
• Exercise daily to the point of breathlessness and mild sweating.
• Get some early morning sun on the body every day possible. Wade and swim in the ocean frequently to access naturally-occurring thyroid minerals.
• Acupressure points: press points on both sides of the spinal column at the base of the neck, 3 times for 10 seconds each.

—Reflexology point:

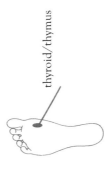

thyroid/thymus

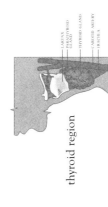

LARYNX
PARATHYROID GLAND
THYROID GLAND
CAROTID ARTERY
TRACHEA

thyroid region

G 399

Common Symptoms: Bulging eyes and blurred vision; fatigue; restlessness and irritability; insomnia; nervous tension; unhealthy weight loss; systolic hypertension, mood swings, and sometimes mental psychosis during a "thyroid storm." Younger victims often have a goiter, older victims have heart palpitations.
Common Causes: Autoimmune traits are thought to be partially inherited; stress; overuse of diet pills; mental burnout and fatigue; zinc deficiency; anorexia syndrome.

See KNOWING YOUR GLANDS page 548 for more. Or call the Thyroid Society 800-849-7643.

Can't find a recommended product? Call the 800 number listed in Product Resources for the store nearest you.

Hair Growth

Healthy Hair, Graying Hair

We all want it... thick, gorgeous hair. Your scalp has at least 100,000 hairs so you have a lot to work with. You normally shed about 25 to 50 hairs a day. Your hair is one of the mirrors of your health. Healthy hair is a mirror of both good nutrition and common-sense care. Natural hair care products are being enthusiastically rediscovered all over America. Hair consists of protein layers called keratin. In healthy hair, the cell walls of the hair cuticle lie flat like shingles, leaving hair soft and shiny. In damaged or dry hair, the cuticle shingles are broken and create gaps that make hair porous and dull. Hair problems are never isolated conditions. They are the result of more basic body imbalances. In fact, changes in hair are often the first indication of nutritional deficiencies.

Diet & Superfood Therapy

—**Nutritional therapy plan for prevention:**

1—Nutrition is the real secret to healthy hair. Feed your hair a high vegetable protein diet. Make a mix of the following hair foods and take 3 TBS daily: wheat germ (oil or flakes), blackstrap molasses, brewer's yeast and sesame seeds.

2—Healthy hair foods: Carrots, green peppers, lettuces, bananas, strawberries, apples, peas, onions, green peppers, cucumbers, sprouts, green tea. Have aloe vera juice in the morning.

3—Avoid saturated fats, sugars and processed, refined foods. They show up.

4—Poor liver function equals unhealthy hair. Too much alcohol, caffeine and drugs put a heavy load on the liver and rob the body of B vitamins.

—**Kitchen cosmetics for hair:** 1) Wet hair, blot, and apply 4 TBS mayonnaise. Wrap in a towel for 30 minutes. Rinse/shampoo. 2) Mix yogurt and an egg. Apply to hair. Wrap in a towel for 30 minutes. Rinse and shampoo. 3) Mix 1 egg yolk with the second shampooing for bounce.

—**Effective superfoods: (choose 1 or 2)**
• Crystal Star SYSTEMS STRENGTH™.
• A low fat protein drink every morning can have a dramatic effect on dry hair texture: Unipro PERFECT PROTEIN, or Solgar WHEY TO GO.
• Red Star NUTRITIONAL YEAST for hair color.

Herb & Supplement Therapy

—**Interceptive therapy plan: (Choose 2 to 3 recommendations)**

1—**Minerals are critical to hair health, especially from herbs and sea greens:**
• Crystal Star HEALTHY HAIR & NAILS™ tea (also a good rinse for shine). **Natural silica boosts hair strength and shine:** *Horsetail* extract; or • Crystal Star SILICA SOURCE™ extract daily, or Flora VEGE-SIL capsules. • *Rosemary* sprigs steeped in wine enhance mineral uptake. **Sea greens minerals are dramatic for hair growth:** • 2 TBS daily dried snipped sea greens like *kelp,* or • Crystal Star IODINE-POTASSIUM™ caps 4 daily, or 6 *kelp* tablets daily; or • Arise & Shine liquid ORGANIC SEA MINERALS; • New Chapter OCEAN HERBS; • Nature's Path TRACE-MIN-LYTE with sea greens.

2—**Protect against early graying:** • Crystal Star ADR-ACTIVE™ to prevent graying. • *Fo-Ti Root,* • *gotu kola* extract, or • Bio-Tech SHEN-MIN caps for 3 months.

3—**EFA's are imperative to hair health:** • *Evening Primrose* oil 2000mg daily. Rub in • Jojoba oil daily until sebum deposits disappear. ♀ • Shampoos rich in EFA's are Hemp or Henna shampoo, Neem Oil shampoo and Babassu Palm shampoo.

4—**Strengthen your hair:** • Cysteine 500mg 2 daily; • Tyrosine 500mg 2x daily; • vitamin C with bioflavonoids 6 daily; • Biotin 600mcg daily. ♂

—**Herbal hair enhancers for oily hair:** use plant-based astringent hair products with *witch hazel* or *lemon balm.* Rinse hair with white vinegar after your shampoo.
—**Herbal hair enhancers for dry hair:** use plant-based astringent hair products with *burdock, nettles* and *rosemary;* Camocare concentrate for dazzle; Home Health *olive oil* and *aloe vera* shampoos. Rinse hair in sea water or kelp water for body.
—**Herbal hair enhancers for damaged hair:** use plant-based astringent hair products with *sage* and *calendula* for body, *wheat germ oil* and *jojoba* for condition.
—**To help restore hair color and growth after illness or radiation treatments:** 1 each daily: PABA 1000mg, molasses 2 TBS, pantothenic acid 1000mg, folic acid 800mcg, B-complex 100mcg with extra B₆ 100mg and folic acid 800mcg, Country Life sublingual B-12, 2500mcg a day. New hair visible noticeably in about 3 weeks.

Lifestyle Support Therapy

—**Bodywork:**
• Massage scalp each morning for 3 minutes to stimulate hair growth.
• Sunlight helps hair grow, but too much sun dries and damages.
• Use alcohol-free stylers, not hair sprays that damage hair and pollute the air.
• Wash hair in warm, not hot water. Rinse in cool water for scalp circulation.
• In light of concern about lead-based hair dyes, is henna a good choice for hair color? Henna is a natural non-carcinogenic plant used for centuries for coloring. It gives body while it colors, often dramatically. Henna works best on thin, light, porous hair.

—**Make a super hair tonic:** Make 8-oz green tea and 8-oz. *rosemary* tea (with fresh sprigs if possible). Strain each. Add 1 TB lemon juice and 1 TB white vinegar. Work through hair and leave on 1 minute. Rinse.

—**Make a hot oil treatment:** Mediterranean women use the fatty acids from olive oil to condition their hair. Just mix olive oil with drops of essential *lavender* and *rosemary* oil and rub in hair. Leave on 5 minutes and rinse.

See next page and DANDRUFF page 362 for more information.

Common Symptoms: Too dry or too oily hair; lots of falling hair; flaky deposits on the scalp; brittle hair with split ends; lack of bounce and elasticity.
Common Causes: Poor diet with several mineral deficiencies; lack of usable protein; poor circulation; recent illness and drug residues; liver malfunction resulting in loss of hair.

Can't find a recommended product? Call the 800 number listed in Product Resources for the store nearest you.

Hair Loss

Alopecia, Male Pattern Baldness

Over 30 million men and 20 million women have thinning or falling hair. Alopecia areata affects 2.5 million people, and may be triggered by a glitch in the immune system. Heavy hair loss may be a sign of an early heart attack. Male pattern baldness affects up to 60% of the male Caucasion population. Female pattern baldness, related to heredity, thyroid disease and hormonal changes, represents 50% of women who have permanent hair loss. Although androgenic alopecia is hereditary and not easily reversible, other factors, both internal and external, are involved in most hair loss that can be improved for thickness and regrowth. Hair health depends on blood circulation and nutrition. Your therapy choice must be vigorously followed. Occasional therapy has little or no effect. Two months is usually the minimum for really noticeable growth.

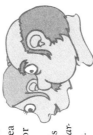

Diet & Superfood Therapy

–Nutritional therapy plan:

1–Most important diet tip: eat sea greens every day for EFA's. 2 TBS dried, snipped sea greens over rice, soup or salad produces real results.

2–Eat foods rich in silica and sulphur: beets, parsley, sea greens, garlic and onions, sprouts, horseradish, green leafy veggies, carrots, bell peppers, eggs, apricots, cucumbers, rice, and seeds.

3–Eat foods rich in iodine and potassium: sea greens and sea foods for growth and thickness.

4–Add soy foods for phyto-hormones, plant protein, EFA's and vitamin E.

5–Add biotin-rich foods: brown rice, lentils, oats, soy foods and walnuts.

6–Drink 6 glasses of water daily.

7–Reduce salt, sugar and caffeine - avoid animal fats, and refined and preserved foods.

–Make a hair protein mix to stop shedding: wheat germ flakes, brewer's yeast, pumpkin seeds, chopped dulse; take 2 TBS daily in food.

–Effective superfoods: (choose 1 or 2)

• Crystal Star SYSTEMS STRENGTH™ drink or caps for absorbable minerals and sea greens.
• ALL 1 MULTIPLE drink with green plant base.
• AMAZAKE rice drinks for B vitamins. ♂
• Beehive Botanicals ROYAL JELLY, POLLEN and SIBERIAN GINSENG drink.

Herb & Supplement Therapy

–Interceptive therapy plan: (Choose 2 to 3 recommendations)

1–**Natural silica and other mineral building blocks boost hair strength:** • Ageless Products NU HAIR, or SILICEA GEL; • Crystal Star SILICA SOURCE™ extract, • *horsetail* tea, or • Flora VEGE-SIL capsules.

2–**Sea greens feed you hair inside and out:** • 2 TBS daily dried snipped sea greens like *kelp*, or • Crystal Star IODINE-POTASSIUM™ caps 4 daily, or 6 *kelp* tablets daily; or • Arise & Shine liquid ORGANIC SEA MINERALS; • New Chapter OCEAN HERBS; • Nature's Path TRACE-MIN-LYTE with sea greens.

3–**EFA's are imperative to hair growth:** • *Evening Primrose Oil* 3000mg or *borage oil* caps, or Omega Nutrition OMEGA PLUS caps; Spectrum high lignan FLAX OIL, 3 caps daily (results usually within 6 weeks). • Omega Nutrition Coconut Butter; • Crystal Star GINSENG/REISHI extract internally. Use • *Rosemary-dulse* tea as a hair rinse.

5–**Stimulate your scalp:** • *Ginkgo Biloba* extract for regrowth; • CoQ-10, 60mg 3x daily; • *Cayenne* extract rub: use directly on scalp before shampooing. Leave on for 30 minutes. • *Ginger* tea rub- leave on 15 minutes; or combine the following scalp stimulant ingredients. Massage into hair for 10 minutes and rinse out: 4 TBS aloe vera gel, 1 TB white vinegar, 1 TB *jojoba* oil, 1 tsp. *rosemary* essential oil, ¹/₄ tsp. *ginger* powder. • *White sage* tea for thinning hair. ♀

6–**Feed your hair amino acids:** • Cysteine 2000mg daily with • zinc 75mg daily, especially if hair loss is related to low thyroid with zinc deficiency.

7–**Treat your prostate to treat your hair loss:** Male pattern baldness emanates from testosterone levels. • Herbal prostate remedies - *saw palmetto*, *potency wood*, and *panax ginseng* or • Crystal Star PROX FOR MEN™ or • Ethical Nutrients MAXI-PROS PLUS.

8–**Hormone balancing herbs can help hair loss in women:** • A *black cohosh, dong quai, burdock* combination, or • Crystal Star EST-AID™ caps. • Crystal Star GINSENG/LICORICE ELIXIR™, use internally and rub on scalp. ♀

9–**B-vitamins help hair growth** (usually noticeable within 4 months): • 2 TBS or more blackstrap molasses daily; • B-complex 150mg daily with extra niacin 50mg daily, PABA 1000mg, pantothenic acid 1000mg, biotin 1000mcg for 2 months.

Lifestyle Support Therapy

–Bodywork:

• Be careful of tight hairstyles and curlers, hot rollers, and chemicals for perming or straightening. Discontinue commercial hair coloring, flat irons, hot hair dryers.

• Stress is clearly a contributor: Get a massage therapy treatment once a week (with scalp massage). Get outdoor exercise every day possible for body oxygen.

• Rinse hair with sea water or vinegar for thickness.

• Aromatherapy oils for alopecia: *sage, cedarwood, rosemary, thyme.*

–Head circulation is a key:

• Finger massage scalp vigorously for 3 minutes every morning.

• Brush dry hair well for 5 minutes daily.

• Rinse for several minutes with alternating hot and cold shower water.

• Use a slant board once a week.

–Effective scalp conditioners: 1) Biotin treatments; 2) Jojoba oil and shampoo to relieve sebum build-up, like Hobe ENERGIZER TREATMENT shampoo; 3) Aloe vera oil.

Common Symptoms: *Thinning or complete loss of hair by either men or women (both male and female pattern baldness occur).*

Common Causes: *Poor circulation; poor diet with excess salt and sugar and too little protein; dandruff or seborrhea; plugs of sebum, high cholesterol; heredity; gland imbalance (especially the thyroid) in women from postpartum changes or discontinuance of birth control pills and overproduction of male sex hormones; hair loss above the temples in women can mean a possible ovarian or adrenal tumor.*

See previous page and Menopausal Hair Loss page 452 for more.

Can't find a recommended product? Call the 800 number listed in Product Resources for the store nearest you.

Hashimoto's Disease

Chronic Lymphocytic Thyroiditis

Hashimoto's is an autoimmune disorder where the immune system suddenly attacks healthy tissue. Hashimoto's is the most frequent cause of hypothyroidism (low thyroid), and the most common cause of enlarged thyroid (goiter) in America. Iodine depletion from X-rays or low dose radiation (like mammograms) may be a prime factor in development of the disorder. Hashimoto's is related to disorders like diabetes, adrenal exhaustion, Graves' disease and vitiligo. At its worst, Hashimoto's can completely destroy the thyroid gland. Most prevalent in menopausal women (usually with high stress lives), almost one in ten women over the age of 65 have early-stage hypothyroidism clearly linked to Hashimoto's! Natural treatments for Hashimoto's focus on rebalancing glandular health, reducing symptoms and normalizing immune response.

Diet & Superfood Therapy

—Nutritional therapy plan:

1—A largely fresh foods, immune-boosting diet full of fruits and vegetables is the mainstay of treatment for this disease. Take a veggie drink (pg. 218) or a potassium broth (pg. 215) several times weekly. (Also see superfoods below.)

2—Avoid "goitrogen" foods that prevent your body's use of iodine, like cabbage, turnips, peanuts, mustard, pine nuts, millet, tempeh and tofu. (Cooking these foods inactivates the goitrogens.) *Note: Cancer of the thyroid has been linked to highly fluoridated water.*

3—Avoid table salt, (use an herb salt instead), but eat plenty of iodine-rich foods: sea greens (2 TBS daily over rice, soup or a salad), sea foods, fish, mushrooms, garlic, onions and watercress.

4—Eat vitamin A-rich foods: yellow vegetables, eggs, carrots, dark green greens, raw dairy.

5—Avoid refined foods, saturated fats, sugars, white flour and red meats.

—Effective superfoods: (choose 1 or 2)
• Crystal Star SYSTEMS STRENGTH™ drink or capsules daily for 2 to 3 months.
• Green Kamut JUST BARLEY.
• Body Ecology VITALITY SUPER GREENS.
• Green Foods MAGMA PLUS drink.
• Su Wellness CHLORELLA drink or tabs daily.
• Transitions EASY GREENS drink.

Herb & Supplement Therapy

—Interceptive therapy plan: (Choose 2 or more recommendations)

1—Raw glandular therapy helps dramatically: • Nutricology TG-100 capsules (highly recommended); • Nutri-PAK thyroxin-free double strength thyroid; • Premier Labs RAW THYROID complex; • Enzymatic Therapy THYROID/TYROSINE COMPLEX; or • Tyrosine 500mg with Lysine 500mg 2x daily; • Country Life ADRENAL COMPLEX w. tyrosine. *Note: If you take thyroid hormone medication for Hashimoto's, do not take iron supplements along with the medicine. Iron binds up the thyroxine, rendering it insoluble.*

2—Balance thyroid function: Your thyroid needs iodine to produce its hormones. Low thyroid invariably means too much estrogen with numerous problems for women. Herbal iodine, especially sea herbs, is effective without side effects. • Crystal Star IODINE SOURCE™ extract or • IODINE/POTASSIUM™ caps 2x daily; • New Chapter OCEAN HERBS; • Enzymatic Therapy ENZODINE; • Morada Research Labs THYROID liquid; • Solaray ALFA JUICE caps; • Kelp tabs 8 daily.

3—Enhance your adrenals: • Crystal Star ADRN™ extract 2x daily (almost immediate energy) or • META-TABS 6 daily; • Sarsaparilla extract tea; • Evening Primrose oil caps 2000mg daily; • Raw Adrenal glandular.

4—Treat constipation: low thyroid can lead to body toxicity and immune system impairment. Gentle bowel cleansers like *aloe vera* or *slippery elm* teas are good choices. • Crystal Star BWL-TONE I.B.S.™ caps, 2 caps 3x daily; • Rainbow Light EVERY-DAY FIBER SYSTEM. Ascorbate vitamin C with bioflavonoids 3000mg daily.

5—Protect your cardiovascular health: Hypothyroidism can accelerate atherosclerosis! Tone with • *Hawthorn* and • *Ginkgo Biloba* extracts; add • CoQ₁₀ 100mg daily and • Country Life sublingual B-12 2500mcg.

6—Boost circulation and repair nerves: • *Gotu kola* extract caps, up to 6 daily; • *Siberian ginseng* extract 2x daily; • *cayenne* caps 3 daily.

—For goiter: apply • BLACK WALNUT extract as a throat paint, and take ½ dropperful 2x daily; apply • *calendula* compresses twice a day for a month.

Lifestyle Support Therapy

—Bodywork:
• Take a brisk half hour walk daily; exercise increases metabolism and stimulates circulation.
• Sun bathe in the morning. Sea bathe and wade whenever possible.
• The drug levothyroxine, frequently given for hypothyroidism can cause significant bone loss. Ask your doctor. Avoid antihistamines and sulfa drugs.
• Avoid fluorescent lights and fluoride toothpaste. They deplete vitamin A in the body. If you work under fluorescents, take Emulsified A 25,000IU 3x daily, or beta carotene 100,000IU daily, with vitamin E 400IU daily.
• For dry skin caused by thyroid malfunction. Apply Herbal Answers, HERBAL ALOE FORCE GEL.

—Acupressure point:
Press hollow at base of the throat to stimulate thyroid, 3x for 10 seconds each.

—Reflexology point:

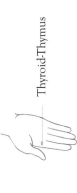

Thyroid-Thymus

Common Symptoms: Generally painless thyroid enlargement; fatigue, weight gain, sensitive to cold, constipation, dry skin and hair, thin falling hair, brittle nails, depression and loss of enthusiasm for life.
Common Causes: An unbalanced thyroid invariably causes over-production of estrogen for women. Hashimoto's hypothyroidism can be easily determined by a simple blood test. Conventional medical treatment has been a lifelong prescription of synthetic thyroid hormone. But for many women, synthroid is linked to severe headaches, insomnia, bone loss and tachycardia (rapid heart contractions). While I don't recommend that Hashimoto's victims reject conventional treatments, shifting the emphasis away from drugs toward natural therapies can greatly raise your own healing capacities.

Can't find a recommended product? Call the 800 number listed in Product Resources for the store nearest you.

Headaches - Vascular
Migraines, Cluster Headaches

Migraines are more than just bad headaches. They're a total body assault. Upwards of 25 million American men and women suffer from migraines. Classic migraines are preceded by an aura, sudden sensitivity to smell and light, nausea, vomiting, diarrhea, chills and fever. Symptoms can last up to 3 or 4 days. Common migraines have no aura, but much of the same visual disturbances, changes in taste and smell, weakness and confusion as well as pain. Cluster headaches are clustered in time, two or more sudden, extremely painful headaches a day, clustered over the eyes or forehead, and usually affect men. (They appear to be connected to testosterone imbalance.) There are no advance warning symptoms. Many vascular headache reactions can be successfully addressed by natural healing methods. Indeed, sometimes these work when nothing else does.

Diet & Superfood Therapy

—Nutritional therapy plan:
Food allergies and intolerances are by far the biggest triggers for migraine headaches.

1—Avoid these known triggers:
• Pickled fish and shellfish, aged and smoked meats and other nitrate foods, aged cheeses, red wines, avocados, caffeine, chocolate, pizza, sourdough bread, sodas and refined sweeteners.

Avoid red meats and dairy products, excess caffeine (withdrawal can be a precipitator), sodas (phosphorus binds up magnesium), MSG, soy sauce, citrus, peanuts, tomatoes and hard liquor.

2—At the first signs of migraine type headache: take 1-2 cups of strong coffee to prevent blood vessel dilation, or a glass of carrot-celery juice.

3—Eat pain preventers:
• High magnesium foods reduce throbbing: leafy greens, fresh sea foods and sea greens, nuts, whole grains, molasses. • Vitamin C rich foods: pineapple for bromelain, broccoli, hot and bell peppers, sprouts, cherries. • Turkey for serotonin.

4—Drink green tea daily or Crystal Star GREEN TEA CLEANSER™ as a preventive.

—Effective superfoods: (choose 1 or 2)
• Crystal Star SYSTEMS STRENGTH™.
• Nutricology PRO-GREENS with EFA's. ♀
• Transitions EASY GREENS drink. ♀
• Aloe Falls ALOE GINGER juice.

Herb & Supplement Therapy

Note: consider a colon cleanse. It's very effective in stopping vascular-type headaches.

—Interceptive therapy plan: (Choose 2 or more recommendations)

1—Help control the pain: For Migraines: • Crystal Star MIGR-EASE™ caps (often works when nothing else does); Ginkgo biloba extract caps 6 daily; • Feverfew extract capsules (Solaray MYGRALEAF) or liquid); • Crystal Star MIGR™ extract with feverfew, or • Quantum MIGRELIEF™ extract. • DLPA 1000mg for pain control - natural endorphins. **For Cluster Headaches:** • Take 1 ginger capsule at first sign of visual disturbance. Then take • Crystal Star STRESSED OUT™ extract, with ♂ • ASPIR-SOURCE™ caps for frontal lobe pain (usually results within 25 minutes). Rub • CAPSAICIN cream on temples or take • Capsicum-Ginger capsules 4 daily, or • Crystal Star MENTAL INNER ENERGY™ with kava kava.

2—Magnesium therapy to check release of pain-producing chemicals: • magnesium citrate 800mg daily; or • Nature's Plus QUERCETIN PLUS 500mg 2x daily with magnesium 500mg 2x daily for nerve twitching. • Glutamine 1000mg 2x daily.

3—Calm stress reactions: • 5-HTP, 50mg daily or • Solgar 5-HTP 100mg; • Crystal Star RELAX CAPS™ for painful spasms. Apply lavender essential oil to temples; • Twin Lab GABA PLUS, or • Country Life RELAXER capsules for brain stress.

4—B-vitamin therapy: • B-2 100mg daily, with • Stress B-complex 100mg; • Country Life sublingual B-12 2500mcg as a preventive. Take • royal jelly, up to 50,000mg daily for the best B-vitamins. • **Niacin for migraines:** up to 500mg daily for normal circulation. (Niacin is not recommended for cluster headaches.)

5—Add EFA's: • Evening primrose oil, 4000mg daily; ♀ Omega-3 flax caps 3 daily.

6—If your migraine is hormone-related: • Crystal Star FEM-SUPPORT™ or DEPRESS-EX™ caps 6 daily. • Transitions PRO-GEST oil, rub into temples.

7—Antioxidants are a key to prevention: • Nutricology GERMANIUM 150mg; • Melatonin, an antioxidant hormone, especially for cluster headaches, .3mg at night, one week on one week off. ♂ • MICROHYDRIN, available from Healthy House, especially for migraines. ♀

Lifestyle Support Therapy

If you have a history of heart problems, ask your doctor before taking migraine medicines that constrict blood vessels.

—Bodywork:
• ICE IT. Chill a head wrap and slip it on; or put an ice pack on the back of the neck to reduce swelling; or put your feet in cold water to draw blood from the head.
• Almost immediate results: a coffee enema to stimulate liver and normalize bile activity; a bowel movement may relieve vomiting.
• **Effective physical therapies:**
–Chiropractic manipulation
–Acupuncture and acupressure
–Massage therapy
–Biofeedback/relaxation training
–Deep breathing exercises
–Fresh air and exercise
–Magnet therapy is effective for migraines.

—Reflexology therapy: 1) Apply pressure to inside base of the big toe 3 times for 10 seconds each time. 2) Massage temples for 5 minutes. Breathe deeply. Do 10 neck rolls. Pull ear lobes for 5 seconds. Rub all around ear shell. 4) Hold hand open, palm down; massage flesh between thumb and forefinger with other hand. Pain begins to recede immediately.

Common Symptoms: Nutritional awareness is a must for preventing migraine-type headaches. Cluster headaches mean severe, localized pain; dilated blood vessels with irritated adjacent nerves; nasal histamine reactions; sensitivity to light; restlessness. Migraines mean constriction/dilation of brain, scalp and face blood vessels, lasting anywhere from 4 hours to two days; recurrent several times a month; a preceding aura, light sensitivity, visual problems; halos around lights; nausea and vomiting, made worse by light and movement; intense, lasting pain, usually on one side of the head; water retention.

Common Causes: Food allergies; too much caffeine, fat and sugar; sticky platelets; birth control pills; H. pylori bacteria or lack of friendly intestinal flora; liver blockage; overuse of drugs; magnesium deficiency.

See the HYPOGLYCEMIA DIET page 427 to help blood sugar regulation.

Can't find a recommended product? Call the 800 number listed in Product Resources for the store nearest you.

Headaches - Stress and Tension

Sinus Headaches, Nervous Headaches

Headaches don't fit into neat little diagnostic boxes. There seem to be as many kinds and pathologies as there are people who have them. **Tension headaches:** muscle contraction headaches of the scalp and back of the head, usually caused by stress or fatigue. They may last for hours or days and your head feels like it's in a vise. Most people find it hard to sleep. Tension headaches respond well to physical treatments like massage, relaxation techniques like acupressure, alternating hot and cold showers, and cold compresses. **Sinus headaches:** congestion and inflammation of the nasal sinuses. Natural remedies work extremely well for most headaches because they balance the body. If you respond well to homeopathic treatment, I recommend consulting with a good homeopath, since the etiology for headaches is so broad.

Diet & Superfood Therapy

—Nutritional therapy plan:

1—Go on a short 24 hour juice fast (pg. 192) to remove congestion. Drink lots of water and lemon, and veggie drinks (pg. 218) or potassium broth. (pg. 215).

2—Follow the next day with an alkalizing diet: apples and apple juice, cranberry juice, sprouts, salads and some brown rice.

3—Make an alkalizing mix of brewer's yeast, lecithin granules, cider vinegar and honey; take 2 TBS daily to restore body balance.

4—Avoid headache trigger foods:
• Additive and chemical-laced foods
• Salty, sugary or wheat-based foods
• Excessive caffeine foods
• Dairy foods, especially cheese
• Condiments, sulfites, MSG
• Too much alcohol, beer, wine

5—Use caffeine: Apply cold black tea bags to the eyes for 15 minutes. Or even just have a cup of black coffee.

6—Add almonds. 12 to 15 when you have a headache are enough to have the salicin kick in.

—Effective superfoods: (choose 1 or 2)
• Nutricology PRO-GREENS w. EFA's
• Solgar EARTH SOURCE GREENS & MORE with EFA's.
• Crystal Star SYSTEMS STRENGTH™ drink.

Herb & Supplement Therapy

—Interceptive therapy plan: (Choose 2 or 3 recommendations)

1—**Relax, soothe and relieve tension:** •Crystal Star STRESSED OUT™ extract; •Bromelain up to 1500mg. Acts like aspirin without stomach upset. • Enzymatic Therapy KAVA-TONE caps; •Valerian-Wild Lettuce or Scullcap extract drops; •Homeopathic Hylands Calms Forte; Morada Research PAIN RELIEF extract.

2—**Enhance nerve health:** Mineral-rich herbs provide key biochemical ingredients for neurotransmission. •Crystal Star RELAX™ caps 2 as needed to help rebuild nerves (relief felt in about 25 minutes). •Nature's Plus QUERCETIN PLUS 500mg 2x daily with magnesium 500mg 2x daily, to prevent nerve twitching. Morada Research NERVOUS SYSTEM nerve food; Medicine Wheel STRESS EASE.

3—**Magnesium and B-vitamin therapy:** •Magnesium citrate 800mg daily with •Country Life MAXI-B with taurine. • Niacin therapy: 100mg or more as needed daily to keep blood vessels and circulation open.

4—**Balance your body with tonics:** •Guayaki YERBA MATÉ green tea, an almost immediate tonic for stress headaches. • Ginkgo Biloba extract capsules 6 daily.

5—**Add EFA's:** •Evening Primrose Oil 2000mg; rub •Chinese WHITE FLOWER oil or • TIGER BALM on forehead and temples.

—For hormone-related headaches: •Crystal Star FEM-SUPPORT™ with ashwagandha. • Chamomile tea as needed; Herbal Magic RELAXA-HERBAL caps.

—For sinus headaches: Crystal Star ANTI-HST™ 2, 3 to 4x daily. Drink rosemary tea, or mix the essential oil in hot water and inhale as an effective steam; or take the extract under the tongue. Rub • CAPSAICIN cream on temples or take • Capsicum-Ginger capsules 4 daily. (Spicy foods, like hot peppers also help open up sinuses.) •Crystal Star ASPIR-SOURCE™ for face pain.

—For stress headaches: •Crystal Star DEPRESS-EX™ caps with St. John's wort. •DLPA 1000mg or a GABA compound like •Country Life RELAXER caps for brain relief. • Crystal Star ANTI-FLAM™ caps ♀ or extract. ♂ •Dip a cold, wet washcloth into cold witch hazel, or catnip-sage tea and use on your forehead.

Lifestyle Support Therapy

—Lifestyle measures:
• Take a brisk walk. Breathe deeply. The more brain oxygen, the fewer headaches.
• Lie down with head higher than the body.
• If you work under fluorescent light, make sure bulbs don't flicker... it can bring on a blinding headache.
• ICE IT. Apply an ice pack on the back of the neck and upper back. Add a hot foot bath and pain reduction is dramatic.
• Apply onion or horseradish poultices to the nape of the neck or soles of the feet to relieve inflammation.
• Have a chiropractic adjustment, shiatsu massage, or massage therapy treatment if headaches are chronic. Take Chondroitin 1200mg daily if spinal misalignment is the cause.

• **Aromatherapy for headaches:**
Apply lavender oil on temples.
Apply peppermint oil on temples.
Apply eucalyptus for sinus headaches.

—**Reflexology pressure point:**

press and/or
apply ice.

See also SINUSITIS page 496 AND STRESS page 508 for more information.

Can't find a recommended product? Call the 800 number listed in Product Resources for the store nearest you.

Common Symptoms: Pain over the eyes, a dull ache in the forehead and temples; inability to sleep; irritability.
Common Causes: Emotional stress; food allergies or sensitivities; eyestrain; muscle tension; pinched nerve; constipation; too much caffeine, salt, sugar or MSG intake; hypoglycemia; artificial sweeteners like Aspartame (NUTRASWEET, EQUAL); water retention; PMS; poor circulation; poor posture; sluggish liver; jawbone misalignment (TMJ); arthritis; Candida albicans; drug toxicity; arteritis (inflammation of the artery); malnutrition as an infant; infant diseases, such as encephalitis, meningitis, or herpes simplex; heavy metal poisoning; nerve malfunction through deficient prostaglandin formation.

Hearing Loss

Tinnitus, Excess Wax, Ear Malfunction

Hearing loss is the third most common health problem for people over 65. For men, it starts much earlier than that. In a new 23 year study, the National Institute on Aging says men start losing their hearing in their twenties; women don't have noticeable hearing loss until their sixties. (A lot of women are right..... their husbands really aren't hearing them.) Today, estimates are that one in ten Americans suffer some hearing problem - 85% associated with tinnitus (ringing in the ears). Much of the rest is noise-induced. The problems addressed here are the result of externally or nutritionally-based causes - as opposed to internal bone fusions that need surgical attention. Lose excess weight. Fat clogs the head, too. See Hypoglycemia Diet pages in this book for additional diet suggestions.

Diet & Superfood Therapy

Nutritional therapy plan:

1—Eat light to hear better - plenty of vegetable proteins, sprouts, whole grains, fruits and cultured foods.

2—Reduce dietary fats, cholesterol and mucous-forming foods. Avoid refined sugars, heavy starches and concentrated foods.

3—Take fresh grated horseradish in a spoon with lemon juice. Hang over a sink to release excess mucous and clear head passages.... almost immediately.

—For ringing in the ears:

• Go on a short 3 day mucous cleansing diet (pg. 196). Then eat fresh foods for the rest of the week. Have plenty of salads and citrus fruits. Have a glass of lemon juice and water each morning.

• Then, for a month, eat a mildly cleansing diet. Avoid all clogging, saturated fat foods. Reduce dairy products. Add plenty of vegetable fiber foods.

• Keep your diet very low in sugars, salt, and dairy foods.

• Drink only bottled water.

—Effective superfoods:

• Sun CHLORELLA drink daily.
• Crystal Star CHO-LO FIBER TONE™.

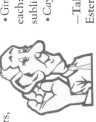

Herb & Supplement Therapy

—Interceptive therapy plan: (Choose 2 to 3 recommendations)

1—Improve blood flow to the hearing apparatus: • Ginkgo Biloba extract 60mg 3x daily for 3 months or more. • Enzymatic Therapy ORAL NUTRIENT CHELATES, two packs daily to open clogged arteries. • Niacin therapy: 500mg daily.

2—Dissolve excess wax and dirt: • Put 6 drops garlic oil and 3 drops goldenseal extract in the ear. Hold in with cotton. Repeat daily for a week. Flush out with vinegar and water. • Or put 4 drops white vinegar and 3 drops 70% isopropyl alcohol in the ear; leave 30 seconds; flush out with water. Repeat daily for a week.

3—Relieve pressure and open ear canals: • Crystal Star ANTI-HST™ caps 4 daily; • Echinacea extract drops and • Siberian Ginseng extract caps 4x daily. • **Mega C therapy:** Use Ester C crystals $\frac{1}{4}$ tsp. every hour to bowel tolerance for 1 week.

4—Silica helps elasticize vascular walls: • Crystal Star SILICA SOURCE™ caps; • Flora VEGE-SIL; • Body Essentials SILICA GEL 1 TB in 3-oz. liquid 3x daily. ◯⁺

5—Antioxidants may prevent hearing loss: • Nutricology GERMANIUM 150mg daily; • Beta carotene 150,000IU daily; • Vitamin C with bioflavonoids, 3000-5000mg daily for 3 months; • PCOs from grapeseed or white pine 100mg 3x daily.

—Ear drops: Dilute in water to use as drops: • Lobelia extract; • Peppermint extract; • Mullein oil drops to relieve pain; • Herbs, Etc. MULLEIN-GARLIC ear drops.

—For ringing in the ears: (A common high-dose aspirin side effect for arthritis sufferers) • Ginkgo Biloba extract 60mg 3x daily for 3 months; • Or, make a tea with 10 drops each: Ginkgo Biloba extract, goldenseal extract, black cohosh extract. • Country Life sublingual B-12 2500mcg with folic acid 400mcg for 1 month. • Licorice extract; • Cayenne-Ginger caps for circulation.

—Take a good hearing vitamin mix - one of each: Emulsified A 25,000IU; Ester C 1000mg with bioflavonoids; Mezotrace MULTIMINERAL; Magnesium 800mg; Glutamine 1000mg; B-complex for regrowth of damaged ear canal hairs.

Lifestyle Support Therapy

—Bodywork:

• Massage neck, ear and temples. Pull ear-lobes - top front and back to clear passages of excess wax or mucous.

• Use diluted 3% H_2O_2 to gently clean out excess ear wax or obstructions. ⚲

• Smoking limits blood flow to the inner ear.

• Avoid continuous loud noise. (Listening to loud rock music through headphones on a regular basis results in major ear problems.)

• Acupressure point:
Squeeze the joints of the ring finger and the 4th toe, covering all sides for several minutes each day.

—For ringing in the ears:

• Avoid high doses of aspirin.
• Massage the ear as above.
• Acupressure: stroke gently downward from the top of the temple to the bottom of the cheek with the nails for 30 seconds on each side.

—Reflexology point:

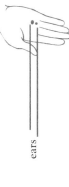

ears

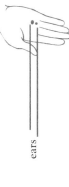

Common Symptoms: Degenerative hearing loss; feeling of fullness and clogging in the ear; obstructed ear passages; no pain, but an extremely annoying ringing sound in the head.

Common Causes: Arteriosclerosis; food allergies; thickening of ear passages or fluid congestion in the middle ear reducing vibration; excess ear wax; mucous clog; infection or inflammation; swelling and congestion; chronic bronchial mastoid and sinus inflammation; hypoglycemia (raised blood insulin causes poor carbohydrate metabolism); a diet with too many mucous-forming foods; poor digestion (low HCL); poor circulation; high blood pressure; imbalance in the inner ear; low immune defenses; raised copper levels, but low calcium levels; metabolic imbalance.

See EAR INFECTIONS page 373 for more information.

Can't find a recommended product? Call the 800 number listed in Product Resources for the store nearest you.

Heart Arrhythmias

Palpitations, Tachycardia, Atrial Fibrillation

Arrhythmias: Electrical disruptions that affect the natural rhythm of the heart. **Palpitations:** the heart beating out of sequence. **Atrial fibrillation:** episodic heart flutter, shortness of breath; the uncomfortable awareness of a racing heart, often accompanied by dizziness or fainting; may predispose a person to having a stroke. **Atrial tachycardia:** too rapid contractions of the heart coming on in sudden attacks; usually associated with coronary artery disease. May increase the risk of congestive heart failure. DIGOXIN, often given for arrhythmias, has side effects that include G.I. irritation, hearing and visual disturbances, headaches and dizziness. Lifestyle and diet change are better ways to avoid arrhythmias. If your pulse is over 80 and remains that way, you should make some diet improvements and get a further heart diagnosis.

Diet & Superfood Therapy

Nutritional therapy plan:

1—Take a green drink once a week esp. during initial healing. (See page 218, or below.) Keep your diet low in fats, salt and calories. Have a fresh green salad and some whole grain protein every day. Add sunflower and sesame seeds, miso soup, rice and oat bran, and green leafy vegetables frequently. Reduce dairy foods.

2—Make a stable heart mix of lecithin granules, toasted wheat germ, brewer's yeast, chopped sea vegetables; sprinkle 2 TBS daily on a salad, soup or protein drink.

3—Drink a bottle of mineral water every day.

4—Arrhythmias can be aggravated by coffee, tea, alcohol, or nicotine. Reduce these stimulants if you are prone to arrhythmias.

—Effective superfoods:

• Crystal Star SYSTEMS STRENGTH™ drink or capsules for daily potassium.
• Solgar WHEY TO GO protein drink.
• Mona's CHLORELLA packets.
• New Moon GINSENG-GINGER WONDER syrup.
• Nutricology PRO-GREENS with EFA's.
• Transitions For Health EASY GREENS.
• Beehive Botanicals ROYAL JELLY-GINSENG drink.

Herb & Supplement Therapy

—Interceptive therapy plan: (Choose 2 to 3 recommendations)

1—**Regulate heart action:** Heart regulating herbs usually work within 1 minute for simple palpitations. • *Hawthorn* extract as needed (about 800mg daily); or HEART STABILIZER available from Healthy House • *Cayenne* extract drops; • *Siberian ginseng* extract drops; • *Valerian* extract. • Crystal Star HEARTSEASE-HAWTHORN™ caps, a preventive. • Magnesium 800mg daily, esp. if you have had heart surgery. • *Ginkgo Biloba* extract helps prevent ischemia-caused fibrillation.

2—**Help remove fatty deposits that cause some arrythmias:** • Berberine-containing herbs, *goldenseal root, Oregon grape root,* or *barberry.* Add • taurine 500mg 2x daily with Ester C 550mg 2x daily.

3—**Normalize circulation:** • *Butcher's broom* tea (for 2 to 3 weeks); • *Rosemary* tea (or rosemary wine sips); • *Ginger* capsules 2 daily; • *Peppermint-Sage* tea. • Solaray CHROMIACIN 3x daily (don't take high doses of isolated niacin).

4—**Calm and stabilize your system:** • Stress B Complex 150mg with extra B-6, 100mg; • Country Life RELAXER capsules and • Country Life CALCIUM-MAGNESIUM-POTASSIUM capsules. • *Cayenne-Ginger* caps or Solaray COOL CAYENNE 2 daily, or • Heartfoods CAYENNE products, to increase your strength gradually. • To deter atrial fibrillation: Rainbow Light CALCIUM PLUS with high magnesium, 4 daily; or Country Life CAL-MAG-BROMELAIN caps.

5—**Essential fatty acids (EFA'S) seem to protect against arrhythmias:** *Evening primrose oil* 2000mg daily, or *Omega-3 flax oils* 3 daily, or Spectrum Organics high lignan FLAX OIL caps 3 daily; Crystal Star IODINE/POTASSIUM caps with sea greens 2 daily.

6—**Antioxidants are key preventives:** • OPC's from white pine or grapeseed 100mg daily; • Future Biotics VITAL K daily; • CoQ-10, 60mg 3x daily; • Carnitine 1000mg 2 daily; • Vitamin E 400IU with selenium 200mcg. daily; MICROHYDRIN, available at Healthy House, helps remove fatty buiid-up on arteries.

Lifestyle Support Therapy

See *How To Take Your Own Pulse* on pg. 548.

—Bodywork:

• Plunge your face into cold water when arrhythmia occurs to stop palpitations.
• Avoid soft drinks. The phosphorus binds up magnesium and makes it unavailable for heart regularity.
• Springlife POLARIZERS help normalize against heart arrhythmias.

—Reflexology points:

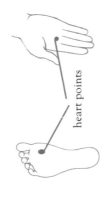

heart points

—Heart action area:

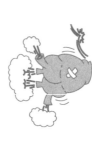

See also ANXIETY-PANIC ATTACK page 313 for more information.

Common Symptoms: Irregular and/or rapid heartbeat; uncomfortable awareness of your heartbeat; skipped heartbeats and shortness of breath; a feeling that you cannot breathe; light-headedness; often chest discomfort.

Common Causes: Poor diet with too much refined sugar and saturated fat; lack of exercise/aerobic strength; obesity; smoking; stressful lifestyle; high blood pressure; diabetes.

Can't find a recommended product? Call the 800 number listed in Product Resources for the store nearest you.

Heart Disease

Cardiovascular Diseases, Angina, Coronary, Heart Attack, Stroke

Heart disease is still the biggest killer of Americans. A million of us die each year because of heart problems. Yet, most heart disease is 100% preventable with changes in diet and lifestyle. Almost unknown before the turn of this century, today, two-thirds of America suffers from some kind of cardiovascular disease - heart attack, coronary, hypertension, atherosclerosis, stroke, rheumatic heart and more. Natural therapies are proving to reduce mortality better than aggressive medical intervention or even the most advanced drug treatment. Heart problems in women are different than those of men; they are hormone-dependent. Beware of calcium channel blockers. They block many body functions and are implicated in aggravated cardiovascular problems. Actively explore magnesium, Nature's calcium channel blocker, with your physician.

Diet & Superfood Therapy

Nutritional therapy plan:

1–Your diet is your greatest asset in preventing heart disease. A healthy heart diet has plenty of magnesium and potassium rich foods: fresh greens, sea foods and sea greens; flavonoids from pitted fruits, green tea and wine, soy, brown rice, whole grains, garlic and onions.

2–Reduce saturated fat to no more than 10% of your daily calorie intake. Especially limit fats from animal sources and hydrogenated oils.

–Pay conscious attention to avoiding red meats, caffeine foods, refined sugars, fatty, salty and fried foods, prepared meats and soft drinks. The rewards are worth the effort.

3–Eat 70% of daily calories from complex carbohydrates like vegetables and grains; 20% of calories from low fat protein sources.

4–Eat less than 100mg per day of diet cholesterol. Keep cholesterol below 160.

5–Add 6 glasses of pure water daily to your diet. It is the best diuretic for a healthy heart. (Chlorinated/fluoridated water destroys vitamin E in the body).

6–A glass or two of wine with dinner can relieve stress and raise HDLs.

7–Make a hearty morning mix of lecithin granules, toasted wheat germ, brewer's yeast, snipped dry sea greens, molasses, take 2 TBS daily.

–Effective superfoods: (choose 1 or 2)
• Crystal Star SYSTEMS STRENGTH™ drink.
• ALOE VERA juice with herbs.
• Beehive Botanicals ROYAL JELLY, POLLEN, SIBERIAN GINSENG drink.

Herb & Supplement Therapy

–Interceptive therapy plan: (Choose several recommendations)

1–**In an emergency:** • 1 teasp. *cayenne* powder in water, or *cayenne* tincture drops in water may help bring a person out of a heart attack; or take liquid carnitine as directed. • One-half dropperful *Hawthorn* extract every 15 minutes; or • HEART STABILIZER available from Healthy House.

2–**Tone the heart muscle:** • NutriCology CoQ-10 with TOCOTRIENOLS (tocotrienols help lower cholesterol). • Ascorbate or Ester C with bioflavonoids, up to 5000mg daily for interstitial arterial integrity-elasticity, and prevent TIA's (little strokes). • EVENING PRIMROSE oil 1000mg 4 daily for EFA's and prostaglandin balance, (prostaglandins regulate arterial muscle tone.); or • Omega Nutrition ESSENTIAL BALANCE caps; • Magnesium rich herbs: *motherwort, parsley;* or • Magnesium 800mg, or • Country Life CALCIUM-MAGNESIUM-BROMELAIN.

3–**Improve blood flow:** • Golden Pride FORMULA ONE oral chelation w. EDTA; • Wakunaga KYOLIC SUPER FORMULA 106; • Crystal Star GINSENG-REISHI extract, • *red sage tea* or *Gingko Biloba* extracts are vasodilators, 2-3x daily; • Natural Balance CREATINE 3000mg daily; MICROHYDRIN, available at Healthy House.

4–**Antioxidants strengthen the cardiovascular system and keep it clear:** • Crystal Star HEARTSEASE-HAWTHORN caps, or • HEARTSEASE-CIRCUCLEANSE™ tea; • Grapeseed PCO's 100mg 3x daily; • Biogenetics BIO-GUARD.

5–**Boost your thyroid to reduce heart disease risk:** • Spirulina, liquid chlorophyll, or Pines MIGHTY GREENS drink; or • 2 TBS dry sea greens daily.

6–**Cardiotonics help the heart beat stronger and steadier:** • CoQ-10, 60mg 3x daily; • Carnitine 1000mg daily; • *Cayenne-Ginger caps* or *Garlic* capsules 6 daily; or • Heart Foods HEART FOOD *Cayenne* caps; • Siberian ginseng caps 2000mg or tea 2 cups daily; • Wheat germ oil caps for tissue oxygen.

7–**Phyto-estrogen heart protective herbs for menopausal women:** • Crystal Star FEMALE HARMONY™, or • *Ginkgo Biloba* extract helps prevent ischemia-caused fibrillation. WOMEN'S HEART PROTECTOR, available at Healthy House; • *Vitex* extract; • *Licorice root tea;* • Crystal Star GINSENG-LICORICE EXLIXIR™ drops.

8–**Heart disease preventives:** • Folic acid to keep homocysteine levels down, with • B-6 100mg and • Country Life sublingual B-12, 2500mcg.

9–**Reduce blood stickiness to prevent a heart attack:** • Bromelain 1500mg regularly increases fibrinolysis; • Chromium picolinate or Solaray CHROMIACIN for arterial plaque and insulin resistance. • Omega-3 fish or flax oils 3x daily.

Lifestyle Support Therapy

–Watchwords:

• Bite down on the tip of the little finger to help stop a heart attack.

• Apply hot compresses and massage chest of the victim to ease a heart attack.

• Chewing an aspirin immediately following symptoms of a heart attack, may be able to reduce mortality through its ability to reduce arterial blockage.

• Take alternate hot and cold showers frequently to increase circulation.

• Smoking constricts arteries and can cause blood pressure to skyrocket, too. Researchers estimate that 150,000 heart disease deaths would be prevented each year if Americans just quit smoking! Is it time for you to quit?

• Take some mild regular daily exercise. Do deep breathing exercises every morning for body oxygen, and to stimulate brain activity.

• Consciously add relaxation and a good daily laugh to your life. A positive mental outlook does wonders for stress.

–Reflexology points:

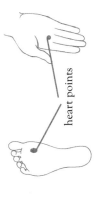

heart points

See the healthy heart suggestions on the following pages for more information.

Can't find a recommended product? Call the 800 number listed in Product Resources for the store nearest you.

Diagnosing Your Cardiovascular Problem

Signs that you are suffering a heart attack or a stroke: 1) sudden weakness or numbness of the face, arm and leg, usually on one side of the body; 2) trouble talking or understanding speech; 3) fluctuating state of consciousness, with tingling sensations; 4) dimness or loss of vision, particularly in one eye; 5) sudden severe headache and dizziness, leading to unsteadiness or a sudden fall. **Call an emergency room immediately if you feel you are having a heart attack of any kind.**

Can Herbs Help in a Heart Attack Emergency?

Sometimes they can. Historically, up through the nineteenth century, tincture of cayenne was a traditional healer's emergency method to bring a person out of a heart attack. About 5 droppersful (approx. 30 drops each) have been able to stop a heart attack. If the victim is unconscious, begin with two droppersful and add more as response begins. Up to 10 or 12 droppersful may be needed, but reports from healers even today are miraculous for this technique.

In addition, studies show that, when taken at the onset of symptoms, the amino acids l-carnitine, 330mg 3x daily, lessens the severity of a heart attack and reduces complications. Stronger, liquid carnitine can sometimes be used in an emergency. Ask your health practitioner. Remember herbs (and most natural healing remedies) are best used for degenerative, chronic ailments. If you live near a clinic of any kind, get there immediately if you or someone close to you is having a heart attack. Modern medicine is at its best in just this kind of emergency.

–ANGINA: A warning sign of a heart attack. **Signs and symptoms:** recurring, sudden, intense chest pains, lasting 30 seconds to 1 minute, with a vise-like grip of pressure across the chest. People usually feel the first angina attacks during physical exertion because one or more arteries are partially clogged, with the blood supply to the heart reduced, functioning inefficiently and painfully. Do not ignore this type of sign as "just indigestion." May also be brought on by emotional stress, exposure to cold, or overexertion.

Alternative healing protocols: Follow a vegetarian diet. •Take 1000mg Carnitine, 2000mg Arginine, Lysine 2000mg daily and vitamin E 800IU daily to scour arteries; •CoQ-10, 60mg 4 daily; •cayenne/ginger caps, 2 daily; •Crystal Star HEARTSEASE-HAWTHORN daily, or •Ginkgo Biloba extract capsules, up to 240mg daily to increase blood flow to the brain; •Omega-3 flax oil 3x daily; •Vitamin C 3-5000mg daily with bioflavonoids; •Bromelain 1500mg daily; •Golden Pride FORMULA ONE, oral chelation w. EDTA 2 packs daily.

–ACUTE MYOCARDIAL INFARCTION, (CORONARY): This is a heart attack, with permanent damage to the heart muscle, or death. As plaque builds up in the coronary arteries, eventually one becomes narrowed to the point of total obstruction. Instantly the part of the heart served from that artery is without blood supply. In five minutes it will suffer damage or even death from the cut off of oxygen. The heart stops beating; the blood supply to the brain is cut off. **Signs and symptoms:** excruciating pain, starting in the lower chest and spreading throughout the upper half of the body, and weak, rapid pulse with perspiring, pale skin. Blood pressure drops dangerously, there is dizziness and then unconsciousness. High fever usually follows this kind of attack. If you feel you're having a heart attack, call 911 immediately and unless you're allergic, chew aspirin. It may save your life.

Alternative healing protocols: Antioxidants are a key (see previous page). •Liquid carnitine for myocardial infarction during an attack. Use •N-acetyl-cysteine, •vitamin C 1000mg daily and •CoQ-10 60mg 4x daily to inhibit heart damage from free radicals after an infarction. Use •Magnesium 400mg 2x daily to help prevent coronary; •folic acid 400 mcg to keep homocysteine levels down, with •B-6 100mg and •Country Life sublingual B-12, 2500mcg •Fo-Ti root to increase heart vigor. •L-Arginine 1000mg daily helps blood vessels widen. •Women might use a DHEA supplement as a preventive after menopause. Take • HAWTHORN extract as needed, especially to normalize heart rate. Take •ginger and garlic 6 each and drink •a cup of green tea daily as preventives. Take regular proteolytic enzymes to prevent inflammation, such as •MICROHYDRIN 3 caps daily, available at Healthy House.

–STROKE: A stroke is a blockage of the blood supply to the brain, similar to that of a coronary, the difference being cell death in the brain. Oxygen-deprived brain tissue dies within minutes. **Signs and symptoms:** from temporary loss of speech or vision, disordered behavior, thought patterns and memory, to paralysis, coma and death. See the top of this page for signs you may be having a stroke. Ask for a stethoscope neck check (for a bruit sound) if you think you are at risk. *Note: Modern medicine suggests regular intake of aspirin to prevent life-threatening strokes. The theory is that aspirin inhibits a specific enzyme, making the blood less prone to dangerous clotting. Ginger not only inhibits the same enzyme, but it does so without side effects.*

Alternative healing protocols: Up to 80% of strokes are preventable. Take •a cup of Japanese green tea, or •Crystal Star GREEN TEA CLEANSER™ each morning. Eat cold water fish twice a week salmon is the best. Add more fruits and vegetables (and less caffeine and alcohol) to your diet. Have a green salad every day. Reduce salty and sugary foods. Add fiber. Snip dry sea greens over any food or eat sushi often (loaded with vitamin K). Take •1000mg carnitine 2x daily and HAWTHORN extract as needed. Use •Golden Pride FORMULA ONE, oral chelation w. EDTA 2 packs a.m./p.m. •Vitamin C 3000mg daily with rutin and bioflavonoids 500mg; •Future Biotics VITAL K PLUS for potassium. Take •B-complex 100mg daily with extra •folic acid mcg; add •vitamin E 400IU; •magnesium 400mg to normalize heart action. Meditation and acupuncture both show success as relaxation techniques against stroke.

–ATHEROSCLEROSIS: Atherosclerosis results in the most common cardiovascular ailment - high blood pressure, page 417. (See Atherosclerosis page 315 and Cholesterol page 349.)

Can't find a recommended product? Call the 800 number listed in Product Resources for the store nearest you.

–**MITRAL VALVE PROLAPSE (MVP):** The mitral valve is one of several gates within the heart that regulates oxygen-rich blood flow. A prolapse (loss of tone) of the gate valve is a heart abnormality thought to be related to rheumatic fever. **Signs and symptoms:** palpitations or rapid heart rate, anxiety attacks or night time panic attacks, shortness of breath, and usually physical weakness. Even though common, the uneven flow of blood increases the likelihood of clot formation in people under 45, who also have a higher rate of stroke during their younger years. 85% of people with MVP have a magnesium deficiency that affects the collagen structures throughout the body. Small, thin women are more likely to have a mitral valve prolapse.

Alternative healing protocols: • 1000mg L-carnitine 3x a day to relieve symptoms; • *Hawthorn* extract as needed; • Crystal Star HEARTSEASE-HAWTHORN capsules or •Solaray HAWTHORN BLEND; • *Gingko Biloba* to normalize circulation; • Crystal Star FEMALE HARMONY™, with phyto-estrogen herbs; • magnesium 400mg daily. Relaxation techniques like mediation, shiatzu and biofeedback are a good idea; along with daily mild exercise, such as leisurely swimming or a brisk walk.

–**CONGESTIVE HEART FAILURE:** CHF occurs when a damaged heart (caused by arteriosclerosis or other disease (hypothyroidism), ceases to pump effectively. Circulation is inefficient; organs and tissues become clogged with blood. **Signs and symptoms:** great energy depletion, dizziness and shortness of breath after exertion. Ankles and feet usually swell, and there is nausea and gas. Later symptoms are greater heart exhaustion and fluid in the lungs. High iron stores after menopause may put a woman at increased CHF risk. Exercise helps the body rid of excess iron.

Alternative healing protocols: •Magnesium, 800mg daily for better muscle performance, or • Country Life CALCIUM-MAGNESIUM-BROMELAIN; • CoQ-10 60mg 4 daily; • CSA (chrondroitan sulfate A), up to 1200 mg; an herbal combination with • *Arjuna* herb, • *Astragalus*, or Ayurvedic • *Coleus Forskohlii* (highly recommended); •vitamin E 800IU daily and •Crystal Star GINSENG-RIESHI extract as immune boosting antioxidants; • *HAWTHORN* extract as needed; • Creatine 100mg 4x daily to improve heart muscle metabolism; •vitamin C 3000mg daily with bioflavonoids; •BILBERRY extract daily. •Stress B-complex 100mg with extra thiamin (B-1), 200 mg and pantothenic acid 250mg daily.

–**CARDIOMYOPATHY:** An insidious type of heart failure with a deadly weakening of an enlarged heart muscle and only a fraction of the blood the body needs being pumped.

Alternative healing protocols: Reduce your risk by reducing caffeine and nicotine. Use • CoQ-10, 100mg 3 daily; • *hawthorn* or *Fo-Ti* (*Ho-Shu Wu*) extract 500 mg daily; • *Ginkgo Biloba* or *ginger* capsules daily to normalize circulation; • magnesium 400mg 2x daily or • Country Life CAL-MAG-BROMELAIN 1500 MG; • L-carnitine 500mg 2x daily; • taurine 500mg daily.

–**ISCHEMIA:** Reduced blood flow to the heart and cell oxygen starvation, caused by atherosclerotic plaques along the artery walls. Ischemia leads to angina, coronary or congestive heart failure. **Signs and symptoms:** high blood pressure; poor circulation; aching feet, legs and muscles, or numbness on one side, speech difficulty, double vision and vertigo.

Alternative healing protocols: • *HAWTHORN* extract as needed; •BILBERRY extract protects integrity of microvessel walls; • CoQ-10, 60mg 4 daily; • *garlic* capsules 6 daily; *ginger* capsules 4 daily to inhibit platelet aggregation; •PHYCOTENE MICROCLUSTERS, potent mixed carotenes, available at Healthy House; •Vitamin E 800IU with selenium 200mcg daily.

–**ARRYTHMIAS: Tachycardia:** heartbeat so rapid that the heart cannot deliver blood efficiently. It can be fatal. **Palpitations:** the heart beating irregularly. **Fibrillation:** more serious than tachycardia, there is a weak, irregular quiver to the heartbeat. See page 406.

Is heart disease contagious?

New research points to the infectious bacteria *Chlamydia pneumoniae*, as a possible factor in heart disease development. *C. pneumoniae* is a different species of the same bacteria that causes the STD, Chlamydia. It's a common cause of pneumonia, sinusitis and bronchitis — most people are infected by it 2 or 3 times during their lives. Blocked blood vessels are 20 times more likely to carry *C. pneumoniae* than unblocked vessels. Further, scientists speculate that *C. pneumoniae* creates inflammation that plays a role in the progression of atherosclerosis, too. Important note: a recent month-long clinical trial found that antibiotic therapy reduced the number of heart attacks and deaths in hospitalized heart patients. Herbal antibiotics are a safe and effective natural alternative. If you are recovering from a heart attack or have coronary heart disease, a month long course of *Echinacea/Goldenseal* extract or Crystal Star's ANTI-BIO™ caps may flush out infectious bacteria trapped in blocked lymph glands and blood vessels.

Better heart care may be a new reason to brush and floss regularly!

People with periodontal disease are 2.7 times more likely to have a heart attack than people with healthy gums! Researchers suspect that gum disease allows toxic bacteria from excess plaque to enter the bloodstream, causing blood platelets to clump up, accelerating atherosclerosis! The National Institutes of Health recently funded a five-year study to explore the link between periodontal disease and heart attacks. If you are already have gum disease or periodontitis, add CoQ-10, 100mg to your daily program, specific for teeth and gums and your heart; and brush with •MICROBRITE powder daily, available at Healthy House.

Can't find a recommended product? Call the 800 number listed in Product Resources for the store nearest you.

Heart Problems for Men and Women are Different

Until very recently, men and women's heart disease was considered largely the same. New research shows that men and women face very different challenges of heart disease. I've worked extensively to create natural healing programs that address the unique heart needs of men and women with heart protecting herbs, healing foods, and lifestyle therapies.

Let's start with men. Men's heart disease has been the focus of conventional medicine. Women have largely been left out of heart census taking. In 1995, over 455,000 men died from heart disease. The good news is that even though the death rate for men is still high, male children today actually have a lower chance of dying from heart attacks than their fathers did.

Many studies point to emotional health as a major factor in men's heart problems. Stress, anger, and overwork are now, (and probably have always been), major triggers of heart attacks for men. A Harvard School of Public Health study shows that men with the highest anger scores on personality tests are three times more likely to develop heart disease.

High blood pressure and atherosclerosis are the top cardiovascular problems that men face. **High blood pressure,** often called "the silent killer", affects 1 in 3 U.S. of all adults. Men are more at risk for HBP than women until about age 55. High blood pressure is most dangerous for African American males. When blood pressure is high, the heart and arteries are over-worked, and atherosclerosis speeds up. Coronary heart disease is 3 to 5 times more likely in people with high blood pressure! Over-consumption of salt, a high stress lifestyle with little "downtime," and smoking are key factors in the development of high blood pressure.

Atherosclerosis (hardening of the arteries) is strongly tied to a diet high in animal fat, especially from butter, red meat, ice cream and eggs, the very foods many men overeat! Atherosclerotic plaques on your arteries restrict blood flow to organs and tissues leading to heart attacks, strokes, even gangrene.

Can donating blood regularly prevent a heart attack for a man? Yes, it can! Men have twice as much iron in their bodies as women. Iron acts as a catalyst in cholesterol oxidation, linked to artery hardening and scarring. Recent studies show that men can cut their risk for heart attack or stroke up to a third by reducing their excess iron when they regularly donate blood.

Does Oral Chelation Reverse Men's Heart Disease? Intravenous chelation therapy with EDTA has largely been ignored by mainstream medicine, but it has been used successfully for blood vessel diseases like arteriosclerosis for over 40 years. Intravenous chelation with EDTA (*ethylenediamine tetra acetic acid, a synthetic amino acid*) binds to and flushes out arterial plaque and calcium deposits that cause artery hardening. Intravenous chelation is a powerful but expensive therapy. Oral chelation is a good option for many people, especially men. It's cheaper and more convenient that IV chelation, yet still improves blood flow and may even reverse some cardiovascular problems. Consider Golden Pride's oral chelation program, FORMULA #1.

A Man's Healthy Heart Program

1) Men tend to overeat- especially fatty foods. For men, a low fat, high fiber diet is an important part of a heart protection plan. It is essential for recovery from existing heart problems. Reduce fatty dairy foods like ice cream and rich cheeses. Cut back on red meat, especially pork. A better choice? Eat seafood at least once a week. An 11 year study covering over 22,000 male physicians found that eating seafood just once a week cuts men's risk of sudden cardiac death by 52%!

2) Use olive oil instead. You can't fry in olive oil, but fried foods are so bad for your heart that this is probably a plus. Olive oil boosts healthy HDL cholesterol levels and removes fats from the blood. I like Spectrum Naturals cold pressed organic extra virgin olive oil.

3) Men at risk for heart disease need more fiber! Fiber has proven in numerous studies to reduce arterial plaque from atherosclerosis. Herbs are a good source of cleansing fiber for the male system. Herbs also help reduce cholesterol and eliminate fatty build-up from the body. I recommend an herbal fiber rich drink mix daily like Crystal Star's CHOL-LO FIBER TONE™.

4) Add healing spices like *garlic, onions, tumeric and cayenne peppers* to your diet. Hundreds of clinical trials show garlic's thins the blood, normalizes blood pressure, helps reduce serum cholesterol and arterial plaque build-up. Both onions and garlic stimulate healthy circulation. Cayenne peppers strengthen all cardiovascular activity, dilate arteries and reduce blood pressure. Tumeric, an anti-inflammatory spice, helps decrease cholesterol levels and prevents progression of atherosclerosis. Don't like spicy recipes? Consider a garlic product like Wakunaga's KYOLIC FORMULA 106, with *garlic, vitamin E, hawthorn and cayenne pepper.* Boost circulation to thin "sticky blood" with Crystal Star HEARTSEASE-CIRCU-CLEANSE™ tea or Futurebiotics CIRCUPLEX.

5) Eat more SUPERGREEN foods, especially spinach, chard and sea greens, for magnesium therapy and EFA's. Magnesium is a key mineral for heart regulation. A magnesium deficiency can contribute to hypertension, irregular heartbeat, even heart failure!

6) Eat vitamin C rich foods like citrus fruits, broccoli or peppers. Low blood levels of vitamin C are linked to progressing atherosclerosis and to increased heart attack risk. A new study shows that men with no pre-existing heart disease who are deficient in vitamin C have 3.5 times MORE heart attacks than men who are not deficient in vitamin C.

7) Herbal stress busters are an excellent choice for men. They can reduce anxiety linked to high blood pressure and heart palpitations. Herbal nervines like *kava kava, passionflower and scullcap* calm acute stress reactions. Especially for men, I recommend *Siberian ginseng,* a primary adaptogen that builds body resistance to stress and restores nervous system health.

 H 410

See this complete HEALTHY HEART SECTION, and information you should know about heart surgery page 547.

Can't find a recommended product? Call the 800 number listed in Product Resources for the store nearest you.

What about heart disease in women?

In 1997 almost 550,000 American women died from cardiovascular disease – over 100,000 more deaths than men! Heart disease deaths accounted for half of all women's deaths! Even more frightening, new studies reveal women receive less medical treatment despite having more cardiac symptoms than men. Heart disease for women is linked to high cholesterol, obesity or too little exercise as it is in men. **It is also clearly hormone-related.** There is no time that a woman's risk for heart disease is higher than during menopause. Risk for heart disease rises noticeably with every year a woman approaches menopause and continues to rise with age. Because of this, hundreds of thousands of new, prophylactic, hormone replacement therapy prescriptions are written every year by doctors trying to protect menopausal women from heart disease.

Yet, the use of hormone replacement therapy or ERT to protect against heart disease is highly debatable. There is also no conclusive evidence that estrogen protects against heart disease. In fact, a 1997 review presented at the International Meeting on Atherosclerosis in Paris concludes that the heart protective benefits attributed to estrogen may result from population selection bias or even changes towards healthier lifestyles during the course of the studies. Studies find hormone replacement therapy does not prevent heart attack or death for women who already have heart disease. I don't think hormone replacement therapy, with its links to uterine and breast cancer, should be considered as a long-term preventive for heart disease. I think there are better solutions for preventing heart disease naturally that don't carry these risks.

If you're thinking about beginning hormone replacement therapy to prevent heart disease, here are new facts you need to know.
1) The most commonly prescribed hormone replacement drug, Premarin, actually suppresses folic acid, contributing to high homocysteine levels, a known risk factor for heart disease.
2) Tests with some estrogen contraceptive pills actually increase a woman's risk of heart disease, heart attack, stroke and serious blood clotting problems.
3) Some reports suggest that SERMs (*selective estrogen receptor modulators*) like Evista may protect against heart disease. But this drug **should not** be taken by women with a history of congestive heart failure. Evista also increases risk of serious blood clots in the legs, lungs or eyes, particularly if you're sedentary for long periods of time.

What Are The Biggest Heart Problems For Women?

—**A heart attack is especially serious for a woman.** Statistics show that a woman is 50% MORE LIKELY to die from a heart attack than a man! Women have heart attacks at older ages when they are in poorer health than men. A woman's arteries are less able to compensate for the partial death of heart muscle caused by a heart attack, so a second heart attack is even more dangerous for women. Heart attack symptoms are also different: Women are less likely to have intense chest pains during a heart attack. (This is why researchers believe they are more reluctant to seek treatment.) Heart attack symptoms women should watch for include shortness of breath, fatigue, even back pain.

—**Congestive Heart Failure is a big problem for menopausal women.** Over two million women alive today have CHF. Congestive heart failure occurs when the heart is unable to efficiently pump blood. In people with CHF, risk for sudden cardiac arrest and death is up to 9 times higher than the general population! High iron stores after menopause may put a women at risk. Symptoms to watch for: extreme fatigue and water retention (particularly bloated ankles). Consider • WOMEN'S HEART PROTECTOR for CHF available from Healthy House and creatine 3000mg daily or • Natural Balance CREATINE 3000 to 5000mg daily as protection.

—**Dangerous Atrial Fibrillation:** Women with this irregular heartbeat are 90% more likely to die than those without. If you're affected by atrial fibrillation, a cardiotonic, herbal heart protector with *arjuna* and *hawthorn* like WOMEN'S HEART STABILIZER can help regulate heartbeat and strengthen your entire cardiovascular system.

Are You Having A Panic Attack or A Heart Attack?

Many women confuse panic attacks with heart attacks during menopause because their symptoms seem so severe. Menopausal heart palpitations and nighttime anxiety attacks are extremely common. When I first went into menopause, I remember waking up terrified that I was having a heart attack, but found out later that it was a panic attack.

Here are the signs to look for:
• hyperventilating or feeling short of breath especially at night.
• racing heartbeat, dizziness or feeling faint.
• bolting upright out of bed in the early morning hours.
• feeling like you're "going crazy" or losing control, or being full of fear that has no basis in reality and the fear interfering in the normal functioning of your life.
If you have these symptoms, you're probably suffering from a panic attack. It will more than likely pass quickly. If symptoms persist, seek out a qualified health practitioner. Herbs offer relief from nighttime panic attacks. I keep heart stabilizing herbs like *hawthorn, arjuna, ashwagandha* and *passionflowers* by my bed at night for immediate relief.

See this complete HEALTHY HEART SECTION, and information you should know about heart surgery page 547.

Can't find a recommended product? Call the 800 number listed in Product Resources for the store nearest you.

A Woman's Healthy Heart Program

1: **Sea greens act as total body tonics to restore female vitality during menopause.** Sea greens are loaded with fat-soluble vitamins like D and K that help our bodies make steroidal hormones like estrogen and DHEA which protect against heart disease during menopause. Sea greens also dissolve fatty deposits in the cardiovascular system that precipitate heart disease.

2: **Phytoestrogen foods like soy help maintain normal vascular function.** Soy foods not only lower cholesterol, but along with herbs, soy is a rich source if phytoestrogens for female vitality and heart protection during menopause. My favorite phytoestrogen heart protector for post-menopausal women is a *dong quai/damiana/ashwagandha* extract combination.

3: **Have cold water fish 2 to 3 times a week for heart-healthy omega-3 oils and EFA's.** Salmon is one of God's gifts, a rich source of omega-3 fatty acids and vitamin E. Salmon is farm-raised now so you don't have to worry about endangerment as we do with swordfish.

4: **Use natural vitamin E (400IU) daily.** Even though it's old news, vitamin E daily still cuts heart attack risk 77%.

5: **Take a daily herbal heart tonic to protect against congestive heart failure, especially if you have reached menopause.** Use a heart tonic combination with herbs like *hawthorn, bilberry, motherwort, ashwagandha, dong quai, gingko biloba, astragalus, red sage, and ginger root* for 6 months as circulatory support; or try HEART FOOD CAPS by Heart Foods.

6: **CoQ-10, 60mg 4 daily, or Real Life Research CoQ 20/20 strengthens the heart muscle and helps it work more effectively.** (CoQ-10 is also a protector against breast cancer.)

7: **EFA's (essential fatty acids) are important to women's heart health, because they are critical for hormone balance,** thought to be a big part of women's heart problems. EFA's help decrease the "stickiness" of blood platelets. *Evening primrose oil* provides top quality EFA's for women. Spectrum Naturals high lignan Organic Flax Oil is a good diet/salad dressing choice.

8: **Eat brown rice regularly for heart smart B vitamins.** Brown rice as a valuable source of fiber, vitamins and minerals is superior to refined grains for heart health.

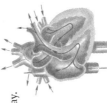

Quick Heart Rehabilitation Check Program

This program is designed especially for those of you who have survived a heart attack, or major heart surgery. Coming back is tough. Beginning and sticking to a new lifestyle that changes almost everything about the way you eat, exercise, handle stress, and even the smallest details of your life, is a challenge. The following mini-rehabilitation program is a blueprint that you can use with confidence. It addresses the main preventive needs - keeping your arteries clear and your blood slippery - goals that clearly can be achieved through a good diet and exercise. This program has proven successful against heart disease recurrence.

—Reduce saturated fats to 10% of your diet; less if possible. Limit polyunsaturated oils to 10%. Add mono-unsaturates (olive oil, avocados, nuts and seeds). Add EFA's (fish, flax oil, etc.).

—Eat potassium-rich foods for cardiotonic activity: spinach and chard, broccoli, bananas, sea greens, molasses, cantaloupe, apricots, papayas, mushrooms, tomatoes, yams, etc. or take a potassium drink (pg 215), Crystal Star SYSTEMS STRENGTH™ drink, or Future Biotics VITAL K. (a serving of high potassium fruits or vegetables offers about 400 mg of potassium, a serving of the above drinks offers approx. 100-1250 mg of potassium).

—Eat plenty of complex carbohydrates, such as broccoli, peas, whole grain breads, vegetable pastas, potatoes, sprouts, tofu and brown rice. Have a green salad every day.

—Have 3 to 4 servings of cold water fish, seafood sea greens soy food like miso every week for EFA's and high omega-3 oils.

—Have a glass of wine at dinner for relaxation and digestion.

—Eat magnesium-rich foods for heart regulation: tofu, wheat germ, oat or rice bran, broccoli, potatoes, lima beans, spinach and chard.

—Eat high fiber foods for a clean system and alkalinity: whole grains, fruits and vegetables, legumes and herbs.

Choose several of the following supplements as your individual daily micro-nutrients:

- **For clear arteries:** Solaray CHROMIACIN; selenium, omega-3 flax or fish oils 3x daily; Formula ONE, oral chelation w. EDTA 2 packs a.m./p.m.
- **For heart regulation-stability:** Mona's CHLORELLA tabs 15 daily; magnesium 400 mg; carnitine 500 mg; HEART STABILIZER, at Healthy House; *hawthorn or gotu kola* extracts.
- **For antioxidants:** Wheat germ oil raises oxygen level 30%; Sun Wellness CHLORELLA tabs; vitamin E 400IU with selenium 200 mcg; CoQ-10, 60 mg, *Gingko Biloba* extract.
- **Cardiotonics:** *Hawthorn* extract; *cayenne* or *cayenne-ginger* capsules; garlic; *Siberian ginseng* extract; *gotu kola* extract; PHYCOTENE MICROCLUSTERS available from Healthy House.
- **For anti-cholesterol-blood thinning:** Ginger or *cayenne-ginger* caps 4 daily; *butcher's broom*; taurine 500 mg; Golden Pride FORMULA ONE, oral chelation w. EDTA 2 packs a.m./p.m.
- **For healthy blood chemistry:** Chromium picolinate; Ester C 500 mg with bioflavonoids daily especially if you have had bypass heart surgery.
- **For preventing TIA's (small strokes):** CoQ-10, 60 mg 2 daily; ascorbate or Ester C with bioflavonoids, up to 500 mg daily for arterial integrity; vitamin E 400IU and selenium 200 mcg.
- **Natural calcium channel blockers:** magnesium 1200 mg daily; parsley caps 2 daily; carnitine 1000 mg daily.

Can't find a recommended product? Call the 800 number listed in Product Resources for the store nearest you.

Let's get to the heart of the matter.

Of all the world's people, Americans are in the highest risk category for heart disease. And if you think conventional medicine will protect you, think again. Many experts think drugs and surgical techniques to "protect" your heart are based on big bucks instead of health. Surgery alone cost Americans over $50 billion each year. (Incidentally, new studies show fish oil capsules after a balloon angioplasty can help prevent re-clogging....a big problem.) Clearly, lives have been saved and extended, but drugs and surgery carry serious risks. Most of us know someone for whom by-pass surgery or a pace-maker began the beginning of the end. My own father-in-law was one of those. New studies show that calcium channel blockers, the top selling blood pressure drugs, increase heart attack risk up to 60%! The research also shows that they raise the risk of suicide.

Many cholesterol-lowering drugs can cause liver toxicity, stomach distress and vision impairment. They also deplete CoQ-10, an essential co-enzyme that strengthens the heart, by up to 50%. By-pass surgery, the most popular surgical heart disease "solution," benefits less than 10% of heart patients. Many don't live 6 or 7 years after their first operation.

Is our 20th century lifestyle so bad that we are literally killing ourselves? Perhaps. First: there's our still sad American diet. Less than 25% of us get the recommended 5 servings of fruits and vegetables a day that protect against heart disease. Even worse, 25% of the "vegetables" we do eat in America are french fries: the most damaging for cardiovascular health! Low fiber is another big problem, (despite all the media attention). The typical American eats less than one-third of the daily fiber recommended for cardiovascular health! Second: there's our sedentary lifestyle. Lack of exercise also makes us a wide open target for heart disease. Regular moderate exercise cuts risk for heart attack and stroke almost in half. Our computers have changed our lives at every level. New statistics from the National Institute of Health show astounding 58% of adult Americans get no exercise at all! Third: Americans are "stressed out." Chronic stress is a part of the American lifestyle, and stress levels are rising. Most Americans feel overwhelmed on a regular basis. Financial or work-related stress in common. A recent survey find that over 25% of the baby boomers (at the peak of their careers and earning power) still feel out of control in their lives! Chronic stress attacks your entire cardiovascular system. It causes coronary arteries to constrict, blood pressure to soar and cholesterol to build on artery walls. It's no wonder our hearts are about to explode!

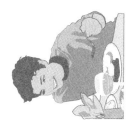

You can carve out heart health with your own knife and fork

The single most influential key to heart health is your diet. Almost all cardiovascular disease can be treated and prevented with improvement in nutrition. In general, refined, high fat, high calorie foods create cardiovascular problems, and natural foods relieve them. Yet Americans get over half their calories from processed foods that are high in calories and low in nutrients. Fried foods, salty and sugary foods, low fiber foods, fatty dairy foods, red meats, processed meats, tobacco and caffeine all contribute to clogged arteries, LDL cholesterol, high blood pressure and heart attacks. The following diet is easy to live with, and has all the necessary elements to keep arteries clear, and heart action regular and strong. It emphasizes fresh, whole fiber foods, high minerals with lots of potassium and magnesium, oxygen-riches from green vegetables, sprouts and wheat germ (wheat germ oil can raise the oxygen level of the heart as much as 30%), and vegetable-source proteins. It all adds up to today's definition of living well. Pleasure is derived from improved health and vitality instead of rich food and drink. The rewards are high; a longer, healthier life, and control over your life.

On rising: A high protein vitamin/mineral drink, like All One MULTIPLE with green plant base or Nature's Plus SPIRUTEIN in orange or grapefruit juice, or a cup of Japanese green tea.

Breakfast: Make an EFA mix of 2 TBS each: lecithin granules, wheat germ, brewer's yeast, hone and sesame seeds. Sprinkle 2 teasp. every morning in fresh fruits or mix with yogurt; and/or have a poached or baked egg with bran muffins or whole grain toast and kefir cheese; or some whole grain cereal or pancakes with a little maple syrup.

Mid-morning: have a veggie drink (see page 218), or Pines MIGHTY GREENS superfood, or Crystal Star SYSTEMS STRENGTH™ drink, or all natural V-8 juice (pg. 218) or a cup of antioxidant tea like *rosemary* or *peppermint* tea; and/or some crunchy raw veggies with kefir cheese or yogurt dip; or a cup of miso soup with sea greens snipped on top.

Lunch: have a cup of *fenugreek* tea with additions with 1 teasp. honey and a healthy pinch of *ginger*; then have a tofu and spinach salad with some sprouts and bran muffins; or a high protein salad or sandwich with nuts and seeds and black bean or lentil soup; or an avocado, low fat cheese or soy cheese sandwich on whole grain bread; or a seafood pasta salad.

Mid-afternoon: have *peppermint* tea, or Crystal Star ROYAL MU™ tonic tea; or a cup of miso soup and a hard boiled egg, or whole grain crackers, or carrot juice or Personal V-8 (pg. 218).

Dinner: have a broccoli quiche with whole grain crust; or baked seafood with brown rice and peas; or a veggie casserole; or a stir fry with soup and rice; or grilled fish or seafood and a green salad and baked potato. A glass of wine before dinner is good for things that help your heart....relaxation, digestion and tension relief. Wine has an enzyme that breaks up blood clots.

Before bed: have another cup of miso soup, or a cup of Sovex nutritional yeast paste broth in hot in water (delicious), apple or pear juice, or chamomile tea.

Notes: 1) Avoid commercial antacids that neutralize natural stomach acid and invite the body to produce even more acid, thus aggravating stress and tension.

2) Preventative heart health works: people who exert themselves for either recreation or work are strikingly free of circulatory diseases. To be effective for heart and artery health, the heart rate and respiration must rise to the point of mild breathlessness for 5 minutes each day. A daily walk, or exercise like dancing or swimming strengthens the whole cardiovascular system. It also reduces stress, the underlying cause of all disease.

Can't find a recommended product? Call the 800 number listed in Product Resources for the store nearest you.

Hemorrhage

Internal Bleeding, Excessive Bleeding, Blood Clotting Problems, Nosebleeds

The suggestions on this page refer to first aid for minor or non-life threatening problems. Obviously, you should get to an emergency room or call an ambulance if there is an emergency situation. Nosebleeds, bleeding gums and urinary tract bleeding are types of bleeding that can be addressed with these remedies. Most remedies are astringents (tighteners) or styptics (stoppers) that may also be used for swollen veins or hemorrhoids. Once the bleeding has been arrested, the idea with natural remedies is, as always, to address the underlying causes (such as weak membranes or capillary structure) that allow the bleeding to be excessive.

Diet & Superfood Therapy

—Nutritional therapy plan:

1—Make a variety of sprouts a regular part of your diet for natural vitamin K to help clotting and optimize healthy intestinal flora.

Other high vitamin K foods: kale, spinach and all dark green veggies, broccoli, cauliflower, and eggs.

2—Take a cup of green tea every morning. (I am prone to excessive bleeding, but since I strated a green tea regimen, the condition has normalized.) Green tea catechins control hemorrhage by activating coagulants.

3—Have a glass of carrot-spinach juice frequently, or take a green vegetable drink (pg. 218) once a week.

4—Eat plenty of papayas. Use citrus peel directly on the bleeding area.

—Superfood therapy: (choose 1 or more)

• Crystal Star BIOFLAV, FIBER & C SUPPORT™ drink with extra bioflavonoids to increase tissue integrity.

• Crystal Star ENERGY GREEN™ drink once a week to build healthier blood balance.

• Green Foods MAGMA PLUS, or liquid chlorophyll 3 teasp. daily.

• Beehive Botanical ROYAL JELLY/POLLEN/ SIBERIAN GINSENG drink for stronger blood.

Herb & Supplement Therapy

—Interceptive therapy plan: (Choose 2 to 3 recommendations)

1—When bleeding just won't stop: • Take capsicum, take 1 teasp. in a cup of hot water to stop bleeding. (Take with an eyedropper on the back of the tongue if it is too hot to swallow); or • take 2 dropperfuls bilberry extract and 2 cayenne capsules and get to a clinic. • Take 2 turmeric extract capsules.

2—For better clotting ability: • Solaray CALCIUM CITRATE caps 4 daily. Make a • clotting tea combo: Licorice root, comfrey root, shepherd's purse, goldenseal root, cranesbill; or make a • clotting paste with crushed plantain leaves and water and apply.

3—Astringents tighten veins and capillaries. (Use externally and internally to check bleeding): • White oak bark or yarrow tea; • Myrrh extract; • Bilberry extract; • Solaray CRANESBILL blend capsules; • Goldenseal extract; • Nettles tea and capsules.

4—For bloody urine: • take 2 to 4 turmeric extract capsules; or make an "astringent tea: plantain leaf, calendula flowers, horsetail, and bugleweed. (May also be used as a compress.)

5—For intestinal and somach bleeding: 2 cups daily • Pau d' arco, or white oak bark tea; • Turmeric extract capsules; • Comfrey root or ginger root tea; or • Shepherd's purse capsules. • Vitamin K 100mcg 3x daily to maintain micro-flora integrity.

6—For nosebleeds: • Arnica ointment (a specific); white willow tea compresses; • Vitamin C 3000mg daily for nosebleeds (especially if you also bruise easily).

7—High flavonoids strengthen veins and capillaries for prevention: • OPCs from grapeseed or white pine 100mg 3x daily; • Quercetin 1000 with bromelain 1000mg, 2 daily; • Vitamin C therapy for collagen and interstitial tissue formation - Ester C or ascorbic acid crystals with bioflavonoids and rutin. Take up to 5000mg daily; or Twin Lab CITRUS BIOFLAVONOID caps.

—Homeopathic remedies, especially for clotting difficulties from dental or cosmetic surgery: • Ferrum Phos. for bright red bleeding; • Arnica for bleeding accompanied by bruising, or nosebleeds; • Phosphorus for persistent bleeding.

Lifestyle Support Therapy

Don't use aspirin or other blood-thinner drugs like Heparin if you are at risk for internal bleeding.

—For a vein or artery: apply direct pressure with cold compresses or ice packs. Get to a doctor and treat for shock.

—Bodywork:

• Acupressure point: Press the insides of the thighs with the fingers just above the knees, for 10 seconds at a time.

• Body pressure points:

—Hold arm in the air on the side of the bleeding to decrease pressure.

—Pull knuckle of the middle finger on either hand until it pops, to lower blood pressure and tension.

—For a nosebleed: blow once vigorously to clear the nose, then pinch the sides of the nose together. Place a cold compress on nose. Apply pressure and hold firmly for 10 minutes.

• Styptics to apply directly:
Cold cloths or ice packs
Plantain and water paste
Witch hazel
Calendula salve or poultice
Propolis tincture
Yarrow

See also SHOCK TREATMENT page 495 for more information.

Can't find a recommended product? Call the 800 number listed in Product Resources for the store nearest you.

Common Symptoms: Inability to clot even small wounds; internal pain as with a rupture or ulcer; easy bruising and ulcerations; broken blood vessels; black stools when there are stomach ulcers. For hemorrhage from an accident to an artery or the head, usually accompanied by nausea, dizziness, enlarged pupil, drowsiness, confusion, even convulsions.
Common Causes: Broken blood vessels; weak vein and vessel walls; internal wounds from an accident; lack of vitamin K in the body, from heredity, or from eating irradiated foods which deplete vitamin K in the system; over-use of aspirin or other blood thinning drugs; accumulation of arterial plague. An English study shows that the process may be prevented from even occurring by taking PCOs.

H 414

Hemorrhoids
Piles, Anal Fissure

Hemorrhoids, also called piles, are swollen, inflamed veins and capillaries around the anus that often protrude out of the rectum. There is usually constipation and thus, because of straining, rectal bleeding. New research also shows a link with diarrhea and hemorrhoids. The pain and discomfort of hemorrhoidal itch and swelling are well known. Anal fissures are often misdiagnosed as hemorrhoids, but they are not swollen veins, but instead tiny tears in the lower part of the intestine. They are very painful and often require surgery (over 40,000 surgeries a year) to fix. A change in diet composition and natural therapies can help you avoid drugs and surgery for either hemorrhoids or anal fissures.

Diet & Superfood Therapy

—Nutritional therapy plan:

1—Diet improvement is the key to permanently reducing hemorrhoids. Avoid refined, low fiber foods, and acid forming foods, such as caffeine and sugar.

2—Take 1 TB olive oil or flax seed oil before each meal. Include plenty of fiber foods in your diet, particularly lots of vegetable cellulose, such as stewed and dried fruits, brans and vegetables.

3—Include sprouts and dark greens for vitamin K to inhibit bleeding.

4—Include plenty of berries and cherries for PCO's to strengthen veins and capillaries.

5—Take 2 TBS cider vinegar mixed with honey each morning.

6—Drink plenty of healthy liquids throughout the day, like juices and mineral water and Guayaki YERBA MATÉ green tea. ♂

7—Keep meals small, so the bowel and sphincter area won't have to work so hard.

8—Apply papaya skins or lemon juice directly to inflamed area to relieve itching.

—Superfood therapy: (choose 1 or more)
• Crystal Star BIOFLAV, FIBER & C SUPPORT™ with bioflavonoids for tissue integrity.
• Y.S. WAKASA CHLORELLA GOLD.
• AloeLife ALOE GOLD drink and apply ALOE SKIN GEL to hemorrhoids.
• Liquid chlorophyll 3 teasp. daily.

Herb & Supplement Therapy

—Interceptive therapy plan: (Choose 2 to 3 recommendations)

1—Relieve inflammation and encourage healing: • Crystal Star HEMR-EASE™ capsules for 2 weeks to (May also be used as a suppository). • Crystal Star HEMR-EASE GEL™; • St. John's wort oil. • Apply calendula ointment and make a hemorrhoid tea: mix equal parts comfrey root, wild yam, and cranesbill. Take internally and apply directly. • Take stone root tea, 3 cups daily for a month. • Use homeopathic remedies: Hylands HEMMOREX, Hippocastanum, or BioForce homeopathic HEMORRHOID RELIEF. Take • Enzymatic Therapy HEMTONE capsules to stop rectal bleeding; • take vitamin E 400IU daily and apply to inflamed area for healing.

2—Encourage vascular tone: • Ginkgo Biloba extract; • Solaray CENTELLA caps for vascular tone. Add • Crystal Star LIV-ALIVE™ tea for sluggishness, and • BWL-TONE IBS™ caps or • butcher's broom tea for gentle healing. • Evening primrose oil caps 4 daily.

3—Strengthen vein and capillary walls with flavonoids: • Vitamin C therapy for collagen and interstitial tissue formation: use Ester C or ascorbic acid crystals with bioflavs. and rutin. Take up to 5000mg daily; (also make a solution in water to apply directly). • Source Naturals activated QUERCETIN with bromelain 4 daily.

4—Herbal suppositories are easy and work almost right away. (use cocoa butter as the delivery medium): • Goldenseal-Myrrh; • Slippery elm; • Garlic-Comfrey; • Cranesbill; • Yarrow; • White oak bark. Use a bee pollen 1000mg tablet as a suppository. Insert 1 daily. • (Use NatureAde SOFT-EX tablets to soften stool short term.)

5—Nutrients that help rebuild colon and rectum health from the inside: • PCOs from grapeseed or white pine, 2 daily; • Bromelain 1500mg caps; lecithin caps 1900gr daily; • Vitamin K 100mcg 2x daily with vitamin B-6 250mg daily.

—For anal fissure: take internally and apply 3—Crystal Star ANTI-BIO™ caps; or apply 3—Crystal Star ANTI-BIO™ gel (with una da gato).

Lifestyle Support Therapy

—Bodywork:
• Take a good half hour walk every day.
• Put feet on a stool when sitting on the toilet to ease strain.

• Effective rectal applications:
  Ice packs
  Witch hazel as needed.
  MotherLove RHOID BALM or SITZ BATH. ♀♂

• Effective enemas to remove congestion:
  Nettles ♀♂
  Chlorella or spirulina
  Cayenne/garlic
  Nutribiotic GRAPEFRUIT SEED extract
  - 20 drops per gallon of water.

• Effective compresses:
  Alternating hot and cool water, or cold water compresses every morning.
  Horsetail tea - frequently
  Elderberry

—Reflexology point:

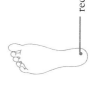
— rectum

H 415

Common Symptoms: Pain, itching and rectal bleeding with bowel movements; inflamed anal fissure; protruding swellings.
Common Causes: Junk food diet with too many refined, fried, fatty, low residue foods and not enough healthy hydrating liquids; constipation with habitual straining; pregnancy; overeating; lack of exercise, too much sitting; Vit. B₆ deficiency; acid/alkaline imbalance, especially from drugs such as anti-depressants and pain killers, or antacids and laxative abuse; liver exhaustion; allergies; obesity; diarrhea.accumulation

See also COLON HEALTH & CONSTIPATION page 357 for more.

Can't find a recommended product? Call the 800 number listed in Product Resources for the store nearest you.

Hepatitis

Severe Viral Liver Infection

There are several types of viral hepatitis. Type A: (infects 200,000 Americans each year) a viral infection passed through blood and feces; Type B: (infects about 1 million Americans each year) a sexually transmitted viral infection carried through blood, semen, saliva and dirty needles; sometimes develops into chronic hepatitis; Type C: (infects 4 million Americans each year) a post-transfusion form. Type D: caused by Epstein-Barr virus and cytomegalovirus; Non-A, Non-B: higher mortality viruses passed through transfusion blood products, which frequently develop into chronic hepatitis. Severity of hepatitis ranges from chronic fatigue to serious liver damage, and even to death from liver failure or liver cancer. Natural therapies have had outstanding success in hepatitis cases, both in arresting viral replication, and in regeneration of the liver.

Diet & Superfood Therapy

—Nutritional therapy plan:

1—Hepatitis Healing Diet:

For 2 weeks: Eat only fresh foods: salads, fruits, juices, bottled water. Take a glass of carrot/beet/cucumber juice every other day. Take a glass of lemon juice and water every morning. Take Sun Welness CHLORELLA granules daily.

Then for 1 to 2 months: Take carrot-beet-cucumber juice every 3 days, and papaya juice with 2 teasp. spirulina each morning. Eat lots of vegetable proteins, with steamed vegetables, brown rice, tofu, eggs, whole grains and yogurt. Avoid red meats.

Then for 1 more month: Take 2 glasses of tomato juice/wheat germ oil/brewer's yeast/lemon juice every day. Take a daily glass of apple-alfalfa sprout juice. Continue with vegetable proteins, cultured foods, fresh salads and complex carbs for strength.

Avoid refined, fried, fatty foods, sugars, heavy spices, alcohol and caffeine during healing.

—Superfood therapy: (choose 1 or more)
• Nutricology PRO-GREENS with EFA's.
• Crystal Star SYSTEMS STRENGTH™ drink.
• Body Ecology VITALITY SUPERGREEN.
• SunWellness CHLORELLA drink.
• AloeLife ALOE GOLD drink with spirulina tabs 6 daily. ♂
• Green Foods WHEAT GERM EXTRACT.

Herb & Supplement Therapy

—Interceptive therapy plan: (Choose 2 to 3 recommendations)

1—Cleanse the liver of toxins: Source Naturals Alpha Lipoic acid 400mg daily; Jarrow SAMe 200, 600mg daily; • Crystal Star LIV-ALIVE™ capsules 4 to 6 daily, with LIV ALIVE™ tea 2 cups daily for 1 month. Reduce dose to half the 2nd month. Liver detox teas: • Oregon grapeseed clover tea; • Pau d'arco-calendula tea. • Take Ascorbate Vitamin C crystals, up to 10,000mg daily in water, to bowel tolerance for 1 month.
• Enzymatic Therapy LIVA-TOX, with THYMU-PLEX caps for thymus strength.

2—Inhibit viral replication: • Echinacea-St. John's wort therapy for lymphatic support: alternate 4 days of echinacea extract and 4 days of St. John's wort extract. • Nutribiotic GRAPE-FRUIT SEED extract 10 drops 3x daily for 1 month in juice. Also apply to lesions.

3—Heal liver tissue: • Phosphatidyl-choline caps, 1000mg daily, • Solaray LIPO-TROPIC PLUS caps; • Rainbow Light LIVA-GEN extract with ADVANCED ENZYME SYSTEM formula; or • Enzymedica PURIFY caps. • L-carnitine 2000mg daily; • vitamin E 400IU daily; • Nutricology GERMANIUM 150mg daily.

4—Normalize liver function with liver tonics for at least 1 month: • Nutricology NAC (N-acety-cysteine) 500mg 3x daily; • Crystal Star GINSENG-LICORICE ELIXIR™ drops; • Maitake mushroom extract caps; or • Dandelion root extract, or • astragalus extract or • lobelia extract drops in tea; or turmeric extract capsules or bayberry-cayenne capsules, 6 daily to control inflammation. • Crystal Star ANTI-HST™ caps to control histamine reactions, for 1 month. Reduce dose to half 2nd month.

5—For long term liver support: Use • Crystal Star BITTERS & LEMON CLEANSE™ THISTLE SEED extract and • Futurebiotics MSM 1000mg; • MILK THISTLE SEED extract and • Crystal Star BITTERS & LEMON CLEANSE™ each morning for 3 months. • Beta carotene 150,000IU daily, with • B-complex 150mg, and • Country Life sublingual B-12 2500mcg or 1 month and extra folic acid 800mcg. Reduce beta carotene to 50,000IU, and B-complex to 100mg daily.

Probiotics help reestablish immunity: • Jarrow DOPHILUS + FOS if detection is early: Take 1 teasp. powder in water 2-3x daily for 7 days; then 1 teasp. 4x daily at meals and bedtime for 7 days. • Natren BIFIDO FACTORS daily for 1 month, with • CoQ10, 60 mg 3x daily as an immune stimulant.

Lifestyle Support Therapy

—Lifestyle measures:
• Count on 2 weeks for emergency detox measures; 1-3 months for healing the liver and rebuilding blood and body strength.
• Get plenty of bed rest, especially during the acute infectious stages.
• Overheating therapy has been effective for Hepatitis. See page 225 in this book. A steam bath or sauna can remove much of the toxicity through the skin.
• Use chlorophyll implants twice weekly for the first two critical weeks of healing to detoxify.
• Avoid all alcohol, amphetamines, cocaine, barbiturates, or tobacco of any kind.
• Use hot castor oil packs over the liver area.

—Reflexology point:

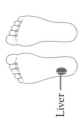

Liver

See LIVER HEALING section page 443 and SEXUALLY TRANSMITTED DISEASES page 491 for more.

Can't find a recommended product? Call the 800 number listed in Product Resources for the store nearest you.

Common Symptoms: All forms of hepatitis are characterized by great fatigue, flu-like symptoms of exhaustion and diarrhea; enlarged, tender, congested, sluggish liver; loss of appetite to the point of anorexia, nausea; dark urine, gray stools; sometimes vomiting; skin pallor and histamine itching; depression; skin jaundice; cirrhosis of the liver.
Common Causes: Infectious hepatitis is largely a lifestyle disease - with almost 90% of intravenous drug users infected. Others at risk include dental and medical workers, and over 25% of people receiving blood transfusions. Hepatitis can lead to liver cancer, cirrhosis and is sometimes itself fatal.

High Blood Pressure

Hypertension

High blood pressure is a major problem in America's fast-paced, high-stress world. Believe it or not, it's the leading health problem for women today. Fewer than half have their blood pressure under control. It causes 60,000 deaths a year and directly relates to more than 250,000 deaths from stroke. It is a silent condition that steals health and foreshadows serious cardiovascular disease that can steal life. Most cases of high blood pressure are caused by arteriosclerosis and atherosclerosis, along with exhausted kidneys - factors that can be brought under control by diet and lifestyle improvement. In fact, clinical studies show that people with hypertension who make good life changes fare much better than those on anti-hypertensive prescription drugs. It is worth noting that vegetarians have less hypertension and fewer blood pressure problems.

Diet & Superfood Therapy

Nutritional therapy plan:

1—Keep body weight down. One of the biggest risk factors is excess fat storage. Go on a juice diet for 1 day every week for 2 months to improve body chemistry and reduce extra blood fats:

2—Have citrus juices or a potassium drink (pg. 215) in the morning. Make a mix of wheat germ, flax oil, brewer's yeast; take 2 TBS daily.

3—Have a veggie green drink (pg. 218), V-8 juice, or carrot juice at mid-day;

4—Have apple, pear or papaya juice before dinner.

5—Chamomile tea or Sovex yeast broth at bedtime.

6—Then follow the High Blood Pressure Diet on the next page: include lots of vitamin C, magnesium and potassium foods: broccoli, bananas, dried fruits, potatoes, seafood, bell peppers, avocados, celery, brown rice and leafy greens.

7—Eat smaller meals more frequently; consciously undereat. Avoid refined foods, caffeine, salty, sugary, fried, fatty foods, prepared meats, heavy pastries and soft drinks. All cause potassium depletion and allow arterial plaque build-up.

—Superfood therapy: (choose 1 or more)

• Sun Wellness CHLORELLA drink daily.
• New Chapter GINGER WONDER syrup.
• Future Biotics VITAL K drink daily.
• Crystal Star BIOFLAV., FIBER & C SUPPORT™ drink.

Herb & Supplement Therapy

—Interceptive therapy plan: (Choose 2 to 3 recommendations)

1—**Help regulate your blood pressure:** •Crystal Star HEARTSEASE H.B.P.™ caps or tea daily, or • America's Finest GUGULIPID - HAWTHORN complex, or •Vitamin E therapy: Take 1 100IU capsule daily for 1 week, then 4 capsules daily for 1 week, then 2 400IU capsules daily for 1 week. Add 1 selenium 200mcg, and 1 Ester C with bioflavs each time, for hypertension caused by toxic heavy metals. Add •PHYCOTENE MICROCLUSTERS available at Healthy House for uptake.

2—**Tone your arterial system with flavonoids:** Take •HAWTHORN extract as needed, especially if you have palpitations. •Ginkgo Biloba extract for extra circulation; •Cayenne-ginger caps 4 daily, or Wakunaga AGED GARLIC extract; •Grifon MAITAKE caps •Bilberry extract or •BD Herbs GRAPESEED organic PCO's 100mg as needed; •Garlic, or onion-garlic caps 6 daily. •Siberian ginseng extract caps, 2000mg.

3—**Naturally reduce edema swelling:** •Crystal Star TINKLE™ caps; •Dandelion extract drops in tea. Most high blood pressure medicines cause potassium-magnesium loss. If you are taking diuretics, take •vitamin C 1000mg daily, potassium 99mg daily (or Crystal Star herbal Potassium-Iodine caps) and •B-complex 100mg.

4—**Reduce your risk of a stroke:** •Crystal Star GREEN TEA CLEANSER™ each a.m. •Rainbow Light CALCIUM PLUS caps w. high magnesium, 6 daily.

5—**Reduce your stress to control hypertension:** Nature's Secret ULTIMATE B daily with extra B₆ 100mg, niacin 100mg 3x daily. Crystal Star RELAX CAPS™ or GINSENG-REISHI drops in water. •Hyland's homeopathic CALMS FORTE tabs. •CoQ₁₀ 60mg 3x daily; •Country Life RELAXER caps with GABA; •Suma caps 6 daily; •Crystal Star ADR-ACTIVE™ caps 4 daily.

6—**Boost your essential fatty acids:** •Omega-3 fish or flax oils 3 daily; •Evening Primrose Oil 3000mg daily.

7—**Digest fats and dairy foods better to help high blood pressure:** •Bromelain 1000mg. daily; •Chromium picolinate 200mcg. daily to combat insulin resistance. •Transformation LYPOZYME; •Planetary TRIPHALA caps as directed. •Golden Pride FORMULA ONE oral chelation a.m. and p.m. with EDTA.

Lifestyle Support Therapy

—Bodywork:

•You have high blood pressure if you have a repeated reading over 150/90mmHg. If you have a high blood pressure problem, monitor your progress often with a home or free drugstore electronic machine reading.

•Avoid tobacco in all forms to dramatically lower blood pressure. Smoking constricts blood vessels, making your heart work harder. Smoking also aggravates high blood sugar levels.

•Phenylalanine (especially as found in Nutra-Sweet) and over-the-counter antihistamines can aggravate high blood pressure.

•Eliminate caffeine and hard liquor. They can cause adrenaline rushes that make blood pressure soar. (A little wine at night with dinner can actually lower stress and hypertension.)

•Exercise is important. Take a brisk 30 minute walk every day, with plenty of deep lung breathing.

•Relaxation techniques are very important. Massage and meditation are two of the best for hypertension.

•Use a dry skin brush all over the body frequently to stimulate better blood flow.

—Reflexology point:

•Pull middle finger on each hand 3x for 20 seconds each time, daily.

Common Symptoms: Headaches; irritability; dizziness and ringing in the ears; flushed complexion; red streaks in the eyes; fatigue and sleeplessness; edema; frequent urination; depression; heart arrhythmia; chronic respiratory problems.

Common Causes: Clogging arterial fats and increased fat storage; calcium and fiber deficiency; thickened blood from excess mucous and waste; insulin resistance and poor sugar metabolism; thyroid imbalance; obesity; lack of aerobic exercise; too much salt and red meat, causing raised copper levels; kidney malfunction; auto-toxemia from constipation; prostaglandin imbalance.

See the HEALTHY HEART pages in this book for more information.

Can't find a recommended product? Call the 800 number listed in Product Resources for the store nearest you.

Do you have to take high blood pressure drugs for life?

Calcium channel blockers inhibit the entry of calcium into heart cells and smooth muscle cells of blood vessels. Without calcium, the cells cannot contract and the result is lowered blood pressure. But calcium is an important mineral for heart health! Calcium regulates the contraction and relaxation of the heart and inhibits heart spasms. Calcium is most beneficial when it is brought into the body with a balanced ratio of magnesium through foods. I always say magnesium is "Nature's calcium channel blocker." Magnesium naturally blocks the entry of calcium into heart muscle cells and vascular smooth muscle cells, reducing vascular resistance to lower blood pressure. Good food sources include: dark green veggies (or sea greens), whole grains, nuts and seeds, beans and poultry.

Beta blockers work to impede the action of the body's beta receptors, adrenaline response modifiers between the heart and brain. The theory is that the brain can't notify the heart to constrict the arteries, so it slows down, regardless of its need.

Americans are being told that if they have high blood pressure, lifetime drug therapy is the best solution. But over the long-term, side effect hazards may outweigh the benefits of these drugs. New studies published in the journal Circulation find that calcium channel blockers increase heart attack risk up to 60%. British studies show they raise the risk of suicide! For men, impotence commonly results. The drugs are also linked to breast cancer and memory loss. Side effects of beta blockers are dizziness, nausea, asthma symptoms, impotence in men and joint pain, to name a few.

Can natural therapies lower blood pressure? The newest information shows that most people don't require medication to control their disease. Millions can reverse high blood pressure with simple diet and lifestyle therapy. 1997 Harvard Medical School research finds a low-fat diet may lower blood pressure as much as drugs. New research from the West Oakland Health Center finds that meditation for 20 minutes, twice daily is as effective as drug therapy to lower blood pressure.

High Blood Pressure Prevention Diet

Eighty-five percent of high blood pressure is preventable without drugs. A diet change is the best thing you can do to control high blood pressure. Reduce and control salt use. (See Low Salt Diet, pg. 176). The key to salt balance in your body is drinking plenty of water. When your body perceives that it is becoming dehydrated, it responds by retaining sodium to reduce further water loss, starting a vicious cycle of cravings for salty foods and liquids that ends in high blood pressure. (Constantly taking diuretics for high blood pressure can aggravate this cycle.) Start by eliminating foods that provoke high blood pressure - canned and frozen foods, cured, smoked and canned meats and fish, commercial peanut butter, soy sauce, bouillon cubes and condiments, fried chips and snacks, dry soups. The rewards are high - a longer, healthier life - and control of your life. Avoid antacids that neutralize natural stomach acid and invite your body to produce even more acid.

On rising: Have lemon water and honey, or a high vitamin/mineral drink such as All One MULTIPLE with green plant base or Crystal Star SYSTEMS STRENGTH™ drink.

Breakfast: Make a mix of 2 TBS each: lecithin granules, toasted wheat germ, brewer's yeast, honey and sesame seeds. Sprinkle some on fresh fruit or mix with yogurt; or have a poached or baked egg with bran muffins or whole grain toast, and kefir cheese or unsalted butter; or some whole grain cereal or pancakes with a little maple syrup.

Mid-morning: Have a veggie drink (pg. 218) or Crystal Star ENERGY GREEN™ drink, or Green Foods GREEN MAGMA, or natural V-8 juice or *peppermint* tea: or a cup of miso soup with sea greens snipped on top, or low-sodium ramen noodle soup; and/or some crunchy raw veggies with a kefir cheese or yogurt dip.

Lunch: Have one cup daily of fenugreek tea with 1 teasp. honey; then have a tofu and spinach salad with some sprouts and bran muffins; or a large fresh green salad with a lemon oil dressing. Add plenty of sprouts, tofu, raisins, cottage cheese, nuts, and seeds as desired; or have a baked potato with yogurt or kefir cheese topping, and a light veggie omelet; or a seafood and vegetable pasta salad; or some grilled or braised vegetables with an olive oil dressing and brown rice.

Mid-afternoon: Have a bottle of mineral water, a cup of *peppermint* tea, or a tea made from Crystal Star GINSENG/LICORICE ELIXIR™ extract, or ROYAL MU™ tonic tea; or a cup of miso soup with a hard boiled egg, or whole grain crackers; or dried fruits, and an apple or cranberry juice.

Dinner: Have a baked vegetable casserole with tofu and brown rice, and a small dinner salad; or a baked fish or seafood dish with rice and peas, or a baked potato; or a vegetable quiche (such as broccoli, artichoke, or asparagus), and a light oriental soup; or some roast turkey and cornbread dressing, with a small salad or mashed potatoes with a little butter; or an oriental vegetable stirfry, with a light, clear soup and brown rice. A little wine is fine with dinner for relaxation, digestion and tension relief.

Before bed: Have a cup of miso soup, or Red Star NUTRITIONAL YEAST broth, apple juice, or some *chamomile* tea.

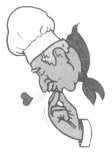

H 418

Can't find a recommended product? Call the 800 number listed in Product Resources for the store nearest you.

Hormone Imbalances - Women

Estrogen Disruption, Hysterectomy Aftermath, Environmental Hormone Effects

A healthy female system works in an incredibly beautiful, complex balance. It is an individual model of the creative universe. A woman is usually a marvelous thing to be, but the intricacies of her body are delicately tuned and can become unbalanced or obstructed easily, causing pain and poor function. From childbearing age, to premenopause, to menopause, to post-menopause, many women are affected by imbalances and fluctuations in their hormones that rattle their lives. Female hormone imbalances are involved in a myriad of health problems including: fibroids, endometriosis, headaches, PMS, depression, low libido and infertility. Hormones help regulate everything from energy flow, to inflammation, to a woman's monthly cycle. Tiny amounts can cause big reactions, both good and bad. Maintaining hormonal balance in today's world is not easy. Every day, we are bombarded with man-made hormones – from widespread hormone-mimicking pollutants, hormone drugs and hormones injected in our foods. A hormone balancing lifestyle program is something most of us can benefit from. Using lifestyle therapy to rebalance hormones ratios gently harmonizes your body, rather than regulating hormones by injection which sometimes stops natural hormone production by the endocrine glands entirely. I find natural, hormone balancing therapies after trauma, stress or serious illness, or after a hysterectomy, childbirth, a D & C, or an abortion allow your body to achieve its own hormone levels and bring itself to its own balance at its deepest levels.

Diet & Superfood Therapy

–Nutritional therapy plan:

1—Eat smaller meals. Overeating can suppress hormone production.

2—Limit consumption of fatty dairy products and meats (especially beef and pork), notoriously high in hormone-disrupting chemicals. Chicken is also an offender. I hear from women who have a 1 to 1 reaction with breast swelling from eating chicken injected with hormones. Look for hormone-free chicken and turkey at health food stores - Petaluma Poultry ROSIE THE ORGANIC CHICKEN, Diestel and Coleman Natural Products.

3—Wash produce thoroughly to reduce hormone disrupting pollutant residues. Use Healthy Harvest FRUIT & VEGETABLE RINSE.

4—Add soy foods (tofu, tempeh, soy milk, etc.) to your diet for hormone normalizing isoflavones.

5—Drink green tea to flush out excess estrogen disrupting chemicals.

6—Especially eat cruciferous veggies like broccoli to help flush excess estrogen out.

–For estrogen balancing effects:
• Crystal Star BIOFLAV., FIBER & C support.
• Ethical Nutrients TRIPLE BALANCE drink.

Herb & Supplement Therapy

–Interceptive therapy plan: (Choose 2 to 3 recommendations)

1—For **female hormone balance:** •Crystal Star FEM-SUPPORT™ extract, or FEMALE HARMONY™ caps or tea, or •Crystal Star PRO-EST BALANCE™ herbal progesterone cream roll-on (quickly effective). Add •Vitex extract or •Y.S. ROYAL JELLY/GINSENG drink or •Dong quai-damiana extract.

For women with abnormal periods: Vitex extract; or Moon Maid POR-MENO wild yam cream, or •Crystal Star PRO-EST BALANCE™ wild yam cream; •Crystal Star DONG QUAI-DAMIANA extract as needed; or •Rainbow Light VITEX-BLACK COHOSH complex...

For hormone boosting after hysterectomy or during menopause: •Royal Jelly-Red Ginseng combo; •Peruvian rainforest herb Maca; •Country Life MAXINE INTIMA FOR WOMEN.

For adult acne or hair growth on face, chest and chin: Saw palmetto extract 160 mg, 2x daily. (Do not use if trying to become pregnant or if on hormone therapy.)

For female nerve and gland health: Black cohosh, licorice, ashwagandha.

2—**Hormone tonics for more energy:** •Crystal Star ADR-ACTIVE™ capsules with FEEL GREAT™ tea; •Optimal Nutrients DHEA or Body Ammo FOUNTAIN of YOUTH creme; •B-complex 100mg daily, extra pantothenic acid 1000mg.

3—**Essential fatty acids normalize hormone production:** •Evening primrose oil, 1000mg, 2-4 daily; •Barleans Organic Oils ESSENTIAL WOMAN; •Long Life IMPERIAL TONIC with royal jelly and EPO; •Nature's Secret ULTIMATE OIL.

4—**Hormone support nutrients for women:** •Calcium-magnesium,1000-2000mg daily, iron, 20 mg; folic acid, 400 mcg; B$_6$ 50 mg; •manganese, 2.5 to 5 mg. Note: If you are taking synthetic hormones, they can destroy vitamin E in the body, increasing risk for heart diseases. Supplement with vitamin E 400IU daily to counteract this.

Lifestyle Support Therapy

–Bodywork techniques for hormone balance:
• Massage therapy reestablishes unblocked meridians of energy and increases circulation.
• Deep abdominal breathing - page 554.
• Yoga stretches every morning.
• Take a good brisk exercise walk every day.
• Get morning sunlight on the body every day possible, on the arms for women.
• Smoking disrupts hormonal activity.
• Muscle Testing (Applied Kinesiology), is useful for determining which hormonal herbs or supplements are specific to your problem. Once you learn the simple technique (see a nutritional consultant, a holistic chiropractor, or a massage therapist) you can easily do it at home to decide which products are right for you.

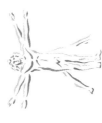

H 419

Common Symptoms: Painful, difficult menstruation, or absence of menstruation; spotting between periods; depression; mood swings and irritability; water retention.
Common Causes: Birth control pills for hormone replacement therapy; adrenal exhaustion due to stress; severe dieting or body building; surgery or long illness; protein or iodine deficiency; calcium deficiency; B Complex or EFA deficiencies.

For saliva hormone testing. Dr. David Zava, Ph.D., ZRT Laboratory, 503-469-0741, fax 503-469-1305, Address: ZRT Laboratory, 12505 NW Cornell Rd., Portland, OR 97229.

Can't find a recommended product? Call the 800 number listed in Product Resources for the store nearest you.

What About Environmental Hormones?

Hormone disrupters are so commonplace in modern society that there is no way to completely avoid them. Hormone disrupters come from pollutants, drugs, hormone-injected meats and dairy products, plastics, and pesticides. All of the Earth's waterways are connected, so chemical pollutants containing environmental hormones reach your food supply wherever you live. The problem is so huge that just last September the Environmental Protection Agency began implementing a congressionally mandated plan to test 87,000 compounds to determine their effect on the reproductive systems of humans and animals.

Estrogen-mimicking pollutants may even be changing the face of human evolution. New reports show the devastating effect of hormone disrupting pollutants on our wildlife and human health. Pallid sturgeons, found only in the Mississippi river, are now condemned to extinction as decades of exposure to pollutant PCB's (polychlorinated biphenyls) and DDT (dichloro-diphenyl-trichloroethane) have resulted in no new species birth for the last 10 years. Studies done on turtles at the University of Texas find that even when environmental factors (like heat) are controlled to determine a male outcome, females or intersex turtles are hatched from just a small amount of PCB's are painted on the eggs.

Hormone disrupters affect your entire endocrine system, all the communication system of your glands, hormones and cellular receptors in your body. They alter the production and breakdown of your own hormones, and the function of your hormone receptors – disrupting hormone balance at its developmental core. They can compete for hormone receptor sites in the body and bind to them in place of natural hormones, causing major fluctuations in hormonal levels in the body. Compounding the problem, these chemicals increase in potency 160 to 1600 times when they're combined inside your body from several different sources, like from hormone-injected meats and pesticide-sprayed produce.

The effects of estrogen disruption mean maintaining female hormone balance is clearly a challenge.

One of the biggest health threats facing the health of women today is the excess estrogen assault from our environment. Man-made estrogens are in pollutants, hormone-injected meats and dairy foods, plastics, pesticides and drugs. (The hormone replacement drug for women, Premarin, is the top-selling drug in America!) Science is just beginning to accept, even though many naturopaths have known for some time, that man-made estrogens can stack the deck against women by increasing their estrogen levels hundreds of times over normal levels. Although many scientists still believe that there is no significant difference between man-made and natural hormones, it seems apparent from the evidence of thousands of women, that even if a lab test can't tell the difference, their bodies can. Nearly HALF of African-American girls and 15% of Caucasian girls now begin to develop sexually by age 8, a clear indicator of hormone disruption. There is grim news about estrogenic chemicals and developing human fetuses, too. Male and female hormones must remain in balance in an embryo for sexual organs to develop normally. In early stages, a fetus is capable of developing either set. Hormone balance determines whether the child will be male or female. Exogenous estrogens can upset this balance, resulting in children with stunted male sex organs or with both sets of sex organs.

There is a link between pesticides and breast cancer. Pesticides, like other pollutants, are stored in body fat areas like breast tissue. Some pesticides including PCB's and DDT compromise immune function, overwork the liver and affect the glands and hormones the way too much estrogen does. One study shows 50 to 60% more dichloro-diphenyl-ethylene (DDE) and polychlorinated bi-phenols, (PCB's) in women who have breast cancer than in those who don't. The quantity of DDT in body tissues is also higher. In fact, some researchers suggest that the reason older women are experiencing a higher rate of breast cancer may be that these women had greater exposure to DDT before it was banned. The dramatic rise in breast cancer is consistent with the accumulation of organo-chlorine residues in the environment. Israel's recent history offers a case study. Until about 20 years ago, both breast cancer rates and contamination levels of organo-chlorine pesticides in Israel were among the highest in the world. An aggressive phase-out of these pesticides has led to a sharp reduction in contamination levels, followed by a dramatic drop in breast cancer death rates.

Some of the diseases associated with chronic exposure to estrogen mimics in the environment:
—breast and reproductive organ cancer, —breast and uterine fibroids, —polycystic ovarian syndrome, —endometriosis, —pelvic inflammatory disease.

Is there any way to reduce your exposure?

First, cut back on fat! Hormone disrupters accumulate in body fat. This is why a high fat diet is a major risk factor for long term exposure to them, and why it may lead to increased risk for hormone-driven cancers.

Second, eat sea greens like wakame, nori and dulse regularly. Algin, a gel like substance in sea greens, protects against chemical overload (often involved in breast cancer) by binding to chemical wastes so they can be eliminated safely from the body.

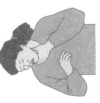

Can't find a recommended product? Call the 800 number listed in Product Resources for the store nearest you.

Are the new designer estrogens, the SERMs (selective estrogen receptor modulators), estrogen disrupters?

SERMs are a part of the new revolution in hormone replacement drugs. It's not about hot flashes anymore because women are finding out they can handle them on their own with herbs and foods, as they have for centuries. SERMs were developed to fight what are perceived as menopausal diseases like osteoporosis, heart disease, even Alzheimer's disease, without increasing breast and uterine cancer risk, like traditional HRT drugs.

Designer estrogen SERMs seem promising at first glance. Some reports suggest that Evista (the most widely prescribed SERM) may prevent breast cancer without increasing risk for other cancers, and may protect against heart disease. Further, studies show Evista does increase bone density in women with osteoporosis. But Evista comes with its own set of drawbacks. Evista may not prevent fractures, the very problem women fear most, and it does not prevent bone loss in the spine. Twenty-five percent of patients in one study reported more hot flashes, a sign of estrogen disruption, while using Evista. Evista also increases risk for serious blood clots in the legs, lungs and eyes - especially for sedentary women. Its effects on circulation are so powerful many women discontinue therapy because leg cramps caused by the drug are so severe. Scientists are even concerned that Evista may increase risk for Alzheimer's disease because it seems to act as an anti-estrogen in the brain, (hot flashes may be a sign of falling hormone levels in the brain). In Alzheimer's, where estrogen appears to provide protection, anti-estrogen activity in the brain is obviously not desirable. Evista should not be taken by women with a history of congestive heart failure (faced by many women after menopause), pregnant women or individuals with active cancers. Drug-resistance to Tamoxifen (an anti-breast cancer drug) may develop if you take Evista because the two drugs are so closely related.

We may have more knowledge about our bodies than we did 50 years ago, but we still don't understand hormones well. Hormones have widespread effects that are poorly understood. Although doctors are ecstatic about SERMs, these drugs still work at the hormone level and may disrupt delicate hormone balance. Phytohormone-containing herbs like *wild yam*, *red clover* and *dong quai* are really natural SERMs, which safely control menopause symptoms and may even help protect women from diseases like osteoporosis or heart disease after menopause.

I believe herbs are still a better choice for hormone balance.

Many of the phytoestrogen containing herbs, like *black cohosh* for instance, are not just natural (instead of chemical) direct estrogens. As living medicines, they can work intelligently with your body. In many cases, these herbs don't compete for receptor sites or have a direct estrogenic activity in the body. In fact, they work mainly as adaptogens which balance glandular activity and normalize body temperature fluctuations. They do what herbs always do best no matter what the problem is ...... they are body normalizers.

—**For hot flashes and night sweats:** •Crystal Star EST-AID™ capsules, 4 to 6 daily; •Moon Maid Botanicals PRO-MENO *wild yam* cream; •Transitions PRO-GEST cream; •VITEX extract; vitamin E 800IU; • *Evening Primrose Oil* caps 3000mg daily; • Nature's Secret ULTIMATE B daily and • Ester C 3000mg daily.

—**For side effects from synthetic hormones or birth control pills:** •Nature's Plus vitamin E 800IU; •Country Life MAXINE capsules daily; •B-complex 100mg daily, with extra B$_6$ 250mg; •Country Life sub-lingual B-12, 2500mg and folic acid 800mcg daily; e •mulsified A & D 25,000IU/1,000IU; •Ester C 550mg with bioflavonoids, 6 daily; •Solaray CALCIUM CITRATE SUPREME capsules, 46 daily; •Crystal Star FEM-SUPPORT™ extract 2-3x daily, or •Nature's Apothecary FEMALE BALANCE..

—To **rebalance prostaglandin formation:** (Prostaglandin imbalance can lead to breast and uterine fibroids, arthritis, eczema, menstrual difficulties, high blood pressure and cholesterol, and a tendency to gain weight.) Avoid saturated fats, especially from red meats and pasteurized, full fat dairy products. Take •high omega-3 oils from cold water fish or flax seed oil 3x daily. Or use • *Evening Primrose* or •Nature's Secret ULTIMATE OIL capsules 46 daily for 3 months.

Is hormone replacement therapy always necessary after a hysterectomy?

More than a half million American women have hysterectomies every year. The surgery is major, sometimes requiring a month or more of recovery time, but still, 1 in 4 women will have their uterus removed by the time they're 60. 1 in 1,000 women actually die as a result. Endometriosis, uterine fibroids, or heavy periods are common reasons for a hysterectomy. The surgical removal of a woman's uterus or ovaries (or both) can mean major disruptions in hormonal health, premature menopause and usually a lifelong prescription of hormone replacement drugs. In many cases, natural therapies can help a woman avert surgery and help her body normalize naturally. Vitex extract and natural progesterone creams help manage heavy, abnormal bleeding.

Herbs are also an excellent choice to boost hormone production by the adrenal glands if surgery has already been done. By supporting endocrine health, rainforest herb *Maca* can control hysterectomy-induced symptoms like depression, low libido constipation and hot flashes. An added bonus: *Maca* is rich in absorbable calcium, magnesium and silica, important for bone strength. Natural Balance INNERGY is an energizing formula with herbs like *tribulus* and *maca* known for balancing hormones and increasing libido.

See endometriosis page 377 and fibroids page 385 for more info.

Can't find a recommended product? Call the 800 number listed in Product Resources for the store nearest you.

Hormone Imbalances - Men

Andropause, Impotence, Environmental Hormone Effects

Low testosterone affects an astounding 1,000,000 American men! Yet in a recent survey, 68% of men cannot name a single symptom caused by low testosterone. Only 15% named low sex drive as a symptom of low testosterone; 6% named fatigue; 3% named a decrease in muscle mass; and less than 1% linked low testosterone to men's osteoporosis. Clearly, many men are in the dark about how hormone imbalances affect their health. Men's hormone changes have been much less publicized and researched than women's, but hormone disruption is as much a part of a man's life as it is a woman's. Some men are more attuned to their hormonal fluctuations than others. Some report clear monthly changes in their energy levels, mood, work and sports performance that they attribute to their equivalent of a "period." Blood levels of testosterone fluctuate dramatically at different times in life from 250 to 1,200 nanograms, and these changes affect a man's performance, mood and sexuality. While a man's hormone fluctuations are less dramatic than a woman's, testosterone levels start to decline around age 40, falling up to 10% each decade. This phenomenon called "andropause" is now recognized by almost eight in ten family physicians as a real condition that affects quality of life for men. More physicians are becoming increasingly interested in TRT, or testosterone replacement therapy for andropausal men, but I find most men benefit the most from a detailed lifestyle program emphasizing natural foods, bodywork therapies and supportive herbs and supplements designed to meet their changing needs. See pg. 266 of this book for more information.

Diet & Superfood Therapy

Nutritional therapy plan:

—1—Eat smaller, more frequent meals. Overeating can suppress hormone production.

2—Limit consumption of fatty dairy products and meats (especially beef and pork), notoriously high in hormone-disrupting chemicals. Chicken is also an offender. Buy hormone-free poultry - Petaluma Poultry ROSIE THE ORGANIC CHICKEN, Diestel and Coleman Natural Products.

3—Wash produce thoroughly to reduce hormone disrupting pollutant residues. Use Healthy Harvest FRUIT & VEGETABLE RINSE.

4—Add soy foods (tofu, tempeh, soy milk, etc.) to your diet for hormone normalizing isoflavones.

5—Drink green tea to flush out fats that harbor hormone disrupting chemicals.

6—Limit your use of microwaves. Microwaving foods kills enzymes. Enzymes are an important tool for glandular and hormone metabolism.

7—Drink in moderation. Heavy drinking can lead to prostate problems and impaired erections.

For male stamina and endurance:

—
• Nature's Secret BEYOND ENDURANCE.
• Crystal Star ENERGY GREEN™ drink mix.

Herb & Supplement Therapy

—Interceptive therapy plan: (Choose 2 to 3 recommendations)

1—For male hormone balance: • L-Glutamine 500mg 4x daily to stimulate rejuvenating growth hormone; • Crystal Star MALE PERFORMANCE™ caps for 3 months. • Siberian Ginseng extract; • Crystal Star GINSENG-LICORICE ELIXIR™.

—Raw glandular therapy: raw pancreas, raw orchic, raw pituitary.

—For low sperm count: • Carnitine 1000mg 2x daily helps sperm cells "swim" to their destination; • B₁₂ 6,000 mcg. daily.

—Effective herbal hormone-balancing combinations for men: • Panax ginseng-Damiana; • Panax ginseng-Sarsaparilla; • Licorice root-Dandelion root.

—Male virility: • Yohimbe extract; • Tribulus terrestris; • Ginkgo biloba; • Catauba.

2—Boost hormone production: • Crystal Star MALE GINSIAC™ extract with fresh panax ginseng roots and potency wood; • Golden Pride REJUVENATE FOR MEN; • CoQ-10, 60mg 3x daily improves physical performance.

3—Hormone tonics for more energy: • Crystal Star ADR-ACTIVE™ extract with • FEEL GREAT™ caps; • Rainbow Light ADAPTO-GEM caps; • Smilax extract 15 drops daily; • Beehive Botanical ROYAL JELLY-GINSENG-POLLEN caps.

4—Essential fatty acids normalize production of steroid hormones: • Evening primrose oil 2000mg daily; • Long Life IMPERIAL TONIC with royal jelly and evening primrose oil; • Twin Lab MAX-EPA; • Nature's Secret ULTIMATE OIL; • Omega Nutrition ESSENTIAL BALANCE OIL, caps and liquid.

5—Boost nutrient intake: • Futurebiotics VITAL SUPPORT FOR PEOPLE OVER 35; • Country Life MAX FOR MEN; • Nature's Herbs MALE VITE; • Cal-mag-zinc 4 daily; • Zinc 75mg daily; • selenium, 200mcg; • vitamin E, 400 IU; • magnesium 750 mg. Note: An extremely low fat diet is disastrous for andropausal health. It may reduce testosterone levels almost to preadolescent levels – bad news for an older man!

Lifestyle Support Therapy

—Bodywork techniques for hormone balance:
• Massage therapy reestablishes unblocked meridians of energy and increases circulation.
• Deep abdominal breathing - page 554.
• Yoga stretches every morning.
• Exercise is vital to male hormone health.
• Get morning sunlight on the body every day possible, on the genitalia for men.
• Smoking disrupts hormones activity.
• Muscle Testing (Applied Kinesiology), is useful for determining which hormonal herbs or supplements are specific to your problem. Once you learn the simple technique (see a nutritional consultant, a holistic chiropractor, a massage therapist), you can easily do it at home to decide which products are right for you.

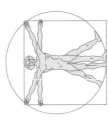

Common Symptoms: Prostate pain and inflammation; lack of abdominal tone; poor urinary and sexual function.
Common Causes: A vasectomy; adrenal exhaustion due to stress; severe dieting or body building; surgery or long illness; protein or iodine deficiency; calcium deficiency; B Complex or EFA deficiencies; synthetic steroid use.

For saliva hormone testing, Dr. David Zava, Ph.D., ZRT Laboratory, 503-469-0741, fax 503-469-1305, Address: ZRT Laboratory, 12505 NW Cornell Rd., Portland, OR

Can't find a recommended product? Call the 800 number listed in Product Resources for the store nearest you.

Andropause

These needs of the male body increase as a man approaches andropause. Men need a high energy diet to keep active as they grow older, plenty of nutrients to retain sexual potency, and proteins to maintain muscle mass. If you're in andropause, consider natural therapies as an effective way to renew vitality. Men I've talked to who are using them report better energy, increased stamina and more sexual satisfaction.

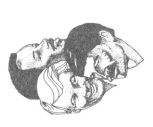

Are you in andropause? Signs to watch for:

—Is your energy unusually low lately? Is your work output or sports performance less than you're used to?

—Have you lost height? Are your shoulders slightly hunching? (a sign of early osteoporosis) Get a side view in your mirror.

—Has your beard or head hair growth slowed? Is your chest hair getting sparse but ear hair increasing?

—Have you lost muscle mass? Has you strength or endurance decreased?

—Is your urination frequent and/or difficult, especially at night? (a sign of an enlarged prostate)

—Are your erections less strong or less frequent? Is your sex drive lower than normal for you?

—Are you anxious about your well-being and your future?

Natural Therapies Renew Male Vitality

—**Diet improvements (even if your diet is okay) are essential.**

1: Reduce fried foods, red meats and fatty dairy foods (full of disrupting hormones), caffeine and sugar – all deplete the adrenals and drain male energy.

2: Don't go too far. An extremely low fat diet is disastrous for andropausal health. Recent studies find it may reduce testosterone levels almost to preadolescent levels – not good news for an older man! Include healthy fats from seafood instead, and lean, hormone-free turkey and chicken regularly. Flax seed oil is a healthy oil to use in salad dressings. (Use about 1 TB)

3: Increase your intake of zinc to renew sexual potency. Zinc, highly concentrated in semen, is the most important nutrient for male sexual function. Eat high zinc foods like liver, oysters, brewer's yeast, nuts and seeds regularly. Add zinc-rich spirulina to your superfood supplement list, and try •Source Naturals OPTI-ZINC caps.

4: Add more high energy foods like complex carbohydrates from whole grains, legumes, and fresh fruits and vegetables. Add a superfood drink each afternoon for concentrated "green" nutrition like •Crystal Star ENERGY GREEN™ drink to reduce any craving for high fat junk foods. •Transitions EASY GREENS is another good choice.

—**Take care of your prostate.** Many men don't realize how much they can relieve prostate problems without drugs. The pharmaceutical industry isn't going to tell them! In Europe, botanical medicines are the first-choice treatments for men instead of drugs. Some prostate drugs, like Proscar, can cause impotence and decreased libido! **For the majority of prostate problem, drugs are unnecessary!** Herbs like *saw palmetto* and *pygeum* show excellent results in wide clinical trials. Here's why: As men grow older they tend to accumulate more of the rogue testosterone, dihydrotestosterone (DHT), which causes cells to multiply and the prostate to enlarge. The Quarterly Review of Natural Medicine finds *saw palmetto* reduces the symptoms of BPH by blocking DHT, inhibiting the enzyme 5alpha reductase related to prostate enlargement. Consider •Crystal Star PRO✗™ FOR MEN or •Morada Research Laboratories PROSTATE to help reduce prostate enlargement and dribbling urine symptoms. (Usually improvement in 48 hours.) Check your alcohol intake. Heavy drinking can lead to prostate problems and impaired erections. Dr. Howard Peiper's book Natural Solutions For Sexual Enhancement, says "alcohol, especially beer, elevates levels of DHT in the body and can be a contributing factor in sexual dysfunction." DHT elevation is linked to testosterone decline and elevation of female hormones.... definitely undesirable for men.

—**Build muscle mass.** Take a high protein drink every morning to build muscle mass and stamina. •Nutritional Tech. ESSENTIAL WHEY has branch-chain amino acids, leucine, isoleucine and valine - ideal for building muscle protein. Before you turn to a drug-based growth hormone supplement, consider L-glutamine 1000mg 3 to 4x daily. It helps your pituitary stimulate your own growth hormone - for some men dramatically. Add a glutamine fortified body builder like Unipro   , to improve muscle tone.

—**Renew sexual potency.** Try the Aurvedic herb •*tribulus terrestris*, to boost libido and impotence in men. Athletes like its benefits of increased strength and stamina. Try •Nutritional Tech. T2 -TRIBULUS TERRESTIS, or •Natural Balance COBRA, or •Crystal Star MALE PERFORMANCE™ caps with a long history of success for enhancing the sexual experience. In one study, 78 healthy, but sedentary men were studied during nine months of regular exercise. The men exercised 60 minutes a day, three days a week. **Every single man** reported significantly enhanced sexuality, including increased frequency, performance and satisfaction. Rising sexuality was even correlated with degree of fitness improvement. The more fitness the men were able to attain, the better their sex life!

—**Don't forget regular exercise.** It's a vital component of male sexuality. It makes your body stronger, function better and endure longer. I've talked to many men over 40, working stressful jobs with major family responsibilities who just can't keep it up anymore because their adrenals are shot from years of abuse. If you tend to eat fast foods on the run, drink a lot of coffee and get little sleep you're setting your body up for an adrenal crash. Adrenal exhaustion for men sometimes precipitates depression and severe stress reactions. Crystal Star •ADRN™ extract has a long history of success in restoring a man's energy and vitality.

—**Feed your adrenals.** Men need healthy adrenals to keep active and energized as testosterone levels begin to decline.

See next page and Prostate Health, page 483 for more information.

Can't find a recommended product? Call the 800 number listed in Product Resources for the store nearest you.

What about environmental hormones and male hormone problems?

Women aren't the only ones endangered by the estrogen-imitating effects of chemicals and pesticides. There is substantial evidence that man-made estrogens threaten male health and fertility, too. An unusually large number of male babies (both animals and human) are showing up with male feminization (small testicles, low sperm count, and miniature penises), a trend many scientists believe is directly related to chemicals in our environment. The dramatic rise in prostate cancer deaths over the last 40 years is another wake-up call to change our environment for health.

While the rate of prostate cancer has doubled since World War II, male sperm counts have declined by half - a trend that has led to speculation that environmental, dietary, and lifestyle changes in recent decades are interfering with a man's ability to make sperm. Semen analysis tests over the last few decades show undeniably that total sperm count as well as sperm quality of the general male population has been deteriorating. In 1940, the average sperm count was 113 million per ml. In 1993 that value had dropped to 65 million. Total amount of semen has also fallen dramatically, from 3.5ml in 1940 to 2.74ml in 1993. Today men have only about 39% of the sperm counts they had in 1940. For the first time in America's history, one in six married couples of childbearing age has trouble conceiving and completing a successful pregnancy.

Pollutants used to be considered strictly estrogenic, like poly-chlorinated bi-phenols (PCBs), as well as dioxin and pesticides used for agriculture. New reports reveal environmental androgens in pollutants (substances that mimic male sex hormone) are much more widespread than previously thought. Vanderbilt University School of Medicine found that of ten pollutants, 5 bound to the androgen receptor while only 2 bound to the estrogen receptor. Men can really benefit from adding more dietary fiber from whole grains, fresh fruits and vegetables that can bind to and eliminate hormone-disrupting pollutants lodged in their bodies. Always wash commercial produce thoroughly to reduce harmful pollutant residues and buy organic whenever possible. The produce sections in health food stores are like gold, not just in terms of taste and local freshness but in the concept that good food really is good medicine!

What about male impotence?

Impotence affects 52% of U.S. men between 40 and 70 years of age? It says a lot for the state of men's bodies today. Viagra was one of the first new designer drugs to be marketed directly to the public through advertising. It was and is promoted as a love aid for impotent men and its phenomenal success says a lot about the state of male reproductive health in our world today. The fact that it is a powerful, potentially dangerous drug has been vastly understated in the public advertising. Viagra is a citrate salt taken orally. It enhances the physical mechanism needed for erection, producing smooth muscle relaxation and increasing circulation to the penis. It is useful for some cases of impotence caused by spinal cord injuries, diabetes or radical prostatectomies. Viagra reached $1 billion in sales in just its first year with a potential of up to $11 billion a year. Viagra's manufacturer is developing faster acting versions of the drug. Other drug companies are developing a Viagra rival to tempt both the male and female libido. **Does Viagra mean better sex?** More than a year into the Viagra craze we see that enhancing sexuality through drug chemistry is not what we thought it was. It's much more in terms of danger and much less in terms of help for impotence. Side effects and risks surfaced almost immediately. At this writing there have been over 130 Viagra-related deaths- from massive cardiac arrest, stroke, cardiovascular complications or drug interactions. Although the company that manufactures Viagra maintains it's safe if used properly, the reports speak for themselves.

Can natural therapies help if you're impotent? Unless you have a clear medical condition, better libido results not from a pill, but from a good lifestyle program. Many sexual difficulties often begin in the dining room, from stress and a poor diet, not the bedroom. Atherosclerosis, clearly related to diet, can block blood supply to the penile artery, is the primary cause of impotence in nearly half of men over 50! Diabetes, smoking, overuse of alcohol or sedatives, and anti-depressant drugs or high blood pressure medicines regularly cause impotence. Sexual function depends on healthy glands and organs to produce sex hormones. Herbs work through the glands to rebalance and nourish. Herbs enhance and enrich sexual feelings and activity, but they do not overwhelm or instigate it, like some drugs. Ginkgo biloba improves circulation, increases vascular strength and reverses atherosclerosis impotence. In one study, ginkgo was 30% more effective than drug injections with 50% of patients showing regained potency. Take the whole herb extract, about 15 drops under the tongue, 2 or 3 times a day.

What about vasectomies?

Science has long debated whether a vasectomy, the contraceptive procedure which severs or seals off the vessel that carries sperm from the testes, increases the risk of prostate cancer in men. New studies on two large groups of men, show that vasectomies do increase risk of prostate cancer. In one study of 73,000 men, 300 of the men developed prostate cancer between 1986 and 1990. The men with vasectomies had a 66% greater risk of prostate cancer than did the men without vasectomies. In a separate study, vasectomies increased the risk of prostate cancer by 56%. As sperm builds up in the sealed-off vas deferens after a vasectomy, the body re-absorbs the cells. This confuses the immune system, making it less alert to tumor cells. Sometimes the body's immune defenses try to mount a response against its own tissue. A vasectomy also affects testical secretions and lowers prostatic fluid. When the natural movement of sperm and hormones is artificially prevented, a host of male health problems result.

See Libido and Sexuality page 488 for more information.

Can't find a recommended product? Call the 800 number listed in Product Resources for the store nearest you.

Uncovering the truth about the new "superhormone revolution."

There is a "superhormone revolution" sweeping the U.S. today. Drug companies are selling hormones like they were vitamins or beauty aids! Every day they tempt us to try new and different hormones. They're selling big promises: Beauty, a long life span or recharged sexuality. Some "hormone authorities" even recommend taking a concoction of several hormones, called a hormone cocktail. Americans are loading up on hormones to deal with today's lifestyle disorders. Thousands of us are swallowing down DHEA, melatonin, pregnenolone, human hGH growth hormone, testosterone, estrogen, progesterone, and thyroid hormone (now, that's a mouthful of hormones!) - all in the hope of finding the "silver bullet" to protect our health.

Drug companies tell us that superhormones will enable us to be healthy and live to the ripe-old age of 120. Some once-conservative medical doctors even say that the money spent on diet, exercise, herbal remedies and drugs is wasted...and that superhormone supplements are the sole pillar for vital health. It's a sensationalized spin that has truly created a hormone circus!

What's driving the superhormone revolution? America's baby boomers are the force behind the billion dollar hormone dance. As they cross the 50-yard line of life, the realities of aging are staring boomers in the face. They're demanding new answers- and lots of change. So it shouldn't come as a surprise that hormones are a megabucks business. The most prescribed drug in the U.S. today is Premarin, an estrogen replacement drug, DHEA, pregnenolone and ANDRO are rising stars in the supplement hormone world, already generating over $325 million in sales annually. Don't be fooled. They may be sold over-the-counter, but these hormones are drugs with hidden dangers and big reactions! Regard them with respect and caution.

There is no doubt that hormones play a dramatic role in human health or that hormone production slows down with age. But I don't believe a cabinet full of superhormone supplements and drugs is the best choice for most people. Hormones are incredibly minute glandular secretions, produced from body chemical substances called steroids which affect the part of the brain that influences sexual behavior. Hormones regulate everything from energy flow, to inflammation, to a woman's monthly cycle, to a man's hair growth. They are tricky, even dangerous, substances to work with. Tiny amounts can cause big reactions, both good and bad. Hormone drugs often disrupt hormone balance further and can lead to many hormone-driven problems including breast and uterine cancer.

Why are our hormones so imbalanced? Hormone imbalance disorders are raging through this country. We see hormone imbalance in women's disorders like PMS, endometriosis and fibroids, and men's disorders like impotence, prostate enlargement, and male andropause. Women with hysterectomies are only beginning to see the harm that removing delicate glands, or treating fragile hormones with drugs can do. Bone loss in both sexes is related to hormone imbalance. The major factors in hormone imbalance disorders are: body assault from hormone disrupting chemicals in foods, drugs and pollutants (nearly 40% of pesticides used in commercial agriculture are suspected hormone disrupters!); trauma, stress or illness; a poorly functioning liver (the liver metabolizes excess estrogen); a high fat diet (excess fat harbors hormones); poor glandular function; and a diet high in refined "non food" refined, chemicalized foods that the body rejects or ignores.

There is plenty you may not know about superhormones...

—**fiction:** *Over-the-counter superhormones like DHEA, melatonin and ANDRO are natural substances.*

fact: ALL over-the-counter hormone supplements are produced in a lab, even when they start out with a plant extraction or animal glandular material.

—**fiction:** *They are safe for regular use.*

fact: Side effects are common with superhormones. Their long range effects on human health are unknown. Deep hormone balance can be affected. Taking hormones as if they were vitamins is playing Russian Roulette with your health, especially for athletes who usually combine more than one highly concentrated, stimulant or hormone (both legal or illegal).

—**fiction:** *Superhormones will make a man a superman or a woman a love slave.*

fact: There are times when taking supplemental hormones is okay, as for an acute situation or a short term need. The proper usage of superhormones can lead to dramatic improvements in health and quality of life. Still, I believe that advertising hormones as cosmetics is both irresponsible and misguided. Carelessly taking high dosages of superhormones may be counterproductive, perhaps even dangerous, as we have seen with Viagra. When you begin mixing hormone-like steroidal substances in your body, you are changing your natural body chemistry. I have seen some of the unpleasant side effects like female chest hair growth and bloody urine for myself. I believe a better choice is subtle, safe foods or herbs that contain plant hormones, especially for healthy people with normal hormone levels. Many are remarkably similar to human hormones and can even be taken up by human hormone receptor sites!

What About Plant or Phyto-Hormones?

Plant or phyto-hormones are remarkably similar to human hormones. They can be accepted by hormone receptor sites in our bodies, and, at $1/400th$ to $1/50,000th$ the strength of human hormones, they are extremely gentle and safe, exerting a tonic effect rather than drug-like activity. Although used for centuries by both men and women, we are just beginning to understand their power for modern needs. Studies on soy foods and herbs such as ginseng, *black cohosh* and *wild yam* clearly show hormone-normalizing effects.

See MENOPAUSE pages for more complete information about both synthetic and phytohormones.

Can't find a recommended product? Call the 800 number listed in Product Resources for the store nearest you.

Hypoglycemia
Low Blood Sugar

Hypoglycemia and diabetes stem from the same causes. Hypoglycemia is regularly a way station on the road to diabetes. Often called a "sugar epidemic" today, hypoglycemia is a condition in which the pancreas overreacts to repeated high sugar intake by producing too much insulin. The excess insulin lowers blood sugar too much as the body strives to achieve proper glucose/insulin balance. This is particularly harmful to the brain, the most sensitive organ to blood sugar levels, which requires glucose as an energy source to think clearly. Hypoglycemia causes a change in the way the brain functions. Small fluctuations disturb one's feeling of wellbeing. Large fluctuations cause feelings of depression, anxiety, mood swings, fatigue even aggressive behavior. Sugar balance is also needed for muscle contractions, the digestive system and nerve health.

Diet & Superfood Therapy

—Nutritional therapy plan:

1—Nutrient deficiencies always accompany hypoglycemia. A healthy diet is critical.

2—Go on a 24 hour liquid diet (pg. 192) if low blood sugar symptoms appear regularly. Add a high nutrient, sugar-free protein powder (see below). A feeling of wellbeing will return rapidly.

3—Avoid all sugary foods, even natural sugars, like honey, molasses or maple syrup until sugar balance is achieved. Reduce dairy foods, fried, fatty foods, fast foods, pastries, red and prepared meats.

4—Eliminate alcohol (the worst for hypoglycemics), refined foods, caffeine, preserved foods and red meats permanently.

5—Complex carbohydrate, high fiber foods, like whole grains, fresh fruits and vegetables, make it easier for the body to handle glucose and help stabilize blood sugar swings.

6—Include some vegetable protein at every meal. Eat low fat dairy products, seafoods, sea greens, soy foods and brown rice frequently. Add cultured foods such as yogurt and kefir for G.I. flora.

—Effective superfoods: protein drinks help build a "floor" under a sugar drop.
• Solgar WHEY TO GO protein.
• Unipro PERFECT PROTEIN drink.
• Crystal Star ENERGY GREEN™ drink.
• Lewis Labs BREWER'S YEAST (B-complex).

Herb & Supplement Therapy

—Interceptive therapy plan: (Choose several recommendations)

1—Help your body rebalance sugar levels: •Crystal Star SUGAR STRATEGY LOW™ capsules and tea; •Crystal Star GINSENG 6 SUPER TEA™ helps remove sugar from the blood; •Crystal Star CHO-LO FIBER TONE™ or other fiber cleanse morning and evening to absorb excess carbohydrates and balance sugar curve. •Vitamin C 3000mg with bioflavonoids or Ethical Nutrients SUPER FLAVONOID C. (Take vitamin C immediately during an attack).

2—Adrenal tonics help the body handle stress: •Crystal Star ADR-ACTIVE™ caps or ADRN™ extract nourishes exhausted adrenals; •Beehive Botanical or Y.S. ROYAL JELLY with ginseng caps or drink; •Gotu kola caps, 2 daily. •Country Life GLYCEMIC FACTORS and MOOD FACTORS capsules; •Transformation ULTRA-ZYME to support adrenals; •Enzymatic Therapy RAW ADRENAL extract; •Evening Primrose Oil caps 2000mg; •B Complex 100mg 2x daily with extra PABA 100mg, and pantothenic acid 500mg.

3—Help stabilize blood sugar swings: •Glutamine 500mg daily. •Crystal Star GINSENG-LICORICE ELIXIR™ drops as needed; •1 teasp. each: spirulina granules and bee pollen granules in a fruit juice, or •Nutrex HAWAIIAN SPIRULINA, between meals. •Take AloeLife ALOE GOLD concentrate 1 teasp. 3x daily before meals (add pinches of cinnamon, ginger and nutmeg to help control cravings).

4—Enzyme therapy is important: Glucose homeostasis depends on using a wide range of micro-nutrients - many of which are in short supply in the American diet. •CoQ-10 60mg 3x daily for 3-6 weeks; •Pancreatin 1200mg with meals; •Prevail GLUCOSE FORMULA; •Alta Health CANGEST before meals for carbohydrate digestion, especially if candida yeast is also a problem.

5—Chromium may be critical: Chromium therapy choices include •GTF Chromium 200mcg; •Solaray CHROMIACIN; •Chromium picolinate 200mcg daily; •Premier Labs VANADIUM, 25mcg; •Country Life DMG B₁₅ 125mg sublingual.

6—Add minerals: •Mezotrace SEA MINERAL COMPLEX daily or •Nature's Path TRACE-LYTE liquid minerals in juice.

Lifestyle Support Therapy

—Lifestyle measures:
• Lifestyle changes for hypoglycemia pay off handsomely for total health, too.
• Eat 6 to 8 mini-meals throughout the day to keep blood sugar levels up. Large meals throw sugar balance way off, especially at night.
• Eat relaxed, never under stress.
• Relaxation techniques that are successful for hypoglycemia include regular massage therapy treatments.

—Bodywork:
Get some exercise everyday to work off unmetabolized acid wastes.
• Some oral contraceptives can cause glucose intolerance and poor sugar metabolism. Ask your doctor.

—Reflexology point:

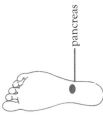

pancreas

See next page and Low Blood Sugar Test on page 544 for more information.

Can't find a recommended product? Call the 800 number listed in Product Resources for the store nearest you.

Common Symptoms: Manic/depressive psychological states; irritability, often violence; restlessness and insomnia; anxiety, depression and a feeling of going crazy; dizziness, general shakiness and trembling; ravenous hunger and craving for sweets; heart problems; lethargy or hyperactivity; nausea; blurry vision; frequent headaches or migraines; unusual night time urination; great fatigue.

Common Causes: Poor diet or excess dietary sugar causing abnormally low levels of glucose in the blood; poor pancreas function; drinking alcohol on an empty stomach; prolonged fasting or dieting for weight loss; food allergies; too much alcohol, caffeine or nicotine; stress; exhausted adrenals, kidney failure or liver damage; hypothyroidism; too large meals.

Hypoglycemia sufferers beware! Sugar and sweeteners are in almost everything you eat today.

Hidden sugars like "high fructose corn syrup," (in almost all commercial sodas and juices today), can be a health hazard if you are hypoglycemic. New studies show that sodas sweetened with high fructose corn syrup, cause mineral loss, especially phosphorous and calcium, which may contribute to osteoporosis. Studies from Israel reveal that rats fed a high fructose diet age faster with premature skin wrinkling and sagging.

Even more frightening, new studies are pouring in on sugar-free artificial sweeteners like aspartame in Equal which many people think are healthier than sugar. These sweeteners are actually chemicals that may be interacting with our normal body processes to set up an environment for illnesses like lupus, multiple sclerosis and Alzheimer's disease. In fact, aspartame sweetener has received more complaints about adverse reactions than any other food ingredient in FDA history. Aspartame's major brand names, NutraSweet and Equal, have taken the place of saccharin in pre-prepared foods and drinks, and that means we get a lot of it. Some people have serious reactions from aspartame – extreme dizziness, headaches, throat swelling, allergic reactions and retina deterioration are just a few documented side effects. The Conference of the American College of Physicians says aspartame is causing a plague of neurological diseases in this country. Pregnant and lactating women, toddlers or allergy-prone children, and those with PKU, should definitely avoid aspartame products.

In 1999, World Environmental Conference scientists presented new information on aspartame's side effects: If aspartame's temperature exceeds 86° F, its wood alcohol converts to formaldehyde. Formaldehyde causes methanol toxicity in the body, accumulating in the retina causing blurred or tunnel vision, visual disturbances like bright flashes or black spots and may cause retinal bleeding. Over time, body methanol toxicity mimics the symptoms of multiple sclerosis (MS), lupus and fibromyalgia. The conference believed that many cases of M.S. and lupus may actually be misdiagnosed "Aspartame disease." Aspartame also alters delicate brain chemistry, leading to memory loss and brain damage, and aggravating Parkinson's disease and increasing Alzheimer's risk. This is especially important news for the elderly who consume chemically sweetened beverages at record levels. Eliminating aspartame offers complete remission of symptoms for some people.

Amazingly enough, Gulf War Syndrome may be directly related aspartame poisoning! Diet sodas sweetened with aspartame were left sitting in the blistering desert heat for weeks at a time for our troops in Desert Storm. By the time, our soldiers drank them, aspartame's chemical structure was so altered by the heat, the soldiers got sick almost immediately.

Brain tumors rates have increased by 10% since aspartame was added to our food supply, statistics adding validation to studies done in the 70's with lab animals who were fed aspartame, then showed unusually high numbers of brain tumors. Sadly, the very people for whom artificial sweeteners are developed are its biggest victims. Aspartame, 200 times sweeter than sugar, keeps blood sugar levels out of control by disrupting the way your body uses insulin. Diabetes and hypoglycemia may progress and worsen. Some diabetic patients have suffered severe reactions after switching to aspartame sweeteners.

Over 5,000 products containing this poison and since the patent has recently expired, you'll more than likely be seeing even more aspartames in foods soon. Read labels carefully!

Diet For Hypoglycemia Control

The key factors in hypoglycemia are stress and poor diet... both a result of too much sugar and refined carbohydrates. These foods quickly raise glucose levels, causing the pancreas to over-compensate and produce too much insulin, which then lowers body glucose levels too far and too fast. The diet on this page supplies your body with fiber, complex carbohydrates and proteins - slow even-burning fuel that prevents the sudden sugar elevations and drops. Eat small frequent meals, with plenty of fresh foods to keep sugar levels in balance. I recommend a diet like this for 2 to 3 months until blood sugar levels are regularly stable.

Other watchwords: 1) Eat potassium-rich foods: oranges, broccoli, bananas, and tomatoes. 2) Eat chromium-rich foods: brewer's yeast, mushrooms, whole wheat, sea foods, beans and peas. 3) Eat high quality vegetable protein at every meal.

On rising: take a "hypoglycemia cocktail:" 1 teasp. each in apple or orange juice to control morning sugar drop: glycine powder, powdered milk, protein powder, and brewer's yeast; or a protein/amino drink, such as Mona's CHLORELLA, Wakunaga KYO-GREEN with EFA's, or Crystal Star SYSTEMS STRENGTH™.

Breakfast: an important meal for hypoglycemia - include ⅓ of daily nutrients; have oatmeal with yogurt and fresh fruit; or poached or baked eggs on whole grain toast with butter or kefir cheese; or whole grain cereal or pancakes with apple juice, soy milk, fruit, yogurt, nuts or fruit sauce; or tofu scrambled "eggs" with bran muffins, whole grain toast and butter.

Mid-morning: have a veggie drink (page 218), Green Foods GREEN MAGMA with 1 teasp. Bragg's LIQUID AMINOS, or Crystal Star ENERGY GREEN™ drink as a liver nutrient; or a sugar balancing herb tea, such as *licorice*, *dandelion*, or Crystal Star SUGAR STRATEGY LOW™ tea; and some crisp, crunchy vegetables with kefir or yogurt cheese;

Lunch: have a fresh salad, with cottage cheese or soy cheese, nuts, noodle or seed toppings, and lemon oil dressing; or a high protein sandwich on whole grain bread, with avocados, low fat cheese; or a bean or lentil soup with tofu or shrimp salad or sandwich; or a seafood and whole grain pasta salad; or a vegetarian pizza on a chapati crust with low fat cheese.

Mid-afternoon: have a hard boiled egg with sesame salt, and whole grain crackers with yogurt dip; or a *licorice* herb tea, such as Crystal Star GINSENG/LICORICE ELIXIR™ in water, another green drink, such as Vibrant Health GREEN VIBRANCE™ with spirulina; or yogurt with nuts and seeds.

Dinner: have some steamed veggies with tofu, or baked or broiled fish and brown rice; or an oriental stir fry with seafood and vegetables; or a vegetable Italian pasta dish with verde sauce and hearty soup (add green beans for pancreatic support); or a Spanish beans and rice dish, or paella with seafood and rice; or a veggie quiche and a small mushroom and spinach salad.

Before bed: have a cup of Sovex nutritional yeast or miso broth; or papaya juice with a little yogurt.

See *Sugars and Sweeteners in a Healing Diet* page 169 for more.

Can't find a recommended product? Call the 800 number listed in Product Resources for the store nearest you.

Hypothyroidism
Sluggish Thyroid, Goiter

Hypothyroidism affects over 5 million Americans, most commonly striking women between the ages 30-50. In infants, malfunctioning of the thyroid gland is called cretinism, marked by mental retardation and dwarfism. In hypothyroidism, the thyroid gland ceases to produce adequate thyroid hormone to meet the body's demands. An amazing 10% of women are deficient in thyroid hormone! New statistics show 15 to 20% of women over 60 have some degree of hypothyroidism. Metabolism slows and virtually every cell in the body is affected. At its worst, this disease can completely destroy the thyroid gland. Conventional treatment for adults is a lifelong prescription of thyroid hormone, levothyroxine (Synthroid), linked to severe headaches, insomnia, bone loss and tachycardia (rapid contractions of the heart).

Diet & Superfood Therapy

—**Nutritional therapy plan:**

1—Follow a 75% fresh foods diet for a month to rebalance metabolism. Have a green salad daily.

2—Eat plenty of iodine-rich foods: sea greens, sea foods, fish, mushrooms, garlic, onions and watercress. Use iodine-rich herb salt or sea greens instead of table salt.

3—Eat vitamin A-rich foods: yellow vegetables, eggs, carrots, dark green vegetables, raw dairy.

4—A veggie drink (pg. 218) or a potassium broth (pg. 215) twice a week. (See superfoods below.)

5—Avoid refined foods, saturated fats, sugars, white flour and red meats.

6—Avoid "goitrogens," foods that prevent the use of iodine: cabbage, turnips, peanuts, mustard, pine nuts, millet and soy products. (Cooking these foods inactivates the goitrogens.)

7—Take 2 TBS lecithin granules daily over whole grain cereal for memory boosting nutrients.

—**Superfood therapy: (choose 1 or more)**
• Crystal Star SYSTEMS STRENGTH™ drink or capsules daily for 2 to 3 months.
• Body Ecology VITALITY SUPER GREEN.
• Pines MIGHTY GREENS.
• Green Foods WHEAT GERM extract.
• Sun Wellness CHLORELLA drink or tabs daily.
• Transitions EASY GREENS drink.
• Wakunaga KYO-GREEN with EFA's.

Herb & Supplement Therapy

Do not take iron with thyroid medication. It binds up the thyroxine, rendering it insoluble.

—**Interceptive therapy plan: (Choose 2 to 4 recommendations)**

1—**Increase thyroid activity:** The thyroid needs body iodine to produce its hormones. An imbalanced thyroid causes excess estrogen production with numerous problems for women. **Herbal iodine sources are effective without side effects:**
• Crystal Star IODINE SOURCE™ extract or • IODINE-POTASSIUM™ caps 2x daily, or • META-TABS 2 daily; • Ethical Nutrients THYRO-VITAL; • Solaray ALFA JUICE caps; • Enzymatic Therapy ENZODINE or THYROID/TYROSINE COMPLEX; or • Tyrosine 500mg with L-lysine 500mg 2x daily, or • Taurine 500mg with L-lysine 500mg 2x daily. • Kelp tabs 8 daily, with cayenne 3 daily.

Natural glandular therapy: Natural thyroid hormone replacement more closely resembles human thyroid hormones. • Nutri-PAK thyroxin-free double strength thyroid. • Nutricology TG100 or • Jones Medical NATURE-THROID. Use under the supervision of a health professional. • Raw Thyroid complex, or • Raw Thymus glandular; • Transitions PRO-GEST natural progesterone cream.

2—**Support your adrenals to help your thyroid:** • Crystal Star ADRN-ACTIVE™ extract 2x daily; or • Country Life ADRENAL COMPLEX with tyrosine. • Evening Primrose oil, 2000mg daily. • Siberian ginseng extract 2000mg daily, or • Rainbow Light ADAPTOGEM, or • Planetary Formulas SCHIZANDRA ADRENAL SUPPORT.

3—**Stop thyroid destruction with antioxidants:** • CoQ$_{10}$ 100mg daily; • Country Life sublingual B-12, 2500mcg daily; • Emulsified A 25,000IU 3x daily; • Vitamin E 400IU daily; • Ascorbate vitamin C with bioflavonoids 3000mg daily.

4—**For goiter:** apply • BLACK WALNUT extract as a throat paint, and take ¹/₂ dropperful 2x daily; apply • calendula compresses twice a day for a month.

5—**Improve memory and mental function with EFA's:** For women, • EVENING PRIMROSE OIL 1,000 mg. 3x daily; For men, • flax seed oil 2 TBS daily. • Ginkgo Biloba extract 2x daily; • Herbal Magic GINSENG-GINKGO REJUVENATOR twice daily. • Country Life Magnesium-potassium-bromelain, 2 daily; • Zinc 75mg daily.

Lifestyle Support Therapy

• The drug levothyroxine, frequently given for hypothyroidism can cause significant bone loss. Ask your doctor. Avoid antihistamines and sulfa drugs.

• Low thyroid levels affect your child's IQ. Studies show children born to mothers with underactive thyroids have IQ's 7 points lower than children born to healthy mothers!

—**Bodywork:**
• Take a brisk half hour walk daily; exercise increases metabolism and stimulates circulation.
• Sun bathe in the morning. Sea bathe and wade whenever possible.
• Color therapy: for hypothyroid, wear orange glasses 30 min; switch to blue for 5 min.
• Avoid fluorescent lights and fluoride toothpaste. They deplete vitamin A in the body.

—**Acupressure point:**
Press hollow at base of the throat to stimulate thyroid, 3x for 10 seconds each.

—**Reflexology point:**

Thyroid-Thymus

H 428

Common Symptoms: Unrelenting fatigue; moderate weight gain; slow heart rate; hands, feet and ears becoming cold easily; yellowish color on hands and feet; swollen thyroid gland (goiter); hair loss; constipation; heavy menses; dry skin and hair; poor memory; depression; and changes in personality. If you think you might have hypothyroidism, a simple blood tests from your physician can confirm diagnosis. Goiter symptoms include enlargement of the thyroid gland, usually a woman's problem.
Common Causes: Hashimoto's thyroiditis; iodine deficiency from X-rays or low dose radiation (such as mammograms); excessive dieting; heredity. Cancer of the thyroid has been linked to highly fluoridated water.

See Taking Your Basal Temperature page 552, HASHIMOTO'S DISEASE page 402 and SLUGGISH THYROID page 537 for more.

Can't find a recommended product? Call the 800 number listed in Product Resources for the store nearest you.

Immune Response
Building Stronger Immunity

Your immune system is your bodyguard. It works both pro-actively and protectively to shield you from anything in your world that threatens your life and limb. The main elements of the immune system are the thymus gland, bone marrow, the spleen, the complement system of enzymatic proteins, and the lymphatic system with white blood cells and lymphocytes, the backbone of immune defenses. Your immune system is ever-vigilant, constantly searching for proteins, called antigens, that don't belong in your body. It can deal with a wide range of pathogens - viruses, funguses, bacteria and parasites. It can even recognize potential antigens, such as drugs, pollens, insect venoms and chemicals in foods, and malignant cells and foreign tissue, such as transplanted organs or transfused blood. (See next page for more.)

Diet & Superfood Therapy

—Nutritional therapy plan for prevention:

1—The American diet of processed foods, 20% sugars and 37% fat, suppresses immunity. Saturated fats in pastries, fried foods, and red meats are the worst culprits. Reduce dairy and sugary foods.

2—Take a protein drink each morning. (pg. 276).

3—Eat plenty of fresh foods, fiber foods, whole grains, sea foods, eggs and cultured dairy foods, like yogurt and kefir for friendly G.I. flora.

4—Food enzymes are basic to immune response. Include a cup of green tea, fresh fruits and vegetables in your diet every day. Especially include enzyme-rich sprouts, garlic, papaya and sea greens.

5—Environmental pollutants, particularly pesticides, lower immunity. Eat organically grown foods whenever possible.

—Immune-enhancing superfoods:

• Green superfoods supply a "mini-transfusion" to detoxify your bloodstream. Mona's CHLO-RELLA, Green Foods GREEN MAGMA, Rainbow Light HAWAIIAN SPIRULINA, *wheat grass, spirulina,* or Crystal Star ENERGY GREEN™.

• Crystal Star BIOFLAVONOID, FIBER & C drink and GREEN TEA CLEANSER™.

• AloeLife ALOE GOLD JUICE.

• Solgar EARTH SOURCE GREENS - MORE.

• Unipro PERFECT PROTEIN.

• BioStrath YEAST ELIXIR w. HERBS.

Herb & Supplement Therapy

—Interceptive therapy plan: (Choose 2 to 3 recommendations)

1—**Stimulate white blood cell activity with natural antibiotics:** • Allergy Research Group LACTOFERRIN caps with colostrum; Olive Leaf extract as directed; • NAC (N-acetyl-cysteine) 600mg daily; • DMG (N-dimethyl-glycine) about 100mg daily.

2—**Immune modulators act as response tonics:** • Crystal Star HERBAL DE-FENSE TEAM™ formulas, or • Natural Balance MODUCARE caps for 2 months.

• *Siberian ginseng, • Panax ginseng or • Suma root;* • Propolis caps 3 to 4 daily during high risk seasons; • Earth's Bounty NONI LIQUID; • Herbal Magic IMMUNE SYSTEM KIT™, • Zand HERBAL INSURE extract; • Future Biotics VITAL K.

3—**Enhance your thymus gland activity to stimulate immunity:** • Raw thymus glandular, or • Nature's Path THY-LYTE, or Enzymatic Therapy THYMULUS; or • Nutricology Organic Thymus. (Tap thymus with knuckles each morning to stimulate.)

4—**Enzymes are basic to immune response:** • Biotec CELL GUARD w. SOD 6 daily, or • Solgar SOD 2000 units for 6 weeks; Enzymedica PURIFY; • Milk Thistle Seed extract; or • *Goldenseal - Oregon grape root; • Licorice root* tea for a month.

5—**Sea plants help your body remove toxins with electrolyte minerals:** Sea greens of all kinds, 2 TBS daily, provide therapeutic iodine, potassium and sodium alginate to help purify your body; or take • Crystal Star SYSTEMS STRENGTH™ caps, or • PO-TASSIUM-IODINE sea plant complex; or • Biotec PACIFIC SEA PLASMA tablets 6 daily; • Mezotrace SEA MINERALS; • Nature's Path TRACE-MIN-LYTE (sea greens).

6—**Probiotics provide a strong immune environment:** • Transformation Enzyme PLANTADOPHILUS; • Dr. DOPHILUS + FOS; • Solaray MULTI-DOPHILUS.

7—**Build foundation immune strength with antioxidants:** • PCO's from grapeseed and white pine, 100mg daily, or • Country Life WELL-MAX with PCO's; • vitamin E 400IU with selenium 200mcg; • vitamin C/Ester C with bioflavonoids 3000mg; and zinc 50mg daily; • CoQ₁₀ 60mg 2x daily; • Nutricology GERMANIUM 150mg; • Source Naturals WELLNESS; • MICROHYDRIN, available at Healthy House.

8—**Medicinal mushrooms enhance interferon production:** Reishi, shiitake and maitake mushrooms; • Planetary Formulas REISHI SUPREME, Grifon MAITAKE.

Lifestyle Support Therapy

—Bodywork:

• Relaxation techniques are immune-enhancers. A positive mental attitude makes a big difference in how the body fights disease. Creative visualization establishes belief and optimism. Biofeedback or massage therapy to reduce stress.

• Regular aerobic exercise keeps system oxygen high, and circulation flowing. Disease does not readily overrun a body where oxygen and organic minerals are high in the vital fluids.

• Tobacco/nicotine in any form is an immune depressant. The cadmium content causes zinc deficiency. It takes 3 months to rebuild immune response even after you quit.

• Stimulate immunity by a few minutes of early morning sunlight every day. Avoid excessive sun. A sunburn depresses immunity.

• Get quality rest, immune power builds the most during sleep.

• Stop and smell the roses. A conscious, free-flowing emotional life is fundamental for inner harmony.

• Aromatherapy immune oils: *lavender or rosemary oil.*

• Eliminate recreational drugs. Reduce prescription drugs, especially antibiotics and cortico-steroids that depress immunity.

See the following pages for more information.

Common Symptoms: *Chronic and continuing infections, colds, respiratory problems; Candida yeast overgrowth; chronic fatigue; chronic allergies.*

Common Causes: *Glandular malfunction, usually because of poor diet and nutrition; staph infection; prolonged use of antibiotics and/or cortico-steroids, (long-term use of these drugs can depress the immune system to the point where even minor illness can become life-threatening.); some immunization shots; Candida albicans yeast overgrowth; great emotional stress; food and other allergies; environmental and heavy metal pollutants; radiation.*

Can't find a recommended product? Call the 800 number listed in Product Resources for the store nearest you.

The immune system is the body's most complex and delicately balanced infrastructure.

We hear so much about immune system breakdown today. Yet, most of us don't know very much about it, or how it works. It's really an amazing part of our bodies. While the workings of other body systems have been well known for some time, the complex nature and dynamics of the immune system have been largely a mystery. One of the problems in comprehending immune response is its highly individual nature. It's a personal defense system that comes charging to the rescue at the first sign of an alien force, such as a harmful virus or pathogenic bacteria. Personal immune response shows us that we are the ultimate healer of ourselves.

Most Americans today don't have good immune response to fight off illness. Pollution, drug overload and nutrient-poor diets compromise our immune health even in good weather. So we're already pre-disposed to a life of frequent colds and flu when bad weather rolls in. Stress is a definite culprit in reduced immune response because it affects the production of interferon, your body's natural antiviral agent. People who are under continuous stress from work or their personal lives are 2 and a half times more likely to get a cold or flu infection than other people. You may think you're protected if you've had a flu shot, but think again. Flu shots are only effective for specific flu viruses..... you may be exposed to a different one, or even a brand new one (flu viruses mutate rapidly). That means your shot won't be effective. In any case, follow-up studies show flu shots are only effective for 30% of the population.

Drugs aren't the answer for immune enhancement. The immune system is not responsive to drugs for healing. Even doctors admit that most drugs really just stabilize the body, or arrest a harmful organism, to allow the immune system to gather its forces and take over. Each one of us has a unique immune response system. It would be almost impossible to form a drug for each person. Antibiotics used to fight infections actually depress the immune system when used long-term. Long courses of tetracycline and erythromycin are some of the most common and some of the worst for immune health. But natural nutritive forces, like healing foods and herbal medicines can and do support the immune system. They enhance its activity, strengthen it, and provide an environment through cleansing and detoxification for it to work at its best.

I believe the only way to stay healthy during high risk times is to prepare your body for the defenses it's going to need. Even if you've improved your diet, take another look at it because a super nutritious diet is imperative when you're under attack.

What does the immune system really do?

Immune defense is autonomic, using its own subconscious memory to establish antigens against harmful pathogens. It's a system that works on its own to fend off or neutralize disease toxins, and set up a healing environment for the body. It is this quality of being a part of us, yet not under our conscious control, that is the great power of immune response. It is also the dilemma of medical scientists as they struggle to get control of a system that is all pervasive and yet, in the end, impossible to completely understand. It is as if God shows us his face in this incredibly complex part of us, where we are allowed to glimpse the ultimate mind-body connection.

Maintaining strong immune defenses in today's world is not easy. Daily exposure to environmental pollutants, the emotional and excessive stresses of modern lifestyles, chemicalized foods, and new virus mutations are all a challenge to our immune systems. Devastating, immune compromised diseases are rising all over the world. Reduced immunity is the main factor in opportunistic diseases, like candida albicans, chronic fatigue syndrome, lupus, HIV, hepatitis, mononucleosis, herpes II, sexually transmitted diseases and cancer. These diseases have become the epidemic of our time, and most of us don't have very much to fight with. An overload of antibiotics, antacids, immunizations, cortico-steroid drugs, and environmental pollutants eventually affect immune system balance to the point where it cannot distinguish harmful cells from healthy cells.

I see traditional medicine as "heroic" medicine. Largely developed in wartime, its greatest strengths are emergency measures - the ability to arrest a crisis, destroy or incapacitate pathogenic organisms, reset and re-attach broken body parts, and stabilize the body so it can gather its healing forces. Because drugs work in an attempt to directly kill harmful organisms, it is easy to see that their value would be for emergency measures, and for short term use.

But, three unwanted things often happen with prolonged drug use: 1) Our bodies can build up a tolerance to the drug so that it requires more of it to get the same effect. 2) The drug slowly overwhelms immune response so the body becomes dependent upon it, using it as a crutch instead of doing its own work. 3) The drug misleads our defense system to the point that it doesn't know what to assault, and attacks everything in confusion. This type of over-reaction often happens during an allergy attack, where the immune system may respond to substances that are not really harmful. Most of the time, if we use drugs wisely to stimulate rather than over kill, if we "get out of the way" by keeping our bodies clean and well nourished, the immune system will spend its energies rebuilding instead of fighting, and strengthen us instead of constantly gathering resources to conduct a "rear guard" defense.

The very nature of immune strength means that it must be built from the inside out. The immune system is the body system most sensitive to nutritional deficiencies. Giving your body generous, high quality, natural remedies at the first sign of infection improves your chances of overcoming disease before it takes serious hold. Powerful, immune-enhancing superfoods and herbs can be directed at "early warning" problems to build strength for immune response. Building good immune defenses takes time and commitment, but it is worth it. The inherited immunity and health of you, your children and your grandchildren is laid down by you.

One more thing: Laughter lifts more than your spirits. It also boosts your immune response. Laughter lowers cortisol, an immune suppressor, allowing immunity to function better.

See my book COOKING FOR HEALTHY HEALING *for a complete diet program for immune health.*

Can't find a recommended product? Call the 800 number listed in Product Resources for the store nearest you.

What depresses immune response?

—Long courses of drugs: antacids (reduce nutrient assimilation), antibiotics (destroy friendly bacteria vital to GI immunity), anti-inflammatory drugs like acetaminophen, aspirin and ibuprofen (inhibit white cells that fight infection).

—Long term exposure to second hand smoke, chemicals and other pollutants (put a strain on the body's natural detoxification system and lead to genetic mutations that cause cancer).

—A diet high in refined, chemicalized "foods in a box," so popular today. I call these foods "non food" foods that your body simply rejects or ignores. Fake fats like olestra that rob cancer-fighting carotenoids are especially disrupting.

—Repeated exposure to allergens (from foods, chemicals or environmental allergens) causes the immune system to take a dive because immune defenses are all channeled to deal with the allergen rather than to fight infection. (In turn, allergies are usually the result of impaired immunity.)

—A diet high in trans fatty acids (in deep fried foods, fast foods, and almost all snack foods), saturated fats or refined sugars. Trans fatty acids increase LDL (bad) cholesterol and decrease HDL (good) cholesterol, and have been found at high levels in women with breast cancer. Saturated fats interfere with prostaglandin E1 which regulates efficient T-cell activity. Eating sugary foods suppresses white blood cell activity for a few hours! Eating these foods regularly may mean your immune system is taking a nose dive all day long!

—Low intake of protective, antioxidant and enzyme-rich fruits and vegetables.

—Excessive dieting or low nutrient intake (depresses interferon activity). Overeating also depresses immune response.

—A lifestyle low on rest. Natural killer cell activity is reduced by as much as 28% when sleep is cut by 4 hours in clinical tests performed at U. California at San Diego School of Medicine.

—Having parents who smoke, drink to excess or abuse drugs. Children born to addicted parents have more genetic predisposition to illness and infections.

—Not being breast-fed as a child. Breast milk is rich in antibodies, essential fatty acids and interferon that strengthen a child's developing immune system.

—A poor outlook on life or severe, long lasting depression. In addition, people who overextend themselves may be unusually susceptible to immune system malfunction.

Does Your Immune System Need A Boost?

It isn't easy to measure immune health. Each one of us is different and the character of immune response varies widely. I've worked for years to develop ways people can communicate with their bodies. Here's a personal quiz to monitor your immune status: If you answer yes to more than 3 of these questions, your immune system is probably sluggish.

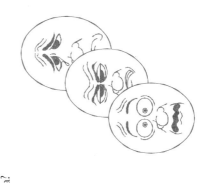

1: Do you suffer from chronic infections, colds, respiratory problems or allergies?
2: Do you have or have you had in the past any immune-deficient diseases, like chronic fatigue syndrome, Hashimoto's or fibromyalgia?
3: Do you have a history of malabsorption problems, like irritable bowel syndrome (I.B.S.), or chronic diarrhea or constipation?
4: Do you have diabetes or liver disease?
5: Do you have bouts of systemic candida or yeast infections that don't seem to go away even after conventional treatments?
6: Do you have a skin disorder like adult acne or Rosacea?
7: Have you recently undergone surgery, chemotherapy or radiation treatment?
8: Have you ever been the recipient of an organ transplant?
9: Have you undergone long-term treatment with antibiotics or steroid drugs?
10: Do you have periodontal disease?
11: Do you drink 2 or more drinks of hard alcohol 4 to 5 times a week or take recreational drugs on a regular basis?
12: Are you a smoker or are you exposed to second-hand smoke on a regular basis?
13: Do you live in area where there is smog or heavy pesticide use?
14: Are you regularly exposed to industrial heavy metals, like cadmium, asbestos or mercury?
15: Do you drink untreated tap water or eat produce sprayed with pesticides?
16: Do you regularly eat meats, like pork or beef that are injected with antibiotics and hormones?
17: Do you have circulation problems or a history of claudication?
18: Do you suffer from chronic stress, anxiety, panic attacks or depression?
19: Do you suffer from chronic insomnia? Are you always tired?.

See my book Cooking For Healthy Healing for a complete diet and lifestyle program to enhance immune response.

Can't find a recommended product? Call the 800 number listed in Product Resources for the store nearest you.

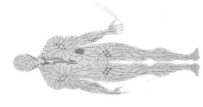

Lymphatic system health is the foundation of good immune response.

The lymphatic system includes lymphatic vessels and nodes, the thymus gland, tonsils and spleen. It's really a network of tubing that drains waste products from tissues, and carries the body's cellular waste to its final elimination organs. The lymphatic system acts as your body's secondary circulatory system. It's made up of millions of tiny vessels, ducts and valves that flush wastes, filter debris and render harmful bacteria harmless. The lymph nodes are also the factory for crucial white blood cells (lymphocytes) that produce the powerful antibodies which form the overall defense of your body against infections. In fact, the lymph system is a key to your body's immune defenses and a major player in your health.

As lymph flows around your body, large, eater cells called macrophages in the lymph nodes engulf foreign particles like harmful bacteria and cellular debris. Swollen lymph nodes are often really infected lymph nodes caused by an overload of pathogens in the lymphatic system that the body cannot keep under control. The lymphatic system doesn't have a pump, like the heart. The valves of the lymph system can keep lymph fluid moving along, but they depend on your breathing and muscle movement to drive them. It's one of the reasons I recommend exercise and deep breathing as an important part of any immune enhancing program. Exercise improves circulation in the lymphatic system so it can remove waste materials that block immune response.

The health of your lymphatic system depends to a large extent on the health of your liver. The liver produces most of the body's lymph, and the performance of the lymph system is highly dependent on special types of macrophages in the liver that filter bacteria like candida yeasts and toxins absorbed by the intestinal tract. Lymph is also a major route for nutrients from the liver and intestines, so it's rich in fat soluble nutrients, like protein, produced in the liver.

Is your body showing signs of lymph congestion?

A lymph-draining cleanse and a healing program for lymphatic health can make a difference if: 1) you are under chronic stress; 2) you are constantly tired (may mean liver exhaustion); 3) your skin is extremely pale; 4) you are extremely thin; 5) your memory is noticeably failing; 6) you get frequent colds; 7) your body looks uncharacteristically soft and pudgy or has newly noticeable cellulite (may mean too many saturated fats and sugary foods).

Alternative healing protocols: Boost nutrients: Poor nutrition is the most frequent cause of a sluggish lymph system. Protein and B_{12} deficiency especially effect lymphatic efficiency. Have a mixed vegetable lymph builder: handful parsley, 1 garlic clove, 5 carrots, and 3 celery stalks. Add 2 teasp. green superfood like •Solgar EARTHGREENS & MORE or •Wakunaga of America KYO-GREEN. Lymph boosting vegetables: cabbage, kale, carrot, bell pepper, collards and garlic. Lymph-enhancing fruits: apple, pineapple, blueberries and grape. Include potassium-rich foods regularly – sea greens, broccoli, bananas and seafood. Spicy foods like natural salsas, cayenne pepper, horseradish and ginger boost a sluggish lymph system. Take a glass of lemon and water regularly in the morning for lymph revitalization. Avoid caffeine, sugar, dairy products and alcoholic drinks. They contribute to lymphatic stagnation.

—**Optimize liver health:** Herbal bitters like *turmeric*, *cardamom* and *lemon peel* regenerate the liver and lymphatic system; or •Gaia Herbs SWEETISH BITTERS ELIXIR or •Crystal Star's BITTERS & LEMON™ extract. •Crystal Star LIV-ALIVE™ tea for liver and lymph; or a •lymph blend tea of *white sage*, *astragalus*, *echinacea root*, *Oregon grape root* and *dandelion root.*

—**Cleanse your lymphatic system for optimum defense against pathoegn invasion:** •*Echinacea*, one of the best herbal lymph cleansers I know, flushes the lymphatic system to keep the body disease free. •*Red root*, a powerful lymphatic cleanser, synergistic with *echinacea*; •*Astragalus* extract is a highly successful lymph cleansing single herb. For deep lymph cleansing for serious immune deficient disease, •Gaia Herbs SUPREME CLEANSE. Electrolyte boosters detoxify the lymph glands: •Nature's Path TRACE-LYTE LIQUID MINERALS.

—**Boost lymphocyte formation:** •Crystal Star ANTI-BIO™ caps; •shark cartilage, about 1400 mg; •Herbs Etc. LYMPHATONIC with *echinacea* reduces lymphatic swelling and congestion,; •Nature's Apothecary LYMPH CLEANSE; •Enzymatic therapy LYMPHOCLEAR; •Gaia Herbs ECHINACEA- RED ROOT SUPREME. Silica, found in high levels in lymph nodes, plays an integral role in lymphatic health. Silica therapy can lead to dramatic increases in phagocytes (the cells that that kill pathogens) and general improvement in lymphatic health. Silica is especially beneficial for people with lymphatic diatheses (malfunction of the lymphatic system). •Eidon SILICA MINERAL SUPPLEMENT; or •Flora VEGE-SIL.

—**Improve lymphatic filtration:** •Zinc picolinate 30mg; •vitamin E, 400 IU; •vitamin C, 1 to 3,000 mg daily. •B-complex, 100mg daily and Country Life sublingual B-12, 2500mcg; •vitamin C, 1 to 3,000 mg daily.

—**Stimulate lymphatic circulation:** •A seaweed bath is one of the quickest ways I know to stimulate lymphatic drainage to rid your body of disease-causing toxins. In a therapeutic bath, the electromagnetic action of seaweed releases excess body fluids and wastes from congested cells through the skin, replacing them with vital, immune boosting minerals. Unpolluted, shoreline waters are hard to find. •Crystal Star offers a blend of prepackaged seaweeds- HOT SEAWEED BATH™ (See page 228 for more information.) •A mineral bath is also effective. Add 1 cup Dead Sea salts, 1 cup Epsom salts, $1/2$ cup regular sea salt and $1/4$ cup baking soda to a tub; swish in 3 drops *lavender* oil, 2 drops *juniper* oil, 2 drops *marjoram* oil and 1 drop *ylang ylang* oil. Stir the water briskly to disperse evenly. •Take an alternating hot and cold hydrotherapy treatment at the end of your daily shower to stimulate lymph circulation. •Lymph supporting therapies: massage therapy (elevate feet and legs for 5 minutes every day, massaging lymph node areas), acupuncture and acupressure are both successful.

Can't find a recommended product? Call the 800 number listed in Product Resources for the store nearest you.

Indigestion and Heartburn

Gas, Bloating, Flatulence

Indigestion plagues up to 40% of Americans. Digestion problems go beyond the symptoms of gas and bloating. Energy is reduced, constipation results from metabolic byproducts that aren't eliminated, allergic reactions, diarrhea and fatigue can all ensue. If you have chronic indigestion, you're probably aging faster than normal, your immune defenses are low, and you may be at risk for infections like candida yeasts and chronic fatigue to take hold. As we age, digestion weakens. Our bodies make less stomach acid (a 65 year old has 85% less HCl than they did at 35). Without enough HCl to activate natural pepsin, proteins don't digest well. You may become deficient in critical amino acids. Acid blocking drugs at any age may mean that important B vitamins (especially B-12), minerals and trace minerals aren't assimilated well either.

Diet & Superfood Therapy

—Nutritional therapy plan:

1—Eat an alkalizing diet, with plenty of cultured foods like yogurt, kefir and miso soup, high fiber foods like whole grains, fresh vegetables, fruits, and enzyme-rich foods like papaya and pineapple.

2—Avoid fatty, spicy, sugary and acid-forming foods. Omit fried foods, red meats, fatty dairy products, dried fruits, sodas and caffeine.

3—Eat smaller meals. Chew food very well.

—Cleanse the digestive system and establish good enzymes:

• Start with a cleansing, pectin mono diet of apples and apple juice for 2 days. Then for 4 days use a diet of 70% fresh foods and steamed brown rice for B vitamins. Add fresh veggies and high fiber foods gradually if digestion is delicate.

- If 1 tsp. cider vinegar in water relieves your heartburn you need more stomach acid.

- $\frac{1}{2}$ tsp. baking soda in water eases bloating.

- Settle a sour stomach with lime juice and a pinch of ginger.

- A glass of wine is OK for better absorption.

—Superfood therapy: (choose 1 or 2)

• Crystal Star ENERGY GREEN™ drink.
• Solgar WHEY TO GO protein drink.
• Sun Wellness CHLORELLA
• Aloe vera juice 2-oz. First signs of heartburn. ♂

Herb & Supplement Therapy

—Interceptive therapy plan: (Choose 2 or more recommendations)

1—**Bitters herbs help the cause of heartburn:** • Crystal Star AFTER MEAL ENZ™ extract in water; • PRE-MEAL ENZ™ before meals; • BITTERS & LEMON CLEANSE™ extract each morning as a preventive. • Gaia Herbs SWEETISH BITTERS.

2—**Get to the heart of heartburn:** • Crystal Star GINSENG/LICORICE ELIXIR™; • L-glutamine therapy 1500mg daily for long-term relief; • Prevail ACID EASE or • Betaine HCl capsules after meals; ♂ • Turmeric extract (curcumin)

3—**Soothe the burn:** • Slippery elm tea or tablets; • marshmallow tea; • Hylands homeopathic Indigestion after meals; • Umeboshi plum paste. For acute indigestion: • Enzymatic Therapy DGL tabs.♀ • Rainforest Remedies BELLY BE GOOD.

4—**For gas and bloating:** • Ginger capsules 2 to 4 as needed; Homeopathic remedies like • Ignatia 6c, or • Dioscorea 6c work for bloating. Take 2 to 4 peppermint oil drops in water. (Also helpful for irritable bowel syndrome). • Homeopathic-BioForce Indigestion Relief, or Nux vomica; • Activated charcoal - short term.♂

Relieve gas quick: • pinches cinnamon, nutmeg, ginger, cloves in water- drink down.

5—**For belching and burping:** • AkPharma BEANO drops; • Prevail BEAN-VEGI formula; • Country Life DIGESTIVE formula; • Morada Research ACID STOMACH.

6—**For cramping and diarrhea:** • Activated charcoal tabs - short term; • Apple pectin tabs; • Crystal Star CRAMP BARK COMBO™ caps.♀

7—**Complete digestion with good digestion teas:** • Peppermint, spearmint or alfalfa-mint tea; • Catnip/fennel/lemon peel tea; • Chamomile tea; • Wild Yam tea, especially if you have eaten too much refined sugar.

8—**Effective enzyme therapy:** • Bromelain 1500mg daily, or • Nature's Plus chewable bromelain 40mg; • Biotec Goods BIO-GESTIN; • American Health PAPAYA CHEWABLES; • Crystal Star SYSTEMS STRENGTH™ drink; • Pancreatin capsules 1400mg; • FutureBiotics VEGETARIAN ENZYMES; • Garlic/parsley caps.

9—**Probiotics for friendly flora:** • Solaray SUPER DIGEST AWAY; • Prof. Nutrit. DR. DOPHILUS + FOS; • Ethical Nutrients INTESTINAL CARE; • Premier Labs MULTI-DOPHILUS caps.

Lifestyle Support Therapy

—Bodywork:

• Commercial antacids neutralize stomach acid, inviting the stomach to produce even more acid, often making the condition worse in the long run. New tests even show that chronic use of aluminum-containing antacids causes bone loss. Avoid over-using antibiotics. They destroy friendly flora in the digestive tract, too.

• Indigestion triggers: late night snacks, chocolates, alcohol, smoking, lots of sugar-free sorbitol candies (cramping and diarrhea).

• Apply ginger compresses to abdominal area.

• For flatulence: take a catnip or slippery elm enema for immediate relief.

• Lie on your back and draw knees up to chest to relieve abdomen pressure.

• Try to eat when relaxed. Meals eaten in a hurry or under stress contribute to poor digestion. Life isn't going to slow down on its own. Make a conscious effort to lessen digestive stress. Try a short walk before eating.

—Reflexology point:

food assimilation

Common Symptoms: Gnawing, burning pain and tenderness occurring directly after food consumption; excess gas and abdominal distention; passing foul gas; poor food assimilation.

Common Causes: Poor food combining; eating too much food, and too many refined, fatty and spicy foods; allergies to sugar, wheat or dairy; enzyme deficiency; candida yeast overgrowth; food allergies; too much caffeine or alcohol are heartburn triggers, sodas and acid-forming foods; chronic constipation from lack of fiber; diverticulitis; vegetable protein deficiency; HCl deficiency.

See page 555 for a Food Combining Chart. See page 127 for a complete discussion of enzyme therapy.

Can't find a recommended product? Call the 800 number listed in Product Resources for the store nearest you.

Infections
Staph Infections, Viral Infections, Bacterial Infections

A staph infection involves a staphylococcus micro-organism, is *usually virulent*, and is often food-borne. Antibiotic measures are effective. **A bacterial infection** involves pathogenic microbial bacteria. Antibiotic agents are normally effective. **A viral infection** involves virus organisms that infiltrate the deepest regions of the body and live off the body's cell enzymes. Virus infections are virulent, deep-reaching and tenacious. Antibiotics are not effective. Antiviral treatment must be vigorous, since viruses can both mutate and move to escape being overcome. All infections regularly cause painful inflammation as the body reacts to overcome them. Chronic recurring infections can indicate low thyroid function.

Diet & Superfood Therapy

—Nutritional therapy plan:

1—**For any infection:** a quick, enzyme therapy detox is effective: use 3 parts water to 1 part fresh pineapple juice; drink 8 glasses in 24 hours.

2—Take 6 glasses of vegetable juices (pg. 218), or potassium broth (pg. 216) over the next 24 hours.

3—Then eat only fresh foods and brown rice for three days to keep the body alkaline and free flowing.

4—Take a glass of lemon juice and water each morning to stimulate kidney filtering.

5—Include vegetable source proteins for faster healing; sea greens and sea foods, whole grains, sprouts, and soy foods.

6—Avoid foods that feed infections: all sugars, refined foods, caffeine, colas, tobacco and alcohol (except for a little wine) during healing.

—Superfood therapy: (choose 1 or 2)

• Crystal Star SYSTEMS STRENGTH™, daily during healing, then ENERGY GREEN™ for strength and body chemistry balance.

• Nutricology PROGREENS with EFA's.♀

• Future Biotics VITAL K drink.

• Aloe vera juice, such as AloeLife ALOE VERA GOLD, morning and evening.

• Green Foods GREEN MAGMA.

• Mona's CHLORELLA.

• Klamath BLUE GREEN SUPREME.♂

Herb & Supplement Therapy

Don't take iron supplements during an infection. They may make the bacteria grow faster.

—Interceptive therapy plan: (Choose 2 to 4 recommendations)

1—Herbs can help infective conditions that are resistant to medical treatment.

For a staph infection: • Nutribiotic GRAPEFRUIT SEED extract, • Olive leaf extract, or East Park OLIVE LEAF extract; and • Echinacea extract, or • Herbs. Etc. ECHINACEA TRIPLE SOURCE; Take down inflammation with • Bromelain 1500mg daily, or • *una da gato* or • *turmeric* extract caps, and • Vitamin C crystals with bioflavs., ¹/₂ teasp. in water every hour, acute stages, reducing to 5000mg daily.

Thymus-immune defense: • raw thymus 3x daily; • Enzymedica PURIFY protease.

For a bacterial infection: Destroy the active microbe with • *Oregano* oil, like Now OREGANO OIL as directed; • CoQ-10, 60mg 4x daily; • *Olive leaf* extract as directed. • Nutribiotic GRAPEFRUIT SEED extract or • Crystal Star ANTI-BIO™ extract or caps. (Use • Crystal Star FIRST AID CAPS™ in acute stages.) Reduce inflammation with • *Turmeric* (curcumin), or • quercetin 1000mg 2x daily and bromelain 1500mg daily and Lysine 1000mg 2x daily. Boost immunity with • *Propolis*, • *Garlic*, • *Echinacea* or • Crystal Star GINSENG/REISHI mushroom extracts, or • Dr. DOPHILUS + FOS; • Colloidal silver or Nature's Path SILVER-LYTE as directed. Flush lymphatic toxins with • Crystal Star BLDR-K™ extract drops every 4 hours, and • Vitamin C crystals with bioflavs 3000mg daily.

For a viral infection: • *Olive leaf* extract caps, or Nutricology PRO-LIVE olive leaf caps; • Crystal Star ANTI-VI™ or ANTI-BIO™, or • *Garlic* (both gram negative and gram positive viruses), • *Goldenseal*, • *Myrrh*, • *Astragalus*, *Propolis* or • *St. John's wort* extracts or • *Oregano* oil as directed; or • vitamin A (not beta-carotene) 100,000IU daily **for 3 days only.** Take down inflammation with • Lane Labs BENE-FIN shark cartilage caps and • Vitamin C crystals with bioflavs., ¹/₂ teasp. in water every hour in acute stages. Limit bacterial harm with • Professional Nutrition DR. DOPHILUS + FOS. Raise immunity with *reishi* or *maitake* mushroom, and echinacea. Restore homeostasis with • Planetary TRIPHALA caps; and • PCO's 100mg daily.

Lifestyle Support Therapy

—Help remove infections through the skin:

• Earth's Bounty O₂-SPRAY, staph infections.

• Crystal Star ANTI-BIO™ gel.

• *Garlic* poultice takes down swelling.

• *Tea tree oil*: both staph and fungal infections.

• Nutribiotic GRAPEFRUIT SKIN SPRAY.

• Green clay packs for inflammation.♀

• Honey keeps skin infections from spreading.

• Herbal Answers HERBAL ALOE FORCE gel.

—Bodywork:

• Overheating therapy is effective in controlling virus replication. Even slight temperature increases can lead to considerable reduction of infection. See page 225 for the technique.

• Use a sauna to raise blood temperature; apply *ginger-cayenne* compresses to affected area.

• Activate kidney cleansing with a *chamomile* or chlorophyll enema.

• Sleep. Healing is at its peak during sleep.

—For children:

• *Osha root* tea or Hylands HYLAVIR tablets.

• Anti-infection aromatherapy for children 1 year and up: 1 drop *tea tree* oil, 1 drop essential oil of *lavender*, 1 drop *calendula* oil in juice.

• Make an anti-infective salve: equal parts *garlic* powder, *goldenseal* powder, zinc powder-mix into *calendula* ointment.

Common Symptoms: *Inflammation, boils, sores, and abscesses; breakdown of tissue into waste matter and pus; sore throat, cough, and headache; high temperature and fever; reduced vitality; chronic fatigue and lethargy.*

Common Causes: *Lowered immunity; over-use of antibiotics; chronically low nutrition diet with too many refined foods and too few green vegetables; food or environmental allergies.*

See also FUNGAL AND PARASITIC INFECTIONS pages 390 & 476 for more information.

Can't find a recommended product? Call the 800 number listed in Product Resources for the store nearest you.

Infections have taken on an uglier face. Are you prepared for the supergerm assault?

Germ warfare is out of control all over the world—and it's no longer just coming in from foreign countries... Supergerms like e. Coli, salmonella, antibiotic-resistant pneumonia and staph infections are a real and present danger in the U.S. today, largely caused by the over-use of antibiotics! Supergerms can attack anyone, anytime. In the last fifteen years, infectious diseases jumped from the fifth leading cause of death to the third leading cause in the U.S.

Deadly flus are killing people in Hong Kong. Mystery respiratory illnesses are claiming the lives of Native Americans in the Southwest U.S. Mad Cow disease from contaminated beef has killed more than 20 people in Britain. Devastating, hemorrhaging Ebola virus have attacked thousands in Africa, clueless that their lives would be claimed within a few short weeks. Many infectious disease experts believe it is just a matter of time before Ebola makes it to the U.S. via an infected airline passenger!

At least 30 new diseases from supergerms have emerged in the last 20 years. Experts believe hundreds more are on the way. Strains of drug-resistant tuberculosis and pneumonia are targeting people with compromised immune systems, especially those with HIV - itself a supervirus unheard of until the 1940s! Staph infections (increasingly acquired during hospital visits), once easily treated by penicillin, are now 95% resistant to conventional treatment! Recent reports show virulent staph organisms are resistant to the most powerful new antibiotics.

Food borne supergerms are leaping on the U.S. radar with a death toll of 9,000 Americans each year. E. coli contaminated beef and other foods have sent thousands to the hospital!! The problem is so severe that FDA food safety inspectors say they can't keep up with demand. Blame is placed on substandard conditions in the agriculture industry, exposure to infected animals and contaminated foods, and low immune respose from pollution, chemical toxins and poor diet. Over-use of antibiotics is one of the biggest offenders. Last year the Institute of Medicine called for a global effort to fight the problem of antibiotic overloading!

Has antibiotic therapy backfired?

The advent of penicillin and antibiotics during World War II was a boon for fighting infectious disease. Clearly antibiotic therapy has saved many lives, from wartime injuries, strep infections, meningitis and pneumonia. But antibiotics are powerful drugs that should not be taken casually or indiscriminately. When they are overused or misused antibiotics can be a recipe for disaster! For example, thousands of antibiotics are prescribed every year to treat the viruses that cause colds and flu. If you're taking antibiotics to get rid of a virus or an allergy-related condition like chronic bronchitis or sinusitis (unrelated to bacterial infection) not only is it ineffective, it also reduces that antibiotic's ability to treat your future bacterial infections.

Germs are getting smarter, mutating into more deadly strains that conventional antibiotics can't touch. Ampicillin and tetracyclin, used extensively in the 30s, are practically useless today. A strange phenomenon is taking place. It appears that the more antibiotics you take, the more a disease strain or infection will try to find a new way to attack! Another problem with grave consequences: Some people, quite understandably, in an effort to limit their antibiotic intake, stop taking their antibiotics before the prescription is completed. If you don't take the full recommended course of antibiotics, you are unknowingly giving germs that haven't been destroyed the opportunity to mutate and form their own defense against the drug. This is one of the big reasons why doctors have to try new and more powerful antibiotics to quell virulent supergerm infections.

Another phenomenon: even Third World countries, without a long history of antibiotic use, are suffering. With the best will in the world, America has sent carloads of antibiotics to these countries in an effort to control some of their virulent infections. The antibiotics were distributed liberally without prescriptions and their overuse has now spurred the development of hundreds of new drug-resistant strains — and the strains are migrating around the world as infected people travel or move.

You may not take antibiotics regularly, but you're not immune. People are getting low dose antibiotics daily from commercial meats, dairy products and produce without knowing it. About 40% of the antibiotics produced in the U.S. each year are fed to cattle, pigs and chickens to fight diseases that break out in unsanitary, overcrowded feed lots. A 1998 Harvard Medical School study shows that an astounding 300,000 pounds of antibiotics was sprayed on fruits like apples and pears to prevent a blight!

Even more worrisome, new household cleaning supplies contain antibiotics to keep your home "germ-free," but when those antibiotics are saturated in your home, otherwise harmless germs may transform into something more dangerous. A study published in the journal Nature finds that triclosan, a widely used antibacterial household chemical, can cause certain bacteria to mutate into new strains resistant to treatment.

What can you do to fight supergerms? 1) Use antibiotics only when needed and use as directed. Don't always accept a prescription for an antibiotic at face value. Ask your physician if an antibiotic is really right for your type of infection. 2) For basic household cleaning, stick with environmentally sound cleaners free of harmful chemicals and antibiotics. Plain old soap and water is still the best choice for personal hygiene. 3) Reduce antibiotic exposure from food. I recommend organic meats and dairy to avoid antibiotic overload. I primarily eat foods from the sea because they aren't as affected by rampant hormone and antibiotic injection as commercial farm animals. Free range turkeys have a more natural diet than commercial animals and their meat is free from antibiotics, too.

Check out my herbal program on the next page to help solve the antibiotic resistant drug problem.

Can't find a recommended product? Call the 800 number listed in Product Resources for the store nearest you.

Herbs To The Rescue! How can herbs, which we think of as so gentle and subtle, work when drugs can't?

Herbal antibiotics may become some of our best weapons against drug-resistant diseases. Herbal antibiotics work differently than antibiotic drugs. In essence: herbs work with each person's individual immune system. Drugs work against the harmful organism. As heroic medicine, they often work best for short time use, to arrest a virulent pathogen and give your body a chance to stabilize so your own immune response can take over. But antibiotic drugs target all bacteria in your body, not just the harmful ones. They wipe out friendly bacteria in the intestines, important for immune strength and protection against Candida yeast overgrowth, E. Coli and Salmonella infections. Antibiotics taken over time also weaken immune response. Research from Baylor School of Medicine reveals that antibiotics actually prevent immune system white blood cells from attacking and killing pathogenic bacteria.

—**Herbs with antibiotic properties work with your body's own immune defenses.** They help flush the lymphatic system of disease toxins, and stimulate immune response so your body can neutralize or eliminate the pathogens through its *own* immune response without harming healthy tissue. Herbs are living medicines that interact with our bodies in a very complex way. We may never understand all their healing power, but one way to see how herbs work is to remember that whole herbs are foods. Herbs work with body enzyme and digestive functions just as foods do. As with foods, you don't get the interactions with drugs like you would when you combine different drugs. Think about it, would you stop eating spinach, for instance, just because you're taking an antibiotic? The healing support pathways are different than drugs - even for those drugs that originally started as plants.

There are the three categories of herbal antibiotics you can use for your natural supergerm arsenal:

1: Immune Boosters are not direct germ killers. They illustrate how herbs like *echinacea* and *astragalus* with antibiotic activity work as opposed to drug antibiotics.

—*Echinacea* is a potent immune system stimulant. *Echinacea* increases levels of the antiviral substance interferon in the body. *Echinacea* increases phagocytosis, the process where your immune system engulfs pathogens. *Echinacea* helps cleanse the blood and boost lymphatic filtration and drainage making it a powerful detoxifier for removing infective organisms, especially when combined with *goldenseal* and *myrrh*. *Echinacea* prompts the thymus, bone marrow and the spleen to produce more immune cells for more protection. *Echinacea* helps cleanse the blood and boost lymphatic filtration and drainage making it a powerful detoxifier for removing infective organisms, especially when combined with *goldenseal* and *myrrh*.

—*Astragalus* also boosts natural killer activity and enhances interferon production against harmful pathogens. It is particularly beneficial for respiratory illnesses because it can promote the regeneration of bronchi cells. *Astragalus* is ideal for travelers who may be more exposed to drug-resistant disease strains. Consider Herbs Etc. Echinacea/Astragalus Complex.

2: Herbal Lymph Flushers work with the lymphatic system, your immune system's circulatory process, to flush, filter and engulf pathogens, rendering them innocuous.

—*Echinacea* flushes the lymphatic system to keep the body disease free. *Echinacea* extract is, by far, one of the best lymph cleansers I know to build body defenses against disease.

—Seaweed baths aren't just a spa weight loss technique, the electromagnetic action of seaweed stimulates lymphatic drainage to rid your body of disease-causing toxins through the skin, replacing them with vital, immune boosting minerals. Crystal Star offers prepackaged seaweeds- Hot Seaweed Bath™.

—Bitters herbs boost the activity of your liver. The liver produces most of the body's lymph, fluid rich in lymphocytes, which form your immune systems primary overall defense. A short course of herbal bitters like *turmeric, cardamom* and *lemon peel* regenerates the liver and lymphatic system to enhance immune response. Consider Gaia Herbs Sweetish Bitters Elixir.

3. Organism Killers are super powerful herbs.... they may be the best or only tool to wipe out supergerms...

—*Olive leaf* extract is effective against 56 different pathogens. Park Research of Henderson, NV finds that olive extract may remedy as many as 120 illnesses. Even serious infections like herpes, tuberculosis and pneumonia respond to *olive leaf*. *Olive leaf* extract is ideal for people traveling to third world countries. Now or Nutricology *Olive Leaf Extract* caps.

—*Tea tree oil* has new studies showing that it can kill antibiotic-resistant staph infections even at low concentrations. Adding 1-3 drops of *tea tree* oil to an infuser and breathing deeply can fight off most respiratory infections. Note: Do not take 100% pure *tea tree oil* internally unless under the guidance of a health professional experienced in the use of essential oils.

—*Garlic* has a powerful antibiotic punch against infections like dysentery and *H. pylori*, responsible for the majority of ulcers, including antibiotic-resistant strains. In one study, immune cell activity increased 140% in people who ate 2 bulbs in a two-day span and 156% in people who took 1800 mg of aged garlic. Consider Wakunaga Kyolic Super Formula 100.

—*Oregano* oil contains over 50 compounds with organism killing actions. It can inhibit candida yeast, bacteria, viruses and parasites. In a study, *oregano* was found to inhibit bacteria on foods, so cooking with it may help prevent food borne illness. Note: Direct contact to pure oregano essential oil can cause mild burns. Allergy Research Group Oregano Oil.

Two more protectors to know:

—Probiotics like acidophilus are a good choice for supergerm protection. New studies find probiotics suppress even virulent strains of E. Coli, staph, candida and salmonella in the intestinal tract. Acidophilus has been found to be as effective as the drug Neomycin Sulfate against E. Coli. Results are even effective against breast cancer. In a study published in Nutrition and Cancer in 1997, the growth of breast cancer cells was slowed by up to 85% by Lactobacillus acidophilus and Bifidobacterium bifidum. Consider Wakunaga Kyo-Dophilus.

—Selenium therapy enhances immune cell defense against super viruses. Experts theorize that HIV and Ebola viruses feed off selenium, weakening the immune system to the point where it can no longer fight off life-threatening infections. In a Chinese study hemorrhagic fever patients (like Ebola virus), death rates decreased from 100% to 36% with selenium! In another study, selenium significantly reduced infections in 74% of AIDS patients. Consider 200mcg selenium for protection daily.

Can't find a recommended product? Call the 800 number listed in Product Resources for the store nearest you.

Infertility

Difficulty Conceiving Children - Men and Women

For the first time in history, incredible numbers of people are having trouble conceiving. An amazing 20% of married couples in the U.S. today are affected by some kind of fertility problem. The fertility industry grosses $2 billion a year! Unfortunately, current conventional fertility treatments have many drawbacks. In vitro fertilization often results in multiple pregnancies and tough decisions for expectant parents. (To correct this problem, a new technique called "blastocyte transfer" is in the works to reduce risk of multiple births.) Evidence also shows Intracytoplasmic Sperm Injection (ICSI), introduced in 1993 to boost sperm count in infertile men, may cause abnormalities in embryos and even slow development in children.

Diet & Superfood Therapy

—Nutritional therapy plan:

1–Diet is all-important. The body does not readily allow conception without adequate nutrition. Consciously follow a healthy diet and lifestyle for at least six months before trying to conceive. See my book "COOKING FOR HEALTHY HEALING" for a complete diet for infertility.

—For women:

• Reduce dairy products, (especially full fat milk), fried and fatty foods, sugary and junk foods.
• Avoid tobacco, alcohol, except moderate wine, caffeine, red meats (they may have synthetic hormones), and chemical-laced foods.

—For men:

Make a mix of brewer's yeast, bee pollen granules, wheat germ, pumpkin seeds; blend 2 teasp. into any superfood drink below.

—For both sexes:

• Eat zinc foods: oysters, wheat germ, onions, sunflower and pumpkin seeds.
• Eat plenty of whole grains, cultured foods like yogurt, sea foods and sea vegetables, fresh fruits and vegetables. Limit fat intake.
• Have a cup of green tea every morning.

—Superfood therapy: (choose 1 or 2)

• Crystal Star BIOFLAV, FIBER & C SUPPORT.
• Green Foods MAGMA PLUS drink.
• Y.S. ROYAL JELLY with Siberian ginseng drink.

Herb & Supplement Therapy

—Interceptive therapy plan: (Choose 2 or 3 recommendations)

1–**For women:** Preconception (normalize menstrual cycle).• *VITEX* extract promotes ovulation;• Crystal Star FEMALE HARMONY™ caps 4 daily with EVENING PRIMROSE OIL for EFAs, 4 daily; or • Crystal Star PRO-EST BALANCE™ roll-on or Moon Maid PRO-MENO *wild yam* cream for 1 month with extra B_6 to reduce chance of miscarriage. • High potency *royal jelly* 2 tsp. daily; • aromatherapy rose oil; or • Histidine 500mg daily for more sexual enjoyment. • *Red raspberry* tea to tone uterus, discontinue after pregnancy achieved. • *Licorice* extract or • Crystal Star GINSENG-LICORICE ELIXIR™, hormone balance for polycystic ovary syndrome.

Women's fertility nutrient boosters: • Enzymatic Therapy NUCLEO-PRO F, or STEREO-PLEX MF, with • RAW OVARY extract and • RAW FEMALE glandular. • Vitamin E 400IU 2x daily; • B-complex such as Nature's Secret ULTIMATE B with extra B_6 100mg, PABA 1000mg and folic acid 800mcg daily. • Country Life sublingual B-12, 2500mcg daily. • Rainbow Light CALCIUM 1200mg with high magnesium 1200mg. • *Cayenne-ginger* caps, *Motherwort* tea, or Hawthorn extract 3-4x daily for a feeling of well-being. • VITAMIN E CLUSTERS from Healthy House.

2–**For men:** Effective ginseng boosters • Crystal Star MALE GINSIAC™ extract, or MALE PERFORMANCE™ caps or • *ginseng/damiana* 4 caps daily. To boost sperm quality and amount • SIBERIAN GINSENG extract (increases almost 30%); • L-carnitine 3000mg daily if subfertile; • Arginine 1500mg daily (unless you have herpes); • Vitamin C 3000mg daily and niacin 500mg for low sperm count or sperm clumping; • chromium picolinate 200mcg daily; and • Zinc 50-75mg daily. To remove heavy metals (esp. lead from pesticides) • Crystal Star HEAVY METAL CLEANZ caps 6 daily, with • Country Life sublingual B-12, 3500 mcg and folic acid 800mcg.

Men's fertility nutrient boosters: • Vitamin E 400IU with selenium 200mcg daily (tests show pregnancies increase 21%); • Enzymatic Therapy NUCLEOPRO M caps or STEREO-PLEX MF; • Solaray MALE CAPS w. orchic extract, or • Country Life MAX w. orchic. • Cal-Mag 1000mg for testosterone balance.

Lifestyle Support Therapy

—Lifestyle measures:

• For both parents: Do not smoke; avoid secondary smoke. Avoid areas with smog and pollutants as much as possible.
• Get regular mild exercise every day.

—Reflexology points:

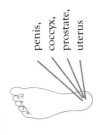

penis,
coccyx,
prostate,
uterus

—For women:

anxiety and infertility are linked. Consciously relax more. Acupuncture, guided imagery, deep breathing (page 554) are successful for women as relaxation techniques.
• Vaginal pH balance douche right before intercourse: use baking soda/honey for over-acid condition, vinegar/water for over-alkaline.
• Alternate hot and cold sitz baths to stimulate circulation.

—For men:

avoid bikini underwear, hot electric blankets, and hot water beds.
• Sun bathe in the early morning, nude if possible for 15 minutes.
• Stress and abnormal sperm production are linked. Relax.

Common Symptoms: Difficulty in both conceiving and bearing a child, a condition of both man and woman.

Common Causes: Poor nutrition and stress are at the base of most fertility problems. For men: zinc deficiency; a fast food diet; heavy metal toxicity; stress; bacterial infections; and too much alcohol or marijuana. For women: anxiety; emotional stress or depression; severe anemia; polycystic ovary syndrome; hormonal imbalance. Hormone mimics from pollutants, chemical residues in food, water, link infertility in both sexes. Type of underwear men wear may not influence fertility as previously thought. 1999 research shows sperm count and testicular temperature is no different in men who wear briefs than in men who wear boxers.

See HORMONE IMBALANCE page 419, HOME HEALING PROCEDURES page 541, HEALTHY BABY section page 236 for more.

Can't find a recommended product? Call the 800 number listed in Product Resources for the store nearest you.

Insect Bites and Stings

Bees, Wasps, Mosquitos, Non-Poisonous Spiders

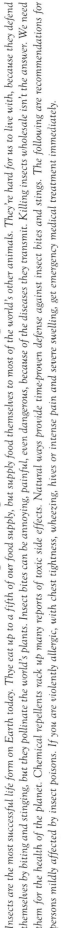

Insects are the most successful life form on Earth today. They eat up to a fifth of our food supply, but supply food themselves to most of the world's other animals. They're hard for us to live with, because they defend themselves by biting and stinging, but they pollinate the world's plants. Insect bites can be annoying, painful, even dangerous, because of the diseases they transmit. Killing insects wholesale isn't the answer. We need them for the health of the planet. Chemical repellents rack up many reports of toxic side effects. Natural ways provide time-proven defense against insect bites and stings. The following are recommendations for persons mildly affected by insect poisons. If you are violently allergic, with chest tightness, wheezing, hives or intense pain and severe swelling, get emergency medical treatment immediately.

Diet & Superfood Therapy

—**Household helpers for insect bites:**
• raw onion slices or vinegar - wasp stings
• raw potato slices
• lemon juice
• vinegar, especially for mosquitoes
• tobacco and water paste
• toothpaste
• cologne or rubbing alcohol
• honey mixed with 1 drop *peppermint* oil
• baking soda mixed with water
• ice packs
• charcoal tabs or burnt toast
• wheat germ oil
• chlorophyll liquid

—**Avoid:**
consuming sugar and alcohol for 24 hours before you are going to be in mosquito territory.
bananas and nuts and other serotonin-rich foods that attract insects.
meats and sweets for faster healing.
alcohol - it causes the skin to swell and flush, aggravating bites and stings.

—**Superfood therapy: (choose 1 or 2)**
• Sun Wellness CHLORELLA to reestablish body balance.
• AloeLife ALOE SKIN GEL - apply.

Herb & Supplement Therapy

—**Interceptive therapy plan: (Choose 2 to 3 recommendations)**

1—**Natural antihistamines take down inflammation:** • Crystal Star ANTI-HST™ 2 to 6 daily, and • ANTI-FLAM™ caps to take down rash or swelling. Take every 4 hours. • Quercetin Plus with bromelain or • Source Naturals ACTIVATED QUERCITIN. Apply *neem* oil. • Vitamin C therapy: Use calcium ascorbate powder. Take 1/4 teasp. every 15 minutes right after the bite, then 1/4 teasp. every few hours until pain and swelling are gone. Also mix some powder to a paste with water and apply directly. • Or take vitamin C capsules 1000mg with Pantothenic acid 1000mg, several times daily as an antihistamine.

Add • Bach Flower RESCUE REMEDY to keep stress from the bite or sting down.

2—**Stop the sting with herbal applications:** • B&T STING STOP gel; • Comfrey leaf poultice; • Turmeric powder paste; • Witch hazel; • Tea tree oil. Dissolve • PABA tablets in water and apply. • Crush papaya tablets with water to a paste and apply.

3—**Draw out the poisons with herbal compresses:** • Hot *parsley* leaf; • Black cohosh; • Chamomile; • crushed fresh *ivy* leaves applied to sting; • green clay packs.

4—**Flush poisons from your system:** • Take a few drops of *cayenne* extract in warm water every 1/2 hour to boost circulatory defenses. Use • ECHINACEA extract or • BD Herbs ECHINACEA extract every few hours to flush lymph glands.

—**For prevention:** Take vitamin B-1, 100mg for children, 500mg for adults, or • Source Naturals COENZYMATE B for a month during high risk seasons. • Rub fresh elder leaves or elder-chamomile tea on area. • Mix 1 teasp. each citronella, pennyroyal, eucalyptus oils in a base of safflower oil and apply to exposed skin (especially against fleas). Or use • Heart Foods TICKWEED PLUS with *neem* oil, or • Quantum BUZZ AWAY (Deet free).

—**Homeopathic remedies:** • Ledum tincture to relieve swelling and stinging; • Apis ointment for puffiness; • Cantharis for inflammation.

Lifestyle Support Therapy

—**Environmental preventives:**
• Sprinkle *garlic* or *eucalyptus* powder around the house.
• Sprinkle *sassafras* tea or dried tomato leaves around the house.
• Sprinkle vanilla water around the house.
• Wear light colors. Avoid flowery perfumes to escape bees. They think you are a source of pollen!

—**Once bitten.....**
• Apply cold or ice pack compresses, and see shock page in this book if reaction is severe.
• To lessen the effect of a bite, keep quiet, and keep the affected area below the level of the heart.
• Pull a bee stinger out sideways with tweezers or by dragging you fingernail across the stinger. Apply a wet mud paste to take down inflammation.

—**Natural repellent oils:** Reapply often - repellency is based on aroma. Don't use on fine fabrics.
• Citronella for mosquitoes, ticks and flies.
• Cedarwood for fleas and ticks.
• Tea tree oil for mosquitos.
• Eucalyptus for most flying insects.
• Lemon-Eucalyptus for mosquitos.
• Lemon grass for a broad range of insects.
• Pennyroyal for fleas (do not use if pregnant).
• Peppermint, rosemary, thyme, geranium and lavender for flies, mosquitos and fleas.

Common Symptoms: Pain, swelling, itching, and redness around the bite area; more severe reactions include nausea, dizziness, headache, chills, fever, allergic and histamine side-effects. Unless allergic, a child can handle about 1 bee sting per pound if there are multiple stings, before it becomes an emergency.

See BRUISES, CUTS & ABRASIONS page 329 for more information.

Can't find a recommended product? Call the 800 number listed in Product Resources for the store nearest you.

Insomnia

Sleep Disorders, Sleep Apnea, Snoring

Sixty-seven percent of adult Americans experience insomnia symptoms on a regular basis. We consume over a million and a half pounds of tranquilizers annually! Yet we sleep 20% less than our ancestors did. Sleep deprivation is a health problem because only during rest do bone marrow and lymph nodes produce substances that empower immune response. Sleep involves nighttime blood glucose levels. A blood sugar drop will awaken you. Commercial sleeping pills interfere with the ability to dream, and interrupt natural sleep patterns. They interact adversely with alcohol and tranquilizers because the nervous system never really relaxes. They lose their effectiveness in as little as 3-5 days of use. Don't worry about "making up" lost sleep. One good night's sleep repairs fatigue. It takes several days of common-sense therapy to establish good sleep patterns.

Diet & Superfood Therapy

—**Nutritional therapy plan:**

1—A carbohydrate rich meal, like pasta with vegetables induces sleep. A meal with both proteins and carbohydrates (adding meat to the pasta) keeps you awake.

2—Eat only a light meal at night. Good latenight "sleepytime" snacks about an hour before bedtime: bananas, celery and celery juice, wheat germ and wheat germ oil, brown rice, a little warm milk, lemon water and honey, brewer's yeast, Sovex NUTRITIONAL YEAST broth, or miso soup with 1 TB Bragg's LIQUID AMINOS in water.

3—Have a glass of wine at dinner for minerals, digestion and relaxation.

4—Have a small glass of bottled mineral water at bedtime.

5—Don't take caffeine drinks except in the morning.

6—Avoid a heavy meal in the evening, especially a heavy protein meal.

7—Avoid salty and sugary foods before bed. Don't eat too late.

—**Effective superfoods: (choose 1 or 2)**

• B&T ALFALCO, homeopathic Alfalfa tonic drink before bed. ♂
• Beehive Botanicals SIBERIAN GINSENG-ROYAL JELLY drink.

Herb & Supplement Therapy

—**Interceptive therapy plan: (Choose 2 to 3 recommendations)**

1—**Nervine relaxers ease tension that causes sleeplessness:** • Crystal Star RELAX CAPS™ 2 as needed; or • NIGHT CAPS™ 4 as needed ♀ or NIGHT ZZZ™ extract, ♂ or • PILLOW TIME™ tea. • *Passionflowers* capsules or extract, especially if weaning away from sleeping pills. • *Gotu kola* caps 2 as needed.

2—**Adaptogens help normalize body functions (especially glands and hormones):** • Crystal Star REISHI-GINSENG extract. • Melatonin, 3mg for sleep disorders, if your melatonin is low, on a temporary basis, to reset your biological clock.

Herbal melatonin sources: • *St. John's wort,* • *feverfew,* and • *scullcap* (especially if you have a headache at bedtime).

3—**Muscle relaxers ease muscle tightness, let you relax:** • Herb Pharm PHARMA KAVA or Jarrow Formulas KAVA caps especially if under a great deal of stress.

For restless legs: • Vitamin E 400IU before bed; • Folic acid 800mcg daily.

4—**Natural sedatives:** • Chamomile tea or tincture; • *Valerian* caps 2 before bed, or Crystal Star VALERIAN-WILD LETTUCE extract; or • Flora FLORA-SED before bed.

5—**Improve sleep quality:** • 5-HTP 50 to 200mg before bed to rebalance serotonin. • If you're in pain, take one each: DLPA 500mg, Calcium-magnesium capsule. • If hypoglycemic, take GABA 500mg and Glycine 500mg capsules before bed.

6—**For better calcium and magnesium balance in the blood:** (so you won't wake up at night and not be able to return to sleep.) • Crystal Star CALCIUM SOURCE™; • Floradix HERBAL REST liquid; • Rainbow Light CALCIUM PLUS with high magnesium; • Rosemary Gladstar's *Valerian-Hops* formula. • B Stress complex 100mg.

7—**For quality sleep and dream recall:** • INCREDIBLE DREAMS™ tea.

8—**For nightmares:** • Nelson Bach Flower Remedies; • B₁ 500mg at night for 1 to 2 months; • Niacinimide 500mg. • *Catnip/lemon balm* tea. ☺

—**Aromatherapy for insomnia:** • *Chamomile* or *lavender* oils on temples, pillow, bottoms of feet. • Or make a hops-rosemary sleep pillow.

—**Homeopathic sleep remedies:** • Hyland's CALMS FORTE; ♀ • *Chamomilla;* • *Nux vomica* if you've over-indulged; ♂ • Boiron QUIETUDE.

Lifestyle Support Therapy

—**Bodywork:**

• Snoring is caused by 1) an obstruction or narrowing of the airway; 2) sleep apnea - breathing ceases because the tongue blocks the throat.
  Get off your back. Elevate your head.
  Lose weight. Cut back on alcohol at night.
  MSM - drip a dilute solution into nostrils beforte bed for up to 80% less snoring.
  Drink chamomile tea before bed.
  Go to bed earlier to control snoring.
  Use BREATHE RIGHT nasal strips.

—**Stress reduction techniques:**

• Biofeedback, yoga, hypnotherapy, and regular massage therapy treatments help.
• Gaze at a lighted candle for 3 minutes before retiring.
• Before bed breathing stretch: take 10 deep breaths; wait 5 minutes; take 10 more.
• Use a "white noise," sleep sound machine.
• Take an epsom salts bath before bed. Enough of the natural magnesium will enter your skin to relax your muscles, help you sleep.
• Exercise in the morning, outdoors if possible; a "sunlight break" promotes sleep 12 hours later, and keeps circadian rhythm regular. Take a "constitutional walk" before bed.

Common Symptoms: Chronic inability to sleep; prematurely ended or interrupted sleep; difficulty falling asleep; snoring and sleep apnea can be a serious disorder, linked to high blood pressure, irregular heartbeat, headaches and excessive fatigue. Long term insomniacs have reduced work productivity, depressed cognitive abilities, impaired memory, are sleepy and irritable in the daytime and get sick more often.

Common Causes: Insomnia itself is due largely to psychological, rather than physical factors. Chronic stress, tension, depression and anxiety; the inability to "turn your mind off;" too much caffeine; pain; hypoglycemia; overeating; too much salt and sugar; B complex deficiency; nicotine or other drugs; asthma; indigestion and toxic liver overload; too high copper levels. Snoring can be caused by poor food digestion.

See also Stress & Tension page for more information.

Can't find a recommended product? Call the 800 number listed in Product Resources for the store nearest you.

Kidney Disease

Nepritis, Kidney Stones (next page), Bright's Disease

Kidney infections are usually severe, serious, and should be attended to immediately. Nephritis involves chronic inflammation of the kidney tissues. In Bright's disease (usually connected with diabetes) the blood becomes toxic from an overload of unfiltered wastes. Inflammation develops with blood in the urine, high blood pressure and water retention. Diabetes is a forerunner of Bright's Disease. Kidney stones are extremely painful, but very preventable. (See next page.) Prevention through improved diet and exercise is the best medicine. Kidney caution - elderly people who chronically use NSAIDS drugs (Advil, Motrin, and Aleve often have high blood levels of creatinine, a sign that kidney function is impaired.

Diet & Superfood Therapy

—Nutritional therapy plan:

1—Below, a short 3 day kidney cleanse to remove toxic infection and help dissolve stones:

Each morning take 2 TBS cider vinegar or lemon juice in water. Take one each of the following juices daily: carrot-beet-cucumber, cranberry, potassium broth (pg. 215), and a green veggie drink (pg. 218).

Take 2 cups watermelon seed tea daily if there are kidney stones.♂♀

Take aloe vera juice before bed.

Take 8 glasses of water each day.

2—Then, a simple low salt, very low protein, vegetarian diet with 75% fresh foods for a week.

3—Avoid all refined, fried, fatty foods, and cola drinks during healing. Avoid salts, sugars, and caffeine-containing foods. Eliminate dairy products. Reduce all animal protein.

4—Add sea greens and bee pollen, 2 TBS each for healing amino acids daily.

Superfood Therapy (choose 1 or 2)
• Crystal Star ENERGY GREEN™.
• Transitions EASY GREENS.
• Rainbow HAWAIIAN SPIRULINA.♂
• Future Biotics VITAL K drink daily.
• Aloe Falls ALOE JUICE with ginger.
• Sun Wellness CHLORELLA 2 pkts. daily.

Herb & Supplement Therapy

Eliminate iron supplements during healing. Avoid L-cysteine, it aggravates crystallization in the kidneys.

—Interceptive therapy plan: (Choose 2 to 3 recommendations)

1—**Control infection:** • Crystal Star ANTI-BIO™ capsules 6 daily 'til infection clears; then • STN-EX™ capsules for a month to help dissolve stones. Then, • GREEN TEA CLEANSER™ or • Herbs Etc. KIDNEY TONIC every morning for another month.

2—**Healthy kidney flushing support:** • Dandelion tea, 2 cups daily; • Crystal Star BLDR-K™ caps or tea; • Uva Ursi, Couchgrass or Watercress tea. (Take Crystal Star IODINE-POTASSIUM caps daily if taking diuretic drugs.)

3—**Normalize kidney activity:** • Cleavers tea; • Parsley-cornsilk tea; • St. John's wort extract caps (especially if incontinent); • Solaray ALFAJUICE caps daily; • vitamin K 100mcg; • Solaray CALCIUM CITRATE 4 daily; • Gotu Kola caps 4 to 6 daily.

4—**Reduce kidney inflammation:** • Quercetin 1000mg daily with bromelain 1500mg daily; • B-complex 100mg; extra B-6, 100mg daily and • magnesium 800mg daily. • Enzymatic Therapy LIQUID LIVER with GINSENG and RENATONE 2x daily. • High omega-3 flax oil daily. • Solaray LIPOTROPIC PLUS daily, or • Choline/Inositol caps 4x daily. • Tranformation Enzyme EXCELLZYME.

5—**Reverse kidney damage:** • GINKGO BILOBA extract as needed; • Spirulina 1 teasp. powder daily, especially from drug damage. • Licorice tea 2 cups daily or • Crystal Star GINSENG-LICORICE ELIXIR™ drops in water; • Evening primrose oil caps 4 daily. • MICROHYDRIN available at Healthy House; • Enzymedica PURIFY caps.

6—**Kidney cleansers and detoxifiers:** • Burdock root tea, 2 cups daily; Echinacea extract 4x daily; • garlic-cayenne caps 8 daily; Alpha Lipoic acid up to 600mg daily; • Dandelion extract especially for nephritis.♀ • Gaia Herbs PLAINTAIN-BUCHU SUPREME; • Golden Pride FORMULA ONE oral chelation with EDTA.♂

Lifestyle Support Therapy

—Bodywork:

• Take a daily brisk walk to keep kidney function flowing.

• Avoid commercial antacids during healing.

• Avoid NSAIDS drugs. They have been implicated in kidney failure cases.

• Avoid smoking and secondary smoke.

• Apply moist heat packs, comfrey compresses, and/or alternating hot and cold compresses on the kidney area.

• Apply Chinese white flower oil or tiger balm to kidney area 2-3x daily.

• Apply compresses to kidney area, like hot ginger/oatstraw, cayenne/ginger, mullein/lobelia.

• Use capsicum, spirulina or catnip enemas 2-3x weekly to stimulate better kidney function.

—Reflexology points:

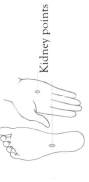

Kidney points

• In addition, press on the back, on the tops of both hip bones, 3x for 10 seconds each.

K 440

Common Symptoms: Kidney disease means painful, frequent urination; chronic lower back pain and fatigue; chills and fever; fluid retention. For kidney stones, there may be no apparent symptoms except a dull ache in the lower back, until the stone blocks the urinary tract, which results in excruciating, radiating pain. Then there is very painful urination, nausea, fever and vomiting.

Common Causes: Excess sugar, red meat, carbonated drinks, sugars and caffeine in the diet; diabetes; allergies; heavy metal poisoning; excess aluminum; EFA deficiency; overuse of prescription or pleasure drugs; B vitamin and magnesium deficiency; overuse of aspirin, salt and chemical diuretics.

See following page for a KIDNEY STONES CLEANSING DIET.

Can't find a recommended product? Call the 800 number listed in Product Resources for the store nearest you.

Do you have kidney stones?

Every decade since World War II, the U.S. has seen a steady rise in kidney stone cases. Today 10% of American men and 5% of American women have a kidney stone by the time they're seventy. Kidney stones are a diet-related illness directly linked to low dietary fiber, high fat and high calcium (usually from dairy sources), and large amounts of animal protein, refined sugar, alcohol and salt. They parallel the rise of the Standard American Diet, full of fat, fried foods, rich dairy products and sugar. Excessive use of antacids and adrenal exhaustion also contribute to kidney stones. Kidney stones form when minerals that normally float free in kidney fluids combine into crystals. When inorganic mineral waste overloads and the body has too little fluid, kidney stones form. There are three types of kidney stones: those composed of calcium salts, the most common type (75-85%), struvite, or non-calcium-containing crystals (10-15%), and uric acid crystals, at about 5-8% occurrence. It takes from 5 to 15 hours of vigorous, urgent treatment to dissolve and pass small stones.

A vegetarian diet, low in proteins and starches, that emphasizes fresh fruits, vegetables and cultured foods to alkalize the system, is the key to avoiding kidney stone formation. This type of diet is high in fiber to reduce urinary calcium waste. It eliminates caffeine foods, salty, sugary and fried foods and soft drinks that inhibit kidney filtering. It avoids mucous-forming foods, like dairy foods, heavy grains, starches and fats, to relieve irritation and inhibit sediment formation. *Note: Do not use TUMS for indigestion. They may increase risk for stone formation.*

Is your body showing signs that it needs a kidney stone cleanse? There may be no apparent symptoms at first except a dull ache in the lower back. When the stone(s) become large enough to block the urinary tract, there is excruciating, radiating pain with extremely painful urination and constant urgency to urinate. The abdomen becomes distended. Women who have heavy menstrual bleeding or anemia, signs of a vitamin K deficiency, should be especially careful since it can lead to stones. As infection sets in, there are chills, nausea, vomiting and fever.

The Kidney Stone Cleanse

Note: Dehydration which causes a reduction in urine volume and an increased rate of excretion of stone constituents is a factor relating to kidney stones. Drink 8-10 glasses of bottled water each day of your cleanse, so that waste and excess minerals are continuously flushed. Stagnate urine flow is a factor in kidney stone formation.

The night before your kidney stone cleanse.... Take a cup of chamomile tea.
The next day.... Take 2 TBS. olive oil through a straw every 4 hours to help dissolve stones.
—**On rising:** take cranberry juice (from concentrate) in water with 1 tsp. honey; or 2 TBS apple cider vinegar in water with 1 tsp. honey; and a cup of chamomile tea.
—**Breakfast:** have a glass of cranberry juice, or fresh watermelon juice, or Crystal Star GREEN TEA CLEANSER™
—**Mid-morning:** take 1 cup watermelon seed tea. (grind seeds, steep in hot water 30 minutes, add honey); or a green drink (page 218); or dandelion tea, or Crystal Star BLDR-K™ tea.
—**Lunch:** have a carrot/beet/cucumber juice, and a spinach salad with cucumbers.
—**Mid-afternoon:** have a cup of chamomile tea; and asparagus stalks and carrot sticks with kefir cheese; or fresh apples with kefir or yogurt dip.
—**Dinner:** have brown rice with steamed veggies or steamed asparagus with miso soup and snipped, dry sea greens; or a baked potato with kefir cheese and a spinach salad.
—**Before Bed:** take a glass of aloe vera juice and another cup of chamomile tea; or miso/ginger soup with sea greens snipped on top.

After your cleanse: When you begin eating solid foods, make sure you eat plenty of fresh fruits and vegetables. Studies show that even meat eaters had a lower incidence of stones when they ate higher amounts of fresh fruits and vegetables. Keep salt and protein low for at least 3 weeks. Establish a diet with plenty of fiber. Vitamin K is an important part of your body's natural inhibitors of kidney stone formation. Eat plenty of spinach and sea greens, high in vitamin K.

Supplements to consider:
Kidney stone cleansers: Ascorbate or Ester C powder in water; ¼ tsp. every hour to bowel tolerance until stones pass - about 5000mg daily; Alpha Lipoic acid 100 to 150mg daily.
Mineral balancers to prevent stones: Flora VEGE-SIL caps 2 daily for kidney stone prevention; Solaray CALCIUM CITRATE 4 daily.
To prevent stones: Vitamin C 3000mg with bioflavonoids for a month to acidify urine; Futurebiotics VITAL K or vitamin K 100mcg daily; quercetin 1000mg daily with bromelain 1500mg.
Enzyme support: Transformation Enzyme EXCELLZYME and PUREZYME (a protease supplement that breaks apart protein-based viscid matter that cements salts into stones).
Dissolve kidney sediment wastes: Enzymatic Therapy ACID-A-CAL caps; chamomile, rosemary, or dandelion/nettles tea - about 5 cups a day for one to 2 weeks; Jean's Greens P.P.T. tea.
Green superfoods inhibit growth of stones: Crystal Star ENERGY GREEN, Transitions EASY GREENS, Aloe Falls ALOE-GINGER, Sun Wellness CHLORELLA 2 pkts. daily.
Fiber supplements reduce risk of stones: All One WHOLE FIBER COMPLEX; Nature's Secret ULTIMATE FIBER.
Heat therapy: Apply wet, hot compresses and lower back massage when there is inflammation flare up, especially lobelia or ginger fomentations.

See my book Cooking For Healthy Healing for a complete kidney healing diet.

Can't find a recommended product? Call the 800 number listed in Product Resources for the store nearest you.

Leukemia

Blood and Bone Marrow Cancer

Leukemias are cancers which originate in the tissues of the bone marrow, spleen and lymph nodes. They are characterized by excessive production of white blood cells and seem to result from a failure of the bone marrow to function adequately. The spleen and liver are infiltrated and damaged by the excess leukocytes. Lymph nodes and nerves are also affected. Thirty-thousand Americans are diagnosed each year with leukemias - 20,000 die as a result of it. New research shows a link between childhood leukemia and parents who smoke. Natural treatments, especially in conjunction with cytotoxic drugs have improved the remission rate of this type of cancer to over 50%. Cortico-steroid drugs given to relieve symptoms of leukemia, over a long period of time greatly weaken immunity and bone strength.

Diet & Superfood Therapy

—Nutritional therapy plan:

1—Food healing value is lost very quickly in this disease. Make sure the diet is very nutritious.

2—Start with a gentle cleansing/detoxification program (pg. 191) for 2 months. Follow with a macrobiotic diet program, using organically grown foods (pg. 333) for 3 to 4 months with no animal protein and lots of alkalizing foods.

3—Vegetable proteins are the key after initial detoxification. Eat lots of green leafy vegetables on a continuing basis for red blood cell formation. Include plenty of potassium-rich foods.

4—To clean vital organs, take a glass of carrot/beet/cucumber juice every day for the first month of healing; every other day for the second month; once a week the third month. Add a potassium broth every other day (pg. 215).

5—Take 2 glasses of cranberry juice daily.

6—Avoid alcohol, junk and chemicalized foods, refined sugars and red meats.

—Superfood therapy: (Choose one)

• Green Foods CARROT ESSENCE and GREEN MAGMA drinks.
• Sun Wakasa GOLD, liquid CHLORELLA.
• Beehive Botanicals ROYAL JELLY with SIBERIAN GINSENG and PROPOLIS 4x daily.
• AloeLife ALOE VERA GOLD daily.
• Rainbow Light HAWAIIAN SPIRULINA.

Herb & Supplement Therapy

—Interceptive therapy plan: (Choose 2 to 3 recommendations)

1—Help detoxify the blood: • Crystal Star DETOX™ caps 2 daily with GREEN TEA CLEANSER™ 2x daily, or 2 cups of burdock tea daily for 1 month. • Crystal Star CAN-SSIAC™ caps or • Natural Energy CAISSE'S TEA or • Pau d'arco tea. • Flora FLOR-ESSENCE Essiac liquid for 2 months. • Vita Carre BOVINE CARTILAGE or • Nutricology MODIFIED CITRUS PECTIN to stimulate glutathione.

2—Help reduce organ swelling: • Turmeric capsules (curcumin) 8 daily; • Crystal Star LIV-ALIVE™ capsules with • MILK THISTLE SEED extract for 2 months to revitalize liver function. • Enzymatic Therapy LIQUID LIVER with SIBERIAN GINSENG 4 daily. • Allergy Reasearch Group LACTOFERRIN with colostrum.

3—Help kill the cancer: • Nutricology GERMANIUM 150mg daily; • American Biologics Colloidal Silver. • Glutathione 50mg 4x daily; • Earth's Bounty O₂ caps as directed. • American Biologics DIOXYCHLOR for detoxification.

4—Help rebuild marrow and red blood: • PHYCOTENE MICROCLUSTERS available at Healthy House. • Folic acid 800mcg daily, especially if taking chemotherapy. • Floradix LIQUID IRON; • Siberian ginseng extract; • Health Aid America SIBERGEN; • Garlic/cayenne caps 8 daily; or Yellow Dock tea; • Crystal Star IRON SOURCE™ extract. • Country Life sublingual B-12, 2500mcg every other day for body balance/strength. • Enzymedica PURIFY caps.

5—Normalize blood cells and lymphatic system: • Nutricology CAR-T-CELL liquid; • Enzymatic Therapy THYMUPLEX tablets; • Crystal Star GINSENG-REISHI extract, or • Crystal Star GINSENG-CHLORELLA extract for 2 months.
• Pau D'Arco or Echinacea extract to normalize the lymphatic system.

6—Strengthen the blood and immune system: • HAWTHORN extract; • Niacin therapy: 250mg 4x daily all during healing with • B Complex 100mg, 4x daily, with extra folic acid, and B₆ 250mg. • New Chapter OCEAN MINERALS 4 daily for needed minerals. • Ascorbate vit. C or Ester C powder, up to 10,000mg daily with bioflavonoids and rutin for several months. • Beta carotene 150,000IU daily with selenium 200mcg; • zinc 50mg. • Vitamin E 800IU with selenium 200mcg; • zinc 50mg.

Lifestyle Support Therapy

—Bodywork:

• Overheating therapy is effective for leukemia. See page 225 in this book.
• Use in conjunction with wheat grass enema or implant therapy for best results.
• Avoid pesticides, X-rays, microwaves, electromagnetic fields from power lines and radiation of all kinds if possible. There seems to be a clear link between these and leukemia, especially in children.
• Chemotherapy treatment for other cancers has sometimes been implicated in the development of leukemia.
• Smoking is linked to leukemia.
• Relaxation techniques, such as meditation, imagery, acupuncture and reflexology are effective for leukemias.

—Lymph-Flow Bath: Put 1/2 pound each baking soda and sea salt in the tub. Soak for 20 minutes. Dunk head 5 times. Drip dry; stay warm; then shower.

Common Symptoms: Increase in white blood cells, with no red blood cell production; extreme tiredness and anemia with symptoms similar to pernicious anemia, like weakness and pallor, easy bruising, bone pain, thinness and weight loss; fever, chills and chronic infections - especially in children; spleen malfunction or swelling of the spleen, liver and lymph nodes; red spots under the skin; swollen, bleeding gums and bone pain.

Common Causes: Indiscriminate use of X-rays and some drugs, especially in children and pregnant women; severe malnutrition with too many refined carbohydrates (especially in children); overfluoridation of the water; thyroid malfunction; deficiencies of vitamin D, iron, B₁₂ and folic acid; chronic viral infections; hereditary proneness. See Cancer causes in this book.

See the CANCER DIET in this book, or COOKING FOR HEALTHY HEALING by Linda Rector-Page for a complete healing diet.

Can't find a recommended product? Call the 800 number listed in Product Resources for the store nearest you.

Liver Health

Renewal and Revitalization

Be good to your liver. A healthy liver is the key to a healthy life! The health and vitality of every body system depends to a large extent on the vitality of the liver. It is the body's most complex and useful organ - a powerful chemical plant that converts everything we eat, breathe and absorb through the skin into life-sustaining substances. The liver is a major blood reservoir, filtering out toxins at a rate of over a quart of blood per minute. It manufactures bile to digest fats and prevent constipation. The liver is a vast storehouse for vitamins, minerals, and enzymes that it releases as needed to build and maintain healthy cells. Fortunately, since we live in an increasingly toxic world, the liver has amazing regenerative powers. A complete liver renewal program takes from three months to a year.

Diet & Superfood Therapy

—Nutritional therapy plan:

1—Keeping fat low in your diet is crucial for liver vitality and regeneration. Optimum nutrition is the best liver protection.

2—Follow an alkalizing, rebuilding diet for a month with high quality vegetable protein. (See Liver Detox, page 205).

3—Take daily during healing: 1 TB each lecithin granules and brewer's yeast, 2-3 glasses cranberry or apple juice and 8 glasses of bottled water.

4—Avoid red meats and other acid-forming foods - caffeine, alcohol, refined starches and dairy products during all healing phases. Reduce sugars, saturated fats and fried foods permanently.

Liver health and support foods:

Vegetable fiber foods that absorb excess bile and increase regularity.

Potassium-rich foods: sea foods, dried fruits.

Chlorophyll-rich foods: leafy greens, sea greens.

Enzyme-rich foods: yogurt and kefir.

Sulphur-rich foods: eggs, garlic and onions.

—Superfood therapy: (Choose one or two)

• Green Foods CARROT ESSENCE.

• Beehive Botanicals ROYAL JELLY, GINSENG, POLLEN drink.

• Crystal Star SYSTEMS STRENGTH™ drink.

• George's ALOE VERA JUICE (high sulphur).

• Sun Wellness CHLORELLA 1 pkt. daily.

Herb & Supplement Therapy

—Interceptive therapy plan: (Choose 2 to 3 recommendations)

1—**Gently cleanse the liver:** SAMe 800mg daily with • Crystal Star LIV-ALIVE™ caps 6 daily and tea, 2 cups daily, with • BITTERS & LEMON CLEANSE™ extract each morning. • Alpha Lipoic Acid 300-600mg daily; • Enzymatic Therapy LIVA-TOX, or • Nature's Apothecary LIVER CLEANSE. • Ascorbate vitamin C 500mg every hour during cleansing stage, then 3000mg daily.

Cleanse your liver to help balance your hormone levels: • Burdock Root tea 2 cups daily. • Source Naturals CO-ENZYMATE B daily with • Country Life PHOSPHATIDYL CHOLINE 600mg or • Solaray LIPOTROPIC PLUS - esp. if taking contraceptives. Or take • AloeLife FIBERMATE powder and mix in 1 teasp. high omega-3 flax seed oil daily. • Country Life sublingual B-12, 2500mcg daily.♀

2—**Prickly herbs heal and enhance your liver:** Take one or a combination of the drops in water 3x daily. • MILK THISTLE SEED extract in aloe vera juice; • ARTICHOKE extract; • DANDELION ROOT extract; • BURDOCK ROOT extract.

3—**Bitters herbs boost liver and bile production:** • Crystal Star GREEN TEA CLEANSER™; • Solaray TURMERIC extract caps (*curcumin*) 4 daily; or • *barberry-turmeric* capsules 6 daily; • Gaia SWEETISH BITTERS; • Enzymedica DIGEST CAPS; • *dandelion extract drops;* • *turmeric-cardamom-lemon peel* added to any drink.

4—**Enhance liver vitality:** • *Pau d'Arco* tea; • *Reishi* or *Maitake* mushroom extracts; • *Bupleurum* extract (especially if immune compromised); • Royal jelly 2 teasp. daily; • Nutricology GERMANIUM 150mg; • Crystal Star GINSENG/REISHI extract.

5—**Replenish liver nutrients:** Liver rebuilding tonic: • Mix 4-oz. *hawthorn berries,* 2-oz. *red sage,* 1-oz. *cardamom.* Steep 24 hours in 2 qts. of water. Add honey. Take 2 cups daily. • Crystal Star GINSENG/LICORICE ELIXIR™ an ongoing liver tonic.

6—**Probiotics help normalize liver function:** • Natren TRINITY, or • Prof. Nutrition Dr. DOPHILUS + FOS, or take • Prevail LIVER FORMULA caps.♂

7—**Boost liver antioxidants:** • Enzymatic THYMU-PLEX; • Carnitine 1000mg; • Beta-carotene 100,000IU, or • PHYCOTENE MICROCLUSTERS from Healthy House; • CoQ₁₀ 100mg daily; • PCO's from grapeseed or white pine 100mg daily.

Lifestyle Support Therapy

—Bodywork:

• The liver is dependent on high quality oxygen coming into the lungs. Exercise, air filters, time spent in the forest and at the ocean, and drinking pure water are important.

• Overheating by raising blood temperature is effective. See pg. 225 in this book.

—Good liver lifestyle practices:

Eat smaller meals, minimize late night eating.

Get adequate, regular sleep.

A daily brisk aerobic walk.

Overusing either saccharin foods or acetaminaphen drugs can cause liver toxicity.

• Take one coffee enema during your detoxification cleanse; (1 cup coffee to 1 qt. distilled water.) Wheat grass implants are also effective.

• Take several saunas if possible during a liver cleanse for faster, easier detoxification.

—Reflexology point:

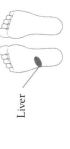

Liver

Common Symptoms: *Sluggish system; general depression and melancholy; unexplained weight gain and great tiredness; poor digestion; food and chemical sensitivities; PMS; constipation and congestion; nausea and shakes; dizziness; dry tongue and mouth; jaundiced skin and/or liver spots; skin itching.*

Common Causes: *Too much alcohol and/or drugs; too much sugar, refined, low nutrition foods, and preservatives; overeating - esp. too much animal protein; low fiber; low vegetable diet; exposure to toxic environmental chemicals and pollutants; stress; hepatitis virus; long-term use of prescription drugs (especially antibiotics and tranquilizers); drip from a chronic sinus infection; candida yeast infection.*

See Liver Detox page 205 for more info.

Can't find a recommended product? Call the 800 number listed in Product Resources for the store nearest you.

Liver Disease
Cirrhosis, Jaundice

Cirrhosis, or scarring, of the liver tissue is a serious, degenerative condition, preventing the liver from its proper function. It is the second biggest killer of people between 45 and 65 in America today. Usually a consequence of alcohol abuse, it is also almost always a part of other severe liver infections, such as hepatitis, EBV, and AIDS related syndromes. Jaundice, the yellow discoloration of the skin and eyelids due to excess concentrations of bilirubin, is a symptom of liver congestion, not a disease. If your diet is nutrient poor, the liver becomes exhausted, and even more serious debilitation results. Note: Smoking is terrible for liver health. Try even harder to quit all forms of tobacco. It almost goes without saying that alcohol must be eliminated.

Diet & Superfood Therapy

Liver congestion is the underlying condition. Optimum nutrition is the key to liver healing.

—Nutritional therapy plan:

1—If condition is acute, go on a 3 day liquid detoxification diet (see Liver Detox, page 205) to clean out toxic waste. Drink 6-8 glasses of pure water daily.

2—Take a carrot/beet/cucumber juice daily for 1 week, then every other day for a week, then every 2 days, then every 3 days, etc. for a month.

3—A glass of lemon juice and water each morning.

4—Include two glasses of carrot juice daily for a month during healing.

5—Eat plenty of fresh fruits and vegetables. Particularly eat plenty of vegetable protein such as sprouts, whole grains, tofu, wheat germ, and brewer's yeast.

6—Avoid all alcohol, fried, salty or fatty foods, caffeine, sugar and tobacco.

7—Make a mix of lecithin, brewer's yeast and wheat germ oil; add 2 tsp. to any drink.

—Superfood therapy: (Choose one or two)
- Crystal Star ENERGY GREEN™.
- Wakunaga KYO-GREEN with EFA's.
- AloeLife ALOE GOLD drink.
- Green Foods GREEN MAGMA.
- Sun Wellness CHLORELLA 1 pkt. daily.
- Solgar WHEY TO GO protein drink.

Herb & Supplement Therapy

—Interceptive therapy plan: (Choose 3 or more recommendations)

1—**Gently cleanse the liver:** • Crystal Star GREEN TEA CLEANSER™ daily for 3 to 6 months. • Garlic capsules 4 daily. • Natren BIFIDO FACTORS 3x daily to cleanse and restore liver tissue; *Dandelion* root extract drops in water. For jaundice: take • *Barberry* tea until clear.

2—**Boost liver metabolism and function:** • SAMe 800mg daily with • TMG (trimethylglycine if desired, 2000mg daily); • Crystal Star LIV-ALIVE™ caps 6 daily with • BITTERS & LEMON CLEANSE™ extract each morning, • or LIV-ALIVE™ tea (3 cups daily for 3 weeks, then 1 cup daily for a month.); • Lipoic Acid 600mg daily; or MRI ALPHA-LIPOIC ACID; • Enzymatic Therapy LIQUID LIVER with *Siberian Ginseng*. • Vitamin C 500mg every hour for cleansing stage, then 3000mg daily. • MILK THISTLE SEED extract 3x daily against alcohol damage.

3—**Help heal internal scarring:** • Crystal Star GINSENG 6 SUPER TEA™; • Solaray CENTELLA ASIATICA 4 daily; or • *Schizandra* extract; • Make a healing liver tea. Take 1 cup daily: 1 TB each: *bilberry, ginkgo biloba, ginger* rt.

4—**Lipotropics prevent fat accumulation in the liver:** • Choline 600mg or • Country Life PHOSPHATIDYL CHOLINE 600mg 4x daily; or • Solaray LIPO-TROPIC PLUS caps; • Choline/inositol 100mg; • Methionine 2x daily; • Lecithin capsules 2 daily.

5—**Powerful antioxidants address critical free radical damage:** Take for 2 to 3 months- • Ascorbate vitamin C crystals 5000mg daily or to bowel tolerance. • Nutricology GERMANIUM 150mg. • CoQ10 60mg 3x daily. • Beta-carotene 150,000IU daily. • Solaray ALFAJUICE caps. • Vitamin E 800IU with selenium 200mcg 2x daily; • Country Life sublingual B-12, 2500mcg daily for energy. • MICROHYDRIN available from Healthy House.

6—**Nutrients to help against severe liver dysfunction:** • Morada Research LIVER to stimulate new liver cells; • Enzymatic Therapy LIVA-TOX caps; • Glutamine 500mg 4x daily; • Carnitine 500mg 2x daily; • Enzymatic Therapy SUPER MILK THISTLE COMPLEX with artichoke; • Enzymedica DIGEST.

Lifestyle Support Therapy

—Signs of liver congestion:
- Indigestion and mild nausea after meals.
- Especially indigestion after fatty foods.
- Unexplained head and body aches.
- Low energy, easy fatigue.
- Distention in the stomach (liver area).
- Slightly yellow look to the skin and eyelids.
- Body fluid retention and swelling.

—Bodywork:
- Take a coffee enema once a week for a month to flush out and stimulate liver activity. (1 cup strong brewed in a quart of water), or chlorella or spirulina implants.
- Take a daily early morning sunbath.

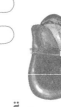

—Reflexology point:

Liver

—Liver area:

L 444

Common Symptoms: Sluggish, reduced energy; constipation alternating to diarrhea; often jaundice; skin itching/irritation; bags under the eyes. Severe symptoms include anemia and large bruise patches. As cirrhosis progresses, there is increasing weakness, jaundice and abdominal distention.

Common Causes: Liver toxicity from excess alcohol and/or drugs; environmental pollutants; excess refined foods and sugars; long term malnutrition.

See also HEPATITIS page 416 and LIVER DETOX DIET page 205.

Can't find a recommended product? Call the 800 number listed in Product Resources for the store nearest you.

Low Blood Pressure

Hypotension, Hypoadrenalism

Even though we hear much less about it, chronically low blood pressure is also a threat to good health. Low blood pressure is generally recognized as 100/60 or below. LBP is abnormal blood pressure due to a variety of causes, from a reaction to drug medication to an electrolyte-loss response to a disease, or an endocrine or nerve disorder. LBP is also a sign that arterial system walls and tissue are weak; blood and fluid can leak and abnormally distend them, and prevent good circulation. Natural treatment works well when there are symptoms such as dizziness or light-headedness upon standing up, or faintness, indicating a reduction of cerebral flow.

Diet & Superfood Therapy

—**Nutritional therapy plan:**

1—Follow a fresh foods diet for a week, with veggie drinks (pg. 218), potassium broth (pg. 215), brewer's yeast, and green salads. Take a lemon and water drink every morning with 1 teasp. honey.

2—Then, follow a modified macrobiotic diet for 2 months, stressing vegetable proteins, green salads with celery, (natural sodium) miso, onions, garlic (natural sulphur) and other alkalizing foods, and dried or fresh fruits. —Include strengthening complex carbohydrates, such as peas, broccoli, potatoes and whole grains.

3—Bioflavonoids are the key for stronger blood vessels: Citrus juices, esp. pineapple juice; grape juice; green tea.

4—Avoid canned and refined foods, animal fats, red meats, and caffeine. Reduce all high cholesterol, starchy foods.

5—Natural salts help hypoadrenalism: sea salt or Knudsen RECHARGE electrolyte drink, or Alacer MIRACLE WATER.

—**Superfood therapy: (Choose one or two)**

• Crystal Star SYSTEMS STRENGTH™ drink or caps for absorbable minerals.

• Protein drinks: Unipro PERFECT PROTEIN or Solgar WHEY TO GO.

• Future Biotics VITAL K, 6 teasp. daily.

• Crystal Star GREEN TEA CLEANSER™.

Herb & Supplement Therapy

Avoid the amino acids phenylalanine and tyrosine if your blood pressure is low.

—**Interceptive therapy plans: (choose 2 or 3 recommendations)**

1—**Normalize blood pressure:** • Crystal Star HEARTSEASE/HAWTHORN™ capsules 2-4 daily for a month, with • 8 garlic caps daily; or Heart Foods CAYENNE HEART FOOD caps. • Vitamin E therapy for 8 weeks: work up from 100IU daily the first week, to 800IU daily, adding 100mg daily each week; or • VITAMIN E CLUSTERS available from Healthy House. • Dandelion root caps 4 daily.

2—**Support better metabolism:** • Crystal Star BITTERS & LEMON CLEANSE™ extract for metabolism support; • Kelp tablets 10 daily, or • Biotec SEA PLASMA tablets 10 daily; or • Siberian ginseng extract caps, 4-6 daily; or • Imperial Elixir SIBERIAN GINSENG.

3—**Boost and regulate circulation:** • Crystal Star HEARTSEASE/CIRCULEANSE™ tea for prevention. • Cayenne/ginger caps 4 to 8 daily. • Magnesium 400mg 4x daily, or • Solaray CAL/MAG CITRATE, 1000mg calcium and 1000mg magnesium, or • Rainbow Light CALCIUM PLUS with high magnesium.

4—**Tone blood vessels with flavonoid-rich herbs:** • HAWTHORN or BILBERRY extracts 2-3x daily; • Gotu kola extract or Rosemary for nerve balance; • Lemon peel, Hibiscus or Rose hips tea. • Vitamin K 100mcg 2 daily for capillary strength.

5—**Normalize adrenal function:** • Crystal Star ADR-ACTIVE™ capsules 2x daily for a month with extra • Ginkgo Biloba or Hawthorn or Licorice extract 4x daily; or • Morada Research ADRENAL GLAND extract; • DHEA 25mg daily for 3 months.

6—**Enhance liver function to normalize blood pressure:** • Enzymatic Therapy LIQUID LIVER with Siberian Ginseng. • B Complex 100mg daily with extra B₁ 100mg and pantothenic acid 500mg. • Floradix LIQUID IRON.

7—**Antioxidants are important:** • PCO's from grapeseed and white pine, 100mg daily, or • BD Herbs GRAPE SEED organic extract for extra high flavonoids. • Germanium 150mg 2x daily. • Vitamin C with bioflavonoids and rutin 3000mg daily or • Ethical Nutrients SUPER FLAVONOID C; • Extra zinc 30mg 2x daily.

Lifestyle Support Therapy

Sometimes tiredness and lack of energy are a sign of low blood pressure. Check out your symptoms.

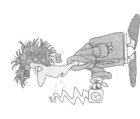

—**Bodywork:**

• Acupressure, chiropractic spinal manipulation and shiatsu therapy are all effective in normalizing circulatory function.

• Alternating hot and cold hydrotherapy (pg. 228) revs up circulation.

• Avoid tobacco and secondary smoke.

• Consciously try to relax the whole body once a day with short meditation, yoga exercises and rest.

• Do deep breathing exercises (page 554) to stimulate circulation and oxygenate the tissues.

• Stand up slowly to allow blood pressure to normalize.

Common Symptoms: Malfunction of the circulatory system's systole/diastol action; thinning of the blood; great fatigue and easy loss of energy; sometimes dizziness and lightheadedness, especially on standing quickly; heat and cold intolerance; nervousness; extreme tiredness after exercise; reduced immunity and susceptibility to allergies and infections, particularly opportunistic disease like candida yeast overgrowth.
Common Causes: Poor diet with vitamin C and bioflavonoid deficiency causing a "run-down" condition; weak adrenal function; kidney malfunction causing system toxemia; emotional problems; anemia; overuse of drugs that lower immunity.

See ADRENAL HEALTH page 300 and CHRONIC FATIGUE SYNDROME page 350 for more information. Call the 800 number listed in Product Resources for the store nearest you.

Can't find a recommended product?

Lung Disease

Tuberculosis, Sarcoidosis, Cystic Fibrosis

Chronic pulmonary diseases have increased dramatically in the last decade. Three that have been part of this unusual rise are discussed here. **Sarcoidosis** is a systemic viral infection with widespread, grainy lesions on tissue or organs. The lungs and liver are both usually affected, with a chronic cough and difficulty breathing. **Tuberculosis** is a highly contagious, bacterial infection that's on the rise in America. It is characterized by bloody sputum, a chronic cough, shortness of breath and fatigue, night sweats, serious weight loss and chest pain. **Cystic fibrosis** is an inherited childhood disease characterized by recurring lung infections and severe malnutrition from lack of nutrient absorption. The abnormality can destroy the lungs and cause serious impairment to the liver and pancreas.

Diet & Superfood Therapy

—Nutritional therapy plan:

1—Go on a short mucous cleansing liquid diet (pg. 196). Then, use the following lung cleansing diet for two weeks:

Lemon or grapefruit juice and water each morning with 1 tsp. honey; or water-diluted pineapple juice as a natural expectorant.

Fresh carrot juice or potassium drink (pg. 215) daily.

Two fresh green salads daily.

Steamed vegetables with brown rice and tofu or seafood for dinner.

Cranberry or celery juice before bed.

2—High quality protein is needed to heal lung diseases. The diet should be high in vegetable proteins and whole grains, low in sugars and starches.

Include cultured foods such as yogurt and kefir for friendly G.I. flora.

Lung specifics- apricots, peaches, plums.

Include brewer's yeast 2 teasp. daily.

Take a protein drink each morning.

—Superfood therapy: (Choose one or two)

- Salute ALOE VERA JUICE with herbs.
- Crystal Star SYSTEMS STRENGTH™.
- Unipro PERFECT PROTEIN.
- Green Foods CARROT ESSENCE.
- Rainbow Light HAWAIIAN SPIRULINA.

Herb & Supplement Therapy

—Interceptive therapy plans: (choose 2 or 3 recommendations)

1—Help control lung infection: • Crystal Star ANTI-BIO™caps 6 daily for 1 week; then 2 daily with • BIO-VI™ extract for 2 months. Then Crystal Star • RESPR™ caps 4 daily • DEEP BREATHING™ tea daily; or • OLIVE LEAF extract caps 3x daily.

2—Help remove pollutants from the lungs: • Crystal Star HEAVY METAL™ caps 6 daily; • Premier Labs GERMANIUM 150mg; • Enzymedica PURIFY.

3—Help heal the lungs: • Pau d'arco tea 3C. daily; • Evening Primrose Oil 6 daily.
• B-complex 150mg, extra B-12, 2500mcg for anemia; • Now OREGANO OIL soft gels.

4—Antioxidants for the lungs: (May give to children in lower dose as protection.)
• Beta-carotene 150,000IU daily; • Lycopene 5-10mg; CoQ-10 100mg 3x daily; • Carnitine 1000mg 2x daily;
• Grape seed or white pine PCOs 100mg 3x daily; • American Vitamin C 5000mg with bioflavonoids daily.

H_2O_2 therapy: • Earth's Bounty OXY-CLEANSE caps, or • American Biologics DIOXYCHLOR for 1 month. Rest for a month; resume if needed. There will be intense and prolonged coughing, as accumulated waste is released. H_2O_2 works to destroy chronic infection in the lungs and provide nascent oxygen to the tissues.

—Natural help for tuberculosis:
• Olive Leaf extract caps; • High potency royal jelly 2 tsp. daily; • Silica is a specific- Eidon SILICA, 6 daily, and Body Essentials SILICA gel chest rub. • Chlorella 20 tabs daily. • Vitamin A 100,000 daily (one month under practitioner). • CoQ-10, 100mg 3x daily; • Quercetin 1000mg with Bromelain 1500 daily; • Vitamin C 5000mg daily or to bowel tolerance.

—Natural help for sarcoidosis:
• Planetary TRIPHALA caps; • Melatonin .3mg to reduce nodules; • FutureBiotics VITAL GREEN tabs; • Garlic caps 8 daily.

—Natural help for cystic fibrosis:
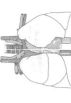 • Transformation PURE-ZYME protease as directed; • CoQ-10 200mg daily; • Echinacea/ goldenseal caps 6 daily or • Crystal Star BIO-VI™ extract drops 4x daily; • Omega-3 flax oil, 2tsp. daily; • Solaray ALFAJUICE caps 6 daily; • Nutricology GERMANIUM 150mg; • Herbal healers: licorice, osha root, astragalus, thyme or coltsfoot; • Natren LIFE START daily.

Lifestyle Support Therapy

—Bodywork:
• Avoid all CFC's. They are as harmful to your lungs as they are to the atmosphere.
• For T.B.: Calendula ointment chest rub.
• Get plenty of fresh air and sunshine, away from air pollution.
• Scratch the arm lightly, for 5 minutes daily, along the meridian line from the shoulder to the outside of the thumb to clear and heal lungs.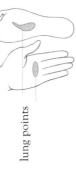
• For cystic fibrosis, use gentle percussion on the chest to keep mucous from clogged airways.
• Take a catnip or chlorophyll enema once a week to clear body toxins out faster.

—Reflexology point

lung points

—Lung area:

Common Symptoms: Constant coughing, inflammation and pain; bloody expectoration; difficulty breathing; difficulty performing even simple activities without shortness of breath. Cystic fibrosis symptoms include very salty sweat from dysfunctional sweat glands.

Common Causes: Environmental and heavy metal pollutants, such as chlorofluorocarbons and smoking; malnutrition, and vitamin A deficiency; suppressive over-the-counter cold and congestion remedies that don't allow the lungs to eliminate harmful wastes properly. Cystic fibrosis is genetically inherited.

See the ASTHMA DIET page 319 or "Cooking For Healthy Healing" for a complete lung healing diet.

Can't find a recommended product? Call the 800 number listed in Product Resources for the store nearest you.

Lupus

Systemic Lupus Erythematosis

Lupus is a multi-system, auto-immune, inflammatory, viral disease affecting over half a million Americans, more than 80% of them black and Hispanic women. The immune system becomes disoriented and develops antibodies that attack its own connective tissue. Joints and connective are affected producing arthritis-like symptoms. Kidneys and lymph nodes become inflamed; in severe cases there is heart, brain and central nervous system degeneration. Orthodox treatment has not been very successful for lupus. Natural therapies help rebuild a stable immune system and relieve some of the associated stress. Our experience shows that you feel worse for 1 or 2 months until toxins are neutralized. Then, suddenly, as a rule, you feel much better. A natural program works, but requires many months of healing.

Diet & Superfood Therapy

—Nutritional therapy plan:

1—Diet therapy, especially eliminating food allergens reduces the symptoms of lupus. Follow the Arthritis Cleansing Diet, page 318 for 3 months:

2—Eat 60-75% fresh foods during this time. Avoid nightshade plants that aggravate lupus, like eggplant, tomatoes, tobacco.

3—A potassium drink, pg. 215 daily for 1 month, then every other day for 1 month, then once a week the 3rd month (sometimes dramatic results).

4—Then follow a modified macrobiotic diet (pg. 333) until blood tests clear, (sometimes 2-3 years, but healing success rate is good). Take aloe vera juice 1 to 2 glasses daily. Drink green tea every morning or Crystal Star GREEN TEA CLEANSER™ to re-establish homeostasis.

5—A low fat, vegetarian diet is strongly recommended to increase essential fatty acids and decrease red meats, sugars, starchy foods.

—Superfood therapy is important: (choose 2 or 3)

• Wakunaga KYO-GREEN drink.
• Crystal Star SYSTEMS STRENGTH™ drink.
• Nutricology PRO-GREENS with EFA's.
• Beehive Botanical ROYAL JELLY with Siberian ginseng; or CC Pollen BUZZ BARS.
• AloeLife ALOE GOLD JUICE 2x daily, or FIBERMATE 2x daily.
• Sun Wellness CHLORELLA 20 tabs daily.

Herb & Supplement Therapy

—Interceptive therapy plan: (Choose 2 to 4 recommendations)

1—**Reduce inflammation and manage pain:** • Homeopathic Hormonegentics HGH 2c-30c; • MSM caps 800mg daily or • Futurebiotics MSM caps or MSM with MICROHYDRIN available at Healthy House; • *Gotu kola* extract or • Solaray *Centella Asiatica* caps 6 daily. • Quercetin 1000mg and bromelain 1500mg daily. • Solaray TURMERIC (*curcumin*) caps for inflammation.

2—**Relieve arthritis-like symptoms:** • Acetyl-L-Carnitine 1000mg daily. • Chondroitin 1200 and Glucosamine 1500mg daily. • *Evening Primrose* oil 3000mg daily for inflammation; • Crystal Star AR-EASE™ caps, very relieving. • *Burdock* tea 2 cups daily, blood cleanser for muscles; • Nutricology GERMANIUM 150mg.

3—**Add magnesium and B-vitamins for muscle pain:** • Magnesium 400mg 2x daily or • Ethical Nutrients MALIC/MAGNESIUM to ease tender points; • B-complex 150mg 3x daily, or • Nature's Secret ULTIMATE B tabs for effective EFA's.

4—**Relieve stress caused by lupus:** • SAMe (*S-adenosyl methionine*) 800mg daily; • *Reishi* mushroom extract or • Crystal Star GINSENG-REISHI extract 4x daily relax without sedation. • *Kava kava* extract or • Crystal Star RELAX™ caps with kava relieves muscle spasms. • *Siberian ginseng* extract or • Crystal Star ADRN-ACTIVE™ caps relieve adrenal stress; • *St. John's wort* 300mg daily for lupus depression.

5—**Heal the liver:** • Crystal Star LIV-ALIVE™ caps and tea daily for 1 month; • *bupleurum* extract 2x daily; • Enzymatic Therapy LIQUID LIVER with *Siberian Ginseng*; • Country Life sublingual B-12, 2500mcg daily. • Enzymedica PURIFY.

6—**Boost immune response against lupus:** • *Astragalus* extract 4x daily; • Nutricology LAKTOFERRIN w. colostrum; • Glutathione 100mg daily; • PCO's from grapeseed 100mg 3x daily; • Vitamin C up to 5000mg daily with bioflavs; • CoQ-10 300mg daily; • Beta-carotene 150,000IU daily; • High potency royal jelly, 40,000mg or more. • Rainforest Remedies STRONG RESISTANCE.

7—**Hormone balancing aids:** DHEA is a specific against lupus: • Nutricology DHEA 50mg daily; • *Dong Quai* and *Sarsaparilla* extract caps; • Crystal Star PRO-EST BALANCE™ roll-on.

Lifestyle Support Therapy

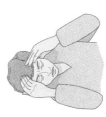

• The risk of lupus has been found to be 40% more likely in users of oral contraceptives than in women who have not used them.

• Birth control pills, penicillin, allergenic cosmetics, and phototoxins from UV rays may result in a flare-up of lupus.

• Over-medication for lupus, especially by cortico-steroid drugs is dangerous; they weaken the bones, cause excess weight gain and eventually suppress immune response.

—Bodywork:

• Get plenty of rest and quality sleep.

• Apply ANTI-BIO™ gel with *una da gato* to heal roughened skin patches.

• Take a walk every day for exercise and stress reduction.

• Effective stress reduction techniques for lupus include biofeedback, meditation, yoga and acupuncture.

Common Symptoms: Great fatigue and depression; rough, red skin patches; chronic nail fungus - red at cuticle base; skin pallor; photosensitivity to light; inability to tear; low grade chronic fever; rheumatoid arthritis symptoms; kidney problems; anemia and low leukocyte count; pleurisy; inflammation, esp. around the mouth, cheeks and nose; seizures, amnesia and psychosis; low immunity.

Common Causes: Viral infection; degeneration of the bods, often caused by too many antibiotics or prescription drugs from Hydrazine derivatives; alcoholism; food allergies; emotional stress; reaction to certain chemicals; latent diabetes; overgrowth of Candida albicans yeasts; chronic fatigue syndrome; triggered by UV sunlight.

See Arthritis page 316 and Immunity sections page 429 for more information.

Can't find a recommended product? Call the 800 number listed in Product Resources for the store nearest you.

Lyme Disease
Lyme Arthritis

Lyme disease is serious illness caused by a micro-organism transmitted to humans by the deer tick, a pest no bigger than a freckle. Almost 100,000 Americans have been infected as of 1999 (about 16,000 yearly). Lyme disease is a serious, steadily debilitating, degenerative disease, with symptoms much like those of arthritis. It is difficult to guard against. Antibiotics are the current medical treatment of choice, and seem to work in the initial phases, symptoms usually recur after the drugs are withdrawn, and they do not work in the later stages at all. Natural therapies (best used after a course of drug antibiotics) that address the disease as if it were a virus have had the best success. Strong immune response is the best defense. Lyme disease is most prevalent in the upper East Coast, upper Midwest, Northern California, and the Oregon coast.

Diet & Superfood Therapy

—**Nutritional therapy plan:**

1—A modified macrobiotic diet (pg. 333) is recommended for 2-3 months to strengthen the body while cleaning out and overcoming the disease.

2—Take a potassium drink (pg. 215) 2x a week.

3—Have a veggie drink (pg. 218) or a fresh green salad every day.

4—Take 1 teasp. each daily: wheat germ oil for body oxygen, EGG YOLK LECITHIN, royal jelly 40,000mg or more.

5—Avoid alcohol, tobacco, all refined and caffeine-containing foods, and sugars. Omit red meat, high gluten and starchy foods.

—**Superfood therapy: (Choose one or two)**

• Green Foods GREEN MAGMA drink.

• Crystal Star ENERGY GREEN™ drink and ZINC SOURCE™ drops.

• Sun Wellnes CHLORELLA, 2 pkts. daily.

• Nutricology PRO-GREENS w. EFA's.

• Morada Research GOD'S GARDEN POWER FOOD blend.

• Solgar WHEY TO GO protein drink.

Herb & Supplement Therapy

Deer ticks also transmit the even more serious pathogen, Ehrlichia, that causes HGE, that can be fatal. Rigorously check for tiny deer ticks if you live in an infested area. Use natural therapy after a course of medical antibiotics.

—**Interceptive therapy plan: (Choose 2 to 4 recommendations)**

1—**Herbal anti-virals show the best effects:** Clean the tick bite with: • tea tree oil, • calendula extract, • echinacea/goldenseal extract, or • St. John's wort extract 2-3x daily. Then take • OREGANO OIL or OLIVE LEAF extract caps, 3x daily, or • Crystal Star BIO-VI™ extract 2x daily, one week on, one week off to overcome the infecting microbe, or • Nutribiotic GRAPEFRUIT SEED extract, 10 drops 3x daily in water. Take • Nutricology GERMANIUM 150mg daily; • Colloidal silver as directed.

2—**Reduce inflammation, repair nerve damage:** • Crystal Star ANTI-FLAM™ caps or extract, or turmeric (curcumin) caps 6 daily. • Crystal Star RELAX CAPS™ to rebuild nerve structure. • Solgar oceanic carotene 100-150,000IU daily with quercetin with bromelain as an anti-inflammatory.

3—**Enhance lymphatic and liver activity:** • Crystal Star ANTI-BIO™ caps or extract 6x daily or echinacea extract to cleanse lymph glands; • Crystal Star LIV-ALIVE™ caps or extract 6x daily to enhance liver activity for a month. • Garlic capsules 6 daily; • Vitamin C or Ester C powder, $\frac{1}{4}$ teasp. every hour to daily bowel tolerance as toxin neutralizer, especially during acute attacks and recurrences.

4—**Boost immune response with:** • N-acetyl-cysteine (NAC) 2000mg daily; • Crystal Star GINSENG/REISHI™ extract or • GINSENG 6 SUPER TEA™ with • suma extract or astragalus extract to re-establish homeostasis. • Lane Labs BENE-FIN shark cartilage to enhance leukocytes with • Enzymatic Therapy THYMULUS complex.

5—**Probiotics reestablish homeostasis:** • Natren LIFE START ⊚ or • Jarrow JARRO-DOPHILUS for damage from long courses of antibiotics and to restore intestinal health. • Solaray pancreatin 1300mg 4x daily on an empty stomach.

—**To repel lyme ticks:** Use • myrrh or pennyroyal oil topically. Apply • Earth's Bounty O_2 gel to the bite.

Lifestyle Support Therapy

DEET chemical repellent, while effective, can be fatal if ingested and can cause adverse reactions in children.

—**Bodywork:** Time is critical. The longer the tick is attached the greater the risks of serious disease. Symptoms show up 3 weeks after tick bite.

• Use natural tick repellents on exposed body areas. A few drops of eucalyptus oil on a tick will cause it to fall out.

• Remove the tick with tweezers as close to the head as possible. Pull straight up. Do not squeeze or twist it. (Gut contents will empty into you.) Never touch the tick with your hands. Apply alcohol to bite area.

—**Prevention is the key:**

• Keep lawns cut short and shrubbery to a minimum where children play.

• When walking through tall grass or brush, wear long-sleeve shirts and pants, and tape pant legs into socks. Wear shoes and boots that cover entire foot.

• Put suspicious clothing in the dryer to kill ticks by dehydration. Just washing clothes is not effective.

• Do a meticulous, daily body inspection if you have been in the woods or live in an infested area. Have a partner inspect for louse-size arachnids or dark freckle-sized nymphs behind knees, in scalp and pubic hair, in armpits and under watchbands.

• Check outdoor pets for ticks regularly.

L 448

Common Symptoms: A large red "bull's-eye" rash with a light center, near the site of the bite that becomes as large as 10 to 20 inches; initial flu-like symptoms of stiff neck, chills and aches; unusual fatigue and malaise, head aches and joint pain, especially in children; later symptoms of heart arrythmia, muscle spasms with racking pain, meningitis (brain inflammation), chronic bladder problems, arthritis, facial paralysis and other numbing nerve dysfunctions, and extreme fatigue. Note: Lyme disease symptoms mimic several other disease conditions. Have a simple test done by a health care clinic if you feel that you are at risk.

Contact www.lyme.org. or American Lyme Disease Foundation (800-886-LYME). Treat Lyme Disease early.

Can't find a recommended product? Call the 800 number listed in Product Resources for the store nearest you.

Measles
Rubella

Measles is a highly contagious viral infection that attacks a lowered immune system. The first symptoms appear as an upper respiratory cold or flu, followed by a red rash. While usually thought of as a childhood disease, measles also affects adults whose immunity to the virus has not been established. Measles is most communicable in the early stages. Rubella (German measles), characterized by swollen lymph glands and then a rash, is a more severe, even more contagious form of viral measles, infecting a wider area of the body. After effects of measles are rare in children but may be permanent in adults. Women are often left with chronic joint pain. Keep immunity high for the best defense. Take great care if you are pregnant. Measles can cause birth defects. Measles vaccinations have a number of side effects for children - be wary.

Diet & Superfood Therapy

—Nutritional therapy plan for prevention:

1—Start with a liquid foods diet for at least 24 hours to increase fluid intake as much as possible. Use fresh fruit and vegetable juices, miso soup, bottled water and herb teas such as catnip, chamomile or rosemary, that will mildly induce sweating and clean out toxins faster.

2—Then follow with a simple, basic diet featuring vitamin A and C-rich fresh fruits and veggies.

3—Give 1 teasp. acidophilus liquid in citrus juice each morning. Offer fresh fruits all through the morning, with yogurt if desired.

4—Have a fresh green salad each day.

5—Have a cup of miso or clear soup with 1 teasp. brewer's yeast and 1 TB snipped sea greens daily.

6—Have a cup of miso (or Ramen) soup each day, and a cup of Red Star NUTRITIONAL YEAST extract broth before bed.

—Superfood therapy: (choose 1 or 2)
• Crystal Star BIOFLAV, FIBER & C SUPPORT™ drink 2x daily.
• BioStrath original LIQUID YEAST.
• New Chapter GINGER WONDER syrup to soothe a sore throat and provide healing benefits.

Herb & Supplement Therapy

—Interceptive therapy plan: (Choose 2 to 3 recommendations)

1—To curb the viral infection: • Crystal Star FIRST AID CAPS™ 2 daily for 2 days to break out the fever and rash, and start the healing process. • Crystal Star ANTI-VI™ tea 2 cups daily, or • St. John's wort extract or capsules, or • mullein-lobelia tincture in acute stage; ⊛ • Crystal Star ANTI-FLAM™ extract drops in water to reduce inflammation; or • Herbs, Etc. PHYTOCILLIN, or • Enzymedica PURIFY.

2—Deal with the skin rash: Use • marjoram, catnip, yarrow or chamomile teas, 3-4 cups daily to break out rash; • raspberry, gotu kola or lobelia tea to heal sores; • apply marjoram tea to sores to soothe; or • PHYCOTENE CREAM from Healthy House.

—Herbal body washes soothe and heal the skin: make into tea, soak a washcloth and wipe down a rashy body. Elder flower; Peppermint; or Ginger root. ⊛

3—For eyestrain and discomfort: Make a dilute tea from • Crystal Star EYE-BRIGHT TEA™; use as an eyewash to soothe.

4—To control an accompanying middle ear infection: • Crystal Star ANTI-BIO™ caps 4 to 6 daily, or extract drops 4x daily to clear infection. (May also be used as ear drops morning and evening.) • Nutribiotic GRAPEFRUIT SEED extract to clear infection fast. Warm • lobelia extract in the ear; • garlic oil caps, 2 daily.

5—For a cough and sore throat: • Crystal Star ZINC SOURCE™ herbal drops for almost immediate sore throat relief. Use • licorice tea or • coltsfoot tea, or • Crystal Star GINSENG-LICORICE ELIXIR™ drops as an expectorant. • Zinc gluconate lozenges, esp. • Zand HERBAL ZINC lozenges for kids. ⊛

6—To speed recovery: Vitamin A therapy is a key: • Emulsified vitamin A & D 10,000IU/400IU for children as soon as rash appears. Use a stronger dose for rubella, up to 100,000IU in divided doses. • Vitamin C therapy is important: • Alacer effervescent EMERGEN-C, 2 to 4x daily in juice, or ascorbate vitamin C, 1/4 teasp. 3 to 4x daily in juice or water. • Enzymatic Therapy VIRAPLEX complex

7—To rebuild immunity: Probiotics: • Natren LIFE START or • Solaray ACIDOPHILUS FOR CHILDREN 3x daily; ⊛ or Source Naturals LIFE FLORA to replace G.I. flora. • Rainforest Remedies STRONG RESISTANCE.

Lifestyle Support Therapy

—Bodywork:
• Use hydrotherapy baths with comfrey or calendula flowers to induce sweating, and neutralize body acids.
• Apply ginger-cayenne compresses to the rash.
• Frequent hot baths will often release poisons through the rash.
• Apply calendula gel to sores.
• Take tepid oatmeal baths to relieve skin itch and rash.
• Eyestrain and photosensitivity are common. Keep child especially in a darkened room.
• Pat aloe vera gel on sores, and also put aloe vera juice in bathwater for skin healing.
• Take a garlic or catnip enema during acute stage to lower fever and clean out infection fast (person should be 8 years or older.)

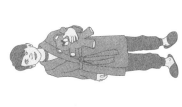

See also CHILDHOOD DISEASES page 245 for more.

Can't find a recommended product? Call the 800 number listed in Product Resources for the store nearest you.

Common Symptoms: Cold and flu-like symptoms of sneezing, runny nose, red eyes, headache, cough and fever; lymph nodes are usually swollen; fever is followed by a red rash on the face and upper body which sloughs off when the fever drops. With rubella, there is heavy coughing and the rash covers the body; light hurts the eyes; white spots appear in the mouth and throat; there is usually a middle ear infection, and sometimes hearing is affected permanently.

Common Causes: Low immunity from a poor diet, or too many immune-depressing antibiotics or cortico-steroid drugs.

Menopause
Women's Change of Life

Menopause is intended by nature to be a gradual reduction of estrogen by the ovaries with few side effects. The body changes and hormonal fluctuations are normal. In a well-nourished, vibrant woman, the adrenals and other glands pick up the job of estrogen secretion to keep her active and attractive after menopause. Unless you are absolutely sure you need synthetic estrogen replacement, choose a natural menopause. Although almost 90% of women experience some menopausal symptoms, most only last a year or two and are not severe enough to interrupt their lives. Many stem from exhausted adrenals and poor liver function where estrogen is not being processed correctly. If you're experiencing a raging hormone roller coaster, with hot flashes, mood swings, vaginal dryness and low libido, check out these pages for the natural way to "keep the change!"

Diet & Superfood Therapy

—Nutritional therapy plan:

1—A good diet is crucial to sailing through the second half of life disease-free and full of vitality. Limit fatty dairy products and meats, especially beef and pork, high in hormone disrupting chemicals. Reduce sugars and alcohol. (A little wine with dinner is fine.) Avoid caffeine. It taxes adrenal glands, upsets hormone levels. Steam and bake foods - never fry.

2—Especially eat cold water fish like salmon, and tuna for EFA's and to cut heart disease risk.

3—Add soy foods like miso and tofu and avoid spicy foods to reduce hot flashes. Balance estrogen levels by boosting boron-containing foods, like green leafy veggies, fruits, nuts, legumes. (Boron also helps harden bones.)

4—Whole grain fiber, fresh fruits and veggies regulate estrogen levels and reduce mood swings.

5—Eat calcium-rich foods: vegetables, non-fat dairy products. Eliminate carbonated drinks loaded with phosphates that deplete calcium. Drink bottled mineral water instead.

—Superfood therapy: (choose 1 or 2)
• Crystal Star BIOFLAVONOID, FIBER & C SUPPORT™ with cranberry.
• Crystal Star ENERGY GREEN™ with sea greens.
• Mona's CHLORELLA with EFA's.
• Y.S. GINSENG/ROYAL JELLY drink.

Herb & Supplement Therapy

—Interceptive therapy plan: (Choose several recommendations)

1—For hot flashes: Crystal Star's program: • EST-AID™ caps 4-6 daily the first month, 2 daily for 2 months, to control hormone imbalances; • CALCIUM SOURCE™ caps for bone weakness accompanying estrogen changes; • Evening primrose oil caps 4000mg daily to handle mood swings. • EASY CHANGE™ caps or roll-on for the years of the change; • ADR-ACTIVE™, or • FEMALE HARMONY™ for a feeling of well-being. Add • GINSENG 6 SUPER™ caps or tea for energy; and • MILK THISTLE SEED extract to help normalize estrogen levels.

More suggestions: Transitions For Health WOMEN'S PHASE II and PRO-GEST CREAM as directed; or • Moon Maid PRO-MENO wild yam cream; • Ester C with bioflavs 4x daily, for hot flashes and excess menses bleeding. • Enzymatic Therapy NUCLEO-PRO F caps, 2 daily. (Chew for fast results), or • Futurebiotics MENOPHASE 1 and II; • Transitions for Women HOT FLASH FORMULA; • Vitex extract (most commonly prescribed menopause remedy in Europe).

2—**Normalize temperature fluctuations:** • Bioflavonoids, structurally similar to the body's estrogen - • Ethical Nutrients SUPER FLAVONOID-C; • Vitamin E 800 daily; • Gamma oryzanol,100 mg 3x daily; • CoQ10 60mg 3x daily.

3—**Bone builders:** • Pioneer Nutr. CALCIUM-MAGNESIUM BONE PROTEIN; vitamin D 400IU; • Trace Minerals Research TRANSCEND for WOMEN.

4—**For sleep disturbances and anxiety:** • 1 gram niacinamide at bedtime to stimulate serotonin; • Nature's Balance RHODIOLA ROSEA; • 5-HTP, 50-100mg or • Crystal Star NIGHT CAPS™ 2 at bedtime; • Homeopathic Nux Vomica; • Kava kava or • Herb Pharm PHARMA KAVA drops (not if drinking alcohol).

5—**Elevate mood and increase energy:** • Ginkgo biloba extract; • Herbal Magic GINSENG-GINKGO REJUVENATOR; • Siberian ginseng extract; • Nature's Secret ULTIMATE B; • Stress B-complex 100mg; • Barlean's high lignan flax oil 3 daily.

6—**Iodine therapy for thyroid -metabolism balance:** • Sea greens, 2 TBS daily or sushi daily to your diet; take • Crystal Star IODINE/POTASSIUM caps or • New Chapter OCEAN HERBS; or • Bernard Jensen LIQUI-DULS; • Kelp tabs 8 daily.

Lifestyle Support Therapy

—Lifestyle changes for better body balance:

• Exercise regularly outdoors to get the advantages of natural vitamin D for bone health. A daily brisk walk keeps the system flowing.

• Do deep stretches on rising and each evening before bed. Yoga for body toning.

• Weight training 3 times a week along with aerobic exercise is a perfect way to keep skin from sagging. Weight training helps you keep the muscle while you lose the fat. In a natural menopause, when estrogen levels drop naturally, so does some body fat and excess fluids.

• Get a massage therapy treatment once a month for energy restoration, a body tune-up and a feeling of well-being.

• Smoking contributes to breast cancer, emphysema, osteoporosis, wrinkling and early menopause. Now is the time to quit!

• 20 minutes in a sauna daily significantly cuts night sweats for menopausal women.

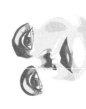

See also OSTEOPOROSIS page 468 for more information.

Can't find a recommended product? Call the 800 number listed in Product Resources for the store nearest you.

Common Symptoms: Erratic estrogen and other hormone secretions by the glands causing hot flashes, insomnia and fatigue; low libido, irritability, calcium imbalance, unstable behavior, mood swings, palpitations; calcium metabolism disturbances causing osteoporosis; skin and vaginal dryness and sometimes atrophy; occasional appearance of male characteristics.
Common Causes: Deficient nutrition and lack of exercise; thyroid imbalance; exhausted adrenals; poor food absorption; B vitamin deficiency; emotional stress.

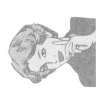

Taking control of your life change

Sixty million women will be menopausal in America by the year 2010. The temperature of the planet may rise from so many hot flashes! More seriously, menopause is intended by Nature to be a gradual reduction of estrogen by the ovaries with few side effects. In a well-nourished, vibrant woman, the adrenals and other glands pick up the job of estrogen secretion to keep her active and attractive after menopause. But our modern stressful lifestyles and poor eating habits mean that many women reach their menopause years with prematurely worn out adrenals, magnifying hormone fluctuations. A women that recognizes the significance of keeping her adrenals healthy, choosing to change her habits to support her adrenal energy holds in her hands the potential for eliminating unpleasant menopausal symptoms.

Adrenal boosting tips for menopausal women to consider: 1: Add Vitamin C 5000mg daily to maintain adrenal integrity and convert cholesterol to adrenal hormones. 2: Add sea greens to your diet, at least 2 TBS dry, chopped sea greens (any kind) daily. Add 6 to 12 pieces of sushi to your weekly diet. Sea vegetables are a rich source of fat-soluble vitamins like D and K which assist with production of steroidal hormones like estrogen, and DHEA in the adrenal glands. 3: The herbs *Licorice, Sarsaparilla* and *Siberian ginseng* work specifically to stimulate the adrenal glands to regulate body energy after menopause. Consider Crystal Star ADRN-ACTIVE™ caps 2 daily. 4: Royal jelly daily is a rich source of adrenal boosting pantothenic acid.

What About Hormone Replacement Therapy?

Premarin, an estrogen replacement drug for menopausal women made from pregnant mare's urine, is the top selling drug of any kind in the U.S. But there is a firestorm of controversy about synthetic hormone replacement. The threat of breast and uterine cancer is dramatically increased with HRT, and the risk increases as a woman ages. In 51 studies covering 21 countries involving more than 52,000 women with breast cancer and 108,000 women without breast cancer, women who used Premarin for 5 years or longer had a 35% higher risk of developing cancer than women who had never been on HRT. (Good news! The higher risk for breast cancer diminished and largely disappeared after about 5 years off HRT treatment.)

The drug companies and much of the medical community, for whom synthetic hormones are an incredibly profitable business, continue to justify these risks because of the perceived advantages to osteoporosis and heart disease protection. Many physicians prescribe HRT as a lifetime drug, believing that it is the only way to prevent heart disease and osteoporosis no matter how good you feel. Yet, the newest research reveals that benefits for these diseases are not validated over the longterm.

Does HRT really protect against menopausal heart disease? Using hormone replacement therapy or ERT to protect against heart disease is highly debatable. There is no conclusive evidence that estrogen protects against heart disease. We do know that beginning HRT at menopause to prevent heart disease carries risks. For example, tests with some estrogen-containing contraceptive pills have actually increased a woman's risk of heart disease, heart attack, stroke and serious blood clotting problems. A 1997 review presented at the International Meeting on Atherosclerosis in Paris concludes that the heart protective benefits attributed to estrogen may result from population selection bias or even changes to healthier lifestyles during the course of the studies. In addition, HRT drugs can deplete folic acid, raising homocysteine levels, a known risk factor for heart disease, and destroy vitamin E, a heart protective antioxidant.

What's the HRT connection to osteoporosis? HRT is still strongly promoted for osteoporosis prevention. Many menopausal women are so afraid of osteoporosis that with a little coaxing from their physicians they begin taking hormone drugs right away. Of those, about 60% discontinue the therapy because of side effects or fear of cancer! There is no question that hormones are involved in bone-building and bone loss, but declining estrogen levels after menopause do not by themselves cause osteoporosis. Although some studies show estrogen inhibits bone cell death, the newest tests reveal that as many as 15% of women on estrogen therapy continue to lose bone! Moreover, estrogen isn't the only hormone involved in bone building. The hormone progesterone actually increases bone density in clinical tests. Low androgen levels of DHEA and testosterone also play a role in bone loss, particularly in men's osteoporosis. Osteoporosis prevention is a program not a pill. See pg. 468 for more.

Are there environmental consequences with so many women on HRT drugs for menopause? The latest studies show there may be. Studies on the high sewage Las Vegas wash reveal high levels of synthetic hormones from human urine in waters where male fish show signs of hormone disruption. In these waters, male carp produce the egg laying protein associated with females. It remains to be seen if HRT or birth control drugs are to blame. If it is, we have a huge problem on our hands. Billions of pounds of supposedly "treated" sewage is released in discharge waters where wildlife make their home! More research is currently being done to determine the long term effects of hormones from human urine on our environment.

Menopause the natural way:

I don't believe hormone replacement is the best course for most women. Beyond increased cancer risk, HRT causes many side effects. Weight gain (especially fatty deposits on the hips and thighs), heavy bleeding (worse than a woman's former period), PMS-like symptoms, migraine headaches, uterine and breast fibroids, and low libido are all reported by women taking hormone drugs. Unless you have specific, extenuating circumstances (only about 6% of American women do), a natural menopause may be the best way. Even women who don't have a symptom-free menopause say they feel younger and more energetic when they address their menopausal changes with natural remedies. If you are about to be confronted with the great Hormone Replacement Therapy choice, consider carefully before you agree. The program on pg. 450 can go a long way to convincing you to want to "keep the change."

See following page for more on specific menopause problems.

Can't find a recommended product? Call the 800 number listed in Product Resources for the store nearest you.

M 451

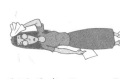

Natural Therapies for Specific Problems Associated with Menopause

Aggravating symptoms which often accompany menopause are due to the body's difficulty in adapting to its new hormone functions. Many are positively influenced with natural therapies.

—**HOT FLASHES and NIGHT SWEATS:** The body's temperature-regulating mechanism becomes unstable during the shifting hormone balance of menopause. As estrogen levels drop, the pituitary responds by increasing other types of hormones to re-establish hormone homeostasis. Hot flashes generally last 2 to 4 years after menstruation ends, and subside as the body adjusts to its new hormone levels. Stress, too much caffeine and alcohol trigger hot flashes. **Alternative therapy protocols:** • Crystal Star EST-AID™ caps 4 to 6 daily, or extract 15 drops under the tongue as needed; • Body Ammo SOY DHEA cream; • Transitions For Women HOT FLASH FORMULA; or Source Naturals HOT FLASH; • Crystal Star PRO-EST EASY CHANGE™ roll-on gel or • Body Ammo SOY DHEA cream, 3 cups daily; • VITEX extract 2x daily; • *dandelion* tea to strengthen the liver; • Spectrum Essentials EVENING PRIMROSE OIL, 1300 mg 3x daily. • GINSENG tea with 2 teasp. high potency royal jelly daily.

—**SAGGING INTERNAL TISSUE and ORGANS:** Herbal compounds are well-suited to elasticizing tissue and toning prolapsed organs. **Alternative therapy protocols:** • Crystal Star WOMEN'S BEST FRIEND™ caps, 6 daily or • *Vitex* extract, or Rainbow Light VITEX SUPERCOMPLEX; • Jarrow GLUCOSAMINE SULFATE; • Sage Woman Herbs CALCIUM/MINERALS; • Schiff PHYTOCHARGED ESSENTIAL FATTY ACIDS; • Ethical Nutrients INJURY TABS to tighten soft and connective tissue.

—**FOR FRIGIDITY, PAINFUL INTERCOURSE or DRY VAGINA:** Reduced estrogen levels can cause vaginal mucous membranes to become dry, resulting in painful intercourse - just at a time of life when you can be more spontaneous, without fear of pregnancy. **Alternative therapy protocols:** • High potency Y.S. or Premier 1 royal jelly 2 teasp. daily; • *panax ginseng* tea 1 cup daily or *panax ginseng* caps 2 daily; • rub on Moon Maid VITAL VULVA salve; • vitamin E 800IU, rub on vitamin E oil or use Vitamin E suppositories; • *Evening Primrose Oil*, 4000 daily for EFAs, with B-6, 250mg. • RubTransitions PRO-GEST cream on abdomen as directed; • Country Life MAXINE capsules, 2 daily; • Crystal Star WOMEN'S DRYNESS™ extract or • LOVE FEMALE™ caps for more responsive libido. • Country Life ADRENAL - TYROSINE, or • Enzymatic Therapy THYROID - TYROSINE caps, 4 daily.

—**DEPRESSION, IRRITABILITY, INSOMNIA and FATIGUE:** Psychological symptoms distress many normally practical, well-balanced women. Many women feel that their lack of energy during menopause is the number one disruption in their lives. **Alternative therapy protocols:** magnesium-rich foods, like leafy greens, almonds, apricots, avocado, carrots, citrus fruits, lentils, and salmon counteract depression and anxiety; reduce caffeine intake (it affects mood more during menopause). • Crystal Star MENTAL INNER ENERGY™ caps with *kava kava* and *ginseng*, offers more energy; • FEM-SUPPORT™ extract with *ashwagandha*, offers balance. • Crystal Star DEPRESS-EX™ with *St. John's Wort*, or • Herbs Etc. DEPRE-ZAC, and • Nature's Secret ULTIMATE B COMPLEX help emotional anxiousness. • Aromatherapy essential oils help menopausal depression: *Bergamot, Geranium, Neroli, Clary Sage,* and *Jasmine* by Wyndemere; • Homeopathics are a good choice: • DEPRESSION, STRESS, EXHAUSTION by Nova; • GOOD MOODS, RESTFUL SLEEP, STRESS RELIEF, by Nature's Apothecary.

—**BODY SHAPE CHANGES AND MENOPAUSAL WEIGHT GAIN:** Women have a gynoid pattern of fat distribution that accumulates fat around the hips and buttocks. It is much harder for women to lose fat in their problem areas than for men. Estrogen in the female body directs the storage of "sex-specific fat", on the buttocks, hips and thighs for the purposes of child-bearing and hormone functions. As women get older, the problem escalates. Estrogen reduction during menopause contributes another change in fat distribution. Menopausal women develop more fat storage in the deep abdominal cavity than menstruating women. The good news is that small changes in diet and lifestyle can help solve the weight problems that women have. See Weight Gain After 40, page 521 for more information and suggestions. **Alternative therapy protocols:** If you haven't been exercising, now is the time- at least 3x weekly to retain muscle and gain body tone; for weight loss results without overstimulation. Weight training along with moderate aerobic exercise and pre-workout stretches three times a week realizes excellent results, along with • Beehive Botanicals ROYAL JELLY/GINSENG drink; • Crystal Star THERMO-CITRIN® GINSENG™ (alternate with APPETITE™ caps); • Nature's Secret THIN SOLUTION or CRAVE LESS - BURN MORE program; • DHEA creams like Body Ammo DHEA cream reduce body fat and increase muscle mass in postmenopausal women.

—**FACIAL HAIR GROWTH/HEAD HAIR LOSS:** Extremely common conditions for menopausal women. Female pattern baldness is a disconcerting problem involving genetics, vitamin-mineral uptake and stress. Changes in hormone production, specifically the slow-down in estrogen production, affect the functioning of hair follicles, result in the head hair loss and facial hair growth women hate. Excess dihydrotestosterone (DHT) in women can cause hair follicles to become dormant as in men. Balanced thyroid hormone production is critical to normal hair growth. Hypothyroidism leads to coarse, lifeless hair which easily falls out. Hyperthyroidism causes soft, thinning hair and hair loss. **Alternative therapy protocols:** • sea greens make a big difference -most women notice better hair growth and texture in 3 to 4 weeks. Take at least 2 TBS daily of dried chopped sea greens, and eat lots of sushi. Reduce animal fats to unclog hair follicles; add soy foods for plant protein (hair is 97% protein!); • *Evening Primrose Oil* 4000 mg daily; • Crystal Star CALCIUM SOURCE™ or a a cal/mag/zinc combination with high magnesium for hair growth. • B Complex 100mg with extra B$_6$ daily; • Country Life sublingual B-12, 2500mcg every other day. Mix fresh blender-ground ginger with aloe vera gel and apply to hair; leave on 15 minutes. • Ethical Nutrients 8 TREASURES; VITEX extract, or Nature's Path TRACE-MIN-LYTE to stimulate hair growth.

—**POOR CIRCULATION/TINGLING IN THE LIMBS:** A common menopausal condition, especially evident when one takes a deep breath. **Alternative therapy protocols:** Make a daily circulation drink for almost immediate improvement: Mix $\frac{1}{2}$ cup tomato juice, $\frac{1}{2}$ cup lemon juice, 6 teasp. wheat germ oil, 1 teasp. brewer's yeast; *Hawthorn* extract or *Ginkgo Biloba* extract as needed; • PCOs from grapeseed or white pine 100mg 2x daily; *gotu kola* or *cayenne/ginger* 4 caps daily; • Sage Woman Herbs CIRCULATION; or • Futurebiotics CIRCUPLEX caps.

See MENOPAUSE page 450 for specific phytohormone product suggestions.

Menstrual Problems

Excessive Flow (Menorrhagia), Inter-period Bleeding (Metrorrhagia)

Progesterone is the factor that assures uniform shedding of the uterine lining - low levels of this hormone result in tissue buildup. At the same time, the relatively high level of estrogen stimulates the uterine lining, causing even more endometrial tissue formation. The combination of these two factors leads to abnormally heavy flow during menstruation, and/or spotting between periods as excess tissue is shed. A low progesterone-to-estrogen ratio also causes PMS symptoms of bloating, irritability and depression during the cycle. Mild to moderate hypothyroidism is almost always involved in menorrhagia; response is often dramatic to herbal iodine therapy.

Note: some contraceptive pills cause breakthrough bleeding. If this is your problem, you might be able to solve it simply by switching prescriptions.

Diet & Superfood Therapy

—Nutritional therapy plan:

1—Consciously work on nutrition improvement, with emphasis on vegetable proteins, mineral-rich foods and high fiber foods.

2—Eat plenty of leafy greens, seafood and fish for EFA's.

3—Increase Omega-3 rich foods: salmon, cold water fish, sea greens, flax seed oil for EFA's.

4—Add sulphur foods like garlic, onions and turmeric spice.

5—Restrict intake of animal foods, especially cheese and red meats (many are loaded with the hormone DES that has an effect on human blood).

6—Reduce fried, saturated fatty foods, sugars, and high cholesterol foods.

7—Avoid caffeine and caffeine-containing foods, hard liquor (a little wine is fine).

8—Make a mix of brewer's yeast flakes, wheat germ flakes, amaranth grain (astringent), lecithin granules; add 2 TBS to the diet daily.

—Superfood therapy: (choose 1 or 2)

• Crystal Star BIOFLAV., FIBER & C SUPPORT™ drink daily for tissue strength.

• Y.S. or Beehive Botanical Royal Jelly/Ginseng.

• Sun Wellness CHLORELLA or Crystal Star ENERGY GREEN™ for breakthrough bleeding.

• Carrot juice or Green Foods CARROT ESSENCE.

Herb & Supplement Therapy

—Interceptive therapy plan: (Choose 2 or more recommendations)

1—**Help curtail the bleeding and shorten periods:** • Enzymatic Therapy RAW MAMMARY COMPLEX caps 2-3 daily for almost immediate results; • Enzymatic Therapy FEM-TROL capsules if periods are too frequent; • Nettles extract, $1/4$ tsp. 2x daily; • Vitamin K 100mcg 2 daily; • Vitamin A normalizes heavy bleeding; up to 100,000IU for 2 to 3 weeks only, then reduce to 10,000IU.

2—**Lengthen luteal phase to curtail long bleeding periods:** • EFA's from *Evening Primrose Oil* 6 daily, or • *Flax Seed Oil* for spotting or • Nature's Secret ULTIMATE OIL for EFA's, 2 daily. • Crystal Star FEMALE HARMONY™ caps 2 daily with 2 *bayberry* capsules, for 2 months to normalize cycle, especially if pre-menopausal.

3—**Balance progesterone:** • Transitions PROGEST CREAM, • Moon Maid PRO-MENO, or • Crystal Star PRO-EST BALANCE™ roll-on applied as directed.

4—**Astringents help moderate blood loss:** • Make an astringent tea - take a cup 3x daily, during and before your period: *shepherd's purse, cranesbill, red raspberry, periwinkle and agrimony,* or • Crystal Star GREEN TEA CLEANSER™ each morning.

5—**Address underlying hypothyroidism:** • Crystal Star IODINE-POTASSIUM caps, or • IODINE THERAPY™ extract; • Bernard Jensen LIQUI-DULS iodine drops or • Premier raw thyroid. • Bee pollen caps 1000mg 2 daily. • Enzymatic Therapy THYROID/TYROSINE, or • Nature's Path TRACE-MIN-LYTE.

6—**Tone the reproductive system:** • Crystal Star WOMAN'S BEST FRIEND™ caps 6 daily, with • VITEX extract as a tissue toner; • Crystal Star FEM SUPPORT™ extract 4x daily with *Ashwagandha*; • MILK THISTLE SEED extract for spotting.

7—**Balance your iron supplies:** • Crystal Star IRON SOURCE™; • Floradix LIQUID IRON. • Country Life B-12, 2500mcg, • folic acid 400mcg - iron uptake.

8—**Strengthen connective tissue with bioflavs and silica:** • Flora VEGE-SIL, or • Crystal Star SILICA SOURCE™ for connective tissue strength; • Twin Labs CITRUS BIOFLAVONOIDS and rutin 500mg. • Rainbow Light CALCIUM PLUS capsules 4 at a time daily. • Nature's Plus Vitamin E 800IU.

Lifestyle Support Therapy

—Bodywork:

• Acupressure: Press on the insides of the legs about 5" above the knees; 5 minutes on each leg to decrease bleeding.

• Apply icepacks to the pelvic area.

• Get extra sleep during this time.

• Get daily regular exercise to keep system and metabolism flowing.

• Avoid drugs of all kinds, even aspirin and prescription drugs if possible. Many inhibit Vitamin K formation.

—Reflexology point:

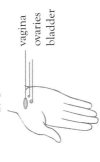

vagina
ovaries
bladder

Common Symptoms: *Excessive bleeding for 2 or more days, with large dark clots, spotting between periods. An abnormal (but non-cancerous) PAP smear may occur.*

Common Causes: *Hypothyroidism, sluggish or lazy thyroid; uterine fibroids; nutrition deficient diet with too much caffeine, salt and red meat, causing hormone and glandular imbalance; uterine fibroids, endometriosis, or pelvic inflammatory disease or hyperplasia; endometriosis; overproduction of estrogen; too much aspirin or other blood-thinning medications; calcium or chronic iron deficiency; underactive, possible polyps; Vitamin K deficiency.*

See Menopause pages 450-452 for more information.

Can't find a recommended product? Call the 800 number listed in Product Resources for the store nearest you.

Menstrual Problems

Suppressed, Delayed, Irregular Flow, Peri-Menopause

Irregular menstrual periods are among the most common disorders women suffer. Most are related to gland health and lifestyle. Intense body building and training for marathon or competition sports affects menstruation (sometimes to the point of cessation) because a woman's body fat is extremely reduced. The body will not slough off tissue when it feels at risk in forming more. In young girls, menses may be delayed because of abnormally low estrogen levels due to low blood calcium levels, or to eating disorders and crash dieting. Irregular menses due to prolonged emotional stress should be addressed with relaxation and exercise techniques.

Diet & Superfood Therapy

–Nutritional therapy plan:

1—Make sure the diet is very nutritious, with plenty of vegetable proteins and complex carbohydrates. (Your body may not menstruate regularly if it is malnourished).

2—Eat brown rice and other B-complex-rich foods like sea greens (loaded with EFA's, too).

3—Avoid red meats. Switch to Omega-3 rich protein foods: salmon, cold water fish, sea greens, flax seed, sesame seeds.

4—Avoid caffeine and caffeine-containing foods, such as chocolate and sodas.

5—Have a green veggie drink (pg. 218), (or see below) several times a week for healthy blood building.

6—Make a mix of toasted wheat germ, lecithin granules, and brewer's yeast; take 2 TBS each daily for adrenal support.

7—Drink plenty of pure water daily.

–Superfood therapy: (choose 1 or 2)
• Crystal Star ENERGY GREEN™.
• Nutricology PROGREENS with EFA's.
• Transitions EASY GREENS.
• Beehive Botanical ROYAL JELLY/GINSENG drink for metabolic balance.
• Rainbow Light HAWAIIAN SPIRULINA; take with B-complex 100mg for best results.
• Green Foods VIBRANT WOMAN.

Herb & Supplement Therapy

–Interceptive therapy plan: (Choose 2 to 4 recommendations)

1—Help normalize flow: • Crystal Star FLOW EASE™ tea 2 cups daily or • FEM-SUPPORT™ extract 2x daily; • Black cohosh caps or Black Haw tea for suppressed menstrual discharge. • Transitions PROGEST CREAM, or • Moon Maid PROMENO wild yam cream (take as directed or periods may be very irregular). • Enzymatic Therapy NUCLEO-PRO F caps, with • THYROID/TYROSINE and • RAW MAMMARY COMPLEX glandulars.

2—Balance hormones to normalize cycle: • Crystal Star FEMALE HARMONY™ caps and tea with • burdock tea 2 cups or • Crystal Star GINSENG/LICORICE ELIXIR™ for hormone balance. • Rainbow Light VITEX-BLACK COHOSH SUPERCOMPLEX for abnormal cycles. • Una da Gato caps for irregular menses. • American Health GLANDULAR TONIC.

–Balancing EFA sources (correlated with irregular, painful periods): • EVENING PRIMROSE oil 4000mg daily, or Spectrum EVENING PRIMROSE oil 1300mg caps; • Flax seed oil 3 daily; • Nature's Secret ULTIMATE OIL.

3—For healthy blood composition: • Crystal Star IRON SOURCE™; • Turmeric (curcumin) extract caps 6 daily help move stagnant blood. • Nature's Plus Vitamin E 800IU. • B-complex 100mg daily, with extra folic acid 400mcg and • Country Life sublingual B-12, 2500mcg every other day.

–Tone uterine tissue: • Blue cohosh caps for 1 month.

4—Support exhausted adrenals: • Crystal Star ADR-ACTIVE™ 2 capsules daily with • BODY REBUILDER™ caps 2 daily; • CC Pollen HIGH DESERT ROYAL JELLYwith ginseng, 2 teasp. daily; • Medicine Wheel FOUNTAIN of YOUTH, or • Planetary SCHIZANDRA ADRENAL SUPPORT.

–For teenage delayed menses: • Dong quai/damiana caps or extract 2x daily, with an herbal calcium formula such as • Crystal Star CALCIUM SOURCE™, or a good • calcium/magnesium supplement with • zinc 50mg daily and • kelp tabs 8 daily for 2 months.

Lifestyle Support Therapy

–Help remove infections through the skin:
• Pelvic compresses: especially seaweed compresses (Crystal Star HOT SEAWEED bath is also indicated and successful in many cases).
  • Horehound compresses
  • Ginger compresses
  • Alternating hot and cold sitz baths to stimulate pelvic circulation.
• Regular mild exercise to keep system free and flowing.
• Do knee-chest position exercises for retroverted uterus.
• Consciously try for adequate rest and a reasonable schedule until periods normalize.
• Acupuncture, meditation and massage therapy treatments have all been effective for irregular menses.

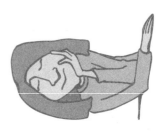

M 454

Common Symptoms: *Absence of menses; delayed menses in young girls; irregular menses; with a feeling of continual heaviness and bloating.*

Common Causes: *Poor health or nutrition; gland and hormone imbalance; too much caffeine and too many carbonated drinks; poor organ and abdominal tone; lack of exercise or too much exercise (marathoner's syndrome); extreme, or very low protein, weight loss diet foods; anorexia or excess dieting for weight loss; hypoglycemia; low blood calcium levels; IUD-caused cervical lesions or cysts; venereal disease; stress, emotional shock or depression; adrenal exhaustion; previous birth control pill use causing irregularity; pregnancy aftermath.*

See PMS page 473 for more information and natural cramps therapy.

Can't find a recommended product? Call the 800 number listed in Product Resources for the store nearest you.

Miscarriage

Miscarriage Prevention, False Labor

Did you know that as many as 1 in 3 of all pregnancies end in miscarriage? Miscarriage mainly occurs in the first 12 weeks of pregnancy, often before a woman even recognizes she's pregnant. Miscarriage is often Nature's way of dealing with an abnormal embryo that could not have lived a normal life if the pregnancy had been brought to full term. Rarely is miscarriage the fault of the mother's actions (such as stress, a fall or exercise), except when her nutrition is very poor, or if she is addicted to drugs or nicotine. Even then, Nature tries hard to avoid conception under dangerous conditions. Spontaneous miscarriage is most likely to occur in the first trimester. Aside from the early discomforts of pregnancy, miscarriage is the greatest threat during this time, especially if the mother is over 35 and has had difficulty becoming pregnant.

Diet & Superfood Therapy

—Nutritional therapy plan:

1—A good prevention/building diet should include plenty of magnesium and potassium-rich foods; leafy greens, brown rice, green and yellow veggies, tofu, sprouts, molasses, etc. Add sea greens for natural vitamin B$_{12}$ and plant protein. Be sure you get enough vegetable protein for the baby's growth: whole grains, sprouts and seeds, low fat dairy foods and sea foods.

2—Limit intake of goitrogen foods that impair thyroid function like cruciferous vegetables, peanuts, mustard, pine nuts, millet and soy products, especially if you're hypothyroid (low thyroid).

3—Avoid alcohol, caffeine, drugs. Reduce sugars and refined foods of all kinds. NO soft drinks; they bind magnesium and make it unavailable.

4—Make a mix of lecithin, 4 teasp. toasted wheat germ, brewer's yeast and molasses; take 2 TBS daily over cereal or in a green drink.

5—Avoid large amounts of ginger if you have a history of miscarriage.

—Effective superfoods: (choose 1 or 2)
•Crystal Star BIOFLAV., FIBER & C SUPPORT™ drink daily for tissue strength.
•Green Foods VIBRANT WOMAN.
•Solaray ALFAJUICE.
•Earthrise NUTRA GREENS.
•All ONE MULTIPLE green plant base daily.

Herb & Supplement Therapy

—Interceptive therapy plan: (Choose 2 to 3 recommendations)

1—For threatened miscarriage: • Have the woman lie very still and give a cup of *false unicorn* tea every $^1/_2$ hour. As hemorrhaging decreases, give the tea every hour, then every 2 hours. Add 6 *lobelia* extract drops as a relaxer to the last cup. • Or give • *hawthorn* extract $^1/_2$ dropperful and bee pollen 2 tsp. hourly or CC POLLENERGY caps (520mg) until bleeding is controlled.

2—To prevent miscarriage: John Lee M.D., says transdermal progesterone 40mg a day can help prevent miscarriage caused by luteal phase failure. Ask your healthcare professional. Whole *wild yam* creams and *sarsaparilla* (herbs with progesterone activity) may also help prevent miscarriage due to hormonal insufficiency. Consider • Transitions PROGEST CREAM, and take emulsified A & D daily.

• Take a *Red Raspberry-Catnip* tea blend, or • Crystal Star MOTHERING TEA™ all through pregnancy 2 cups daily, and kelp tabs 6 daily. • Vitamin E 400IU and vitamin K 100mcg 2 daily during pregnancy protect against miscarriage. Take • *black haw* tea in small doses throughout danger period to prevent spontaneous abortion.

3—Tone the uterus and nourish the reproductive system: Use • *blue cohosh, squaw vine* and *false unicorn* root or Herbal Magic FEM-BALANCE as uterine tonics. Use • *motherwort* tea to reduce anxiety, nourish the female reproductive system. Low selenium levels are implicated in first trimester miscarriage. Take • vitamin E 100IU with selenium 200mcg.

4—Vitamin C and bioflavonoids strengthen veins and blood vessels: 45% of chronic aborters have low levels of vitamin C. • Vitamin C or Ester C with bioflavs. and rutin strengthen, 2-3000mg daily. • Alacer SUPER GRAM C II or III; • Solaray QBC with bromelain and C; • Twin Lab CITRUS BIOFLAVS. with rutin 500mg.

5—For false labor: To help stop bleeding, take • 2 caps *each* *cayenne* and *bayberry*; or • take *lobelia* and *cayenne* extracts together and *nettles* tea. Get to a hospital or call your midwife immediately. • Take Crystal Star ANTI-SPZ™ caps 4 at a time, or CRAMP BARK COMBO™ extract, for pain. • Take *blue cohosh* for afterpain.

Lifestyle Support Therapy

Take a prenatal formula all through pregnancy for a healthier baby and to help prevent miscarriage.

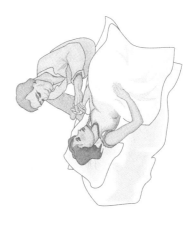

—Environmental preventives:
• To determine if the fetus is still alive: take body temperature first thing upon waking, Have a thermometer by the bed, already shaken down, move as little as possible, and take temperature before getting up. The fetus is alive if body temperature is 98.6 or above, unless normal body temperature is low due to abnormally low thyroid metabolism).

• Don't smoke. Smokers are twice as likely to miscarry and have low birth weight babies as non-smokers.

• Avoid X-rays; they can damage the fetus.

See HAVING A HEALTHY BABY in this book for more information.

Can't find a recommended product? Call the 800 number listed in Product Resources for the store nearest you.

Common Symptoms: *Spotting to profuse bleeding during pregnancy, usually with cramps, lower back pain and severe abdominal pain.*
Common Causes: *Development of extra fetal chromosomes; chronic infections; latent diabetes; deficient uterine muscle tone; weak blood vessels and capillaries; lack of protein and sufficient nutrition for both mother and child; improper fixing of the fetus to the womb walls; allergic reaction to drugs; overload of prescription and/or recreational drugs.*

Mononucleosis
Epstein-Barr Virus Infection

Mononucleosis was one of the first acute, infectious diseases to be recognized as an immune-compromised group of symptoms in young adults. Today, mono is associated with the Epstein-Barr virus or the cytomegalovirus (both herpes-type viruses). Mono is a chronic fatigue syndrome; the first symptoms are severe tiredness. Respiratory and lymphatic systems are affected early with severe flu-like infection. Glands, lymph nodes, bronchial tubes, liver and spleen are all debilitated. The virus is virulent and highly infectious. Immune response is very weak. Fatigue is long term, even after acute symptoms have been overcome. Medical antibiotics are not effective for this virus. Liver, lymph and spleen systems are the main organs involved in healing. Concentrate your efforts on revitalizing these areas. At least three months of rebuilding are needed for restoration of strength.

Diet & Superfood Therapy

—Nutritional therapy plan:

1—High quality vegetable proteins are a key to healing. Begin healing with plenty of cleansing/flushing fruit juices and bottled water for 1 week to relieve fever and sore throat. Do not fast. Strength and nutrition are too low.

2—Particularly use apple/alfalfa sprout, papaya/pineapple, and pineapple/coconut juices for strength and enzyme enhancement.

3—Follow with a week of green drinks, potassium broth (pg. 215), and vegetable juices to cleanse, strengthen and rebuild liver function.

4—Eat a diet high in vegetable proteins; (brown rice, tofu, nuts, seeds, sprouts, etc.), and cultured foods: (yogurt, kefir, etc.) for friendly flora.

5—Add vitamin A and vitamin C rich foods, like fruits and vegetables.

6—Take your choice of superfood drinks during entire 3 month healing time.

—Effective superfoods: (choose 2 or more)
- AloeLife ALOE GOLD drink.
- Sun Wellness CHLORELLA WAKASA GOLD.
- Crystal Star SYSTEMS STRENGTH™ drink.
- Nutricology PRO-GREENS with EFA's.
- YS or Beehive Botanical ROYAL JELLY/GINSENG drink.
- Future Biotics VITAL K drink daily.
- Solaray ALFA-JUICE.

Herb & Supplement Therapy

—Interceptive therapy plan: (This program has had notable success.)

1—**Address the viral infection:** • Crystal Star ANTI-VI™ extract drops in water 6x daily for 2 weeks, then • ANTI-BIO™ caps or extract, 6x daily for 2 weeks; • OLIVE LEAF extract and • OREGANO OIL are effective. • Echinacea/goldenseal rt. and garlic clear lymph glands of infection. • Crystal Star CLEANSING & PURIFYING™ tea helps normalize blood composition. • Vitamin C powder with bioflavonoids, ¼ teasp. every 2 hours in water or to bowel tolerance daily for 1 month. (Reduce dosage in the 2nd and 3rd month, but continue the C program.) • MICROHYDRIN available at Healthy House; • Earth's Bounty OXY-CAPS daily.♂

2—**Cleanse and enhance liver and spleen functions:** • Alpha lipoic acid 300-600mg daily, • Crystal Star LIV-ALIVE™ caps 6 daily; • MILK THISTLE SEED extract 3-4x daily for 3 months. • Enzymatic Therapy LYMPH-SPLEEN complex.

3—**Rebuild adrenal response:** Take 2 each daily, • Crystal Star ADR-ACTIVE™ caps and • BODY REBUILDER™ caps.♀ Then add • GINSENG 6 SUPER TEA™ for body homeostasis.♂

4—**Re-establish body strength:** • Nutricology GERMANIUM 150mg; • Country Life sublingual B-12, 2500mcg daily for 1 month, then every other day for a month; • Crystal Star FEEL GREAT™ tea♀ or • GINSENG SUPER 6™ caps♂ 2 daily for 2 months; or • PHYCOTENE MICROCLUSTERS available at Healthy House daily.

5—**Enhance immune response:** • Siberian ginseng extract; • Astragalus extract; • Cordyceps extract; • Reishi mushroom capsules, • Crystal Star REISHI/GINSENG extract or • Planetary REISHI MUSHROOM SUPREME. • Biotec CELL GUARD 6 daily. • Enzymatic Therapy THYMULUS and THYROID/TYROSINE capsules.

6—**Natural amino acids help rebuild body essentials:** • Full spectrum amino acids like • Anabol Naturals AMINO BALANCE for critical essential protein. • Bee pollen capsules, 8 daily; • Biotec Pacific SEA PLASMA tabs 10 daily.

7—**Proteolytic enzymes and probiotics re-establish deep body health:** • Transformation PURE-ZYME as directed. Take • CoQ₁₀ 60mg 4x daily. Add • Natren BIFIDO FACTORS, or • Prof. Nutrition DR. DOPHILUS, ¼ teasp. in water.

Lifestyle Support Therapy

—Bodywork:
• Bed rest during the acute stages, and regular mild exercise during the rebuilding stages are critical to successfully overcoming mono.

• Get early morning sunlight on the body every day possible.

• Overheating therapy has been effective for mono in curbing the advance of the virus. See page 225 for correct home technique.

• Biofeedback has also been successful.

• Avoid all pleasure drugs, caffeine and chemical stimulants. These are often the substances that reduce immunity to its infective point.

—Reflexology point:

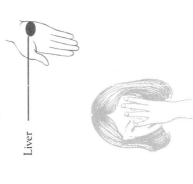

Liver

Common Symptoms: Symptoms occur in 4 to 7 weeks of exposure with severe flu/pneumonia/lung symptoms; swollen lymph nodes in the neck; high fever and sore throat; loss of appetite and extreme fatigue. A totally run-down condition; spleen enlargement; pallor; pain on the upper left side of the abdomen; jaundice as the liver throws off body poisons. Sometimes skin rashes or bruises around the mouth.
Common Causes: An opportunistic disease allowed by a weak immune system and contagion (often sexual) from an infected carrier; overuse and abuse of pleasure drugs and/or alcohol; liver malfunction.

See LIVER CLEANSING DIET suggestions and CHRONIC FATIGUE SYNDROME for more information.

Can't find a recommended product? Call the 800 number listed in Product Resources for the store nearest you.

Motion Sickness
Jet Lag, Inner Ear Imbalance

Motion sickness happens when the brain can't respond properly to a motion it doesn't understand. Inner ear imbalance is usually at the root of motion sickness symptoms. Deaf people do not get motion sickness. Jet lag is the inability of the internal body rhythm to rapidly resynchronize after sudden shifts in sun time. Our internal clocks are set by hypothalamus-controlled hormonal rhythm and by the pineal gland's sensitivity to light. Our bodies instinctively try to maintain stability by resisting time change, causing psycho-physiological impairment of wellbeing and performance. Natural remedies are highly successful without the side-effects of standard Dramamine-type drugs. Get enough sleep and don't drink alcohol before traveling. Stay between the left and right sides of a boat to minimize the rocking motion.

Diet & Superfood Therapy

—Nutritional therapy plan:

1—Before departure: Take a cup of miso soup with 2 pinches of ginger added; or a bowl of brown rice mixed with 3 TBS brewer's yeast; Or take a cup of strong green tea.

2—During the trip: Suck on a lemon or lime during the trip whenever queasiness strikes. Munch on soda crackers to soak up excess acids. Take sugar-free, carbonated sodas. Avoid fried, salty, sugary or dairy foods. They can cause digestive imbalance.

3—For jet lag: Drink water, juices and herb teas to combat dehydration on a flight - but avoid alcohol when flying. It can upset nervous system biochemistry. During re-adjustment, eat high vegetable protein meals when you are trying to stay awake; high carbohydrate meals when you are trying to sleep. Eat complex carbohydrates if you are traveling to high altitudes. For irregularity, have a salad two or three times a day.

—Superfood therapy: (choose 1 or 2)
• New Moon GINGER WONDER syrup. ☺
• Crystal Star BIOFLAV, FIBER & C SUPPORT™ drink before departure. ♂
• Nature's Secret ULTIMATE GREEN tabs, 6 to 10 daily. ♀

Herb & Supplement Therapy

—Interceptive therapy plan: (Choose 2 to 3 recommendations)

1—Prepare your body's equilibrium before a trip: • Crystal Star GREEN TEA CLEANSER™ each morning for a week before a trip, and during a trip for stomach enzyme balance. • Ginger caps, 4 capsules before a trip, 2 to 4 during a trip; or ginger/cayenne caps - better than Dramamine. • Crystal Star TRAVELERS COMFORT™ extract before and during the trip. • GINKGO BILOBA extract before and during traveling for inner ear balance. Take • Biotec Foods JET STRESS, and wear a • SpringLife POLARIZER. (Excellent results for chronic sufferers.)

2—Soothe nerve stress: Take • Crystal Star MINERAL SPECTRUM™ caps, about a month before a trip for best body balance. Take • Peppermint or chamomile tea; • Crystal Star MENTAL INNER ENERGY™ caps with kava kava and ginseng, or • Enzymatic Therapy KAVA-TONE. ♂ • Homeopathic Hyland's Calms Forte. ♀

3—Ginseng is effective for body balance: • Siberian ginseng extract before and as needed during a trip; • Crystal Star GINSENG/LICORICE ELIXIR™ as needed.

4—B's are for better balance: • Vitamin B-1, thiamine, 500mg, acts like Dramamine before a trip. ♀ • Vitamin B-complex 100mg for several weeks prior to travelling, extra folic acid 400mcg, and • Country Life sublingual B-12, 2500mcg.

5—Soothe your digestion: • Nutribiotic GRAPEFRUIT SEED extract helps overcome the effects of bad food and water or a trip.

—For jet lag: Before a long flight: Take • Glutamine 500mg and 1 echinacea/goldenseal cap, 2 vitamin C with bioflavonoid tablets, 1 beta-carotene capsule, 1 GINKGO BILOBA extract capsule for inner ear balance. Take a few drops of • GINGER extract in water for almost immediate relief during or after a flight. • Tyrosine 500mg 2 to 3 daily a few days before a trip and during the trip as needed. • Melatonin therapy: take 3mg before retiring on your trip and for two to three days after for best results. • Medicine Wheel MOTION STOP drops as needed.

—During your trip take • GINKGO BILOBA extract drops as needed, and
• 6 vitamin C 500mg chewables with • B-complex 100mg daily.

Lifestyle Support Therapy

—Bodywork: During an attack:
Massage knee caps for 3 minutes.
Massage little finger for 10 minutes.
Massage back of head at base of skull, and behind ears on mastoids.
Massage legs and extremities frequently on a long plane flights.
Breathe deeply for 1 minute. Get fresh air and oxygen as soon as possible.

—Reflexology point:

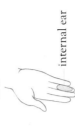

internal ear

—For jet lag:
• Shift your sleep/wake cycle in advance to the new time. Schedule a stop-over if you can.
• Stay away from secondary smoke in the airport. It can keep you toxic for hours.
• Walk about in the plane to promote circulation and prevent blood stagnation.
• As soon as you arrive, get out in the sunlight to help reset your biological clock.

Common Symptoms: *For motion sickness: upset stomach and/or vomiting, bad mood and increased heart rate during a vehicle trip; queasiness; cold sweats; sleepiness; dizziness; poor appetite. For jet lag: fatigue; lethargy; poor performance; dehydration; inability to sleep well. Within 48 hours of landing, some people experience chronic low-grade fever, cough and headaches.*
Common Causes: *For motion sickness: inner ear imbalance; mineral deficiency; fear or stress about the trip; lack of oxygen at heights. For jet lag: circadian rhythm upset when traveling over more than 2 time zones.*

See also VERTIGO and DIZZINESS page 511 for more information.

Can't find a recommended product? Call the 800 number listed in Product Resources for the store nearest you.

Multiple Sclerosis
M.S. and A.L.S. (Amyotrophic Lateral Sclerosis)

For 500,000 Americans, multiple sclerosis is a progressive, central nervous system disease in which the myelin sheath that wraps the nerves is damaged. It seems to be triggered in a strange way by an auto-immune reaction (where the immune system attacks itself) to viruses like herpes or Epstein Barr virus. After fighting these viruses, the immune system creates antibodies to the brain's myelin which bears an uncanny resemblance to the viruses. M.S. must be treated vigorously. A little therapy does not work, but long lasting remission is possible. Natural therapies take 6 months to a year. Strong immune defense is essential. A.L.S. (Lou Gehrig's disease) is a disease of the skeletal muscle nerves that results in progressive muscle wasting as the muscles lose their nerve supply. Treat both M.S. and A.L.S. for nerve damage first, then work on restoring muscle function and immune health.

Diet & Superfood Therapy

–Nutritional therapy plan:

1–Malnutrition and stress often precede M.S. Follow a cleansing diet for 2 months, similar to one for Candida albicans (see pg. 341). Then, follow a modified macrobiotic diet (pg. 333) for 6 months. Take potassium broth (pg. 215) 2x a week.

2–The diet should be 70-80% fresh foods, with plenty of salads and green drinks; 15-20% fresh fruits; and 5-10% vegetable proteins from sprouts, legumes and seeds. Eat a bowl of brown rice every day for B vitamins. Eat fish and sea greens with the rice at least three times a week for EFA's. *Kombucha* mushroom drink, along with a mild detox report several cases of marked improvement.

3–Keep sugar levels low. Avoid all refined and fried foods, full-fat dairy foods, and caffeine foods. Eliminate meats except fish. Reduce high gluten foods. Eliminate pectin-containing candies.

–Superfood therapy: (choose 1 or 2)

• All One GREEN PHYTOBASE for pain.
• Mona's CHLORELLA to stim. B and T cells.
• Crystal Star BIOFLAV, FIBER & C SUPPORT™ drink to rebuild nerve tissue.
• Green Foods WHEAT GERM extract.
• Solgar WHEY TO GO protein drink.
• Nutricology PROGREENS with EFA's.
• CC Pollen ROYAL JELLY 2 teasp. daily.
• Crystal Star SYSEM STRENGTH with EFA's.

Herb & Supplement Therapy

–Interceptive therapy plan: (Choose 2 to 3 recommendations)

1–Rebuild strong nerve structure: • Crystal Star RELAX caps with St. John's wort (highly successful); • CoQ$_{10}$, 60mg 4x daily; • Ginkgo biloba extract for tremor; oatseed tea for nerve pain. • Chondroitin sulfate-A 1200mg for spine improvement, with magnesium 400mg 3x daily; • Pacific BioLogic ADAPTRIN (Padma 28).

2–Preserve brain cells with amino acid therapy: • NADH - 10mg in the morning; • Phosphatidyl serine 100mg 3 daily/ 3 months; • Lysine 500mg daily; • Carnitine 500mg or • Source Naturals Acetyl-L-Carnitine 1000mg; • Country Life AMINO MAX with B-6; • Threonine for spasticity.

3–Essential fatty acids are a key: • EVENING PRIMROSE OIL caps 4-6; • Nature's Secret ULTIMATE OIL or Omega-3 rich flax oil 3x daily. • Crystal Star PRO-EST BALANCE™ a *wild yam* source for DHEA boost; • DHA 200mg daily, or Source Naturals FOCUS DHA, with • Beta carotene 150,000IU. • Jarrow EGG YOLK LECITHIN and cold water fish oils 3x daily, helpful for M.S.-related eye damage.

4–A mild liver detox cleans out trigger toxins: • Alpha lipoic acid 300-600mg; • Crystal Star LIV-ALIVE™ caps 6 daily and LIV-ALIVE™ tea; • Vitamin C, $^1/_4$ teasp. every hour to bowel tolerance, daily for a month; reduce to 5000mg daily.

5–Boost B-vitamins: • Country Life sublingual B-12, 2500mcg 2x daily for 1 month, then every other day for 2 months; • Nature's Secret Ultimate B or B-complex 150mg daily; • extra folic acid 400mcg 2x daily. • **Niacin therapy:** 500mg 3x daily, with B$_6$ 500mg. • Country Life DMG B$_{15}$ SL.

6–Enhance the adrenals: • Vitamin K 100mcg daily; • American Biologics SUB-ADRENE; • Crystal Star ADRN- ACTIVE with sea greens 2 to 4 daily.

7–Antioxidants rebuild immune strength: • MICROHYDRIN available from Healthy House; • Grifon MAITAKE D-FRACTION; • Nutricology GERMANIUM 150mg; • Glutathione 100mg daily. • Transformation PUREZYME as directed.

–For A.L.S.: Amino acid therapy slows the rate of deterioration up to 75% (better than drugs). A combination of leucine, isoleucine and valine test well. I recommend a full spectrum formula like • Anabol Naturals AMINO BALANCE 3x daily.

Lifestyle Support Therapy

–Bodywork:

• Overheating therapy is effective for M.S. See page 225 in this book for home technique.
• As with other motor-brain-nerve disorders, accumulations of aluminum may be a factor. Avoid it in pots and pans, deodorants and commercial condiments.
• Remove mercury amalgam fillings.
• Sunlight and vitamin D influences the remission of M.S. There are far less incidences of the disease in sun-belt regions.
• Take a *catnip enema* or *spirulina* implant once a week for several months.
• Avoid emotional stress and excessive fatigue, keep your diet healthy to keep from triggering the onset of M.S. attacks.
• Avoid smoking and secondary smoke. You need all the oxygen you can retain.
• Mild daily exercise, guided imagery, massage therapy and mineral baths are useful in controlling M.S. and A.L.S.

–Reflexology points:

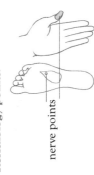

nerve points

M 458

Common Symptoms: *Symptoms result from damage to the brain and spinal cord. Initial onset usually occurs between age 30 and 45. More women than men are affected. Numbness, tingling sensations, and often eventual paralysis; great fatigue; visual loss, preceded by blurring, double-vision and eyeball pain; breathing difficulty; slurred speech; mental disturbance; poor motor coordination/staggering gait; tremors; dizziness; bladder and bowel problems; sexual impotence in men; nerve degeneration; many symptoms mimic Lyme disease.*

Common Causes: *Poor food assimilation and toxemia from poor bowel health; lead or heavy metal (mercury fillings) poisoning; hypoglycemia; B vitamin deficiency; food allergies; Candida albicans overgrowth.*

See Nerve Health page in this book for more information.

Can't find a recommended product? Call the 800 number listed in Product Resources for the store nearest you.

Muscle Cramps, Spasms and Twitches
Leg Cramps

Muscle spasms, cramps, twitches and tics are usually a result of body vitamin and mineral deficiencies or imbalances. Most cramping occurs at night as minerals move between the blood, muscles and bones. A good diet and natural supplements have been very successful in fortifying and strengthening the body against nutrient shortages. Improvement is noticeable within one to two weeks. Leg cramps are usually the result of poor circulation.

Diet & Superfood Therapy

—**Nutritional therapy plan:**

1—Eat vitamin C-rich foods; leafy greens, citrus fruits, brown rice, sprouts, broccoli, tomatoes, green peppers, etc.

2—Eat potassium-rich foods; bananas, broccoli, sunflower seeds, beans and legumes, whole grains and dried fruits.

3—Add sea greens to your daily diet for iodine and potassium. A difference in about a week

4—Eat magnesium-rich foods; lettuce, bell pepper, green leafy vegetables, molasses, nuts and seafoods. Take a veggie drink (pg. 218) 2x a week.

5—Drink plenty of healthy liquids. Muscles need fluids to contract and relax.

6—Take an electrolyte drink often, like Knudsen's RECHARGE for good mineral salts transport.

7—Avoid refined sugars, processed and preserved foods. Food sensitivities to these are often the cause of twitches and spasms.

—**Superfood therapy: (choose 1 or 2)**
• Crystal Star SYSTEMS STRENGTH™ drink.
• Green Foods GREEN MAGMA/barley grass.
• Crystal Star ENERGY GREEN™ drink.
• Green Kamut JUST BARLEY.
• Sun Wellness CHLORELLA with 1 tsp. kelp.
• Future Biotics VITAL K 3 teasp. daily. ♀
• Rainbow Light HAWAIIAN SPIRULINA. ♂

Herb & Supplement Therapy

—**Interceptive therapy plan: (Choose 2 to 3 recommendations)**

1—**Reduce cramping:** • Crystal Star ANTI-SPZ™ caps 4 at a time; or • CRAMP BARK COMBO™ extract. • Alacer EMERGEN-C drink; *Lobelia* extract drops for cramping; • Crystal Star VALERIAN-WILD LETTUCE or Medicine Wheel SERENE drops to calm muscle spasms; • Floradix HERBAL IRON for leg cramps.

Homeopathic remedies for muscles: • Hyland's *Mag Phos* to reduce pain. • *Arnica Montana* for recovery.

2—**Reduce inflammation:** • Quercetin 1000mg with bromelain 1500mg • Acetyl -L-Carnitine 1000mg daily. • Glucosamine-chondroitin, 1500/1200mg 6 daily; • American Biologics INFLAZYME FORTE or • Enzymedica PURIFY for muscle inflammation; • Crystal Star ANTI-FLAM™ caps daily, 4 at a time as needed.

3—**Reduce pain and aches:** • MSM caps 800mg daily or • Futurebiotics MSM caps; • Crystal Star GINSENG/LICORICE ELIXIR™, cortisone-like properties without side effects. • Aromatherapy: apply *rosemary* or *juniper* essential oils.

For men: • Country Life LIGATEND as needed, • MAXI-B COMPLEX w/ taurine; Nature's Path CAL-LYTE with electrolytes; • Magnesium/ potassium/bromelain 3 daily, with • zinc 75mg, and chromium 100mcg to rebuild muscle strength.

For women: • Solaray CAL/MAG CITRATE 4-6 daily, with vitamin D 1000IU; • Magnesium 400mg 2x daily or • Ethical Nutrients MALIC/MAGNE-SIUM to alleviate tender points; • CoQ-10, 60mg, 3x daily.

4—**Restore nerve health:** • Crystal Star RELAX CAPS™ daily 4 to 6. • *EVENING PRIMROSE OIL* 4 daily for EFAs; • *Passionflowers* or *Scullcap* tea as needed.

5—**Help rebuild strong muscle tissue:** • Crystal Star SILICA SOURCE™ caps or • Flora VEGE-SIL silica caps 3-4 daily for collagen and tissue regeneration; • *Horsetail/oatstraw* tea; • Solaray ALFA-JUICE caps. • Vitamin C or Ester C, up to 5000mg daily with bioflavonoids for collagen formation.

—**For leg cramps at night:** • B-complex 100mg daily, with extra B₆ 250mg and pantothenic acid 250mg for nerve repair. Take extra B₆ before bed at night as needed; • Calcium/Magnesium 1000/500mg; • Vitamin E 400IU; • PCO's 50mg 2x daily.

Lifestyle Support Therapy

Note: *If you take high blood pressure medicine and have continuing muscle spasms, ask your doctor to change your prescription. Some have sodium imbalance that upsets mineral salts in the body.*

—**Bodywork:**

• Take vinegar or epsom salts baths, or apply a hot salt pack. To make: heat sea salt in pan, funnel into an old sock; apply directly to affected area.

• Topical applications:
–*Arnica* tincture
–*Lobelia* extract

• For leg cramps: Massage legs; elevate the feet; slap soles and legs with palm to stimulate circulation.

• Use alternating hot and cold hydrotherapy, or hot and cold compresses applied to the area to ease pain, promote circulation and healing.

• Shiatsu and massage therapy are effective in re-aligning the body's "electrical" impulses, and relieving muscle cramps.

• Acupressure is highly successful. See Acupressure page 31 in this book.

• Take brisk walk every day to relieve leg cramps at night.

Common Symptoms: *Uncontrollable spasms and twitches of the legs, facial muscles, etc.; unexplained leg cramps at night.*
Common Causes: *Metabolic insufficiency of calcium, magnesium, potassium, iodine, trace minerals, and vitamins E, D and B₆: lack of sufficient HCL in the stomach; vitamin C and silicon deficiency causing poor collagen formation; food allergies to preservatives and colorants.*

See also SPORTS INJURIES page 506 for more information.

Can't find a recommended product? Call the 800 number listed in Product Resources for the store nearest you.

Muscular Dystrophy
Spina Bifida

Muscular dystrophy is a term for several disorders where there is severe weakening of the muscles and nerve growth due to abnormal development. MD disorders affect about 40,000 people in the U.S., mostly young children. In children, muscle and nerve degeneration prohibits the ability to support body weight. Spina bifida is a condition where there is a genetic defect in the nerve growth and development of the spinal column. Children born with spina bifida have poor motor ability and coordination, and are essentially paralyzed from the waist down. Sometimes spina bifida is undiagnosed until adulthood. Natural therapies have been successful in increasing nutrient assimilation, in overcoming EFA deficiency, in rebuilding nerve and muscle tissue, and sometimes in arresting progressive muscle wasting.

Diet & Superfood Therapy

—Nutritional therapy plan:

1—Go on a 7 day brown rice cleansing diet to release toxins and for healing B vitamins (pg. 197).

2—Then follow an intensive macrobiotic diet for degenerative disease for 2 months, and a modified macrobiotic building diet (pg. 333) for 6 months or more.

3—Take a potassium drink (pg. 215) daily for the first 6-8 weeks of healing. Reduce to once a week for the next 6 months. Add one veggie drink (pg. 218) every week.

4—2 TBS daily of dried, chopped sea greens in a soup or salad for rebuilding mineral and enzyme strength.

5—Mix some lecithin granules, nutritional yeast, wheat germ: take 2 TBS daily.

6—Avoid all refined foods, caffeine foods, and highly salted foods.

7—Eat plenty of leafy greens for folic acid to prevent birth defects like spina bifida.

—Superfood therapy: (choose 1 or 2)

• Crystal Star SYSTEMS STRENGTH™.
• Pines MIGHTY GREENS drink.
• Future Biotics VITAL K up to 6 teasp. daily.
• Crystal Star ENERGY GREEN™ drink.
• Herbal Answers ALOE FORCE JUICE.
• Green Foods WHEAT GERM extract.
• Nutricology PRO-GREENS w. flax oil EFA's.

Herb & Supplement Therapy

—Interceptive therapy plan: (Choose 2 to 3 recommendations)

1—**Help repair and rebuild nerve damage:** • Crystal Star RELAX CAPS™ 4 to 6 daily as needed (excellent empirical results); • Highest potency royal jelly up to 100,000mg 2 teasp. daily; *Scullcap* extract as a healing nervine; • Phosphatidyl choline (PC55) 4 daily, or • EGG YOLK LECITHIN daily to help neuro-transmission.

2—**Help rebuild stronger muscles:** • CoQ₁₀ 100mg 3x daily to help regeneration of myelin sheath and halt muscle wasting progression; • Creatine as directed; • MSM caps 800mg daily or • Futurebiotics MSM caps; • GINKGO BILOBA extract caps 4 daily; • Country Life GLYCINE 500mg with • CARNITINE 2000mg daily, and • Country Life sublingual B-12, 2500mcg for muscle weakness; • Crystal Star BODY RE-BUILDER™ caps to overcome muscle atrophy.

For muscle pain: Glucosamine-Chondroitin combo 1500/1200mg daily;

3—**Stimulate circulation:** • HAWTHORN extract 2-4x or as needed daily; • *Cayenne/ginger* caps 6 daily; • BILBERRY extract for circulatory tone; • Golden Pride FORMULA ONE oral chelation with EDTA; • niacin 500mg for increased circulation; • *Siberian ginseng* extract or • Health Aid America SIBERGIN.

4—**Add magnesium and B-vitamins:** • Magnesium 400mg 2x daily or • Ethical Nutrients MALIC/MAGNESIUM to alleviate tender points; • B-complex 150mg 3x daily, or • Nature's Secret ULTIMATE B tabs.

5—**Essential fatty acids are a key:** • Evening primrose oil caps 2000mg daily; • Omega-3 flax oil, or • Omega Nutrients OMEGA-PLUS caps 3 daily; • Nature's Secret ULTIMATE OIL, • Spectrum organic ESSENTIAL MAX EFA oil.

6—**Antioxidants are a key:** • Ascorbate vitamin C or Ester C powder with bioflavonoids, ¹/₄ teasp. every 3 hours during main healing period. Then reduce to 3 to 5000mg daily; • Nutricology GERMANIUM 150mg; • MICROHYDRIN available at Healthy House has reports of nerve restoration. • Vitamin E 800IU to protect against cell membrane damage; • PCOs 50mg. 3x daily.

—**For spina bifida:** take folic acid during pregnancy 400-800mcg daily, and give if there is suspected spina bifida in adulthood.

Lifestyle Support Therapy

—Bodywork:

• Regular massage therapy treatments are notably helpful for both nerve and muscle normalization.

• Overheating therapy has been successful in controlling muscular dystrophy. See page 225 in this book.

• Avoid tobacco and alcohol. Question high blood pressure drugs containing sodium. Chemical drugs of all kinds, taken to excess, can lead to increased lethargy and dependency.

• Use hot and cold hydrotherapy to stimulate circulation (pg. 228).

• Use mineral baths like BATHERAPY for cleansing and muscle support.

• Get early morning sunlight on the body every day possible to rebuild muscle strength.

—Reflexology point:

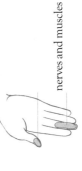

nerves and muscles

See next page for more information.

Can't find a recommended product? Call the 800 number listed in Product Resources for the store nearest you.

Common Symptoms: Muscle weakness and atrophy; nerve damage and atrophy; tremor and palsy; degenerating ability to walk, with frequent falling and stumbling; deep tendon reflexes are usually lost early; occasional loss of bladder control. There may be mild mental retardation in some types of muscular dystrophy.

Common Causes: Muscular dystrophies seem to be a result of an inherited defective gene - often because of folic acid, or other micronutrient deficiency in the mother; poor diet/food assimilation causing deficient minerals during pregnancy; EFA and prostaglandin deficiency. Spina bifida may be congenital or the result of the mother's nutritional status during pregnancy, and nutrient intake during infancy.

M 460

Myasthenia Gravis

Muscle Wasting Disease, Facial Tics (Bell's Palsy)

Myasthenia gravis is a debilitating muscle disease, now thought to be an immune disorder, because immune antibodies that normally fight infection instead turn against normal tissue. Largely a woman's problem, it is characterized by progressive weakness and rapid fatigue, beginning with the muscles and nerves of the lips, tongue and face. Breathing and swallowing are also affected. Complete exhaustion and paralysis are a final result. Many of the symptoms as well as successful treatments are the same as for muscular dystrophy. Remission has shown marked success from an improved diet. Bell's palsy is a non-progressing facial nerve disorder characterized by facial paralysis, beginning with muscle weakness on one side of the face and the inability to close one eye.

Diet & Superfood Therapy

—Nutritional therapy plan:

1—Avoid nightshade plants: tomatoes, eggplant, white potatoes, green peppers, etc.

2—Eat vitamin C-rich foods; leafy greens, citrus fruits, brown rice, sprouts, broccoli, tomatoes, green peppers, etc.

2—Eat potassium-rich foods; bananas, broccoli, sunflower seeds, beans and legumes, whole grains and dried fruits.

3—Add sea greens to your daily diet for iodine and potassium. A difference in about a week

4—Eat magnesium-rich foods; lettuce, bell pepper, green leafy vegetables, molasses, nuts and seafoods. Take a veggie drink (pg. 218) 2x a week.

5—Take 2 teasp. wheat germ oil daily in juice or water.

—Superfood therapy: (choose 1 or 2)

• Crystal Star ENERGY GREEN™ with barley grass.

• Pines MIGHTY GREEN BLEND.

• Sun Wellness CHLORELLA packets or tabs.

• All One GREEN PHYTOBASE drink for pain.

• Green Kamut JUST BARLEY.

• Aloe Life ALOE GOLD drink.

• Solgar EARTH SOURCE GREENS.

• Y.S. ROYAL JELLY/GINSENG drink.

Herb & Supplement Therapy

—Interceptive therapy plan: (Choose 2 to 3 recommendations)

1—**Help rebuild stronger muscles:** • MSM caps 800mg daily or • Futurebiotics MSM caps with chromium picolinate 200mcg; or MSM with MICROHYDRIN, available at Healthy House. • Crystal Star RELAX CAPS™, 6 daily as needed.

2—**For more rapid improvement, balance thyroid activity:** • Transitions PROGEST CREAM as directed, with a thyroid glandular like • Enzymatic Therapy THYROID/TYROSINE complex; ♀ add • Crystal Star IODINE/POTASSIUM™ caps for more thyroid help. • Country Life DMG sublingual.

3—**EFA's help repair neurotransmitters and nerves:** • EVENING PRIMROSE OIL caps 4-6 daily; • NADH - 10mg in the morning; • Twin Lab EGG YOLK LECITHIN 2-3x daily. Excellent results. • Choline 600mg. • Phosphatidyl choline (PC 55), or • Phosphatidyl serine (PS) 100mg 3 daily/ 3 months, or • DHA 200mg daily with magnesium 400mg 3x daily; • High potency royal jelly 40-50,000mg 2 teasp. daily. • Biotec PACIFIC SEA PLASMA tabs 8 daily; • Glycine 500mg daily.

4—**Increase circulation:** • GINKGO BILOBA extract 2-3x daily if there is muscle tremor. Apply • cayenne and ginger compresses to affected areas to help prevent atrophy or cayenne/ginger capsules 2 at a time as needed. • SIBERIAN GINSENG extract 3-4x daily. ♂

5—**Relieve pain:** • Acetyl-L-Carnitine 1000mg daily. • Glucosamine-chondroitin, 1500/1200mg 6 daily; • Vitamin E 800mg. • Biochemics PAIN RELIEF lotion.

6—**Proper elimination is important to release toxins:** • Crystal Star FIBER & HERBS CLEANSE™ caps 4-6 daily for 3 weeks.

7—**Add magnesium and B-vitamins:** • Magnesium 400mg 2x daily or • Ethical Nutrients MALIC/MAGNESIUM to alleviate tender points; • B-complex 150mg 3x daily, or • Solaray MEGA B STRESS 100mg daily, with extra pantothenic acid 500mg and B₆ 250mg daily and extra • Solaray 2000mcg B₁₂ or • Source Naturals Dibencozide 10,000mcg.

8—**For eye tics:** CoQ₁₀ 100mg daily, or Real Life Research CoQ 20/20.

Lifestyle Support Therapy

—Bodywork:

• Avoid smoking, secondary smoke, and oxygen-depleting pollutants as much as possible.

• Get some mild outdoor exercise every day for fresh air, and aerobic lung and muscle tone.

• Relaxation techniques are helpful because stress aggravates myasthenia gravis symptoms.

• Massage therapy and shiatsu are both effective in increasing oxygen use and strengthening nerves and muscles.

—Reflexology points:

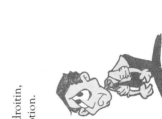

nerves and muscles

See also MUSCULAR DYSTROPHY page 460 for more.

Common Symptoms: Severe muscle weakness and fatigue, especially in the upper body; facial muscle weakness (drooping eyelids); inability to perform even small tasks because of lack of strength; progressive paralysis and exhaustion; double vision; poor articulation and speech. Emergency symptoms include great difficulty in breathing and swallowing.

Common Causes: Immune disorientation; chemistry failure between the nervous system and the muscles; choline and prostaglandin deficiency causing poor neurotransmission; chronic constipation causing poor elimination of toxins; chronic sugar regulation imbalances.

Can't find a recommended product? Call the 800 number listed in Product Resources for the store nearest you.

Nails

Nail Health, Nail Fungus

Nails can be very useful as an "early warning system" in diagnosing illness and evaluating health. If the eyes are the "windows of the soul," the nails are considered the "windows of the body." They are one of the last body areas to receive the nutrients carried by the blood, and show signs of trouble before other better-nourished tissues do. Healthy nails are pink, smooth and shiny. Changes in their shape, color and texture signal the presence of disease in the body. Disorders of the blood, glands, circulation and organs as well as nutritional deficiencies (most nail problems are diet-related) all show up in nail conditions. Give yourself 3 to 6 months to achieve nail health. Note: Griseofulvin™ tabs for nail fungus can affect liver function.

Diet & Superfood Therapy

—Nutritional therapy plan:

1—Good nutrition is the key for nail health. Give your program a month to show improvement. I find that nothing seems to happen for 3 weeks; noticeable changes appear in the 4th week.

2—Eat plenty of vegetable protein and calcium foods, like whole grains, sprouts, leafy greens, molasses, and seafood to strengthen nails.

3—Eat sulphur-and-silicon-rich foods, like onions, sea vegetables, broccoli and fish.

—Foods for nails:

For color and texture; mix honey, avocado oil, egg yolk, and a pinch of salt. Rub on nails. Leave on 1/2 hour. Rinse off.

For brittle nails: massage castor oil into nails.

For discolored nails; rub fresh lemon juice around nail base. Take chewable papaya enzymes.

For weak nails; soak daily for 5 minutes in warm olive oil or cider vinegar.

For splitting nails; take 2 TBS brewer's yeast, or 2 teasp. wheat germ oil daily for a month.

—Superfood therapy: (Choose one or two)
• Rainbow Light Hawaiian SPIRULINA for zinc.
• Mona's CHLORELLA.
• Lewis Labs BREWER'S YEAST.

Herb & Supplement Therapy

—Interceptive therapy plan: (Choose 2 or 3 recommendations)

1—**Plant minerals are the best choice for mineral deficiency nail problems:** Silica is a key: For 2 months, take • Horsetail or dandelion tea or extract 3x daily; or • Crystal Star SILICA SOURCE™ extract; or • Flora VEGE-SIL caps; or • Body Essentials SILICA GEL, internally as directed; apply directly daily.

2—**To strengthen nails and encourage growth:** • Futurebiotics HAIR, SKIN and NAILS tabs 2 daily; • Crystal Star MINERAL SPECTRUM™ caps or • Nature's Path TRACE-MIN-LYTE (both with sea greens) 2 daily, or • Cal/mag/zinc caps 4 daily with boron for better mineral up-take. • Nature's Plus ULTRA NAILS, with extra biotin 600mcg daily for splitting nails.

—**Herbal nail soaks for strength** (may also be taken internally): • Dulse-oatstraw tea; • Pau d'arco tea; • kelp tea (also take 6-8 tabs daily); mix a • mud face mask in water and apply (don't take internally.); white vinegar soak.

3—**EFA's nourish nails:** • Evening primrose or borage oil caps 4 daily for a month.

4—**For nail fungus:** Apply • castor oil or • tea tree oil daily for 6 weeks; soak nails in • Nutribiotic GRAPEFRUIT SEED EXTRACT solution, 3 to 4 drops in 8-oz. water until fungus clears (usually 4 weeks); soak nails in • American Biologic DIOXY-CHLOR or • Earth's Bounty O₂ SPRAY; use • Nature's Pharmacy MYR-E-CAL fungus spray. Massage in • oregano oil; or use • 1 part diluted DMSO solution mixed with 1/2 part oregano oil and 1/2 part olive oil - clean nails, then rub all around nail.

—Special supplements for nail problems:
• Zinc 50mg daily for spots/poor growth; • Vitamin E 400IU or jojoba oil for broken nails or hangnails; • Vitamin A & D for poor growth, ridges and crusty skin around nails; • Betaine HCl and vitamin A for brittleness, splitting and white spots; • Raw thyroid extract for spots or chipping; • A green clay poultice draws out a nail infection; • use wild alum (cranesbill herb) paste with water to relieve inflammation from ingrown or hangnails.

Lifestyle Support Therapy

—Bodywork:

• Nail enamels are among the most toxic environmental polluters. Fake nails or tips add weight to the nails and prevent them from thickening naturally. Nail color dyes penetrate the nail to the skin, often causing allergic reactions. A simple manicure without polish - with beeswax spread on the nails and buffed to a shine leaves your nails naturally beautiful.

• If you polish your nails, don't keep them constantly polished. Allow them to breathe at least 1 day a week. Buff instead. To tint nails naturally: make a thin paste of red henna powder and water. Paint on and let dry in the sun. Rinse off for pretty pink nails with no chipping.

• Do a paraffin (from beauty supply stores) hand dip to restore nail and skin elasticity. When wax hardens, put on old mittens or socks for ten minutes. (Wax does not adhere.) Peel off for satiny hands and feet.

• Acupressure treatment: Press 3x for 10 seconds on the moon of each nail to stimulate circulation and bring up color.

Nail Signs: White spots: zinc, thyroid or HCl deficiency; **White bands on nails:** zinc/protein deficiency; **White bands on nails:** vit. B₁₂ deficiency, kidney or liver problems; **Discolored nails:** vit. B₁₂ deficiency, possible heart disease, or liver problems; **Yellow nails:** vit. E deficiency, poor circulation, lymph congestion, too much polish; **Green nails:** bacterial nail infection; **Too white nails:** liver malfunction, poor circulation, anemia, mineral deficiency; **Blue nails:** lung and heart problems, drug reaction, blood toxicity from too much silver or copper; **Black bands on nails:** low adrenal function, chemotherapy or radiation reaction; **No half moons or ridged nails:** vit. A deficiency, kidney disorder, protein deficiency; **Splitting, brittle or peeling nails:** Vitamin A & D deficiency, poor circulation, thyroid problems, iron, calcium or HCl deficiency; **Poor shape:** iron-zinc deficiency; **Thick nails:** poor circulation; **Dark, spoon-shaped nails:** anemia, B₁₂ deficiency; **Pitted, fraying, split nails:** vitamin C and protein deficiency; **"Hammered metal" looking nails:** hair loss; **Down-curving nails:** heart and liver disorders; **White nails with pink tips:** liver cirrhosis.

Can't find a recommended product? Call the 800 number listed in Product Resources for the store nearest you.

Narcolepsy

Chronic Sleeping Disorder, Sleeping Sickness

Narcolepsy is a chronic, neurological sleep disorder involving sleep-wake mechanisms in the brain. Victims are unable to control their sleep spells, and suddenly fall asleep. Sleeping attacks are erratic, recurrent, overwhelming, and can happen at any time - day or night, no matter what the person is doing. Sufferers are easily awakened, although they fall asleep again within an hour or two. Narcoleptics may also experience complete loss of muscle control. There may be up to 200,000 people in the U.S. with narcolepsy (men and women equally). There are two types of the disorder - DDD (dopamine dependent depression), and a type a involving a B$_6$ deficiency of the dopaminergic system and poor use of body oxygen.

Diet & Superfood Therapy

—Nutritional therapy plan:

1—Food allergies are thought to be involved with narcolepsy. A rotation/elimination diet may be helpful. See a nutritional health professional, and start by eliminating common allergens like wheat, corn, potatoes, eggs and dairy food. See Food Allergy page 309.

2—The diet should be low in fats and clogging foods, such as dairy products and animal proteins; high in light cleansing foods, such as leafy greens and sea vegetables.

3—Eat nutritional yeast and other foods high in B vitamins, like brown rice, on a regular basis.

4—Eat tyrosine-rich foods, such as wheat germ, poultry, oats and eggs for better brain connection.

—Superfood therapy: (Choose one or two)

• Sun Wellness CHLORELLA 2pkts daily for natural germanium.

• Nature's Life SUPER GREEN PRO-96 or Nutricology PRO-GREENS, both with EFA's.

• Rainbow Light Hawaiian SPIRULINA drink.

• Morada Research GOD'S GARDEN POWER FOOD blend.

• Y.S. ROYAL JELLY/GINSENG drink.

Herb & Supplement Therapy

—Interceptive therapy plan: (Choose 2 to 3 recommendations)

1—**Boost circulation to the brain:** • *Ginkgo biloba* extract or • Wakunaga GINKGO BILOBA PLUS as needed; • *Rosemary* aromatherapy applied on the temples.

2—**Ginseng helps regulate sleep patterns and are key brain nutrients:** • Crystal Star GINSENG 6 SUPER™ tea and • GINSENG 6 SUPER™ cap are effective. • GINSENG/LICORICE ELIXIR helps balance critical sugar use; • (• chromium picolinate 200mcg daily, and • Magnesium 800mg daily also regulate sugar); or use • SIBERIAN GINSENG extract drops or • Imperial Elixir SIBERIAN GINSENG.

3—**Normalize serotonin levels:** • *St. John's wort* extract as needed; • Enzymatic Therapy THYROID/TYROSINE caps, 4 daily as an anti-depressant. • For bad moods, add 5-HTP 50mg at night for serotonin connection. • Stress B-complex 150mg daily, with extra B$_6$ 200mg daily; or • Country Life AMINO MAX caps with B$_6$ daily for at least 2 months for additional brain protein.

4—**EFA's help body "electrical" alignment and neurotransmission:** • EVENING PRIMROSE OIL caps 4-6 daily; • Omega 3 flax oils 3-4x daily; • Twin Lab EGG YOLK LECITHIN 2-3x daily. Excellent results. • Choline 600mg, or Phosphatidyl serine (PS) 100mg 3 daily/ 3 months; • High potency royal jelly 40-50,000mg 2 teasp. daily. • Biotec PACIFIC SEA PLASMA tabs 8 daily; • Glycine 500mg daily.

5—**Normalize body chemistry:** • Crystal Star GINSENG-REISHI extract; • *gin-seng-gotu kola* caps 4 daily; • MICROHYDRIN from Healthy House as directed. • Transformation EXCELLZYME; Nutricology ANTI-OX II.

6—**Antioxidants are critical for brain balance and energy:** • Alpha Lipoic Acid neutralizes toxins and recycles glutathione for better use. (or take • Glutathione 100mg daily.) • NADH 5 to 15mg daily; • Nutricology GERMANIUM 150mg; • CoQ$_{10}$ 60mg 2x daily; (Take with vitamin E 400IU for best results.) • PCOs 100mg 4x daily; • Country Life DMG B$_{15}$ daily or • Unipro DMG liquid, under the tongue.

7—**Support thyroid and adrenal functions:** • Crystal Star META-TABS™ or • IODINE-POTASSIUM SOURCE™ caps with ADR-ACTIVE™ caps 2 each daily • Enzymatic Therapy ADRENAL COMPLEX.

Lifestyle Support Therapy

—Bodywork:

• Establish regular circadian rhythms (day/ night) for your body. Regular sleep habits are important for a person with narcolepsy. Soothing *chamomile* aromatherapy or *lavender* baths can help at first.

• Take regular daily exercise for circulation and tissue oxygen.

• Biofeedback and chiropractic adjustment are both effective in correcting the "electrical - shorts" involved in brain-to-motor transmission.

• Avoid hallucinogenic drugs - they aggravate frightening nightmares and the experience of sleep paralysis where a narcoleptic person is unable to move even though awake. Sometimes a dangerous panic reaction sets in.

• Hallucinations and dreams are so real in narcolepsy that the person often cannot tell fantasy from reality.

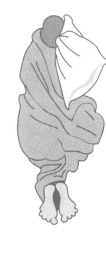

See FOOD ALLERGY page 309 HYPOGLYCEMIA page 427 and THYROID HEALTH page 428 for more.

Can't find a recommended product? Call the 800 number listed in Product Resources for the store nearest you.

Common Symptoms: Symptoms usually begin during the teens with uncontrolled, excessive drowsiness and inappropriate, erratic periods of sleep; longer than normal sleep during regular sleep hours; loss of muscle control (cataplexy) when awake sometimes triggered by strong emotions, and sleep paralysis, where the person is unable to move while awake; memory loss; dream-like hallucinations.

Common Causes: Irregular work/sleep schedules that throw off the body clock; hypoglycemia; food allergy; vitamin B$_6$ or tyrosine deficiency; low thyroid function and metabolism; heredity; constant exposure to physical or mental stress; brain infection; depression accompanying poor brain and adrenal function; poor assimilation and use of body oxygen.

Nausea

Vomiting, Upset Stomach, Morning Sickness, Infant Colic

Nausea can be caused by many factors - motion sickness, vertigo, exposure to toxic chemicals or even psychological shocks. Over 50% of pregnant women experience high frequency morning sickness nausea during the first trimester. While it is quite understandable that the wide variety of sudden hormone and metabolic changes is contributing to morning sickness, there are also many natural treatments that can lessen the severity. Infant colic and other nausea causes that involve allergic reactions, infection or nervous reactions can also be helped with natural, soothing therapies.

Diet & Superfood Therapy

—**Nutritional therapy plan:**

—**For nausea:** A 24 hour diet of plenty of mild liquids and herb teas. Mix $1/4$ teasp. baker's yeast in warm water to quell non-pregnancy nausea. Take lemon and maple syrup in water. Cultured foods like yogurt or Rejuvenative Foods VEGI-DELITE.

—**For morning sickness:** Keep soda crackers or dry toast by the bed; take before rising to soak up excess acids; eat ice chips to calm spasms; drink a little fresh juice for alkalinity. Cucumbers soaked in water and eaten relieve stomach congestion fast.

For breakfast, slowly sip orange juice or ginger ale sweetened with honey; then a little bran cereal. Or take vanilla yogurt in the morning; friendly flora settle digestive imbalance.

Take 2 TBS brewer's yeast flakes in juice or on a salad daily for absorbable, non-toxic B vitamins. Get fiber from vegetables and whole grains to keep bowels clean and flowing.

—**For colic:** A nursing baby's digestion is dependent on yours. Avoid cabbage, brussels sprouts, onions, garlic, yeast breads, fried or fast foods. Refrain from red meat, alcohol, refined sugar and caffeine until a colicky child's digestion improves.

Chronic colic in an infant indicates a dairy allergy. No cow's milk; goat's milk or soy milk are better alternatives. Give papaya or apple juice.

Herb & Supplement Therapy

—**Interceptive therapy plan:** (Choose 1 or 2 recommendations)
—**For morning sickness:** Take • ginger caps or extract on rising, or make ginger tea or • ginger/peppermint tea (or homemade ginger ale, page 224), sip slowly with crackers. • Acidophilus powder, $1/4$ teasp. 3x daily, or • chewable papaya enzymes to settle gastrointestinal imbalance. • Stress B complex 50mg daily, with • magnesium 400mg.
• Vitamin B$_6$ shots are sometimes effective for severe morning sickness.

Rebalance your hormones: • Crystal Star FEMALE HARMONY™ or MOTHERING tea daily; or • red raspberry tea daily. (Helpful all during pregnancy). • Premier One or Y.S. ROYAL JELLY, one teasp. each morning on rising.

Decongest your liver: • MILK THISTLE SEED extract; • Dandelion/yellow dock root tea. • Rose hips tea daily. • Catnip tea with 1 goldenseal cap on rising.

—**For nausea:** • New Chapter GINGER WONDER syrup does wonders for any kind of stomach upset; or make a • ginger tea or • ginger/peppermint tea and drink slowly with crackers. Other anti-nausea teas: • Peppermint or spearmint tea with a pinch of ginger, or • catnip/peppermint tea; • sweet basil tea, or • alfalfa/mint tea. Take $1/4$ teasp. umeboshi plum paste, especially from over-indulgence in sweet, rich foods. • Activated charcoal tabs 500-1000mg as needed. • Vitamin B$_6$ 50-100mg daily; • Acidophilus powder - $1/4$ teasp. 3x daily, or chewable papaya enzymes to settle gastrointestinal imbalance. • Homeopathic Nat. Sulph.; Nux Vomica.

—**For infant colic:** • Apply warm ginger compresses to the stomach and abdomen; • give very dilute fennel tea or catnip tea, 1 tsp. in water with a little maple syrup. • Natren LIFE START $1/4$ teasp. in water or juice 2-3x daily, or • Solaray BIFIDO-BACTERIA powder for infants; • Solaray BABY LIFE for mineral and B Complex deficiency; • Hyland's Homeopathic Colic or Mag. Phos. tabs; • small doses of papaya enzymes dissolved in juice. • B-complex liquid for children, dilute doses in water about once a week.

Lifestyle Support Therapy

—**Bodywork:**
—**For morning sickness:**
• Deep breathing exercises every morning, and a brisk deep breathing walk every day for body oxygen.
• Acupressure points: Press the hollow of each elbow 3x for 10 seconds each.
• Biofeedback and hypnotherapy have been effective. See a qualified chiropractor or massage therapist, esp. if nerve reactions are part of the cause.
• Soft classical or new age music in the morning will help calm you and the baby.

—**For simple nausea:**
• Massage the abdomen with aromatherapy oils like peppermint, chamomile or lavender.
• Mix pinches from your spice cupboard in a cup of water - nutmeg, ginger, cinnamon, turmeric, basil, mace, etc. Drink straight down.

—**For infant colic:**
• Give a catnip enema once a week, or as needed for instant gas release.

See MOTION SICKNESS page 457 for more.

N 464

Common Symptoms: Morning Sickness: nausea and vomiting morning or night during the first trimester of pregnancy; gland and hormone upset causing digestive imbalance; sensitivity to food substances. **Colic:** Excess gas and abdominal discomfort; incessant crying; burping; hiccups.
Common Causes: Morning Sickness: gland and hormone imbalance as the body adjusts to a new biorhythm; congested liver if yellow bile is vomited; low blood sugar. **Colic:** poor food absorption; chronic constipation; or poor food combining; introduction of protein foods too soon (may form lifelong allergies); mother's acidity during breast feeding; mineral deficiency; enzyme deficiency; candida albicans yeast.

Can't find a recommended product? Call the 800 number listed in Product Resources for the store nearest you.

Nerve Health

Nervous Tension, Anxiety

Along with the brain, your nervous system is the chief means of receiving input messages from your body parts and the outside world. It consists of the central nervous system - brain and spinal cord, peripheral nerves that run from your CNS to all other parts of the body and your autonomic nervous system, and the nerves to your blood vessels, organs and glands. We live in a world of frayed nerves today, because the nervous system is the first to be affected by stress, tension and emotion, all aggravated forces in our lifestyle. Poor nerve health can spawn a host of physical disorders, such as Alzheimer's and Parkinson's disease, inflammatory reactions like meningitis, loss of muscular movement and control, and impaired coordination. The nervous system also affects mental balance - weak nerves result in neuroses, tension or anxiety.

Diet & Superfood Therapy

—Nutritional therapy plan:

1—Diet improvement is a key factor in controlling nerve health: Add to the diet regularly, high fiber foods, fresh greens, vegetable proteins, and natural sulfur foods, like onions, garlic, oat bran, lettuce, cucumbers, and celery.

2—B vitamin foods are important for nerves; eat brown rice, whole grains and leafy greens.

3—Keep your diet low in salt and saturated fats.

4—Avoid acid forming foods, such as red meats, caffeine, carbonated drinks - the phosphorus binds up magnesium, making it unavailable.

5—Magnesium is a key mineral in nerve health. Eat plenty of leafy greens - a salad every day.

—Special foods for nerves:
•Nutritional yeast for calming B vitamins.
•Sunflower seeds and molasses for thiamine and iron.
•Carrot/celery juice for nerve restoration.
•Veggie drinks (pg. 218) for chlorophyll.
•Wheat germ oil 1 teasp. daily.
•Garlic capsules 6 daily.

—Superfood therapy: (Choose one or two)
•Crystal Star SYSTEMS STRENGTH™.
•Sun Wellness CHLORELLA packets or tabs.
•Aloe Life ALOE GOLD drink.
•CC Pollen DYNAMIC TRIO.

Herb & Supplement Therapy

—Interceptive therapy plan: (Choose 2 to 4 recommendations)

1—**Nerve relaxers and restorers:** • Crystal Star RELAX™ caps and tea as needed, STRESSED OUT™ extract 2 to 3x daily; • Deva Flowers ANXIETY drops; *Catnip tea*; • Crystal Star HEARTSEASE-H.B.P.™ caps 4 daily; ♂ • *Black Cohosh* extract drops in water 2x daily for 1 month. ♀ • Aromatherapy nerve relaxer: *lavender oil*.

2—**Calm nerve spasms and tics:** • *Turmeric-bayberry* capsules 4 daily; • TYROSINE 500mg 2x daily. • Nutramedix CALM X.

3—**Nerve toning herbs:** • *Chamomile tea*; • *Rosemary* or • *Scullcap* tea or capsules; • *Ginkgo Biloba* extract 2x daily for motor nerves; • *Hawthorn* extract drops under the tongue. • Herbal Magic RELAXA-HERBAL; • Aromatherapy oils of *peppermint or cinnamon*.

4—**Rebuild and regenerate nerves:** • Crystal Star MENTAL INNER ENERGY™ extract with *ginseng* and *kava kava*; • *Gotu kola or ginsenggotu kola* caps 4 daily; • *Siberian ginseng* extract; • *Reishi mushroom* extract; • Bee pollen, 2 teasp. daily; • Country Life MAXI B complex with taurine daily, and extra B_1 100mg and B_6 100mg daily; • Ester C 3-5000mg daily with bioflavonoids and rutin 500mg each for collagen development.

5—**Minerals are dynamic nerve nourishers:** • Nature's Plus MAGNESIUM-POTAS-SIUM-BROMELAIN caps; • Rainbow Light CALCIUM PLUS with high magnesium, 4 daily; • Crystal Star MINERAL SPECTRUM with sea greens; • Nature's Path TRACE-MIN-LYTE daily. • Morada Research NERVOUS SYSTEM nerve food.

6—**EFA's repair nerves:** • Evening primrose oil caps 4-6 daily; • EGG YOLK LECITHIN 3x daily, excellent results. • Omega Nutrition ESSENTIAL BALANCE caps 3 daily, or • DHA 200mg daily with magnesium 400mg 3x daily; • Royal jelly 40-50,000mg 2tsp. daily. • Biotec 8 daily; • Glycine 500mg daily. • PACIFIC SEA PLASMA tabs

Lifestyle Support Therapy

—Bodywork:
•Tobacco and obesity both aggravate nerve disorders and tension. Lose weight and stop smoking.
•Wear acupressure sandals for a short period every day to clear reflexology meridians.

—Relaxation techniques are effective:
•A brisk walk with deep breathing every day for body oxygen.
•Techniques like yoga, meditation and massage therapy are wonderful for the nerves.
•Take baths with baking soda or sea salt.
•Regular massage therapy treatments.
•Gardening, crossword puzzles, hobbies, artwork, etc. can all relieve tension and anxiety.
•Laughter is the best relief of all.

—Reflexology points:

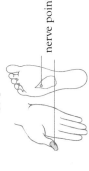

nerve points

See next page and DIABETIC NEUROPATHY page 369 for more information.

Common Symptoms: Extreme nervousness and irritability, often with high blood pressure; inability to relax; lack of energy; chronic headaches and neck stiffness; dizziness and blurred vision, palpitations and heart disease proneness.

Common Causes: Too many refined foods, especially sugars; smoking; unrelieved mental or emotional stress; hyperthyroidism and metabolic imbalance; attack from viral or bacterial infections; prostaglandin imbalance; exposure to damaging chemicals in solvents. Bottle fed babies have a 46% higher risk of developing neurologic abnormalities than breast-fed babies.

Can't find a recommended product? Call the 800 number listed in Product Resources for the store nearest you.

Nerve Damage
Numbness, Nerve Paralysis

Widespread suspension or permanent loss of function and sensation of the motor neurons. If there has been an accident or body trauma, there is often cerebral damage as well.

Diet & Superfood Therapy

—Nutritional therapy plan:

1—Go on a short 24 hour liquid diet (pg. 192) to lighten the circulatory load and clean out wastes.

2—Then, eat only fresh foods for 3 or 4 days to alkalize and clean the blood. Drink 2 cups green tea daily.

3—Then add lightly cooked foods to your 75% fresh foods diet for the rest of the week. Make a mix of nutritional yeast and unsulphured molasses and take 2 TBS daily in any juice.

4—Follow with a modified macrobiotic diet (pg. 333) for 3 weeks, emphasizing whole grains and vegetable proteins, until condition clears.

—Superfood therapy: (Choose one or two)

• Green Foods WHEAT GERM ESSENCE.
• Crystal Star ENERGY GREEN™.
• Green Foods GREEN MAGMA, 2 packets daily; add 1 teasp. kelp granules to each drink for nerve restoration.
• Biostrath original LIQUID YEAST.
• Futurebiotics VITAL K drink 2x daily.
• Crystal Star SYSTEMS STRENGTH™ drink for absorbable potassium, carotenes and iodine.
• Beehive Botanical ROYAL JELLY/GINSENG drink.
• Sun Wellness CHLORELLA drink with extra kelp added, 1 teasp. daily.

Herb & Supplement Therapy

—Interceptive therapy plan: (Choose 2 to 3 recommendations)

1—**Help repair and restore nerves:** • Crystal Star RELAX CAPS™ 2-4 at a time to help rebuild nerves, with • Gotu kola caps 4 daily for nerve repair; • St. John's wort extract to help regenerate nerve tissue; • Ginger/oatstraw tea; • Siberian Ginseng extract; Aromatherapy: • Rosemary essential oil. • Vitamin C up to 5000mg daily with bioflavonoids and rutin to help rebuild nerve connective tissue; or • Morada Research NERVOUS SYSTEM neve food; or • Enzymedica PURIFY. Effective herbal nervine tonics: • Passionflowers or • scullcap tea.

2—**Strengthen circulation:** • Butcher's broom tea or Crystal Star HEARTSEASE/CIRCU-CLEANSE™ tea daily for 1 month to clean out circulatory wastes; • GINKGO BILOBA or • HAWTHORN extract, 2 to 4x daily, or Heart Foods HEART FOOD PLUS; • Cayenne/ginger caps 4 daily, or • Crystal Star GREEN TEA CLEANSER™ 2 cups daily with • cayenne/ginger caps 3 daily for 2 months. ♂
• Golden Pride FORMULA ONE, oral chelation with EDTA, a.m. and p.m. ♂

3—**Reduce nerve inflammation:** • Devil's claw extract drops in water 2x daily; • Rainbow Light CALCIUM PLUS caps with high magnesium, 4 daily.♀

4—**Essential fatty acids nourish the nervous system:** Evening Primrose oil 4000mg daily; Phosphatidyl Choline (PC55); Twin Lab EGG YOLK LECITHIN 3x daily.

5—**Topical nerve help applications:** Rub on capsaicin creme, or • Nature's Way CAYENNE PAIN RELIEVING OINTMENT; • Cayenne/ginger compresses; • St. John's wort oil. • Apply B&T TRIFLORA analgesic gel.

—Neurotransmitter nutrients are critical:
• Crystal Star RELAX caps with St. John's wort (highly successful); • CoQ_{10}, 60mg 4x daily; • Ginkgo biloba extract for tremor; • L-Glutamine 1000mg daily. • Chondroitin sulfate-A 1200mg for spine improvement; • Country Life RELAXER with GABA 100mg and taurine, or • Twin Lab GABA PLUS supplying 500mg GABA; • B-complex 150mg with extra B_6 500mg daily, if numbness is from nerve interference or a stroke and extremeties are periodically numb; • Wakunaga NEURO-LOGIC; or • Niacin therapy: 500mg daily.

Lifestyle Support Therapy

—Lifestyle measures:

• Avoid alcoholic drinks - symptoms seem to worsen.

• Use alternating hot and cold hydrotherapy (pg. 228) to boost circulation.

• Stress reduction techniques: Biofeedback for neuro-muscular feedback, acupuncture, massage therapy, shiatsu, and chiropractic adjustment have all shown excellent results.

—Reflexology points:

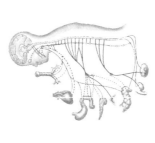

nerve points

—Autonomic nervous system:

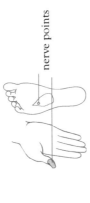

Common Symptoms: Lack of feeling in various parts of the body; hands, legs, itching fingers and toes "going to sleep" or tingling; temporo-mandibular joint misalignment; sporadic auditory or visual disturbances, such as double vision or a blind spot in the visual field; sometimes personality changes; lower back pain.
Common Causes: Poor circulation; thyroid deficiency; pinched nerve or spinal lesions; stroke and brain dysfunction; psychic inhibition, such as from hysteria; multiple sclerosis type nerve damage; nerve damage from a blow or an accident like a whiplash injury; poor diet with too many mucous-forming foods.

See PARKINSON'S DISEASE page 477 for more information.

Can't find a recommended product? Call the 800 number listed in Product Resources for the store nearest you.

Neuritis
Trigeminal Neuralgia

Generally regarded as a syndrome of motor, reflex and sensory nerve symptoms, neuritis (peripheral neuropathy) is an inflammation of a nerve or nerves. It is usually a degenerating process, and often part of a chronic, degenerating illness, such as diabetes or leukemia. Trigeminal neuralgia is sudden, sharp, severe pains shooting along the course of a nerve often as a result of pressure on the nerve trunks, or poor nerve nutrition and an over-acid condition.

Diet & Superfood Therapy

—Nutritional therapy plan:

1–Go on a short 24 hour liquid diet (pg. 192) to rebalance body acid/alkaline pH.

2–Then, for the rest of the week eat mostly fresh foods, with plenty of leafy greens, sprouts, celery, sea vegetables, and enzyme foods such as apples and pineapple. Take a glass of lemon juice and water every morning. Have a potassium broth or essence (pg. 215) every other day.

3–Make a mix of lecithin granules, sesame seeds, brewer's yeast, and wheat germ; take 2 TBS daily.

4–Add essential fatty acids from the sea for nerve restoration: sea foods and sea greens daily for at least 2 months.

5–Drink 6 glasses of water with a slice of lemon, lime or cucumber daily.

6–Keep salts, saturated fats and sugars low. Avoid caffeine especially (a trigger), hard liquor and soft drinks (bind up magnesium).

—Superfood therapy: (Choose one or two)

• Crystal Star ENERGY GREEN™ drink.
• Vibrant Health GREEN VIBRANCE.
• Beehive Botanicals ROYAL JELLY, Siberian ginseng and bee pollen drink.
• Mona's CHLORELLA 1 teasp. daily.
• Future Biotics VITAL K 3 tsp. daily.
• Biostrath LIQUID YEAST with herbs.

Herb & Supplement Therapy

—Interceptive therapy plan: (Choose 2 or more recommendations)

1–**Help repair and restore nerves:** • Crystal Star RELAX CAPS™ as needed for rebuilding nerve sheath, 4 daily; • Crystal Star IODINE/POTASSIUM caps 2 daily for nerve restoration. • BILBERRY extract for tissue-toning flavonoids or • Ascorbate or Ester C with bioflavonoids and rutin, 5000mg daily, to rebuild connective tissue. • Country Life LIGATEND as needed.♂

2–**Relieve nerve spasms:** • GINKGO BILOBA extract for facial neuralgia; • Crystal Star BACK TO RELIEF™ or ANTI-SPZ™ caps for spasmodic pain; • DLPA 750mg as needed for pain. • Homeopathic: Hylands *Calms* or *Calms Forte* tabs.♀

3–**Reduce nerve inflammation:** • Solaray Curcumin (*turmeric* extract) or • Crystal Star ANTI-FLAM™ caps 4 daily to take down inflammation; • *Devil's claw* extract drops in water 2x daily; • Rainbow Light CALCIUM PLUS caps with high magnesium, 4 daily; • Quercetin 1000mg; Bromelain 1500mg daily, or • Transformation PUREZYME for protease. • Homeopathic *Aranea Diadema* - radiating pain or • *Mag. Phos.* for spasmodic pain, or • *Hypericum* if nerve injury.

4–**Topical nerve help applications:** Rub on capsaicin creme, or • Nature's Way CAYENNE PAIN RELIEVING OINTMENT; • *Cayenne/ginger* compresses; • St. *John's wort* oil. • Apply B&T TRIFLORA analgesic gel.

5–**Effective herbal nerve tonics:** • Lobelia extract drops; • *Passionflowers* or *scullcap* tea; • *valerian/wild lettuce* extract, a powerful nerve relaxant; or make a nerve soothing tea: *St. John's wort, peppermint, lavender, valerian, lemon balm, blessed thistle.* Hylands Nerve Tonic. • Niacin therapy: 500-1500mg daily to stimulate circulation.

6–**Essential fatty acids nourish the nervous system:** • Evening Primrose oil 4000mg daily; • Barleans high lignan flax oil, or • Omega Nutrients OMEGA-PLUS caps 3 daily; • Phosphatidyl Choline (PC55); • Twin Lab EGG YOLK LECITHIN 3x daily.

7–**Neural nutrients for long term restoration:** • Country Life sublingual B-12, 2500mcg daily; and • Stress B-complex 100mg with extra B₆ 250mg and folic acid 400mcg; • Taurine 500mg daily.

Lifestyle Support Therapy

—Bodywork:

• Get some regular mild exercise every day for body oxygen and circulation.

• Use hot and cold hydrotherapy to stimulate nerve circulation (pg. 228).

• Do 10 neck rolls as needed at a time to relieve nerve trauma.

• Stress management techniques should be a part of any healing program:

• Acupuncture, chiropractic adjustment, shiatsu, and massage therapy are all effective in controlling nerve disorders.

—Reflexology points:

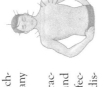

nerve points

Common Symptoms: *Muscle weakness and degeneration; burning, tingling, numbness in the muscles or nerve area; motor and reflex weakness; facial tics; nerve inflammation.*
Common Causes: *Spinal pinch or lesions; excess alcohol or prescription drugs; prostaglandin and/or B vitamin deficiency; diabetic reaction; herpes; poor circulation; multiple sclerosis-type weakness and numbness; kidney and gallbladder malfunction; arthritis; lupus; migraines; heavy metal poisoning.*

See my book Cooking For Healthy Healing for a complete diet for nerve health.

Can't find a recommended product? Call the 800 number listed in Product Resources for the store nearest you.

Osteoporosis
Osteomalacia, Ankylosing Spondylitis

Osteoporosis is a disease that robs bones of their density and strength, making them thinner and more prone to break. Eventually, bone mass decreases below the level required to support the body. Long considered a woman's problem, because of its female hormone involvement, osteoporosis affects up to 35 to 50% of women in the first 5 years after menopause. Osteoporosis also affects men, just at a later age and with less ferocity. Over 35 million Americans suffer from osteoporosis today, and for women, osteoporosis is greater than the combined risks of breast, uterine and ovarian cancers. **Osteomalacia** involves lowered calcium in the bone. **Ankylosing spondylitis** is a type of osteoporosis where spine vertebrae fuse together in bone spurs. Nutritional therapy offers a broad base of both treatment and protection.

Diet & Superfood Therapy

Vegetarians have lower risk of osteoporosis, with denser, stronger bones after menopause, and in later life.
—**Nutritional therapy plan:**

1—Eat vitamin C foods like kiwis, oranges, grapefruit and potatoes for collagen production.
2—Add sea greens like nori, wakame, dulse, kombu or kelp (2 TBS daily, snipped on salads, soups, rice, pizzas), for bone minerals and vitamins D and K that boost hormones like estrogen, progesterone and DHEA, prime bone supports.
3—Eat calcium, magnesium and potassium-rich foods - broccoli, fish and seafood, eggs, yogurt, kefir, carrots, dried fruits, sprouts, miso, beans, leafy greens, tofu, bananas, apricots, molasses, etc.
4—Reduce protein intake from red meat and dairy foods. They disrupt pH balance and lead to mineral loss. Get protein from fresh fish, legumes, vegetables and sea greens instead. (Note: pasteurized milk is not a good source of absorbable calcium, and can actually interfere with mineral assimilation.) Drink juices like carrot and orange instead. One 8-oz. glass of fresh carrot juice has 400mg bioavailable calcium. An 8-oz. glass of fortified milk has 250mg with low assimilation.
5—Avoid sugar, high salt foods (snackfoods and processed foods), alcohol (esp. hard liquor), caffeine foods, tobacco, and nightshade plants that interfere with calcium absorption.

—**Superfoods are important:**
• Crystal Star ENERGY GREEN™ with EFA's.
• Nutricology PRO GREENS with EFA's.
• Ethical Nutrients FUNCTIONAL GREENS.
• Y.S. ROYAL JELLY-POLLEN-GINSENG drink.

Herb & Supplement Therapy

—**Interceptive therapy plan: (Choose 2 or 3 recommendations)**

1—**Balance your hormones (don't just add estrogen):** • Ipriflavone 600mg daily, or • Metabolic Response Modifiers OSTEO-MAX 200mg ipriflavone with 200mg MCHC (microcrystalline hydroxyapatite concentrate). Plant hormones are effective: • Crystal Star OSTEO DEFENSE, 4 daily. (Use with • evening primrose oil 3000mg daily, for maximum mineral absorption and hormone balancing EFAs); • Crystal Star PRO-EST OSTEO™ roll-on, or • Transitions EMERITA PRO-GEST as directed. Take with • Nutricology GERMANIUM 150mg daily for best results.

2—**Boost your minerals (not just calcium):** • Calcium citrate 1500mg / magnesium 1000mg and boron 3mg for absorption (too much boron alone actually causes bone loss.) • Flora VEGE-SIL for 6 mos.; or • Ethical Nutrients BONE BUILDER with silica. • Crystal Star CALCIUM SOURCE™ and • SILICA SOURCE™ extract (silica helps collagen-calcium production). • Mezotrace SEA MINERAL COMPLEX, with Betaine HCl for absorption; • Morada Labs BONES/CALCIUM caps; • Enzymatic Therapy OSTEOPRIME; ♀ • Nature's Path CAL-LYTE. ♂ • Nature's Path TRACE-MIN-LYTE (contains 500mg sea plants and electrolytes).

Boost mineral absorption vitamins: • Vitamin D 1000IU; • marine carotenes 100,000IU, and • zinc 30mg daily; and • vitamin K 100mcg.

3—**Boost bone health with EFA's:** • Crystal Star Evening Primrose oil with E, 6 daily; • Spectrum Naturals 1300mg Evening Primrose oil; • high omega-3 flax oil 3x daily, or • Barlean's OMEGA TWIN flax-borage combo; or • Nature's Secret ULTIMATE OIL.

4—**Add more enzymes to boost nutrient absorption:** Men especially benefit from enzyme therapy; • Herbal Products Dvlpt. POWER PLUS ENZYMES; ♂ • Prevail OSTEO FORMULA; or • Pioneer Nutr. CALCIUM-MAGNESIUM BONE PROTEIN ♀ daily. Note: Low stomach acid diminishes calcium absorption. Herbal "bitters" encourage the body to produce more stomach acid.

5—**Bioflavonoids - important for their hormone-like activity:** • Vitamin C or Ester C with bioflavs. up to 5000mg daily for collagen development and connective tissue; or • HAWTHORN, • BILBERRY, or • GINKGO BILOBA extracts.

6—**B vitamins are important:** • B-complex 100mg daily with extra B_6 250mg;
• Country Life sublingual B-12, 2500mcg daily.
7—**For bone pain:** • Glucosamine 1500mg /chondroitin 1200mg combo, or • DLPA 750mg for bone pain.

Lifestyle Support Therapy

—**Bodywork:**
• Smoking cigarettes causes bone loss in women. Smoking a pack a day during adulthood results in a 10% loss in bone density, leaving bones more subject to fracture than than those of non-smokers. Smoking also appears to interfere with estrogen production.
• Get early morning sunlight on the body every day possible for vitamin D.
• Avoid fluorescent lighting, electric blankets, aluminum cookware, non-filtered computer screens, etc. All tend to leach calcium from the body.
• Exercise is a nutrient in itself. Weight-bearing exercise is a good way to build bone and prevent bone loss. Duration of exercise is more important than intensity. Note: if you already have low bone density, I suggest starting on a weight bearing exercise program after improvements from diet changes are seen in your bone scans in order to avoid injury. I've found the best ones are often water workout exercise. The water limits overdoing it, and is very forgiving to fragile bones. Consult with a qualified health professional to find out what exercises are right for you.

—**Reflexology point:**

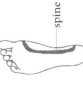
spine

O 468

See also BONE HEALTH page 326 for more information.

Can't find a recommended product? Call the 800 number listed in Product Resources for the store nearest you.

You can arrest or avoid post-menopausal bone loss

Osteoporosis is far more complex than was thought even just 5 years ago. Bone and cartilage are an ever-changing infrastructure. Bone is living tissue, and like other body systems requires a wide variety of nutrients. Osteoporosis is partially a result of reduced nutrient (particularly mineral) absorption, which is highly bound to enzyme activity. High levels of phosphorous in meat, soft drinks and other common processed foods deprive the body of calcium. Lack of vitamin D from sunlight, and too little exercise also contribute to bone porosity. **You don't have to let osteoporosis steal your health!** The good news is that you can start today to build up your bones, even if you've already been diagnosed with the disease. I've seen natural therapies literally transform people crippled by osteoporosis who are living active, full lives after rigorously following natural therapies. After more than 15 years of working with osteoporosis, I find the most successful treatment involves not only balancing (normalizing) hormone levels, but also improving lifestyle and dietary habits that we know accelerate bone loss. It's not just a case of adding estrogen. Successful osteoporosis treatment is a complete lifestyle program, not just a pill!

—**What about calcium?** It's a cornerstone of medical world treatment for osteoporosis. Calcium is the most abundant mineral in the body, and 98 percent of all calcium is stored in the bones. But osteoporosis is the result of much more than a calcium deficiency, so calcium isn't the whole answer, or even the only mineral involved in bone health. Osteoporosis involves both mineral and non-mineral components of bone, so your bones need a full range of supportive nutrients. Getting your minerals from mineral-rich veggies like broccoli, kale and collard greens, and herbs like *oatstraw, kelp, dulse, burdock, dandelion, borage seed and lobelia* may be a better choice. Unlike dairy foods, mineral-rich herbs and veggies come without heavy protein, and they offer many more nutrients for bone building, particularly high levels of vitamin K, which helps calcium attach to bone tissue, and magnesium and potassium. I recommend ditching high fat dairy products and considering more veggies for bones of steel.

Still there are always two sides to everything. We know modern farming techniques leech minerals from the soil, so hardly anyone gets enough minerals from foods. Massive water fluoridation across the U.S. means many Americans are losing some calcium with every sip of their tap water. Today, I'm a firm believer in high quality plant mineral supplements for maximum bone building. Calcium supplements can't stand on their own as a viable treatment. In fact, bone strength is best enhanced when calcium is used with other nutrients, such as B vitamins, magnesium, silica, manganese and boron. How do you know if you have a calcium deficiency? Calcium deficiencies show up pre-menstrually as back pain, cramping, or tooth pain. (Take a calcium supplement before your period to see if this is your problem.... supplementation helps these symptoms disappear.) But, women who think they are helping themselves by taking calcium-containing antacids may be doing just the opposite. Antacids are linked to easy fracture because they block stomach acids, causing, some specialists say, reduced bone growth.

There is a clear relationship between high protein consumption and osteoporosis, too. Amino acids from excess protein enter the kidneys and cause loss of water and excretion of large amounts of minerals, especially calcium, which is released from bone material to neutralize the acidity of the protein amino acids. Protein from animal sources is an even bigger danger for osteoporosis. Studies of vegetarians and non-vegetarians from age 60 through 90, reveal that the mineral content in meat eater's bones decreased 35% over time, while mineral content of a vegetarian's bones decreased only 18%. High levels of phosphorous in meat, soft drinks and other common processed foods also deprive the body of calcium.

How do hormones fit into the bone building picture? A man's testosterone supply protects against osteoporosis. For a woman, osteoporosis involves thyroid malfunction, and poor collagen protein as well as progesterone/estrogen balance. We know that progesterone is a key factor in laying down and strengthening bone. Many doctors prescribe a combination of Premarin, (from pregnant mare's urine), conjugated man-made estrogens, and Provera, a synthetic progesterone, to address menopausal bone loss. (See also page 421 on the new SERM drugs for osteoporosis.) However, new research shows that neither Premarin nor Provera prevent osteoporosis. Taken orally, the drugs pass through the liver where much of the substance is lost or altered. For this reason, and because hormones are readily absorbed through the skin, the estrogen patch has become popular. Our experience has been that neither work as well as natural, plant-derived progesterone therapy, delivered in herbal combinations. Early tests on women over 60 show that plant progesterone, such as that found in wild yam, along with an appropriate diet and supplements, may even reverse osteoporosis, something no synthetic hormone in any combination has been able to demonstrate.

What about progesterone creams derived from wild yam roots? Can they really stave off osteoporosis? In a recent study on women with osteoporosis, a bone scan showed up to 5% new bone density in an eighteen month period after the women used a natural wild yam progesterone cream, along with a good nutritional program. A 4 year study shows that plant-derived progesterone creams increased bone density anywhere up to 40% for women from 45 to 60 years of age. Results were even better when a germanium supplement was added orally.

Is crash dieting bad to the bone? A recent study shows that for each 10% decrease in weight, there is a two-fold increase in the risk of hip fractures in older women. When blood calcium levels become too low from crash dieting, your bones release their calcium to keep the rest of the body running smoothly. In addition, women who diet to excess regularly show up with estrogen deficiency, also involved in bone loss. Even taking calcium supplements was not enough to maintain bone mass during dieting. The test was very discouraging because almost all the women gained all of the weight back. Better results were obtained for dieters when minerals were added to the weight loss diet via green drinks and vegetable juices. Women who took in minerals from these sources didn't gain the lost weight back, either as quickly or as much. Since a majority of American women admit to being on a weight control diet most of the time, it seems maintaining a broad spectrum of low fat foods, and adding high mineral drinks from food or herb sources to avoid bone loss while dieting is a better choice.

Can't find a recommended product? Call the 800 number listed in Product Resources for the store nearest you.

Are you at risk for osteoporosis? Check the following risk factors.

1) post-menopausal small-boned white or Asian women, with a family history of osteoporosis, especially those who have not had children; 2) women over 75 years, especially those with a history of calcium and vitamin D deficiency; 3) women who have a consistently high consumption of tobacco, caffeine and animal proteins; 4) women who over use cortico-steroid drugs. If you are taking long courses of cortico-steroid drugs, consider reducing your dosage. Research indicates that over a long period of time these drugs tend to leach potassium from the system, weakening the bones; 5) women with long use of synthetic thyroid. The drug Synthroid can increase risk for both osteoporosis and high cholesterol, and may also aggravate weight problems; 6) hormone imbalances, especially for women who had their ovaries removed before menopause, or who had an early menopause, before 45 years old, or those with a history of irregular or no menstrual periods. Hormone and calcium deficiencies appear regularly in women with irregular menstrual cycles, notably when they result from excessive exercise or eating disorders.

These risk factors really affect a lot of women, because over 50% of American women suffer from calcium deficiency alone. You can test yourself for probable osteoporosis. Use pH paper (sold in most health food stores), and test your urine. A habitual reading below pH 7 (acid) usually means calcium and bone loss. Above pH 7 (alkaline) indicates a low risk.

Is your lifestyle putting you at risk for osteoporosis?

A low nutrition, processed foods diet sets the stage for bone loss.

—Low mineral intake means a lack of structural support and impaired digestion. Minerals are critical for a strong skeletal system, and they are the bonding agents between you and your food. A lack of minerals means low thyroid function and poor collagen protein development, also part of osteoporosis.

—Osteoporosis is highly bound to food-enzyme activity. It is at least in part, a result of poor digestion and enzyme deficiency. If you don't eat enough fresh plant foods, you probably have low enzymes and poor digestion. I find this is especially true for older men who try to correct digestive problems with handfuls of antacids.

—Too much protein.... There is a clear relationship between high protein consumption and osteoporosis. According to *The Journal of the American Dietetic Association* when protein consumption is doubled, calcium loss increases 50%!

—Over-acid blood from overeating red meats, sodas, caffeine foods and alcohol puts you at risk for bone loss. Soda warning: USDA research finds that men who consume five cans of cola a day for three months absorb less calcium, increasing risk for bone deterioration and injuries or breaks!

Beyond diet, your lifestyle influences osteoporosis.

—Too little exercise stunts healthy bone development. Too little sunlight means less vitamin D is available for bone building.

—Smoking interferes with your body's calcium and estrogen production. Women smokers have 10% lower bone density and are more vulnerable to fractures than non smokers.

—Depression may cause bone loss. Research shows that people with a history of severe depression have 15% less bone density in their lower spines than non-depressed people.

—Overusing steroids, antibiotics or tobacco, and too much alcohol severely reduces mineral absorption.

—Drinking fluoridated water is a risk factor! New studies link hip fractures to fluoridated water. Here's why: Fluoridated water literally leeches calcium from the bones.

—Ovary removal puts you at greater risk for osteoporosis.

You can check for early warning signs of osteoporosis:

1: Bone loss is greatest in the spine, hips and ribs, so osteoporosis begins to show up as chronic back and leg pain. Bone pain may also occur in the spine, affecting the cranial nerves.

2: Look for loss of bone in the jaw and tooth sockets. Bone may draw away from the teeth, causing them to loosen, or fall out. Look for unusually frequent dental problems, too.

3: Vision defects or facial tics may also occur due to bone marrow obliteration.

Note: Natural food stores have an osteoporosis urine test. Use pH paper (drugstores sell it too). A habitual reading below pH 7 usually means calcium and bone loss. Above pH 7 indicates a low risk.

Can pumping iron stop bone loss? Studies find people who do regular weight bearing exercises have denser bones than those who don't. It seems your bones can rebuild themselves, but only when they're used. A sedentary lifestyle increases osteoporosis risk. Power walking is good for bones, so are aerobic workouts, like Tae Bo, or weight bearing exercise 3-4 times a week (especially for men and women under 35 whose bone mass is still growing). You can use your own body weight in bone building exercises, especially outside in the sun to increase production of bone building vitamin D. Here's two of my favorites: 1: For your upper arms - do mini push up against the wall. Just stand at arm's length away from a wall, with your hand flat against the wall. Then just lean in and push back about 10 or 12 times for each arm. 2: For your lower back and legs. Stretch as high as you can. Then lean over as far as you can toward your toes and hold for 5 seconds.

Can't find a recommended product? Call the 800 number listed in Product Resources for the store nearest you.

Ovarian Cysts

Polycystic Ovary Syndrome, Type II PAP Smear, Small Tumors

Ovarian cysts, officially called polycystic ovary syndrome, are showing up in record numbers, especially in women with menstrual difficulties, in women who have irregular or no periods, and for women who have excessive bleeding during their periods. The cysts are small, non-malignant, chambered sacs filled with fluid. As with so many women's problems, they are thought to be hormone-driven, usually from too much estrogen, and hypothyroidism. But they are often painful, especially during intercourse, and can cause excessive menstrual bleeding and inter-period spotting. Medical treatment involves hormone therapy or removal, with accompanying hazards. Alternative treatment focuses on dietary measures and herbal medicines.

Diet & Superfood Therapy

—Nutritional therapy plan:

1—Reducing dietary fat intake is the first, best step to reducing cyst growth. High fats mean high circulating estrogen. Too much estrogen is the most common cause of cysts. Saturated fats from red meats and dairy foods are the worst offenders. Get protein for healing vegetable sources, whole grains, sprouts, soy foods and seafoods.

2—Over-acidity sets up an environment for ovarian cyst development. B vitamin rich foods, like leafy greens and other fresh vegetables, miso, brown rice, wheat germ, brewer's yeast, sea greens and green drinks (page 218) alkalize the system.

3—Especially avoid fried, salty foods, during menses. Eliminate heavy starches, full fat dairy products, and hard liquor.

4—Eat iodine rich foods from the sea to overcome hypothyroidism. Avoid caffeine and refined sugars which deplete your body of iodine, a nutrient you need for healthy thyroid activity.

5—Drink bottled water. Chlorinated water tends to leach vitamin E from the body.

—Superfood therapy (choose 1 or 2):
• Crystal Star SYSTEMS STRENGTH™.
• Transitions EASY GREENS.
• Nutricology PRO GREENS with EFA's.
• Green Foods VIBRANT WOMAN.
• Pines MIGHTY GREENS.

Herb & Supplement Therapy

—Interceptive therapy plan: (Choose 2 to 3 recommendations)

1—**Help reduce and dissolve cysts:** • Crystal Star WOMAN'S BEST FRIEND™ caps, 4 daily for 3 months, with • ANTI-FLAM™ caps for inflammation pain.• Lane Labs BENE-FIN SHARK CARTILAGE as an anti-infective; • Black cohosh extract or • Enzymedica PURIFY helps dissolve adhesions. • Transitions PROGEST CREAM: rub on abdomen. Results in approximately 3 months.

Draw out infection: • Make an effective vaginal pack with powders of echinacea, goldenseal root, white oak, cranesbill, chaparral and red raspberry in water and glycerine to make a solution. Soak a tampon in a strong water solution of these herbs. Insert in the vagina at night (wear a sanitary napkin to prevent leakage). Rinse vagina in the morning with a goldenseal-myrrh tea with 1 TB vinegar. Use 1 week on and 1 week off for 6 weeks. Use with a blood cleansing combination like • Crystal Star DETOX!™ caps, or a daily blood cleansing tea like • dandelion-parsley root-raspberry-ginger tea. Often works in 6 weeks to dissolve small cysts.

2—**Add EFA's and take down inflammation:** • Crystal Star Evening Primrose oil with E, 6 daily; • Spectrum Naturals 1300mg Evening Primrose oil; • high omega-3 flax oil 3x daily, or • Barlean's OMEGA TWIN flax-borage combo; or • Nature's Secret ULTIMATE OIL. • QUERCETIN 1000mg with BROMELAIN 1500mg daily.

3—**Iodine therapy helps hypothyroidism, often effective in 3-4 months:** (Take with vit. E, an estrogen antagonist, for best results.) • Bernard Jensen LIQUI-DULS; • Crystal Star IODINE/POTASSIUM™ caps or • IODINE SOURCE™ extract. • Two TBS dry sea greens snipped over rice, salad, soup or a pizza are a therapeutic dose.

4—**Love your liver to better handle** estrogen and flush out excess estrogen secretions. • Milk Thistle Seed extract; • Dandelion tea; • B-complex 100mg daily; • Sun Wellness CHLORELLA 1 pkt. daily; Pancreatin 1300mg for fat metabolism.

5—**Antioxidants that help:** • PCOs from grapeseed,100mg 3x daily; • Nutricology germanium 150mg; • Vitamin E 400IU as an estrogen antagonist; or VITAMIN E CLUSTERS available from Healthy House; • Vitamin C 5000mg daily with bioflavonoids (for estrogen-like effects to balance estrogen-progesterone ratio).

Lifestyle Support Therapy

—Lifestyle notes: An IUD, too much caffeine, a high fat diet, some birth control pills, synthetic hormones, and being overweight aggravate ovarian cysts. Frequent radiation treatments and X-rays that you may undergo for other problems may change cell structure and set up an environment for ovarian cyst growth.

Diabetes, especially alcohol-induced diabetes, is a high-risk factor. A stressful lifestyle that encourages an over-acid system and poor waste elimination, sets up unhealthy body chemistry for cysts.

—Reflexology point: Reflexology has documented success in dissolving cysts.

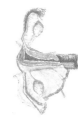

uterus
ovaries

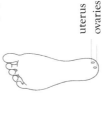

—Ovary region:

Common Symptoms: Pain in the fallopian tubes or ovaries; the inability to conceive; an erratic, painful menstrual cycle; unusual swelling and discomfort in the lower abdomen and breasts; often profuse uterine bleeding because of endometrial hyperplasia that results from unbalanced estrogen stimulation; painful intercourse; heel pain; fever and coated tongue; excess hair growth because of an imbalance between estrogen, progesterone and testosterone levels; unusual weight gain because of low thyroid activity.
Common Causes: Lifestyle habits: using an IUD; too much caffeine; a high fat diet; frequent radiation treatments or X-rays; birth control pills; synthetic hormone replacement; obesity.

See ENDOMETRIOSIS page 377 for more information.

Can't find a recommended product? Call the 800 number listed in Product Resources for the store nearest you.

You may not need surgery for ovarian cysts

Ovarian cysts are showing up in record numbers, especially in women with menstrual difficulties (see previous page). Endometriosis can also cause endometrial cysts on the ovaries. These are called "chocolate" cysts because they contain oxidized blood with the appearance of chocolate syrup. Endometrial cysts cause almost incapacitating pain in the uterus, lower back, and organs in the pelvic cavity prior to and during the menses. Painful intercourse, excessive bleeding, including the passing of large clots and shreds of tissue during the menses, and infertility are some of the other symptoms. Ovarian cysts are not cancerous and the need for surgery removal arises not because of malignancy, but because the pedicle of the cyst becomes twisted and gangrenous, or because of painful pressure on surrounding organs. Natural therapy focuses on normalizing hormone levels and correcting the unhealthy body chemistry. It has been quite successful, and offers you a choice before jumping into surgery. Give yourself from 4 to 6 months of healing on an herbal, hormone-balancing regimen for ovarian cysts.

Do you think you might have ovarian cysts? They are difficult to diagnose without a medical exam. Here are the signs to look for:

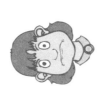

—acute or chronic pain in the fallopian tubes or ovaries and usually the inability to conceive.
—an erratic menstrual cycle with unfamiliar pain, unusual swelling and discomfort in the lower abdomen.
—often profuse uterine bleeding because of endometrial hyperplasia that results from unbalanced estrogen stimulation.
—painful intercourse, heel pain, and constantly swollen breasts.
—unusual abdominal gas, fever and coated tongue.
—Some women also experience excess hair growth due to an imbalance between estrogen, progesterone and testosterone levels, and unusual weight gain because of low thyroid activity.

What about Type 2 PAP smears?

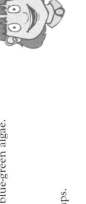

They can be a sign of ovarian cysts as well as cervical dysplasia and endometriosis. Herbal medicines can help stop these problems before they become full blown. An herbal program for a Type 2 PAP smear should be begun immediately upon learning about the smear results.

1: Take one herbal chlorophyll source drink with *Chlorella* or *Spirulina*, or Crystal Star ENERGY GREEN™ drink daily. Chlorophyll is so close to human plasma in its composition, it is a prime agent for immune enhancement, especially as it naturally occurs in medicinal plants, such as green grasses and blue-green algae.
2: Take four Benefin SHARK CARTILAGE capsules daily.
3: Take four PCO tablets daily, from grape seed oil or white pine about 400mg daily.
4: Take four 1000mg EVENING PRIMROSE OIL daily.
5: Take antibiotic, anti-inflammatory herbs like Crystal Star WOMAN'S BEST FRIEND™ caps 6 daily, or *goldenseal/echinacea/myrrh* caps.

Can you prevent ovarian cysts from returning?

Preventive measures call for balancing estrogen levels as naturally as possible. Look to phyto-hormone-containing herbal compounds first. Phytoestrogen-rich herbs can prevent a woman's own or other estrogens from attaching to cell receptors. Phytoestrogens have $1/400$ or less the estrogenic activity of human hormones. They can be used to "jam" the cellular receptor sites for estrogen, to prevent it from stimulating the cells. Soy foods, such as tofu and soy milk, buckwheat, citrus, and flax are also good sources of estrogen-blocking flavonoids.

As the cysts and pain reduce, and normalization begins, continue with a three month preventive program.
1: Take two capsules daily of a body balancing phytohormone-rich herbal combination like Crystal Star FEMALE HARMONY™.
2: Keep fat intake to 15% of your diet. Keep your diet 50% fresh fruits and vegetables. Have a green salad daily for chlorophyll and fiber. Avoid hard alcohol, tobacco and caffeine.
3: Take vitamin E 400IU daily, as an estrogen antagonist. Take B-complex 100mg daily to help the liver metabolize estrogen. Take *evening primrose* oil 1000mg. daily, as an EFA.
4: Take vitamin C 2000mg daily with bioflavonoids. Bioflavonoids have estrogen-like effects to help balance the body's estrogen-progesterone ratio.
5: Take an herbal iodine source twice daily, like Crystal Star IODINE-POTASSIUM caps. Eat iodine-rich foods, like sea greens, sea foods, fish, mushrooms, garlic, onions, watercress.
A hot seaweed bath using sea plants may be used for iodine therapy. The skin is the body's largest organ of ingestion. Iodine from sea vegetables is easily absorbed through the pores during a seaweed bath. Hypothyroidism is a matter of blocked iodine utilization. Some foods, called goitrogens, contain substances that hang up the body's use of iodine. Some of these are cabbage, turnips, peanuts, mustard, and pine nuts. They should be eaten cooked to inactivate the goitrogenic substances.

Can't find a recommended product? Call the 800 number listed in Product Resources for the store nearest you.

P.M.S.

Pre-Menstrual Syndrome, Cramps, Dysmenorrhea

PMS is by far the most common women's health complaint. It is estimated that a whopping 90% of all women between the ages of 20 and 50 experience some degree of PMS. For some women, it disrupts their whole lives. Over 150 symptoms have been documented - new ones are being added all the time. The hormone shift in estrogen/progesterone ratios during the menstrual cycle is the major factor in PMS symptoms. (Women report the most symptoms in the two week period before menstruation, when the ratios are the most elevated.) The modern women's lifestyle seems almost made to order for stress and imbalance. Our foods and our environment are full of chemicals that clearly affect delicate hormone balance. Natural therapies work well for most women because they address the full spectrum of factors involved, but they need time to work.

Diet & Superfood Therapy

Improve your diet first to control PMS. Women with severe PMS symptoms eat 60% more refined carbohydrates, 280% more sugars, 85% more dairy products, and 80% more sodium than women who don't get PMS.

–Nutritional therapy plan:

1–A low fat, vegetarian diet with regular sea food clearly diminishes symptoms. Add soy foods like miso, tempeh and tofu, and cruciferous veggies to reduce excess estrogen linked to PMS.

2–Try a mood swing, anti-constipation drink: 2 cups fresh peaches, chunked; 2 frozen bananas, chunked; 1 cup apple juice.

3–Keep the diet low in salt and sugar. Eat plenty of cultured foods, like yogurt and kefir for friendly flora. Eat brown rice often for B vitamins. Eat smaller meals often for blood glucose balance.

4–Avoid caffeine, red meat, sugars and saturated fat animal products. Eliminate dairy products during PMS days.

5–Drink 6 glasses of bottled water daily. Have fresh apple or carrot juice every day during PMS.

–Superfood therapy: (Choose one)
• Crystal Star SYSTEMS STRENGTH™ drink for iodine-balancing sea greens.
• Transitions EASY GREENS.
• Solgar WHEY TO GO protein.
• Red Star NUTRITIONAL YEAST.

Herb & Supplement Therapy

–Interceptive therapy plan: (Choose 2 or 3 recommendations)

1–Normalize hormone fluctuations: Crystal Star's 2-month program is highly successful: • FEMALE HARMONY™ capsules 2 daily each month, with EVENING PRIMROSE oil 6 daily the 1st month, 4 daily the 2nd month. Before your period, drink green tea or • Crystal Star GREEN TEA CLEANSER™ each morning as a mini detox. Take • TINKLE TEA™ or caps for 5 days prior to your period to relieve pre-period edema. Use • FEM SUPPORT™ extract for stress and to tonify; • PRO-EST BALANCE™ roll-on to prevent cramping and pain. During your period use ANTI-SPZ™ caps, 4 at a time; FLOW EASE™ tea, or CRAMP BARK COMBO™ extract as needed. (Apply • LYSINE/LICORICE™ gel for PMS mouth sores.)

2–Relieve estrogen build-up: • Crystal Star IODINE/POTASSIUM caps; • Herbal Magic FEMSTRUATION, Pioneer PMS FORMULA, or Futurebiotics HERBAL HARMONY; • Mood Maid PRO-MENO *wild yam cream*; • vitamin E 400 IU daily. Rebalance hormone levels with • *Burdock tea* 2 cups daily.

3–Relieve cramping: • *Chamomile tea*; • *Ginger tea* or • New Chapter DAILY GINGER extract drops in water; • Transitions PRO-GEST CREAM - rub on abdomen; • Homeopathic *Mag. Phos.*; • Calcium/magnesium to relax the uterus.

Pelvic applications for cramps: Ice packs to pelvic area; • *Ginger compresses* on pelvic area. • New Chapter ARNICA GINGER gel. • Aromatherapy compress: one drop each; oils of *chamomile, marjoram, juniper* and *helichrysum* in a quart of cool water.

4–Ease mood swings: • 5-HTP, 50mg; • Crystal Star DEPRESS-EX™ caps; • Now SAMe caps. • Nature's Secret ULTIMATE B; • GABA 2000mg daily; • Crystal Star RELAX CAPS™; • Vitamin C up to 5000mg daily to neutralize heavy metal toxins.

5–Relieve excessive flow: • *Bayberry capsules* 4 daily; • *Cranesbill/red raspberry tea*; • Vit. C 3000mg w. bioflavonoids or • *Bilberry* for bioflavonoids, • vitamin K 100mcg.

6–Relieve breast soreness and fluid retention: • Crystal Star TINKLE™ tea; • *Dandelion tea*; • *Ginkgo Biloba* or *Vitex extract*; • *Evening Primrose Oil* 3000mg daily.

7–Relieve lower back pain: • Barleans Omega-3 rich flax oil 3 daily; • quercetin 1000mg and bromelain 1500 mg.

Lifestyle Support Therapy

–Bodywork:

• Treat yourself to a good massage or shiatsu session before your period to release clogging mucous and fatty formations. Massage breasts and ovary areas to relax reproductive organs.

• Exercise is a must for female balance. Exercise improves the way your body assimilates and metabolizes nutrients, especially hormones. It changes food habits, and decreases craving for alcohol or tobacco. It boosts beta endorphin levels in the brain. It improves circulation to relieve congestion. It encourages regularity for rapid elimination of toxins.

• Stretching/relaxation exercises such as yoga with deep breathing and tai chi help. Acupuncture and reflexology are also effective.

• End your shower with a cool rinse to stimulate circulation and relieve lymph congestion.

• Meditate to banish PMS. Harvard studies show 57% improvement for women with PMS who meditate twice daily for 15-20 minutes. Be sparing with your schedule during premenstrual days. Give yourself some slack, take some time to read, listen to music and relax.

• Light is linked to PMS. Get out in the sunshine at least 20 minutes a day.

• Stop smoking and avoid second-hand smoke. Nicotine inhibits hormone function.

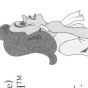

Common Symptoms: *Mood swings, tension, irritability, and depression; argumentative, aggressive behavior; water retention, bloating, and constipation; headaches; lower back pain; sore, swollen breasts; nausea; heavy cramping; low energy; food cravings for salt and sweets; acne and skin eruptions. Mouth sores with mood swings mean there is probably low progesterone or thyroid level.*

Common Causes: *Prostaglandin imbalance; estrogen excess or imbalance because of poor liver malfunction; thyroid insufficiency; lack of regular exercise; lack of B vitamins, mineral and protein deficiencies; endometriosis; too much salt, red meat, sugar and caffeine; stress and emotional tension. Switch from tampons to pads if you are very congested. Some research also shows that tampons may raise the risk of endometriosis.*

See next page, LIVER CLEANSING page 205 and HYPOGLYCEMIA DIET page 427 for more information.

Can't find a recommended product? Call the 800 number listed in Product Resources for the store nearest you.

What's really going on with PMS?

The intricacies of a woman's body are delicately tuned, and can become unbalanced or obstructed easily, causing pain, poor function, and lack of "oneness" that often results in physiological and emotional problems, especially during the menstrual cycle. PMS seems to be partially a consequence of the modern woman's emancipation. In times past, women were a silent, long-suffering lot, who felt that female disorders were just part of being a woman. Women were not out in the high profile workplace with men, and they could go to bed and suffer alone. In addition, our diets consisted of more whole and fresh foods than they do today. And our environment wasn't full of chemicals, nor our foods full of junk.

Today, up to 90% of premenopausal American women suffer from P.M.S. Symptoms like headaches, acne, food cravings, bloating, constipation or diarrhea, and mood swings can last anywhere from 2 days to as long as 2 weeks! Some women say their cycles make them feel out of control all month! While most women try to "grin and bear" the aggravation of PMS, 5 to 10% have symptoms serious enough for them to seek professional help. Low brain serotonin, excess estrogen, prostaglandin imbalance, and a diet loaded with sugar and caffeine are all implicated in PMS. But drugs and chemical medicines, standing as they do outside a woman's natural cycle, usually do not bring positive results for women. Indeed the medical establishment, with its highly focused "one-treatment-for-one-symptom" protocols has not been successful in addressing PMS. For example, contraceptive drugs, regularly given to reduce symptoms, make PMS worse for some women. Antidepressant drugs like Prozac, the new rage for PMS treatment, mean insomnia and shakiness for many patients. Natural treatment is much more gratifying. It emphasizes a highly nutritious diet, herbal tonifiers and balancers, and naturally-derived vitamins to encourage the body to provide its own balance for relief.

PMS symptoms tend to get worse for most women in their late thirties and beyond. They are often magnified after taking birth control pills, after pregnancy, and just before menopause because of hormone imbalances. But, with such a broad spectrum of symptoms affecting every system of the body, there is clearly no one cause and no one treatment. A holistic approach is far more beneficial, and self care allows a woman to tailor treatment to her own needs.

The Natural Keys To Controlling P.M.S.

Menstruation is a natural part of our lives. PMS is not. Women can take control of PMS naturally and effectively.

A woman can expect a natural therapy program for PMS to take at least two months, as the body works through both ovary cycles with nutritional support. The first month, there is noticeable decrease in PMS symptoms; the second month finds them dramatically reduced. Don't be discouraged if you need 6 months or more to gently coax your system into balance. Even after many of the symptoms are gone, continuing with the diet recommendations, and smaller doses of the herb and vitamin choices makes sense toward preventing the return of PMS.

—**Essential fatty acids balance prostaglandins.** Prostaglandins are vital hormone-type compounds that act as transient hormones, regulating body functions almost like an electrical current. Foods like ocean fish, olive oil, and herbs like • Evening Primrose, normalize prostaglandins by balancing your body's essential fatty acid supply. Too much saturated fat from meats and dairy products inhibits prostaglandin balance and proper hormone flow. Arachidonic acid in animal fats tends to deplete progesterone levels and strain estrogen/ progesterone ratios. • Evening Primrose oil 2000mg daily, especially along with a broad spectrum herbal balancing compound, shows excellent results for many women.

—**Love your liver to balance estrogen and progesterone levels:** Lower your fat intake and reduce dairy foods to help your liver do its job. A high-fat diet hampers liver function. Many dairy foods are a source of synthetic estrogen from hormones injected into cows. If the thyroid does not have enough iodine, insufficient thyroxine is produced and too contribute to estrogen stores. Focus on high quality vegetarian protein to improve estrogen metabolism. On PMS days, avoid dairy products altogether. A cup of green tea, or a green tea blend like • Crystal Star GREEN TEA CLEANSER™ each morning can go a long way toward relieving organ congestion and detoxifying the liver. Non-fat yogurt is a good choice because it also contains digestive lactobacillus. Reduce caffeine to one cup of coffee or less a day. Caffeine tends to deplete the liver and lowers B vitamin levels, contributing to anxiety, mood swings, and irritability. Fifteen to 30% of women with breast tenderness find relief by stopping caffeine use. A little wine is fine, but hard liquor should be avoided to control PMS. Strong alcohol compromises liver function by lowering B vitamin levels, reducing its ability to break down excess estrogen. Consider • MILK THISTLE SEED extract or a • dandelion tea daily.

—**Enhance your thyroid to reduce PMS:** Estrogen levels are controlled by thyroid balance. If the thyroid does not have enough iodine, insufficient thyroxine is produced and too much estrogen builds up. Herbs from the sea are an excellent choice for thyroid balance because they are rich in potassium and iodine. Two tablespoons daily in a soup or salad, or over rice, or six pieces of sushi a day, are a therapeutic dose. Or try • Crystal Star POTASSIUM/IODINE™ caps, • Bernard Jensen LIQUI-DULS, or • New Chapter OCEAN HERBS.

—**Phytohormone-rich herbal compounds help balance body estrogen levels:** Phyto-estrogens are remarkably similar to human hormones. They can help raise body estrogen levels that are too low by stimulating the body's own hormone production, or by attaching to estrogen receptor sites. Remarkably enough, plant estrogens can also lower estrogen levels that are too high. Even though they are only ¹/₄₀₀th or less of the strength of the body's own circulating estrogens, they are able to compete with human estrogens for receptor sites. When the weaker estrogens attach to receptors, the net overall effect is a lowering of the body's estrogen levels. Phytohormone-rich plants such as soybeans and wild yams, and hormone-rich herbs like black cohosh, panax ginseng, licorice root and dong quai, have a safety record of centuries. A broad-spectrum herbal combination like • Crystal Star FEMALE HARMONY™ tea or capsules or • Futurebiotics PMS FORTE may be taken over a long period of time, as a stabilizing resource for keeping the female system female, naturally. Natural, whole, wild yam creams also show success against PMS as transdermal sources of plant progesterone for estrogen/progesterone ratio balance.

Can't find a recommended product? Call the 800 number listed in Product Resources for the store nearest you.

Pain Control

Using Pain's Information for Better Healing

Pain is a mechanism our bodies use to draw attention to a problem. Pain signals us to consciously attend to its underlying cause. Pain is almost completely individual. Every person feels and reacts differently to pain. It can stem from large pain centers that control certain areas of the body, and from specific local areas that demand pinpoint action. There are different kinds of pain: physical, emotional, chronic, local, intermittent, throbbing, dull, spasmodic, sharp, shooting, etc. Pain can be your body's best friend. It alerts you when something is wrong and needs your attention. It identifies the location, severity, and type of problem, so that you can treat the right area. Pain can be your body's worst enemy. Continuous, constant pain saps strength and spirit, causes irrational acts and decisions, and alters personality. Pain killers allow you to think clearly, work and live, while addressing the cause of the problem. But pain killing drugs, while strong, afford relief by masking pain, or deadening certain body mechanisms so that they cannot function. Herbal pain managers have much broader actions than analgesic drugs. They are more subtle and work at a deeper level, to relax, soothe and calm the distressed area. Herbs let you use pain's information about your body, yet not be overwhelmed by the trauma to body and spirit. There are four basic pain centers in the body: 1: the cerebro-spinal area, (neural affliction, lower back pain and cramping); 2: the frontal lobe area, (earaches, toothaches, and headaches over the eyes); 3: the base of the brain (migraines, tension headaches); 4: the abdominal area, (menstrual cramping, digestive and elimination pain).

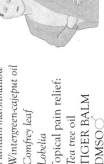

Diet & Superfood Therapy

—Nutritional therapy plan:

1—A vegetarian diet, low in fats, high in minerals is best for all kinds of pain - back and menstrual pain, migraines, arthritis, muscle aches.

2—Eat plenty of complex carbohydrates and vegetable proteins for strength: whole grains, broccoli, peas, brown rice, legumes, sea foods, etc.

3—Add anthocyanin foods like cherries and berries as anti-inflammatories (often up to 10 times better than aspirin).

4—Add high mineral foods to the diet for solid body blocks. Emphasize magnesium and calcium foods for muscle strength. Include bioflavonoid-rich foods, like fresh fruits and vegetables.

5—Have a vegetable drink (pg. 218), and a green leafy salad every day.

6—Avoid caffeine, salty and sugary foods that to avoid an overacid condition.

—Superfood therapy: (choose 1 or 2)

• Crystal Star SYSTEMS STRENGTH™.
• Crystal Star BIOFLAV, FIBER & C SUPPORT™ drink for bioflavonoids.
• Wakunaga KYO-GREEN.
• Sun Wellness CHLORELLA 1 pkt. daily.

Herb & Supplement Therapy

—Interceptive therapy plan: (Choose 2 to 3 recommendations)

1—Herbal pain management: • Kava Kava extract for stress relief; • Lobelia drops for cramps; • Valerian/Wild Lettuce extract, a sedative and anti-spasmodic; • White willow, anti-inflammatory/ analgesic; • Cramp bark, cramping and spasms; • Passionflowers or scullcap, gentle sedatives; • St. John's wort, nerve damage; • Wild yam and cat's claw for inflammation; rub on • Capsaicin cream for nerve pain; • Myrrh, an analgesic; • Calendula for injury pain; • Black cohosh and cayenne for neck pain.♀

Crystal Star herbal pain relievers work better than single herbs for pain: • Crystal Star ANTI-FLAM™ for inflammation; • BACK TO RELIEF™ caps for lower back/cerebro-spinal pain; • ASPIR-SOURCE™ for headache, tooth and face pain; • ANTI-SPZ™ caps, or • CRAMP BARK extract for spasms-muscle pain; • STRESSED-OUT™ tea or extract, and • RELAX™ caps for nerve pain; • AR EASE™ caps and tea for joint pain.

2—EFA's and enzymes reduce inflammation: Use proteolytic enzymes: • Enzymedica PURIFY; • bromelain 1500mg; • papain. Combine enzymes with • Quercetin 1000mg and • ascorbate vitamin C with bioflavs and rutin 5000mg daily. • MSM, 1000mg, or • Futurebiotics MSM or • MICROHYDRIN with MSM from Healthy House; • Evening Primrose Oil caps 3000mg daily; Earth's Bounty NONI caps.

3—Natural pain killers: • Glucosamine 1500mg-chondroitin 1200mg complex as needed; • DLPA 1000mg daily; • PCO's from grapeseed or white pine 100mg 3x daily. • Country Life LIGATEND capsules as needed daily; • Twin Lab GABA PLUS caps daily; • DLPA 1000mg as needed; • CoQ10 60mg 3x daily; • Magnesium for muscle cramping pain, 800mg daily. • Vitamin K 100mcg daily for chronic pain.

4—Magnet therapy for pain is effective: Try • MagnaLyfe products. • Spring Life POLARIZERS also show effective pain relief over a long period of time.

Lifestyle Support Therapy

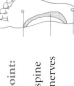

—Bodywork:

• Acupressure: pinch and massage webs between the thumb and index finger.
• Chiropractic adjustment, biofeedback, acupuncture, or Nature's Way massage therapy control pain.
• Pain-relieving compresses:
   Plantain-marshmallow
   Wintergreen-cajeput oil
   Comfrey leaf
   Lobelia
• Topical pain relief:
   Tea tree oil
   TIGER BALM
   DMSO♀
   Chinese WHITE FLOWER oil.
   Biochemics PAIN RELIEF lotion.
   Capsaicin creme, or Nature's Way CAYENNE PAIN RELIEVING ointment.
   B&T ARNI-FLORA homeopathic gel.

—Reflexology point:

   spine
   nerves

Common Symptoms: Sharp shooting twinges or a dull ache; muscle wasting; poor reflexes; numbness; soreness in the sensory nerves, particularly the lower back.

Common Causes: Poor posture; poor nutrition with lack of green vegetables and calcium-rich foods; an over-acid diet that eats away protective mucous membrane and nerve sheathing; poor muscle development; adrenal and pituitary gland exhaustion; recovery from disease, injury or surgery; flat feet; obesity; internal or external tumors or growths.

For many people natural therapies are superior to drugs and their side effects. See ARTHRITIS page 316 for more.

Can't find a recommended product? Call the 800 number listed in Product Resources for the store nearest you.

Parasite Infections

Intestinal Worms, Amoebic Dysentery, Giardia

Worm and parasite infestations can range from mild and hardly noticeable to serious and even life-threatening in a child. Worms are parasites that live and feed in the intestinal tract. Amoebas cause dysentery, acute, unremitting diarrhea, and are usually contracted from parasite infested water or food in third world or tropical countries. Other parasites seem to be able to move all over the body, including the brain, weakening the entire system. Nutritional therapy is a good choice for thread and pin worms, but is very slow in cases of heavy infestation. Short term conventional medical treatment is often more beneficial for masses of hook and tape worms and blood flukes. A strong immune system is the best defense for parasites, many of which have become drugresistant. Note: New research shows that liver flukes may be a cause of cancer.

Diet & Superfood Therapy

—Nutritional therapy plan:

1—Go on an apple juice fast and mono diet for 4 days. (One day for a child). Take 8 garlic caps daily during the fast and chew fresh papaya seeds mixed with honey. **On the 3rd day**, add papaya juice with 1 TB *wormwood* tea, and 1 TB molasses. **On the 4th day**, add 2 cups *senna/peppermint* tea with 1 TB castor oil, and eat raw pumpkin seeds every 4 hours. A high resistance diet must be followed to prevent recurrence. Eat lots of onions and garlic. Avoid all sweets, pasteurized milk and refined foods. Amaranth grain helps remove parasites. Eat a daily green salad. No junk foods!

2—**Herbal fast to expel tapeworms:** Mix 4-oz. cucumber juice with honey and water. Take only this mixture for 24 hours. Follow with 3 cups *senna/pumpkin seed* tea. Drink down at once.

3—**For amoebic dysentery:** Take carrot/beet/cucumber juice once a day for a week to clean the kidneys. Take a lemon juice/egg white drink each morning. Take 2 TBS epsom salts in a glass of water to purge the bowels. Then eat a high vegetable protein diet with cultured foods, such as yogurt.

—Superfood therapy: (Choose one or two)
• Mona's CHLORELLA -2 teasp. daily.
• AloeLife ALOE GOLD juice daily.
• Crystal Star CHO-LO-FIBER TONE™.

Herb & Supplement Therapy

—Interceptive therapy plan: (Choose 2 to 3 recommendations)

1—**Release and cleanse the parasites:** • Crystal Star VERMEX™, or Herbal Magic PARASITE KIT; • Arise & Shine WORM SQUIRM liquid or • Farmacopia IMMUN-NEEM capsules, 4 daily with 2 *garlic* capsules, after every meal for 2 weeks, and 4 cups *fennel* tea daily. (Or take garlic oil capsules in the morning. Refrain from eating or drinking until bowels have moved. Repeat for 3 days.) Then take • Creation's Garden PARASINE and keep intestines cleansed and flushed with • Crystal Star BITTERS & LEMON CLEANSE™ or Enzymedica PURIFY caps each morning. • Ayurvedic TRIKHATU tablets; • Uni-Key VERMA PLUS.

Anti-infectives: • Crystal Star ANTI-BIO™ caps 4 daily as a lymph flush; • *Black walnut hull* or • *Myrrh* extract; • *Una da gato* caps 6 daily; *Basil tea*; • *Cayenne/Garlic* capsules 8 daily; • *Witch hazel leaf* tea or • *dandelion* tea, 4 cups daily. • Uni-Key PARA-KEY or • East Park OLIVE LEAF EXTRACT, a potent paraciticide.

2—**Relax bowels to release worms:** • *Valerian* caps 4 daily; • *Slippery elm* tea 2 cups daily; • Magnesium 400-800mg daily.

3—**Remove putrefactive fecal matter and mucous build-up:** • Solaray GARLIC/BLACK WALNUT caps; • Nature's Way HERBAL PUMPKIN; • Ayurvedic Concepts BITTER MELON; • Homeopathic *Ipecac* as directed.

4—**Especially for giardia:** Nutribiotic GRAPEFRUIT SEED extract internally; BLACK WALNUT or MYRRH extract, 10 drops under the tongue every 4 hours, or *tea tree* oil, 4 drops in water 4x daily, or goldenseal extract in water for 10 days.

5—**Immune enhancers against parasites:** • Morada Research PARASITIC KILL #1 as directed; • Earth's Bounty OXY CAPS. • Floradix HERBAL IRON liquid for strength during healing; • Beta carotene 50,000IU daily as an anti-infective; • B-complex 50mg daily. ☺

6—**Probiotics are important to re-establish intestinal health:** • Prof. Nutrition Dr. DOPHILUS +FOS; • Alta Health CANGEST or • Natren TRINITY powder, 1/2 teasp. 3x daily.

Lifestyle Support Therapy

—Lifestyle risk factors you can avoid:
• Frequently eating raw or smoked fish.
• Eating prosciutto or homemade sausages.
• Kissing pets.
• Not properly washing hands after using the restroom.
• Drink only bottled water.

—Bodywork:
• Take *garlic* enemas daily during healing.
• Take a high colonic irrigation to clean the colon fast.
• Drink extra water at least 8 to 10 glasses a day to flush out dead parasites.
• Apply zinc oxide to opening of anus. Then take a warm sitz bath using 1 1/2 cups epsom salts per gallon of water. Repeat for 3 days. Worms will often expel into the sitz bath.
• For crabs and lice - apply around anus:
  Thyme oil, (dilute with a carrier oil) ☺
  Sassafras oil
  Tea tree oil
  Myrrh extract and tea tree oil mixed.

Common Symptoms: *Round worms: fever, intestinal cramping. Hookworms: anemia, abdominal pain, diarrhea, lethargy; Blood flukes: lesions on the lungs, hemorrhages under the skin - typical in AIDS cases; Protozoa, (amoebae): arthritis-like pain, leukemia-like symptoms, uncontrollable running of the bowels, pain, and dehydration. They coat the lining of the intestine to prevent nutrient absorption. Tapeworms: intestinal obstruction (even from a single worm). Giardia: diarrhea, weakness, weight loss, cramping, bloating and fever.*

Common Causes: *Low immune defenses; poor diet (low nutrition = low immunity); poor hygiene; fungal and yeast overgrowth conditions; infested, poorly cooked, or spoiled meat.*

See next page, DIVERTICULITIS, COLITIS AND CROHN'S DISEASE pages for more.

Can't find a recommended product? Call the 800 number listed in Product Resources for the store nearest you.

Parkinson's Disease

Central Nervous System Dysfunction

Parkinson's disease is a debilitating neurological disorder caused by dopamine depletion in the brain, characterized by a slowly spreading tremor, muscular weakness and body rigidity. Normal posture becomes stooped, walking becomes shambling, motion is trembling and lifespan is shortened. The victim, whose thinking processes often remain normal, feels frozen, unable to make any voluntary movements. Parkinson's affects men and women equally, usually between the ages of 50 and 75; about 500,000 cases are found in the U.S. It is thought that a neuro-toxin causes oxidative damage to the basal ganglia in the brain that controls muscle tension and movement. L-dopa, the drug of choice for Parkinson's, has hallucinatory side effects and causes leg cramps. Natural therapy helps re-establish normal biochemistry.

Diet & Superfood Therapy

—Nutritional therapy plan:

1—Go on a completely fresh foods diet for 3 days to cleanse and alkalize. Use organically grown foods when possible.

Then, follow a modified macrobiotic diet (pg. 333) for 3 to 6 months until condition improves. Eat smaller meals more frequently. Keep meat protein low. Eliminate alcohol, caffeine and refined sugars.

2—Go on short 24 hour juice fast (pg. 192) every two weeks during healing, with aloe vera juice each morning to accelerate toxin release. Drink unfluoridated bottled water.

3—Live cell therapy from green drinks and chlorella has been notably successful in reducing symptoms. Take vegetable drinks (pg. 218) at least twice a week, and/or Sun CHLORELLA once a day.

4—Make a nerve mix of lecithin granules, toasted wheat germ, almonds, sunseeds, sesame seeds and brewer's yeast and take 2 TBS. daily.

—Superfood therapy: (Choose one or two)

• Crystal Star SYSTEMS STRENGTH™ drink.
• AloeLife ALOE GOLD each morning.
• Now NUTRITIONAL YEAST (Red Star).
• Lewis Labs high potency LECITHIN and BREWER'S YEAST.
• Sun Wellness CHLORELLA for 2 months.
• Green Foods WHEAT GERM extract.

Herb & Supplement Therapy

—Interceptive therapy plan: (Choose 1 or 2 recommendations)

1—**Rebuild nerve strength to ease tremor:** • Crystal Star RELAX CAPS™ 2 as needed, and • STRESSED OUT™ extract to ease shakiness (help within an hour); • Twin Lab GABA plus, or • Country Life RELAXER caps. • Threonine fights spasticity.

2—**Nourish brain and nerves: Ginseng therapy is effective:** • Crystal Star MENTAL CLARITY™ caps 1 daily; • Beehive Botanicals GINSENG/ROYAL JELLY, 4 daily; • Imperial Elixir SIBERIAN GINSENG • Beehive Botanicals ROYAL JELLY/GINSENG capsules or drink. • Rainbow Light ADAPTO-GEM ginseng complex.

3—**Increase body's dopamine biosynthesis:** • NADH, 5-10mg in the morning; • Tyrosine 1000mg daily or • Enzymatic Therapy THYROID-TYROSINE daily; • Lysine 500mg daily; glutathione 100mg daily. (Parkinson's victims usually low.) • Country Life full spectrum AMINO MAX, or • Wakunaga NEURO-LOGIC daily.

4—**Enhance neurotransmitter activity:** • Phosphatidyl serine (PS) 100mg 3x daily; • Solaray EUROCALM to aid in serotonin formation, or • Metabolic Response Modifiers NEURO-MAX; **Niacin therapy:** 500mg 2x daily, with B-complex 100mg, extra B_6 500mg daily if not taking L-dopa (if taking L-Dopa, do not take vitamin B_6; it can block L-Dopa to the brain), and • B-12, sublingual 2500mcg every other day. • Magnesium 800mg daily. Creatine 3000mg daily for neuroprotection.

5—**Increase circulation:** • HAWTHORN extract as needed; • GINKGO BILOBA extract for leg cramps and tremor. • Solaray CAYENNE/GINSENG formula; • Golden Pride FORMULA ONE oral chelation with EDTA as directed.

6—**Critical EFA's for the nerves and brain:** • EVENING PRIMROSE OIL 46 daily; DHA 200mg daily or Neuromins DHA as directed; • Barleans lignan-rich flax oil 3x daily; • Nature's Secret ULTIMATE OIL.

6—**Help overcome Parkinson's depression:** DLPA 500-750mg.

7—**Antioxidants are critical in overcoming oxidative damage to the brain:** • PCO's from grapeseed or white pine 100mg 3x daily. (also helps side effects from Sinemet) • Vitamin E 1000IU 2x daily **WITH** • Vitamin C 5000mg daily with bioflavonoids; (as an ascorbic acid flush, pg. 234 for the initial 2 weeks).

Lifestyle Support Therapy

—Bodywork:

• Relaxation techniques like chiropractic treatment, massage therapy, acupuncture and acupressure have had notable success in reversing early Parkinson's.

• Regular aerobic exercise is critical for outlook and muscle health. A brisk walk every day is highly recommended.

• Use catnip enemas once a month during healing to encourage liver/kidney function.

• Avoid aluminum (cookware, deodorants with aluminum chloride, condiments with alum, etc.)

—Reflexology point:

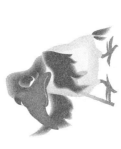

nerve points

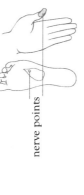

Common Symptoms: Signs begin with a slight tremor in the hands or slight dragging of the foot, pronounced with stress or fatigue; then voluntary movement becomes increasingly difficult; walking becomes stiff and slow; lethargic movement with speech difficult to follow, often with vision problems; the face becomes expressionless and drooling develops because of muscle rigidity; there is numbness and tingling in the hands and feet; depression (which can show dramatic improvement with supplementation) often sets in.

Common Causes: Poor diet of chemicalized foods; hyperthyroidism; aluminum/heavy metal toxicity; pesticide residues; overuse of some psychotropic drugs; allergy reaction to sugary foods and raw meat.

Call (800) 457-6676 for the latest Parkinson's information and practitioner referral. See Personal Ailment Analysis Section page 529.

Can't find a recommended product? Call the 800 number listed in Product Resources for the store nearest you.

Phlebitis

Thrombo-Phlebitis, Embolism, Arterial Blood Clot

Phlebitis is vein inflammation, usually in the legs. It is a relatively common condition. An **embolism** is the obstruction of a blood vessel by a foreign substance or blood clot. **Thrombophlebitis** is the existence of a blood clot within the vascular system. **Deep vein thrombosis** is life-threatening because the clot can break free and occlude a vessel or lodge in the lung. Get medical help immediately!

Diet & Superfood Therapy

—Nutritional therapy plan:

1—Take one glass of each every other day:
Black cherry juice
Fresh carrot juice
A veggie drink (pg. 218), or see below.
2—Have a daily cup of green tea.
3—Have a leafy green salad every day.
4—Eat plenty of onions, garlic and other high sulphur foods. Have an onion/garlic broth at least 2-3x week.
5—Drink 6 glasses of bottled water daily.
6—Make a circulation mix of lecithin granules and nutritional yeast and take 2 TBS daily.
7—Avoid all starchy, fried and fatty foods. Avoid refined sugars, caffeine and hard liquor.

—Superfood therapy: (Choose one or two)
• Crystal Star BIOFLAV., FIBER & C SUPPORT™ drink for venous integrity.
• Sun Wellness CHLORELLA 1 packet daily.
• Wakunaga KYO-GREEN.
• Aloe Life ALOE FIBER MATE drink.
• Crystal Star ENERGY GREEN™ drink.
• Green Foods WHEAT GERM extract.
• Solgar WHEY TO GO protein drink to lower cholesterol.

Herb & Supplement Therapy

—Interceptive therapy plan: (Choose 2 or more recommendations)

1—**Help normalize blood composition and circulation:** • Crystal Star HEARTSEASE-CIRCU-CLEANSE™ tea with butcher's broom or • Butcher's broom capsules or tea for 1 month. • Crystal Star HEARTSEASE/HAWTHORN caps or HAWTHORN extract 2-4x daily for 3 months to normalize circulation. • Natural Balance CARDIO-TMG converts homocysteine to methionine. • Glucosamine 1500mg and chondroitin 1200mg capsules for anti-thrombogenic and anti-coagulant activity. • Enzymedica PURIFY, protease, a powerful blood purifier. • Reishi mushroom extract capsules or • Crystal Star GINSENG/REISHI extract to rebuild immunity.

Niacin therapy: 500mg 3x daily, with • Chromium picolinate 200mcg♀ or Solaray CHROMIACIN daily♂.

2—**Take down inflammation:** • Bromelain 1500mg daily with Quercetin 1000mg as an anti-inflammatory and clot inhibitor for fragile veins. • Crystal Star GREEN TEA CLEANSER™ each morning on rising with ANTI-FLAM™ caps 4 as needed;
• EVENING PRIMROSE oil 4-6 daily; • Barleans lignan-rich flax oil 3x daily;

3—**Strengthen veins and capillaries with flavonoids:** • Crystal Star VARI-VAIN™ caps and roll-on with grapeseed PCO's and horse chestnut, or • PCO's from grapeseed or white pine 100mg 3x daily to strengthen arterial system. • GINKGO BILOBA or BILBERRY extract capsules 6 daily. • Solaray CENTELLA-VEIN 3x daily.

Apply effective herbal compresses right to the legs: • St. John's wort and St. John's wort oil; • Yarrow flowers and • Calendula flowers.

4—**Cleanse infection:** • Nutricology GERMANIUM 150mg daily (highly effective); • USNEA extract, or • Crystal Star BIO-VIT™ extract 4x daily; • ECHINACEA extract combats bacterial infection, always present in phlebitis; • Ascorbate vitamin C crystals with bioflavs and rutin, ¼ teasp. daily to bowel tolerance for 2 weeks. • Biotec CELL GUARD 8 daily to scavenge free radicals.

5—**Help intermittent claudication** (atherosclerosis affecting the legs): • Pacific BioLogic ADAPTRIN (Ayurvedic Padma 28) as directed. • Vitamin E therapy, 800IU; • GINKGO BILOBA extract drops as needed. Rapid improvement often noted.

Lifestyle Support Therapy

• Elevate legs whenever possible. No prolonged sitting. Consciously stretch and walk frequently during the day.
• Believe it or not, even too tight underwear or jeans can constrict circulation in the abdomen and groin where deep-vein phlebitis originates. Keep your weight down to relieve pressure on circulatory system instead of squeezing into tight clothes.
• Take a brisk half hour walk daily.
• Avoid smoking and secondary smoke. It constricts blood vessels and restricts oxygen use.
• Avoid chemical anti-coagulants and oral contraceptives unless absolutely necessary.
• Take alternating hot and cold sitz baths, or apply alternating hot and cold ginger/cayenne compresses to stimulate leg blood circulation.

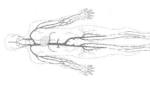

—Effective applications:
B&T ARNICA
CALIFLORA gel
Earth's Bounty O₂ spray

—Effective compresses:

Plantain
Witch hazel
Fresh comfrey leaf
Alcohol compresses

Common Symptoms: Swelling, inflammation; redness and aching in the legs; fever with blood clots in the legs; pain and tenderness along course of a vein; swelling below obstruction.
Common Causes: Clogged and toxic bloodstream from excess saturated fats, especially from too much red meat and fried food; inactivity, lack of daily exercise, and sedentary lifestyle; poor circulation from constipation, obesity or weak heart; oral contraceptive side effect; prolonged emotional stress. Watch out for too tight underwear.

See the HEALTHY HEART DIET page 413 for more information

Can't find a recommended product? Call the 800 number listed in Product Resources for the store nearest you.

Pneumonia

Bacterial Pneumonia, Viral Pneumonia, Pleurisy

Pneumonias and pleurisy are inflammatory lung diseases caused by a wide array of viruses and other pathogenic organisms. **Bacterial pneumonia,** *contracted most often by children, is caused by staph, strep or pneumo-bacilli; it responds to antibiotics, both medical and herbal.* **Viral pneumonia** *is an acute systemic disease caused by a variety of virulent viruses which does not respond to antibiotics. Herbal antivirals have shown some success.* **Pleurisy** *is an inflammation of the pleura membrane surrounding the lungs, and often accompanies pneumonia. Pneumonias drastically weaken the immune system. Typically, it can take 2 to 3 months to recover strength and up to 2 years to be able to resist a cold or flu without falling victim to another bout of pneumonia.*

Diet & Superfood Therapy

—Nutritional therapy plan:

1—Go on a mucous-cleansing liquid diet for 1 to 3 days during the first and acute stages. (pg. 196). Drink plenty of fruit juices, herb teas and bottled water to thin mucous. Avoid alcohol.

2—Take a hot lemon and honey drink with water each morning, or a cup of green tea, or an aloe vera juice drink. Or have a fresh carrot juice, a potassium broth (pg. 215) or see below.

3—Then follow a largely fresh foods, cleansing diet for 1-2 weeks.

4—Then eat a diet high in vegetable proteins, low in meat, dairy and animal fats, to allow lungs to heal easily. Add cultured foods: Rejuvenative Foods VEGGIE DELITE, yogurt and kefir.

5—As an emergency measure, take fresh grated horseradish root in a spoon with lemon juice. Hang over a sink immediately to expel large quantities of mucous.

—Superfood therapy: (Choose one or two)
• Crystal Star SYSTEMS STRENGTH™.
• Nature's Life PRO GREENS 96.
• AloeLife ALOE GOLD drink.
• Crystal Star BIOFLAV., FIBER & C SUPPORT™ drink daily for 6 weeks of healing.
• Sun Wellness Chlorella WAKASA GOLD.
• Klamath BLUE GREEN SUPREME.
• New Moon GINGER WONDER syrup. ☜

Herb & Supplement Therapy

—Interceptive therapy plan: (Choose 2 to 3 recommendations)

1—**Control the infection:** • Olive leaf extract capsules 2 to 6 daily; • Oregano oil 3 capsules, 3x daily; • MICROHYDRIN, available at Healthy House; • Crystal Star ANTI-BIO™ caps or extract (or ANTI-VI™ extract or tea for viral pneumonia) 6x daily to flush toxins, with • FIRST AID CAPS™ 3x daily to sweat out mucous.

—**After crisis has passed,** take • Crystal Star RESPR™ caps and tea with • ANTI-HST™ extract drops, to encourage oxygen uptake. Add • Crystal Star ANTI-SPZ™ caps 6 daily, or • *cayenne/ginger/goldenseal* caps 6 daily,♀ or *garlic* 8 caps daily,♂ or *mullein/lobelia* extract drops in water ☜ as broncho-dilating anti-spasmodics. **Boost circulation for better oxygen uptake:** • *Hawthorn* or *Ginkgo Biloba* extract. **Diuretics help reduce lung fluid:** • *Uva Ursi/Cornsilk* tea; • *Senna/Dandelion.*

1—**Expectorants help remove excess mucous from the lungs:** • *Pleurisy* root tea or • *slippery elm* tea; • Crystal Star X-PEC™ tea with extra ginger pinches.

1—**Take powerful antioxidants:** • Carnitine 1000mg 3x daily for 1 month; NAC (N-acetyl-cysteine) 500mg 3x daily; • CoQ-10, 60mg 4x daily; • Nutricology germanium 150mg 2 daily. • Beta carotene 150,000IU with extra lycopene 5-10mg; • PCO's from grapeseed or white pine 100mg 3 daily.

1—**Protect your lungs against further infection:** • Vitamin C/antioxidant therapy: • Ascorbate vitamin C crystals with bioflavonoids and rutin, ¹/₄ teasp. every hour to bowel tolerance, daily for 2 weeks; then every 2 hours for 2 weeks; then 3000mg daily for a month; or use • EXTA-CEE available at Healthy House for 100% availability. • Zinc picolinate 4x daily, or • Source Naturals OPTI-ZINC 30mg daily; • Vitamin E 400IU 2x daily; • Crystal Star GINSENG/LICORICE ELIXIR™ as a demulcent and adaptogen.

1—**For pneumonia with pleurisy** (burning lungs, difficulty taking a deep breath, great fatigue even on a short walk): • Turmeric (*curcumin*), anti-inflammatory; • Earth's Bounty O₂ CAPS as directed and rub O₂ SPRAY rubbed on the chest twice daily; • Thyme extract drops in water as a decongestant. ☜

Lifestyle Support Therapy

—Lifestyle measures:

• Do not risk your health if you experience major difficulty in breathing. Short term heroic medicine may be necessary. Newer broad spectrum drugs can sometimes give your body a "breather" from the infection trauma and are less harmful to normal body functions than most primary antibiotics. Ask your physician.

• Get plenty of rest. Do conscious diaphragmatic breathing, especially during recovery. Breathe in, pushing abdomen out, then from chest to completely fill upper and lower lungs.

• Apply a hot *cayenne/ginger* poultice: Mix powders - ¹/₂ teasp. *cayenne,* 1 TB *lobelia,* 3 TBS *slippery elm,* 2 TBS *ginger* and enough water to make a paste. Leave on chest 1 hour.

• Apply a mustard plaster to chest to stimulate lungs and draw out poisons: Mix 1 TB mustard powder, 1 egg, 3 TBS flour and water to make a paste. Leave on until skin turns pink.

• Take an oxygen bath. Use 1 to 2 cups 3% H₂O₂ to a tub of water. Soak 20 minutes.

• Overheating therapy is effective, especially for viral pneumonia to quell virus replication. See page 225 for home method.

• Take hot and cold showers to stimulate lung circulation (pg. 228). Then use chest or back percussion with a cupped hand front and back to loosen matter.

Common Symptoms: *Inflamed lungs and chest pain; aggravated flu and cold symptoms, worsening after 5 days; swollen lymph glands; difficult breathing; heavy coughing and expectoration; back, muscle and body aches; chills and high fever; sore throat; inability to "get over it"; fluid in lymph and lungs; great fatigue which remains for six to eight weeks even after recovery.*

Common Causes: *Low immunity from poor nutrition; gum disease; a preceding respiratory infection from a virus or bacteria; clogged lymph nodes; chemical sensitivity or allergy, especially to pesticides and herbicides; body stress and fatigue, especially from a long day outdoors in winter.*

See LUNG DISEASE page 446 for more information.

Can't find a recommended product? Call the 800 number listed in Product Resources for the store nearest you.

Poisoning, Environmental Illness

Heavy Metals, Radiation, Chemical Contaminants, Gulf War Syndrome

Heavy metal poisoning is becoming a major problem of modern society. There seems to be no way to avoid toxic exposure. Chemical pollutants and toxic byproducts affect every facet of our lives, from our water and food supply to the workplace and our homes. Their toxic effects are serious... allergies, birth defects, even cancer. The main effect of an unhealthy environment is on immune response, especially in the way that our filtering organs, the liver and kidneys, are impacted. Periodic detoxification needs to be a part of life so that the body can use its own cleansing mechanisms to maintain healthy immunity. A hair analysis is very helpful in determining nutrient deficiencies caused by environmental toxins.

Diet & Superfood Therapy

—Nutritional therapy plan:

1—Do not go on an all-liquid diet when trying to release heavy metals or chemicals from the body. They enter the bloodstream too fast and heavily for the body to handle, and can poison you even more.

2—Go on a seven day brown rice and vegetable juice diet (pg. 197) to start releasing poisons from the body. Have a glass of fresh carrot juice, a potassium broth (pg. 215), and miso soup daily.

3—Green drinks are a key as detoxifiers and blood builders, (page 218) or see below.

4—Eat a diet full of leafy greens, and other mineral-rich foods, like sea greens. Eat organically grown foods as much as possible. Avoid canned foods. Drink only bottled or distilled water.

5—Make a mix of $1/4$ cup each: wheat germ, molasses, lecithin granules and brewer's yeast, and take 2 TBS daily.

6—Avoid fried foods, red meats, pasteurized dairy products, fatty and sugary foods. Avoid caffeine - it inhibits liver filtering.

—Superfood therapy: (Choose one or two)
- Crystal Star ENERGY GREEN™.
- Green Foods GREEN MAGMA.
- Aloe Answers ALOE FORCE juice with herbs.
- Future Biotics VITAL K drink.
- Sun Wellness CHLORELLA drink, especially against radiation.

Herb & Supplement Therapy

Avoid commercial antacids - they interfere with enzyme production, and the ability of the body to carry off heavy metals. Use plant enzymes instead.

—Interceptive therapy plan: (Choose 2 or more recommendations)

1—Release contaminants from the body: • Crystal Star HEAVY METAL CLEANSE™ or • DETOX™ caps for 2-3 months. • For lead poisoning in children: take vitamin C with • CLEANSING & PURIFYING™ tea daily; or • Crystal Star FIRST AID™ caps - to release toxins through sweat; also source of white pine PCOs, a preventive formula taken at 2 daily over 3 months. • Golden Pride FORMULA ONE, oral chelation with EDTA daily. For radiation poisoning: vitamin C powder with bioflavonoids $1/2$ teasp. every hour to bowel tolerance as a tissue flush.

2—Enhance and stimulate liver activity: • Lipoic Acid 600mg daily for 2 months. • Crystal Star LIV-ALIVE™ caps with • MILK THISTLE SEED extract; • Dandelion extract; • Crystal Star LIV-ALIVE™ tea or • Enzymatic Therapy LIVATOX caps; • EVENING PRIMROSE oil caps 4 daily; • Biostrath LIQUID YEAST.

3—Boost thyroid balance and function: Crystal Star IODINE THERAPY™ extract or IODINE/POTASSIUM™ caps 2-6 daily, or Kelp 8-10 tabs daily, especially against suspected radiation poisoning. Solaray ALFA-JUICE caps; J.R.E. IOSOL.

4—Build strong immune defenses with herbal immune enhancers: • Astragalus extract; • Propolis extract or lozenges; • Garlic 6-8 caps daily; • Siberian ginseng extract caps; • Spirulina 2 teasp daily, or • Spirulina MICROCLUSTERS, available at Healthy House (especially for radiation/chemotherapy toxins); • Mona's CHLORELLA 2 teasp. daily for chemical toxins.

5—Protect yourself with powerful antioxidants: • Carnitine 1000mg 3x daily for 1 month; • NAC (N-acetyl-cysteine) 500mg 3x daily; • CoQ-10, 60mg 4x daily; • Nutricology GERMANIUM 150mg daily. • Beta carotene 150,000IU with extra lycopene 5-10mg; • PCO's from grapeseed or white pine 100mg 3 daily; • Vitamin E 400IU with selenium 200mcg; • Glutathione 100mg daily; • MICROHYDRIN available at Healthy House; • Source Naturals OPTI-ZINC 30mg daily, and CHEM-DEFENSE; • Enzymatic Therapy THYMUPLEX. • Biotec CELL GUARD 8 daily.

Lifestyle Support Therapy

—Lifestyle measures:

• Protect against radiation syndromes: avoid foods labeled irradiated or electronically pasteurized.

• Use an inside air filter to remove toxins in the air. Use vinegar, baking soda and salt as cleansers if you are very sensitive.

• Protect yourself from EMF fields: avoid non-filtered computer screens, cellular phones, electric blankets, microwave ovens. (Don't use plastic wrap in the microwave, Its heat can drive the molecules into the food.) Look at EMF info on appliances.

• Avoid smoking and secondary smoke, pesticides (sprinkle pepper on anthills instead) and herbicides, phosphorus fertilizers, fluorescent lights, aluminum cookware and deodorants.

• Get plenty of tissue oxygen. Take a walk every day, breathing deeply. Do deep breathing exercises on rising, and in the evening on retiring to clear the lungs and respiratory system.

• Earth's Bounty O_2 SPRAY on soles of feet every 2 days to keep tissue oxygen high.

• Take a hot seaweed bath, or a sweating bath, such as Crystal Star POUNDS OFF BATH™. Use a dry skin brush before and after the bath to remove toxins coming out on the skin.

• Spring Life POLARIZERS have notable success against environmental pollutants.

Common Symptoms: Signs you may be chemically toxic: you may wake up each morning just feeling lousy for no reason; you smell things far better than most people. Perfumes and strong cleansers bother you. You don't tolerate alcohol well or certain medication; even some vitamins make you feel worse. You feel worse in certain stores. Your reaction time when driving is noticeably poorer in city traffic. You may even experience schizophrenic-like, psychotic behavior; memory loss and senility; infertility and impotency; insomnia; small black spots along gum line; bad breath and body odor.
Common Causes: Buildup of pollutants and toxic chemicals; insecticides; amalgamated dental fillings; fluoridated water; hair dyes; aluminum cookware and deodorants; smoke, smog; zinc depletion.

See page 44 on neutralizing the effects of chemotherapy and radiation.

Can't find a recommended product? Call the 800 number listed in Product Resources for the store nearest you.

Poisoning, Food

E. Coli, Salmonella, Botulism, Arsenic

Each year, more than 2 million Americans report cases of food poisoning. The actual number may be far higher since food poisoning signs mimic flu and diarrhea symptoms. Even with government inspections, better packaging, refrigeration and chemical preservatives, food poisoning is on the rise (mostly in children and the elderly). It's one of the places scientists point to for the fast development of antibiotic-resistant disease strains. **Botulism** is poisoning by a micro-organism similar to that causing tetanus. (Do not give honey to infants for fear of botulism.) **Salmonella** is widespread (a new strain DT104 is now responsible for nearly 10% of food poisoning cases) coming from bacteria found in hormone-injected beef and poultry. **E coli,** a bacterial infection that attacks the kidneys sickens as many as 20,000 American annually and kills several hundred.

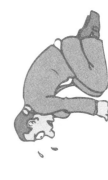

Diet & Superfood Therapy

—Nutritional therapy plan:

1—Take $^1/_2$ cup olive oil very slowly through a straw to remove poison from the stomach or a glass of warm water with 1 teasp. baking soda.

2—Take no milk, juice, alcohol or vinegar until poisons have moved from the stomach.

3—Eat high fiber foods, citrus fruits, wheat germ, whole grains, green and yellow vegetables. These foods act as protectors against pesticides and poisons in food.

—Toxin neutralizing foods:

1-2 heads of iceberg lettuce
Bamboo shoots
Strong black or green tea
Burnt toast
2 raw eggs
Lemon water
Apple pectin caps

—Superfood therapy: (Choose one or two)

• George's high sulphur ALOE VERA JUICE morning and evening for a week after poisoning.

• Take a green drink every 4 hours to normalize body chemistry: Crystal Star ENERGY GREEN™ or Mona's CHLORELLA 1 teasp. in water.

• Balance your intestinal structure with Solgar WHEY TO GO protein drink.

• Future Biotic VITAL K, 2 teasp. daily.

Herb & Supplement Therapy

—Interceptive therapy plan: (Choose 2 or more recommendations)

1—If you think you have food poisoning: Take •Activated charcoal tabs to absorb poison; 3 to 5 every 15 minutes, or •Solaray CLAY & HERBS caps or bentonite clay powder as directed to absorb poisons. Take •vitamin C powder, $^1/_2$ teasp. every $^1/_2$ hour (or vitamin C caps 500mg every hour) to bowel tolerance to flush and alkalize the tissues. •Niacin therapy helps sweat out poisons; 250-500mg every hour until improvement is felt (about 3-4 capsules).

2—Normalize your stomach and intestines: Take •Crystal Star CLEANSING & PURIFYING™ tea 3 times daily, with •Sun Wellness CHLORELLA tabs, 10 every 4 hours to neutralize toxins and normalize body chemistry. Use •Nelson Bach RESCUE REMEDY for rebalance. Take •Garlic caps 2 with each meal. For salmonella: take •Guarana water extract. For e. coli and salmonella: take •bee pollen granules. For arsenic poisoning: take •Yellow dock-nettles tea.

3—Detoxify your liver: •MILK THISTLE SEED extract is primary, (even used in Europe to fight liver disease caused by Amanita, death cap mushrooms). •Alpha Lipoic Acid 300-600mg daily; •Enzymatic Therapy LIVA-TOX caps 3 daily or •SAMe 800mg daily with •Crystal Star LIV-ALIVE™ caps 6 daily and tea, 2 cups daily; •Crystal Star BITTERS & LEMON CLEANSE™ extract each morning.

4—Sea greens are primary poison protectors: •Crystal Star SYSTEMS STRENGTH™ caps 8 daily; Kelp tabs 12 daily. Nature's Path TRACE-MIN-LYTE with sea greens, 4 daily. Toxin neutralizing teas: Plantain, Scullcap, Wormwood tea.

5—Probiotics produce fatty acids and acidify the bowel to inhibit pathogenic micro-organisms, including salmonella: •Prof. Nutrition DOCTOR DOPHILUS + FOS, or •Natren BIFIDO FACTORS. Take with •Crystal Star ANTI-BIO™ extract for extra stomach cleansing anti-infective bitters.

6—Protective supplements against food poisons: •Vitamin E 400IU with selenium 200mcg; •Vitamin C, 3000mg daily; •Glutathione 100mg daily; •mixed carotenes PHYCOTENE MICROCLUSTERS available from Healthy House; •Biotec CELL GUARD 6 daily; •Nature's Life CAL-MAG LIQUID, phos. free.

Lifestyle Support Therapy

—Bodywork:

• Discard all bulging food cans.

• Use an emetic of Ipecac, or strong lobelia tea with $^1/_4$ - $^1/_2$ teasp. cayenne to vomit up poisons and empty the stomach. Follow with white oak tincture to normalize the stomach.

• Use a coffee or catnip enema to flush the bowel and stimulate liver detox function.

• Sweat out pesticides and chemical poisons from food in a long, low heat sauna. Or use home overheating therapy is effective. See page 225 in this book for correct technique.

• Spring Life POLARIZERS have notable success against food-borne pollutants.

• Use American Biologics DIOXY-CHLOR or NutriBiotic GRAPEFRUIT SEED extract in water as directed to decontaminate produce or Healthy Harvest VEGETABLE RINSE.

Common Symptoms: Salmonella infects the intestines with the classic symptoms of diarrhea, nausea, cramps and vomiting. Many people get cold sweats after eating; severe abdominal pain and flatulence; severe headache; chills and fever; rashed skin. Botulism signs are weak, limp muscles 12 to 36 hours after eating, double vision, dry mouth, speech difficulty, vomiting, stomach cramps, even respiratory failure can result.
Common Causes: Harmful bacteria in food; pesticides and fungicide residues in food; additives and preservatives in food; sulfites and MSG reactions; food allergy reaction; breathing noxious fumes; lack of proper cleaning of cutting boards and food preparation areas in both restaurants and homes.

Call the POISON CONTROL CENTER Hotline, 800-764-7661, if you need emergency information.

Can't find a recommended product? Call the 800 number listed in Product Resources for the store nearest you.

Poison Oak
Poison Ivy, Sumac

Urushiol, the toxic oleoresin responsible for the poison oak/ivy reaction, is one of the most potent external toxins on earth! Its toxicity can survive for 100 years after the plant is dead. Irritating resins are carried in smoke when the plant is burned. Even sap that has been diluted 50 million times can induce toxicity. **One quarter ounce of urushiol has the potential to affect everyone on earth.** Poison oak, poison ivy and sumac all react with the body's immune system T-lymphocytes to produce the itchy rash. Over 2 million people a year get a poison oak or ivy reaction; more than 60% of American are sensitive to it. Sensitivity during childhood is highest, but once you lose your sensitivity, an immunity sets in and remains for life.

Diet & Superfood Therapy

—Nutritional therapy plan:

1—Apply cider vinegar, denatured alcohol, or a cornstarch paste to blisters to control itching and neutralize acid poisons.

2—Follow a fresh foods diet during acute blistering to cleanse systemic poisons out of the bloodstream. No junk or fried foods.

3—Apply oatmeal paste to rash areas to neutralize toxins. ☞

4—Take several veggie green drinks during acute phase (pg. 218 or see below).

—Superfood therapy: (Choose one or two)

• Alkalize your body with ALOE VERA juice and apply aloe vera gel.

• Green Foods GREEN ESSENCE.

• Mona's CHLORELLA.

Herb & Supplement Therapy

—Interceptive therapy plan: (Choose 2 or more recommendations)

1—**Stop the itch:** •Crystal Star P.O. #1 and P.O. #2 capsules alternately as directed to calm the itch and help neutralize the systemic poison. (Excellent results.) Apply •Crystal Star ANTI-BIO™ gel as needed. •Homeopathic *Rhus Tox.*

1—**Reduce swelling, promote healing:** •Nutribiotic GRAPEFRUIT SEED extract caps as directed, or SKIN SPRAY as needed (sometimes works overnight);

•Enzymedica PURIFY, protease breakes down poison oak proteinaceous matter.

•Emulsified vitamin A & E oil; •Nature's Pharmacy GOLDEN MYRE-CAL lotion with *goldenseal*; or apply •a paste of honey and *goldenseal* powder; cover with a bandage. •Vitamin E oil decreases healing time.

1—**Calm the histamine reaction and soothe the nerve endings:** •Crystal Star ANTI-HST™ capsules 6 daily until clear, to help curb the histamine allergy reaction. •Vitamin C therapy is a natural antihistamine: take vitamin C crystals, ¼ teasp. every hour to bowel tolerance, until itching lessens, then reduce to ¼ teasp. 4x daily until clear. Take •magnesium 400mg 2x daily. Take •zinc 30mg daily.

1—**Strengthen the adrenal glands against sensitivity:** •Crystal Star ADRN™ extract or ADR-ACTIVE™ caps 2x daily. •Hylands homeopathic *Poison Oak* tabs to build resistance protection.

—Effective topical healers:

•*Jewelweed* tea, a specific, apply locally, take internally.

•*Tea tree oil,* which sloughs off old, affected tissue, and leaves healthy tissue intact; •*Comfrey/aloe salve;* •B &T CALIFLORA gel; •*Calendula* ointment or *calendula-goldenseal* ointment, or *Goldenseal* solution in water; •*Witch hazel;* •Bioforce ECHINACEA cream; •Fresh *plantain* leaves, crush and rub on affected areas; •*Sassafras* tea; •*Black walnut* tincture, apply locally, take internally; •*Oregon grape root, yerba santa or yellow dock root washes;* •Nature's Life CAL-MAG liquid.

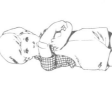

Lifestyle Support Therapy

—Bodywork:

• *Artemesia* (mugwort) grows in the same vicinity as poison oak, and appears to be a naturally-occurring protective plant against it. Rub fresh mugwort leaves on any exposed skin before you go out in the woods or brush.

• Cover all exposed skin before going out.

• Wash within 30 minutes of contact in cold water with a non-oil soap. (Oil soaps spread the urushiol.)

• Swim in the ocean if possible for effective, neutralizing therapy.

—Effective bath additions:

1 cup Epsom salts with 4 TBS green clay added and a few drops of peppermint oil
   Apple cider vinegar
   Baking soda or cornstarch
   Oatmeal

—Effective applications: wash affected area in cold water first.

   Aloe vera gel
   Earth's Bounty O₂ spray
   Chinese WHITE FLOWER OIL ♀
   Witch hazel
   Rubbing alcohol ♂
   Wet black tea bags

Common Symptoms: Allergic reactions to the allergen in poison oak range from an annoying itch to a life-threatening condition. Itching blisters on the skin ooze, erupt and spread the systemic plant poisons. There may be throat swelling, cramps and diarrhea. People with sun-sensitive skin are most susceptible. Allergic reaction takes place within 72 hours after contact.

Common Causes: The resin responsible for the allergic skin reaction must touch the skin or clothing of the person to cause the reaction. Resins can even be carried in smoke of the burning plant, so don't burn it or try to uproot it. Kill poison oak and ivy with a systemic herbicide for best results. The blisters don't contain the oleoresin; you can't "pass it on."

See SKIN, ITCHING, page 500 for more information.

Can't find a recommended product? Call the 800 number listed in Product Resources for the store nearest you.

Prostate Enlargement

Benign Prostatic Hypertrophy, Prostate Inflammation

A large number of men suffer from prostate enlargement problems. Disorders usually begin after age 35 and by age fifty, over 25 percent of all men have an enlarged prostate. By 70, it's over 50% and by age 80, over 80% percent. Lifestyle causes, such as obesity, and hormonal changes, such as increased estrogen levels and altered testosterone levels, are at the root of the problem. Drugs like PROSCAR and PROSGUARD report side effects of decreased potency and libido - in some cases it is stifled entirely. But men can help themselves easily and naturally to manage prostate problems without the highly adverse side effects (often as bad as the prostate problem itself), and limited success of the drug approach. Watchwords should be: less fat, more fiber, stay fit. Avoid chemical antihistamines. Overuse impairs liver and prostate function.

Diet & Superfood Therapy

–Nutritional therapy plan:

1–Take lemon juice and water every morning for two weeks to cleanse sediment; then cider vinegar and honey in water daily for a month to prevent sediment recurrence. Add green tea daily.

2–Follow a fresh foods, low fat, high fiber diet for 1 week, with plenty of green salads, fresh fruits, juices and steamed vegetables.

3–Add whole grains, soy foods, sea foods and sea greens (2 TBS daily) for EFA's for 3 weeks.

4–Make a prostate health mix of lecithin granules, toasted wheat germ, pumpkin seeds, oat bran, brewer's yeast, sesame seeds, and crumbled dry sea greens; take 4 TBS daily over rice or miso soup.

5–Drink 6 glasses of water or cleansing fluids daily. Especially add 2 glasses of cranberry juice. Have a vegetable drink (pg. 218) every day during healing.

6–Avoid red meats, caffeine, hard liquor, carbonated drinks, especially beer, during healing. Limit spicy foods that irritate your bladder. Avoid tobacco, all fried, fatty and refined foods forever.

–Superfood therapy: (Choose one or two)

• Crystal Star SYSTEMS STRENGTH™ drink for iodine and potassium nutrients.

• Nutricology PRO GREENS with EFA's.

• Y.S. ROYAL JELLY/GINSENG drink.

• Wadell Creek fresh organic BEE POLLEN.

• Sun Wellness CHLORELLA 1 pkt. daily.

Herb & Supplement Therapy

–Interceptive therapy plan: (Choose 2 or more recommendations)

1–**A highly successful anti-inflammatory herbal program:** •Crystal Star PROX™ caps 6 daily, (or extract for 1 month), then 4 daily for 1 month; •Crystal Star RE-LAX™ caps to ease urination; •EVENING PRIMROSE oil 4000mg daily for 1 month, then 2-4 daily for 1 month with •bee pollen caps 2 daily, and •ANTI-BIO™ caps 4 daily for 1 month. •Nature's Plus Bromelain 1500mg for fast healing.
Follow-up: •Crystal Star MALE PERFORMANCE™ for regeneration, •IODINE/POTASSIUM™ caps, or kelp tabs 10 daily for prevention, •GINSENG/LICORICE ELIXIR™ to guard against prostate cancer. Take •vitamin E 400IU; or white oak bark tea, or •Melatonin 3mg at night to decrease size of prostate.

2–**Flush sediment and congestive residues:** •Vitamin C crystals, $\frac{1}{2}$ teasp. every hour to bowel tolerance for 2 weeks, then $\frac{1}{2}$ teasp. 4x daily for 2 weeks, then 3000mg daily for 1 month. •Glycine 1000mg for sediment control; •Enzymedica PURIFY to dissolve lesions.. Use •Uva Ursi tea, •Una da Gato caps; •Nettles extract or •horsetail-nettles tea to reduce prostate swelling rapidly. •GABA to relieve frequent urination and fight infection. •Vitamin E 800IU daily.

3–**Soothe the pain with EFA's:** •Evening Primrose oil 4000mg daily; •Barleans lignan-rich flax oil 3x daily; •Crystal Star ANTI-FLAM™ caps 2 as needed.

4–**Flavonoids are protective:** (help keep cancer-causing hormones from latching onto cells) •PCO's from white pine or grapeseed 100mg 3x daily; •Bilberry extract 2x daily, or •vitamin C 5000mg with protective bioflavs. daily.

1–**Rid the body of pathogens:** •Echinacea/goldenseal extract drops 4x daily; •Garlic caps 8 daily, or •Pau d'arco tea 3 cups daily; •mixed carotenes 100,000IU.

1–**Follow a two-month prevention program:** •Zinc 100mg daily for 1 month, then 50mg daily for 1 month; •B-6, 200mg daily; •Glutamine 1000mg daily;

1–**For prostatitis:** A saw palmetto/pygeum formula, like •Solaray PYGEUM or PROSTA-GEUM, with •Barleans lignan-rich flax oil 3x daily; •Bromelain 1500mg daily, •zinc 50mg 2x daily, •vitamin E 800IU daily, •Crystal Star CHLORELLA-GINSENG extract to guard against prostate cancer.

Lifestyle Support Therapy

Some studies show that a man should think twice before having a vasectomy, because of the increased risk of prostate cancer among vasectomized men. As sperm builds up in the sealed-off vas deferens, the body reabsorbs it and sometimes tries to mount an autoimmune response to its own tissue. In addition, the testes are a powerful focal point of the life force of a man. When something interferes with the movement of sperm, energy flow is blocked, eventually resulting in stagnation and degeneration. A vasectomy can also result in liver blockage that leads to prostate inflammation, leg cramps, abdominal pain and irritability.

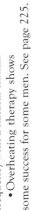

–Bodywork:

• Sexual intercourse during prostatitis irritates the prostate and delays recovery. After recovery, sex life should be normal in frequency with a natural climax.

• Overheating therapy shows some success for some men. See page 225.

• Use chamomile tea enemas (pg. 539) once a week during healing as an acid cleanser. Or take warm chamomile sitz baths for 20 minutes at a time morning and evening.

• Apply ice packs to reduce pain.
• A brisk daily walk helps.
• Warm baths soften and relax.

See PROSTATE CANCER page 336 for more information.

Common Symptoms: With BPH, the disease is basically the symptoms - see below. Inflamed, swollen, infected prostate gland (under the scrotum and testes); frequent, painful desire to urinate with reduced flow of urine; incontinence in severe cases; fever; lower back and leg pains; impotence, loss of libido, and/or painful ejaculation; reduced immune response; unusual insomnia and fatigue.

Common Causes: A high fat diet puts a man at greatest risk, as does a poor diet with too little fiber and too many over-acid, or spicy foods; too much alcohol and caffeine; EFA and prostaglandin depletion; exhausted lymph system from too many over-the-counter antihistamines; internal congestion and poor circulation; lack of exercise; zinc deficiency; venereal disease.

Can't find a recommended product? Call the 800 number listed in Product Resources for the store nearest you.

Rheumatic Fever

Severe Systemic Inflammation, Roseola

Rheumatic fever is a serious inflammatory condition following a strep infection. It normally affects small children between 3 and 12 years old. The severe inflammation of full blown rheumatic fever can affect the heart or brain; arthritis-like pain and stiffness often settle in the joints. Rheumatic fever can be prevented if the strep virus is killed within ten to twelve days of infection, because it will not have become virulent enough in that time to overwhelm the body's immune defenses. However, once the disease has been contracted, recurrence is common, and treatment must be maintained for months, even years so that rheumatic heart disease does not develop. Natural treatment focuses on rebuilding immune response. **Roseola**, often called scarlet fever, is a similar young child's infectious disease accompanied by high fever, nausea and a similar skin rash.

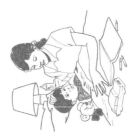

Diet & Superfood Therapy

—Nutritional therapy plan:

1—Adhere to a fresh juice and liquid diet for the first bedridden stages of healing to reduce body work and strain.

2—Take potassium broth or essence, (page 215), and apple/alfalfa sprout juice daily during the acute period.

3—Take Red Star NUTRITIONAL YEAST or MISO broths, or miso soup with snipped sea greens daily for B vitamins and strength.

4—Then eat fresh and mildly cooked foods, including plenty of seafoods and vegetable protein from whole grains, tofu, sprouts, etc. Eat only small meals. Drink bottled water.

5—Avoid all sugars, salty, refined foods during healing. Keep fats low. No fried foods, caffeine or carbonated drinks during healing.

—Use superfoods to rebuild immunity:

• Crystal Star SYSTEM STRENGTH™ for iodine, potassium and broad spectrum nutrient support. (Excellent results.)
• Sun Wellness CHLORELLA 1 pkt. daily.
• Wakunaga KYO-GREEN drink.
• Pines MIGHTY GREENS drink.
• Amazake RICE DRINK for healing protein.
• AloeLife ALOE GOLD drink.

Herb & Supplement Therapy

—Interceptive therapy plan: (Choose 2 to 3 recommendations)

1—Overcome the infection: • Crystal Star ANTI-BIO™ caps 4 daily for at least a month; • Garlic tabs 6 daily; • Bene-Fin SHARK CARTILAGE caps 2 daily as an antiviral; • Colloidal silver as directed; ⊛ • Beta carotene 50-100,000IU daily.

2—Reduce inflammation: • Evening primrose oil caps 4 daily; • Lobelia or dandelion extract; elderberry tea 2 cups daily; or • Herbs, Etc. ECHINACEA TRIPLE SOURCE.

3—Ease arthritis symptoms: • Crystal Star AR-EASE™ tea or • ANTI-FLAM™ extract drops for pain and stiffness; • America's Finest BOSWELLIN; • High potency royal jelly 2 teasp. daily; Take • wintergreen leaf/white willow tea internally.

4—Normalize cardiopulmonary activity: • CoQ₁₀ 60mg 2x daily; • Crystal Star HEARTSEASE/HAWTHORN™ caps, or • HAWTHORN extract drops in water; ⊛ or Heart Foods HAWTHORN PLUS to normalize circulation.

5—Strengthen against recurrence: • Crystal Star GINSENG/CHLORELLA extract drops in water or • GINSENG 6 SUPER TEA™. Effective antioxidants include: • Vitamin E 4800IU daily; • PCOs from grapeseed or white pine 50mg 3x daily; ⊛ • Germanium 30mg 3x daily; ⊛ • Solaray B₁₂ 2000mcg daily during healing. • Rainforest Remedies STRONG RESISTANCE.

6—Flush the glands, especially the lymphatic system: • Ascorbate vitamin C crystals with bioflavonoids, ¼ teasp. every hour in juice, or until stool turns soupy during acute periods, then reduce dosage to 3-5000mg daily.

7—Probiotics are important to replace friendly flora after lengthy antibiotic courses. • Prof. Nutrition DR. DOPHILUS ¼ teasp. in water 4x daily. • Enzymatic Therapy THYMU-PLEX caps for immune stimulation.

—Homeopathic treatment is very effective in the initial phase. See a homeopathic physician. Homeopathy may be used even if chemical medications are already being taken. Remember to reduce doses for children.

Lifestyle Support Therapy

—Bodywork:

• Plenty of bed rest is a key. Treatment may take months, or even years.
• Yoga and mild muscle-toning exercises, and/or massage therapy during confinement (which can last for several weeks) will prevent loss and atrophy of body strength.
• Take a catnip enema once a week to remove infection and reduce fever. ⊛
• Do not use aspirin as an anti-inflammatory. ⊛
• Notify dentist of rheumatic heart disorder if having an extraction or anesthesia for any reason.
• Apply a tea tree oil rub on sore joints. ⊛
• Apply wintergreen oil compresses to chest.

Common Symptoms: After an initial moderate fever, there is chronic extreme weakness; heart weakness may result; there is often a skin rash; poor circulation, shortness of breath and a continuing sore throat. The most common symptom of full-blown rheumatic fever is arthritis. Roseola symptoms include a high fever for 3 or 4 days, and sometimes convulsions. A rash often covers the chest, arms and tummy.

Common Causes: Inflammation of the main circulatory system causing holes in the heart ventricles; allergic reaction; low immunity, especially in children; often accompanied by acute viral disease; toxic exposure to harmful chemicals, environmental pollutants, or radiation.

See INFECTIONS page 434 for more information.

Can't find a recommended product? Call the 800 number listed in Product Resources for the store nearest you.

R 484

Schizophrenia

Psychosis, Mental Illness, Tardive Dyskinesia

Schizophrenia is a psychosis with severe perception disorder, characterized by hallucinations, delusions, extreme paranoia, and disturbed thought content. Personal relationships are abnormal, work is almost impossible. The schizophrenic often withdraws emotionally and socially. Anti-psychotic (neuro-leptic) drugs may do more harm than good. Tardive dyskinesia is a side effect disorder, with slow, rhythmical, involuntary movements, caused exclusively by neuroleptic drugs used to treat schizophrenia and psychosis. It is bizarre in that the symptoms themselves are similar to a psychosis. Over 70% of the patients taking antipsychotic drugs develop this grim disorder which almost totally isolates them socially. Natural therapies have been successful treating schizophrenia and in reversing TD. Avoid yohimbe in all herbal supplements - it may aggravate schizophrenia.

Diet & Superfood Therapy

—Nutritional therapy plan:

1–A diet for hypoglycemia has been very successful in controlling schizophrenia. Improving body chemistry is a key:

2–Start with a short 3-day juice cleansing diet to normalize blood composition (pg. 191). Minimize fruit juices if hypoglycemia is involved.

3–Then, eat largely fresh foods for the remainder of the week. Eat niacin-rich foods like broccoli, carrots, potatoes and corn.

4–Gradually add vegetable proteins, gluten-free grains (like brown rice, millet and amaranth), fish (like salmon, tuna, halibut), and sunflower seeds. Turkey is a good, calming tryptophan source.

5–Eliminate all refined sugars, caffeine, red meats, food with additives and preserved foods. Especially eliminate arginine foods like peanut butter and nuts. They can be toxic to a schizophrenic's brain.

—Effective superfoods: (choose 1 or 2)

• Crystal Star CHO-LO-FIBER TONE™ with organic flax seed oil for EFA's.
• Unipro PERFECT PROTEIN drink.
• Pines MIGHTY GREENS.
• Nutricology PRO GREENS with EFA's.
• Beehive Botanicals GINSENG/ROYAL JELLY.
• Crystal Star SYSTEMS STRENGTH™ with EFA's.
• Lewis Labs LECITHIN and BREWER'S YEAST.

Herb & Supplement Therapy

—Interceptive therapy plan: (Choose 2 to 3 recommendations)

1–**Enhance neurotransmitter activity:** • Crystal Star DEPRESS-EX™ caps 6-8 daily; • NADH, 10mg in the morning; • EGG YOLK LECITHIN 3x daily; • Country Life PHOS. CHOLINE COMPLEX softgels; • Wakunaga NEURO-LOGIC as needed, or • Phosphatidyl serine (PS) 100mg 3 daily for 3 months; • High potency royal jelly 50,000mg or more, 2 teasp. daily. • Magnesium 800mg 2x daily.

2–**For better cerebral circulation:** • Ginkgo Biloba extract; • Siberian Ginseng extract; • Crystal Star MENTAL CLARITY™ caps - 1 daily; • zinc 50mg 2 daily.

Niacin - vitamin C therapy: 1-3000mg daily or use • Solaray CHROMIACIN daily. (A baby aspirin before taking removes niacin flush). Take with • vitamin C powder with bioflavonoids and rutin, $1/4$ teasp. every 2 waking hours to bowel tolerance for the first month of healing for withdrawal from tranquilizers and drugs.

3–**EFA's lift mood, nourish the brain:** • DHA 200mg, 2 daily; • Source Naturals FOCUS DHA ,3 daily; or • Neuromins DHA. • Evening Primrose Oil 4000mg daily; • Nature's Secret ULTIMATE OIL; • Crystal Star IODINE SOURCE™ drops, • Biotec PACIFIC SEA PLASMA, or kelp tabs 8 daily for ocean EFA's.

4–**Nerve stability against depression and anxiety:** • Crystal Star RELAX CAPS™ for nerve rehabilitation; • St. John's wort extract or • Country Life MOOD FACTORS for depression; • Gotu kola to restore nerves; • Valerian, scullcap or VALERIAN-WILD LETTUCE extract to calm. • Crystal Star FEEL GREAT™ caps or tea for balance.

5–**Balance body chemistry with amino acid therapy:** • Glutamine 1000mg 3x daily; • Tyrosine 1000mg 2x daily; • Glycine 1000mg 2x daily; • GABA 500mg 2x daily; • Country Life MAX AMINO caps w. B_6 • Crystal Star ANTI-HST™ to balance body histamine levels; • Enzymatic Therapy THYROID-TYROSINE.

6–**B vitamins are key:** • Stress B-complex 150mg; extra B_6 500mg and folic acid 800mcg daily. • Real Life Research TOTAL B; • Premier GERMANIUM w. DMG.

—For tardive dyskinesia: • Evening Primrose oil 4000mg daily; • Crystal Star WITH-DRAWAL SUPPORT™ caps. •CoQ-10 200mg daily; • Niacin 500mg 3x daily (flush-free OK); • Stress B-complex 200mg; •Vitamin E 800IU with selenium 200mcg.

Lifestyle Support Therapy

New research shows that the herb rauwolfia serpentina (an Ayurvedic anti-psychotic remedy), works almost as well as reserpine, the drug for schizophrenia derived from it, with far fewer side effects like tardive dyskinesia.

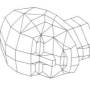
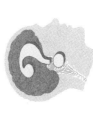

—Bodywork:

• Get some exercise every day, especially running, walking or jogging. The oxygen will do wonders for your head.

• Take ocean walks for sea minerals; a visit to a mineral-rich spring and spa are also effective.

• Regular massage therapy and spinal adjustment have had some success.

• Try to stick to an interesting daily schedule so you don't drift and lose the days to inertia.

• Avoid all pleasure drugs, and as many prescription drugs as possible. For many people, permanent brain change and psychosis can result.

Common Symptoms: Severe mental depression; lethargy; emotional swings, often to violent actions; delusions and hallucinations; detachment from reality; the brain is without thought much of the time. What remains is scattered and chaotic like random shotgun fire. Tardive dyskinesia: social withdrawal, slow, shuffling gait, lethargy; grimaces and outbursts.

Common Causes: Develops from both genetic and environmental factors - hypoglycemia or diabetes; severe gluten or dairy allergies; chemical toxicity; too high copper levels; nutrient deficiency from too many junk foods and refined sugars; prescription or pleasure drug abuse; vitamin B-12 or iodine deficiency; elevated histamine levels; hypothyroidism; gland imbalance or a gene fluke, especially in the nicotine receptor.

See the HYPOGLYCEMIA DIET suggestions page 427 for more information.

Can't find a recommended product? Call the 800 number listed in Product Resources for the store nearest you.

Sciatica

Neuritis of the Sciatic Nerve

Sciatica is neuritis of the sciatic nerve which runs from the low back across the buttocks, into the leg, calf and foot. Sciatic pain is caused by a compression of the sciatic nerve, characterized by sharp, radiating pain running down the buttocks and the back of the thighs. The inflammation is arthritic in nature - extremely sensitive to weather change and to the touch.

Diet & Superfood Therapy

—Nutritional therapy plan:

1—A mineral rich diet is important: Take a potassium broth (pg. 215) every other day for a month to rebuild nerve health. Add iodine foods like sea greens, sea foods, shellfish.

2—Have a leafy green salad every day. Take a little white wine with dinner to relieve tension and nerve trauma.

3—Eat calcium and magnesium rich foods, such as green vegetables, sea greens, spinach, tofu, whole grains, molasses, nuts and seeds.

4—Take a good natural protein drink, such as one from page 276, or see below.

5—Drink bottled mineral water, 6-8 glasses daily.

6—Avoid caffeine foods, refined sugars, especially chocolate.

—Effective superfoods: (choose 1 or 2)
• Crystal Star ENERGY GREEN™ drink.
• Wakunaga KYO-GREEN one packet daily for nerve rebuilding.
• Unipro PERFECT PROTEIN drink.
• Pines MIGHTY GREENS.
• Nutricology PRO GREENS with EFA's.
• Beehive Botanicals GINSENG-ROYAL JELLY drink.
• Crystal Star SYSTEMS STRENGTH™ drink for electrolyte minerals.
• Future Biotics VITAL K , 3 teasp. daily.

Herb & Supplement Therapy

—Interceptive therapy plan: (Choose a recommendation in each category)

1—**Help repair and restore nerves:** • Crystal Star RELAX CAPS™ as needed for rebuilding nerve sheath, 4 daily; • Crystal Star IODINE/POTASSIUM caps 2 daily for nerve restoration. • BILBERRY extract for tissue-toning flavonoids or • Ascorbate C or Ester C with bioflavonoids and rutin, 5000mg daily, to rebuild connective tissue. • Country Life LIGATEND as needed. ♂

2—**Relieve nerve spasms:** • GINKGO BILOBA extract for facial neuralgia; • Crystal Star BACK TO RELIEF™ or ANTI-SPZ™ caps for spasmodic pain; • DLPA 1000mg as needed for pain. • Homeopathic- Hylands *Calms* or *Calms Forte* tabs. ♀

3—**Reduce nerve inflammation:** • Solaray Curcumin (turmeric extract) or • Crystal Star ANTI-FLAM™ caps 4 daily to take down inflammation; • *Devil's claw* extract drops in water 2x daily; • Rainbow Light CALCIUM PLUS caps with high magnesium, 4 daily; • Quercetin 1000mg; • Bromelain 1500mg daily or • Enzymedica PURIFY for protease. • Homeopathic *Aranea Diadema* - radiating pain or • *Mag. Phos.* for spasmodic pain, or • *Hypericum* if nerve injury.

4—**Thyroid therapy is important:** • Crystal Star POTASSIUM-IODINE™ caps or IODINE SOURCE extract; or Nature's Path TRACE-LYTE with sea greens 4 daily.

5—**Effective herbal nerve tonics:** • *Lobelia* extract drops; • *Passionflower* or *scullcap* tea; • *valerian/wild lettuce* extract, a powerful nerve relaxant; Hylands *Nerve Tonic.* • Niacin therapy: 500-1500mg daily to stimulate circulation. ♂

6—**Essential fatty acids nourish the nervous system:** • *Evening Primrose* oil 4000mg daily; • Omega-3 oils like flax and fish oils 3x daily • Phosphatidyl Choline (PC55); • Twin Lab EGG YOLK LECITHIN 3x daily; Vitamin E 400IU daily.

7—**Neural nutrients for long term restoration:** • Country Life sublingual B-12, 2500mcg daily; and • Stress B-complex 100mg with extra B$_6$ 250mg; • Anabol Naturals AMINO BALANCE; • Taurine 500mg daily; *Black cohosh* extract drops. ♀

8—**Topical nerve help applications:** Capsaicin creme, or • Nature's Way CAYENNE PAIN RELIEVER ointment; • America's Finest BOSWELLIN CREAM; • *Cayenne/ginger* compress; a cold compress of chamomile or lavender essential oils.

Lifestyle Support Therapy

—Lifestyle measures:
• Treatment should focus on removing the pressure on the nerve - via chiropractic or massage therapy treatments.
• Apply ice packs or wet heat to relieve pain.
• Take hot epsom salts baths to relax nerve.
• Apply alternating hot and cold, (finishing with cold), or hops/lobelia compresses to stimulate circulation.
• Effective topical applications:
TIGER BALM
Chinese WHITE FLOWER oil
B&T TRIFLORA analgesic gel
St. John's wort oil
Mix *wintergreen, cajeput, rosemary* oils. Massage into area.
• Gentle morning and evening stretches, and daily yoga exercises are effective.

—Reflexology point:

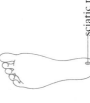

sciatic nerve

Common Symptoms: Severe sometimes debilitating pain in the leg along the course of the sciatic nerve - felt at the back of the thigh, running down the inside of the leg; lower back pain; muscle weakness and wasting; reduced reflex activity.

Common Causes: Sciatic nerve compression resulting from a ruptured disc or arthritis, or an improper buttock injection; poor posture and muscle tone; poor bone/cartilage development; exhausted pituitary and adrenal glands; menopause symptoms; obesity; lack of exercise; high heels; protein and calcium depletion; not enough green vegetables; flat feet.

See BACK PAIN page 321 AND NEURITIS/NEURALGIA page 467 for more information.

Can't find a recommended product? Call the 800 number listed in Product Resources for the store nearest you.

Seasonal Affective Disorder

S.A.D., Winter Blues, Pineal Gland Imbalance

S.A.D. makes people sad. Wintertime means depression for 35 million Americans. Over 80% of the people affected are women (researchers think women produce less serotonin a mood enhancing brain chemical than men). Work productivity noticeably declines, and relationships suffer. S.A.D. begins to manifest itself after the autumn equinox as sunlight hours lessen. The disorder is latitudinal : in Mexico, Florida and Texas, only 1.4% of the population suffers from acute S.A.D. In the Northeast U.S., up to 50% of the population has noticeable winter mood shifts. The unusual appetite and low energy aspects of S.A.D. show our ancient ties to seasonal rhythms, psychological well-being and nutritional factors as they affect our nervous system and behavior.

Diet & Superfood Therapy

—Nutritional therapy plan:

1—Conscious diet improvement is the main key to reducing SAD symptoms. A diet for hypoglycemia has been effective.

2—Make sure you are following a balanced diet with natural foods, rich in complex carbohydrates, (to shift the distribution of amino acids in the blood), and low in fats and sugars.

3—Include B-vitamin and mineral-rich foods, such as brown rice and fresh vegetables. Whole grains, legumes and soy products will help control sugar cravings. Take Red Star NUTRITIONAL YEAST as a source of B vitamins and chromium.

4—Eat more vitamin D-rich foods: eggs, fish, seafoods and sea greens (2 TBS chopped dry sea greens or 6 pieces of sushi a week) for absorbable vitamin D and beta carotene.

—Effective superfoods: (choose 1 or 2)

• Beehive Botanicals or Y.S. GINSENG/ROYAL JELLY.
• Rainbow Light HAWAIIAN SPIRULINA, with B-complex 100mg to balance sugar use.
• Crystal Star SYSTEMS STRENGTH™ drink for electrolyte minerals.
• Biostrath original LIQUID YEAST.

Herb & Supplement Therapy

—Interceptive therapy plan: (Choose 2 or more recommendations)

1—**Relieve depression:** •SAMe 400mg daily; •Crystal Star DEPRESS-EX™ extract with •St. John's wort through winter; or •Allergy Research Group PROZA-PLEX caps; •HAWTHORN extract, or MICROHYDRIN available at Healthy House elevate mood. •Rainbow Light CALCIUM PLUS with high magnesium; •Stress B-complex 100mg daily; •Natural Labs Deva Flower DEPRESSION-GLOOM.

2—**Neurotransmitter normalizers:** •Crystal Star RELAX CAPS™ for nerve rehabilitation; •Country Life MOOD FACTORS for depression; •Gotu kola to restore nerves and overcome mental dullness. Rub •Rosemary essential oil on the temples.

3—**Vitamin D is a key:** Take natural •vitamin D 400 to 1000IU daily all during the winter; or •American Biologics EMULSIFIED A & D 2x daily; or •Twin Labs ALLERGY D, or •Solaray A & D 25,000/1,000IU.

4—**Pineal/pituitary stimulation is a key:** •Glutamine 100mg daily in water; •Crystal Star MEDITATION™ tea; •Parsley/sage tea; •GINKGO BILOBA extract 3x daily; or •Metab. Resp. GINKGO BILOBA caps.

5—**Thyroid health is critical:** •Crystal Star IODINE SOURCE™ extract or •IODINE-POTASSIUM™ caps 2x daily, or •Nature's Path TRACE-MIN-LYTE with sea greens, or •Kelp tabs 8 daily, with cayenne 3 daily; •Solaray ALFA JUICE caps, or •alfalfa tabs 10 daily; •Enzymatic Therapy ENZODINE or •THYROID/TYROSINE COMPLEX; or •Tyrosine 500mg with L-lysine 500mg 2x daily.

6—**EFA's help normalize the body's electrical connections, nourish the brain:** •EVENING PRIMROSE oil 4 daily; •Nature's Secret ULTIMATE OIL; •Omega-3 flax oil 3x daily. •Royal jelly 2 teasp. daily.

7—**Ginsengs have key nutrients to control sugar cravings:** •Crystal Star GIN-SENG-LICORICE ELIXIR™ or FEEL GREAT™ caps or tea; or Imperial Elixir GINSENG-ROYAL JELLY; •Ginseng/gotu kola capsules. Take with •Chromium picolinate 200mcg daily to control sugar levels and normalize brain chemistry.

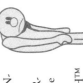

Lifestyle Support Therapy

•Light therapy is a widely accepted treatment for S.A.D., more effective than antidepressant drugs. Indoor or fluorescent light is not effective. Only full-spectrum light shuts off melatonin secretion and reduces SAD symptoms. Exposure for 2 to 3 hours of full-spectrum light offers a 35% reduction in symptoms in 1 week.

•Light boxes have not been approved by the FDA but have shown definite effectiveness. Depression typically begins to lift about a week after "photo-therapy" begin. Consider Environmental Lighting Concepts OTT-LITE (800-842-8848). You'll probably need to use light therapy from mid-fall until spring.

•Going south for a winter vacation helps relieve symptoms temporarily, and helps sufferers function more normally for 3 to 4 weeks after they return. People who use this therapy say they can get through a whole winter with three or four southern trips.

•Get an outdoor exercise walk every day, especially running, walking or jogging. An active lifestyle, especially in winter sports like skiing, means you'll be less disturbed by winter.

•Spend regular time in a greenhouse during the winter if possible. Light does wonders for your pineal gland. Plant oxygen does wonders for your head.

Signs and Symptoms: • Do you oversleep frequently or struggle to get out of bed, even when you get enough sleep? • Do feel lethargic or have poor concentration throughout the day? • Do you suffer from more eyestrain or headaches during the winter? • Do normally simple tasks seem overwhelming or difficult to complete in the winter? • Are you more anxious about things than normal? • Do you have unusually strong cravings for sweets or heavy starches? • Do you gain weight (up to 10-15 lbs.) in the winter, even when you think your diet has stayed the same? • Do feel depressed or low-energy in the winter? Do short periods of sunlight noticeably lift your spirits? • Do you experience a "summer high" starting around June where you feel elated and full of energy?

Common Causes: Not enough full spectrum light during winter months; a result of the pineal gland not receiving enough light stimulation to stop secreting melatonin; hormone and body rhythm imbalance.

Can't find a recommended product? Call the 800 number listed in Product Resources for the store nearest you.

Sexuality
Lack of Normal Sexual Libido

We tend to think our modern era is the only one beset with libido-lowering elements. Certainly there is no question that our nutrient-poor, high fat diets, overuse of drugs and stimulants, and rushed, high-pressured lifestyles lead to low energy and lack of time for love. But the reality is that humanity in every era has felt the need for help in the sexual and reproductive area. After all, this part of our lives is at the most basic, elemental center of our being. The recommendations presented on this page are revitalizers for sexual energy as well as effective natural treatments for the major sexual problems affecting men and women today like impotence and low libido. I recommend looking at herbs first. Herbs have a centuries-old reputation for effectiveness in working with the body toward sexual health and enhancement.

Diet & Superfood Therapy

—**Nutritional therapy plan:** Hormone-disrupting chemicals in commercial produce and hormone-injected meats and dairy foods can wreak havoc on sexual health. Junky, chemicalized foods are part of a body not feeling "up to it." Avoid red meats; keep fats, salt and sugar low.

—**For women:** 1) Increase soy foods for a mild, natural estrogenic effect. 2) Eat foods rich in EFA's - sea foods, sea greens, leafy greens, whole grains, nuts, legumes and seeds. 3) Eat vitamin E foods for more body moisture - soy foods, wheat germ, seeds, nuts and vegetable oils, and beta carotene foods like apricots, mangoes and carrots. 4) Boost adrenal energy with vitamin B foods like brown rice. 5) Eat magnesium-rich foods, like almonds, green leafy vegetables, avocado, carrots, citrus fruits, lentils, salmon and flounder counteract depression and anxiety. 6) Foods from the sea nourish an underactive thyroid for increased libido.

—**For men:** A man's sex drive is dependent on testosterone and a good blood supply to the erectile tissue, factors that rely on good nutrition and exercise. 1) Eat zinc source foods: liver, oysters, nuts, seeds and legumes. 2) Dopamine (L-Dopa) is intimately associated with sex drive in men. One16-oz. can of fava beans has almost a prescription dose! 3) Add mineral-rich foods like shellfish, greens and whole grains; EFA's from flaxseed and sea greens. 4) Eat fiber-rich foods like legumes, fruits and vegetables to avoid atherosclerosis of the penis. 5) Drink in moderation. Heavy drinking can lead to reduced erections. Two or three alcoholic drinks can delay orgasm in women or decreases its intensity.

Herb & Supplement Therapy

—**Interceptive therapy plan: (Choose 2 or more recommendations)**
—**Revitalize the male system:**

1—Ginseng and ginseng-like herbs are primary tonics for male sexual virility: •Ethical Nutrients TRUE ENERGY. •*Yohimbe* caps 750-1000mg to stimulate testosterone (*Do not take yohimbe if you take diet products with phenylpropanolamine, or have heart, kidney, liver disorders.*) •Crystal Star LOVE MALE™ caps, •MALE GINSIAC™ or •LOVING MOOD FOR MEN™ extracts, •MALE PERFORMANCE™ caps or •PRO-EST PROX™ roll-on for longer erections.

2—EFA's boost healthy seminal fluids: Highest potency •royal jelly 60,000-120,000mg daily. •Heart Foods KEEP IT UP tabs. •*Ginkgo Biloba* for erectile dysfunction. •Unipro B₁₅ DMG liquid or tablets. •Premier GERMANIUM with DMG. •Zinc 50mg 2x daily with lecithin caps 1900mg.

3—For a stronger erection: •Liquid niacin before sexual intercourse; •Arginine 3000mg 45 minutes before sex for more penile blood flow (not if you have herpes) •Carnitine 1000mg 2x daily; •Life Enhancement PRO-SEXUAL PLUS. •Nutritional Tech. T2 -TRIBULUS TERRESTIS, or •Natural Balance COBRA, or •Crystal Star MALE PERFORMANCE™ caps; •Enzymatic Therapy NUCLEO-PRO M.

—**For women:** •Crystal Star LOVE FEMALE™ caps for 3 days before a special weekend. •*Yohimbe* 500mg caps for a tingle. (*See above for contra-indications.*); •Crystal Star WOMEN'S DRYNESS™, or •Moon Maid VITAL VULVA, or •vitamin E, 800IU for vaginal fluids. •Transitions PROGEST cream, or •Crystal Star PRO-EST BALANCE™ roll-on. •Long Life IMPERIAL TONIC with *royal jelly* and EPO; •Enzymatic Therapy THYROID/TYROSINE. •Enzymatic Therapy KAVATONE. Highest potency •Y.S. royal jelly 60,000-120,000mg. daily.

—**For both:** •2 *cayenne-ginger* capsules for enhanced orgasm, or •4 *Ginseng/damiana* caps. Montana Big Sky LOVING MOOD, or •Crystal Star CUPID'S FLAME™ or •GINSENG 6 SUPER tea or caps; •100mg niacin - 30 minutes before sex to enhance sexual flush, mucous membrane tingling and the intensity of the orgasm.

—**Effective superfoods: (choose 1 or 2)** •Unipro PERFECT PROTEIN; •Hsu's WILD AMERICAN GINSENG tabs; •Crystal Star SYSTEMS STRENGTH™ drink, or Nature's Path TRACE-LYTE drink for electrolyte minerals.

Lifestyle Support Therapy

—**Bodywork:**
•Environmental estrogens in hormone-injected food animals, herbicides and pesticide affect male sperm counts and female hormone balance. Avoid hormone-injected meats and dairy products, and herbicide-sprays to avoid environmental estrogens (see page 420 for more).
•Exercise can increase sex drive, especially exercise with your mate. Regular exercise such as dancing, walking and swimming stimulates circulation and increases body oxygen.
•Hypnotherapy has been effective when the problem is psychologically based.
•Try aromatherapy oils dotted on your sheets: both sexes turn on to *ylang-ylang, jasmine, and sandalwood.*

—**Lifestyle habits affect male sexual health:**
•Check your prescription drugs; some have the side effect of impaired sex drive.
•Prolonged recreational drug use inhibits sperm production.
•Heavy metal or radiation damages sperm and chromosome structure.
•Sexually transmitted diseases scar the vas deferens and testes, obstructing sperm delivery to the penis; infertility results.
•Smoking, because the cadmium contained in cigarette papers interferes with the utilization and absorption of zinc.

See next page for more information.

Can't find a recommended product? Call the 800 number listed in Product Resources for the store nearest you.

Is your libido low? If you've lost your interest in sex, you might want to check out some of the natural answers to low sexuality.

—If you're a woman in menopause have you gained unusual weight (low thyroid and metabolism) or lost your normal energy (adrenal exhaustion)?
—If you're a man in andropause (see page 423), have erections become slow and difficult (atherosclerosis) or painful (prostate swelling, poor circulation)?
—Have you become dissatisfied with the path your life is taking? Are you depressed?
—Do you feel unattractive or that you've lost your looks as you've aged?
—Have you been under a lot of emotional stress for a long period of time?
—Is there unusual tension in your job? Is your personal relationship unhappy?
—Has your diet deteriorated to fast foods on the run? Are you getting exercise every week?
—Was your childhood marked by physical abuse or great trauma? (sometimes the feelings don't surface for years)
—Have you resorted to too many prescription (or pleasure) drugs to get through your day?

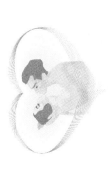

Some answers to individual sexuality and libido problems

For men:

—**For low libido and impotence:** •*Catauba* 4000mg, •Optimal Nutrients POTENT POTION •*Muira Pauma* 4000mg as needed; •*Pipsissewa*, low libido in older men. Take •5-HTP 100mg an hour before sex; •Histidine 500m with B-6 and niacin. The extraordinary popularity of Viagra is a wake-up call for men. But better sex through drugs may not be the best way to go. Natural therapies correct underlying causes of most impotence - poor circulation and atherosclerosis of the penile artery. Herbal fiber reduces cholesterol and eliminates fatty build-up that contributes to impotence. •Crystal Star's CHOL-LO FIBER TONE™ (takes about 3 months). •*Ginkgo Biloba* helps impotence caused by atherosclerosis. In a recent study, *ginkgo* was actually more effective than drug injections. 50% of patients showed regained potency- compared to 20% using injections. •*Yohimbe*, 1000mg helps for more rapid erections. (*Do not take if you have high blood pressure, are taking high blood pressure medicine, or diet products containing phenylpropanolamine, or have heart, kidney or liver disorders.*) •Arginine 3000mg daily boosts nitric oxide involved in the erection mechanism. •Life Enhancement PROSEXUAL PLUS. Acupuncture - a new study shows 20 out of 29 men overcame impotence after acupuncture treatment. If you smoke, quit! Smoking just 2 cigarettes a day can inhibit an erection. 4,400 Vietnam vets showed a 50% higher rate of impotence in smokers compared to non-smokers.
—**To prolong erections and reduce premature ejaculation:** for both older and younger men. •Crystal Star PRO-EST PROX™ roll-on; •Morada Research Labs PROSTATE (a prostate tonic for prostate-related sexual problems); •*horsetail-nettles* tea helps reduce prostate swelling rapidly. *Saw palmetto*, a tissue building steroid-like herb, reduces premature ejaculation. •Crystal Star MALE PERFORMANCE™ with *saw palmetto* has a long history of success; •Crystal Star PROX roll-on is especially effective for younger men; or •homeopathic *Conium* and *Selenium*.

For women:

—**Tonify the female system with adaptogen herbs.** •Crystal Star FEEL GREAT™ caps, 2-3 caps daily; •Herbal Magic GINSENG/GINKGO REJUVENATOR caps 2 caps twice daily.
—**Libido-enhancers:** •Peruvian *Maca*, •Nutramedix INVOGOREX; •Futurebiotics MAXATIVA for women; •*Dong Quai/Damiana* extract; •Alive ROYAL JELLY vials boost acetylcholine for sexual response; •Histidine 500mg with B-6 100mg.
—**Essential fatty acids improve aging skin tone, and lubricate your body internally and externally:** •Nature's Secret ULTIMATE OIL. •EVENING PRIMROSE OIL 3000 mg daily; •Ginkgo Biloba improves low libido in women caused by anti-depressant drugs in a new study.
—**For depression-related libido problems:** •*St. John's wort*, or 5-HTP to increase serotonin; •*Ginkgo Biloba* improves low libido in women caused by anti-depressant drugs in a new study.
—**For vaginal dryness:** A common problem after menopause. Intercourse may become painful and some women experience vaginal infection. For immediate relief: Apply natural •vitamin E oil, sesame seed oil, •aloe vera gel or •Moon Maid VITAL VULVA to vaginal opening. (Take vitamin E internally for long term relief - improves blood supply to the vaginal walls). Take •Crystal Star WOMEN'S DRYNESS™ extract to produce more membrane fluid; or Ayurvedic •*Shatavari* (*Asparagus racemosus*)- a primary sexual tonic for women with vaginal atrophy.

—**For men and women:** Surprise... wild oats helps both sexes! The Institute for Advanced Study Of Human Sexuality shows 300mg of wild oats extract three days a week leads to a dramatic increase in multiple orgasms for women! Results are very good for men in frequency of intercourse and orgasm. •Gaia Herbs OATS, WILD MILKY SEED. *Tribulus terrestris* (Indian puncture vine), increases female sex drive without the side effects of hormone drugs. In one study, ²/₃ of women treated with tribulus report renewed sexual interest! Tribulus also has a long history of success for reducing male impotence and is believed to raise testosterone levels by activating luteinizing hormone (LH) in the pituitary gland. •Nutritional Technologies T2-TRIBULUS TERRESTRIS. ANDRO may boost a waning libido, enhance energy and promote muscle growth for men and women with a proven testosterone deficiency. Use under the supervision of a health professional. Aromatherapy stimulates a loving mood. Sexuality-enhancing aromatherapy oils for men include: *cinnamon, sandalwood, lavender, patchouli, coriander, jasmine* and *cardamom*. Sexuality-enhancing oils for women are: *ylang ylang, rose, clary sage, neroli* and *rosewood*.

See HORMONE *pages 419-425 for more information.*

S 489

Can't find a recommended product? Call the 800 number listed in Product Resources for the store nearest you.

A New Look at Contraception, Fertility and STD protection

Every method of contraception has risks, but the risk of contracting a sexually transmitted disease, and unwanted pregnancy are obviously greater. Both partners, but especially women, need to earnestly evaluate their lifestyles, sexual discipline and partner's attitudes to make a responsible choice. Unless you are in a long-term relationship, absolutely make sure that your partner is monogamous, take precautions against STD's. Even if you know your partner is monogamous, be careful. Once a virus gets into your system, it never goes away. Sometimes people carry STD's from previous relationships and don't know it, or don't want to share the fact with a new partner. Don't forget that HIV and AIDS can kill you; herpes and HPV, (the virus that induces genital warts) are permanent. These STD's may become dormant, but they do not leave the body. STD's are especially dangerous to an unborn child because they can be transferred during birth. Even STD's that are not permanent cause a great deal of pain and can leave you permanently infertile.

—**BARRIER METHODS:** condom, diaphragm, cervical cap and vaginal sponge, are the most popular contraceptive devices since the advent of the AIDS epidemic. The latex (not lambskin) **condom** is the method that offers almost complete protection from STD's. It encourages couples to share responsibility for birth and disease control. However, failure rate from breakage, heat or wear is almost 15%. Use a back-up spermicide with a condom. Since the pill shifted the responsibility for contraception from men to women, condom use has become less common - especially among teenagers, where the greatest STD infection is being experienced. The new **female condoms**, polyurethane ringed sheaths that fit over the cervix, are comfortable, and can be inserted ahead of time, but they are clumsy, and unromantic, hanging slightly outside the vagina. The female condom also has twice the failure rate of the male condom with an estimated 21 in 100 women becoming pregnant in the first year of use. However, they give the woman a choice if the man refuses to wear a condom, and they do protect against STD's. The **diaphragm**, fitted correctly, used with spermicide, without any tiny holes or cracks is an effective, unobtrusive method of birth control, and provides some protection against STD's. Many sensitive women get bladder infections from the diaphragm rubbing against the urethra, and yeast infections from the spermicide. The **cervical cap** with spermicidal jelly creates a seal that prevents sperm penetration and inactivates sperm, is effective for 48 hours of birth control, but is not effective against STD's. The **vaginal sponge** is impregnated with spermicide, inserted in the back of the vagina; it is effective for 24 hours. It is not a good choice for women who have had children, or for sensitive women who become irritated from a large dose of spermicide. It may become a cause of toxic shock syndrome when the women is unable to remove the sponge or when fragments remain.

—**SPERMICIDES:** creams, jellies, suppositories and foams, are put into the vagina to kill or immobilize sperm. They have some ability to kill sexually-transmitted viruses, but should always be used with a barrier method of contraception since they have up to 21% failure rate. *Some tests show that Nonoxynol-9 contraceptive gel can put both men and women at more risk for STD's.*

—**HORMONAL CONTRACEPTIVES:** today's pills have much lower doses of hormones, but many women are still sensitive to the synthetic estrogen impact and wary of breast and uterine cancer risk. High blood pressure, migraine headaches, depression, water retention, thrush, gum inflammation, increased fibroid growth, weight gain, breast enlargement, low libido, and changes in skin pigmentation are still frequent side effects - and of course the pill does not protect against STD's.

—**HORMONE IMPLANTS:** (Norplant) surgically inserted into a woman's upper arm, release tiny doses of hormone into the bloodstream. Even these small amounts of synthetic hormones show side effects of irregular menstruation, intra-period spotting, headaches, depression. They are effective birth control for five years, but do not protect against STD's. They are painful and leave an unsightly scar when removed.

—**DEPO-PROVERA:** (progestin) injections, used every 13 weeks, prevent egg release by the ovaries to protect against unwanted pregnancy. The injections are highly effective against unwanted pregnancy, but I advise caution. The drug can accelerate bone loss and elevate breast cancer risk. It causes changes in bleeding patterns, breast soreness, headaches and weight gain for many women. Some women even report autoimmune problems similar to fibromyalgia that last months after Depo-Provera use is discontinued. —**The "mini pill" is a progestin only birth control pill that can be used while breast-feeding. It has a high success rate, but must be used at the same time every day to be effective, making it inconvenient for the majority of users. In addition, side effects like weight gain, irregular periods, breast soreness and nausea are common. The "mini pill"** can also increase risk for ovarian cysts in susceptible women.

—**EMERGENCY CONTRACEPTIVE KITS: (the "morning after pill")**, prevents ovulation to safeguard against pregnancy. **Morning-after contraception can be used within three days of unprotected sex to prevent an unwanted pregnancy, but do not affect pregnancies that have already occurred.** Nausea, dizziness and cramping are common side effects.

—**MALE BIRTH CONTROL** pills and injections are the newest hormonal contraceptives. Male birth control uses testosterone to lower sperm counts in order to prevent pregnancy. Side effects include: infertility, low libido, impotence, depression and PMS like symptoms. The male birth control pill will not be available for another 5-10 years as studies evaluate its safety.

—**STERILIZATION,** is the most rapidly rising form of contraception in American women. **Tubal ligation** means hormones, ovulation and menstruation continue as usual, but the egg disintegrates in the tubes and is absorbed by the bloodstream. Side effects are irregular bleeding, increased menstrual pain and excessively heavy periods, (a hysterectomy may be necessary to stop the bleeding) Some women report bone loss, back pain, incontinence, loss of libido, hot flashes and night sweats as a result of tubal ligation. Male sterilization is rising, too. Half a million American men undergo a **vasectomy** to become sterile every year. The tubes that carry the sperm to the penis are cut and tied. The man can continue to ejaculate semen without sperm, but many questions about side effects and long-term hormone imbalances are now being raised. Some evidence suggests that vasectomy raises risk of prostate cancer. No sterilization form protects against STD's. Note: A **no-scalpel vasectomy** is recommended. An NSV reduces body trauma and speeds recovery time. Instead of making two half-inch incisions in the scrotum to reach the vas deferens, in a NSV, the doctor makes one small hole in the scrotal sack to draw out the tubes that carry sperm.

—**IUDs** have fallen from favor because of their many complications, increased risk of infertility, adverse health effects and high risk for STD's.

Can't find a recommended product? Call the 800 number listed in Product Resources for the store nearest you.

Sexually Transmitted Diseases

Venereal Infections, Vaginosis,

Sexually transmitted diseases are a factor today in every choice we make about our sexuality and our reproductive lives. No treatment for impotence, no questions about fertility or sterility, no decision about child conception can be made without considering the STD quotient. Sexually transmitted diseases are more prevalent, more insidious and more dangerous than ever before. Experts say that one out of every five Americans has a sexually transmitted infection. Vaginosis, a little-known bacterial vaginal infections, puts women at risk for far more serious pelvic inflammatory disease (PID), even for contracting AIDS. Whether you believe our culture is paying for years of sexual freedom, (which is turning out not to be free, after all), or whether you believe that STD's are the result of irresponsible behavior and misinformation, they can't be ignored.

Diet & Superfood Therapy

–Nutritional therapy plan:

1–Follow a very cleansing liquid diet for 3 days (pg. 191) during acute stages. Take one each of the following juices daily: Potassium broth (pg. 215), fresh carrot juice, vegetable drink (pg. 219, or see below), apple/parsley juice to alkalize.

2–Then continue with a cleansing fresh foods diet to alkalize. Include several bunches of green grapes daily (an old remedy that still works).

3–Avoid refined, starchy, fried and saturated fat foods. Avoid red meats, pasteurized dairy products, and caffeine during healing.

–Effective superfoods: (choose 1 or 2)

•Crystal Star ENERGY GREEN™.
•Herbal Answers ALOE FORCE JUICE before meals.
•Mona's CHLORELLA 2 pkts. daily.
•Nutricology PRO-GREENS with EFA's.
•Wakunaga KYO-GREEN.
•Green Foods CARROT ESSENCE.

Herb & Supplement Therapy

–Interceptive therapy plan: (Choose 2 to 3 recommendations)

Note: Many STD's benefit from using GRAPEFRUIT SEED extract or SKIN SPRAY first. •Crystal Star ANTI-BIO™ or ANTI-VI™ formulas 6x daily, with •Crystal Star WHITES OUT 1 and WHITES OUT 2 capsules alternate 3x daily for a month. ♀ •Now OREGANO OIL soft gels. Add •Beta carotene 150,000IU daily; •Vitamin C crystals ½ teasp. every hour to bowel tolerance during acute phase, reduced to 5000mg daily for a month.

2–For Chlamydia (4 million new cases per year): •Crystal Star DETOX™ caps with goldenseal. (also open and apply to sores). •Mix powders of *goldenseal, barberry, Oregon grape root* and *garlic* with vitamin A oil and apply directly to the cervix via an all-cotton tampon. •Premier Labs GERMANIUM 150mg; •CoQ₁₀ 60mg 4x daily; •Vitamin E 400IU 2x daily; or •Am. Biologics emulsified A & E; •Lane Labs BENE-FIN SHARK CARTILAGE 4 caps daily, or East Park OLIVE LEAF extract caps as anti-viral agents.

3–For Trichomonas (3 million new cases per year): •Crystal Star WHITES OUT ♀ #1™ and WHITES OUT #2™ capsules for 2 months (alternate every 2 hours), with •ZINC SOURCE™ extract internally or Zinc 50mg 2x daily (also apply topically). •Bathe sores several times daily in a *goldenseal/myrrh* or *gentian* herb solution. •Use a TEA TREE oil vaginal suppository nightly. •Beta carotene 150,000IU daily; •Vitamin C crystals ½ teasp. every hour to bowel tolerance during acute phase, reduced to 5000mg daily for a month.

4–For Syphilis (up to 100,000 new cases per year): After antibiotics, use: •Crystal Star DETOX™ with goldenseal; •Sarsaparilla extract for 4 months; •ECHINACEA extract 4x daily; *Pau d' arco* tea or *Calendula* tea 3 cups daily. •*Calendula* ointment; •CoQ₁₀ 300mg daily; •Nutricology GERMANIUM 150mg; •MICROHYDRIN available at Healthy House, or Prof. Nutrition DOCTOR DOPHILUS +FOS.

5–For Vaginosis: •Vitamin E cream and 400IU internally daily; •B-complex 100mg daily; rebalance with •Crystal Star WHITES OUT 1 and WHITES OUT 2.♀

Lifestyle Support Therapy

Beware: Nonoxynol-9 contraceptive gel can put both men and women at more risk for STD's.

–Bodywork:

•Strong doses of antibiotics are the usual medical treatment, but the most recent outbreaks (especially in teenagers) are showing resistance or non-response to these drugs.

•Overheating therapy is very effective in controlling virus replication. Even slight body temperature increases can lead to considerable reduction of infection. See page 225 in this book for effective technique.

•Smoking and a poor diet increase risk because they reduce immune defenses to create an environment for infection. Smokers are 3 times more at risk than non-smokers.

•Oral contraceptives are known to potentiate the adverse effects of nicotine, and to decrease the levels of key nutrients like vitamins C, B-6, B-12, folic acid, and zinc. In addition, some oral contraceptives aggravate the formation of pre-cancerous lesions because of their imbalancing estrogen content.

–For crabs (pubic lice): wash pubic hair thoroughly; tweeze out die-hards; comb through a vinegar-water solution.

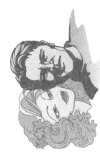

Common Symptoms: *Symptoms usually appear two to three weeks after sexual contact.* **Gonorrhea:** *cloudy discharge for both sexes; frequent, painful urination, yeast infection symptoms; pelvic inflammation.* **Syphilis:** *First contagious stage; sores on the genitalia, rash and patchy, flaky tissue, fever, mouth sores and chronic sore throat.* **Chlamydia:** *thick discharge in both men and women, urethritis; pelvic pain, sterility. Can cause birth defects if present during pregnancy. Constant douching may put you more at risk.* **Trichomonas:** *caused by a parasite, found in both men and women, usually contracted through intercourse, severe itchiness and thin, foamy, yellowish discharge with a foul odor.* **Vaginosis:** *vaginal discharge; unpleasant odor.*

Can't find a recommended product? Call the 800 number listed in Product Resources for the store nearest you.

Call the National STD Hotline (800) 227-8922 for more information.

Sexually Transmitted Diseases

Herpes Genitalis

Herpes Simplex 2 Virus is the most widespread of all STD's, affecting 60 to 100 million Americans (up to 500,000 new cases per year). It is a lifelong infection that alternates between virulent and inactive stages. It may be transmitted even when there are no symptoms, by direct contact with infected fluids from saliva, skin discharges or sexual fluids. Babies can pick up the virus in the birth canal, risking brain damage, blindness, even death. Recurrent outbreaks may be triggered by emotional stress, poor diet, food allergies, menstruation, drugs and alcohol, sunburn, fever, or a minor infection. Men are more susceptible to recurrence than women. Outbreaks are opportunistic in that it takes over when immunity is low and stress is high. Optimizing immune function is of primary importance.

Diet & Superfood Therapy

Nutritional therapy plan:

1—Good nutrition is critical against herpes - body chemistry balance is essential. A lysine-rich/arginine-poor diet has some merit. Especially increase your fresh fish (rich in lysine). Arginine-containing foods aggravate herpes. Avoid them until blisters disappear: chocolate, peanuts, almonds, cashews, and walnuts; sunflower and sesame seeds, coconut. Eat wheat, soy, lentils, oats, corn, rice, barley, tomatoes, squash with discretion. Avoid citrus during healing.

2—Have fruit juices, and a carrot/beet/cucumber juice or potassium broth (pg. 215) each day.

3—Then keep the diet consciously alkaline with miso soup, brown rice and vegetables often. Add cultured vegetable protein foods such as tofu and tempeh for healing and friendly G.I. bacteria.

4—Reduce dairy intake, especially hard cheeses, and red meat. Eliminate fried foods, nitrate-treated foods, and nightshade plants like tomatoes and eggplant.

—Effective superfoods: (choose 1 or 2)

• Crystal Star ENERGY GREEN™ drink.
• Nutricology PROGREENS with EFA's.
• George's ALOE juice every morning.
• Green Foods GREEN MAGMA.
• AloeLife FIBERMATE - internal cleansing.

Herb & Supplement Therapy

—Interceptive therapy plan: (Choose 2 to 3 recommendations)

Herbs have had remarkable success against herpes- remitting symptoms, reducing outbreaks.

1—**Control the infection:** Olive leaf extract or • Nutricology PRO-LIVE olive leaf extract as directed; • Take *Lemon balm* extract drops in water; apply *lemon balm* extract or tea directly to sores (remarkable anti-herpes activity); or • Enzymatic Therapy HERPILYN caps and ointment (with *lemon balm*). Take • Crystal Star ANTI-VI™ with St. *John's wort*, (proven against HSV2). • Vibrant Health DUMONTIACEAE red algae, or • Source Naturals INTRACEPT with red algae.

2—**Reduce the inflammatory outbreaks:** • Crystal Star HRPS™ capsules 4 daily; take • Quercetin 1000mg with bromelain 1500mg instant relief; and • Ascorbate vitamin C or Ester C powder $1/4$ teasp. every hour in water up to 10,000mg or to bowel tolerance daily during an attack. Drink plenty of • *peppermint* tea (a specific against herpes).

Here's how lysine therapy works: the HSV2 virus needs the amino acid arginine to replicate. Both lysine and arginine look similar to the virus. If it's available, lysine essentially ambushes the virus into taking it instead of arginine, blocking virus growth and keeping it from reactivating. Apply lysine cream frequently. Take lysine 500mg capsules 6 daily until outbreaks clear.

3—**Heal the sores:** Take • Crystal Star ANTI-BIO™ caps 6 daily, and apply opened capsules to sores, or mix with aloe vera gel and apply. Apply • Crystal Star LYSINE/LICORICE GEL™ or • ANTI-BIO™ gel with *una da gato* (both work well). Take • Diamond HERPANACINE caps 4 daily. ♀ • Apply • St. *John's wort* oil. Take • ECHINACEA extract- 1 dropperful orally every 2 hrs; apply • *echinacea* powder to sores. Apply a • wet black tea bag for 5 minutes at a time for 4 days til lesion crusts over. Apply • Nutribiotic GRAPEFRUIT SEED skin spray.

4—**Rebalance body chemistry:** Biotec CELLGUARD with SOD 6 daily. • *Garlic* 8 capsules daily; • Crystal Star GINSENG/REISHI extract.

5—**Prevent future outbreaks:** • Take selenium 500-600mg daily for a month. • Premier Labs LITHIUM .5mg arrests viral replication (mix an opened capsule with water and apply to sores). • MICROHYDRIN available at Healthy House.

Lifestyle Support Therapy

Steroid drugs taken over a long time for herpes weaken both the immune system and bone density.

—Bodywork:

• Apply ice packs to lesions for pain and inflammation relief. Ice may also be applied as a preventive measure when the sufferer feels a flare-up coming on.

• Get some early morning sunlight on the sores every day for healing Vitamin D.

• Take hot baths frequently for overheating therapy to arrest the virus (pg. 225).

• Wear cotton underwear that breathes.

• Practice stress reduction techniques like biofeedback, meditation and imagery to prevent outbreaks. Acupuncture is effective for herpes.

• Eliminate immune-suppressing drugs, alcohol, and tobacco from your lifestyle.

• If you have an outbreak don't touch the sores; wash hands if you do touch them. Don't touch your eyes if you have touched the sores.

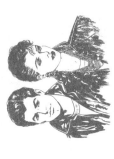

Common Symptoms: *The first herpes outbreak is usually the most potent. It is accompanied by swollen glands and fever, as the body's immune system rallies to fight the infection. A cluster of painful blisters appears below the waist, over the groin, the thighs and buttocks, accompanied by a low grade fever, flu-like symptoms, and swelling of the groin lymph glands. There is headache, stiff neck, fever, pain, swelling, genital itching and blisters that swell and fester, and shooting pains through the thighs and legs. Blisters rupture after 1 to 3 days, then slowly heal in another 3 to 5 days.*

Common Causes: *Transmitted from kissing, oral sex, intercourse; excess arginine in the body; too many drugs; an acid-forming diet; hormone imbalance related to the menstrual cycle.*

Call the Herpes Hotline (919) 361-8488 for more information.

Can't find a recommended product? Call the 800 number listed in Product Resources for the store nearest you.

Sexually Transmitted Diseases

Cervical Dysplasia, Condyloma, Venereal Warts (HPV)

Cervical dysplasia, precancerous cervical lesions is being called the newest sexually transmitted epidemic. It is silent, often unknown by the infected person. Researchers suspect that two sexually transmitted viruses, Human Papilloma Virus (Condyloma warts), the most common STD in the U.S., and Herpes Simplex II are involved, because these viruses also play a role in cervical cancer. They are extremely contagious. Both conditions are the result of risky lifestyle habits and low immunity. Both can result in a abnormal PAP smears (as can long use of some birth control pills). Natural treatments deal with the causes of genital warts and require strong commitment and significant lifestyle changes, with positive outlook for immune support. If there are mouth sores, treat as for thrush. (see page 343), or chew Enzymatic Therapy DGL tablets.

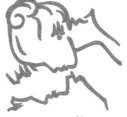

Diet & Superfood Therapy

—Nutritional therapy plan:

1–A diet to encourage strong immune response against dysplasia: Increase fresh fruits, vegetables (especially cruciferous veggies), and high fiber complex carbohydrates as protective factors. Add high folic acid foods like lima beans, whole wheat and brewer's yeast. Add vegetable juices and/or green drinks (pg. 218) for immune support and supplementing vitamin deficiencies.

2–Add 2 TBS chopped sea greens daily for ocean carotene. Add cold water fish like salmon for omega-3 oils. Add leafy greens for folacin. Eat cultured foods to normalize intestinal flora.

3–Reduce dietary fat, especially from animal foods. Reduce caffeine and hard liquor. Particularly avoid foods that aggravate herpes-type infections like sugary junk foods and fried foods.

4–Avoid red meat and poultry foods. These may have been contaminated with estrogens or other hormone treatments.

—Effective superfoods: (choose 1 or 2)

• Sun Wellness CHLORELLA, 2 pkts. daily.
• Crystal Star SYSTEMS STRENGTH™ drink.
• Solgar EARTH SOURCE GREENS & MORE.
• Beehive Botanical ROYAL JELLY with Siberian ginseng 2 teasp. daily.
• George's ALOE VERA juice 2x daily.
• Red Star NUTRITIONAL YEAST.

Herb & Supplement Therapy

—Interceptive therapy plan: (Choose 2 to 3 recommendations)

1–**Control the infection:** •Crystal Star ANTI-VI™ extract or tea to deal with the virus; for 1 month, give your body an ascorbic acid flush with ¼ teasp. vitamin C powder with bioflav. every 2 hours until the stool turns soupy. Then take • vitamin C 5000mg daily with bioflavonoids for a month. Use •Quercetin 1000mg with bromelain 1500mg daily.

2–**Detoxify the blood and liver:** Crystal Star •DETOX™ capsules for one month as a blood cleanser, followed by •FIBER & HERBS CLEANSE™ to rid the colon of re-infection. Drink 2 cups daily of •burdock or dandelion root tea, and take •MILK THISTLE SEED extract for 2 months.

3–**Flush lymph glands:** Echinacea extract, mullein or burdock tea; cayenne caps 2 daily; Enzymatic Therapy THYMULUS. •Crystal Star ANTI-BIO™ caps 6 daily.

4–**For venereal warts** (up to 1 million new cases per year): Take dilute •oregano oil, 6 drops daily (1 part oregano oil to 4 parts olive oil); apply •castor oil cervix packs or East Park OLIVE LEAF extract cream. Make up •Goldenseal/chaparral vaginal suppositories (powders mixed with vitamin A oil)- extremely helpful for women with venereal warts or dysplasia, rendering many disease-free. Take •Crystal Star ANTI-VI™ capsules 4 daily, with FIRST AID CAPS™ to raise body temperature during acute stages; one week off and one week on until improvement. •Steep 4 garlic cloves in 4-oz. of aloe vera juice and apply 2x daily.

5–**For cervical dysplasia:** high levels of folic acid mean lower rates of cervical dysplasia. Take •B-complex with extra 800mcg folic acid daily and sublingual B-12, 2500mcg daily; a •vitamin C flush (see above); •vitamin A up to 100,000IU for a month (not if pregnant), or •beta-carotene 200,000IU. Take •Crystal Star CALCIUM SOURCE™ caps or •black cohosh extract to prevent pre-cancerous lesions from becoming cancerous.

6–**Antioxidants are immune tonics:** •OPC's from grapeseed or pine bark 100mg 3x daily. •Nutricology germanium 150mg; •Vitamin E 800IU with selenium 400mg daily. •Nutricology N-acetyl cysteine 1000mg; •Zinc picolinate 50mg daily.

Lifestyle Support Therapy

—Lifestyle measures:

• High risk lifestyle factors must be eliminated for permanent improvement and prevention of further invasive lesions. Eliminate smoking, oral contraceptives and multiple sexual partners. Use a barrier contraceptive to prevent new contact with HPV or HVS II. Recurrence often occurs after standard surgery alone.

• Avoid surgery by using vaginal packs, Nutribiotic GRAPEFRUIT SEED extract, Body Essentials SILICA GEL, or chlorella powder paste, placed against the cervix draws out toxins and sloughs abnormal cells. Abstain from sexual intercourse during vag pack treatment. (See page 234 for a pack to make yourself.)

• Alternating hot and cold hydrotherapy promotes healing activity to the pelvic area.

—For venereal warts: Earth's Bounty O₂ SPRAY daily for a month; then rest for a month, and resume if necessary. If noticeable improvement occurs in this first month, returning to treatment may not be necessary. The body's defense forces will have taken over.

Common Symptoms: *Heavy painful periods; bleeding between periods; pain during intercourse; genital warts or herpes; chronic gonorrhea or any unusual vaginal discharge; fever and often, infertility. Symptoms of Venereal Warts (HPV): the most common STD, infects ovaries, fallopian tubes, cervix, and uterus. Chronic yeast infection with heavy, pus-filled discharge; painful intercourse; painful, infected sores in the genital area; high fever during infection.*
Common Risk Factors: *Early age of first intercourse, multiple sexual partners; lower socio-economic class with its traditionally nutrient-poor diet, smoking, and oral contraceptives.*

See the previous pages for more information.

Can't find a recommended product? Call the 800 number listed in Product Resources for the store nearest you.

S 493

Shingles
Herpes Zoster, Hives, Angioderma

Shingles are the eruption of acute, inflammatory, herpes-type blisters on the trunk of the body along a peripheral nerve. It is an acute central nervous system infection caused by the Herpes Zoster virus, and the blisters are infectious. Since the virus is the same as that causing chicken pox, there is proneness to shingles if one had chicken pox as a child. Hives are the same type of itching blisters, but are caused by an allergic reaction to a chemical, medication or food. The most common cause of shingles for adults is a reaction to certain medications. Both are very painful, inflammatory skin conditions. Note: Avoid acetaminophen pain killers such as Tylenol, that can aggravate the blisters.

Diet & Superfood Therapy

Nutritional therapy plan:

1—Go on a short 3 day cleansing diet to eliminate acid wastes and alkalize the blood (pg. 191).

2—Take a carrot-beet-cucumber juice, and a natural cranberry or carrot juice each day. Take an apple juice or celery juice each night.

3—Then, eat only fresh foods for 1-2 weeks, with lots of salads and fruits.

4—Avoid arginine-forming foods (see page 355).

5—Keep the diet alkaline, with miso soup, whole grains, vegetables and leafy greens. Eat foods high in B vitamins, such as brown rice, green vegetables and nutritional yeast. Include cultured foods, such as yogurt and kefir for friendly G.I. flora.

6—Avoid acid-forming foods: red meats, cheese, salty foods, eggs, caffeine, fried foods, and sodas.

7—Avoid refined foods, sugars, aspirin, tetracyclines, and meats that may contain nitrates, nitrites and antibiotics.

8—Eliminate allergen foods, like those with preservatives, flavorings, additives and colorings.

—**Effective superfoods: (choose 1 or 2)**
• Herbal Answers ALOE FORCE aloe juice.
• Crystal Star BIOFLAV. FIBER & C SUPPORT.
• Red Star Nutritional Yeast or Bio-Strath original LIQUID YEAST.
• Green Foods CARROT ESSENCE.
• Crystal Star SYSTEMS STRENGTH™.

Herb & Supplement Therapy

—**Interceptive therapy plan: (Choose 2 to 3 recommendations)**

1—**Control eruptions:** •Crystal Star ANTI-HST™ capsules 4 to 6 daily to help produce normalizing antihistamines and open air passages. Add •HRPS™ capsules to help calm itchy blistering. Pat •THERADERM™ tea on blisters to neutralize acids coming out through the skin. •Vibrant Health DUMONTIACEAE red algae, or •Source Naturals INTRACEPT with red algae interfere with herpes virus.

Vitamin C controls eruptions: Use Ester C powder with bioflavs., $1/4$ teasp. every hour in water up to 10,000mg or bowel tolerance during an attack, then reduce to 5000mg daily until blisters heal. Or use EXTA-CEE from Healthy House.

2—**Reduce inflammation and relieve pain:** •Quercetin 1000mg with bromelain 1500 for rapid action. •Emulsified A & D 50,000/1,000IU 2x daily, with •Vit. E 400IU and selenium 200mcg 2x daily. •Apply E oil directly. •Cayenne caps, 2 daily to relieve pain, or •DLPA 750mg for pain. •Enzymatic Therapy HERPILYN caps. Effective homeopathics: •B & T CALIFLORA gel. •B&T SSSTING STOP gel. •Arsenicum. Apply •Crystal Star LYSINE/LICORICE™ skin gel.

3—**Heal the blisters:** •Diamond HERPANACINE caps 4 to 6 daily; or take MSM with MICROHYDRIN available at Healthy House (notable results). Take •Lysine 1000mg internally, and apply LYSINE cream to blisters. Apply •Lemon Balm cream or lemon balm extract directly; or •capsaicin cream or •calendula ointment. Apply •BioForce ECHINACEA cream; •Aloe Answers ALOE FORCE skin gel, or an •aloe vera/goldenseal solution.

4—**Help control the virus:** Take •East Park OLIVE LEAF extract caps. Spray lesions with •Earth's Bounty O₂ SPRAY several times daily; •Crystal Star ANTI-VI™ tea 2-4 cups daily, with •Echinacea extract to flush lymph glands and •Omega-3 flax oil 3 teasp. daily. •Lane Labs BENE-FIN shark cartilage, 6 daily.

5—**Rebuild strong nerves:** •Crystal Star RELAX CAPS™ 4 to 6 as needed; •Stress B-complex 200mg with extra B₆ 250mg and B₁₂ 2000mcg sublingual 2x daily; •Scullcap extract drops; •St. John's wort extract; •Red clover/nettles tea; •Reishi mushroom extract or •Crystal Star Ginseng-Reishi extract; •Magnesium 800mg 2x daily.

Lifestyle Support Therapy

Corticosteroid drugs are frequently prescribed for shingles. Remember that corticosteroid drugs taken over a long period of time for shingles, weaken the immune system, allowing future attacks.

—**Bodywork:**
• Effective topical applications for pain: Petroleum jelly.
Ice compresses.
CAPSAICIN cream or Nature's Way CAYENNE PAIN RELIEVING OINTMENT.
Biochemics PAIN RELIEF eucalyptus lotion.
Epsom salt baths or oatmeal baths or compresses to neutralize acids.
Flax seed compresses.
• Get early morning sunlight on the body for healing vitamin D.
• Relaxation and tension control techniques are effective. Stress creates an acid body condition, and erodes protective nerve sheathing.
• Acupuncture can often relieve even the most stubborn cases of shingles.

See HERPES page 355 and 492 for more information.

S 494

Common Symptoms: Preliminary symptoms include chills, fever and an uncomfortable feeling before swollen, red skin blisters develop, usually around the upper part of the body; pain radiating along one or several nerves preceding outbreaks; attacks last from 2 days to 2 weeks, leaving irritated nerves even after blisters are gone; accompanied by fever, weakness, chills and nausea.
Common Causes: Food allergies, esp. to dairy products, shellfish, wheat, MSG, food additives and preservatives; reaction to antibiotic drugs like penicillin; over-chlorinated drinking water; stress; adrenal and/or liver exhaustion; histamine reaction; acidosis and HCl depletion; poor circulation and constipation; too many prescription drugs; too much caffeine or hard liquors.

Can't find a recommended product? Call the 800 number listed in Product Resources for the store nearest you.

Shock and Trauma Control

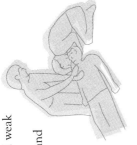

Shock is the condition that develops when blood flow is reduced below the levels needed to maintain vital body functions. Obviously, shock and trauma can happen during serious injuries or illnesses when a great deal of blood and other body fluids are lost. But it can also occur during severe infections, allergic reactions (anaphylactic shock), and nervous system malfunction (a severe reaction to a poisonous insect or snake bite). Major burns, heat prostration, loss of blood in a severe accident, a serious head injury or bone break, or sprains or falls.... every significant injury is accompanied by some degree of shock, because the autonomic nervous system responds to the trauma of injury by altering blood flow. It is usually wise to treat any severely injured person for shock in addition to treating them for the injury. If there is lots of bleeding, severe burns, or a head wound, treatment for shock should be very high priority.

Do you recognize shock? Here are the common signs:

Victim is weak, restless and unresponsive, with irregular deep breathing; the skin is cold, pale and damp to the touch; the pupils are dilated; a rapid weak heartbeat; heart attack or stroke, sometimes with nausea; reduced alertness and consciousness; shallow breathing and confusion.

Have the person lie down with legs elevated slightly above the head. Don't bend the legs. Loosen clothing. Protect the person from extremes of warmth and cold. If there is a chance of serious or life-threatening injury, do not move the person. Give small sips of fluids only if fully conscious - no solid food.

Get medical care immediately!

The following emergency measures are beneficial until medical help arrives:

—Deva Flowers FIRST AID remedy, or Nelson Bach RESCUE REMEDY; 2-4 drops on the tongue every 5 minutes until breathing normalizes.

—Dilute cayenne extract or powder in water (1-3 teasp. or 2-4 capsules); give with an eyedropper on the back of the tongue if necessary every 10 minutes to restore normal heart rate.

—Consciousness-reviving herbs such as strong incense, camphor, bay oil or musk can be used under the victim's nose as aromatherapy for revival.

—GINKGO BILOBA extract - a few drops in water, given on the tongue helps with stroke and allergic reactions such as dizziness, loss of balance, memory loss or ringing in the ears.

—*Arnica Montana* drops are usually the first homeopathic remedy to give for injury; every half hour to 1 hour on the tongue.

—Bromelain 500mg, or Quercetin with bromelain to control body trauma - open 1-2 capsules in water and give in small sips. Acts like aspirin, anti-inflammatory without stomach upset.

—Hops/*valerian* tincture, or Crystal Star VALERIAN/WILD LETTUCE; 5-6 drops in water. Give in small sips every 10-15 minutes for calmness.

You need to know CPR. Cardiopulmonary resuscitation (CPR) is an important medical emergency procedure, if a person's heart or breathing has stopped; CPR is essential in order to avoid brain damage, which usually begins in 4 to 6 minutes after cardiopulmonary arrest.

1. Be sure the person is truly unconscious. If tapping, shouting or shaking does not wake him or her, call immediately for help, giving precise directions and telephone number.

2. Lay the victim flat on the back on a straight, firm surface. If you have to roll the person over, roll him or her towards you with one of your hands supporting the neck as you turn.

3. Open the airway so the tongue is not blocking it. If you feel the person may have a neck injury, use your fingers to move the tongue out of the airway. If not, use the following procedure. Place one of your palms across the forehead, and using your other hand, lift the chin up and forward. At the same time, gently push down the forehead. This head and chin-tilt movement lifts the chin but does not fully close the mouth. As the jaw is tilted, the tongue will move out of the airway. Remove any dentures if present.

4. Check to see if the victim is breathing. Opening the airway may be all that is needed. If no signs of breathing are detected, move the tongue out of the airway again.

5. Begin mouth-to-mouth resuscitation. Remove your hand from the forehead and pinch the victim's nostrils together. Take a deep breath and place your open mouth over the victim's mouth. Exhale completely into the victim's mouth. Take your mouth away; inhale quickly, and repeat four times.

6. Check the pulse on the side of the neck. You should feel the pulse of the carotid artery here. Move your fingers around if you don't feel it at once, and keep trying for 10 to 15 seconds. If there is no pulse begin chest compression to maintain circulation until medical help arrives.

• Kneel next to the victim's chest, midway between the shoulder and waist. Find the tip of the breastbone, and place your hands one over the other, palms down on this point.

• Shift your weight forward, and with your elbows locked, bear down on the victim's chest, compressing it 1½ to 2 inches.

• Compress the chest for half a second, then relax for a half second. Repeat. Count "1 and 2 and 3 and 4 and 5." Each time you reach 5 you should have done 5 compressions.

• After 15 compressions, take your hands off the chest and place them on the neck and forehead as before. Pinch the nostrils and administer 2 strong breaths into the victim's mouth.

• Do 15 more chest compressions. After 4 cycles of chest compressions and mouth-to-mouth breathing, check again for pulse and breathing.

• If neither pulse nor breathing have returned, resume until medical help arrives, or the victim revives, or you can no longer continue. Don't give up too soon!

Thanks and credit to EVERYBODY'S GUIDE TO HOMEOPATHIC MEDICINES *for this section. It is a needed family reference.*

Can't find a recommended product? Call the 800 number listed in Product Resources for the store nearest you.

Sinus Infections
Sinusitis

For 92 million Americans (1 in 3), a chronic sinus infection is a daily energy drain. The sinuses are thin, air-filled chambers in the cartilage around the nose, sides of the forehead, between the nasal passages, the eye sockets and in the cheekbones. When sinus openings are obstructed, mucous and infected pus collect in these pockets causing pain and swelling. Sinusitis is an inflammation of the sinus mucous membranes; chronic sinusitis may cause nasal polyps and scar tissue. New research shows that chronic sinusitis may be a fungal infection. Suppressive over-the-counter sinus medications can both trigger an infection by not allowing the draining of infective material, and aggravate it by driving the infection deeper into the sinus cavities. Natural healing methods revolve around relieving the cause of the clogging and inflammation.

Diet & Superfood Therapy

Nutritional therapy plan:

1–Go on a short 3 day mucous cleansing liquid diet. (pg. 196). Take a glass of lemon juice and water each morning to thin mucous secretions. Take an onion/garlic each day or mix fresh grated horseradish root with lemon juice in a spoon. Take and hang over a sink to expel lots of mucous all at once.

2–Add fresh carrot juice the 1st day. Add a pineapple/papaya juice, or dilute pineapple juice the 2nd day. Add a glass of apple juice the 3rd day.

3–Then, eat only fresh foods for the rest of the week to cleanse encrusted mucous deposits. Drink 8 glasses of healthy liquids, including broths, herb teas and water to relieve congestion.

4–Add plenty of garlic, onions and mustard to your diet. Slowly add whole grains, vegetable protein, and cultured foods like Rejuvenative Foods VEGI-DELITE to your own tolerance.

5–Avoid heavy starches, red meats, pasteurized dairy products, caffeine and refined sugars for at least 3 months.

–Effective superfoods: (choose 1 or 2)
• CC Pollen DYNAMIC TRIO drink/capsules.
• Crystal Star ZINC SOURCE™ drops in water as a nasal rinse or on back of the tongue.
• Mona's CHLORELLA regenerates immunity.
• Herbal Answers ALOE FORCE juice.

Herb & Supplement Therapy

–Interceptive therapy plan: (Choose 2 to 3 recommendations)

1–**Address the infection:** • Crystal Star ANTI-BIO™ caps and • FIRST AID CAPS™ 2-3x daily each for a week. Then • ALRG™ caps, • ALR-HST™ tea, or • ALRG-HST™ extract for 1 week. Or use • Nutribiotic GRAPEFRUIT SEED extract diluted as directed - antibiotic nasal rinse. • Osha root tea, gentle anti-viral; ⊛ Nutricology PRO-LIVE olive leaf extract tabs as directed.

2–**Relieve congestion:** • Vitamin C therapy: Use Ester C powder with bioflavonoids, $1/4$ teasp. every hour to bowel tolerance during acute phase. And dissolve vitamin C crystals in water and drip into nose with eye-dropper. • *Echinacea* extract 15 drops 4x daily; • *Ephedra* tea; • *Lobelia* extract drops in water; • Zand DECONGEST HERBAL; • Nature's Path NASAL-LYTE; • Prevail SINEASE.

3–**Reduce inflammation:** • Quercetin 1000mg with bromelain 1500mg daily or • Source Naturals ACTIVATED QUERCETIN. • Propolis tincture drops ⚥ or high potency royal jelly 2 teasp. daily. ♀

4–**Cleanse the lymph system and sinus passages:** *Fenugreek/thyme* tea; *nettles* tea.

–**Cleanse sinuses with sea salt water:** make a solution of $1/4$ teasp. sea salt to 1 cup warm water. Close one nostril and inhale enough solution through other nostril to be able to spit it out your mouth. Repeat daily for 1 month; or use • *Calendula* tea as a nasal wash.

–**For nasal polyps from sinus infection:** Make a water solution of *goldenseal*, *echinacea* and *myrrh* powders - snuff up the nose to thoroughly rinse nasal sinuses.

5–**For long term relief:** use • USNEA extract, or • Crystal Star BIO-VI™ extract; *garlic* caps 4 to 6 daily; • CoQ$_{10}$ 60mg 3x daily. Add • Beta carotene 50,000IU and • N-acetyl-cysteine (NAC) 500mg, each 2x daily. Add • zinc picolinate 50mg, or • zinc lozenges or • Source Naturals OPTI-ZINC. • *Astragalus* extract drops. • B-complex 100mg with pantothenic acid 500mg, and B$_{12}$ 2000mcg sublingually daily. Biotec CELLGUARD 6 daily during high risk seasons.

–Homeopathic remedies: • Boiron SINUSITIS tabs; • BioForce SINUS RELIEF drops; • *Euphorbium* nasal spray; • *Euphrasia*; • *Kali bichromium*.

Lifestyle Support Therapy

–Bodywork:
• Take a hot sauna for 20 minutes daily during acute phase.
• Steam face and head with *eucalyptus/mullein*, or a *chamomile* steam.
• Mix several drops of *tea tree oil* in a vaporizer. Use at night for clear morning sinuses.
• Apply hot compresses to sinus area: 1) *ginger*; 2) *comfrey/fenugreek*; 3) *mullein/lobelia*. Alternate with cold compresses for best results.
• Apply TIGER BALM or Chinese WHITE FLOWER OIL to sinus area.

–**Acupressure points:** (Acupuncture is effective for chronic sinusitis.)

Massage under the big toes for 1 minute.

Squeeze ends of each finger and thumb hard for 20 seconds.

Press your thumb and index finger gently on the top of your nose on either side for 5 seconds. Repeat 3 times.

–Reflexology points:

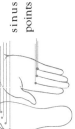

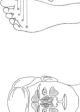

sinus points

Common Symptoms: *Difficult breathing; pressure headaches, a mucous-clogged head; acute throbbing pain in the upper jaw and forehead; runny nose and inflamed nasal passages; post-nasal drip with greenish discharge coughed up; sore throat; indigestion because of mucous overload; facial pain, earaches, toothaches, pain behind the eyes; loss of smell and taste; bad breath from low grade infection.*

Common Causes: *Fungal, viral or bacterial infection, often triggered by an allergy condition; too many mucous-forming foods, like pasteurized dairy products and refined sugar; too many salty, fried foods; poor food combining; lack of green vegetables; constipation and poor circulation; lack of exercise and deep breathing; sometimes overuse of nose drops from the benzalkonium chloride preserver in the drops.*

See my book COOKING FOR HEALTHY HEALING for a complete diet for respiratory health.

Can't find a recommended product? Call the 800 number listed in Product Resources for the store nearest you.

Skin

Health and Beauty

Beautiful skin is more than skin deep. The skin is the body's largest organ of both nourishment and elimination. The skin's protective acid mantle inhibits the growth of disease-causing bacteria. Skin mirrors our emotional state and our hormone balance, and is a sure sign of poor nutrition. (Allergies show up first on the skin.) Skin problems reflect a stressed lifestyle almost immediately. Our skin is the essence of renewable nature...it sloughs off old, dying cells every day, and gives a chance for a new start. Herbal nutrients are great for skin - packed with absorbable minerals, antioxidants, EFA's and bioflavonoids to cleanse, hydrate, heal, alkalize, and balance. Relaxation, nourishment and improved nutrition also show quickly in skin health and beauty.

Diet & Superfood Therapy

—Nutritional therapy plan:

1—Great skin starts with a good diet: Eat potassium-rich foods if your skin is dry: leafy greens, spinach, bell peppers, bananas, broccoli, sesame and sunflower seeds, fish and sea greens.

2—Eat cultured foods: yogurt, tofu and kefir.

3—Eat cleansing foods: fresh fruit, vegetable and fruit juices, celery, cucumbers. Eat vitamin C, E, carotene-rich foods: sea foods and fresh greens.

4—Drink 6 glasses of water every day. Drink watermelon juice when it is available - rich in natural silica to keep the system flushed and alkaline.

6—Eliminate red meats, fried, fatty and fast foods. Reduce caffeine, dairy foods and salty, sugary foods. They show up on your skin.

—Kitchen cosmetic face lifts: apply, leave on 30 minutes and rinse off.

Yogurt to balance pH

Oatmeal to exfoliate

Egg whites for wrinkles

•Make your own AHA wrinkle treatment with a mix of honey and red wine. Smooth on; leave on 20 minutes. Rinse off.

—Effective superfoods: (choose 1)

•Crystal Star BIOFLAV, FIBER, C SUPPORT™.

•Herbal Answers HERBAL ALOE FORCE juice.

•Premier ONE ROYAL JELLY/GINSENG.

Herb & Supplement Therapy

—Interceptive therapy plan: (Choose 2 to 3 recommendations)

1—Essential fatty acids are critical for dry skin: Eat •chia and sunflower seeds; •Evening primrose oil 4000mg daily; •Nature's Secret ULTIMATE OIL; •Sesame seed oil, nourishes while cleaning off eye make-up; •Aloe vera gel; •Barleans flax oil caps 3 daily. •Zia ULTIMATE MOISTURE; •Vitamin A & D 25,000/1,000.

2—Blood cleansers: •Crystal Star SKIN THERAPY #1™ and SKIN THERAPY #2 caps; •Herbs Etc. DERMATONIC; •Sarsaparilla extract; •Dandelion caps 4 daily.

3—Plant enzymes keep free radical damage from showing up on your face: •Enzymedica PURIFY; Nature's Apothecary SKIN SUPPORT; •Crystal Star BEAUTIFUL SKIN gel; •Rosemary extract drops; •Nature's Path SKIN CREAM LYTE.

4—Smoothing/hydrators for skin: •MSM, 1000mg daily for soft, pliable skin; •Cysteine 1000mg for smooth skin. Pat on •Lavender to reduce puffiness; Rose hips tea-lemon juice blend to tighten; •Chamomile tea to tone; •Sandlewood or rose essential aromatherapy oils to hydrate. •**Make my sea plant facial for rapid moisture and tone:** sprinkle about 1 teasp. kelp granules in a small bowl. Blend with 1 tablespoon aloe vera gel. Apply to face and neck. Leave on 10 minutes, rinse.

5—Balancers for too oily, shiny skin: •Earth's Bounty O₂ SPRAY. •Lavender essential oil; •Zia OIL CONTROL extract; •Jojoba oil; •a green clay mask.

6—Total skin support: •Dr. Diamond HERPANACINE 2 daily; •Biotec AGELESS BEAUTY 6 daily; •Crystal Star BEAUTIFUL SKIN™ tea; internally and externally (pat on problem spots); •Ester C with bioflavs., 3000mg daily; •Crystal Star GREEN TEA CLEANSER™ each morning. **Collagen support for supple skin:** •Flora VEGESIL 3 daily; •PCO's 150mg daily; apply •CC Pollen PROPOLIS SKIN CREAM •Derma-E PYCNOGENOL MOISTURIZER; •Jason ESTER C lotion.

Vitamins feed the skin, so nutrition deficits don't show up on the skin. Use •Orjene 7 VITAMIN TREATMENT CREAM; or **Make a vitamin facial once a week:** •Prick open and squeeze 1 vit. A & D 25,000IU, and 1 vitamin E 400IU cap. Grind up 1 zinc 30mg tab and 1 PABA 100mg tab. Mix with 2 teasp. wheat germ oil, flax or jojoba oil and pat on face. Let dry and rinse off.

Lifestyle Support Therapy

—Bodywork:

•Use a gentle, balancing mask once a week. Follow with a blend of aloe vera gel and vitamin E oil.

•Swirl 3TBS honey in bath water for silky skin.

•Apply body lotion after your shower **before** you dry off for the most moisture to your skin.

•Get 20 minutes of early morning sunlight on the skin for Vitamin D.

•Get daily exercise for better skin tone.

•Cosmetic acupuncture and acupressure treatments are effective for skin problems.

•**My own nourishing make-up remover:** Mix in a dark bottle, avocado, almond and sesame oils - makes your skin feel wonderful.

—Exfoliate for glowing skin:

•Loofa sponge, ayate cloth, dry skin brush

•Rub with cucumber or papaya skins

•Rub with a honey/almond/oatmeal scrub

•Crystal Star LEMON BODY GLOW™

—Skin detox cleansers and pH balancers:

•Zia SEA TONIC with aloe.

•Crystal Star HOT SEAWEED BATH™.

•Lemon juice to restore acid mantle.

•Olive oil soap.

•CamoCare FACIAL THERAPY.

•Sage or Burdock root tea.

•Aubrey BLUE-GREEN ALGAE cleanser.

•Jason SUMA moisturizer.

•Herbal Answers ALOE FORCE gel.

Common Symptoms: Unbalanced skin and acid mantle, with sores, spots, cracks, oiliness or dryness, scaling, itching, chapping, redness and rashes.

Common Causes: Emotional stress; poor diet of excess refined foods and sugars; too many saturated fats; caffeine overload; food allergies that cause redness; too high copper levels causing blotching; poor digestion and assimilation; PMS; too much sun; irritating cosmetics; essential fatty acid and bioflavonoid depletion; liver malfunction.

See the following pages for more information about skin problems.

Can't find a recommended product? Call the 800 number listed in Product Resources for the store nearest you.

Skin - Aging

Dry, Wrinkled Skin, Brown Age Spots and Liver Spots

Skin aging is due to: skin cells overloaded with toxins; poor circulation preventing oxygen delivery; dehydration; shrunken skin tissues from lack of fatty acids and muscle tone. Age spots are an external sign of waste accumulation, especially in the liver, (shows up as sallow skin), and of free radical damage in skin cells. Lipofuscin is the age-related skin pigment that oxidizes to actually appear as brown age spots. Wrinkles, lines and rough skin texture are a sign of poor dermal collagen health. When collagen becomes hard and crosslinks with neighboring collagen fibers, skin can't hold moisture or maintain elasticity. It collapses on itself, forming a fish net below the surface of the skin, seen as wrinkles. Crosslinking occurs from free radical attacks on skin cell membranes, collagen and elastin proteins, resulting in wrinkles, dry skin and sagging skin contours.

Diet & Superfood Therapy

—Nutritional therapy plan:

1—Age spots and a yellowish, old skin look are signs that the liver is throwing off metabolic wastes through the skin. Go on a short liver detox cleansing diet (pg. 205) to cleanse accumulated toxins. Then drink carrot/beet/cucumber juice once a week for the next month to keep the liver clean.

2—The continuing diet should include lots of vegetable proteins from whole grains, seafoods, sprouts and soy foods; mineral-rich foods, like leafy greens, onions, cruciferous vegetables and molasses; and foods rich in beta carotene, vitamin E and C, like carrots, greens, sea greens, broccoli.

3—Make a skin food mix of lecithin granules, wheat germ, brewer's yeast, molasses; take 2 TBS daily in juice.

4—Drink 8 glasses of water or healthy liquids daily; include a glass of lemon juice and water; apply lemon juice to age spots.

5—Avoid refined sugars, red meats, and caffeine containing foods. They dry out your skin. Avoid rancid nuts and oils.

—Effective superfoods: (choose 1)

• Herbal Answers ALOE FORCE juice.
• Crystal Star BIOFLAV. FIBER & C SUPPORT™.
• Red Star NUTRITIONAL YEAST or Bio-Strath original LIQUID YEAST for skin B's.
• Crystal Star SYSTEMS STRENGTH™.

Herb & Supplement Therapy

—Interceptive therapy plan: (Choose 2 to 3 recommendations)

1—For age spots: • Ginkgo Biloba extract helps prevent lipofuscin build-up; • Arginine blocks enzyme glycosylation 2000mg daily. Apply • Dong Quai extract to to spots; or • Licorice root lightens age spots; • Reviva BROWN SPOT REMOVER; • Crystal Star ADR-ACTIVE™ caps for freckling. Apply • Earth's Bounty O₂ SPRAY gel to age spots before bed. Results in 1 to 3 months. • Try 2% hydroquinone cream-reacts with your skin's enzymes to block melanin production of spots.

2—For wrinkles: • Apply chamomile tea or • CamoCare Gold AM and PM; • CoQ-10, 100mg 3x daily and apply • CoQ-10 gel; • PCO's 100mg daily and apply • Derma-E PYCNOGENOL MOISTURIZER. Apply • Transitions PRO-GEST CREAM 2x daily for 3 months; • MSM, 1000mg daily for soft, pliable skin; • Aubrey Organics BLUE GREEN ALGAE moisturizer; • Alta Health SILICA with BIOFLAVS. **Vitamins help take out wrinkles:** Take • Vitamin E 400IU; or apply 1 teasp. aloe vera gel mixed with 1 teasp. vitamin E oil; Carotenes are critical for collagen: • PHYCOTENE MICROCLUSTERS available at Healthy House. • Earth Science micro-encapsulated ANTIOXIDANT TONER; • Biotec AGELESS BEAUTY 8 daily.

3—Combat sun aging with EFA's: sea greens rehydrate your skin and hold moisture. • Eat 2 TBS dry, snipped sea greens over rice, soup or salad, or 6 pieces of sushi a day, (noticeable in 3 to 4 weeks). • Evening primrose oil caps 4 daily; • Spectrum ESSENTIAL MAX EFA oil for eye skin; • Zia ULTIMATE C-SERUM; • Abra Therapeutics GREEN TEA PHYTO-SERUM. • Steam face with a mix of EFA herbs: chamomile, eucalyptus, rosemary and nettles for tone.

4—Renew skin elasticity: Estrogen-collagen helps. Effective phyto-estrogen herbs: • Crystal Star EST-AID™ caps 4 daily; CC Pollen ROYAL JELLY skin cream; • Earth Science BETA GINSENG cream; • Crystal Star GINSENG SKIN REPAIR gel™; • Premier One ROYAL JELLY 2 teasp. daily; or • Earth Science GINSIUM-C cream. **5—AHA's have new benefits:** even skin tone, less wrinkles, brown spots and skin scaliness, less oiliness, normalize too thin skin. • Zia EVEN SMOOTHER or • CITRUS NIGHT REVERSAL; • Nonie of Beverly Hills PROTEIN CONDITIONER.

Lifestyle Support Therapy

—Lifestyle measures:

• Reduce your stress with relaxation techniques. Massage therapy releases toxins from lymph glands and tones facial muscles. Softening skin massages oils: jojoba oil, sesame oil, wheat germ oil, or aloe vera gel.

• Avoid tobacco. Tar and nicotine deprive skin of oxygen, causing shriveling, wrinkling.

• Use sunscreen regularly - SPF 15 or greater. Sunscreens prevent age spots from darkening.

—For facial rejuvenation:

• Get plenty of fresh air; exercise at least three times a week.

• Cosmetic acupuncture treatments.

• A seaweed facial once a week for velvety skin sprinkle about 1 teasp. kelp granules in a small bowl. Blend with 1 TB aloe vera gel. Apply to face and neck. Leave on 10 minutes, rinse.

• Anti-wrinkle food facials, like rubbing the insides of fresh papaya skins on the face, or patting on a mix of whipped egg white and cream. Let dry 20 minutes. Rinse off.

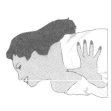

See the following pages for more information on other skin problems.

Can't find a recommended product? Call the 800 number listed in Product Resources for the store nearest you.

Common Symptoms: Brown mottled spots on the hands, neck and face. Sallow, old-looking skin; dry skin with evident lines and wrinkles.

Common Causes: Free radical damage caused by smog and environmental pollutants, too much sun exposure, especially with a thinned ozone layer; stress, poor diet, liver malfunction and exhaustion; skin dehydration often caused by hormone (estrogen) depletion; too much tobacco, fried foods, caffeine, and alcohol; broken capillaries; weak vein walls; long term use of hair colors and permanents; some birth control.

Skin, Cellulite

Fatty Deposits Showing through the Skin

Cellulite is a combination of fat, water and trapped wastes beneath the skin - usually on otherwise thin women. When circulation and elimination processes become impaired, connective tissue loses its strength. Unmetabolized fats and wastes become trapped in vulnerable cells just beneath the skin instead of being expelled through normal means. Over time, the waste materials harden and form the puckering skin effect we know as cellulite. Because it is unattached material, dieting and exercise alone can't dislodge cellulite. An effective program for cellulite release should be in four parts: 1) Stimulate elimination functions; 2) Increase circulation and metabolism; 3) Control excess fluid and waste retention; 4) Reestablish connective tissue elasticity.

Diet & Superfood Therapy

—Nutritional therapy plan:

1—Your diet can help empty fat cells and carry off wastes.

2—Eat fruits and juices in the morning. Have 2 fresh or steamed vegetables at every meal. Have a fresh salad and brown rice once a day.

3—Add flushers every day: pineapple (bromelain), apples and berries (pectin fiber) and citrus (vitamin C) to free trapped toxins. Drink 6 to 8 glasses of water, juices and green tea every day.

4—Balance estrogen: add cruciferous veggies like broccoli to keep excess estrogen flushed. Have Omega-rich fish and seafood twice a week. Have 2 TBS snipped dried sea greens 3 or 4 times a week in a soup, salad or rice; or 6 pcs. sushi daily.

5—Graze - eat smaller, more frequent meals, instead of 2 to 3 large ones.

—The cellulite blacklist:

• All fried and fatty foods; • High caffeine, carbonated sodas, hard liquor; • Red meats; • Full-fat, pasteurized dairy foods; • Extra salty foods (use herbal seasoning).

—Effective superfoods: (choose 1)

• Crystal Star BIOFLAV., FIBER & C SUPPORT for collagen support.

• Carrot/beet/cucumber juice, to clean the liver so it can metabolize fats better.

Herb & Supplement Therapy

—Interceptive therapy plan: (Choose 2 to 4 recommendations)

1—**Release trapped fats and shrink cellulite cells:** • Crystal Star HOT SEAWEED BATH™ stimulate circulation and potentiate lipolysis. • Crystal Star THERMO-CEL-LEAN™ roll-on gel with CEL-LEAN™ caps (also helps balance hormones) or CEL-LEAN RELEASE™ tea before meals. • Biotec AGELESS BEAUTY tabs dissolve, flush rancid fats and wastes. • Nonie of Beverly Hills AHA SKIN CLEANSER.

2—**Stimulate the liver to metabolize fats better instead of storing them:** • Crystal Star LIV-ALIVE™ tea and AMINO-ZYME caps; • Milk Thistle Seed extract; • Source Naturals SUPER AMINO NIGHT caps; • Rainbow Light TRIM-ZYME. • Bromelain 1500mg daily to break down proteins and help metabolize fats.

3—**Raise metabolic rate to burn cellulite fat:** • Crystal Star THERMO-CITRIN GINSENG™ caps, or • Co-enzyme A Technology BODY IMAGE for thermogenesis assistance; • Crystal Star META-TABS capsules to stimulate thyroid function.

4—**Essential fatty acids speed fat digestion, improve skin texture:** • Evening Primrose Oil 3000mg daily; • Soy lecithin caps 1400mg 4x daily; • Borage oil caps 1000mg 2x daily (also reduces swelling); • Omega Nutrition ESSENTIAL BALANCE caps.

5—**Repair / tighten connective tissue to free trapped wastes:** • Crystal Star SILICA SOURCE™ extract for collagen support; • Body Essentials SILICA GEL internally, 1 TB in 3-oz. liquid, externally on problem areas; • Solaray CENTELLA VEIN caps; • Bilberry extract; • grape seed PCO's 100mg 2x daily; • Eidon SILICA moisturizer.

6—**Stimulate circulation to cellulite areas and strengthen capillary network:** • Ginkgo Biloba extract, 120mg daily; • Grape seed extract caps 100mg 2x daily.

—Rub-on cellulite-fighting essential oils:

• Antioxidant oils rosemary and thyme.
• Peppermint oil to increase metabolism.
• Juniper to stimulate circulation.
• Apply Earth's Bounty O₂ SPRAY to fatty areas. (In some cases the fat globules release by coming out through the skin in little white bumps.)

Lifestyle Support Therapy

—Bodywork:

• Kneading massage: from periphery toward the heart. Use a dry skin brush, loofa or ayate cloth to stimulate lymph glands.

• Regular stretching exercise: burns fat, tones muscles, increases circulation and maintains underlying tissue integrity. An arm-swinging daily walk, especially after a large meal helps maintain a slim subcutaneous fat layer.

• Get a spa body wrap: It's a rapid fluid and a inch-loss treatment. While you're at the spa get a massage treatment. It helps release even more trapped fats.

• Take a seaweed bath to release trapped toxins in the cells.

—Do thigh creams work? Some of them do. Natural products don't have the risky side affects. Choose one with AHA's, herbal antioxidants and theophyllisilane for better skin tone. • Jason THIGH THERAPY NIGHTTIME, and THIGH Rx DAYTIME gel and body spray. • Chae BODY THERAPY.

—Reflexology point:

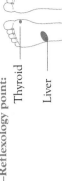

Thyroid

Liver

S 499

Common Symptoms: Lumpy, rippled skin around thighs, hips and love handles; trapped waste and fluid in pockets beneath the skin. When regular fat is squeezed the skin appears smooth - cellulitic skin will ripple like an orange peel, or have the texture of cottage cheese. Tightness, heaviness in the legs; soreness and tenderness when tissue is massaged.

Common Causes: Sometimes a family trait, more often poor nutrition resulting in liver exhaustion and reduced fat metabolism. Inadequate exercise; poor elimination and sluggish circulation; insufficient water intake; imbalanced estrogen activity; crash dieting with rapid regain of weight. Smoking impedes both circulation and metabolism. Be careful of too much sun. UV rays contribute to cellulite.

See WEIGHT LOSS, pages 518-522 or my book Cooking For Healthy Healing for more.

Can't find a recommended product? Call the 800 number listed in Product Resources for the store nearest you.

Skin - Infections

Dermatitis, Inflamed Itches and Rashes, Ulcerations

Dermatitis is an external skin condition caused by a systemic reaction to an allergen - usually in cosmetics, jewelry metals, drugs or topical medications. It can also be the body's reaction to emotional stress, or to a severe deficiency of essential fatty acids. Its systemic nature means that it can and does spread, and can become quite severe. Inflamed skin with itch and rash symptoms can come from a wide variety of causes, ranging from systemic to emotional stress, from food allergies to an infective reaction to cosmetics. Investigate the cause of your symptoms thoroughly before you attempt treatment to get best results.

Diet & Superfood Therapy

—Nutritional therapy plan:

1—Rashes are often symptoms of food allergy, avoid common allergens, such as milk and wheat products, eggs, meats (that usually have nitrates), refined foods, sugar and fried foods.

2—Go on a short 3 day juice cleanse (page 191) to clear acid waste from the system. Drink lemon water in the morning to neutralize acids if the condition is chronic body imbalance.

3—Then eat a diet full of leafy greens, and other mineral-rich foods, such as sea vegetables to re-build healthy tissue and good adrenal function.

4—Use poly or mono-unsaturated oils. Reduce both dietary fats and total calories.

5—Eat cultured foods frequently for healthy G.I. flora.

6—Avoid fried foods, red meats, caffeine, chocolate, pasteurized dairy products, and sugary carbohydrates.

7—Make a skin mix of ¼ cup each: wheat germ, molasses and brewer's yeast; take 2 TBS daily.

—Effective superfoods: (choose 1 or 2)
- Crystal Star BIOFLAV., FIBER & C SUPPORT™ drink.
- Green Foods CARROT ESSENCE and WHEAT GERM concentrates for liver support.
- George's high sulphur ALOE juice.
- Solgar WHEY TO GO protein drink.

Herb & Supplement Therapy

—Interceptive therapy plan: (Choose 2 or 3 recommendations)

1—**Control the infection:** •Crystal Star ANTI-BIO™ gel as needed, and •ANTI-BIO™ caps 6 daily. •Nutribiotic GRAPEFRUIT SEED extract, or mix 4 drops in 5-oz. water and apply directly, or use the spray; •St. John's wort oil, or •Nature's Apothecary HERBAL FIRST AID oil; •Nutricology GERMANIUM 150mg; •GINKGO BILOBA extract 3-4x daily; •Allergy Research OREGANO OIL as directed.

2—**Form new smooth skin:** •Flora VEGE-SIL for healthy new growth. •Crystal Star SILICA SOURCE™, or •Alta Health SILICA with BIOFLAVONOIDS for collagen formation. •MSM, 1000mg daily; •Vitamin C therapy: ascorbate C powder; mix with water to a solution. Apply to area, and take 1 teasp. every hour for collagen-connective tissue growth. •Stress B-complex 100mg 2x daily with extra Biotin 600mcg. ♂

3—**For inflamed skin rash and eruptions:** Crystal Star ANTI-HST™ capsules, 4-6 daily to relieve a typical histamine weal-type rash. Very effective. Homeopathic *Urtica urens*, or *Natrum muriaticum*. •Burdock tea 3x daily; make a paste of •vitamin C powder and aloe vera juice and apply. •Place cold wet *chamomile* tea bags on inflamed area or a compress of cold *chamomile* tea; •mix 3 drops of lavender essential oil in 4 TBS aloe vera gel and apply. •*devil's claw* extract; •Crystal Star THERADERM™ or •BEAUTIFUL SKIN™ capsules, 4 daily. Apply to rash and drink •HERBAL ITCH TEA: *dandelion root, burdock root, echinacea root, kelp, yellow dock root, chamomile*. •Quercetin 1000mg daily with bromelain 1500mg daily; •Zinc 50mg. 2x daily. ♂

4—**Essential fatty acids for smooth skin:** •Evening primrose oil 4 daily; •Barleans lignan rich omega-3 flax oil 3 daily; •Nature's Secret ULTIMATE OIL •Apply wheat germ oil; •*Suma* caps 3-4 daily. ♂ •Country Life MAXIMUM SKIN CARE.

5—**Effective skin healing applications:** •*Aloe vera* gel mixed with goldenseal powder. •Crystal Star BEAUTIFUL SKIN TEA™ - apply to neutralize acids coming out on the skin; apply •BEAUTIFUL SKIN™ gel to a minor rash (sometimes overnight results). •PHYCOTENE CREAM available at Healthy House. •Apply A, D & E oil, take emulsified A & D oil caps; •Prime Pharm. PRIMADERM cream.

6—**For pH balance:** •Prof. Nutrition Dr. DOPHILUS; •Pancreatin 1300mg.

Lifestyle Support Therapy

—Lifestyle measures:
- •Get early morning sunlight on the skin every day possible for healing vitamin D.
- •Take an oatmeal bath for itchy skin.
- •Avoid detergents on the skin. Use mild castile soap. Avoid perfumed cosmetics.

—Effective skin healers:
- •B & T CALIFLORA gel
- •Body Essentials SILICA GEL
- •*Calendula* gel for ulcerations
- •Enzyme Therapy DERMA-KLEAR cream
- •Crystal Star LYSINE/LICORICE™ gel
- •Earth's Bounty O₂ SPRAY
- •Fresh *comfrey* leaf compresses
- •*Tea tree* oil if fungus is the cause
- •PCO's 100mg daily and apply Derma-E PYCNOGENOL MOISTURIZER
- •Aubrey Org. COLLAGEN therapy cream
- •Beehive Botanicals DERMA CREAM

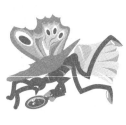

S 500

See FUNGAL SKIN INFECTIONS page 390 for more information.

Can't find a recommended product? Call the 800 number listed in Product Resources for the store nearest you.

Common Symptoms: Inflamed, dry, thickened skin patches; oozing skin blisters; scaby, lumpy skin; itching skin. Tingling, unpleasant skin prickling; redness, eczema-like rash; scaling and bumps on the skin.
Common Causes: EFA deficiency; allergic skin reaction to cosmetics, acid-forming foods like dairy products, pleasure or prescription drugs, or topical medications; emotional stress; poor liver activity resulting in poor metabolism. Liver malfunction or exhaustion; allergic reaction; stress and anxiety; detergents; over-acid system; drug after-effects and side-effects; poor diet with too many refined and chemical foods.

Skin - Damaged
Scars, Sunburn, Stretch Marks

For every sunburn you get that blisters, you double your risk of skin cancer. Even on a cloudy day, 80% of the sun's harmful UV rays come through. Sun damage is cumulative over a lifetime. Moderation is the key. Sunlight can help you avoid breast and prostate cancer (new research shows that a lack of protective vitamin D provided by sunlight may be involved). People who get almost no sun exposure are at higher risk for melanoma than those who get regular, moderate early morning sunshine. Practice good sun sense so that you don't fry now and pay later. Note: I don't recommend tanning beds as an alternative. They may seem safe, but have actually been implicated in accelerated aging of the skin, cataracts and immune system disorders.

Diet & Superfood Therapy

—**Nutritional therapy plan:**

1—Have a veggie drink 3x a week during healing stage. (pg. 218 or see below).

2—Eat a high vegetable protein diet for faster healing. Include plenty of whole grains, sprouts, tofu, and a protein drink every morning, (see below). Eat avocados for skin elasticity.

3—Make a healing skin mix of brewer's yeast, wheat germ, lecithin granules; take 2 TBS daily.

4—Drink 6-8 glasses of mineral water daily to rehydrate from within.

—**Electrolytes for sunburn healing / skin fluid replacement:** Effervescent C 2 packets daily, such as Alacer EMERGEN-C; Potassium broth (pg. 215); Crystal Star SYSTEMS STRENGTH™; Knudsen's ELECTROLYTE drink. No alcoholic beverages - they dehydrate.

•For sunburns: apply yogurt, black tea, oatmeal compresses or vinegar to burned areas. Apply grated apple to burned eyelids for fast relief.

—**Effective superfoods: (choose one)**
•Crystal Star ENERGY GREEN™ drink.
•Nutricology PRO-GREENS with EFA's.
•AloeLife ALOE GOLD juice.
•Beehive Botanicals or Y.S. GINSENG/ROYAL JELLY. Take and also apply.

Herb & Supplement Therapy

—**Interceptive therapy plan: (Choose 2 to 3 recommendations)**

1—For scars: •Transformation PROTEASE caps as directed (excellent results); •Crystal Star GINSENG SKIN REPAIR GEL with vitamin C for 2 to 3 months; •GOTU KOLA (*centella asiatica*) extract caps 4 daily; apply •fresh pineapple to scar and take Bromelain 1500mg daily for 3 months. •Aloe vera or *calendula* gel; Phyto-estrogen herbs like *dong quai, vitex, black cohosh* stimulate better estrogen supply for skin healing. •Vitamin E 400IU daily; prick a capsule and apply externally.

Heal the skin with minerals: •Nature's Path TRACE-LYTE with sea greens; •Nutricology GERMANIUM 150mg, for at least a month. Silicon skin healing treatment takes 3 to 4 months: •Alta Health SILICA with BIOFLAVONOIDS; •Crystal Star SILICA SOURCE™ drops; apply •Body Essentials SILICA GEL.

2—Apply and take EFA's: •Herbal Answers ALOE FORCE skin gel; •Evening Primrose Oil 4000mg daily; •Omega Nutrition ESSENTIAL BALANCE, 2 daily.

3—Sunburn protection: •Alpha lipoic acid 400-600mg daily shields from oxidative damage; •vitamin A 50,000IU WITH calcium 500mg; •Zinc 50mg daily; apply zinc oxide cream. Prevention is the key. If your tissues are loaded with carotene A, vitamin C, E and B complex, your skin stands much less chance of damage by the sun. •B-complex 100mg daily with extra PABA caps 1000mg and PABA cream.

Effective herbal topicals for sunburns: •*Sea buckthorne* oil (also heals radiation burns); •shea butter cream; •CamoCare CHAMOMILE OINTMENT; •Beehive Botanicals PROPOLIS & HONEY; •*Tea tree* oil (with natural SPF); •*Calendula* gel; •Apply a wheat germ oil, A & D oil, *comfrey* leaf and honey poultice (good for stretch marks, too). •CC Pollen PROPOLIS SKIN CREAM •AHA's reduce sunburn wrinkling, like Noni of Beverly Hills PROTEIN CONDITIONER.

4—Antioxidants protect skin: •*Ginkgo biloba* extract 100mg daily; •PCO's 100mg daily and apply •Derma-E PYCNOGENOL MOISTURIZER; •Beta carotene 100,000IU; •Vitamin C therapy, up to 5000mg during acute stage; pat a C solution on burned areas. •Take MSM with MICROHYDRIN available from Healthy House to repair age, sun-damaged skin. •Tyrosine 1000mg daily, is a tan activator.

Lifestyle Support Therapy

—**Sun sense skin burn prevention:**
•Minimize exposure to mid-day sun.
•Wear sunglasses with 100% UV filters.
•Use a sunscreen with SPF 15 or more. Make sure it contains Vitamin E.
•Wear a lip balm with sunscreen.
•Drink plenty of water before, after and during exposure to replenish and moisturize your skin from within.

•Avoid photo-sensitive drugs: antibiotics, diuretics, hypoglycemia drugs, soaps w. hexa-chlorophene, and Phenergan in creams. Check labels.

•For sun damage take a cool bath immediately (no soap or hot water); apply cold compresses to really burned areas.

—**For stretch marks:** Massage aloe vera gel mixed with vitamin E oil on stomach. Some women have success with shea butter or AHAs.

—**For scars:** Massage the scar thoroughly to bring up healthy circulation and skin tone.
•Home Health SCAR-GO.
•Mtn. Ocean MOTHER'S BLEND oil.
•Earth's Bounty O₂ SPRAY.
•Sesame oil, wheat germ oil or avocado oil.

See page 45 for a facial surgery scar healing program.

Common Symptoms: Non-healing or slow healing skin wounds, often with continuing redness, roughness, and irregular weals. Sunburned, dehydrated skin: overreaction to heat and sun exposure; loss of skin elasticity; headache; numbness; high blood pressure and/or rapid pulse. Stretch marks: from post-pregnancy stretching or serious weight-loss dieting.
Common Causes and High Risk Factors: Having had frequent sunburns as a child; living at high altitude; being on immuno-suppressive therapy; heavy use of sun lamps or a tanning bed; having light-colored eyes and hair, fair or freckled skin; moving from a northern climate to the south; working all day outdoors. Protein, vitamin A & D deficiency, zinc and other mineral deficiency.

Can't find a recommended product? Call the 800 number listed in Product Resources for the store nearest you.

Therapy For Other Skin Problems

Your skin heals from the inside out. Don't forget the importance of diet and nutrition to skin regeneration.

—**WHITE HARD BUMPS ON UPPER ARMS and CHEST: Effective natural therapies:** •Vitamin A 25,000IU 2 daily, •zinc picolinate 50mg daily; •Ester C 550mg with bioflavonoids 3 daily. Dab with pineapple juice and take •bromelain 1500mg daily. Take •EFA's: *Evening Primrose oil*, Omega-3 flax oil 3x daily, or Spectrum EVENING PRIMROSE 1300mg. Use a dry skin brush on the areas morning and night until skin is pink from increased circulation. This gives your skin oxygen, sloughs off dead cells and speeds up cell renewal.

—**VITILIGO (leukoderma):** A progressive immune system disorder causing depigmentation of the skin when the body stops making melanin. Some effectiveness has been shown when treated as for radiation poisoning after 6 to 9 months of treatment (see page 44). **Effective natural therapies:** The newest treatment is •phenylalanine 1000mg one hour before exposure to UV light, •high dose vitamin C 3-5grams daily, • sublingual B-12 10,000mcg daily, and • folic acid 800mcg daily. Good reports from •PABA 1000mg with 2 TBS molasses daily as an iron source, • pantothenic acid 1000mg; •magnesium 1500mg daily; •Solaray TURMERIC capsules 4 daily; • Flora VEGE-SIL tabs; • Biotec AGELESS BEAUTY capsules 6 daily; •Crystal Star IODINE SOURCE™, •astragalus caps and •sea greens to stimulate the thyroid. •Evening Primrose oil caps 6 daily; •KHELLA caps are the herb of choice in Europe (sometimes available here); and • Ginkgo Biloba extract. •Calendula gel is a good topical. Beware long use of steroid drugs for vitiligo; some repigmentation, but higher risk of skin cancer.

—**ULCERATIONS:** Keep the diet simple and alkaline during healing. Add more fresh fruits and vegetables. Consciously add vegetable protein sources for faster healing - from whole grains, soy foods, sea foods and cultured foods. Include beta carotene-rich foods for both healing and prevention, from carrots, sweet potatoes, yellow-orange vegetables and sea vegetables. Include vitamin C-rich foods for collagen and interstitial tissue health. Include silicon-rich foods from vegetables, whole grains and seafoods to build healthy connective skin tissue. Take a skin healing mix of 1 teasp. each, wheat germ oil and brewer's yeast in a glass of aloe vera juice 2x daily. Drink 6-8 glasses of bottled water or other healthy liquids like juices and herbal teas daily to keep acid wastes flushed. Avoid saturated fats, sugars, caffeine and caffeine-containing foods.

Effective natural therapies: Hot •comfrey compresses, dry mustard plaster, tea tree oil, propolis tincture, a •green clay poultice, • B & T CALIFLORA gel. Apply •Earth's Bounty O₂ SPRAY to affected area, and on soles of feet (usually a noticeable change in 3 weeks). Make a •paste of *aloe vera* gel and *goldenseal* powder and apply frequently, add a few drops of *tea tree* oil for anti-infective properties. Take •Bromelain 1500mg; •Barleans lignan-rich Omega-3 flax oil 3x daily. Take •Crystal Star BEAUTIFUL SKIN™ caps and apply Crystal Star GINSENG SKIN REPAIR GEL™, or ANTI-BIO™ gel if there is infection. Make a lesion healing tea: •Steep *burdock* and *dandelion* root and add 15 drops per cup of *echinacea* EXTRACT; take 3 cups daily. For open ulcers, use •*calendula* gel, • PABA 500-1000mg, • Flora VEGE-SIL for connective tissue regrowth.

—**SCLERODERMA:** A runaway healing process where the body inexplicably begins and continues to produce too much collagen and connective tissue, replacing normal cell structure, and causing scar tissue to build up on skin, lungs and circulatory organs. It begins with discolored skin, followed by lesions, swelling and horrible pain. **Effective natural therapies:** Drink fresh carrot juice at least twice a week. Take baths with *aloe vera* gel and avocado oil added to the water. Take •MSM, 1000mg daily for soft, pliable skin. Take •*gotu kola* (centella asiatica) extract caps 4 daily and •PABA 1000mg daily for significant skin softening. Apply •*calendula* gel to lesions and take •Bromelain 1500mg daily to reduce swelling. Get regular aerobic exercise to increase perspiration, stimulate metabolism, and rid the body of carbon dioxide build-up. Stop smoking and avoid secondary smoke. Add antioxidants: •CoQ₁₀ 60mg 3x daily, •beta carotene 150,000IU daily, • 2 TBS sea greens (any kind) daily to resmoisturize, •vitamin C with bioflavonoids, 5000mg daily, •glutathione 50mg daily, PCO's from grapeseed or white pine 50mg 4x daily, •B₆ 250mg daily, and • zinc 30mg daily. Keep nutrition at highest possible level with a protein drink like • Nutricology PRO-GREENS with EFA's every day.

—**STRAWBERRIES, EXCESS PIGMENTATION: Effective natural therapies:** Reduce too high copper levels by adding more zinc and iron-rich foods. Reduce clogging waste with a gentle herbal laxative. Apply •B&T CALIFLORA ointment, take •pantothenic acid 1000mg, B₆ 500mg and alpha lipoic acid 600mg.

—**SKIN PROTECTION FROM ENVIRONMENTAL POLLUTANTS: Effective natural therapies:** •Alpha Lipoic acid 300-600mg daily enhances the effectiveness of all other antioxidants and improves skin's integrity. • Nutricology GERMANIUM 150mg, *suma* root capsules 4 daily, • Biotec AGELESS BEAUTY capsules 6 daily, • Vitamin E with selenium 400IU; •*ginkgo biloba* extract - photo-protective; •PCO's 100mg daily and apply •Derma-E PYCNOGENOL MOISTURIZER inhibits collagen deterioration.

—**ROSACEA:** Redness of the central face, small red bumps and enlarged blood vessels on face, neck and chest. Rosacea triggers: tomatoes, chocolate, meat marinades, hot drinks,citrus fruits, vinegar, red wine and red meats. **Effective natural therapies:** Take •Dr. Diamond HERPANACINE capsules (excellent results) Add •EFA's to your diet - EVENING PRIMROSE oil caps 4 daily or Nature's Secret ULTIMATE OIL, or add Omega-3 rich flax oil in your salad dressings. Add •B complex vitamins 100mg daily. Take •PHYCOTENE MICROCLUSTERS available at Healthy House, •vitamin E 400IU with selenium 200mcg. Add •sea greens to your diet 2 TBS daily, or take •Crystal Star IODINE SOURCE™ caps for thyroid stimulation and minerals, or •Nature's TRACE-LYTE with sea greens. Apply •GRAPEFRUIT SEED extract and also take GRAPEFRUIT SEED extract capsules internally. Mix •2 teasp. *tumeric* powder and 6 teasp. *coriander* powder with enough milk to make a paste. Apply and leave on 10 minutes when you see a breakout. Or use •Zia10-minute CRANBERRY PEEL. Drink •*echinacea-pau d'arco* tea 3 cups daily to flush fats from the blood stream. Add probiotics like •Prof. Nutrition DOCTOR DOPHILUS and B-12, up to 5000mcg daily. Rosacea HOTLINE (888) 662-5874.

Can't find a recommended product? Call the 800 number listed in Product Resources for the store nearest you.

Smoking - How to Stop
Second-Hand Smoke, Smokeless Tobacco

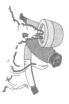

Each cigarette takes 8 minutes off your life; a pack a day takes 1 month off your life each year; 2 packs a day, takes 12-15 years off your life. Cigarettes have over 4000 known poisons, any of which can kill in high enough doses. One drop of pure nicotinic acid can kill a man. Depending on the age that you quit, your life expectancy can increase from 2-5 years. Secondhand or passive smoke, (now the third leading cause of preventable death in the U.S.), and chewing tobacco are just as dangerous, especially for women. Passive smoke reduces fertility, successful pregnancies, and normal birth weight babies. It increases the instance of cervical, uterine and lung cancer, heart disease and osteoporosis in women and men. Don't be discouraged. Quitting is hard work, but it gets easier every day, as the body loses dependence on nicotine.

Diet & Superfood Therapy

—Nutritional therapy plan:

1—There must be a lifestyle and diet change for permanent success against smoking. Start with a 3 day liquid cleansing diet (pg. 191), with fresh fruit and vegetable juices and miso soup to neutralize and clear the blood of nicotinic acid and to fortify blood sugar. Include lots of vegetable proteins. Add magnesium-rich foods like dark leafy veggies, whole grains, seafoods, sea vegetables and legumes.

2—Then, follow with a fresh foods only diet for 3 days, with carrot juice, plenty of carrots and celery, leafy green salads, and lots of citrus fruits to promote body alkalinity. (pH 7 and above readings show decreased desire for tobacco.)

3—Avoid junk foods and sugar that aggravate cravings. Avoid oxalic acid-forming foods like chocolate and cooked spinach or rutabaga that bind up magnesium in the body.

4—Take a cup of green tea or Crystal Star GREEN TEA CLEANSER™ daily to reduce body carcinogens.

—Effective superfoods: (choose 1)
• New Chapter GINGER WONDER syrup.
• Crystal Star AMINO ZYME™ caps to control craving/weight gain after quitting.
• Nutricology PRO-GREENS with EFA's.
• Mona's CHLORELLA for nicotine toxicity.

Herb & Supplement Therapy

—Interceptive therapy plan: (Choose 2 to 3 recommendations)

1—**Control the cravings:** • Crystal Star NIC-STOP™ tea, (with *lobelia*), or • *Lobelia* tea or • *oats/scullcap* tea 2 cups taken over the day in sips to keep tissues flooded with elements that discourage the taste for nicotine. (Add a pinch of *ginger*, or • New Chapter Enzymatic Therapy NICO-STOP for at least 2 months; • Homeopathic Natra-Bio SMOKING WITHDRAWAL RELIEF; or Medicine Wheel NICO-FREE extract; or • Make a tobacco addiction-fighting tea to lessen desire, support nervous system, strengthen adrenals, and cleanse lungs. One part each: *Oatstraw and seed, lobelia seed and leaf, licorice root, calamus root, sassafras.*

2—**Flush the nicotine out of the lymph system and lungs:** • *Echinacea,* flush lymph; • *Ephedra* tea or • Crystal Star DEEP BREATHING™ tea cleanse lungs.

3—**Help neutralize cancer-causing compounds:** Solaray TURMERIC caps 6 daily.

• **For nico-toxicity take daily:** 2 Cysteine 1000mg, 2 Glutamine 1000mg, 4 Vitamin C 1000mg, 4 *Evening primrose oil*, 20 Sun Wellness CHLORELLA tabs.

4—**Calm the nerves:** • Crystal Star RELAX CAPS™ 6 daily, or • WITHDRAWAL SUPPORT™ caps to calm tension; • Magnesium 800mg daily; • Stress B-complex 100mg daily; • VALERIAN/WILD LETTUCE drops in water.

5—**Protect against heart and artery problems with EFA's:** • EVENING PRIMROSE 4000mg daily; • Barleans high-lignan flax oil caps, 3 daily; • Biotec PACIFIC SEA PLASMA sea greens 6 daily; • Natures Path TRACE LYTE with sea greens.

6—**Ginseng helps normalize and control cravings:** • Crystal Star GINSENG/LICORICE ELIXIR™, also helps blood sugar balance; • Crystal Star GINSENG 6 SUPER™ caps help rebuild nerves; • Imperial Elixir AMERICAN GINSENG.

7—**Guard against secondary smoke:** • Glutathione 50mg daily; • Ascorbate vitamin C powder with bioflavonoids, 1/2 teasp. in water every hour to bowel tolerance during acute withdrawal stage, then reduce to 5000mg daily; • PCO's 100mg daily.

8—**Antioxidants are lung protectors against tobacco:** • Premier Labs GERMANIUM 150mg; • Twin Labs LYCOPENE 10mg for lungs; • CoQ 10 60mg 3x daily; • Niacin therapy: 500-1000mg daily, with • Beta-carotene 200,000IU daily.

Lifestyle Support Therapy

—Bodywork:
• Do deep breathing exercises for more body oxygen whenever you feel the urge for tobacco until the desire decreases - about 4 minutes.
• To help curb craving for chewing tobacco, chew *licorice* root sticks or cloves.

Info you may not know about smoking:

—If your parents smoke, you may inherit an addiction even before birth. Fetuses absorb nicotine, CO_2 and tar in the womb (some even pull away from the uterine wall), and second-hand smoke from both parents. The family of a heavy smoker has lung damage and lung cancer risk equal to smoking 1 to 10 cigarettes a day! 1.2 million Americans under 18 become daily smokers every year in the late 1990's.

—Smokers are prone to heartburn and ulcers. Smoking inhibits a protective bicarbonate secretion in the small intestine that neutralizes acid. Cigars are even worse than cigarettes.

—Smoking is a big contributor to high blood pressure because smoke narrows arteries. Nicotine revs up heartbeat when the body calls for more oxygen-laden blood the arteries can't deliver it. Slow suicide.

—Smoking reduces the size of a man's erection. All muscles (not just the penis) grow slower and need longer recovery time if you smoke.

Common Symptoms: Chronic bronchitis; constant hacking cough; difficult and shortness of breath; lung and respiratory depletion and infection; emphysema and dry lungs; often eventual lung cancer and other degenerative diseases; adrenal exhaustion and fatigue; poor circulation affecting vision; high blood pressure; premature aging and wrinkled, dehydrated skin with poor color and elasticity (smoke decreases blood flow to the skin); stomach ulcers; osteoporosis; low immunity; etc. The cost of smoking-related illness is over 50 billion dollars today in medical bills alone.

Common Causes: System stress and disease from nicotine poisoning; emotional insecurity; hypoglycemia; dietary deficiencies; nicotine addiction.

See POISONING, HEAVY METAL page in this book for more information.

Can't find a recommended product? Call the 800 number listed in Product Resources for the store nearest you.

Snake Bite

Poisonous Spider Bites, Scorpions

Get emergency medical help immediately! Time is critical. The methods below are to be used only until this help arrives. There is anti-venin for snake bites, but it is often snake-specific and carries the risk of anaphylactic shock. Buy a snake bite kit before you go on any trip where you can't reach medical help in a reasonable time. Know what poisonous snakes are native to your area. If you can't identify a snake, treat it as if it is poisonous. Only 2 spiders in the U.S. are poisonous - the black widow and the brown recluse. There is anti-venin for black widow spiders, but none for brown recluse spiders. Shock and convulsions may occur.

Diet & Superfood Therapy

Nutritional therapy plan:

1—For snake bite: wash bite with soap and water. No ice compresses for snake bite.

2—Give the victim only small sips of water. No alcoholic drinks. The poison will spread faster.

3—Make a tobacco and saliva poultice and apply to bite.

4—Plant onions and garlic around the house to keep snakes away. Eating daily onions before going into snake country is also thought to be a preventive against the poison of some bites.

—Effective superfoods: (choose 1 or 2)
• Mona's CHLORELLA 2 packets daily.
• Crystal Star SYSTEMS STRENGTH™ for iodine/potassium therapy.
• Nutricology PRO-GREENS with flax EFA's.
• Aloe vera juice to detoxify.

Herb & Supplement Therapy

—Interceptive therapy plan: (Choose 2 to 3 recommendations)

1) **In a life-threatening situation,** where the victim may go into cardiac arrest, *cayenne* may save the person's life. • *Cayenne,* 2 capsules or 8-10 drops of *cayenne* extract in warm water, as a shock preventive to strengthen the heart.

2) **In a life-threatening situation,** where the victim may go into shock or convulsions, massive doses of vitamin C may save the person's life. Use • Calcium ascorbate vitamin C powder, ¼ teasp. in water every 15 minutes as a detoxifier during acute reaction phase.

Use • *Echinacea* extract drops under the tongue or in water in either case to flush poisons from the lymph glands.

3—**Reduce swelling:** Take • Crystal Star ANTI-HST™ caps to help calm a histamine reaction. Take • *yellow dock* tea with *echinacea* extract every hour until swelling goes down. Apply • *Black cohosh* tea or Enzymedica PURIFY as an antidote to venom.

Effective compresses to reduce swelling: • *Plantain;* • *Rue;* • *Fresh comfrey leaf,* • *Slippery elm.*

4—**After the bite crisis has passed, and AFTER poison is out of the body:** Use • Golden Pride ORAL CHELATION therapy with EDTA or alpha lipoic acid 600mg to detoxify the system. Use • Niacin therapy: up to 500mg daily, to dilate and tone blood vessels.

5—**Heal skin from the bite:** • *Aloe/comfrey* salve or *Aloe vera* gel; • *Comfrey* tea; • *Calendula* gel; • Chinese WHITE FLOWER OIL; • Vitamin E 400IU -take internally; • Vitamin A & D 25,000IU - take internally; prick capsule and apply locally; use • Morada Research WOUND SALVE.

Lifestyle Support Therapy

—Bodywork:

• Take precautions if you are going on a camping trip, tropical hike, or working around snake havens like sheds and outhouses. Wear heavy boots and leggings that fangs can't penetrate.

• Keep victim still and calm. Immobilize the bite area and keep it lower than the heart.

• Until medical help arrives, put a constricting band 2 to 4" above the bite. Don't cut off circulation. Move band up if swelling reaches the band.

• If you can't get to medical help within 15 minutes, and swelling is rapid and pain severe, make a small cut with a sharp knife up and down, not across, through each fang mark. Use suction by mouth or a suction cup for at least 30 minutes, repeatedly. Spit out blood. Rinse mouth immediately.

• Do not pour alcohol on a bite. It is useless and may speed up the venom; ice packs are no good either because they may damage tissue.

• A Springlife POLARIZER if used immediately may reduce swelling and adverse reactions.

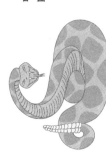

Common Symptoms: Snake bite: *slow upward spreading red lines as poison moves toward the heart; swelling, sometimes severe pain and nausea; sweating, increased heartbeat, dizziness, weakness and fainting, breathing difficulty.* **Black widow bite:** *severe chest and abdominal pain, labored breathing, headache, swollen face, fever, chills, profuse sweating and shock.* **Brown recluse bite:** *within a few days to a week after the bite, a small red, raised blister will form. Then an ulcer that lasts for weeks or even months. There is general weakness, nausea, hive breakouts and kidney problems. California scorpions are not poisonous unless you are allergic. Texas/Southwest scorpions are poisonous. Get medical help.*

See SHOCK & TRAUMA page 495 for more emergency information.

Can't find a recommended product? Call the 800 number listed in Product Resources for the store nearest you.

Spinal Meningitis
Encephalitis

Meningitis is an infectious, viral disease that causes inflammation of nerves, spine, and brain tissue. It is characterized by deficient blood supply to these areas and therefore deficient oxygen to the brain. Children are especially at risk for permanent brain damage or paralysis. Coma or death may ensue if prompt treatment is not undertaken. Medical treatment has been successful with meningitis if received early. However, unfortunately meningococcus microbe is becoming resistant to antibiotics. Nutritional therapies increase the healing rate substantially. **Encephalitis** is a rarer form of the viral infection, with many of the same symptoms. Adults experience severe mental disturbance, disorientation and coma. Acute bacterial meningitis can be rapidly fatal, especially for infants or the elderly. Get emergency help right away for acute symptoms.

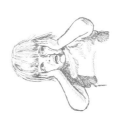

Diet & Superfood Therapy

Nutritional therapy plan:

1—There must be diet and lifestyle change for there to be permanent improvement.

2—A 24 hour liquid diet (pg. 192) should be used one day each week to keep the body flushed and alkaline.

3—The diet should be 50-75% fresh foods and vegetable juices, with fresh carrot juice and a potassium broth (pg. 215) or veggie drink (pg. 218) 2 to 3x a week.

4—Add cultured foods, such as yogurt and kefir, for friendly G.I. flora establishment.

5—Drink only healthy liquids, 8 glasses daily; take 1 to 2 electrolyte drinks daily.

6—Reduce mucous-forming foods, such as dairy products, red meats, caffeine-containing and refined foods.

7—No sugar, fried, or junk foods at all.

—**Effective superfoods: (choose 1 or 2)**
• Green Foods CARROT ESSENCE drink.
• Crystal Star SYSTEMS STRENGTH™.
• Omega Nutrition ESSENTIAL BALANCE JR.
• CC Pollen ROYAL JELLY-HONEY drink.
• Monas CHLORELLA.
• CC Pollen BUZZ BARS- bee pollen energy.
• Nutricology PRO-GREENS w. flax oil.
• Nature's Path TRACE-LYTE for electrolytes.
• Knudsen's ELECTROLYTE DRINKS.

Herb & Supplement Therapy

—**Interceptive therapy plan: (Choose 2 to 3 recommendations)**

1—Reduce infection and help overcome the virus: •Crystal Star ANTI-VI™ extract one week on, one week off, alternating with •ANTI-BIO™ extract to control infection. •ECHINACEA extract 3 to 4x daily to help flush lymph glands and fight infection. •Ascorbate vitamin C or Ester C powder with bioflavonoids, ¼ teasp. every hour during acute phase. Reduce by ½ for maintenance until remission. •Vitamin A therapy is a key: Emulsified vitamin A & D 10,000IU/400IU for children as soon as the rash appears.

For encephalitis: •Homeopathic *Belladonna* 200c, and •Alacer EMERGEN-C electrolyte replacement. •Beehive Botanical or CC Pollen ROYAL JELLY; Long Life IMPERIAL TONIC (Royal Jelly/EPO); •Germanium 150mg, in divided doses. •Enzymatic Therapy VIRAPLEX 4 daily to help overcome the virus.

2—Reduce inflammation: •Quercetin 1000mg with bromelain 1500mg with meals; or Nature's Plus QUERCETIN with Vitamin C and bromelain; •Enzymedica PURIFY; •Fresh *comfrey* leaf tea 5 cups daily. •Crystal Star ANTI-FLAM™ caps.

3—EFA's help normalize brain and nerve health: •Evening *Primrose* oil or •Nature's Secret ULTIMATE OIL caps 4 daily; •High omega-3 flax oil 3 teasp. daily; •Kelp tabs 6-8 daily.

4—For nerve support: •Gotu Kola caps 4 daily; •Scullcap tea daily; •Herbs Etc. NERVINE TONIC; •Lobelia extract drops in water.

5—Enhance your immune system with antioxidants for treatment and prevention: •Enzymatic Therapy THYMU-PLEX caps; •Garlic 6 to 8 capsules daily; •PCO's from grapeseed or white pine 50mg 3x daily; •Solgar OCEANIC carotene 50,000IU; •Chondroitan up to 1200mg for degeneration. •Zinc lozenges 1 to 2 daily.

6—Nourish the brain tissue: •Phosphatidyl choline (Twin Lab PC 55); •B Complex 50mg, with extra B₆ 100mg, and •Solaray B₁₂ 2000mcg daily.

7—Increase blood flow to the brain: •Golden Pride FORMULA ONE oral chelation with EDTA; •Niacin therapy: 100-500mg daily. (If a child, use no flush niacin; if adult, use a baby aspirin first to avoid niacin flush).

Lifestyle Support Therapy

Corticosteroid drugs taken over a long period of time for meningitis weaken both bone structure and immunity.

—**Bodywork:**
•Immerse back of the head in warm epsom salts solution several times daily to draw out inflammation.

•Alternate hot and cold packs on the neck and back of the head to stimulate circulation to the area.

•Use catnip enemas to reduce fever, during acute phase and to clear body quickly of infection.

•Avoid aluminum cookware, deodorants, and other alum containing products.

•Get some fresh air and early morning sunshine every day.

•Get plenty of rest during healing.

Common Symptoms: *Early signs include: lethargy, slow thought and movement; sore throat; a stiff neck and fever; a dark red skin rash, chronic colds with chills; light sensitivity, severe headaches, nausea. (Infants: bulging soft spot on the skull.) Emergency symptoms include: stupor, coma, (change in temperature and sleep patterns may precede a coma), and convulsions with acute inflammation of the brain and spinal cord.*
Common Causes: *Infection by a wide array of viruses, possibly insect-borne; nutritional depletion, especially in children; dehydration is often involved; heavy metal or chemical poisoning; constipation; cerebrovascular disease; psychological trauma.*

Can't find a recommended product? Call the 800 number listed in Product Resources for the store nearest you.

Sports Injuries

Torn Ligaments, Sprains, Muscle Pain, Tendonitis

A strain or pulled muscle is any damage to the tendon that anchors the muscle. **A sprain** is caused by a twisting motion that tears the ligaments that bind up the joints. It takes much longer to heal than a strain. **Tendonitis** is the painful inflammation of a tendon, usually resulting from a strain, and developing as a dull, dragging sensation after exercise. You can help yourself prevent sports injures. Start your workout slowly; warm your body up at least 2 degrees before you start pushing yourself; end your workout with a cool down period to prevent lactic acid buildup.

Diet & Superfood Therapy

—Nutritional therapy plan:

1—A good diet helps you avoid injuries. During healing eat about 50% fresh foods. You need vegetable proteins for faster healing. Muscles need complex carbs from green foods to heal.

2—Eat chromium-rich foods such as lobster, low fat cheeses, brewer's yeast.

3—Eat silicon-rich foods such as rice, oats, green grasses and leafy greens.

4—Drink electrolyte replacements: Knudsens RE-CHARGE, Twin Labs CARBO FUEL powder. Drink extra water and fluids.

5—Eat magnesium-rich foods, like whole grains, nuts, beans, squashes for muscles.

6—Eat high vitamin C foods - a drink of lemon juice/honey/water at night; grapefruit or pineapple juice in the morning.

7—Avoid foods like red meats, sugars, caffeine and carbonated drinks during healing.

8—Antioxidant bars have a place in injury prevention, especially as a source of MCT's. Check out your natural food store for healthy ones.

—Healing superfoods: (choose 1 or 2)
- Green Kamut JUST BARLEY.
- Crystal Star ENERGY GREEN™ drink.
- Green Foods MAGMA PLUS™.
- Nutricology PRO-GREENS with EFA's.
- Esteem SUPER PRO with DMG.

Herb & Supplement Therapy

—Interceptive therapy plan: (Choose 2 to 3 recommendations)

1—**Reduce trauma; reconstruct cartilage:** •Glucosamine 1500mg-Chondroitin 1200mg (safe alternative to NSAIDS drugs); •Crystal Star SILICA SOURCE™ or •Flora VEGE-SIL caps 4 daily, for collagen and tissue regrowth. •Crystal Star BODY REBUILDER™ caps for new tissue; •Vitamin E 800IU for torn cartilage.

2—**Reduce inflammation, swelling:** •St. John's Wort oil, or •Nature's Apothecay HERBAL FIRST AID oil; •Crystal Star HIGH PERFORMANCE™ caps 4 for lactic acid buildup; •Peppermint oil rub (rapid action); •Country Life LIGATEND 4 daily.

3—**Enzyme therapy heals soft tissue:** Enzymedica PURIFY protease; ginger extract (New Moon DAILY GINGER) or capsules, a protease component. •quercetin 1000mg and bromelain 1500mg (Nature's Plus); •Biotec CELL GUARD, 6 daily.

4—**Speed recovery:** •Creatine 1000mg for muscles and joint injuries; ♂ Chromium picolinate 200mcg daily; Vitamin C crystals with bioflavs, ½ teasp. in water, or Alacer EMERGEN-C every hour for collagen and connective tissue healing.

—Healing topicals: •Earth's Bounty O₂ spray; •Herbal Answers ALOE FORCE skin gel; or make a healing paste: mix one part each; goldenseal, comfrey root and slippery elm powders in 2 parts aloe vera gel; apply. •Morada WOUND SALVE for blisters; •Miracle of Aloe MIRACLE FOOT REPAIR for cracked feet.

5—**For muscle pulls, leg cramps:** •Arnica Montana; •Biochemics PAIN RELIEF lotion; •Magnesium 800mg daily; •Stress-B-complex 100mg daily with extra B-6 250mg. •Kava kava relaxes muscles; •Crystal Star ANTI-SPZ™ or •CRAMP BARK COMBO™ extract for pain. Spring Life POLARIZERS promote rapid healing.

6—**Ginseng and sports medicine:** •Siberian ginseng extract for lactic acid buildup; •Crystal Star GINSENG 6 SUPER ENERGY™, •Hoshouwu for ligament, nerve healing. •Crystal Star GINSENG SKIN CARE™ gel w. C/germanium for abrasions, blisters.

—Homeopathic sports remedies: •Arnica for dislocations, sprains, bruises; •Bryonia alba for red, swollen joints; •Ruta Graveolens for pulled tendons; •Hypericum for damaged nerves; •Rhus Tox. for swelling; Boiron Sportenine for tendonitis; •Silicea strengthens ligaments; •Bellis Perennis for repetitive strains; •Hylands Arnicaid.

Lifestyle Support Therapy

—Bodywork:

• Elevate the injured area; apply ice packs immediately. Leave on for 30 minutes. Remove for 15 minutes. Repeat process for 3 hours to decrease internal bleeding from injured vessels.

• Wrap sprains with an ACE bandage (over the ice if necessary) to limit swelling.

• Apply alternating hot and cold packs the next day for circulation, to take down swelling and relax cramps. Elevate legs and slap them hard with open palms to stimulate circulation.

• Massage affected areas frequently. Massage therapy and shiatsu are effective treatments.
- Acupuncture and acupressure help.
- Take a hot bath with 8 drops rosemary oil.

—Healing applications for sports injuries:
- Nature's Way CAYENNE PAIN RELIEVING ointment.
- DMSO liquid roll-on.
- B&T TRIFLORA rub gel
- TIGER BALM analgesic rub
- Tea tree oil.
- Chinese WHITE FLOWER oil.
- Calendula ointment.

Hot salt pack: Heat 1 lb. salt in a heavy cotton pan. Pour in a heavy cotton sock, about ³/₄ full. Place on painful area for 30 minutes. Remarkable.

Common Symptoms: Wrenched knees; twisted ankles; sprained wrists; shin splints; tennis elbows; torn ligaments; muscle pulls; arthritis-like symptoms; bruises; tendon inflammation; Achilles heel; shooting ankle, foot and knee pains. Cramping and soreness during and after muscle exertion; painful joints and nerve endings; limited range of motion; leg cramps at night.

Common Causes: Conditions that allow too many sports injuries - calcium, magnesium, and general mineral deficiency; poor diet, high in acid-forming foods, low in green vegetables and whole grains; too much saturated fat and sugar; HCL depletion; poor circulation.

See ATHLETES' NEEDS page 268 and MUSCLE PAIN page 459 for more information.

Can't find a recommended product? Call the 800 number listed in Product Resources for the store nearest you.

Strep Throat

Sore Throat, Swollen Glands, Laryngitis, Hoarseness

Here are the differences between a strep throat and a sore throat irritation from a cold: Onset of strep throat is rapid; a cold is slow. Throat is very sore with strep throat, not so sore with a cold. You have a fever and aches with strep throat; mild achiness with a cold. You have swollen, tender lymph nodes with strep throat; not with a cold. There are usually complications with strep throat, like streptococcal pneumonia or middle ear infections; sinusitis with a cold. Antibiotics work for strep throat, not usually for a cold. Hoarseness, the result of inflammation of the vocal chords, is typically the result of a virus, or extensive yelling. Laryngitis, rasps, breathy voice, is often due to voice fatigue from a cold.

Diet & Superfood Therapy

—Nutritional therapy plan:

1—Go on a short 24 hr. liquid cleansing diet (pg. 192), or a 3 day mucous cleansing diet (pg. 196). Take garlic syrup. Soak a chopped garlic bulb in 1 pt. honey and water overnight; take a teasp. every hour. Take grapefruit or cranberry juice throughout the day.

2—Take lemon juice and honey in hot water with a pinch of *cayenne* pepper each morning, and a potassium broth (pg. 215) daily. Then eat mainly fresh foods during healing. Have plenty of leafy greens. Eat plenty of plain yogurt. Take Red Star NUTRITIONAL YEAST or miso broth at night before retiring.

3—Avoid all dairy foods, sugary, fried and fatty foods during healing.

—Effective gargles: 1) Lemon juice and brandy; 2) black tea; 3) liquid chlorophyll in water with pinches of *cayenne;* 4) lemon juice and sea salt in water; 5) cider vinegar and honey in water every hour until relief.

—Effective superfoods: (choose one)
• New Chapter GINGER WONDER syrup - use a s a gargle.
• ALoeLife ALOE GOLD juice.
• Wakunaga KYO-GREEN drink.

Herb & Supplement Therapy

—Interceptive therapy plan: (Choose 2 to 3 recommendations)

1—Control the infection: •Crystal Star ANTI-BIO™ extract every hour, or • ANTI-VI™ or •FIRST AID CAPS™, 6x daily, and • ECHINACEA extract to flush lymph glands for at least 7 days. • Enzymatic Therapy ESPERITOX chewables and VIRAPLEX caps as directed. • Lane Labs BENE-FIN SHARK CARTILAGE caps as directed. •Nutribiotic GRAPEFRUIT SEED extract in water, or capsules for infection. •Colloidal silver drops as needed for a week, or • Nature's Path SILVER-LYTE liquid; •Garlic capsules 8 daily or • Wakunaga KYOLIC RESERVE. • Solaray MULTIDOPHILUS or •Nature's Plus JUNIOR DOPHILUS chewables.

2—Reduce inflammation: •Alacer EMERGEN-C every few hours. Hold in the mouth as long as possible for best absorption, and/or • Vitamin C chewable 500mg every hour during acute stages.

For chronic low-grade strep infection: •Crystal Star ZINC SOURCE™ drops (apply directly on throat); take • Enzymatic Therapy THYMU-PLEX caps with vitamin C 5000mg daily, and • Lysine 500mg; add • Zinc lozenges as needed daily.

3—Soothe the throat tissues: •Crystal Star GINSENG-LICORICE ELIXIR™ drops in water as needed, or •COFEX™ tea; or • thyme tea as needed; • Hylands SORE THROAT AND C Plus tabs; • Chamomile tea.

Good lozenges: •Zand HERBAL INSURE lozenges; •Zinc gluconate or propolis lozenges every 2 hours as needed; •Olbas lozenges; •Thayers ROSE HIPS AND C or Wild cherry lozenges.

4—Remove congestion: •Crystal Star X-PEC TEA™ 2x daily; or a •Salt-sage gargle: make 2 cups sage leaf tea; strain, and add 1 teasp sea salt. Gargle to relieve pain and remove mucous. •Herbal Magic CONGEST-EASE.

Natural gargles remove excess phlegm (about every ½ hr.): •Goldenseal/myrrh solution or • Myrrh tincture, ½ teasp. in water; •Fenugreek/honey in water; •Liquid chlorophyll ½ teasp. in water; white oak bark tea.

—For laryngitis and hoarseness: •Licorice root; •Alacer EMERGEN-C. •Beehive Botanical PROPOLIS throat spray; •Gargle tea tree oil, 3 drops in water.

Lifestyle Support Therapy

—Bodywork:
•Effective throat applications:
  Hot ginger compresses.
  Eucalyptus steams.
  Color therapy glasses: wear blue.
  Hot parsley compresses on the throat.
  Drip *black walnut* extract in throat.

•Take hot 20 minute saunas daily.
•Stick tongue out as far as it will go. Hold for 30 seconds. Release and relax. Repeat 3 times to increase blood supply to the area.
•Take a catnip enema to cleanse infection from a strep throat.

—For laryngitis and hoarseness:
•Apply ginger/*cayenne* compresses to throat.
•Don't whisper. It's throat-abrasive.
•Take a hot mineral or epsom salts bath.
•Stop smoking; avoid secondary smoke.
•Hum a little to reduce swelling.

—Reflexology pressure points:

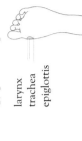

larynx
trachea
epiglottis

S 507

Common Symptoms: *Sore, aching, inflamed, throat and tonsils; swollen throat tissues; difficult talking; laryngitis (inability to speak above a whisper because of swollen throat tissues).*
Common Causes: *Viral or strep infection (if chronic, it may be mononucleosis); tonsillitis; beginnings of a cold or flu; consequence of smoking; lack of sleep; too many mucous-forming foods; adrenal exhaustion; stress.*

See COLDS & FLU, AND VIRAL, STAPH AND BACTERIAL INFECTION pages for more information

Can't find a recommended product? Call the 800 number listed in Product Resources for the store nearest you.

Stress

Low Energy, Tension, Nerves

Are you stressed out? Is your energy at all-time low? Over 20 million Americans suffer from health problems linked to chronic stress. New statistics show that up to 95 percent of visits to health care professionals are stress-related. Everyone is affected by varying degrees of stress.... people who work in polluted atmospheres, people at control desks with machines or instruments demanding continual attention, people who travel coast to coast constantly, people with mundane, boring jobs, etc. At best, stress causes useless fatigue; at worst, it is dangerous to health. Profound stress, such as that caused by job loss or the loss of a loved one takes a serious physical toll. The human body is designed to handle stressful situations, even to thrive on some of them. You can never avoid all stress, but you can maintain a high degree of health to handle and survive stress well.

Diet & Superfood Therapy

—Nutritional therapy plan:

1—Good nutrition is a good answer to stress. As stress increases, protein needs increase. Protein and mineral-rich foods are the best choice - vegetable proteins from whole grains, sea greens, seafoods, soy foods, eggs and sprouts.

2—Have fresh carrot juice and fresh fish or seafood at least once a week.

3—Add magnesium-rich foods from green vegetables and whole grains.

4—Eat B vitamin-rich foods like brown rice and other whole grains.

5—Reduce caffeine intake. Drink green tea instead for energy and antioxidants.

6—Take a glass of wine before dinner. No liquids with meals. Drink bottled water.

7—Make an anti-stress mix of brewer's yeast, toasted wheat germ, sunflower seeds, molasses, flax oil; take 2 TBS daily in food. Take miso soup before bed to relax.

8—Feed your adrenals with foods like sea greens and green drinks (see below).

—Effective superfoods: (choose one)

• Y.S. or Beehive Botanicals ROYAL JELLY/GINSENG and honey tea,

• Crystal Star SYSTEMS STRENGTH™

• ProLogix GREEN SUPREME drink.

• Nutricology PRO-GREENS with EFA's.

• CC Pollen DYNAMIC TRIO.

Herb & Supplement Therapy

—Interceptive therapy plan: (Choose 2 to 3 recommendations)

1—Feed your nerves: •Crystal Star RELAX CAPS™- nerve repair; or •STRESSED OUT™ extract or tea as needed; •Gotu kola or Ginseng/gotu kola caps - nerve support; •Ginkgo Biloba extract - a feeling of wellbeing. •Flora NERVE GUARD drops; Country Life sublingual B-12, 2500mcg daily for 2 months; •5-HTP 50-100mg daily for 2 months. •Vitamin C with bioflavonoids, 3000mg daily. •B complex 150mg with extra B-6 250mg daily. •Stress B Complex 100mg 2-3x daily, with extra B-6 250mg and pantothenic acid 1500mg; •Niacinamide for valium-like activity.

2—Feed your adrenals: •Crystal Star ADR-ACTIVE™ caps/extract; •Licorice root extract, or •Crystal Star GINSENG/LICORICE ELIXIR™ drops; or •Planetary SCHIZANDRA ADRENAL support; •Country Life RELAXER tabs for fast relief.

3—Amino acids boost your brain energy: •SAMe 400mg daily (important in synthesizing brain chemicals); •Glutamine 1000mg daily; •Country Life MOOD FACTORS capsules or •Ananbol Naturals AMINO BALANCE; •Tyrosine 500mg; •DLPA 1000mg as needed; •GABA 1000mg to mimic valium without sedation.

4—Stabilizing minerals: •Crystal Star RELAX™ tea or •CALCIUM SOURCE™ caps. •Magnesium 1200mg daily, or •Rainbow Light CALCIUM PLUS with high magnesium. •Nature's Path TRACE-LYTE with sea greens.

5—Fight depression with essential fatty acids: •Evening Primrose oil 1000mg 2x daily; omega-3 flax oil 2 TBS daily; or •Omega Nutrition OMEGA PLUS caps.

6—Adaptogens strengthen resistance to stress: •Siberian ginseng extract, astragalus or schizandra extracts have fast results; or try •Crystal Star MENTAL INNER ENERGY™ with kava kava, astragalus and suma; •Una da gato caps for immune response.

7—Calm your mind: •Bach RESCUE REMEDY drops; •Rub St. John's wort oil on the temples. •Kava Kava extract or •Herb Pharm PHARMA-KAVA drops.

8—Fight fatigue with antioxidants: •CoQ10, 100mg 4x daily, and •Alpha Lipoic Acid 600mg daily, increase ATP chemical energy. •NADH 5 to 10mg if you're tired all the time. Ascorbate vitamin C with bioflavonoids, 500mg every 4 hours during acute periods, or take Alacer EMERGEN-C; •Premiere Labs GERMANIUM with DMG.

Lifestyle Support Therapy

—Watchwords:

• You have to unwind before you can unleash. Work addiction is the health hazard of our time. Take a break to..... strengthen family and friendship ties; celebrate your life's rituals; build a good diet, adequate rest and exercise into your life; develop creative pastimes (not computer games); delegate at least some responsibilities; live for today.

—Stress reduction / relaxation techniques:

• Massage therapy once a month. Hypnotherapy, aromatherapy, and shiatsu have all shown effective results against stress.

• Quiet your mind with deep, rhythmic deep breathing exercises every day.

• Walk your dog.

• Get regular exercise for tissue oxygen.

• Don't smoke. Nicotine constricts the blood vessels, causing increased stress.

• Go on a short vacation. Take a long weekend. It will do wonders for your head.

• Take a rest period every soft music. Do 3 minutes of neck rolls.

• Have a good laugh every day.

and relaxation day. Listen to Meditate.

S 508

Common Symptoms: *Four levels of stress symptoms: 1) losing interest in everything, eye-corner sagging, forehead creasing, becoming short-tempered, bored, nervous; 2) tiredness, anger, insomnia, paranoia, sadness; 3) chronic head and neck aches, high blood pressure, upset stomach, looking older; 4) skin disorders, kidney malfunction, frequent infections, heart disease, nervous breakdown.*
Common Causes: *Emotional problems; overuse of drugs; work addiction; lack of rest; too much tobacco, caffeine or alcohol; allergies; hypoglycemia; mineral depletion; environmental pollutants; overcrowding; unemployment or job pressure; poverty; marital, social problems.*

See my book STRESS AND ENERGY for more information.

Can't find a recommended product? Call the 800 number listed in Product Resources for the store nearest you.

Taste and Smell Loss
Deviated Septum

There are a broad variety of reasons for this dysfunction, including a deviated septum and response to several common drugs people take today for colds and flu. In addition, nerve endings may be damaged from arthritis or osteoporosis (one of the reasons this problem afflicts older people more than younger people). The natural healing emphasis on overcoming nutritional deficiencies is often able to successfully address many of the root causes. Aromatherapy is gaining importance for taste and smell problems because what we call "taste" (as much as 90%) is actually smell. In most cases, if total atrophy has not developed, at least partial taste and smell can be restored.

Diet & Superfood Therapy

—**Nutritional therapy plan:**

1—A mineral-rich, low fat, low salt diet is a key. Keep your diet free of mucous-clogging foods, such as heavy starches, red meats and pasteurized dairy foods.

2—Add plenty of fresh, crunchy, high texture foods like celery and apples. Have a fresh green salad every day.

3—Eat zinc-rich foods: sea foods and fish, and sea greens snipped over your salads, rice, pizza, soups.

4—Eat magnesium-rich foods: whole grains and green leafy vegetables.

5—Boost minerals and B-vitamins: Have some brown rice, miso soup, and sea greens every day for at least 3 months.

6—Make sure the diet is low in salt and refined sugars. Use herbal salt-free seasonings.

7—Think green! Green tea and green drinks (see below) can sometimes do wonders. Use them for at least 3 months to see results.

—**Superfood therapy: (Choose one or two)**
• Nutricology PRO-GREENS with EFA's.
• Monas CHLORELLA drink.
• Crystal Star SYSTEMS STRENGTH™ drink daily, for at least 3 months.
• Beehive Botanical ROYAL JELLY/GINSENG. ♂
• Rainbow Light HAWAIIAN SPIRULINA. ♀♂

Herb & Supplement Therapy

—**Interceptive therapy plan: (Choose 2 to 3 recommendations)**

1—**Boost your minerals to enhance your sense of smell:** •Magnesium 1200mg daily; •Zinc, up to 100mg daily. Most people with sensory, especially taste, loss have a zinc deficiency. •Crystal Star MINERAL SPECTRUM™ capsules 4 daily, for natural foundation minerals; •Solaray CAL/MAG CITRATE capsules 4-6 daily.

2—**Boost your circulation:** •GINKGO BILOBA extract 4x daily, a primary sensory aid. Add •Country Life sublingual B-12, 2500mg daily (acts on taste), with B-complex 100mg daily, with extra B₆ 100mg and flush-free niacin 100mg for best results. ♀•Cayenne caps or ginger-cayenne caps; •Rosemary aromatherapy applied on the temples; ♀•Gotu kola caps 6 daily for better nerve feeling (make a difference).

3—**Enhance your thyroid activity:** Add •Sea greens, 2 TBS chopped dry, daily over soup, salad or rice (or 6 pieces of sushi a day); •Solgar OCEAN CAROTENE up to 100,000IU daily, or •PHYCOTENE MICROCLUSTERS mixed carotenes available from Healthy House. •Take Kelp tabs 8 daily for 3 months or Bernard Jensen LIQUI-DULS; •New Chapter OCEAN HERBS, or •Nature's Path TRACE-LYTE with sea greens, 2 daily; or •Arise & Shine LIQUID ORGANIC SEA MINERALS; •Ester C 550mg with bioflavonoids 4-6 daily.

4—**Boost your neurotransmitters:** phosphatidyl choline 3000mg, GABA 1000mg or Choline 600mg. (If your choline levels are low, try Huperzine A 50mg to allow levels to rise.) •Take ¼ teasp. each: Glutamine powder and Glycine powder; or Glutamine 1000mg 2 daily, •Evening primrose oil 2-4 daily.

5—**Herbal adaptogens like ginseng help normalize body systems:** Imperial Elixir Siberian ginseng and royal jelly capsules 3-4 daily; or •Siberian ginseng extract capsules 2 daily; •Superior ginseng/royal jelly vials 1 daily. ♀ •Twin Lab propolis extract under the tongue 3-4x daily. ♀♂

6—**Green supplements:** •Nature's Secret ULTIMATE GREEN; •Pines MIGHTY GREENS caps; •Liquid chlorophyll, 1 teasp. before meals in water; •Green Kamut JUST BARLEY; •Solaray ALFAJUICE caps. ♀♂

Lifestyle Support Therapy

—**Bodywork:**
• Use a catnip or chlorophyll enema to cleanse clogging mucous.
• Regular exercise with deep diaphragmatic breathing to keep passages clear (see page 554).

—**Reflexology point:**

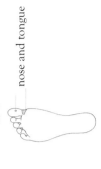

nose and tongue

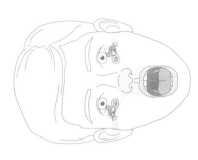

Common Symptoms: Inability, or only partial ability to smell odors or taste foods.
Common Causes: Zinc and other mineral deficiencies; too many antibiotics, causing zinc excretion; thyroid deficiency; side effect of chemotherapy; deviated septum; chronic low grade throat and sinus infection; poor circulation and mucous clogged system; atrophied nerve endings; high blood pressure medicine; over-the-counter cold medicines; chemical diuretics; gland imbalance and poor hormone secretions; hereditary proneness, but most frequent cause is environmental.

See the LOW SALT DIET pg.176 for more information.

Can't find a recommended product? Call the 800 number listed in Product Resources for the store nearest you.

Teething

Children's Tooth and Mouth Pain

Although it may seem like an ailment to every parent who soothes a fussy child on numerous sleepless nights, teething is a natural process of the first baby teeth breaking through the gums. Normally beginning around the seventh or eighth month, a baby will add another tooth about every month, until the complete set of 20 teeth comes in - usually around thirty months. Pain from teething can be minimized with natural methods. Gentle herbs have been used for centuries to help children over this rough growing patch in their lives. (Teething is also a natural reminder to Moms that it's time to wean the child from breast feeding.) Many of the same remedies apply for wisdom teeth breakthrough.

Diet & Superfood Therapy

—Nutritional therapy plan:

1—Include vitamin A-rich vegetables, vitamin D-rich eggs, fish and sea greens and high bioflavonoid foods in the child's diet.

2—Feed plenty of chilled foods; fresh fruits, yogurt, etc. to relieve discomfort.

3—Give lots of cool water daily.

—Chilled food chews:

Cold, hard cookies or bagels.

Let child chew on cold raw carrot sticks.

Give a teething ring that has been kept in the fridge.

—Effective food applications on gums:

Garlic oil rub if there is infection.

Sea salt and honey mix.

Dilute wine or brandy if there is swelling.

—Superfood therapy: (Choose one or two)

• New Moon GINGER WONDER syrup. Put a few drops in juice and rub on gums with a cotton swab.

• Give a dilute solution of Crystal Star BIO-FLAVONOID, FIBER & C SUPPORT™ drink several times a week.

Herb & Supplement Therapy

—Interceptive therapy plan: (Choose 2 to 3 recommendations)

1—Reduce infection and inflammation: Make a weak *goldenseal and honey solution* with water. Give with an eye dropper on back of the tongue. Rub on gums as an anti-infective; •*Myrrh extract drops;* or •*Bilberry extract,* or •*Gaia Herbs BILBERRY* alcohol free extract, an anti-inflammatory; •*Ascorbate vitamin C powder* with bioflavonoids - a weak solution in water. Give internally and apply to gums every few hours. •*Prevail CHILDREN'S VITASE* formula for enzyme therapy.

Effective rub-ons: •*Licorice root extract;* or let the child chew on natural licorice sticks; or Gaia LICORICE ROOT alcohol free extract. •*Lobelia extract or* •*Peppermint oil* - use only a drop or two of these extracts or oil; blend the oils with a few drops of flax oil to dilute; blend the extracts with a little water. •*Clove oil* is especially good (for cutting wisdom teeth, too); •Soak *yarrow flowers* in bran and water for 3 days. Strain and rub on gums as needed. Apply •*aloe vera gel* to gums as needed.

2—Soothe pain naturally: Make weak teas: give internally and pat on with a soft cloth. •*Slippery elm;* •*Chamomile;* •*Raspberry;* •*Catnip;* •*Peppermint;* •*Fennel seed.*

3—Give minerals for stronger teeth: •Chewable Mezotrace CHILDREN'S SEA MINERAL complex. (Break in half or dissolve in juice.)

4—Homeopathic remedies are a good, fast-working choice: •Hylands *TEETHING* tabs; •Natra-Bio TEETHING drops; •*Calcarea carbonica;* •*Chamomilla;* •Hyland's *Calc.-Phos.* tabs (dissolve in juice); rub •*Plantago Majus* tincture on tender gums.

Lifestyle Support Therapy

—Bodywork:

• Massage child's gums lightly with a little honey or propolis (like Beehive Botanical PROPOLIS & HERB SPRAY).

• Make a weak *tea tree oil* solution with water, and rub on gums for swelling or infection.

• Let the child play in the sun for 15 to 20 minutes every morning for full-spectrum vitamins - especially sunlight vitamin D.

—Reflexology point:

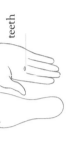

teeth

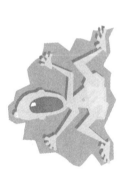

See CHILDRENS REMEDIES page 245 for more information.

Common Symptoms: *Sore, inflamed gums where teeth are pushing through the skin; often slight fever and infection; crying, and often difficulty sleeping; irritability and discomfort. There is usually lots of drooling, with consequent redness and chapped cheeks. The child will want to chew or suck on anything and everything. There may also be periodic diarrhea, skin rashes, runny nose and loss of appetite which might indicate infection beyond just teething.*

Can't find a recommended product? Call the 800 number listed in Product Resources for the store nearest you.

Tinnitus

Inner Ear Malfunction, Meniere's Syndrome, Vertigo

Tinnitus literally means "ringing in the ears," and more than 50 million Americans suffer from it. It starts as a low ringing, like the humming of a transformer. It eventually becomes permanent and robs you of sleep every night. **Meniere's syndrome** is a recurrent and usually progressive group of symptoms that include ringing and pressure in the ears usually with some hearing loss and dizziness. Natural therapies have been successful. **Vertigo** is a result of equilibrium (inner ear) disturbance with the sensation of moving around in space, or of having objects move around you. It occurs when the brain and central nervous system get conflicting messages from the body sensors that affect and maintain balance - the ear, eyes, and skin pressure receptors. Rest, relaxation techniques and proper nutrition are the key to preventing vertigo attacks.

Diet & Superfood Therapy

—Nutritional therapy plan:

1—Attain ideal body weight for better body balance. The diet should be low in saturated fats and cholesterol, high in vegetable proteins and B vitamin foods, such as brown rice, broccoli, tofu, sea foods, and sprouts.

2—Have a potassium broth (pg. 215) or a green drink like those below once a week.

3—Make a mix of nutritional yeast and wheat germ (or 2 teasp. wheat germ oil), take 2 TBS daily on a fresh salad.

4—Eliminate common allergy foods: wheat, corn, dairy products, sprayed foods like oranges and lettuce.

5—Avoid salty, fried foods, chemical-containing foods and preserved foods.

6—Avoid caffeine, especially full-strength coffee.

—Superfood therapy: (Choose one or two)

• Crystal Star ENERGY GREEN™ drink.
• New Moon GINGER WONDER syrup daily.
• Wakunaga KYO-GREEN with EFA's.
• Beehive Botanicals or Y.S. ROYAL JELLY/GINSENG drink.
• Future Biotics VITAL K drink daily.
• Aloe Falls ALOE juice with ginger.
• Lewis Labs NUTRITIONAL YEAST.
• Mona's CHLORELLA.

Herb & Supplement Therapy

—Interceptive therapy plan: (Choose 2 to 3 recommendations)

1—**Boost your circulation:** •GINKGO BILOBA extract drops 3 to 4x daily to promote circulation to the brain, for at least 3 months; •Ginger capsules 4 daily for 3 months; •CoQ-10 100mg 3x daily for 3 months, or •Real Life Reasearch CoQ 20/20 liquid; •Hawthorn extract 3x daily. •Metabolic Response Modifiers CARDIO-CHELATE with EDTA, MSM and NAC; or •Source Naturals TOCOTRIENOLS 34mg Glutamine 1000mg daily. •Butcher's broom tea, or •Crystal Star HEARTSEASE/CIRCU-CLEANSE™ tea with butcher's broom. •Niacin therapy to clear circulation blocks: 250mg 3x daily. For circulation balance: •Catnip tea; •St. John's wort extract; •Cayenne/ginger capsules; •Peppermint tea if there is nausea.

2—**Help repair nerves:** Crystal Star RELAX CAPS™ for nerve rebuilding, and MEDITATION TEA™ to restore mental equilibrium; Black cohosh extract drops 3x daily. Premier GERMANIUM with DMG B$_{15}$ daily. Vitamin E 800IU daily; Rose hips vitamin C or Ester C with bioflavonoids and rutin, up to 5000mg daily.

3—**Reduce your cholesterol and triglyceride levels:** •Crystal Star CHOL-EX™ caps, 3 daily for 2 months; •Crystal Star GINSENG-REISHI extract. •Red yeast rice.

4—**Relieve pain and congestion:** Crystal Star ANTI-HST capsules 4 to 6 daily; •Lobelia extrtact drops in water 2x daily; or •Mullein/Lobelia tea, acts as an expectorant for congestion. •Excess fluid elimination tea: 1 part each - uva ursi, parsley leaf, red clover, fennel seed, flax seed.

5—**Boost your B-vitamins:** Especially B-12. •Country Life sublingual B-12, 2500mcg daily; B-complex 100mg with extra B-6 100mg or Real Life Research TOTAL B liquid. Bee products are a specific: •Superior ROYAL JELLY/GINSENG vials; •Beehive Botanicals ROYAL JELLY/GINSENG capsules; •High potency Y.S. or Premier One ROYAL JELLY 2 teasp. daily; •Ginseng/royal jelly and honey in water as a daily drink.

6—**Silica helps strengthen vascular walls:** •Crystal Star SILICA SOURCE™ caps 4 daily, or •Horsetail/oatstraw tea or •Eyebright tea, or •Flora VEGE-SIL caps daily.
•Add sea greens to your diet, 2 TBS dried, snipped, daily (any kind).

Lifestyle Support Therapy

—Bodywork:

• A series of cranial treatments from a good massage therapist have notable results for TMJ (and therefore tinnitus) sufferers. Chiropractic adjustment and shiatsu massage also show improvement for both tinnitus and vertigo.

• You can mask tinnitus ringing with white noise or soothing sounds from a machine at night. The machines are available everywhere today.

• Practice stress management or relaxation techniques, such as meditation, soft music, yoga and body stretches.

• Take preventive measures: Remove stress from your life as much as possible.

—Acupressure point:

• Pinch between the eyebrows 3x for 10 seconds each time during an attack.

• Press top of the arm, just above the wrist line for 15 seconds at a time.

—Reflexology points:

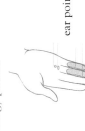

ear points

See DENTAL PROBLEMS - TMJ page 364 and MOTION SICKNESS page 457 for related info.

T 511

Common Symptoms: 80% of people with hearing problems also frequently have hearing loss and nausea. Vertigo victims also frequently have tinnitus. Starting with ear pain, ringing, pressure, and a feeling of faintness and lightheadedness upon standing quickly; the victim has a feeling of falling, a lack of steadiness and feels off-balance. Avoid alcohol, marijuana, methamphetamines, cocaine, hallucinogens, and balance-changing drugs. **Common Causes:** The greatest cause of tinnitus is unrelenting loud noise. Aspirin, wax build-up and TMJ disorder have also been implicated. For vertigo: poor circulation and blood pressure imbalance (which shows up if you stand or move too quickly); lack of brain oxygen or brain tumors; food and chemical allergies; neurological disease; chronic stress and anxiety; hypoglycemia; excess ear wax; B vitamin deficiency.

Can't find a recommended product? Call the 800 number listed in Product Resources for the store nearest you.

Tonsillitis

Tonsil Lymph Inflammation

The tonsils are part of the lymphatic gland tissue on either side of the entrance to the throat. They strain and process poisons from the body. (Unnecessary removal of these glands reduces your ability to respond to pathogens taken in by mouth.) Tonsillitis is tonsil inflammation, usually caused by streptococcal organisms. While the infection itself may not be serious, it always indicates a deeper immune response let-down, and can lead to serious problems, like rheumatic fever and nephritis. Scar tissue accumulates with every tonsillitis attack. If your tonsils do need conventional medical attention, ask about partial laser operation that just trim the tonsils with a carbon-dioxide laser. It's an inexpensive, out-patient procedure that leaves you with a minor sore throat instead of a major trauma, and leaves some tonsil-straining ability of the body intact.

Diet & Superfood Therapy

—Nutritional therapy plan:

1—Go on a 24 hr. (pg. 192) or 3 day liquid cleansing diet (pg. 191) to clear out body toxins. Then eat only fresh foods for the rest of the week during an attack. Get plenty of vegetable protein for healing.

2—Have lemon juice and water each morning with plenty of other high vitamin C juices throughout the day, such as orange, pineapple, and grapefruit juice.

3—Take a potassium broth or essence (pg. 215) once a day.

4—Have an onion/garlic broth each day.

5—Avoid sugars, pasteurized dairy products especially, and all junk foods until condition clears.

6—Drink 6-8 glasses of bottled water daily to keep the body flushed.

—Superfood therapy: (Choose one or two)

•Crystal Star BIOFLAV., FIBER & C SUPPORT™ drink.

•Nutricology PRO GREENS with EFA's.

•Solaray ALFAJUICE caps

•Aloe Falls ALOE GINGER juice, sip as needed - very soothing - or Herbal Answers ALOE FORCE JUICE.

•Beehive Botanicals GINSENG-ROYAL JELLY tea for EFA's.

Herb & Supplement Therapy

—Interceptive therapy plan: (Choose 3 or more recommendations)

1—Control the infection: •Crystal Star ANTI-BIO™ caps 4-6 daily, or •ANTI-VI™ extract drops to flush lymph glands and clear infection, with •FIRST AID CAPS™, 4-6 daily during the acute phase. •Garlic oil, or swab •Black walnut extract directly on throat. Use Herbs, Etc. PHYTOCILLIC, and spray throat with •Nutribiotic GRAPEFRUIT SEED extract as a gargle as directed, for anti-infective activity. •Nature's Plus CHEWABLE ACEROLA C 500mg with bioflavonoids, 1-2 every hour during acute stages (especially if there is constipation which there often is if a dairy allergy is involved).

2—Soothe throat pain and swelling: •Enzymatic Therapy ESBERITOX chewables; •Crystal Star ANTI-FLAM™ caps or extract drops to take down inflammation; •Crystal Star ASPIR-SOURCE™ caps to relieve head and throat pain. •Echinacea extract or cleavers tea as lymphatics to clear lymph tissue. •Licorice root or •Crystal Star GINSENG/LICORICE ELIXIR™ extract. •Nature's Path THROAT-LYTE; •Solaray pantothenic acid 1500mg with B_6 250mg to take down swelling. •Quercetin 500mg with •bromelain 500mg to relieve inflammation.

3—Help clear sinus and throat congestion: •Crystal Star cold COFEX™ tea as a soothing throat coat. •Mullein or •lobelia tea as a throat compress; •Thyme tea as a gargle. •Zinc gluconate throat lozenges as needed. •Propolis lozenges or tincture as needed.

4—Enhance immune response: •Beehive Botanical PROPOLIS SPRAY. •Lobelia drops if there is high fever. •Enzymatic Therapy VIRAPLEX caps 4 daily; or •THYMULUS extract. •Nutramedix IMMUN-X for long term support.

—Note: Investigate raw glandular extracts; they offer biochemical nutritional support for stress and fatigue affecting glands. They can improve gland health dramatically by delivering cell-specific and gland specific factors.

Lifestyle Support Therapy

—Bodywork:

•Take a garlic or catnip enema during an attack to clear body poisons.

•Chill the throat with a towel wrapped around crushed ice.

•Get plenty of bed rest during acute stage.

—Effective gargles:

Weak tea tree oil solution in water every 2-3 hours to counter inflammation.

Warm salt water gargles 3x daily.

Slippery elm tea to soothe.

Liquid chlorophyll 1 tsp. in water.

Goldenseal/myrrh solution in water.

—Hot mineral salts baths frequently.

—Reflexology point:

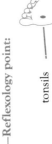

tonsils

See STREP THROAT page 507 for more information.

Common Symptoms: Swollen tonsils and lymph glands on either side of the jaw; difficulty swallowing; fever, chills, and tender sore throat; aches and pains in the back and extremities; bad breath because of the infection; ear infection and hearing difficulty because of the swollen glands; vomiting sometimes.

Common Causes: A strep infection; poor diet that aggravates a sporadic infection; too many starches, sugars, and often an allergy to pasteurized dairy foods and wheat; not enough green vegetables and soluble fiber foods; constipation causing toxic build-up; poor digestion, and non-assimilation of nutrients.

Can't find a recommended product? Call the 800 number listed in Product Resources for the store nearest you.

Tumors

Malignant Tumors, Brain Tumors

Malignant tumors should be addressed as soon as possible to control spreading to other tissues. Tumors may be internal, as brain, gland or organ tumors, or external. Brain tumors should especially be acted upon immediately, because both malignant and benign tumors can cause irreversible neurological damage. Brain tumors are likely to return if not completely excised. Immune enhancement is the key in natural treatment. A whole foods diet and natural supplementation program has been successful in both reducing and in some cases, completely eliminating tumors.

Diet & Superfood Therapy

–Nutritional therapy plan:

1–Go on a short mucous cleansing liquid diet (pg. 196.) Then, for 1 month, have one each of the following juices daily:
-Potassium broth (pg. 215)
-A veggie drink (pg. 218), or see below.
-Cranberry/pineapple juice

2–Add whole grains, high fiber foods and steamed vegetables during the 4th week. Eat primarily fresh foods, especially sprouts, for the next month.

3–Add high sulphur foods: Garlic, onion and cruciferous vegetables or Schiff GARLIC/ONION capsules and AloeLife ALOE VERA juice with herbs.

4–Avoid heavy starches, refined sugars, and all fried foods. Keep the system clean and the liver functioning well with a diet high in greens, and low in dairy products and saturated fats.

5–Drink only distilled bottled water- 6-8 glasses daily to quickly clear toxic wastes.

–Superfood therapy: (Choose one or two)
• Crystal Star ENERGY GREEN™ for iodine, potassium and green therapy.
• Sun Wellness CHLORELLA drink.
• Transitions EASY GREENS, especially for hormone driven tumors.
• Green Foods GREEN MAGMA, 2 pkts daily.
• Herbal Answers ALOE FORCE JUICE drink.

Herb & Supplement Therapy

–Interceptive therapy plans: (choose 2 or 3 recommendations)

1–**Reduce tumor size and growth:** • Nutricology MODIFIED CITRUS PECTIN to reduce tumor spread. Take • Quercetin 1000mg with bromelain 1500mg; • Vitamin K 100mcg to inhibit growth; • CoQ_{10} 60mg 6x daily and Enzymedica PURIFY. • Take histidine, 1000mg 3x daily. • Add vitamin E 400IU and selenium 200mcg. Take • Nutricology GERMANIUM 150mg, and apply a •germanium-water solution daily. •PHYCOTENE MICROCLUSTERS available at Healthy House (clinically proven), or •beta carotene 200,000IU. • Apply Crystal Star ANTI-BIO™ gel; Take •pycnogenol PCO's 100mg 3x daily; • Natural Balance creatine 3000-5000mg daily (for a short time); • Natural Energy Plus CAISSE'S TEA.

2–**Iodine therapy is important:** • Crystal Star IODINE SOURCE™ extract, or •IODINE/POTASSIUM caps 4 daily; or • Kelp tabs 10 daily; • Vitamin E 800IU with selenium 200mcg; or • Nature's Path TRACE-LYTE with sea greens.

3–**EFA's are important balancing nutrients:** •EVENING PRIMROSE OIL 6 daily; • Nature's Secret ULTIMATE OIL especially for radiation/chemical caused tumors. Add • shark cartilage capsules, up to 1400mg, or Nutricology CAR-T-CELL emulsified shark cartilage as directed. • Also open a shark cartilage capsule and mix with $^1/_4$ teasp. vitamin C crystals; or use MSM with MICROHYDRIN available at Healthy House, or • MSM 1000mg daily. Results usually in 3 to 4 weeks.

4–**Certain herbs can reduce tumors:** • Reishi, shiitake, or maitake mushroom capsules, 6 daily, or Grifon PRO-MAITAKE D-Fraction caps; or • Crystal Star GINSENG-REISHI extract; • Tea tree oil; • Comfrey tea 4-5 cups daily; • Pau d'arco/butternut bark tea for natural quercetin (also apply pau d'arco extract, and echinacea extract drops mixed into aloe vera gel). Use • Calendula gel, or make an • escharotic calendula ointment through which tumor cells can exit: equal parts garlic powder, goldenseal powder, zinc powder - mix into calendula ointment. Apply daily for 4 weeks. The commercial product is •HERBAL VEIL 8 by Lenex Labs.

Tumor-reducing poultices: •Chaparral - good results from poultices and 4 capsules daily. •Una da gato, or •Crystal Star ANTI-BIO™ gel with una da gato.

Lifestyle Support Therapy

There has been an enormous increase in numbers of brain tumors reported in the last decade.

Can NutraSweet cause brain tumors? Studies from its own labs show that NutraSweet produced a high incidence of brain tumors at all concentrations examined, and was the reason that the FDA first rejected NutraSweet for human consumption. The more NutraSweet consumed, the more likely tumors would develop. High dose NutraSweet caused a 47X increase in brain tumors over control animals.

A breakdown product of NutraSweet, DKP (diketopiperizine), appears to cause the tumors. As time passes more NutraSweet breaks down into DKP. Soft drink companies now date their colas. Heating NutraSweet also speeds up the DKP breakdown. Using in hot beverages or for cooking is especially hazardous. There also appears to be some proof that NutraSweet further breaks down into formaldehyde.

—**For brain tumors:** Phosphatidyl choline (PC 55) 4 daily; carnitine 2000mg daily; Vitamin C therapy: see column 2; B Complex 150mg daily, with extra pantothenic acid 500mg, and folic acid 400mcg for neuroblastoma to help deter spread of cancerous cells; Natren BIFIDO FACTORS, $^1/_2$ teasp. with meals; Vita Carte BOVINE TRACHEAL CARTILAGE as directed.

Common Symptoms: Growing and mutating lumps and nodules; often inflamed, weeping, and painful; many times with adhesions to other tissue. Brain tumor signs include: chronic headaches; unexplained vomiting; weakness and lethargy; personality changes; double vision; recent incoordination and intellectual deterioration; sometimes seizures and stupor.

Common Causes: Poor diet with years of excess acid and mucous-forming foods; environmental, heavy metal or radiation poisoning; X-rays and low grade radiation tests, such as mammograms, causing iodine deficiency and thyroid malfunction; viral infection such as Epstein-Barr, herpes simplex and Kaposi's sarcoma.

See CANCER pages 332-340 for more information.

Can't find a recommended product? Call the 800 number listed in Product Resources for the store nearest you.

Varicose Veins

Spider Veins, Peripheral Vascular Problems

Peripheral vascular problems like varicose veins are more than a cosmetic nuisance. They're a result of leaky valves and they can be painful, cause unusual fatigue and heaviness, and leg and ankle swelling and cramping. Varicose veins develop when a defect in the vein wall causes dilation in the vein and damage to the valves. When the valves are not functioning well, the increased pressure results in bulging. Spider veins are thin, red, unsightly lines on the face, upper arms and thighs. Vasculitis is an inflammation of the peripheral blood vessels. Women are affected four times as frequently as men. Vein fragility increases with age due to loss of tissue tone, muscle mass and weakening of vein walls.

Diet & Superfood Therapy

—Nutritional therapy plan:

1—Keep weight down to relieve heaviness on the legs. Go on a 24 hour (pg. 192) liquid diet to clear circulation. Eat fresh foods for the rest of the week - plenty of green salads and juices. Add a glass of cider vinegar and honey each morning.

2—Then follow a vegetarian, high fiber diet for the rest of the month. Varicose veins are rarely seen in parts of the world where high fiber diets are consumed. Boost your fiber with fresh fruits and vegetables and whole grains. Include sea foods, beans, whole grain cereals, brown rice, and steamed vegetables.

3—Have a high vitamin C juice every day, to strengthen capillaries, like pineapple, carrot, citrus, fruit, or a veggie drink (pg. 218), or see below.

4—Eat foods with high PCO's, like cherries, berries, currants and grapes.

5—Reduce dairy foods, fried foods, prepared meats, red meats and saturated fats of all kinds. Avoid salty, sugary and caffeine foods.

—Superfood therapy: (Choose one or two)
• Crystal Star ENERGY GREEN™ drink.
• Crystal Star BIOFLAV., FIBER & C SUP-PORT™ drink for venous integrity.
• Mona's CHLORELLA 1-2 teasp. daily.
• Crystal Star CHO-LO FIBER TONE™ drink or capsules morning and evening.

Herb & Supplement Therapy

—Interoceptive therapy plan: (Choose 2 to 3 recommendations)

1—Strengthen vascular fragility and stimulate circulation: •Crystal Star VARI-VAIN™ Kit, roll-on gel and capsules for 3 months (with *horse chestnut* and grape seed PCOs). •GINKGO BILOBA extract caps 2 to 4 daily; •*Gotu kola* caps 4 daily, (especially for spider veins); or •Solaray CENTELLA VEIN capsules help maintain connective tissue. • Crystal Star HEARTSEASE/HAWTHORN™ caps 3 daily.
•Enzymatic Therapy CELLU-VAR cream and capsules to improve venous tone. ♀

2—Boost your flavonoids for vein tone: •*Horse Chestnut* cream •Quercetin 1000mg daily; •Bromelain 1500mg daily, or •Solaray QBC caps 2 daily. •HAW-THORN extract or •BILBERRY extract 4x daily for 1 to 2 months, or •Golden Pride Formula #11 PHYTO-GUARD. Take •PCO caps from grapeseed or white pine, 100mg 3 daily. •Vitamin C crystals with bioflavonoids and rutin, $1/2$ teasp. every 4 hours to bowel tolerance daily for 1 month, for connective tissue and collagen formtion.

3—Reduce pain and heaviness: •Crystal Star CRAMP BARK COMBO™ 4 daily;
•Apply Earth's Bounty O₂ SPRAY to the legs and feet, 2x daily for 2 months; Take •B₁₅ DMG sublingual daily, or •Premier GERMANIUM with DMG. Homeopathic remedies: •BioForce *Varicose Veins Relief* tincture; •B&T CALIFLORA gel; or •*Hamamelis* for swelling.

Effective leg compresses: Apply •*Witch hazel* compresses 2x daily. Apply •*Calendula* compresses morning and evening; Apply •*Ginger* compresses and take 4 capsules Ginger daily. Drink •*Butcher's broom* tea and compresses for circulation increase.

4—Reduce inflammation: •Nature's Plus BROMELAIN 1500mg daily to help break down fibrin. •Take vitamin E 400IU with •Zinc 30mg daily, and apply a mix of $1/4$ teasp. vitamin E oil and 2 TBS liquid lecithin. (The feet and legs tingle and feel hot as if thawing out). Take •*Capsicum* caps 4 daily; or •*Capsicum-Ginger* root caps, 6 daily; or •Schiff GARLIC/ONION capsules; •Vitamin K 100mcg daily and vitamin K cream for spider veins.

Lifestyle Support Therapy

—Bodywork:

• Walk every day; swim as much as possible, for the best leg exercises. Walk in the ocean whenever possible for strengthening sea minerals. Walk in the early morning dewy grass.

• Elevate the legs when possible. Avoid standing for long periods. Go barefoot, or wear flat sandals. Do not use knee high hosiery. The elastic band at the top impedes circulation.

• Sitting for long periods of time is the worst for varicose veins and hemorrhoids. Take short, frequent breaks in your work schedule. Sit with a stool to prop your feet on.

• Massage feet and legs every morning and night with diluted *myrrh* oil.

• Take an epsom salts bath once a week.

• Use alternating hot and cold hydrotherapy (pg. 228) daily.

• Apply aloe vera gel, or Crystal Star CEL-LEAN™ gel. Elevate legs while application soaks in.

—Effective compresses:

White oak bark. (Also take 8 white oak capsules daily.)
Fresh comfrey leaf or *plantain* leaf
Bayberry bark
Marshmallow root
Cider vinegar

See Circulation page in this book for more information.

Can't find a recommended product? Call the 800 number listed in Product Resources for the store nearest you.

Common Symptoms: Distended, swollen, painful, bulging leg veins; legs feel heavy, tight and tired, sometimes with numbness and tingling; thin red, unsightly spider veins; muscle cramps.
Common Causes: Low-fiber, meat and dairy based diet with too many refined foods; vitamin E, C, and A deficiency; EFA (essential fatty acid) deficiency; constipation and straining at the stool; pressure on the veins from excess weight or pregnancy; weakness of vascular walls due to weak connective tissue; poor posture and circulation; liver malfunction; long periods of standing or heavy lifting; damage to veins from inflammation and blood clots in the vein.

Vaginal Yeast Infections

Leukorrhea, Bacterial Vaginosis (BV), Vulvitis

Trichomonas - caused by a parasite, found in both men and women, usually contracted through intercourse. **Leukorrhea** - a yeast type infection occurring during low resistance times and when normal vaginal acidity is disrupted. **Bacterial Vaginosis** (formerly called gardnerella) - thrives when vaginal pH is disturbed. **Vulvitis** - an inflammation of the vulva, caused by allergic reaction, irritation, bacterial or fungal infection. Natural therapies are very successful for most vaginal yeast infections, but a long-term cure is not likely unless dietary/lifestyle changes are made. Be kind to your mate: many of these infections bounce back and forth between sexual partners. Avoid sex during an infection, or at the very least, use barrier protection. Reconsider if you are using birth control pills (they have been implicated in some infections).

Diet & Superfood Therapy

—Nutritional therapy plan:

1—The diet should be primarily fresh foods during healing. Have a large green salad with alfalfa sprouts every day. Keep meals very light, without heavy starches, fatty foods, sugars, or dairy foods.

2—Eat plenty of fermented foods, such as yogurt and kefir, and Rejuvenative Foods VEGI-DELITE for friendly G.I. lactobacilli, especially if you have been taking antibiotics.

3—Normalize your body chemistry: drink 3-4 glasses of cranberry juice from concentrate daily.

4—Avoid red meats, hard liquor, sugar and caffeine while clearing.

5—Schiff GARLIC/ONION caps 6 daily with watermelon seed tea especially if there is also a bladder infection.

—Effective douches

• Cider vinegar - 2 TBS to 1 qt. water. Add $\frac{1}{4}$ teasp. cayenne or 2 TBS green clay if desired.
• Diluted mineral water.
• Baking soda 2 tsp./honey 1 tsp./1 qt. water.
• Chlorophyll liquid 1 tsp. to 1 qt. water.

—Superfood therapy: (Choose one or two)

• Green drinks-use both orally and as douches:
• Crystal Star ENERGY GREEN™ drink.
• Mona's CHLORELLA 1-2 teasp. daily.
• Wakunaga KYO-GREEN drink.

Herb & Supplement Therapy

—Interceptive therapy plan: (Choose 2 to 3 recommendations)

1—Rebalance normal vaginal biochemistry: •Crystal Star WOMAN'S BEST FRIEND™ caps 6 daily, with •Crystal Star WHITES OUT DOUCHE™ for 4 days for a mild infection. Use •Crystal Star WHITES OUT™ #1 and #2 capsules for more severe problems. Use •Crystal Star WHITES OUT™ caps 6 daily or an *Oregon grape root-goldenseal* root compound to boost effectiveness. Drink •*Pau d' arco tea* 3 cups daily; •*Garlic* 8 caps daily; or •*Black walnut hulls* extract 2x daily (also effective in a douche). For recurrent infections- •American Biologics DI-OXYCHLOR, Creation's Garden CANDISINE-1, or Enzymedica PURIFY.

Vitamin therapy effective for vaginal yeast infections: •Zinc 50mg daily is primary (usually results in 3 weeks even when drugs have not been effective against trichomonas). •Beta carotene 100,000IU daily. •Vitamin E 400IU 2x daily. •Vitamin C (ascorbic acid) crystals, $\frac{1}{2}$ teasp. every 2 hours during healing, up to 5000mg daily. A weak water solution may also be used as a douche. •B complex 100mg daily, with extra B$_6$ 100mg. •Vitamin K 100mcg 3x daily.

2—Phyto-estrogen herbs show body-balancing effects against yeast infections: •Crystal Star EST-AID™ caps and tea as a douche, or other formula containing *licorice, dong quai, squaw vine, alfalfa,* like Esteem TOTAL WOMAN.

3—Vaginal herbal suppositories: •Mix powders of *cranesbill, goldenseal, echinacea root, white oak bark,* and *raspberry* with cocoa butter to bind. Roll into suppositories and chill. Insert at night. Seal with a napkin or tampon. Especially for chronic vaginitis - more than a yeast infection. •*Garlic-goldenseal* powders mixed with a little yogurt and smeared on a tampon. •Nutribiotic GRAPEFRUIT SEED concentrate 20 drops in 1 gal. water. May also use orally as directed. Use vitamin A: prick an oil capsule and smear on a tampon, or simply insert the capsule into vagina (it will dissolve), 2x daily.

4—Probiotics are critical: •Transformation PLANTADOPHILUS, •Wakunaga KYO-DOPHILUS, or other acidophilus - $\frac{1}{2}$ tsp. or contents of 5 capsules in 1 TB yogurt. Smear on a tampon and insert upon retiring. Douche in the morning with $\frac{1}{4}$ teasp. acidophilus in water. Take $\frac{1}{4}$ teasp. in water orally, or 6 capsules daily.

Lifestyle Support Therapy

—Bodywork:

• Effective vaginal douches: Add 1-oz. herbs to 1-qt. water. Steep 30 min., strain.
Calendula - esp. for candida infections
Tea tree oil
Witch hazel bark/leaf or chaparral leaf
Sage or white oak bark in white vinegar
3% H$_2$O$_2$, 1 TB in 1 qt. water.

• Vaginal packs and suppositories to rebalance vaginal pH: Apply on a tampon, or mix with cocoa butter or simply insert.
Dilute *tea tree oil* or *calendula* oil.
Natren GY-NA-TREN.
Plain yogurt or a yogurt and water douche.
Acidophilus powder or capsules
Boric acid/alternate with acidophilus.
Dolisos homeopathic *Yeast Clear.*

• For vulvitis:Crystal Star FUNGEX™ gel. Don't use fluorinated cortisone creams. They cause thinning and atrophy of the skin.

• For BV and trichomonas: Drink cranberry juice, insert *tea tree oil* suppositories for 14 days, alternate salt water and vinegar douches for a week, and take vitamins B-complex and C daily each.

• For trichomonas and candida infections: Be sure to treat your sexual partner with a penis soak as well.

Common Symptoms: A yeast infection smells like bread or beer; a bacterial discharge has a fishy odor. **Leukorrhea:** itchy, irritated, inflammation of vaginal tissues; foul, "cottage cheese" discharge; painful sex. **Trichomonas:** severe itchiness; thin, foamy, yellowish discharge with a foul odor. **Bacterial Vaginosis:** foul, fishy odor, white discharge, moderate itchiness. **Vulvitis:** itching, redness, swelling, with fluid-filled blisters. **Common Causes:** Often a condition, not a disease, in which vaginal pH is imbalanced. Causes range from long exposure to antibiotics, to a weakened immune system, and hormone imbalances. The active chemical in many spermicidal creams, nonoxynol-9, aggravates recurrent cystitis and Candida yeast infections, and also kills friendly lactobacilli that protect the vagina against disease-causing micro-organisms.

See SEXUALLY TRANSMITTED DISEASES and CANDIDA ALBICANS healing suggestions for more information.

Can't find a recommended product? Call the 800 number listed in Product Resources for the store nearest you.

Warts
Moles, Skin Tags

Moles are congenital, discolored growths elevated above the surface of the skin, and may appear because of a liver or lung condition. They are harmless unless continually irritated. **Warts** are single or clustered, soft, irregular skin growths found on the hands, feet, arms and face, ranging in size from a pinhead to a small bean. They can also occur on the throat or voice box and affect the speaking voice tone. Usually caused by a virus, they are contagious and will spread if picked, bitten, or nicked through shaving. **Skin tags** are merely excess skin growths. Though some people merely cut or scrape them off, the procedure is quick, painless and infection-free from a clinic or dermatologist.

Diet & Superfood Therapy

—Nutritional therapy plan:

1—Add vitamin A rich foods to the diet, such as yellow and green fruits and vegetables, eggs, and cold water fish.

2—Add sulphur-containing foods, such as asparagus, garlic and onion family foods, fresh figs, citrus fruits and eggs.

3—Include high vitamin C foods with bioflavonoids: citrus fruits, broccoli

4—Add yogurt and other cultured foods to the diet.

5—Take a vegetable drink (pg. 218) or see below.

—Effective food applications:

• Use very soft brown-black bananas. Place a small section of peel (inside down) on the wart. Cover with a bandage and leave on 24 hours. Repeat until wart is gone.

• Apply a mixture of lemon juice, sea salt, onion juice and vitamin E oil.

• Papaya skins

• Raw potato

—Superfoods are very important:

• Crystal Star ENERGY GREEN™ drink with sea vegetables, every day for a month.

• Crystal Star BIOFLAV, FIBER & C SUPPORT™ drink.

• AloeLife ALOE GOLD drink.

Herb & Supplement Therapy

—Interceptive therapy plan: (Choose 2 or 3 recommendations)

1—**Address the infection:** •Crystal Star ANTI-BIO™ caps 6 daily or •BIOV™ extract with *usnea* if there is inflammation or bacterial infection. •For warts, use ANTI-VI™ extract 3x daily and apply ANTI-VI™ tea directly for warts. Apply •Crystal Star GINSENG SKIN REPAIR™ GEL with germanium, vitamin C and bioflavonoids; or •ANTI-BIO™ gel with *una da gato*. Or apply •*tea tree oil or oregano oil*, or •Allergy Research Oregano Oil religiously for 1-2 months, 3-4 times daily. Wonderful results. Take •Nutribiotic GRAPEFRUIT SEED extract caps as directed.

2—**High dose vitamin therapy is sometimes effective:** The high dosages recommended here should be used for no longer than 2-3 months at a time. •Zinc 75mg daily. •Emulsified A 100,000-150,000IU or •PHYCOTENE MICROCLUSTERS available at Healthy House, as an anti-infective. (Nothing seems to happen for 1 to 2 months, then growths may disappear in a week or so, all at once.) •B-complex up to 200mg daily, with extra B$_6$ 250mg daily. •Vitamin C crystals with bioflavonoids; take internally, $^1/_2$ teasp. in water every 4 hours daily. Apply locally to affected area. Also important for immunity against warts.

3—**Boost immune response:** •Enzymatic Therapy VIRAPLEX; or Nutramedix IMMUN-X; •Flora VEGE-SIL 4 daily. •N-acetyl cysteine 2000mg daily. •MICROHYDRIN from Healthy House (fights both viral and bacterial infections).

4—**Applications for warts and moles:** •Put several drops of *lomatium* extract and several drops of castor oil on a bandaid and apply; or •Crystal Star ANTI-VI™ extract drops (with *lomatium*) on a bandaid. Open and apple contents of a •Grifon MAITAKE MUSHROOM capsule daily. •*Celandine* paste or *bloodroot* paste mixed with castor oil. •Martin PYCNOGENOL GEL. •*Garlic* oil 2x daily or *garlic/parsley* caps 6 daily. •Apply a paste of garlic cloves directly and cover with a plastic strip. Use vitamin E oil on surrounding skin so it doesn't burn; also take Vitamin E 800IU daily. Usually takes a week for the wart to fall off. For wart and moles caused by a virus: (not HPV-caused warts). •Rough up a viral wart with the smooth side of an emery board and apply a drop of 3% H$_2$O$_2$ to kill the virus. ♂

Lifestyle Support Therapy

—Bodywork:

• Hypnosis therapy has been successful in controlling warts and moles.

• Some skin therapists now use an electric current passed through a wart to make it shrink.

• For plantar warts: soak foot in the hottest water you can stand about 30 minutes daily for a month. Apply Earth's Bounty O$_2$ SPRAY or H$_2$O$_2$ 3% solution.

• Rough up the wart with the smooth side of an emery board. Make a blend of essential oil of thuja and castor oil (equal parts). Apply 1 or 2 drops to wart twice daily. Wart or mole will slowly shrink and slough off. Do not squeeze or pick.

• **Soak warts** in hot water first. Then apply:

—NutriBiotic GRAPEFRUIT SEED extract full strength, or SKIN SPRAY 2 to 3x daily.

—Castor oil.

—Herbal Answers ALOE FORCE gel.

—Lysine cream applications, and take lysine capsules 500mg 3-4x daily.

—*Calendula* ointment, or B&T CALIFLORA ointment. ♂

• **For moles:** Dilute frankincense essential oil with castor oil and apply. Or, mix one to two drops frankincense oil in tea tree oil and apply.

Common Symptoms: Warts are flat or raised nodules on the skin surface, with a rough, pitted discolored surface, sometimes causing pain and discomfort when rubbed or chafed; if virally caused, warts are often contagious. Moles are generally smooth and rounded.

Common Causes: Vitamin A and mineral deficiencies; viral infection; widespread use of antibiotics and vaccinations that depress normal immunity.

See GENITAL WARTS page 493 and CYSTS, WENS & LIPOMAS page 361 for more information.

Can't find a recommended product? Call the 800 number listed in Product Resources for the store nearest you.

Water Retention
Bloating, Edema

Water retention, the excessive accumulation of fluid in body tissues and cavities, is often a problem of not enough water - a condition of body imbalance. If we don't get sufficient water, fluid levels go out of balance, and the body begins to retain more water in an effort to compensate. Kidney, liver, blood pressure, circulation, pre-menstrual and pregnancy problems are all associated with water retention. Dieting can take away foods that previously provided water. Medical diuretics, alcoholic drinks and other drugs can dehydrate, or you may just not be drinking enough healthy fluids. A natural healing program should concentrate on balancing body chemistry rather than simply releasing water.

Diet & Superfood Therapy

—**Nutritional therapy plan:**

1—Reduce salt and salty foods intake.

2—Eat largely fresh foods for 3-5 days to increase your body's food water content without density.

3—Have a leafy green salad every day with plenty of cucumbers, parsley, alfalfa sprouts and celery.

4—Eat potassium-rich foods like broccoli, seafoods and sea greens for fluid balance.

5—Avoid starchy, sugary, foods. Reduce meats, dried foods and dairy foods that demand more water to dissolve.

6—Drink at least 6-8 glasses of bottled water daily for free flowing functions, waste removal, and appetite suppression. Caffeine drinks are diuretic, but should be avoided by women with pre-period edema.

7—Take electrolyte drinks daily like Alacer MIRACLE WATER or Knudsen's RECHARGE, or Nature's Path TRACE-LYTE liquid electrolytes.

—**Superfoods are important:** Green drinks can provide both needed minerals and body acid/alkaline balance:
• Pines MIGHTY GREENS.
• Green Foods GREEN MAGMA.
• Future Biotics VITAL K 2-4 teasp. daily.
• Crystal Star SYSTEMS STRENGTH™ drink with sea greens for potassium.

Herb & Supplement Therapy

If taking prescription diuretics, be sure to include a potassium supplement in your daily diet.

—**Interceptive therapy plan: (Choose 2 to 3 recommendations)**

1—**Non-depleting, natural fluid balancers:** •Crystal Star BLDR-K™ caps (with anti-infective activity), or •TINKLE CAPS™, 4-6 daily, and/or •BLDR-K™ flushing tea; or Herbal Magic DIURET. •Dandelion leaf tea or •Cornsilk/dandelion tea, 3 cups daily; or •Juniper/parsley/uva ursi tea or uva ursi extract drops in water. •Crystal Star TINKLE TEA™ 2x daily for pre-period edema. •Ascorbic acid therapy: Vitamin C crystals with bioflavonoids and rutin, $1/2$ teasp. in water or juice every 2-3 hours until relief. Then 3-5000mg daily for prevention. •Flora VEGE-SIL as a natural diuretic; •Richardson Labs CHROMA SLIM.

2—**Enhance adrenal activity to regulate salt and water balance:** •Crystal Star ADR-ACTIVE™ caps 2-4 daily; •Arise & Shine LIQUID ORGANIC SEA MINERALS; or •Nature's Path TRACE-MIN-LYTE with sea greens for mineral balance - very important if you have low adrenal function with water retention

3—**Tone and strengthen genito-urinary tissue:** •BILBERRY or HAWTHORN extract as needed daily for tissue tone and to increase circulation. Nature's Apothecary KIDNEY SUPPORT or Herbs, Etc. KIDNEY TONIC.

4—**Enhance liver function:** •Crystal Star CEL-LEAN™ caps 3-4 daily for 1-3 months. •Enzymatic Therapy KIDNEY/LIVER COMPLEX. •B Complex 100mg daily with extra B_6 250mg 2x daily.

5—**Achieve hormone balance to achieve fluid balance:** •Crystal Star FEMALE HARMONY™ caps and tea have proven effective. •ECHINACEA extract, 10 drops in 2 cups daily of burdock tea to flush lymph glands and balance hormones. •Solaray ALFAJUICE 4 daily caps for hormone balance and as a detoxifier.

6—**Proteolytic enzymes correct nutrient assimilation leading to body balance:** •Bromelain 750mg 2x daily for a month, or •Enzymedica PURIFY.

Lifestyle Support Therapy

—**Bodywork:**
• Be careful of overusing chemical/medical diuretics. They can cause potassium and mineral loss, and eventually muscle weakness and fatigue.
• Take hot 20 minute saunas often.
• Crystal Star POUNDS OFF™ bath as a strong diaphoretic for sweating once a week.
• Exercise every day to keep circulation and body metabolism free-flowing.
• Elevate head and shoulders for sleeping.

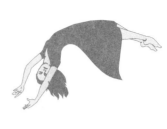

See PMS page 473 for more information about pre-period edema.

Common Symptoms: Swelling of hands, feet, ankles and stomach; PMS symptoms; headache and bloating.

Common Causes: Too much salt, red meat or MSG; kidney or bladder infection; oral contraceptives reaction; hypothyroidism; PMS symptoms; adrenal exhaustion; protein and B Complex deficiency; hormonal changes, especially estrogen output; climate changes; allergies; poor circulation; potassium depletion; allergies; corticosteroid drug reaction; obesity; constipation; lack of exercise. Persistent edema is linked to kidney, liver, bladder and circulatory problems.

Can't find a recommended product? Call the 800 number listed in Product Resources for the store nearest you.

Weight Loss

Weight Control, Excess Fat Retention

The latest statistics are shocking. One out of every two Americans is overweight. This doesn't count kids who are rapidly becoming an overweight generation. Right now, two-thirds of Americans are trying to lose weight. Amazingly, of those, only 20% are actually reducing their calories or exercising. Next to smoking, obesity is the second leading preventable cause of death in the United States, contributing to an excess of 300,000 deaths each year. The natural recommendations presented on this page can be used successfully for a wide variety of men and women struggling with their weight. Notes: Yo-yo dieting increases the risk of gallstones. For the best results, start slowly on your weight loss program and stick with it. The four keys to an effective weight control diet: low fat, high fiber, regular exercise, lots of water.

Diet & Superfood Therapy

—Nutrition diet watchwords:

1—Changing diet composition is the key. The importance of cutting back on saturated fat cannot be overstated. Saturated fats are hard for the liver to metabolize. Focus on healthy fats from seafood, sea greens, nuts and seeds which curb cravings by initiating a satiety response.

2—Fat isn't all bad. It's your body's chief energy source. Most overweight people have too high blood sugar and too low fat levels. This causes constant hunger, the delicate balance between fat storage and fat utilization is upset, and your ability to use fat for energy decreases. Eating fast, fried, or junk foods particularly aggravates this imbalance. You wind up with empty calories and more cravings. Fat becomes non-moving energy; fat cells become fat storage depots. But don't replace fats with fat substitutes like Olestra. Eating a one ounce portion of olestra potato chips on a daily basis reduces blood carotene levels by 50%! Fake fats fool your tastebuds, not your stomach. In one study, people who replaced 20% of their fat with fake fats were still hungry at the end of the day and they ate twice as much food as normal!

3—Water can get you over diet plateaus. Dehydration slows resting metabolic rate (RMR) and can cause waste products like ketones to build up in tissues. Drink juices or green tea in the morning to wash out waste products.

4—A little caffeine after a meal raises thermogenesis (calorie burning) and boosts metabolic rate. Use fat burning spices like ginger, cinnamon, garlic, mustard and cayenne.

5—High fiber fruits and veggies are a key to successful body toning. Have an apple every day!

Herb & Supplement Therapy

—Interceptive therapy plan: (Choose 1 or 2 recommendations)

1—**Stimulate BAT (brown adipose tissue) thermogenesis:** •Evening Primrose oil 1000mg 3x daily; •Carnitine 1000mg 3x daily; Arginine/ornithine 1000mg at bedtime. •Crystal Star THERMO-CITRIN® GINSENG™ caps; •Source Naturals DIET PHEN; •Pep Products ULTRA DIET PEP; •Nature's Secret ULTIMATE WEIGHT LOSS; •Diamond Herpanacine DIAMOND TRIM.

Deficiencies can lead to food binges: •B-complex with extra B-6 200mg (boosts serotonin and metabolizes carbohydrates); lack of minerals can lead to sugar craving: •Crystal Star MINERAL SPECTRUM™ or ZINC SOURCE™ caps.

2—**Control food cravings:** •Crystal Star EXTRA-STRENGTH APPE-TIGHT™ caps; •Nature's Secret THIN SOLUTION; •phenylalanine 500mg before meals (unless sensitive to phenylalanine); •5-HTP as directed; •chromium picolinate (400mcg); •L-glutamine 2000mg or •gymnema sylvestre (for sugar cravings); •Spirulina and bee pollen for energy proteins and blood sugar balance. •Rainbow Light SPIRULINA HERBAL DIET COMPLEX, or Gold Star POWERTHIN. •Wild yam caps balance sugar and boost DHEA, an appetite suppressor.

3—**Natural fat blockers:** •CLA (conjugated linoleic acid) up to 2000mg daily; fat digesting enzymes, like •Prevail FAT ENZYME; garcinia cambogia in formulas like Now's CITRI-MAX with ginseng and kelp, or •Natrol CITRI-MAX PLUS. Pyruvate to aid in the transformation of blood sugar into energy, 5 grams daily; •Twin Lab PYRUVATE FUEL. Chitosan to reduce absorption of dietary fats and cholesterol in the intestines; •Natural Balance FAT MAGNET. Note: Gastrointestinal problems may result from excessive use of pyruvate or chitosan.

4—**Good fats help burn bad fats:** •Barleans omega-3 flax oil or Omega Nutrition ESSENTIAL BALANCE help overcome binging; Co-enzyme A Technology BODY IMAGE. •Richardson Labs CHROMA-SLIM - a lipotropic-carnitine formula.

5—**Boost metabolism:** •Enzymatic Therapy THYROID/TYROSINE caps; for compulsive eating, tyrosine 1000mg with zinc 30mg daily. •Ayurvedic guggulsterone, like Ayurvedic Concepts GUGGUL caps; •Enzymatic Theraply 7-KETO NATURAL LEAN; •CoQ-10 (200mg daily turns fat into energy); L-carnitine (500-4000mg daily). Add •Nature's Plus Bromelain 1500mg 3x daily for maximum metabolism.

—**Superfoods make you feel full:** •Transitions EASY GREENS (women); •Crystal Star ENERGY GREEN™ (men); Nutritional Technologies ESSENTIAL WHEY; •Esteem Products GREEN HARVEST; •All One MULTIPLE w. green plant base.

Lifestyle Support Therapy

—Bodywork:

•Daily exercise is the key to permanent, painless weight control. Exercise releases fat from the cells. (Exercising early in the day can raise metabolism as much as 25%! Exercising before breakfast is best because the body dips into its fat stores for quick energy.)

•Even if eating habits are just slightly changed, you can still lose weight with a brisk hour's walk, or 15 minutes of aerobic exercise.

•One pound of fat represents 3500 calories. A 3 mile walk burns up 250 calories. In about 2 weeks you'll lose a pound of real extra fat. That's 3 pounds a month and 30 pounds a year without changing your diet. It's easy to see how cutting down even moderately on fatty, sugary foods in combination with exercise can still provide the look and body tone you want.

•Exercise promotes an afterburn effect, raising metabolic rate from 1.00 to 1.05-1.15 per minute up to 24 hours afterwards. Calories are used up at an even faster rate after exercise.

•Weight training exercise increases lean muscle mass, replacing fat-marbled muscle tissue with lean muscle. Muscle tissue burns calories; the greater the amount of muscle tissue you have, the more calories you can burn. This is very important as aging decreases muscle mass. Exercise before a meal raises blood sugar levels and thus decreases appetite, often for several hours afterward.

•Deep breathing exercises increase metabolic rate. See pg. 554 of this book.

See the following pages and SKIN, CELLULITE CONTROL page 499 for more.

Can't find a recommended product? Call the 800 number listed in Product Resources for the store nearest you.

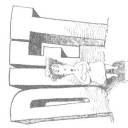

The Six Most Common Weight Loss Blockers

There are almost as many different weight loss problems as there are people who have them. I've identified six of the most common and developed comprehensive programs to address them. Each of the six plans has years of observed success behind it. Once you make the decision to be a thin person, analyze what your weight loss block really is. See **"Can You Diagnose Your Weight Problem?" on pg 525.** Identify your most prominent weight control problem, especially if there seems to be more than one. As improvement is realized in the primary area, secondary problems are often overcome in the process. If lingering problem spots still exist, they may be addressed with additional supplementation after the first program is well underway and producing noticeable results.

1: Lazy Metabolism and Thyroid Imbalance. If you've experienced weight gain after 40 or after menopause, thyroid malfunction and lowered metabolism may be to blame. Huge new studies reveal that as many as 1 in 10 women over 65 have the early stages of hypothyroidism! Fortunately, boosting metabolism and supporting your thyroid is easy. Add seaweeds like kelp, dulse and nori, rich in natural iodine, to your diet as a mainstay. Sea greens are also available in capsules or extracts, like •New Chapter OCEAN HERBS and •Crystal Star's IODINE SOURCE™. Add thermogenic spices like *cinnamon, cayenne, mustard and ginger* to speed up your fat burning process. Try dipping raw veggies in mustard throughout the day. One teasp. of mustard can increase metabolism 25% for up to 3 hours! Note: if you have the slightest tendency to wheat or gluten allergies (you'll bloat when you eat them), avoid breads and pastries.

2: Overeating Fat and Calories. Overeating or eating too much fat are big reasons why it's so hard for people to lose weight, particularly men. Men are often encouraged to dip into second, even third helpings as a sign of manliness or approval for the cook. Men also tend to overeat when they're under stress, fatigued or on-the-run....circumstances under which many American men eat today. Our lifestyles don't help. 45% of every food dollar is spent on eating out, and restaurant portions are bigger than ever as consumers demand more food for their money. Control your portions so you don't overeat. Reduce fats to no more than 20% of your food intake. (Don't replace fats with fat substitutes like Olestra.) An herbal appetite suppressant with St. *John's wort* can curb cravings for fatty foods. Hypericin, one of St. John's wort's constituents, makes the user feel full, much the same way the drug fenfluramine does, but without the hazards of heart valve damage. •Crystal Star EXTRA-STRENGTH APPE-TITE™ caps, •Natural Balance ULTRA DIET PEP or •Source Naturals DIET-PHEN are good choices.

3: Sugar Craving and Blood Sugar Imbalances. Sweets may be your weight loss block. If you are on a very low fat diet, you may be trying to make up for the fat missing in your diet by adding more sugar for better taste. Increase your intake of healthy essential fatty acids (EFA's) especially from sources like seafood, sea greens, flax seed oil to reduce those cravings. •Spectrum Essentials EVENING PRIMROSE OIL is an easy-to-use EFA source, 3000mg daily. You can also target excess sugar in the blood with herbs for weight loss. •Crystal Star GINSENG/LICORICE ELIXIR™ or •Herbal Magic HYPOGLY-HERBAL.

4: Liver Malfunction and Cellulite Formation. Your liver is responsible for fat metabolism. Most of us have a liver that's overloaded with toxic build-up today and it can be responsible for a weight control problem. Cellulite is a body shape problem related to liver malfunction. Women are hardest hit by cellulite because their skin fibers are thinner and more delicate than a man's. Fatty wastes can become lodged beneath the skin's surface more easily in a woman when the liver or lymphatic system is sluggish. Try a 2 week course of herbal bitters to regenerate the liver by increasing bile production: •Crystal Star BITTERS & LEMON™ Extract or •Gaia Herbs SWEETISH BITTERS ELIXIR. Detox your liver with •Monas CHLORELLA. Add B complex to assist with liver detoxification and fat metabolism: •Nature's Secret ULTIMATE B. Cellulite Tip: Seaweed body wraps are especially good because they also squeeze cellulitic waste back into the working areas of the body so it can be eliminated. Check out your nearest day spa for a good program. See page 499 for more on cellulite.

5: Poor Circulation and Low Energy. A sedentary lifestyle with little exercise slows down circulation, metabolism and elimination, factors which impede successful weight loss. For circulation stimulation: •Rosemary Gladstar BUTCHER'S BROOM caps, or •Futurebiotics CIRCUPLEX. Add •CoQ₁₀ - 60mg daily for antioxidant enzyme activity. Mineral electrolytes turn body energy circuits back on: •Nature's Path TRACE-LYTE. Dry brush your skin before showers to speed up your circulation and improve energy for the day. (Great for cellulite, too!)

6: Poor Elimination. If your colon is sluggish (chronic constipation), your body hangs on to toxins and wastes and your weight loss program. This build-up of waste materials in your blood and bowel slows down all systems and your weight loss program. Try an easy make-it-yourself fiber drink. Take 2 TBS of aloe vera juice in the morning for effective relief. Add 2 teasp. of an herbal formula like •Crystal Star FIBER & HERBS CLEANSE™ caps or •Herbal Magic COL-LIV HERBAL. Use massage therapy on your lower back (near the kidneys) to relieve colon congestion. If you get backaches when you're constipated, your transverse colon is probably blocked up by impacted wastes. Sometimes a little light massage work can help to break up the congestion and release the accumulated materials.

See my small library series book WEIGHT LOSS & CELLULITE CONTROL for more info.

Can't find a recommended product? Call the 800 number listed in Product Resources for the store nearest you.

Weight Control For Kids

Today's children are becoming an overweight generation. America's adults may be paying more attention to their diets, but statistics show that U.S. kids are the fattest they've ever been. An estimated 14% of children over the age of 6 are obese. Until the 1960's, weight control wasn't much of a problem for kids. But the fifties ushered in the fast food era - refined, chemicalized foods that changed people's metabolism and cell structure. As the fifties kids became parents, they passed on immune defense depletions and digestion problems to their kids who are now the parents of the overweight, undernourished kids of today. It's only the beginning. T.V. food advertising especially targets kids who are eating an ever widening array of chemical-laced, genetically altered foods, and junky foods with too much fat, salt, sugar and calories. Some kids eat out of a box most of the time!

U.S. schools have dropped the ball for children's health, offering kids more fatty, nutrient-starved meals and less physical exercise. The telecommunications age has brought kids computers, T.V.'s, and video games - and a lot less active playtime. (Today's kids get less exercise and outdoor play than any previous generation.) P.E. classes in U.S. schools, most sports and many extra-curricular activities have been dropped, and our kids are paying the price. Most kids attend only 1 or 2 physical education classes a week. Forty percent of boys 6-12 can't touch their toes; American girls actually run slower today than they did 10 years ago. P.E. teachers have been reassigned to other classes in a full three-quarters of U.S. schools.

Nineties kids watch up to 24 hours of TV a week. By the time U.S. kids reach their senior high school year, they've spent over 3 years of their lives watching TV. Even more alarming, heart disease is now traceable to early childhood. U.S. doctors are discovering that many American teens (even some 3 year olds) already have fatty deposits on their coronary arteries. Today's kids rely on junk foods. Children are rewarded with food for good behavior or denied food for punishment from an early age. As they grow older, kids tend to continue that cycle by rewarding themselves with salty, sugary, fatty snacks, soft drinks, and nitrate-loaded lunch meats before parents even come home from work.

Overweight children face early diseases, low self-esteem, depression and rejection by peers. Getting weight problems under control at an early age is the best choice for later health. As an obese child grows older, he or she doubles the likelihood of adult obesity. But, crash diets are not the solution for kids (or adults). Changing the focus to health, to having a fit body instead of a thin body can make all the difference in a weight management program. Kids need mineral-rich building foods, fiber-rich energy foods, and protein-rich growth foods.

I recommend a light detox to start a good weight control program for an overweight child, who usually has a "toxic overload" from too many chemical-laced foods. A gentle detox normalizes body chemistry. My **JUNK FOOD DETOX FOR KIDS** is a 3 day diet. Avoid all highly processed, junky foods, red meats and dairy foods, except yogurt during this detox.

—**On rising:** give citrus juice with 1 teaspoon of acidophilus liquid, or a glass of lemon juice and water with honey or maple syrup.
—**Breakfast:** offer fresh fruits, such as apples, pineapple, papaya or oranges. Add vanilla yogurt or soymilk if desired.
—**Mid-morning:** give fresh carrot juice. Add ¼ teasp. ascorbate vitamin C or Ester C crystals to neutralize body toxins.
—**Lunch:** give fresh raw crunchy veggies with a yogurt dip; or a fresh veggie salad with lemon/oil or yogurt dressing.
—**Mid-afternoon:** offer a refreshing herb tea, such as *licorice* or *peppermint* tea with honey.
—**Dinner:** give a fresh salad, with avocados, carrots, kiwi, romaine and other high vitamin A foods; and/or a cup of miso soup or other clear broth soup.
—**Before bed:** offer a relaxing herb tea, like *chamomile* tea, or •Crystal Star GOOD NIGHT TEA™. Add ¼ teasp. vitamin C or Ester C crystals; or a cup of MISO broth for strength.

Once the light detox is over, begin a healthy diet. Breakfast is a key for weight loss for kids. A high fiber breakfast cuts a child's calories by up to 200 calories a day and holds a child til lunchtime. Add fresh plant, enzyme-rich foods to the child's diet. Many of today's diet don't work because they rely on microwaved foods - a process that kills the enzymes. Enzyme dead foods create a nutritional gap for our kids (some experts say we would die if all we ate was micro-waved foods). For some children, this also means weight gain and constipation, a major problem for kids that eat a lot of dairy foods like milk, cheese and ice cream. 20% of Caucasian children and 80% of black children don't produce lactase, the enzyme necessary to digest milk.

Here are two enzyme rich juice recipes that even the pickiest of kids will ask for again and again.

#1 **GREEN DRINK FOR KIDS:** Make it in a juicer. Make it easy. Use any fresh veggies that your child likes most. Include green leafy vegetables like spinach, sunflower greens and lettuces. I find that kids like baby veggies. Consider baby bok choy, baby carrots and sprouts. Don't forget sweet tasting veggies like cucumbers, celery and tomatoes.

#2 **ENERGIZING FRUIT SMOOTHIE:** Use fresh fruit, not canned or frozen. Blend 1 banana and 1 orange with apple juice. Add half a papaya or or one-quarter of a fresh pineapple.

If you don't have a juicer, give your child a good plant enzyme supplement to keep his metabolism going strong, like •Prevail's CHILDREN'S DIGESTION FORMULA, or •Transformation's powdered DIGEST ZYME, both quality products I've worked with. Check out my small library series book WEIGHT LOSS & CELLULITE CONTROL for a complete kid's weight loss diet and more tips. It has passed many tests for foods overweight and "couch potato" kids will eat. It focuses on good nutrition, so your child will have less craving for junk foods.

Can't find a recommended product? Call the 800 number listed in Product Resources for the store nearest you.

Weight Control After 40

There's no doubt about it. Weight loss gets more difficult after 40. The latest figures show that body fat typically doubles between the ages of 20 and 50. Everybody goes through a change of life, and those middle years affect our body shapes, too....for both men and women. One of the worst problems America's fitness oriented population faces in their 40's and 50's is a disconcerting body thickening and a slow, steady rise in weight. It seems to happen with everybody, even people who have always been slim, who have a good diet, and who regularly exercise.

For women, a primary calorie-burning process grinds to a halt after menopause. Here's why: A woman's menstrual cycle consumes extra calories. Some experts theorize that the metabolic rise in the last two weeks of the menstrual cycle accounts for 15,000-20,000 calories per year. Those calories really start to add up when menstruation ceases! While a woman needs to work a little harder to lose that extra fat later in life, once her body adjusts to its new hormone levels, weight gain stabilizes, becomes manageable, and, in many cases, falls back to premenopausal levels. Lower testosterone levels in andropausal men can mean a decrease in muscle mass and increase in fat storage. But, by cutting back on fat and adding more fiber to their diets most men can lose the middle-age spread.

I've been working for several years to develop natural weight control techniques for people trying to maintain slimness and tone after their metabolism changes. The program shows promise and results. For weight loss after 40, begin with two starting points: 1) Improve body chemistry at the gland and hormone level; 2) Re-establish better, long-lasting metabolic rates.

#1 LOVE YOUR LIVER. The liver is your body's chemical plant responsible for fat metabolism. It is intricately involved with hormone functions, so it is the prime target to optimize for weight loss after 40. Weight gain and energy loss signal a liver that has enlarged through overwork, alcohol exhaustion and congestion. A good thermogenesis (calorie-burning) herbal formula with ginseng works extremely well. I have used •Crystal Star's THERMO-GINSENG™ extract for many years with success. •Gaia Herbs GINSENG SUPREME is a good choice; or add liver tonics: fresh vegetable juices, dandelion greens, *milk thistle seed extract* (accelerates liver regeneration by a factor of four); •Enzymatic Therapy SUPER MILK THISTLE COMPLEX with artichoke; •Herbs Etc. LIVER TONIC; or a liver tonic tea: *4oz hawthorn berries, 2-oz. red sage, and 1-oz. cardamom seeds.* Steep 24 hours in 2 qts. water. Add honey. Take 2 cups daily.

#2 CONSCIOUSLY EAT LESS. As metabolism slows, you don't need to fuel it up as much, because your body doesn't use up nutrients like it once did. If you eat like you did in your 20's and 30's, your body will store too much, mostly as fat. New research shows that moderate food intake may extend lifespan by as much as ten years!

• **Make sure you are eating a low fat diet.** Even with all the fat-conscious foods on the market today, Americans still consume one-third of their calories as fat. Your fat intake should be about 20% for weight control, 15% or less for weight loss. But remember: no-fat is not good for weight loss, either. Your body goes into a survival mode if you eliminate all fat, shedding its highly active lean muscle tissue to reduce your body's need for food. When lean muscle tissue decreases, fat burning slows or stops.

• **Control your food portions.** Portion control is a cornerstone of weight control. Even though your diet is healthy and the foods you eat reasonably low in fat, there's no way you can eat all you want of anything. Eat smaller meals every two to three hours to keep your appetite hole from gnawing, and to keep metabolic rate high. Small meals virtually prevent carbohydrates and proteins from being converted into fat.

• **Control hunger with safe herbal appetite suppressants.** Serotonin is the brain chemical linked to mood and appetite. Serotonin balancers like *St. John's wort*, 5-HTP, and *evening primrose oil* can help stabilize mood and reduce food cravings. Herbal weight loss combinations help because they can address almost every individual problem of weight control. Superfood herbs like *barley grass, spirulina, sea greens* and *alfalfa* can be a key to controlling appetite. A green drink with these low-calorie foods can be taken mid-afternoon to rapidly decrease a craving for high-calorie foods. Crystal Star's ENERGY GREEN™ drink can raise both metabolic rate and activity levels.

• **Control your cravings:** The herb *gymnema sylvestre* can help control sugar cravings. Gymnema binds with sugar receptors in the mouth, causing sugary foods to lose their appealing sweet flavor, an effect can last for up to 2 hours. Seven different clinical studies show *garcinia cambogia* or HCA (hydroxycitric acid) reduces food intake an amazing 46% when taken orally. Gaia Herbs combines gymnema and HCA in their product •ELIM/SLIM SUPREME.

#3 RAISE YOUR METABOLISM. A higher metabolic rate means you burn more fat, lose weight easier, and maintain your ideal body weight more comfortably.

• Don't skip meals.... especially breakfast. Breakfast is the worst meal to skip if you want to raise metabolism. It sends a temporary fasting signal to the brain that food is going to be scarce. So stress hormones increase, and the body begins shedding lean muscle tissue in order to decrease its need for food. By the time you eat again, your pancreas is so sensitized to a lack of food, that it sharply increases blood insulin levels, your body's signal to make fat. Eating early in the day, when your metabolism is at its best, with hours of activity ahead of you to burn fats is the best for weight loss. Reduce both sugars and fats - they slow metabolism. Fats have twice the calories, gram for gram, as protein and complex carbohydrates. They also use only 2% of their calories before the fat storage process begins. Protein and carbohydrates burn almost 25% of their calories before storing them as fat. Limit alcohol consumption, even wine, to two glasses or less a day. With seven calories per gram, alcohol sugars shift metabolism in favor of fat depositing; too much alcohol burdens the liver and stimulates the appetite.

Can't find a recommended product? Call the 800 number listed in Product Resources for the store nearest you.

• **Eat fat-burning foods.** Foods that raise metabolism are fresh fruits and vegetables (full of enzymes), whole grains and legumes. Eat fruits for breakfast or between meals. If you eat them with or after meals, the fructose is likely to be converted to fat by the liver. Sea greens work especially well for women to recharge metabolism and balance thyroid activity. Sea greens are also a rich source of fat-soluble vitamins like D, and K which help balance estrogen, and DHEA. I like toasted nori, wakame, dulse and sea palm, to recharge metabolism after menopause. Two tablespoons a day are a therapeutic dose. Add them chopped and dried to any salad, soup, rice dish or omelet. Or, add 6 pieces of sushi daily to your diet.

• **Re-activate your fat-burning systems with herbs.** Herbal adaptogens like *panax* and *Siberian ginseng*, *suma*, *gotu kola*, and *licorice root* normalize body homeostasis; *ginkgo biloba* and *hawthorn* boost circulation; *bee pollen*, *alfalfa*, and phytohormone-containing herbs like *sarsaparilla* and *black cohosh* support the liver; spices and sea greens like *cayenne*, *ginger*, *kelp* and *spirulina* help the thyroid govern metabolism. •Crystal Star FEEL GREAT™ caps are a whole body tonic to enhance fat burning and well-being.

• Amino acids boost metabolism and keep lean muscle. —L-Phenylalanine (LPA), suppresses appetite, boosts energy and reduces food craving. (Avoid phenylalanine if you are taking anti-depressant medication, have high blood pressure, or are pregnant.) —L-Tyrosine is a thyroid precursor and reduces appetite. —L-Carnitine suppresses appetite, accelerates fat metabolism and helps control sugar levels. Amino acids and appetite-control herbs combined in a formula like •Crystal Star's AMINO ZYME™ work extremely well. Other amino acid metabolic products I have worked with to assist weight maintenance include •MYOPLEX LITE by EAS, and •AMINO BALANCE by Anabol Naturals.

• **Drink plenty of water.** Drink at least six 8-oz servings of water daily, even if you're not thirsty. Water naturally suppresses appetite, helps maintain a high metabolic rate, promotes good digestion and regular bowel movements, and actually reduces fat deposits. Water may be the most important catalyst for increased fat burning, because it increases the liver's main functions of detoxification and metabolism to process more fats. Don't be concerned with fluid retention. High water intake actually decreases bloating, because it flushes out sodium and toxins. Studies show that decreasing water intake causes increased fat deposits. Expert dieters drink eight glasses of water a day. They know each pound of fat burned releases 22 ounces of water which must be flushed away along with the metabolic by-products of fat breakdown.

#4 **EXERCISE FOR SURE.** Regular exercise is a standard we should all strive for. The newest studies find that getting regular exercise extends life-span and cuts the risk for heart attack in half! But, recent statistics from the National Institutes of Health find that 58% of adult Americans get no or little exercise. Daily exercise is the key to permanent, painless weight control. No diet will work without exercise; with it, almost every diet will. Exercise before a meal raises blood sugar levels, increases metabolism and decreases appetite, often for hours afterward. Even if you just slightly change your eating habits, you can still lose weight with a brisk hour's walk. Aerobic exercise, combined with a low fat, low calorie, fresh foods diet is particularly good for women. One study shows that overweight women who cut their calories and added an aerobic exercise program significantly reduced their PMS problems like mood swings and poor concentration. They also had lower blood levels of monoamine oxidase (an enzyme linked to PMS).... and they lost an average of 36 pounds.

• **Get moderate doses of sunlight.** The sun receives a lot of criticism today, but sunlight in moderation increases metabolism and food digestion. One of the best choices is to eat outdoors. Sunlight can produce metabolic effects in the body similar to that of physical training.

Thermogenesis is Critical To Weight Loss After 40. Thermogenesis is about fat burning. About 75% of the calories you eat work to keep you alive and support your resting metabolic rate. The rest are stored as white fat, or burned up by brown adipose tissue, (BAT), your fat-burning factory. Brown fat is the body's chief regulator of thermogenesis, so the more active your brown fat is, the easier it is to maintain a desirable weight. Dieters who rely solely on restricting their calorie intake usually end up disappointed with the results, because extreme calorie restriction lowers the rate of thermogenesis. Your body actually burns less fat than it did before you started dieting. People who yo-yo on and off low calorie diets have even more problems. When a yo-yo dieter begins to increase calorie intake after dieting, their metabolic rate does not return to pre-diet levels, so they store more calories as fat than they did before they started!

Middle-aged spread means too little thermogenesis after you eat. Everybody increases metabolism after eating, but the amounts of heat (calorie burning) vary widely. Lean people experience a 40% increase in heat production after a meal. Overweight people may have only an increase of 10%. Obesity occurs primarily when brown fat isn't working properly, only a little thermogenesis takes place, and the body deals with the excess calories by storing them as fat. During our mid-life years, starting in our early 40's, a genetic timer shuts down the thermogenic mechanism. Turning this timer back on is the secret to re-activating thermogenesis and a more youthful metabolism. Here's how brown fat works to stimulate thermogenesis: A protein, called uncoupling protein, breaks down, or uncouples, the train of biochemical events that the cells use to turn calories into energy. Brown fat cells continue to convert calories into heat as long as they are stimulated, and as long as there is white fat for them to work on. Brown fat activity is also self-perpetuating, because it energizes more uncoupling proteins, produces more brown fat cells, and results in substantially more excess calories being burned off as heat through thermogenesis.

Research into the genetic basis of obesity shows that some people are not born with enough brown fat. People who eat lightly but still can't lose weight, gain more weight at middle age because the little brown fat they did have is reduced even further. Thermogenesis research demonstrates that it is possible to reverse this abberation. Thermogenic herbs have been successful at reactivating brown fat in middle age. They can increase calorie burning without additional support of diet changes or exercise, although these things offer additional benefits. • Thermogenic herbs increase blood flow to lean muscle tissue, so it works faster and longer. • Thermogenic herbs suppress appetite. You eat less with less effort. • The longer you take thermogenic herb formulas, the more effective they tend to become, because they help your body produce enough thermogenic activity to make a difference.

Weight loss is not easy in today's lifestyle. Reaching your ideal weight is a victory. Keeping it requires vigilance.

Can't find a recommended product? Call the 800 number listed in Product Resources for the store nearest you.

Personal Ailment Analysis
Home Healing Procedures

A How-To Section

One of the most valuable assets of conventional medicine is its diagnostic arsenal of medical tests and laboratory analyses. Without taking any of the authority away from these important medical tools, there are many personal information techniques that you can use a home to determine your body's status during a health crisis or a healing program.

Most of these methods have been part of traditional natural healing for centuries, but seem to have been forgotten, or underestimated in our society's current enchantment with high tech science.

This new section includes Dr. Page's recently completed, innovative work in personal analysis of health problems. These are Signs and Symptoms Alert Tests you can do yourself. They can take you a long way toward understanding how your body works when it's under a disease attack. The knowledge gained can show you a clearer pathway to the natural healing procedures you can use to maximize your restorative program.

Also included are some therapeutic techniques you can use to chart your improvement over the course of the healing process....an interesting part of watching your body and immune system at work.

A CORRECT FOOD COMBINING chart is included as a guide so you can maximize your nutrient assimilation.

New Personal Illness Analysis
Healthy Healing - 11th Edition!

Ailment diagnosis has traditionally been the unchallenged prerogative of conventional protocol. The medical world has maintained that only its complex, expensive and sometimes painful testing procedures can correctly diagnose health problems. But is this actually the case?

Many people feel that much diagnostic testing has little to do with necessary diagnosis, being instead a lawsuit preventive measure, or the result of the enormous, profit-driven establishment between health care providers and health care insurers. People trying to take more responsibility for their health are annoyed, and sometimes overwhelmed by a seemingly endless round of expensive, often invasive tests.

Can you correctly diagnose your own health problems?

I believe in many cases, you can appraise the status of your well-being, especially in uncovering health conditions that are based in your life-style and nutrition choices. Key questions in my self appraisal tests can point you in the right direction to determine your healing needs for certain health problems.

Note: If you have more than half of the "signs and symptoms" listed after each problem, you are probably at risk for that deficiency or health problem. If you have one-quarter of the symptoms, you are probably slightly deficient or have a tendency toward the health problem. Refer to the specific health problems in the AILMENTS SECTION of this book to learn more about each and how to get help in healing yourself with your diet, herbs, supplements and bodywork.

Do you have an eating disorder?

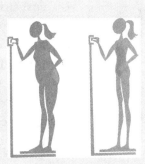

Signs and symptoms of an eating disorder:
- Do you constantly feel fat regardless of your actual weight?
- Have you repeatedly tried and failed to lose weight?
- Do you ever fast or put yourself on incredibly strict diets?
- Are you preoccupied with food?
- Do you eat when you are under stress or depressed?
- Do you try to hide your eating habits from others?
- Is there a relationship between eating and your self-esteem? Do you feel you have lost control?
- Do you sometimes binge, or eat large amounts of food in a short period of time?
- Have you ever tried to "undo" the damage of eating by vomiting, taking laxatives or fasting?
- Do you exercise compulsively? Do you feel guilty or fat if you miss a regular exercise schedule?
- Are you a vegetarian solely to be thin, or for other reasons?
- Do you feel guilty when you eat meat and dairy, or even caloric and high-fat vegetarian foods?
- Do you prepare food for others but refuse to eat it yourself? Do you have a rigid eating routine?
- Do you still think you're fat even after losing a substantial amount of weight?
- How do your weight loss goals compare with what weight charts suggest for your height?

Analyzing your weight problem:

There are almost as many different weight loss problems as there are people who have them. These weight loss problem symptom lists can help you analyze what your weight loss block really is.

1. Lazy Metabolism and Thyroid Imbalance: Is your metabolism is low?
- General weakness and fatigue (especially in the morning)
- Digestive disturbances like heartburn and indigestion
- Unusual depression and anxiety
- Breast fibroids
- Hair loss (especially in middle-aged women)

2. Overeating Fat and Calories: Empty calories like junk food are the downfall of dieters.
- Binging on junk foods, especially fatty and sugary foods, about every ten days
- Eating all your calories at one meal and then trying to eat nothing for the rest of the day when you're dieting. (Most people can't do it.)
- Having second and third helpings at a meal but still feeling hungry

3. Sugar Craving And Blood Sugar Imbalances: Dieters who drastically lower their fats often replace them with empty carbohydrates like sugar and starches. But, sugary foods raise insulin levels too much — your body's signal to make fat, no good for weight loss. Here are the signs:
- Moodiness, being easily frustrated with a tendency towards crying spells
- Great fatigue (especially after sugar binges)
- Having a wired feeling that is only relieved by eating sweets

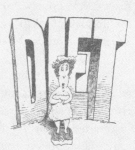

4. Liver Malfunction And Cellulite Formation: Liver malfunction is directly related to sugar metabolism as a cause of weight problems. Further, a poorly functioning liver is almost always involved in cellulite formation. Signs of liver malfunction and cellulite formation:
- Extreme, unrelenting fatigue; unusual depression and sadness
- Unexplained weight gain
- Poor digestion (worsens after fatty meals); chronic constipation and heartburn
- Food and chemical sensitivities
- Bulging, dimply, skin on hips, buttocks, thighs and knees (women); torso and stomach (men)

5. Poor Circulation And Low Energy: For some dieters, initial weight loss is rapid, but then a plateau is reached and further weight loss becomes difficult because restricted food intake slows down metabolism, reduces energy and can affect circulation. Here are signs to watch for:
- Hands, feet, face and ears becoming cold easily
- Poor memory
- Ringing in the ears

6. Poor Elimination: An astounding 30 million Americans have chronic constipation.... and it can be a major factor in weight control. Signs of elimination problems:
- frequent bad breath, body odor and coated tongue
- infrequent bowel movements

I've developed comprehensive programs to successfully address each of the six weight loss blockers covered here. See page 519, or my *Healthy Healing Guide To Weight Loss & Cellulite Control*.

Do you have allergies?

Substances that cause allergy reactions are called allergens.

—Allergies to environmental allergens like air pollutants, asbestos or heavy metals, and seasonal allergens to dust, pollen, spores and mold, are called Type 1 allergies. This type of allergy develops more easily if your body has excess mucous accumulation to harbor the allergen irritants. Drugstore medications for environmental allergies only mask symptoms, often cause drowsiness and have a rebound effect. **The more you use them, the more you need them.** Steroid drugs for environmental allergies, especially if taken over a long period of time, depress immune defenses and impede allergen elimination. Environmental allergens frequently interact in the bodies of allergy sufferers, both activating and aggravating other offending irritants. When this is the case, even the most powerful drugs do not relieve symptoms.

Signs and symptoms that you may have a Type 1 environmental or seasonal allergy:

- Do you have chronic sinus congestion with itchy, watery nose and eyes?
- Do you get headaches with sneezing, coughing and scratchy throat?
- Does your face swell up, with itchy, rashy skin? Do you have a skin rash on your arms or torso?
- Do you have trouble sleeping at night? Are you unusually tired during the day?
- Do you have unusual menstrual pain and congestion?
- Do you have hypoglycemia?

Spore and pollen allergens produce congestion as the body tries to seal them off from its regular processes, or tries to work around them. Extra mucous is formed as a shield around the offending substances, so you feel the allergy symptoms of sinus clog, stuffiness, headaches and puffy eyes. Sometimes the body tries to throw this excess off through the skin, and you get skin irritations or a scratchy sore throat. An allergic response to pollen also causes a histamine release that swells nasal passages and sensitive membranes, producing symptoms like runny, itchy nose and eyes, sneezing and coughing attacks, sore throat, bronchial and sinus infections, itchy skin rashes, asthma, insomnia, menstrual disorders and hypoglycemia.

—Allergies to chemicals and contaminant allergens are called Type 2 allergies. Reactions to chemicals are frequently a defense mechanism, the body's attempt to isolate an offending substance by storing it in fatty tissue. An allergic reaction of this type only occurs after the second exposure to the irritant when your body's histamine response is alerted. Repeated exposures set off massive free radical reactions as the body's contaminant toleration levels are reached; toxic overload results and a severe allergic reaction sets in. Worse, chemical sensitivities initiate other allergy reactions, so that the sufferer becomes allergic to nearly everything else.

Signs and symptoms that you may have a Type 2 allergy to chemicals and contaminants:

- Unexplained migraine headaches? Usually with nausea or diarrhea?
- Frequent skin rashes for no explained reason?
- Low energy? Feel "under the weather" regardless of how much sleep you get?
- Hear your ears ringing, especially at night?
- Frequent colds and flu, or chronic respiratory inflammations?
- Frequently moody and depressed for no reason?
- Gained or lost weight recently for no reason? (Chemical allergies may cause poor metabolism.)
- Do friends and family tell you that your personality changes?
- Are often space-y? Is your memory is getting unusually bad?
- Do you have a child that's chronically hyperactive or who has difficulty learning?

Common chemical-contaminant irritants vary, from a wide range of petrochemicals and estrogenic chemicals, to combustion residues from household appliances and heating systems, to various kinds of sprays, paints and exhaust fumes. Other culprits include: chlorine bleach, moth balls and insect repellents, dry cleaning chemicals, and clothes that have been chemically treated.

—Allergies, intolerances and sensitivities to foods or food additives are the fastest growing form of allergic reactions in the U.S. today, as people are more exposed to chemically altered foods. Food intolerances are often confused with food allergies. **A food allergy** is an antibody reaction — an immune system response to a food your body views as a pathogen or parasite. Food allergies may be hereditary; a child is twice as likely to develop food allergies if one parent has them, or four times as likely if both parents have them. **A food intolerance** is an enzyme deficiency to digest a certain food. For example, people with a lactose intolerance experience the bloating, cramping and diarrhea of an allergy reaction, but the symptoms are really due to a deficiency of the enzyme lactase, which helps digest milk sugar. Common food intolerances include those to wheat, dairy foods, fruit, sugar, yeast, mushrooms, eggs, corn and greens. These foods may be healthy in themselves, but they are often heavily sprayed or treated; in the case of animal products, also injected with antibiotics and hormones. **Food sensitivities** are similar to allergy reactions, but differ in that no antigen-specific antibodies are present. A food sensitivity is usually not a permanent allergy response.

Signs and symptoms that you may have a Type 2 food allergy or intolerance:
- Are you unable to eat normal amounts of a food? Are you nauseated after eating?
- Do you get cyclical headaches with mental fuzziness after eating?
- Do you get heart palpitations, with sweating, rashes or puffiness around the eyes after eating?
- Does your abdomen become excessively swollen after eating with heartburn or stomach cramps?
- Have you gained significant weight even though your diet hasn't changed?
- Do you have Crohn's disease?
- Do you have hypothyroidism or hypoglycemia?
- Do you have a child that's irritable, flushed and hyperactive after eating?

If you answer yes to most of these questions, you may have an allergy, intolerance or sensitivity to certain foods or food additives, another kind of Type 2 allergy. Regardless of the food, the reaction symptoms are similar. Inflammation occurs from histamine release into tissue mast cells, walling off the affected body area until immune response agents can restore health. But this process takes time. If the body is re-exposed before health is renewed, inflammation and symptoms, especially mucous congestion, become chronic.

Do you have asthma?

Asthma is the most serious Type 1 allergy reaction. Twenty million people in the U.S. alone have asthma, up from 10.4 million reported by the National Institute of Health in 1990. Asthma is a chronic, breathing disorder characterized by bronchial spasms which restrict the flow of air in and out of the lungs. A person with healthy lungs can empty air in about 2-3 seconds. An asthmatic's lungs take 6-7 seconds! During an asthma attack, a person has extreme difficulty breathing with especially great difficulty in exhaling because the lungs cannot breathe air out. The bronchioles, tubes which carry air through the lungs, become thick with mucous, causing muscular spasms and choking. Asthma attacks are critically serious, sometimes even fatal — about 5,000 people die of asthma every year. Almost 2 million people need emergency room care for asthma at a cost of over $200 million!

Sadly, asthma is the most common chronic disease of childhood and it's on the rise. The number of children hospitalized for asthma has increased fivefold over the past 20 years! Kids miss 10 million school days each year from asthma-related problems. Children have smaller lungs and bronchial tubes, and less breathing reserves during an asthma attack than adults. They also have more respiratory infections which trigger asthma attacks. Heredity, diet and lifestyle are all involved with asthma's development and symptom severity. A child whose mother has asthma is more likely to develop it than other children. Exposure to tobacco smoke, cockroaches and dust mites, food allergies or sensitivities, hormonal changes and viral infections are linked to asthma.

527

Signs and symptoms that you might have asthma:
- Frequent wheezing, shortness of breath, chest tightness (worse during physical activity or stress)
- Harsh cough with choking that sounds like seals barking with excess phlegm and mucous
- Difficult breathing, particularly difficulty in exhaling (sometimes with heart palpitations)
- Highly reactive to allergens: animals, dust mites, molds, pollen, strong odors or food additives
- Reduced immune response; frequent cold and flu infections

Is the fluoride in your water and toothpaste poisoning you?

I was shocked when I read the new studies on fluoride toxicity and its deadly effects on health, especially for postmenopausal women, young children and developing babies. I was even more shocked to find out that big business, with the help of government officials, is still dumping this hazardous waste, under the guise of its health benefits, into the public water supply. Europe paid attention to those studies and is now 98% fluoridation-free. Many U.S. cities are also beginning to reject fluoride legislation.

Most of us have been brought up to believe fluoride was good for teeth. Fluoride has been added to the water supply and toothpastes for decades, because studies conducted by our Public Health Services determined fluoride had health benefits for teeth. Newer large-scale studies *show no difference* in decay rates of permanent teeth in fluoridated and non-fluoridated areas. In addition, *fluoride sources* were different decades ago. They weren't a by-product of the phosphate fertilizer industry as they are today; they were a product of the aluminum industry, sodium fluoride. Today, the type of fluoride that's added to almost 70% of our water supply is *hydrofluosilicic acid*... much more problematic than the sodium fluoride of years ago. Hydrofluosilicic acid is only 40-50% fluoride. The rest is heavy metals, like arsenic, lead, aluminum, and uranium-238. It's full of waste pollutants, sludges and chemicals that are virtually untreated by the scrub system used to process it before it is dumped into our water. If airborne, this substance can kill humans, plants and animals.

Signs and symptoms of fluoride toxicity:
- bone damage — early signs of osteoporosis, too-easy bone fractures
- dental fluorosis, a first sign of fluoride poisoning is marked by pitted teeth or white specked teeth
- higher than normal birth defects or cancer in an area
- nervous system malfunctions; a tendency to kidney problems
- learning disabilities; lower than normal IQ scores in children (fluoride is more toxic than lead)
- cardiovascular problems like arrthymias
- signs of early Alzheimer's disease

The dedicated people from Citizens for Safe Drinking Water work hard to protect the water supply from mandatory water fluoridation. For more information, you can contact them @ 1-800-728-3833.

Is your liver exhausted?

Your liver is an amazing organ. It is the key to your body's natural detoxification process, and maintaining optimum immune response; it is at the seat of energy production. Your liver converts everything you eat, breathe and absorb through the skin into life-sustaining substances. It manufactures bile to digest fats and prevent constipation. It metabolizes proteins and carbohydrates, and secretes hormones and enzymes. The liver has amazing regenerative powers, but in today's world, protecting your liver from toxic overload and exhaustion is not easy. In the United States, liver disorders, largely a result of a lifestyle that includes lots of toxins, are responsible for more than 50,000 deaths annually.

Signs and symptoms that your liver may be exhausted:

- Liver disease such as cirrhosis or chronic hepatitis, or unusually high cholesterol levels
- Unexplained fatigue and headaches
- Thick, coated tongue (yellowish or white), usually accompanied by chronic constipation
- Jaundice or yellowish tint to the skin, eczema, psoriasis, acne rosacea or several age spots
- Gas or discomfort that worsens after a fatty meal. (The liver is responsible for fat metabolism.)
- A man who is thin everywhere else but who has a protruding stomach
- Frequent cold and flu infections, and a high incidence of allergic reactions
- Eating rich foods like heavy meats and cheeses, excessive drinking and using prescription drugs —especially non steroidal anti-inflammatory drugs and acetaminophen for pain.

Do you have signs of Alzheimer's or Parkinson's disease?

Alzheimer's disease is a progressive, degenerative condition that attacks the brain, forming neurofiber tangles and plaques that result in dementia symptoms—impaired memory, decreased intellectual and emotional function, and, ultimately, complete physical breakdown. It's a devastating, relentless assault that's rising at a rapid rate in industrialized countries worldwide. Increased oxidative damage from free-radicals plays a prominent role in the development of Alzheimer's. Genetic factors may also be involved, but environmental exposure to harmful chemicals, aluminum or inorganic silicon are thought to be a key. Some Alzheimer's victims are really victims of too many drugs.

Parkinson's disease, often a risk factor for Alzheimer's, is the progressive deterioration of specific nerve centers in the brain. The disease changes the balance of acetylcholine and dopamine, two brain chemicals essential for transmission of nerve signals. The altered balance of these neurotransmitters results in a lack of control of physical movements. Although orthodox medicine has been unable to make a difference in these diseases, natural therapies have been successful in slowing deterioration of brain and nerve function.

Signs and symptoms of Alzheimer's and Parkinson's disease:

- A noticeable loss of ability to think clearly or remember familiar names, places or events?
- Loss of touch with reality, difficulty in finishing thoughts or following directions?
- Are there clear, unexplained personality or behavior changes with confusion or poor judgement?
- Is there a slight tremor in the hands with numbness and tingling in the hands and feet?
- If you noticed a hand tremor, has it become more evident with shaking of the head as well?
- Is there slight dragging of the feet, pronounced with stress or fatigue?
- If movement is lethargic, has speech also become slow and difficult to follow?
- Has the face lost expression, with muscle rigidity? Is there slight drooling? Is vision impaired?
- Is there unexplained depression? (Supplementation may offer dramatic improvement.)

Do you know your cancer risk?

Do we know what causes cancer? Even though there are many types of cancer, diet is always the first place to look, both for help and for causative reasons. The latest estimates list nutritional factors as accounting for 60% of women's cancers and 40% of men's. Extrapolating from that number means that good food choices could have helped prevent 385,000 to 700,000 new cancer cases, and between 170,000 to 325,000 cancer deaths in 1994 in the United States alone.

Hormone-driven cancers like ovarian, breast, uterine, kidney, bladder, prostate and colon cancers are closely related to the kind of protein and fat we eat, especially protein and fat from meats, and oxidized fats from junk foods and fried foods. Dietary factors are also directly linked to cancer of the rectum, stomach, intestines, mouth, throat, esophagus, pancreas, liver and thyroid.

Yet, there is encouraging evidence that certain dietary factors also act as anti-carcinogens, preventing tumor development and growth, inhibiting tumor metastasis of cancerous growths, and helping to normalize cancer cells. Nutritional therapy for cancer relies on re-establishing metabolic balance. Whole food nutrition allows the body to use its built-in restorative and repair abilities.

Signs and symptoms that you may be at increased risk for cancer:
- Immune strength is your key protection against cancer. Do you have recurrent or long term infections?
- Do you catch colds easily? Even mild colds are signs of weak immune response.
- Do you get frequent cold sores or have genital herpes?
- Do you have swollen, sore lymph glands?
- Is your circulation poor?
- Do you have chronic indigestion?
- Do you take large amounts of antacids on a regular basis?

Do you have signs of Arthritis?

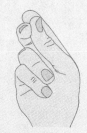

Arthritis isn't a simple disease in any form, affecting not only the bones and joints, but also the blood vessels (Reynaud's disease), kidneys, skin (psoriasis), eyes and brain. Because its causes are rooted in immune response as well as wear-and-tear effects, conventional medicine has not been able to address arthritis successfully. Making diet and lifestyle changes to normalize body chemistry, is the most beneficial thing you can do to control an arthritic condition. I have personally seen notable reduction of swelling, and deformity even in long-standing cases.

Arthritis is unique in its close ties to emotional health. Emotional stress frequently brings onset of the disease. Acid-causing, emotional resentments and negative obsessive-compulsive actions aggravate arthritis. Most arthritis sufferers have a marked inability to relax (relaxation techniques are essential to arthritis healing). Many have a negative attitude toward life that locks up the body's healing ability.

By far the greatest number of arthritis sufferers are menopausal women. Although the focus of diagnosis has been on organic mineral (especially calcium) depletion as a cause of arthritis, I find that hormone imbalance and adrenal exhaustion are the keys to repair therapy.

Signs and symptoms of Arthritis:
- Do you notice marked stiffness and swelling in your fingers, shoulders or neck in damp weather?
- Are you unusually stiff when you get up in the morning, especially when the weather is damp?
- Have you noticed bony bumps on your index fingers? Or bony spurs on any other joints?
- Are your joints starting to crack and pop?
- Are you anemic? Is your skin unusually pale? Have you lost weight lately but weren't on a diet?
- Is your digestion poor? Do you have food allergies or intolerances?
- Do you experience back or joint pain when you move? Does it get worse with prolonged activity?
- Are you more than 20 pounds overweight and feel the extra weight in your knees and hips?
- Do you have long-standing lung and bronchial congestion?
- Are you usually constipated? Do you suffer from ulcerative colitis?
- Do you take more than 6 aspirin a day on a regular basis? Are you on a long-term prescription of corticosteroid drugs? *Either of these may eventually impair the body's own healing powers.*

Is your body full of mucous congestion?

Your body needs some mucous. We're taught that mucous is a bad thing because it obstructs our breathing during a sinus infection, asthma or a cold. But mucous is also a needed lubricant and an important body safeguard. We take about 22,000 breaths a day. Mucous gathers up irritants like dirt, pollen, smoke and pollutants we take in along with our oxygen to protect mucous membranes in the respiratory system. Foods that putrefy quickly inside your body are the ones most likely to produce excess mucous like meat, fish, eggs and dairy products. These foods also slow down transit time through your gastrointesinal tract. Some of us carry around as much as 10 to 15 pounds of excess mucous!

Signs and symptoms of excess mucous congestion:
- Labored breathing, wheezing, coughing, choking and difficulty in exhaling
- Respiratory congestion, sinus congestion, runny nose and sneezing
- Overusing over-the-counter drugs for allergy or asthma
  may drive congestion deeper into lungs.
- Allergies and asthma mean extra mucous in the respiratory system and colon.
  Chronic bronchitis means excess mucous in the bronchi.
- If you catch every infection that goes around, remember excess mucous is a breeding ground.
  for infectious pathogens that cause colds and flu.

Have you become a victim of antacids?

A new survey finds that 15 million Americans have heartburn on a daily basis. Americans spend $1.7 billion on indigestion remedies each year! But antacids are designed to provide temporary relief. Evidence is piling up that excessive use of over-the-counter antacids may wreak havoc on digestive health. They may even themselves become a health problem because they radically change your digestive chemistry.

Do any of these problems pertain to you?

1) **The tolerance effect:** The more you use antacids, the more you need them. Antacids neutralize stomach HCl (*hydrochloric acid*), that you need for digestion, or they block it, confuse the body and disrupt its normal processes. If you take a lot of antacids, your body overcompensates, producing excess stomach acid.

2) **Antacids disrupt your pH balance:** Optimum pH is between 7.35 and 7.45. If you take lots of antacids, your GI tract fluctuates between over alkaline and over acid, leading to problems like diarrhea or constipation, gallbladder problems, hiatal hernia, even malnutrition. A friend thought his heartburn symptoms would improve if he doubled up on his acid blocker dosage. He ended up in the bathroom all night, passing completely undigested food. Disrupting body pH alters your bowel ecology, too, potentially causing dramatic overgrowth of harmful microorganisms.... like candida yeasts.

3) **Pernicious ingredients:** Many antacids contain aluminum which causes constipation and bone pain. Others overdose you on magnesium causing diarrhea. Some contain both aluminum and magnesium, confusing your body with alternating constipation and diarrhea. Antacids full of sodium may cause water retention. Most are laden with chemical coloring agents that can cause allergic reactions in some people or lead to "mood changes" and "mental alterations" if taken regularly. And that's the way many people take them.

4) **Some drugs interact with antacids:** People on drug therapy for HIV know antacids decrease their HIV drug absorption by up to 23%. Oral contraceptives like "the pill" may lose their effectiveness if taken with antacids. People using NSAIDS drugs for arthritis along with antacids suffer $2\frac{1}{2}$ times more serious gastrointestinal complications than those taking a placebo! Antacids not only block drug absorption, they also block your food absorption of nutrients, especially B_{12}, necessary for virtually all immune responses.

5) **Some antacids build up in the body, impeding body processes:** I know a woman who was hospitalized three times for kidney stones until her physician finally advised her to stop taking her over-the-counter antacids because the unabsorbed calcium in them was causing the kidney stone formation.

Do you have a Candida infection?

Candida albicans yeast is common, normally living harmlessly in the gastrointestinal and genito-urinary areas of the body. When immunity and resistance are low, the body loses its intestinal balance and candida yeasts multiply too rapidly, voraciously feeding on excess sugars and carbohydrates in the digestive tract. Candida is an immune-compromised condition, extremely hard to overcome. Unless you assist your body's weakened defenses, candida colonies will flourish and keep releasing toxins into the bloodstream.

Watch out for these lifestyle factors that promote Candida infection:

1) Poor diet — especially excessive intake of sugar, starchy foods, yeasted breads and chemicalized foods. 2) Repeated use of antibiotics — long term use of antibiotics kill protective bacteria (that keep candida under control) as well as harmful bacteria. 3) Hormone medications like corticosteroid drugs and birth control pills. 4) A high stress life, too much alcohol, little rest.

Candida may infect virtually any part of the body. The most commonly involved sites include the nail beds, skin folds, feet, mouth, sinuses, ear canal, belly button, esophagus, intestine, vaginal tract and urethra. Candida also infects deep internal organs, which sometimes results in serious disease. Likely sites of infection include the thyroid and adrenal glands, kidneys, bladder, bowel, esophagus, uterus, lungs and bone marrow.

Signs and symptoms that you may have a candida infection:

- Do you have recurrent digestive problems, gas, bloating or flatulence?
- Do you have rectal itching, or chronic constipation alternating to diarrhea?
- Do you have a white coating on your tongue (thrush)?
- Have you been unusually irritable or depressed?
- Are you bothered by unexplained frequent headaches, muscle aches and joint pain?
- Do you feel sick, yet the cause cannot be found? Do your symptoms worsen on muggy days?
- Is your memory been noticeably poor? Do you find it hard to concentrate or focus your thoughts?
- Do you have chronic vaginal yeast infections or frequent bladder infections?
- If you are a woman, do you have serious PMS, menstrual problems or endometriosis?
- If you are a man, do you have abdominal pains, prostatitis, or loss of sexual interest?
- Do you have chronic fungal infections like ringworm, jock itch, nail fungus or athlete's foot?
- Do you have hives, psoriasis, eczema or chronic dermatitis?
- Do you catch frequent colds that take many weeks to go away?
- Are you bothered by erratic vision or spots before the eyes?
- Are you oversensitive to chemicals, tobacco, perfume or insecticides?
- Do you crave sugar, bread, or alcoholic beverages?
- Have you recently taken repeated rounds for 1 month or longer, of antibiotics or corticosteroid drugs, like Symycin, Panmycin, Decadron or Prednisone, or acne drugs?

Do you have Chronic Fatigue Syndrome?

Latest estimates reveal that between 800,000 to 2 million Americans are struggling with chronic fatigue syndrome right now. Although anyone (even children) can be affected by CFS, it strikes women more often and much harder. Women under 45 are at the highest risk. Clearly it seems, the overworked, overstressed "superwomen" of the 90s are paying the price of their hectic lifestyles in terms of health.

Variations of CFS have been known since the 1800s. As we know it today, Chronic Fatigue Syndrome, is most prevalent in the Western industrialized countries where a 40-60 hour work week, single parent households and raising children is the norm. At the root of CFS development is immune system malfunction (often from a highly toxic environment), a lifestyle that dramatically outruns personal energy reserves and the presence of a virus or group of viruses.

Signs and symptoms that you may have Chronic Fatigue Syndrome:
- Debilitating fatigue (lasting 6 months or more unrelated to other illness)
- Flu-like sore throat and painful lymph nodes in the neck or armpits
- Mental spaciness
- Muscle pain and low grade fever
- Poor sleep quality
- Headaches

Are you suffering from estrogen disruption?

Estrogen disrupters are so commonplace in modern society that there is no way to completely avoid them. All of the Earth's waterways are connected, so chemical pollutants containing environmental hormones reach your food supply wherever you live. Estrogen disrupters are in pollutants, drugs, hormone-injected meats and dairy products, plastics and pesticides. Nearly 40% of pesticides used in commercial agriculture are suspected hormone disrupters!

Man-made estrogens can stack the deck against women by increasing their estrogen hundreds of times over normal levels. Scientists may believe there is no significant difference between man-made and natural hormones, but thousands of women say that even if a lab test can't tell the difference, their bodies can. Women aren't the only ones endangered by the estrogen-mimics. Substantial evidence shows that man-made estrogens threaten male health with reproductive disorders, too. The most alarming statistics relate to sperm count and hormone driven cancers.

Are the new designer estrogens, the SERMs, (*selective estrogen receptor modulators*) estrogen disrupters? SERMs, under the name reloxifene, (brand name Evista) are the new generation of estrogen replacement drugs, developed to address the serious health concerns of menopausal women. Preliminary report suggest these drugs, like traditional HRT drugs (Premarin), still disrupt a woman's delicate hormone balance.

Signs and symptoms that you may have estrogen disruption:
- Breast inflammation and pain that worsens before menstrual periods
- Weight gain (especially in the hips)
- Head hair loss — facial hair growth
- Hot flashes (a sign of estrogen disruption in the brain)
- Heavy, painful periods
- Early puberty (nearly half of African-American girls and 15 % of Caucasian girls are beginning to develop sexually by age 8, a clear indicator of estrogen disruption.)
- Breast, uterine and reproductive organ cancer (A new study shows up to 60% more DDE, DDT and PCB's, known estrogen disrupters, in women with breast cancer.)
- Breast and uterine fibroid development; ovarian cysts
- Endometriosis and pelvic inflammatory disease

Note: You may be especially exposed to estrogen disrupters if you live in a high agricultural area; you eat a high fat diet — fatty areas of your body store these chemicals; you eat hormone-injected dairy foods or meats regularly; you're on prescription HRT drugs or birth control pills.

What does your skin rash mean?

Our skin is the mirror of our lifestyle. Deep body imbalances often reveal themselves as skin disorders. Many skin problems start with internal toxicity, allergies, hormone imbalance and poor digestion. Stress and a poor diet clearly aggravate and contribute to skin disorders. The following symptom list is designed to point you in the right direction in determining what a skin rash may mean.

Eczema is an increasingly common but aggravating skin condition related to food allergies (particularly eggs, soy foods, wheat and milk), an EFA deficiency, low hydrochloric acid in the stomach causing poor digestion, leaky gut syndrome and emotional stress. Atopic dermatitis is a severe type of eczema usually caused by allergies to chemicals, plants, clothing, topical medications, or jewelry metals. Eczema and dermatitis, both systemic, spread. Both conditions are usually temporary and can often be reversed by eliminating the offending allergen, improving digestion and boosting EFA intake.

Signs and symptoms that you may have eczema or dermatitis:
- Reddish, angry patches of skin (frequently on the cheeks, ankles or wrists)
- Crusting and tiny blisters on the skin
- Tingling, unpleasant skin prickling
- Itching, weeping skin
- Bumps and scaling on the skin

Psoriasis is a troublesome and mysterious chronic skin disorder, affecting 6.4 million Americans. Psoriasis is caused by an abnormal growth of skin cells. Normal skin cells mature within about a month, but a psoriatic skin cell takes only three to six days. Heredity plays a role in psoriasis development, but a recent study links psoriasis to immune system malfunction. Psoriasis isn't contagious and its effects can range from mild to severe. Every year, about 400 people die from complications due to severe psoriasis. (In extreme cases, large areas of skin are lost, leaving the body susceptible to severe secondary infections.) Natural therapies focus on stress reduction and herbal anti-inflammatories for symptom relief. EFA supplementation with omega-3 fatty acids has produced good results for psoriasis relief in clinical studies.

Signs and symptoms that you may have psoriasis:
- Inflamed skin lesions with white scales (usually on the scalp, knees, elbows, hands and feet)
- Intense skin sloughing (severe erythrodemic psoriasis)
- Joint inflammation with arthritic pain (10% of people with psoriasis have psoriatic arthritis)
- Pitting of the nails can be a sign of psoriasis

Rosacea is a skin disorder related to adult acne occurring mainly in middle-aged people of Celtic descent. There is no known cure for acne rosacea. Doctors treat it in much the same way as other forms of acne, with oral and topical antibiotics. Eliminating food triggers, particularly spicy foods and alcohol, and avoiding excessive emotional stress, sun, and environmental pollutants is key to control of rosacea breakouts.

Signs and symptoms of rosacea:
- Flushing and redness of the cheeks, chin, nose, and forehead
- Acne-like bumps and pimples
- Dilated blood vessels on the face
- A red, bumpy nose
- Bloodshot eyes or gritty feeling in eyes
- Small, hard bumps on both eyelids

Is your lymphatic system congested?

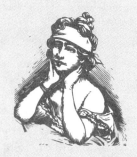

The lymphatic system includes the lymphatic vessels, the lymph nodes, the thymus gland, the tonsils and the spleen. Your lymphatic system acts as the body's secondary circulatory system, flushing waste, filtering and engulfing pathogens and rendering them innocuous. The health of your lymphatic system depends to a large extent on the health of your liver. Lymphatic vessels not only drain waste products from tissues, they are also a major route for body nutrients from the liver and intestines. The liver produces most of the body's lymph, fluid found in lymphatic vessels rich in lymphocytes, special white blood cells which form the overall defense of the body. A sluggish liver invariably means a congested lymphatic system. Your lymphatic system plays a key role in immune defense against cancer and infections.

Signs and symptoms that your lymph system is congested:

- Appearance of cellulite (Inadequate lymph flow is a key factor in cellulite development.)
- Frequent colds and flu (A congested lymphatic system means reduced defense against pathogens that cause infections.)
- Extreme sluggishness, low energy or poor memory
- Chronic exposure to aluminum puts a strain on lymphatic health. If you use aluminum cookware, consume alum-containing foods, or apply alum-containing deodorants on a regular basis, your lymphatic system may be congested.
- If you eat a diet high in saturated fat and refined carbohydrates, your lymphatic system may be congested because these foods compromise glandular health.
- If you live a very sedentary lifestyle with little or no exercise, your lymph system may be congested. Optimum lymphatic flow depends on regular physical activity.

Do you have gallstones?

In the United States, high bile cholesterol levels are the main cause of gallstones, with most stones (80%) composed of cholesterol and varying amounts of bile salts, bile pigments and inorganic calcium salts. When bile in the gallbladder becomes supersaturated with cholesterol, it combines with other sediment matter present and begins to form a stone. Dietary factors like high blood sugar, high calorie and saturated fat intake that lead to obesity are also involved. A stone may grow for 6 to 8 years before symptoms occur. Continued formation of gallstones is dependent on either increased accumulation of cholesterol or reduced levels of bile acids or lecithin. It's easy to see that diet improvement will deter, even arrest, gallstones.

Signs that you may have a tendency to gallstones:

- Do you have periods of nausea, vomiting, fever and intense abdominal pain that radiates to the upper back? These may be signs of cholocystitis (gallbladder inflammation). 95% of people suffering from cholocystitis have gallstones. If these symptoms sound like you, seek medical help immediately. Gallstones can be serious. Ultrasound provides a definitive diagnosis.
- If you are overweight, gallstone risk increases three to seven times.
- Having high cholesterol levels contributes to increased gallstone risk.
- Low vitamin C intake — vitamin C plays a key role in the breakdown of cholesterol.
- Are you a yo-yo dieter? A recent study in *Annals of Internal Medicine* finds that women whose weight fluctuates by 10 to 19 lbs. at a time have a 31% higher risk of developing gallstones. When weight fluctuated more than 19 lbs. at a time, gallstone risk was 68% higher!
- Chronic heartburn, gas and pain after eating, especially fried foods, eggs and cow's milk.

Are your homocysteine levels too high?

Homocysteine is certainly in the news. But the connection between heart disease and homocysteine is not new. Homocysteine is a body substance that helps manufacture proteins and assist with cellular metabolism. It's a harmless amino acid, but in excess, it can cause blood platelets to clump together and vascular walls to break down, leading to atherosclerosis and coronary artery disease. Research linking heart disease to elevated plasma levels of homocysteine began as early as 1969, when Dr. Kilmer McCully, a Harvard pathologist, found rare cases of severe atherosclerosis in children with very high homocysteine levels.

Here's what we know about high homocysteine today: A recent New England Journal of Medicine study shows that people with high homocysteine levels are $4\frac{1}{2}$ times more likely to die of heart disease than other people. New estimates are that 1 in 5 cardiac cases can be attributed to high homocysteine levels. High homocysteine levels may be especially dangerous for women. Women with high homocysteine levels and low folic acid in the blood are twice as likely to have a heart attack than women with normal levels.

Factors that contribute to high homocysteine levels:

— **Eating too much protein:** Protein-rich foods contain the amino acid methionine which converts to homocysteine. This may be a factor to consider if you are on one of the very high protein "Zone" diets so popular in the tabloids today.

— **Vitamin B deficiency:** (especially B_6, B_{12} and folic acid which are needed by the body to break down homocysteine).

— **Prescription drugs deplete B vitamins:** Methotrexate, diuretics used to treat high blood pressure, the cholesterol-lowering medicine Questran, nitrous oxide, azaribine, most oral contraceptives, and even aspirin suppress folic acid and B vitamins that keep homocysteine levels balanced.

— **Genetic defect:** A defect in a reductase enzyme triggers a need for more folic acid than is normally required to prevent elevated homocysteine levels.

— **Aging:** Homocysteine levels increase by about one micromole per liter for every 10 years of age.

— **Thyroid hormone deficiency:** usually leads to rises in homocysteine levels.

— **Smokers:** have higher levels of homocysteine.

— **Caffeine:** evidence from Norway suggests heavy coffee drinking elevates homocysteine levels.

Balance your homocysteine levels naturally.
A simple 4 point program shows protection in one to three months.

1: B vitamins can come to your rescue. A high intake of folic acid and B_6 lowers risk for cardiovascular disease 45% in women (February 1998 issue of the Journal of the AMA). Try B Complex, 100mg daily. Add 50mg extra of B_6 and 400mcg extra of folic acid to help break down homocysteine.

2: Four garlic capsules (1200mg a day) maintain aortic elasticity.

3: Take daily ginger. Many Americans take plain aspirin to prevent a stroke or heart attack because aspirin inhibits a specific enzyme that makes the blood prone to dangerous stickiness. Ginger not only inhibits this same enzyme but it does so without aspirin's side effects like gastric bleeding.

4: Red wine with dinner. Red wine contains resveratrol which has antioxidant and anticoagulant properties to help protect against cardiovascular disease.

Are you depressed?

At some point in their lives, one in five Americans will experience a depressive episode. Over twenty-eight million Americans take anti-depression drugs or anxiety medications to control depression symptoms. Many drugs do seem to relieve symptoms at least temporarily, but they can have disturbing side effects.

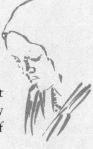

An astounding 20 million prescriptions have been filled for Prozac since its market debut in 1987. Low libido, dry mouth and eyes, dizziness, nausea, headaches and insomnia are only some of Prozac's side effects. Even more frightening, in a 1990 study published in Journal of American Psychiatry, Prozac use led to "intense, violent suicidal preoccupation"!

Signs and symptoms of major depression:
— Poor appetite with weight loss or increased appetite with weight gain
— Insomnia or sleeping excessively (hypersomnia); unusual irritability
— Hyperactivity (going a mile a minute) or doing almost nothing all day
— Loss of interest or pleasure in usual activities, decrease in sexual drive
— Low energy — great tiredness; lowered work productivity
— Feelings of worthlessness, self-reproach or inappropriate guilt
— Diminished ability to think or concentrate
— Recurring problems with friends and family members
— Isolation from others with recurrent thoughts of death or suicide

Depression is a serious disorder that requires serious attention. We all get the blues from time to time, but major depression is different. The American Psychiatric Association says you probably are depressed if you have five of the following eight symptoms for at least a month. I've found the lifestyle program offered on pg. 366 of this book is highly effective for a wide range of people. If you have depression, consult with a healthcare professional to find out what natural therapies are right for you.

Is your thyroid low and metabolism poor?

Your thyroid gland, located where the collarbone comes together with the neck, governs metabolism. Metabolism is still something of a mystery; we may never know exactly how it functions. We do know it provides vital energy resources to every part of the body. Since World War II, an above average number of people have thyroid problems. Researchers speculate that the enormous amount of chemicals that came into our culture during and after the war (some not well-tested for safety) affected thyroid health. Today, thyroid disease affects 13 million people, most of whom are women. Hypothyroidism (low thyroid) is a common problem, aggravated by the strain pollutants in our environment put on glandular health. *Note: Iron supplements render thyroid medicine insoluble and can aggravate hypothyroid symptoms.*

Signs and symptoms of hypothyroidism and low metabolism:
• great fatigue (especially in the morning) and muscular weakness
• hormonal imbalances (like PMS, delayed or absent menstruation)
• bloating, gas and indigestion immediately after eating
• unusual depression, usually with markedly reduced libido
• unexplained hair loss in women, often accompanied by breast fibroids
• unexplained obesity, with frequent constipation
• unusually sensitivity to cold; poor immune response
• unusually high LDL "bad" cholesterol levels
• appearance of goiter (swelling of the thyroid gland)
• puffy face and eyelids, unusually dry or itchy skin
• memory loss
• low selenium levels

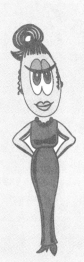

Dr. Page's new Ailment Analysis section is intended as an educational tool to offer information about your alternative healing and health maintenance options today. The recommendations are not intended as a substitute for the advice and treatment of a physician or other licensed health care professional. In many cases, they are effective adjuncts to professional care. Education is the key to making wise health decisions. Part of the job of taking more command of your own health is using common sense, intelligence, and adult judgement based on the knowledge of your own body observations. Ultimately, you must take the responsibility for your choices and how you use the information presented here.

Home Healing Procedures
A hands-on reference for healing techniques and self diagnosis methods

Giving your body an ascorbic acid flush:

This procedure accelerates detoxification programs, changing body chemistry to neutralize allergens and fight infections, promoting more rapid healing, and protecting against illness.

1. Use ascorbate vitamin C or Ester C powder with bioflavonoids for best results.
2. Take $1/_2$ teasp. every 20 minutes until a soupy stool results. Note: Use $1/_4$ teasp. every hour for a very young child; $1/_2$ teasp. every hour for a child six to ten years old.
3. Then reduce amount of C taken slightly so that your bowel produces a mealy, loose stool, but not diarrhea. The body continues to cleanse at this point. You will be taking approximately 8-10,000mg daily depending on your body weight. Continue for one to two days for a thorough flush.

Bentonite clay colonic cleanse:

Bentonite clay is a mineral substance with powerful absorption qualities; it can pull out suspended impurities in the body. It helps prevent proliferation of pathogenic organisms and parasites, and sets up an environment for rebuilding healthy tissue. It is effective for lymph congestion, cellulite in fatty tissues, blood cleansing and reducing toxicity from environmental pollutants. It may be used orally, anally, or vaginally. It works like an internal poultice, drawing out toxic materials, then draining and eliminating them through evacuation. For best results, avoid refined foods, especially sugars and flour, and pasteurized dairy products during this cleanse.

1. To take as an enema, mix $1/_2$ cup clay to an enema bag of water. Use 5 to 6 bags for each enema set to replace a colonic. Follow the normal enema procedure on page 230, or the directions with your enema apparatus.
2. Massage across the abdomen while expelling toxic waste into the toilet.
    Note: Bentonite clay packs are also effective applied to varicose veins and arthritic areas.

Coca's Pulse Test:

Dr. Arthur Coca, an immunologist, discovered that when people eat foods to which they are allergic, there is a dramatic increase in the heartbeat — 20 or more beats a minute above normal. Pulse rate is normally remarkably stable, not affected by digestion or ordinary physical activities or normal emotions. Unless a person is ill or under great stress, pulse rate deviation is probably due to an allergy. By performing COCA'S PULSE TEST one can find and eliminate foods that harm.

1. Take your pulse when you wake in the morning. Using a watch with a second hand, count the number of beats in a 60-second period. A normal pulse reading is 60 to 100 beats per minute.
2. Take your pulse again after eating a suspected allergy food. Wait 15 to 20 minutes and take your pulse again. If your pulse rate has increased more than 10 beats per minute, omit the food from your diet.

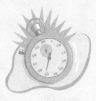

How to use muscle kinesiology:

Muscle kinesiology attributes can be used to determine an individual's response to a food or substance. Muscle testing is a personal technique to use before buying a healing product, because it lets you estimate the product's effectiveness for your own body needs and make-up. You need a partner for the procedure.

1: Hold your arm out straight from your side, parallel to the ground. Have a partner take hold of the arm with one hand just below the shoulder, and one hand on the forearm. Your partner should then try to force down towards your side, while you exert all your strength to hold it level. Unless you are in ill health, you should easily be able to withstand this pressure and keep your arm level.

2: Then, simply hold the item that you desire to test against your diaphragm (under the breastbone) or thyroid (the point where the collarbone comes together below the neck). The item may be in or out of normal packaging, or in its raw state, like a fresh food.

3: While holding the item as above, put your arm out straight from your side as before and have your partner try to press it down again. If the substance or product is beneficial for you, your arm will retain its strength, and your partner will be unable to force it down. If the substance or product is not beneficial, or would worsen your condition, your arm can be easily pushed down by your partner.

How to follow a food elimination diet for allergies:

Find out what foods you're allergic to by following an elimination diet. For one week, eat foods like brown rice, sweet potatoes, all cooked vegetables, and non-acidic fruits - foods that are less likely to cause reactions. When symptoms improve, add other foods one at a time to see if they aggravate symptoms. For best results eat each new food three times a day for 2 days. Foods that trigger symptoms are likely allergens.

How to take an enema:

Enemas are an important therapeutic aid for any mucous or colon congestion cleansing program. They accelerate the release of old, encrusted colon waste, encourage discharge of parasites, freshen the G.I. tract, and cleanse your body more thoroughly. They are helpful during a healing crisis, or after a serious illness or drug-treated hospital stay to speed healing. Some headaches and inflammatory skin conditions can be relieved with enemas. Herbal enemas can immediately alkalize the bowel area, help control irritation and inflammation, and provide local healing action for ulcerated tissue.

Helpful herbs for enemas. Use 2 cups very strong brewed tea or solution to 1 qt. of water per enema.
—**Garlic:** helps kill parasites and cleanse harmful bacteria, viruses and mucous. *Blend six garlic cloves in 2 cups cold water and strain. For small children, use 1 clove garlic to 1 pint water.*
—**Catnip:** helps stomach, digestive problems and cramping; also for childhood disease.
—**Pau d' arco:** body chemistry imbalances, as in chronic yeast and fungal infections.
—**Spirulina:** is effective when both blood and bowel are toxic.
—**Lobelia:** counteracts food poisoning, especially if vomiting prevents antidotes taken by mouth.
—**Aloe vera:** helps heal tissues in cases of hemorrhoids, irritable bowel and diverticulitis.
—**Lemon Juice:** an internal wash to rapidly neutralize an acid system, cleanse the colon and bowel.
—**Acidophilus:** helps gas, yeast, and candidiasis infections. Mix 4-oz. powder to 1-qt. water.
—**Coffee enemas:** have become a standard in natural healing for liver and blood related cancers. Caffeine used in this way stimulates the liver and gallbladder to remove toxins, open bile ducts, encourage increased peristaltic action, and produce necessary enzyme activity for healthy red blood cell formation and oxygen uptake. Use 1 cup of regular strong brewed coffee to 1 qt. water. Also effective for migraines.

How to take a detoxifying, colonic enema:

Place warm enema solution in an enema bag. Hang the bag about 18 inches higher than the body. Attach the colon tube, and lubricate its attachment with vaseline or vitamin E oil. Expel a little water to let out air bubbles. Lying on your left side, slowly insert the attachment about 3 inches into the rectum. Never use force. Rotate attachment gently to ease insertion. Remove kinks in the tubing so liquid will flow freely. Massage abdomen, or flex and contract stomach muscles to relieve any cramping. When all solution has entered the colon, slowly remove the tube and remain on the left side for 5 minutes. Then move to a knee-chest position with your body weight on your knees and one hand. Use the other hand to massage the lower left side of the abdomen for several minutes.

Massage loosens old fecal matter. Roll onto your back for 5 minutes; massage up the descending colon, over the transverse colon to the right side and down the ascending colon. Move onto your right side for 5 minutes, to reach each part of the colon. Get up and quickly expel into the toilet. Look for sticky grey-brown mucous, small dark crusty chunks or tough ribbony pieces to be loosened and expelled during an enema. These poisonous looking things are toxins interfering with your normal body functions. An enema removes them. You may have to take several enemas until there is no more evidence of these substances.

How to use an herbal implant:

Implants are concentrated enema solutions which can be used for serious health problems, such as colitis, arthritis or prostate inflammation. Prepare for the implant by taking a small enema with warm water to clear out the lower bowel, allowing you to hold the implant longer. Then mix 2 TBS of your chosen powder, such as spirulina, or wheat grass, in $1/2$ cup water. Add the mixture to a 4 ounce capacity syringe.

Lubricate tip of the syringe with vaseline or vitamin E oil, get down on your hands and knees and insert the nozzle into the rectum. Squeeze the bulb to insert the mixture, but do not release pressure on the bulb before it is withdrawn, so the mixture will stay in the lower bowel. Hold as long as you can before expelling.

How to take an Arthritis elimination sweat:

A surprising amount of toxic material that aggravates arthritis inflammation can be eliminated by the body via the skin. An arthritis sweat bath with Epsom salts or Dead Sea salts, along with herbs with diaphoretic action, can work almost immediately. Use herbs like *elderflowers*, *peppermint*, or *yarrow*, take them as a tea (as hot as possible before the bath), and continue during the sweat.

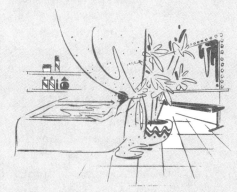

Here's how:

Taking an arthritis sweat before retiring produces the best results. Use about 3 pounds of Epsom salts or the amount directed for Dead Sea salts. Add to very hot bath water. Rub affected inflamed joints with a stiff brush in the water for 5 - 10 minutes; try to stay in the bath for 15 to 25 minutes. On emerging, do not dry yourself. Wrap up immediately in a clean sheet and go straight to bed, covering yourself with several blankets. The osmotic pressure of the Epsom salt solution absorbed by the sheet draws off heavy perspiration, (for this reason the mattress should be protected with a sheet of plastic). The following morning the sheet will be stained with products excreted through the skin - sometimes the color of egg yolk.

Improvement after an Epsom salt bath experience is notable. Continue treatment once every two weeks until the sheet is no longer stained, a sign that your body is cleansed. Drink plenty of water throughout the procedure to prevent dehydration and loss of body salts. (Take care if you have a weak heart or hypertension.)

Purchase the following home tests at most pharmacies.
Ask if you don't see it on the shelf.

Home Ovulation Predictors:

An ovulation test can help women to get pregnant. Pregnancy can only occur during part of the monthly menstrual cycle, for a week or so after ovulation. Ovulation occurs about the midpoint between periods, but many women have irregular cycles, making it difficult for them to know when they are fertile. Ovulation predictors enable women to pinpoint their fertile days by measuring the concentration of luteinizing hormone (LH) in urine. The level of LH increases significantly 12 to 24 hours before ovulation.

Ovulation tests instruct women to test their urine daily for several days early in the menstrual cycle with activating strips. The strips turn a color, which establishes an LH baseline. When LH concentration rises, shortly before ovulation, the test strip turns a different color. A woman can then better plan sexual intercourse for procreation.

Home Bladder Infection Tests:

Bladder infections develop when bacteria ascend the urine tube (urethra) and enter the bladder where they reproduce and infect. Bladder infections most commonly appear in women, and cause painful, overly frequent urination, sometimes back and groin pain, and fever. A bladder infection increases the concentration of nitrites in urine. A home test can detect the nitrites with dip strips that change color when urine comes in contact with the impregnated chemicals. You can purchase a product called DIP-STICK from your pharmacy. It contains a chemical re-agent to indicate the presence of a bacterial infection when dipped in urine. If you are at frequent risk for bladder infections, check yourself weekly so you can nip the infection at the beginning with natural remedies.

Note: Some women develop symptoms of a bladder infection, but don't show the expected amounts of bacteria or nitrites in their urine. If your test results conflict with symptoms of infection, an alternative practitioner gives more weight to your symptoms than to the test. You should too. If you experience symptoms of bladder infection, but your home test turns out negative or marginally positive, call your practitioner. Treatment is usually recommended regardless of test results, because of the risk of kidney infection.

Home Blood Pressure Monitor:

Chronic high blood pressure, or hypertension, is a major risk factor for heart disease and stroke, which together account for almost half of U.S. deaths. If you are more than 30 pounds overweight, have a history of hypertension, heart disease, or stroke, or have a family history of cardiovascular disease, you might give serious thought to investing in a home blood pressure monitor for peace of mind.

For some people, home blood pressure testing is more accurate than professional testing, because the anxiousness of being in a doctor's office raises their blood pressure. Home testing eliminates this "white coat hypertension," and the medications that might be unnecessarily prescribed to treat it.

Simply slip your arm into the provided cuff and fill it with air using the bulb-shaped hand pump. When you release the air, the monitor determines your pressure electronically and displays it digitally. (Although available and more convenient, finger cuffs are not as accurate as the arm cuffs.)

Home Blood Glucose Monitor:

Blood glucose monitors have become indispensable for people with diabetes. Glucose is the simple sugar that fuels the body, but diabetics can't process it properly because they lack the hormone insulin, or can't use the insulin they produce. Glucose monitoring at home allows diabetics to adjust their insulin and-or their diet to control their blood glucose level. (Urine glucose testing, also available for home use, is easier, but gives a less accurate blood glucose reading.)

A drop of blood is placed on a test strip and inserted into the monitor, which electronically measures the glucose level. Calibrations differ; you may need to match your monitor's calibration to that of a test lab.

Home Colorectal Cancer Screening Tests:

All colorectal cancers can not be detected by this test. False positives are not uncommon. A variety of factors besides cancer can introduce small amounts of blood into the stool. Aspirin, hemorrhoids, gastrointestinal problems, as well as some foods, like popcorn, may cause blood in the stool. To reduce the risk of false results, follow package directions scrupulously.

The test is based on the fact that early-stage colorectal tumors release a tiny amount of blood, which becomes incorporated into the stool. Some tests rely on chemically impregnated toilet paper to detect the blood. If the toilet paper changes color after use, it indicates a positive result. Others require the user to place a sheet of test paper in the toilet bowl following a bowel movement. If a color change appears on the paper, blood is present in the stool.

Home pH Testing:

The degrees of acidity or alkalinity of a substance are expressed in pH values. The neutral point, where a solution is neither acid or alkaline, is pH 7. Water has a pH of 7.0. Anything with a pH below 7.0 is acid while anything with a pH above 7.0 is alkaline. The ideal pH range for saliva and urine is 6.0 to 6.8. Our bodies are naturally mildly acidic. Therefore, values below pH 6.3 are considered too acidic; values above pH 6.8 are too alkaline. Maximum acidity is pH 0 and maximum alkalinity is pH 14.

Saliva and urine pH can be measured on litmus paper. Normal saliva pH is 6.4. If saliva pH is above 6.8, it could indicate digestive problems, while a saliva reading below 6.0 might mean liver and blood toxicity. Urine pH cycles from a low of 5.5 to 5.8 in the morning, to a high of 7.0 during the day, averaging 6.4 in a 24 hr. period. If it is too acid, below 6.0, it can indicate dehydration as well as over-acidity.

Colon pH is a critically important area. It should be in a narrow range of 6.8 to 7.0. If it is too alkaline (above 7.0), yeasts and pathogenic bacteria grow. To lower the pH of the colon, implant a good L. bifidus colon culture. Most of the bacteria in the colon is bifidus.

You can determine whether your body fluids are either too acidic or too alkaline, causing acidosis or alkalosis. Purchase nitrazine paper, available at any drugstore, and test your saliva or urine. Perform the test either before eating or at least one hour after eating. The paper will change color to indicate if your system is overly acidic or alkaline. If your test indicated one extreme or another, omit either acid-or alkaline-forming foods from your diet until another pH test shows that you have returned to normal body balance.

Home use protocol for food grade hydrogen peroxide:

See ALTERNATIVE ARSENAL page 100 for how to use H_2O_2 orally (always dilute first):

For external use, purchase 35% food grade H_2O_2, or magnesium peroxide from your local health food store. Do not use household, beauty supply or any other form of peroxide for internal use - many of these products have added chemicals to stabilize the H_2O_2. You will also need an eye dropper.

Watchwords for using H_2O_2:
—Do not use with carrot juice, carbonated drinks or alcohol. Take on an empty stomach 1 hour before or 3 hours after meals.
—If you get the 35% H_2O_2 on your skin, rinse it under running water a few minutes.
—Do not **ever** take 35% H_2O_2 internally. Buy 3% H_2O_2 from the health food store instead.
—If your stomach is upset at any level from 3% H_2O_2, go back one level for a day or two. Then proceed with your daily dosage again.

You may experience slight nausea. In addition, as dead bacteria or various forms of poisons are released from your tissues, many people experience a cleansing effect as they are eliminated through the skin, lungs, kidneys and bowels. Some reactions to the cleansing effect could include skin eruptions, nausea, headaches, sleepiness, unusual fatigue, diarrhea, head or chest congestion, ear infections, boils or other ways the body uses to loosen toxins. This is natural cleansing of the body and should be of short duration.

In most applications, especially those where anti-infective and antifungal properties are needed, I find it more beneficial to use H_2O_2 in an alternating series - usually 10 days of use, and then 10 days of rest, or 3 weeks of use, and 3 weeks of rest, in more serious cases.

Here's an easy chart to determine number of days, drops and times per day to take H_2O_2:

Count Day	Number of drops	Times per day
1	3	3
2	4	3
3	5	3
4	6	3
5	7	3
6	8	3
7	9	3
8	10	3
9	11	3
10	12	3
11	13	3

Douche: mix 6 TBS. of 3% solution to a quart of warm distilled water. Do not exceed this amount.
Colonic enema: add 1 cup 3% solution to 5 gallons warm water. Do not exceed this amount.
Regular enema: add 1 tablespoon of 3% solution to a quart of warm distilled water.
Detox bath: add about 2 quarts 3% H_2O_2 to a tub of warm water.
Foot soak: add 3% H_2O_2 to a gallon of warm water as needed.
For animals: 1-oz. of 3% H_2O_2 can be added to 1 qt. of your pets drinking water if they are ill.
Humidifiers and steamers: mix 1 pint 3% solution to 1 gallon of water.
Laundry: add 8-oz. of 3% to your wash in place of bleaches.

Vegetable soak: add $\frac{1}{4}$ cup 3% H_2O_2 to a sink of cold water. Soak light skinned vegetables (like lettuce) 20 minutes, thicker skinned (like cucumbers) for 30 minutes. Drain, dry and chill to prolong freshness. If time is a problem, spray produce with a solution of 3%. Let stand for a few minutes, rinse and dry.

To freshen kitchen: use a spray bottle of 3% to wipe off counter tops and appliances. It will disinfect and give the kitchen a fresh smell. Works great to clean refrigerator and kids' school lunch boxes.

Sprouting seeds: add 1 oz. 3% to 1 pint of water and soak the seeds overnight. Add the same amount of H_2O_2 each time you rinse the seeds.

House and garden plants: put 1-oz. of 3% in 1 quart water. Mist plants with this solution.

Insecticide spray: mix 8-oz. black strap molasses or sugar and 8-oz. 3% H_2O_2 to 1 gallon of water.

For topical therapeutic use: at a 3% solution, H_2O_2 can effectively be used externally. Make a 3% solution by mixing 1 part 35% H_2O_2 with 11 parts of water. Place in a spray bottle or dip a cotton ball in the solution and use as a facial freshener after bathing, being careful to avoid the eyes, eyebrows and hair.

Earth's Bounty O_2 GEL, combined with aloe vera juice, vegetable glycerine and red seaweed extract, is also useful for general application as a topical antiseptic and antifungal. It may be applied to affected areas on the skin, or massaged into the soles of the feet where the pores are large.

How to check for low blood sugar:

The importance of correct diagnosis and treatment of sugar instabilities is essential. The human body possesses a complex set of checks and balances to maintain blood glucose concentrations within a narrow range. Blood sugar control is influenced by the pituitary, thyroid and adrenal glands, as well as the pancreas, liver, kidneys and even the skeletal muscles. Hypoglycemia symptoms are often mistaken for other problems. Low blood sugar is the biological equivalent of a race car running on empty. It is not so much a disease as a symptom of other disorders. Some of the symptoms can be improved right away by eating something, but this does not address the cause.

Hypoglycemia in children is widely indicated as a cause of both hyperactivity and learning disorders. Chronic negativism, mood swings, aggressive behavior, and obstinate resentment to all discipline are reasons for at least taking the self-test below, as well as a Glucose Tolerance Test from a physician. I find that for children, the condition can only be managed by a diet from which all forms of concentrated sugars have been removed, including fruit juices.

The following questionnaire is for self-determination, reprinted from the Enzymatic Therapy Notebook. It can help you decide, in cooperation with a health care professional, whether you need low blood sugar support, and whether other professional help is necessary.

Mark the following symptoms as they pertain to you: (1) for mild symptoms, occurring once or twice a year; (2) for moderate symptoms, occurring several times a year; (3) severe symptoms, occurring almost constantly. A score of 6 or more signifies a need for sugar balancing and nutritional support. A score of 12 -18 indicates a need for therapeutic measures several times daily.

( ) Irritability
( ) Anti-social behavior
( ) Craving for sweets
( ) Blurred vision
( ) Heart palpitations
( ) Rapid pulse

( ) Mental confusion, spaciness, forgetfulness
( ) Constant phobias, fears
( ) Constant worry, nervousness and anxiety
( ) Nightmares
( ) Cold sweats and shaking
( ) Frequent headaches
( ) Faintness, dizziness, trembling
( ) Poor concentration
( ) Crying spells
( ) Weak spells
( ) Extreme fatigue, exhaustion
( ) Lots of sighing and yawning
( ) Insomnia; inability to return to sleep after awakening
( ) Twitching, involuntary muscle jerks
( ) Digestive problems
( ) Indecisiveness
( ) Unexplained depression
( ) Nervous breakdown
( ) Suicidal intent

Reprinted with permission from the Enzymatic Therapy Notebook.

How to read a blood panel:

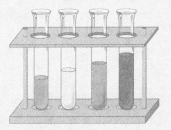

Blood work is an important part of medical diagnostic protocol, but how many of us really understand what it's telling us about our health. The following is a brief guide to the basics of how to read a blood panel and make the most of the results. Note: Fasting, required for 24 hours before blood panel, is done to diagnose serious diseases like diabetes and monitor nutrient levels.

—The **blood glucose level check** is the primary test for diabetes. Average range should be between 70 mg to 105 mg. If your fasting blood glucose level is over 105 mg, you may have diabetes. Boost fiber intake especially from vegetables and whole grains like oats and brown rice to stabilize diabetic blood sugar swings. Regular exercise is another key to successful diabetes control.

—The **urea nitrogen check** determines how well your kidneys break down protein. Average range is between 7 and 22; optimum range is between 7 to 15. Most Americans have high levels of protein byproducts in their blood, largely a result of a diet high in animal proteins. High urea levels can lead to kidney malfunction, arthritis and gout. If this is the case for you, reduce meat and dairy intake; focus instead on high quality protein from legumes and vegetables.

—The blood **calcium** check is especially important for menopausal women who may be at risk for osteoporosis. Although calcium isn't the whole answer for bone health, it plays an important role in bone building. Optimum calcium range is between 8.4 to 10.

Note: A high protein diet tends to leach calcium from the body and is a contributing factor to osteoporosis development. If your calcium levels are below normal, you may want to reduce your protein intake and add a calcium-magnesium supplement. Calcium and magnesium appear together in Nature and work the best therapeutically as a combination.

545

What else does a blood panel check for?

A blood panel looks for **blood enzyme elevations** related to liver damage, hepatitis and gall bladder disease. **Cholesterol and triglyceride levels,** linked to heart disease, are checked. **High uric acid levels,** linked to joint inflammation, are measured as a risk factor for heart disease.

Test results include your **levels of electrolytes** like potassium, sodium and magnesium. Low levels of potassium and magnesium, and high levels of sodium cause elevations in blood pressure, aggravate weight control problems and increase diabetes and heart disease complications.

Note: People who take diuretic drugs are most at risk for low electrolyte levels because these drugs deplete magnesium and potassium in the body.

A complete blood panel is quite extensive. I've only covered some of the highlights of what you may find in your results. Having blood work done is good idea for anyone who wants a better understanding of their health status. Be sure to go over your results and any questions with your physician.

What level should your cholesterol be?

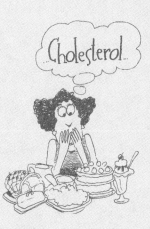

High cholesterol affects as many as 60 million Americans, and it is a major factor for coronary heart disease. Cholesterol screening is recommended for all adults, but test results can be complicated. Here's a rundown of what is tested in today's cholesterol screening and what it can mean for your health.

LDL (low density lipoprotein), is the "bad" cholesterol, which carries cholesterol through the bloodstream for cell-building, but leaves behind the excess on artery walls and in tissues. Ideal LDL levels are less than 130 mg/dL. Levels between 130 mg/dL to 159 mg/dL are borderline high. Levels 160 mg/dL and over are high. Pay close attention to your results here. High LDL cholesterol accumulated on arteries walls can eventually block the flow of blood to your heart or brain, resulting in a heart attack or stroke.

New research points out new concerns. Almost half of all heart diseases patients have pattern-B LDLs, smaller and more dense than normal LDLs. Pattern-B LDLs make their way into blood vessels 40% faster than normal LDLs, so fat is deposited on artery walls faster than it can be removed. Quebec studies show people with more than 25% of pattern-B LDL cholesterol have three times the normal risk of heart diseases — even when their total LDL count is normal! The future of cholesterol screening may involve more precise tests which show the level of pattern-B LDL cholesterol you have.

HDL (high density lipoprotein), is the "good" cholesterol that helps prevent narrowing of the artery walls by transporting excess LDL cholesterol to the liver for excretion as bile. Ideal HDL cholesterol levels should be 60 mg/dL and above. Levels below 35 mg/dL are too low.

Triglycerides increase the density of LDL cholesterol molecules. Ideal triglyceride levels are less than 200 mg/dL. 200 to 399 mg/dL is considered borderline. Levels 400 mg/dL and above are too high and dangerous to health.

Total cholesterol levels: Should be less than 200 mg/dL. Levels 200 to 239 mg/dL are borderline high. Anything over 240 mg/dL is high and puts you at an increased risk for heart disease. Low cholesterol levels (below 180) affect 10% of Americans and can be dangerous, too. According to a new study done by the University of Washington, low cholesterol is a risk factor for hemorrhagic stroke!

If your cholesterol levels are high, the cholesterol reduction program on pg. 349 of this book has been successful for hundreds of people.

Side effects of cholesterol-lowering drugs like Zocor, Mevacor and Pravachol include liver toxicity, stomach distress and vision impairment. According to a study in Journal of Clinical Pharmacology, these drugs also deplete CoQ_{10} by up to 50%, an essential co-enzyme that strengthens the heart and arteries.

Are you considering heart surgery? Here are the risks:

Heart surgery procedures cost Americans over $50 billion each year. They are highly invasive, expensive, traumatic procedures. Many are questioning some of the techniques as a case of the cure being worse than the disease. It's true that sometimes heart surgery can be the beginning of the end of a normal, natural, lifestyle. The latest study from New England Journal of Medicine reveals heart surgery patients fare worse than heart patients who only undergo medical therapy. In fact, heart disease patients actually have 98.4% chance of survival WITHOUT surgery. Most of us know someone for whom bypass surgery or a pacemaker was the beginning of the end. My late father-in-law was one. Here is information you should know about commonly performed heart surgeries.

—**Pacemaker Implant Surgery:** For people who suffer from a slow heart rate — $25,000. Pacemakers are battery-powered devices implanted just under the skin that send out electrical impulses to stimulate heart beat. Research from the Mayo clinic and The Heart Institute in St. Petersburg shows electrical devices like cell phones, medical equipment, even security devices at shopping malls interfere with pacemaker activity, creating fluctuations in heartbeat that can lead to drowsiness, shortness of breath or blackouts. And, the battery in a pacemaker eventually wears out, so it must be continually monitored for effectiveness.

—**Angiogram:** Used to diagnose the severity of coronary artery disease — $11,000. A liquid, containing material visible to an X-ray device is injected into the coronary artery, allowing doctors to locate blockages. According to experts at The Non-Invasive Heart Center of San Diego, angiogram results only cover 25% of total coronary blood flow. Blockages in smaller vessels can be completely overlooked. The angiogram procedure itself can cause stroke, heart attack, or even death.

—**Bypass Surgery:** For people with blocked coronary arteries — $45,000. In this procedure, blocked portions of the coronary arteries are bypassed with grafts taken from veins in the legs. But, the veins of the leg aren't designed to withstand the high pressure blood flow from the heart. There's just too much wear and tear, so many patients don't live beyond 6 or 7 years after their first operation. Only a small percentage of heart disease patients (less than 10%) actually benefit from bypass surgery. According to Julian Whitaker M.D. in his newsletter Health & Healing, nearly 1 in 25 people die during the bypass surgery itself. Bypass surgery is still the most popular heart disease surgery with over 573, 000 operations performed on men and women each year.

—**Balloon Angioplasty:** A balloon-tipped catheter is used to "inflate" or open up blocked arteries — $15,000. An angioplasty causes a heart attack in 4% of people having the procedure. In 5%, the blockage is actually made worse. Statistics show that 35% of "treated" blockages actually return to their pre-op severity in less than a year. I personally know two people who had to have another angioplasty within a year. Doctors from the University of Texas hope to improve angioplasty success rates by using clot busting drugs directly on clot-prone areas during the procedure which may help prevent future blockages.

If you're considering heart surgery, talk to your doctor at length and get all the information about your prospective procedure — the advantages, the healing risks and requirements, and the long term problems. Many natural therapies improve your heart health. See my program for heart health on pg. 412.

How to take your own pulse:

The term "pulse" refers to the number beats your heart has per minute. Taking your own pulse is an easy home healing protocol which can help tell you whether you're at risk for tachycardia, atrial fibrillation or other types of irregular heartbeat.

Take your pulse in the morning.
1: Place your index and middle finger around the back of your wrist.
2: Use your index and middle finger to locate the radial artery in your wrist. Use light pressure to feel for your pulse. It should be easy to find.
3: Count the number of beats your pulse has in 30 seconds. Multiply those results by 2 to calculate your pulse rate per minute. Follow the procedure a second time. Note irregularities like pauses between beats, or beats that come closer to the preceding beats than the following ones and report them to your physician immediately. These may be warning signs of undiagnosed heart abnormalities.

A normal resting pulse reading for adults and teens ranges between 60 to 100 beats per minute. Pulse readings for children and infants are slightly higher. Children ages 7-10 range between 70 to 110 beats per minute; A normal infant pulse rate may reach up to 150 beats per minute. Most physicians advise NOT allowing your heart rate to reach more than 200 beats per minute.

Knowing your glands:

There are two types of glands in the body — exocrine (glands regulated by the hypothalamus, that secrete their fluids through ducts, like the salivary and mammary glands; and endocrine (glands that emit their secretions directly as hormones into the bloodstream). Endocrine glands are involved with almost every body function. They are integral to hormone balance, proper metabolism, high energy and immune response. The health of the endocrine system even interacts directly with our foundation genetics, determining genetic potential.

Deep body balance is dependent on the vitality of your glands. Invariably, your glands suffer the most from a lifestyle high in stress and low in rest and nutrition. Glandular malfunction leads to a wide array of health problems today: from thyroid malfunction, to hair loss, to exhaustion, to diabetes. This section gives you an overview of the major endocrine glands with specific recommendations for maintaining their health.

•**ADRENALS:** the adrenal glands lie just atop the kidneys, and are composed of two distinct parts — the adrenal medulla and the adrenal cortex. The medulla secretes the hormones epinephrine (adrenaline) and norepinephrine in the "fight or flight" response. Adrenal hormones also maintain involuntary functions like heart rate, breathing and digestion. The adrenal cortex secretes corticosteroid hormones, formed from cholesterol. An herbal formula to stimulate some of these corticosteroid hormone effects might include *licorice root, wild yam root, panax ginseng, bupleurum, Siberian ginseng* and *turmeric*. See page 300 for a complete discussion of adrenal health.

•**HYPOTHALAMUS:** located just behind the pituitary gland. Hormones secreted by this small group of nerve cells are involved in breast milk production, body temperature, sleep and wakefulness, water balance and smooth muscle contraction. Adaptogen herbs like *gotu kola, panax ginseng, astragalus* and *Siberian ginseng* help keep the hypothalamus balanced.

•**LYMPH:** the lymphatic system includes the lymphatic vessels, the lymph nodes, the thymus gland, the tonsils and the spleen. It is often called the body's other circulatory system, because it collects tissue fluid that is not needed by the capillaries or the skin and returns it to the heart for recirculation. It is also a key to the body's immune defenses and to cancer protection. The small lymph glands that stud the lymph system contain disease-fighting white blood cells, called lymphocytes, and macrophages which protect our cells against damage. Most lymph fluid is rich in nutrients produced in the liver, especially protein. Lymphatic vessels not only drain waste products from tissues, they are also a major route for body nutrients from the liver and intestines.

  –*Quick Tip:* To revitalize your lymph system with diet, take a glass of lemon juice and water regularly in the morning, and a glass of papaya juice in the evening. Include plenty of potassium-rich foods regularly, such as sea vegetables, broccoli, bananas and seafood. Avoid caffeine, sugar and alcohol during healing.

  –*To stimulate lymph flow:* 1) activate muscles with regular exercise and stretching. Start every exercise period with deep, diaphragmatic breathing. 2) elevate feet and legs for 5 minutes every day, massaging lymph node areas. 3) take a hot and cold hydrotherapy treatment at the end of your daily shower. Mini-trampoline exercise clears clogged lymph nodes. Both acupuncture and acupressure have been successful. Eliminate aluminum cookware, food additives, and alum-containing foods and deodorants.

  –*Lymph system therapy recommendations:* Crystal Star ANTI-BIO™ caps or extract for white blood cell formation, Crystal Star REISHI/GINSENG™ extract to enhance immune health. A good lymph tea blend: *white sage, astragalus, echinacea root, Oregon grape root* and *dandelion root.*

  –*Supplement recommendations:* Enzymatic Therapy LYMPHO-CLEAR, Lane Labs BENE-FIN shark cartilage for leukocyte production, EVENING PRIMROSE OIL caps, and Flora VEGE-SIL.

• PANCREAS: the pancreas is located just behind the stomach. The pancreas is both an exocrine and an endocrine gland which secretes hormones into the bloodstream and digestive enzymes into the small intestine. Its hormone, glucagon, controls blood sugar levels and digestive enzymes. Today, pancreas glandular therapy is used for digestive disorders, low blood sugar and heart problems, and as an antimicrobial and anti-inflammatory. The Islets of Langerhans are tiny glandular clusters in the pancreas that produce insulin. Their destruction or impairment results in diabetes or hypoglycemia.

  Alcoholism, excessive use of prescription drugs, and poor nutrition can lead to pancreatitis, a painful condition related to gallbladder problems that may become critical. In addition, one-third to one-half of unexplained pancreatitis might be triggered by the genetic defect linked to cystic fibrosis. Sugary foods should be avoided if you have a weak pancreas. Nutrients to help maintain pancreatic health include chromium picolinate 200mcg daily, phosphatidyl choline to aid in fat digestion, and pancreatin, a digestive enzyme.

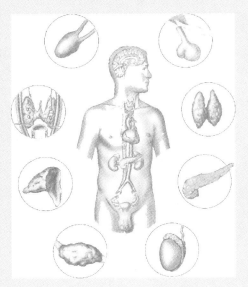

• OVARIES: the ovaries on either side of the pelvic cavity, produce the female eggs for reproduction, and two hormones, estrogen and progesterone, responsible for maintaining secondary sexual characteristics, and preparing the uterus and breasts for the reproductive cycle. See Hormone Health and Balance pages for specific balancing recommendations.

• PINEAL GLAND: Lies just under the pituitary gland, behind the eyes. The pineal gland is highly responsive to light waves; it is the body's light meter. Many health problems result from our modern day indoor lifestyle, in which we receive distorted light waves from sunglasses, eyeglasses, window glass, fluorescent lights and contact lenses. Both pineal and pituitary glands benefit from 20 minutes a day of early morning sunlight. The pineal helps balance the endocrine system, regulating our body rhythms, sleep patterns, fertility and the development of consciousness.

• **PITUITARY:** the pituitary is called the body's master gland, regulating all glandular activity. The major symptoms of pituitary deficiency involve a stressed nervous system, mental processes (especially mental burn-out brought on by stress), poor healing, erratic blood sugar levels and body fluid imbalance.

–*Dietary recommendations:* include plenty of green leafy vegetables. Have a veggie drink (pg. 218) or Future Biotics VITAL K drink, or Crystal Star ENERGY GREEN™ drink once a week. Eat complex carbohydrates like broccoli, potatoes, sprouts, peas, dried fruits, whole grains and brown rice. Take fresh fruit juices each morning. Drink 6 glasses of bottled water daily. Avoid beer, sweet wines, refined foods, sugar, heavy pastries, and canned foods. Avoid all MSG-containing foods and preserved foods.

–*Supplement recommendations:* include a multi-mineral, like MEZOTRACE sea mineral complex, vitamin C or Ester C with bioflavonoids and rutin, Country Life sublingual B-12 2500mcg every other day, Glutamine 500mg 4x daily for growth hormone, B-complex 100mg daily, with extraB-6, 250mg and PABA 1000mg daily, Flora VEGESIL caps and Enzymatic Therapy RAW PITUITARY caps.

–*Herbal recommendations for pituitary/pineal health:* Crystal Star GINSENG 6 SUPER™ TEA or GINSENG-LICORICE ELIXIR™ twice daily; IODINE-POTASSIUM™ caps, or Solaray ALFA-JUICE caps; Beehive Botanicals royal jelly and honey drink mix daily, and *gotu kola-damiana* caps. Sea greens of all kinds work synergistically with the pituitary in glandular formulas.

–*Acupressure points:* press for 10 seconds, 3x each, over the left eyebrow for pituitary stimulation; on the forehead where the eyebrows meet for pineal stimulation.

• **PROSTATE:** the prostate is a large male gland that lies just below the neck of the bladder, and around the top of the urinary tract. The primary function of the prostate is to help the semen move through the urethra during ejaculation. It also produces an alkaline fluid which carries the sperm from the testes into the vagina. This fluid greatly enhances the chances of fertilization because it balances the acid environment of the uterus for the sperm. The prostate enlarges during sexual arousal. If there is prolonged arousal without ejaculation, the pressure from the prostate on the testicles becomes very uncomfortable. See Benign Prostatic Hyperplasia on page 483 for more information.

• **SPLEEN:** the spleen is the largest mass of lymphatic tissue in the body. It produces lymphocytes, destroys worn-out blood cells, and serves as a blood reservoir. During times of great stress or hemorrhage, the spleen can release its stored blood to prevent shock. Depletion symptoms include anemia, pallor, extreme slimness, poor memory and sluggishness.

–*Dietary recommendations for spleen health:* Take a carrot-beet-cucumber juice every day for 1 week, then every other day for another week to "spring clean" these glands of stored toxins. Then, build up red blood cells with a potassium broth (pg. 215), a veggie drink (pg. 218), Green Foods GREEN ESSENCE drink, or Crystal Star ENERGY GREEN™ drink, and a leafy green salad every day. Include brown rice and alfalfa sprouts frequently.

–*Herbal recommendations for spleen health:* Crystal Star HEARTSEASE-HAWTHORN™ caps with *hawthorn* or *yellow dock root* extract for blood building and tone, GINSENG 6 SUPER™ tea or *red root* tea for continued enhancement. Spleen enhancing tea: *4-oz. hawthorn, 1-oz. cardamom, 1-oz. safflowers, 1-oz. lemon balm, 1-oz. red sage*; take 2 cups daily.

–*Supplement recommendations for spleen health:* Enzymatic Therapy LIQUID LIVER with GINSENG, LYMPH-SPLEEN COMPLEX, or GOLDEN SPLEEN 500, Vitamin E 400IU daily for red blood enhancement, marine carotene 50-100,000IU daily, liquid chlorophyll 3 teasp. daily with meals, zinc picolinate 30mg daily and Natren TRINITY probiotics, $^1/_2$ teasp. in water 2x daily.

• **TESTES:** the male gonads, are located in the scrotum. The testicles are the workhorses of the male reproductive system, producing the sperm and the male hormone testosterone. Testosterone causes the development of male secondary characteristics - face and body hair (and the male pattern receding hairline), body odor, voice change, enhanced muscles, male sexual organs and the increased oiliness and coarseness of a man's skin (a factor that means men's skin ages about ten years behind the skin of women). Testosterone also establishes the male sex drive, but has nothing to do with male erection. Some men do experience a decrease in testosterone production as they age, especially if his diet and lifestyle are not conducive to healthy gland function. The symptoms of this endocrine imbalance are similar to a woman's menopause and are called andropause. See pg. 266 for a complete lifestyle program for Male Andropause.

•**THYMUS:** the thymus lies between the thyroid gland and the heart. Known as the "master gland" of the immune system, the thymus gland is vital to the production of T-lymphocyte cells and thymic hormones, critical to cell-mediated immunity. The thymus gland shrinks with age and is easily damaged by oxidation and free radicals. Therapeutic uses of thymus glandular extracts include help against chronic infections, food allergies, auto-immune disorders, hair loss and cancer therapy.

Anti-oxidants are necessary for thymus health: vitamin E with selenium and beta-carotene can help protect the thymus. Zinc, vitamin B_6 and vitamin C help produce thymic hormones.

Herbal recommendations for thymus health: *Echinacea root* and *echinacea-goldenseal-myrrh* compounds are prime herbals for increasing the activity of white blood cells and stimulating the production of interferon. *Panax ginseng* and *licorice* are effective adaptogens for regulating thymus acivity. Crystal Star GINSENG-LICORICE ELIXIR™ acts synergistically with the thymus.

•**THYROID:** the thyroid gland folds around the front and sides of the windpipe at the base of the neck. It secretes the high iodine hormone thyroxin involved in growth, digestion, metabolism (which provides vital energy resources for every body activity), body temperature, reflexes, and heartbeat. The two most common thyroid disorders are hypothyroidism, (as in Hashimoto's disease) where the thyroid is not producing enough thyroxin (a problem that is increasing in our heavily polluted, nutrient-poor environment), and hyperthyroidism, caused by the secretion of too much thyroxin (as in Grave's Disease).

Signs of an underactive thyroid include depression, unusual fatigue, hair loss (especially in women), obesity, intolerance to cold, breast fibroids and poor immune response. Signs of overactive thyroid include: feeling "wired" for no reason, rapid heartbeat, diarrhea, insomnia, bulging eyes or double vision, light menstrual period, feeling warm, and unexplained weight loss. Iodine and potassium, rich in sea greens and herbs are some of the best nutrients to take for thyroid health.

The parathyroid glands are four small glands embedded in the thyroid gland which help maintain the proper level of nutrients in the body. The parathyroid glands produce parathyroid hormone which raises calcium levels in the blood. Raised calcium levels caused by excess parathyroid production can contribute to kidney stones and kidney failure.

Note: see pages 402 and 428 for information about Thyroid diseases.

Monitoring your thyroid performance at home:

The thyroid gland produces hormones which increase protein synthesis in all body tissues, as well as some important enzymes that influence the rate at which fat is burned for energy. If the thyroid is not functioning properly, slow metabolism results. Many people with underactive thyroids also have weight problems. Thyroid dysfunction is almost always involved with women's problems.

A common method for testing thyroid function is to place a basal thermometer under the arm for ten minutes before getting out of bed in the morning. The thermometer must read to tenths of a degree. Normal body temperature ranges for this test are between 97.8 and 98.2 degrees Fahrenheit. A reading below 97.8 may indicate hypothyroid activity (low thyroid); a reading above may indicate hyperthyroid activity (excess thyroid). Some of the factors which can cause thyroid problems, and decrease the rate at which the body burns calories, include malnourishment because of nutrient deficiencies, thyroid and/or pituitary exhaustion because of over-stimulation from caffeine, sugar, or other stimulants, and the presence of substances which inhibit thyroid function, such as hard liquor.

Taking your basal body temperature:

Body temperature reflects metabolic rate, largely determined by hormones secreted by the thyroid gland. Thyroid health can be measured by basal body temperature. You will need a thermometer.

1. Shake down thermometer to below 95°F and place it by your bed before going to sleep at night.

2. On waking, place the thermometer in your armpit for a full 10 minutes. Lie quietly with your eyes closed, making as little movement as possible for the best results.

3. After 10 minutes, read and record the temperature and date.

4. Record temperature for at least 3 mornings. Menstruating women must perform the test on the 2nd, 3rd, and 4th days of menstruation. Men and post-menopausal women can perform the test any time. Normal basal body temperature is between 97.6° and 98.2°.

Use your stool as a tool to tell your body state:

Few of us are comfortable talking about what goes on (or doesn't go on) in our private moments in the bathroom — even with our own physician. That's too bad because your stool can be surprisingly revealing about your health status.

Elimination varies from person to person, but for optimum health, you should eliminate 2-3 times a day (one time for each meal). And, healthy bowel movements should be brown to light brown, light enough to float, bulky (not compacted), and easy to pass. Although it is normal for stool to have some odor, it shouldn't be strong or pungent (signs of increased bowel transit time and a diet too high in animal proteins and saturated fat). If you don't fit this model, you're not alone. Most Americans have some degree of colon toxicity, largely as a result of our diets high in refined, chemicalized foods and low in fiber-rich whole grains, and fruits and vegetables. Your stool can be an important tool to help you assess your digestive health. Here are a few things to watch for:

—Bloody or mucous-covered stools can be a sign of Crohn's disease, ulcerative colitis or even colon cancer. It can also be a sign of hemorrhoidal inflammation and irritation. Report symptoms like these to your physician right away.

—Thin, ribbonlike or flattened stools are usually the sign of an obstruction like a polyp that narrows the elimination pathway. It can also be a sign of Irritable Bowel Syndrome or spastic colon.

—Stools that are large, messy and leave a film in toilet water can be a sign of malabsorption. If the problem is chronic, consider consulting with a qualified health professional. Malabsorption problems can lead to nutritional deficiencies.

—Abnormally fatty stools may be a sign of pancreatitis, inflammation of the pancreas that can lead to diabetes.

—Extremely foul-smelling stools may mean you have a deficiency of "friendly bacteria" that inhabit your intestines, a diet too high in red meat protein, or Candida yeast overgrowth.

—Greenish stools may mean you should cut down on sugar. If you are a vegetarian who doesn't consume a lot of sugar, it may mean you need more whole grains in your diet.

—Pale, greyish stools can be a sign of liver or gallbladder problems.

—Black, tar-like stools may mean you have bleeding in your upper digestive tract. Report these symptoms to your physician right away.

—Reddish stools are usually the result of eating a lot red foods. Beets are the frequent cause here.

—Dark brown stools can be the result of too much salt in the diet.

Are You Trying To Quit Smoking?

Here's the best motivational chart I've ever seen to graphically illustrate the benefits for your body and your life once you really quit.

What happens after you quit smoking?

Within 20 minutes of smoking, your body begins a series of changes that continues for years.
All benefits are lost by smoking just one cigarette a day according to the American Cancer Society.

20 MINUTES:
- Blood pressure drops to normal
- Pulse rate drops to normal
- Body temperature of hands and feet rises to normal

8 HOURS
- Carbon monoxide level in blood drops to normal
- Oxygen level in blood increases to normal

24 HOURS
- Chance of heart attack decreases

48 HOURS
- Nerve endings start regrowing
- Ability to smell and taste is enhanced

2 WEEKS TO 3 MONTHS
- Circulation improves
- Walking becomes easier
- Lung function increases up to 30%

1 to 9 MONTHS
- Coughing, sinus congestion, fatigue, and shortness of breath decrease
- Cilia regrow in lungs, allowing lungs to handle mucous, keep clean and reduce infection.
- Body's overall energy rises

1 YEAR
- Risk of coronary heart disease is half that of a smoker

5 YEARS
- Lung cancer death rate for average former smoker (a pack a day) decreases by almost half
- Stroke risk is reduced to that of a nonsmoker five to 15 years after quitting
- Risk of cancer of the mouth, throat, and esophagus is half that of a smoker's

10 YEARS
- Lung cancer death rate is similar to that of a nonsmoker
- Precancerous cells are replaced
- Risk of cancer of the mouth, throat, esophagus, bladder, kidney, cervix, and pancreas decreases

15 YEARS
- Risk of coronary heart disease of that of a nonsmoker

Sources: The American Cancer Society; Centers for Disease Control

Home fertility test:

There are natural ways to stay informed about your ovulation cycle. The PFT 1-2-3, invented by Karen and Ed Porrazzo, is a completely natural personal fertility and reproductive health system. It allows you to find out when you're the most fertile by licking a tiny slide and viewing crystallization patterns which determine your fertile periods with a microscope. Watching your reproductive cycle from your own home can be informative, interesting and easy. Right now, the product is undergoing extensive medical testing so it can be registered by the FDA in the U.S. For more information on the PFT 1-2-3, contact Personal Fertility Technologies @ 888-573-8123, or visit http://pft123.com. (Product should be available Jan. 2000.)

Deep breathing for stress relief and rejuvenation:

Deep breathing activates relaxation centers in the brain, reducing overall body stress and increasing creative mental energy. When you are tense, your breathing is shallow. When you are emotionally distressed, your oxygen levels decrease. When you are angry or fearful, your breathing rate increases (normal breathing is about16 times per minute). When body fluid and congestion builds up, your breathing is probably restricted because breathing affects the circulation of lymph.

Breathing is controlled by two sets of nerves — the involuntary (autonomic) nervous system, and the voluntary nervous system. An imbalance of the autonomic nervous system contributes to health problems. Improving your breathing enhances the autonomic nervous system and many of its involuntary functions.

Use your breathing as a stress release meditation:

1: Shift your focus away from your racing mind and your stressed emotions. There is a basic connection between your breath and your state of mind. Sit quietly and focus on your breath.

2: Consciously take slow, deep, and regular breaths... your mind will become more calm.

3: Recall a positive, pleasant past experience. Feel appreciation and thankfulness about the good things and people you have in your life. Shifting your focus to positive feelings helps neutralize the stress.

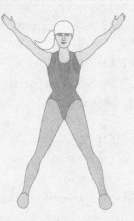

Breath and Body Stretch:

1: Stand tall and raise your hands above your head. Stretch your arms and fingers as if you are reaching for the sky — pretend you are trying to climb up with your hands and arms. As you reach, inhale deeply through your nostrils while rising on your toes.

2: Exhale slowly, and gradually return to the starting position, with your arms hanging loosely at your side. Repeat this at least 5 times. This is a great warm-up to a brisk walk.

Filling a Balloon:

1: Breathe in through the nose and imagine that the in-coming breath is filling a balloon in your belly, then continues up your torso and fills your entire upper body with air.

2: After you are completely filled up with air, exhale, let go and feel the balloon emptying. Do a few of these deep breaths. Relaxation is just a breath away.

Correct Food Combining Chart
A reference tool for a good healing diet

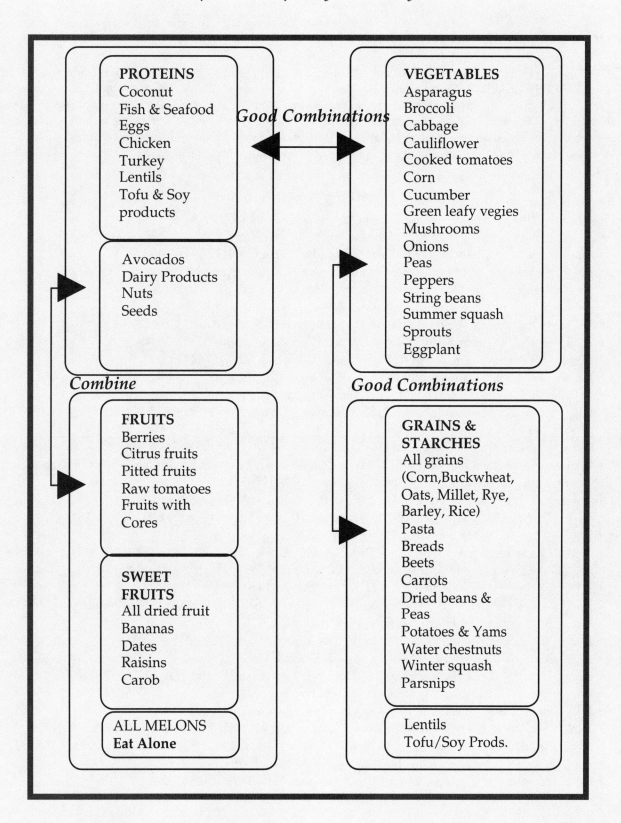

PROTEINS
Coconut
Fish & Seafood
Eggs
Chicken
Turkey
Lentils
Tofu & Soy
products

Avocados
Dairy Products
Nuts
Seeds

Good Combinations

VEGETABLES
Asparagus
Broccoli
Cabbage
Cauliflower
Cooked tomatoes
Corn
Cucumber
Green leafy vegies
Mushrooms
Onions
Peas
Peppers
String beans
Summer squash
Sprouts
Eggplant

Combine

Good Combinations

FRUITS
Berries
Citrus fruits
Pitted fruits
Raw tomatoes
Fruits with
Cores

**SWEET
FRUITS**
All dried fruit
Bananas
Dates
Raisins
Carob

ALL MELONS
Eat Alone

**GRAINS &
STARCHES**
All grains
(Corn,Buckwheat,
Oats, Millet, Rye,
Barley, Rice)
Pasta
Breads
Beets
Carrots
Dried beans &
Peas
Potatoes & Yams
Water chestnuts
Winter squash
Parsnips

Lentils
Tofu/Soy Prods.

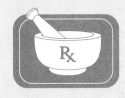

PRODUCT RESOURCES

Where you can get what we recommend.....

The following list is for your convenience and assistance in obtaining further information about the products I recommend in HEALTHY HEALING. The list is unsolicited by the companies named. Each company has a solid history of testing and corroborative data that is invaluable to me and my staff, as well as empirical confirmation by the stores that carry these products who have shared their experiences with us. We hear from thousands of readers about the products they have used. I consider their information with every edition of HEALTHY HEALING. I realize there are many other fine companies and products who are not listed here, but you can rely on the companies who are, for their high quality products and good results.

- Alacer Corp., 19631 Pauling, Foothill Ranch, CA 92610, 800-854-0249
- All One, 719 East Haley St., Santa Barbara, CA 93103, 800-235-5727
- Aloe Life International, 4822 Santa Monica Ave. #231, San Diego, CA 92107, 800-414-2563
- Alta Health Products, Inc., 1979 E. Locust Street, Pasadena, CA 91107, 626-796-1047
- America's Finest, Inc., 140 Ethel Road West, Suites S & T, Piscataway, NJ 08854, 800-350-3305
- Anabol Naturals, 1550 Mansfield Street, Santa Cruz, CA 95062, 800-426-2265
- Arise & Shine, P.O. Box 1439, Mt. Shasta, CA 96067, 800-688-2444
- Barleans Organic Oils, 4936 Lake Terrell Rd., Fern Dale, WA 98248, 800-445-3529
- BD Herbs, 14000 Tomki Road, Redwood Valley, CA 95470, 800-760-3739
- Beehive Botanicals, Route 8, Box 8257, Hayward, WI 54843, 800-233-4483
- Biotec Foods / BioVet Internat'l, 5152 Bolsa Ave. Suite 101, Huntington Beach, CA 92649, 800-788-1084
- Boericke & Tafel Inc.,(B & T) 2381 Circadian Way, Santa Rosa, CA 95407, 800-876-9505
- Bragg/Live Food Products, Inc., Box 7, Santa Barbara, CA 93102, 805-968-1028
- CC Pollen Co., 3627 East Indian School Rd., Suite 209, Phoenix, AZ 85018-5126, 800-875-0096
- Champion Nutrition, 2615 Stanwell Dr., Concord, CA 94520, 800-225-4831
- Coenzyme-A Technologies Inc., 12512 Beverly Park Road B1, Lynnwood, WA 98037, 425-438-8586
- Country Life, 28300 B Industrial Blvd., Hayward, CA 94545, 510-785-1196
- Creations Garden, 25269 The Old Road, Suite B, Newhall, CA 91381, 805-254-3222
- Crystal Star Herbal Nutrition, 4069 Wedgeway Court, Earth City, MO 63045, 800-736-6015
- Dancing Paws, 8659 Hayden Place, Culver City, CA 90232, 888-644-7297
- Dr. Diamond/Herpanacine Associates, P.O. Box 544, Ambler, PA 19002, 888-467-4200
- Dr. Goodpet, P.O. Box 4547, Inglewood, CA 90309, 800-222-9932
- EAS, 555 Corporate Circle, Golden, CO 80401, 800-923-4300
- East Park Research, Inc., 2709 Horseshoe Drive, Las Vegas, NV 89120, 800-345-8367 (orders)
- Eidon Silica Products, 9988 Hibert St. #104, San Diego, CA 92131, 800-700-1169
- Enzymatic Therapy, Dept. L, P.O. Box 22310, Green Bay, WI 54305, 800-783-2286
- Enzymedica, 1970 Kings Hwy., Punta Gorda, FL 33980, 888-918-1118
- Earth's Bounty/Matrix Health Products, 9316 Wheatlands Road, Santee, CA 92071, 800-736-5609
- Esteem Products Ltd., 15015 Main St., Suite 204, Bellevue, WA 98007, 800-255-7631
- Ethical Nutrients/Unipro, 971 Calle Negocio, San Clemente, CA 92673, 714-366-0818
- Flint River Ranch, 1243 Columbia Avenue B-6, Riverside, CA 92507-2123, 888-722-4589
- Flora, Inc., 805 East Badger Road, P.O. Box 73, Lynden, WA 98264, 800-446-2110, (Info.) 604-451-8232
- Futurebiotics, 145 Ricefield Lane, Hauppauge, NY 11788, 800-367-5433
- Gaia Herbs, Inc., 12 Lancaster County Road, Harvard, MA 01451, 800-831-7780
- Golden Pride, 1501 Northpoint Pkwy., Suite 100, West Palm Beach, FL 33407, 561-640-5700

- Green Foods Corp., 320 North Graves Ave., Oxnard, CA 93030 800-777-4430
- Green Kamut Corp., 1542 Seabright Ave., Long Beach, CA 90813, 800-452-6884
- Grifron/Maitake Products, Inc., P.O. Box 1354, Paramus, NJ 07653, 800-747-7418
- Halo-Purely For Pets, Inc. 3438 East Lake Road #14, Palm Harbor, FL 34685, 813-891-6328
- Healthy House, P.O. Box 436, Carmel Valley, CA 93924, 888-447-2939
- Heart Foods Company, Inc., 2235 East 38th Street, Minneapolis, MN 55407, 612-724-5266
- Herbal Magic, Inc., P.O. Box 70, Forest Knowlls, CA 94933, 415-488-9488
- Herbal Products & Development, P.O. Box 1084, Aptos, CA 95001, 831-688-8706
- Herbs Etc., 1340 Rufina Circle, Santa Fe, NM 87505, 505-471-6488
- Herbs For Life, P.O. Box 40082, Sarasota, FL 34278, 941-362-9255
- Imperial Elixir, P.O. Box 970, Simi Valley, CA 93062, 800-423-5176
- Jarrow Formulas, 1824 South Robertson Blvd., Los Angeles, CA 90035, 310-204-6936
- Jones Products Int'l, Inc./ Sport Star, 4069 Wedgeway Court, Earth City, MO 63045, 800-736-6015
- MagneLyfe/Encore Technology, Inc., 80 Fifth Ave., Suite 1104, New York, NY 10011, 877-624-6353
- Maine Coast Sea Vegetables, RR1 Box 78, Franklin, Maine 04634, 207-565-2907
- Maitake Products, Inc., P.O. Box 1354, Paramus, NJ 07653, 800-747-7418
- Medicine Wheel, P.O. Box 20037, Sedona, AZ 86341-0037, 800-233-0810
- M.D. Labs, 1719 W. University, Suite 187, Tempe, AZ 85281, 800-255-2690
- Mendocino Sea Vegetable Co., P.O. Box 1265, Mendocino, CA 95460, 707-937-2050
- Metabolic Response Modifiers, 2633 W. Coast Hwy, Suite B, Newport Beach, CA 92663, 800-948-6296
- Mezotrace Corporation, 415 Wellington St., Winnemucca, NV 89445, 800-843-9989
- Monas Chlorella, 8815 South Decatur Blvd., Las Vegas, NV 89139, 800-275-0343
- Moon Maid Botanicals, 13870 SW 90 Ave., MM104, Miami, FL 33176, 877-253-7853
- Morada Research Laboratories, 22959 Bayshore Rd., Charlotte Harbor, FL 33980, 941-766-1801
- Motherlove Herbal Co., P.O. Box 101, Laporte, CO 80535, 970-493-2892
- MRI (Medical Research Institute), 2160 Pacific Ave., Suite 61, San Francisco CA 94115, 888-448-4246
- Natren Inc., 3105 Willow Ln., Westlake Village, CA 91361, 800-992-3323
- Natural Animal Health Products, Inc., 7000 U.S. 1 North, St. Augustine, FL 32095, 800-274-7387
- Natural Balance (Pep Products), 3130 N. Commerce Ct., Castle Rock, CO 80104-8002, 303-688-6633
- Natural Energy Plus, 4630 N. Paseo De Los Cerritos, Tucson, AZ 85745, 888-633-9233
- Natural Labs Corporation (Deva Flowers), P.O. Box 20037, Sedona, AZ 86341-0037, 800-233-0810
- Nature's Apothecary, 6350 Gunpark Drive #500, Boulder, CO 80301, 800-999-7422
- Nature's Path, P.O. Box 7862, Venice, FL 34287, 800-326-5772
- Nature's Plus, 548 Broadhollow Road, Melville, NY 11747-3708, 516-293-0030
- Nature's Secret/Irwin Naturals, 10549 West Jefferson Blvd., Culver City, CA 90232, 310-253-5305
- Nature's Way, 10 Mountain Springs Parkway, Springville, UT 84663, 800-962-8873
- Nelson Bach, Wilmington Technology Park, 100 Research Dr., Wilmington, MA 01887, 800-319-9151
- New Chapter, P.O. Box 1947, Brattleboro, VT 05302, 800-543-7279
- Noah's Ark, 6166 Taylor Road #105, Naples, FL 34109, 800-926-5100
- Nonie of Beverly Hills, Inc., 16158 Wyancotte Street, Vans Nuys, CA 91406, 310-271-7988
- Nova Homeopathic Therapeutics, 5600 McLeod NE, Suite F, Albuquerque, NM 87109, 800-225-8094
- NOW, 395 S. Glen Ellyn Rd., Bloomingdale, IL 60108, 800-999-8069
- Nutramedix Inc., 212 N. Hwy One, Tequesta, FL 33469, 800-730-3130
- NutriCology /Allergy Research Group, 30806 Santana St., Hayward, CA 94544, 800-545-9960
- Omega Nutrition/Body Ecology, 6515 Aldrich Road, Bellingham, WA 98226, 800-661-3529
- Orthomolecular Specialties, P.O. Box 32232, San Jose, CA 95152-2232, 408-227-9334
- Oshadhi, 1340 G Industrial Ave., Petaluma, CA 94952, 888-674-2344
- Pines International, Inc., 992 East 1400 Road, Lawrence, KS 66044, 800-697-4637
- Planetary Formulas, P.O. Box 533 Soquel, CA 95073, 800-606-6226
- Premier Labs, 27475 Ynez Rd., Suite 305, Temecula, CA 92591, 800-887-5227

- Prevail Corporation, 2204-8 NW Birdsdale, Gresham, OR 97030, 800-248-0885
- Prime Pharmaceutical Corp.,1535 Yonge St. Suite 200, Toronto, Ontario, Canada M4T 1Z2,800-741-6856
- Professional Nutrition, 811 Cliff Dr. , Suite C-1, Santa Barbara, CA 93109, 800-336-9301
- Quantum, Inc., P.O. Box 2791, Eugene, OR 97402, 800-448-1448
- Radiant Life Formulas, 31-B Vista Calabasas, Santa Fe, NM 87501, 888-348-7587
- Rainbow Light, P.O. Box 600, Santa Cruz, CA 95061, 800-635-1233
- Rainforest Remedies, Box 325, Twin Lakes, WI 53181, 800-824-6396
- Real Life Research, Inc., 14631 Best Ave., Norwalk, CA 90650, 800-423-8837
- Rejuvenative Foods, P.O. Box 8464, Santa Cruz, CA 95061, 800-805-7957
- Solaray, Inc., 1104 Country Hills Dr., Suite 300, Ogden, UT 84403, 800-669-8877
- Sonne's Organic Foods, Inc., P.O.Box 2160, Cottonwood, CA 96022, 800-544-8147
- Source Naturals Inc., 23 Janis Way, Scotts Valley, CA 95066, 800-777-5677
- Spectrum Essentials, 133 Copeland St., Petaluma, CA 94952, 707-778-8900
- Springlife Inc., 4630 N. Paseo De Los Cerritos, Tucson, AZ 85745, 888-633-9233
- Sun Wellness, 4025 Spencer St. #104, Torrance, CA 90503, 800-829-2828
- Transformation Enzyme Corporation, 2900 Wilcrest, Suite 220, Houston, TX, 800-777-1474
- Transitions For Health, 621 SW Alder, Suite 900, Portland, OR 97205, 800-888-6814
- Vibrant Health, 432 Lime Rock Rd., Lakeville, CT 06039, 800-242-1835
- Waddell Creek Organic Bee Pollen, 654 Swanton Road, Davenport, CA 95017
- Wakunaga of America / Kyolic, 23501 Madero, Mission Viejo, CA 92691, 800-421-2998 / 800-825-7888
- Wisdom of the Ancients, 640 South Perry Lane, Tempe, AZ 85281, 800-899-9908
- Wyndmere Naturals, Inc., 153 Ashley Road, Hopkins, MN 55343, 800-207-8538
- Y.S. Royal Jelly and Organic Bee Farm, RT. 1, Box 91-A, Sheridan IL 60551, 800-654-4593
- Zand Herbal Formulas, P.O. Box 5312, Santa Monica, CA 90409, 310-822-0500
- Zia Natural Skincare, 1337 Evans Ave., San Francisco, CA 94124, 800-334-7546

There's More......

Coming Soon!
Watch for it!

Dr. Linda Page's

State by State

AMERICAN DIRECTORY of HOLISTIC HEALERS

available early Spring 2000

My offices have received thousands of requests for this directory! It is the only one of its kind we know of. No matter what alternative or holistic healing discipline you're interested in, this directory has a qualified, professional practitioner available for you. Each healer has been checked by our staff for certification, qualifications, specialty and years of practice. We called each practitioner's office to make sure they can take new patients.

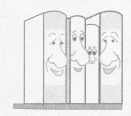

BIBLIOGRAPHY

Your Health Care Choices Today

Mowrey, Daniel B., Ph. D. *The Scientific Validation of Herbal Medicine.* 1986

Krizmanic, Judy. "The Best of Both Worlds." Vegetarian Times. 1995

Mowrey, Daniel, Ph.D. *Next Generation Herbal Medicine.* 1990

Ruch, Meredith Gould, "Feeling Down?" Natural Health. 1993

Grimm, Ellen. "Increase Your Energy with Self-Massage." Natural Health. 1994

Blate, Michael. "Headaches & Backaches." Healthy and Natural Journal. 1994

Weiss, Rick. "Medicine's Latest Miracle Acupuncture." The Natural Way. 1995

Steefel, Lorraine R.N, M.A. "The Use of Acupuncture for Detoxification."Alternative & Complementary Therapies. 1995

Bowles, Willa Vae. "Enzymes for Energy,"Total Health. 1993

Cichoke, Anthony J., D.C. *Enzymes & Enzyme Therapy.* 1994

Cichoke, Anthony J., D.C. "Enzyme Therapy." Let's Live. 1993

Cichoke, Anthony J., D.C. *The Complete Book of Enzyme Therapy.* Avery Publishing Group. 1999

Gregory, Scott J. *A Holistic Protocol for The Immune System.* 1995

Valnet, Jean, M.D. *The Practice of Aromatherapy.* 1990

Tisserand, Robert. *Aromatherapy to Heal and Tend the Body.*1988

Price, Shirley. *Practical Aromatherapy, How to Use Essential Oils to Restore Vitality.* 1987

Robbins, John. *Diet For A New America.* 1987

Gates, Donna. *The Body Ecology Diet.* 1993

Liberman, Jacob, O.D., PhD *Light, Medicine Of The Future.* 1991

Myss, Caroline, Ph.D & C. Norman Shealy, M.D., Ph.D. *The Creation of Health.* 1993

McClennan, Sam (with Tom Monte). *Integrative Acupressure.* A Perigee Book. 1998

International Institute of Reflexology, PO Box 12642, St. Petersburg, FL 33733-2642

Kunz, Kevin & Barbara. "Understanding the Science and Art of Reflexology," Alternative & Complementary Therapies. April/May 1995

Schneider, J. Report from reflexologists: A look at what people do. *Reflexions* 6 (1), 1985

Whitaker, Julian. *199 Health Secrets,* 1993

Godfrey-June, Jean. "Reflexology: The Body's Mini-health Map," The Natural Way, June/July 1995

Herbal Healing

Chen, Ze-lin M.D. & Mei-fang Chen, M.D. *Comprehensive Guide to Chinese Herbal Medicine.* 1992

Reid, Daniel. *Chinese Herbal Medicine.* 1993

Yen-Hsu, Hong. *How to Treat Yourself with Chinese Herbs.* 1993

Frawley, David, M.D. "Ayurveda, the Science of Life." Let's Live. 1993

Weil, Andrew, M.D. *Spontaneous Healing.* 1995

Treadway, Scott Ph.D. & Linda Treadway Ph.D. *Ayurveda & Immortality.* 1986

Zucker, Martin. "Women's Health - Ayurveda Offers Ancient Solutions for Modern Times."Let's Live. 1995

Werbach, Melvyn R., M.D. *Nutritional Influences On Illness - A Sourcebook Of Clinical Research.* 1988

Baar, Karen. *The Real Options in Healthcare.* 1995

Marshall, Lisa Anne. "The Roots of Western And Herbal Medicine."Natural Foods Merchandiser. 1994

Wolfson, Evelyn. *From the Earth To Beyond the Sky - Native American Medicine.* 1993

Hultkrantz, Ake. Shamanic Healing & Ritual Drama. 1992

Fillius, Thomas J., et al. "Chief Two Moons Meridas: Indian Miracle Man?" HerbClip-ABC. 1995

Colbin, Annemarie. *Food and Healing.* 1986

Laux, Marcus. *Cures from the Rainforest Pharmacy.* 1995

Arnold, Kathryn. "Rain Forest Medicine."Delicious! 1994

Schwontkowski, Donna. *Herbal Treasures from the Amazon.* 1995

Mendelsohn, Robert & Michael J. Balick. "More Drugs Await Discovery in Rainforests."ABC. 1995

Baar, Karen. *The Real Options in Healthcare.* 1995

Mehl-Madrona, Lewis E., M.D., Ph.D., "Coyote Medicine Heals Body and Spirit," Let's Live, Sept. 1999

American Herbal Products Association. *Botanical Safety Handbook.* CRC Press, 1997

Duke, James A., Ph.D. *The Green Pharmacy.* Rodale Press. 1996

Page, Linda, N.D., Ph.D. *Reduce Stress-Boost Energy.* 1999

Murray, Michael, N.D. and Joseph Pizzorno, N.D., *Encyclopedia of Natural Medicine.* Prima Publishing, 1998

The Alternative Health Care Arsenal

Howard Loomis, D.C. "Indigestion, *Why HCL, Antacids, and Pancreatin Are Not The Answer,*" American Chirop., April 1988

"Cooked vs. Raw," Natural Health 1999

Haas, Elson, M.D. *Staying Healthy with Nutrition.* 1992

Page, Linda, N.D., PhD. *How To Be Your Own Herbal Pharmacist.* 1997

Murray, Michael T., N.D. *Encycl. of Nutritional Supplements.*1996

Murray, Michael T., N.D. "Introducing Coleus Forskholii." The Doctor's Prescription for Healthy Living, Vol. 3, No. 2

Kirschman, G.J. and John D. *Nutrition Almanac.* 4th ed., 1996

Foods for Your Healing Diet

Hausman, Patricia & Judith Benn Hurley. *The Healing Foods.* Rodale Press, 1989.

Berdanier, Carolyn D. *CRC Desk Reference For Nutrition.* CRC Press, 1998.

Ensminger, Konlande, Robson. *The Concise Encyclopedia of Foods & Nutrition.* CRC Press, 1995.

Editors of Vegetarian Times. *Vegetarian Times Complete Cookbook*. Macmillan, 1995

Murray, Michael T., N.D. *Encyclopedia of Nutritional Supplements*. 1996

Onstad, Dianne. *Whole Foods Companion*. Chelsea Green Pub. 1996

Madison, Deborah. *Vegetarian Cooking For Everyone*. Broadway Books, 1997

Carper, Jean. *The Food Pharmacy*. Bantam Books, 1988

Carper, Jean. *Food- Your Miracle Medicine*. Harper Collins, 1993

A Basic Guide to Detoxification

Larson, Joan Mathews, Ph.D. *Seven Weeks To Sobriety*. 1992

Jensen, Bernard, D.C. *Tissue Cleansing Through Bowel Management*. 1981

Cassata, Carla. "How To Balance Body Chemistry." Let's Live. March 1995

Schechter, Steven, N.D. *Fighting Radiation & Chemical Pollutants with Foods, Herbs & Vitamins -Documented Natural Remedies that Boost Your Immunity & Detoxify*. 1994

Baker, Elizabeth & Dr. Elton. *The Uncook Book - Raw Food Adventures To A New Health High*. 1983

Benninger, Jon. "Detox."The Energy Times. July 1994

Thomson, Bill. "Rejuvenate Yourself in Three Weeks." Natural Health. January 1993

Langer, Stephen, M.D. "Keeping Environmental Toxins At Bay,"Better Nutrition For Today's Living. July 1993

Hobbs, Christopher. "Tonics, Bitters, Digestion, and Elimination." Let's Live. August 1990

Easterling, John. "Rainforest Bio-Energetics."Healthy & Natural Journal. October 1994

Rogers, Sherry A., M.D. "Doctors' Dialogue - Toxic Encephalopathy."Let's Live. March 1995

Hobbs, Christopher. *"Herbs For Health - Losing Addictions Naturally."*Let's Live. April 1993

Murray, Michael, N.D. and Joseph Pizzorno, N.D. *Encyclopedia of Natural Medicine*. Prima Publishing, 1998

"Nutrients and Herbs for the Recovering Addict."Health World. July 1992

Duncan, Lindsey, C.N. "Internal Detoxification."Healthy & Natural Journal. October 1994

Blauer, Stephen. *Rejuvenation*. 1980

Airola, Paavo, Ph.D. *How To Get Well*. 1974

Walker, Norman, D.SC., Ph. D. *Colon Health*. 1979

Goldberg, Burton. "Detoxification Therapy."Alternative Medicine - The Definitive Guide. 1993

Lewallen, Eleanor and John. *Sea Vegetable Gourmet Cookbook & Wildcrafter's Guild*. 1996

Markowitz, Elysa. *Living With Green Power - A Gourmet Collection of Living Food Recipes*.1997

Kennedy, David C. DDS, June, 18, 1998 Letter & Paper (Addressing Fluoride's Relationship to Dental Fluorosis, Hip Fracture, Cancer, & Tooth Decay Costs Savings).

Gates, Donna. *The Body Ecology Diet*. 1996

Haas, Elson M., M.D. *The Detox Diet*. 1996

Harrison, Lewis. *30 - Day Body Purification. How To Cleanse Your Inner Body & Experience the Joys of Toxin-Free Health*. 1995

Anderson, Dr. Richard, N.D., N.M.D. *Cleanse & Purify Thyself*. 1994

Walker, N.W. D. Sci. *Raw Vegetable Juices*. Jove Books. 1987

Healing Programs for People with Special Needs

"Are germs killing your sperm?' Men's Health. March, 1999

Lee, John. R., M.D. The John R. Lee M.D. Medical Letter. July 1999

"An E-asy Answer To Infertility Problems." Natural Foods Merchandise. March 1998

Morien, Krista,"Herbs in the News: Results Of Fertility Study Unfruitful." Herb Research Foundation Vol.3, No 1

"Tea for Two." Men's Health, Dec. 1998

"Massage Delivers Babies." Natural Health, Nov/Dec 1998

"True Life Story of the Effect of Aspartame on the Unborn Child." Leading Edge Research, 1996

Murray, Michael T., N.D. "Evaluating Magnesium." American Journal of Natural Medicine. Dec. 1996

White, Linda, M.D. "Can You Take Herbs During Pregnancy?" Delicious! May 1997

Mars, Brigitte, " Herbs To Know About During Pregnancy." Let's Live. Feb. 1991

Lee, John, M.D. "Getting Pregnant and Staying Pregnant." The John R. Lee M.D. Medical Letter, Sept. 1998

"Good News on SIDS." Time. June 22, 1998

Zand, Janet , LAc, OMD, et al. *Smart Medicine For a Healthier Child*. 1994

Denda, Margare E. & Phyllis S. Williams. *The Natural Baby Food Cookbook*. 1982

"Children's Dietary Needs Go Unmet." Nutrition Science News. February 1998

"Brain Function Harmed." Allergy Hotline. Nov 1998

"Pesticides Residues: Cause For Concern." Health News. April 15, 1999

"Nature's Medicine." Nutrition News 1996, Vol XX, No. 12

King, Frank, Jr. Ph.D. "Homeopathic Answers for Vaccination." Healthy & Natural Journal ,Vol. 6, Issue 4.

Wigmore, Ann. Recipes for Longer Life. 1978

Bauman, Edward, Ph.D. *Eating For Health - A Regenerative Five Food Group System*. 1994

Tunella, Kim, C.D.C. "Enzymes...The Spark of Life." 1994

Howell, Dr. Edward. *Enzyme Nutrition - The Food Enzyme Concept*. 1985

Peiper, Howard & Nina Anderson. *Over 50 Looking 30!* 1996

Murray, Michael T., N.D. *The Healing Power of Foods*. 1993

Jones, Susan Smith. *The Main Ingredients of Health & Happiness*. 1995

Murray, Michael T., N.D. *Healing Power of Herbs*. 1992

Fontaine, Darryl & David Minard. *Forever Young - How To Energize Your Body Naturally*. 1993

Murray, Michael T., N.D. *The Complete Book of Juicing*. 1992

Passwater, Richard A., Ph.D. *The New Super Nutrition*. 1991

Hoffman, Dr. Jay M. Hunza - *15 Secrets of the World's Healthiest & Oldest Living People*. 1979

Hobbs, Christopher. *Ginkgo - Elixir of Youth*. 1995

Batmanghelidj, F. , M.D. *Your Body's Many Cries for Water*. 1996

Kugler, Hans, Ph. D. "Interview." Nutrition & Healing. 1995

Samuels, Mike, M.D. & Nancy Samuels. *The Well Adult.* 1988

Brown, Donald J., N.D. *Herbal Prescriptions for Better Health.* 1995

Loehr, Dr. James E. & Dr. Jeffrey A. Migdow. *Take A Deep Breath.* 1986

Siegel, Bernie, M.D. *How To Live Between Office Visits.* 1993

Dossey, Larry, M.D. *Healing Words.* 1993

Borysenko, Joan & Miroslav. *The Power of the Mind to Heal - Renewing Body, Mind & Spirit.* 1994

Pizzorno, Lara. "Longevity." Delicious! May 1994

"Does Sugar Make You Old Before Your Time?" Natural Health. Jan/Feb 1993

Province, MA, et al: The effect of exercise on falls in elderly patients. A preplanned meta-analysis of the FICSIT trials. JAMA 273: 1341-7, 1995

Barela, Sharon. "The Secrets of Longevity." Veggie Life 1997

Walford, Roy L. Calorie Restriction: Eat Less, Eat Better, Live Longer." Life Extension. Feb 1998

"Healthy Eating After 70." Health News. 1999

"Nutrition Supplement- Vitamins, Minerals, and More." Herbs for Health Sept/Oct. 1999

"Improve Energy Fight Aging with Alpha Lipoic Acid." Herbs for Health Sept./Oct. 1999

"Vitamin E in the Golden Years." Vegetarian Times Oct. 1997

Khalsa, Siri. "Beat the Clock." Nutrition News. Vol XX1, 1997

Kervran, Louis Ph.D."Silica-Secret To Longevity." Flora Herbal Medicine Research Report. Winter 1998, Vol. 1, No. 1.

"Health News: Thanks for the Memories, Lecithin!" Natural Health. Sept/Oct 1995

Kidd, Parris M., Ph.D. Phosphatidylserine offers nutritional support for brain function. Vitamin Retailer Magazine, Jan 1996

Shuman, Jill M., M.S., R.D. "Healthful Aging." NFM's Nutrition Science News April 1996

"Cat's Claw." The Healthy Cell News. Fall/Winter 1997

Khalsa, Siri, "Cat's Claw: The Claw of the Jungle." Nutrition News. 1996

"Walking reduces women's heart attack risk." cnn.com Aug. 15, 1999

Fitzgerald, Frances, "Working On Muscles Without Bulking Up." Health Counselor. Vol. 9, No. 1

"Let's Get Physical," Whole Foods, Feb. 1998

Burke, Edmund R., Ph.D. "What To Do When Exercise Is Through." Nutrition Science News. May 1999

"Protection Against Dirty Air." Men's Health Dec. 1998

"Vitamin E Prevents Muscle Damage After Weight Lifting." Quarterly Review of Natural Medicine Summer, 1998

Colgan, Dr. Michael. *Optimum Sports Nutrition.* 1993

Phillips, Bill. Supplement Review. 1996 (Athletes & Bodybuilders)

Burgstiner, Carson B., M.D. "You Are What You Eat." Health Counselor. 1991

Hobbs, Christopher. "Herbs For Fitness."Let's Live. 1991

Peiper, Howard & Nina Anderson. *Are You Poisoning Your Pets?* 1995

Pitcairn, Richard H., D.V.M., Ph.D. & Susan H. Pitcairn *Natural Health for Dogs & Cats.* 1995

Stein, Diane. *Natural Healing for Dogs & Cats.* 1993

"Learn2 Take a Pulse," Learn2.com

Orey, Cal, "Top Dog- Good Nutrition for Healthy Pets." Let's Live Nov. 1997

"Fat Cats and Big Dogs," Vegetarian Times. Jan 1999

Krastek, Caroline."Pet Power." Whole Foods. March 1998

Anderson, Nina and Howard Peiper, Ph.D. "Essential Fatty Acids Important To Pets." Healthy & Natural Journal. Volume 4, Issue 6

Anderson, Nina and Howard Peiper, Ph.D., "Bad Scraps, Vegetarian Pets, and Ringworm." Healthy & Natural Journal. Vol. 4, Issue 5

"The Natural Way To Take Care of Your Pet." Whole Foods. April 1995

Aillment Analysis and Procedures

"Patients Taking Cholesterol Drugs May Need Extra Co-enzyme Q." NFM's Nutrition Science News, March 1996

"The Dangers of Cholesterol-Lowering Drugs." Dr. Julian Whitaker's Health & Healing. Sept. 1998

"Food for Thought: The Role of Triglycerides," Science News Online, Sept. 21, 1996

"Low Cholesterol Can Be Too Low." Alternative Medicine. July 1999

"The Truth About Cholesterol." First For Women, 7/28/97

"The New Cholesterol Tests." American Health. Sept. 1999

The $35.00 Blood Panel: A Guide For Patients

"The Non-Invasive Heart Center: Angiograms," www.heartprotect.com

"Health Bulletin: Heart Stopping Cell Phones." Men's Health. Nov. 1997

Anton, Rein, M.D., Ph.D. "Reversing Heart Disease Through Oral Chelation."

"For patients- What is a Pacemaker?" www.ccspace.com/PAT/patinf.html

"Too Many Bypasses." Men's Health. March 1998

"Quiz: Are You Depressed?" Depression.com

Lohn, Martiga, "The Bowl Turn." Natural Health. April 1999

Golin, Mark. "Morning Forecast - A 14 Point Health Checklist." Men's Health. July 1995

Stein, Diane. *The Natural Remedy Book For Women.* 1995

Gottlieb, Bill (Editor-in-Chief Prevention Magazine Health Books). *New Choices in Natural Healing - Over 1,800 of the Best Self-Help Remedies from the World of Alternative Medicine.* 1995

Medline (The Physician's National Medical Research Database). Physical Conditions Affected By A Deficiency Of The Metabolic Catalysts. Hawaii Medical Library, Inc.

Herbal Research Publications. *The Protocol Journal Of Botanical Medicine.* 1995

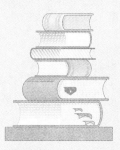

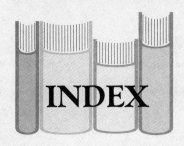

INDEX

D

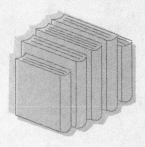

COOKING FOR HEALTHY HEALING

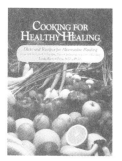

by Linda Page, N.D., Ph.D.   Diets & Recipes For Alternative Healing

The foods we eat change not only our weight but our mood, the texture and look of our bodies, our outlook on life—indeed, the entire universe for us (and consequently, our future). This companion to *Healthy Healing* addresses today's need for food that's healthy, quick to prepare, and delicious. The 900 plus recipes come from the Rainbow Kitchen and the more defined, lifestyle diets Linda has since developed from healing results. The food therapy sections of the book include 33 cleansing, rebuilding and maintenance diets and recipe programs that can be tailored to individual needs. Everything is cross-referenced in three indexes so that diet and menu can be expanded as health improves, and the foods and recipes for other conditions can be included.

HOW TO BE YOUR OWN HERBAL PHARMACIST

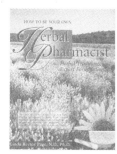

by Linda Page, N.D., Ph.D.   Herbal Traditions - Expert Formulations

There are plenty of books on the market that describe the benefits of specific herbs, but few, if any, show how to combine herbs to address all aspects of specific ailments. This fascinating reference features a "materia medica" on each herb including primary and secondary applications, various part uses, and contraindications; work pages with several herb choices to aid the body in healing itself; examples of how to combine herbs in an effective formula; and suggestions on administering the formula. New to this edition are updated herbal recommendations; an expanded index with more cross referencing; a section about herbal cosmetics; information on using herbal remedies vs. drugs; growing pesticide-free herbs and companion planting; and remedies for children and pets.

DETOXIFICATION

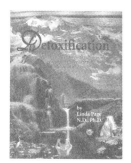

by Linda Page, N.D., Ph.D.   All You Need to Know to Recharge, Renew
                                    and Rejuvenate Your Body, Mind and Spirit

More than 25 thousand new toxins enter our environment each year. Detoxification and body cleansing is a necessary commitment ~ a way of life ~ for good health. In this complete encyclopedia-guide of detailed instructions for detoxification and cleansing, Dr. Page discusses why body cleansing is necessary in today's world. She shows you: what you can expect when you detox; what a good cleanse really does; how to direct a cleanse for best results. Also included: detailed detox charts for special needs; step by step instructions that guide the reader through every detox program; extensive "Green Cuisine" recipe section; Materia Medica - detox herbal supplement directory with over 90 herbs; Glossary of detox terms; list of detox-spa centers in America; recommended product listing; and more.

STRESS & ENERGY

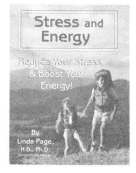

by Linda Page, N.D., Ph.D.   Reduce Your Stress & Boost Your Energy!

From Dr. Page's "Anti-Stress Diet" — to special herbal formulas — to mind/body exercises, the solution to stress is a program, not a pill! Dr. Linda Page presents the very latest in stress reduction techinques and healing programs to help you strengthen your body's ability to adapt to stress. Also included is a special section on stress related diseases like depression, arthritis and heart disease with specific healing programs.

PLEASE TURN PAGE FOR A COMPLETE LIST OF BOOKS BY LINDA PAGE, N.D., PH.D.

Healthy Healing Publications
Books

(Book availability and prices subject to change.)

HEALTHY HEALING - *Eleventh Edition, A Guide to Self Healing for Everyone* - by Dr. Linda Page, N.D., Ph.D. - A 576 page alternative healing reference used by professors, students, health care professionals and private individuals. $32.95 - ISBN 1-884334-89-X
• New - Spiral bound version! $34.95 - ISBN - 1-884334-88-1

COOKING FOR HEALTHY HEALING - *Diets and Recipes for Alternative Healing* - by Dr. Linda Page, N.D., Ph.D. - Over 900 recipes and 33 separate diet and healing programs. 698 pages $29.95 - ISBN 1-884334-56-3

HOW TO BE YOUR OWN HERBAL PHARMACIST - *Herbal Traditions, Expert Formulations* - by Dr. Linda Page, N.D., Ph.D. A complete reference guide for herbal formulations and preparations. 256 pages $18.95 - ISBN 1-884334-78-4

DETOXIFICATION - *All You Need to Know to Recharge, Renew and Rejuvenate Your Body, Mind and Spirit!* - by Dr. Linda Page, N.D., Ph.D. A complete encyclopedia-guide of detailed instructions for detoxification and cleansing. 264 pages $19.95 - ISBN 1-884334-54-7

PARTY LIGHTS - *Healthy Party Foods & Earthwise Entertaining* - by Dr. Linda Page. N.D., Ph.D., and Doug Vanderberg - A party reference book with over 70 parties and more than 500 original recipes you can prepare at home. 358 pages $19.95 - ISBN 1-884334-53-9

THE BODY SMART SYSTEM - *The Complete Guide to Cleansing & Rejuvenation* - by Helene Silver - A complete 21 day regimen and guide that includes diet, relaxation techniques, massage and bath, exercise programs and recipes. 242 pages $19.95 - ISBN 1-884334-60-1

NEW! VHS "UNLEASHING THE HEALING POWER OF HERBS" - Dr. Page presents information about herbs in this beautifully produced, educational, hour long video program. $19.95 ISBN 1-884334-95-4

NEW EXPANDED LIBRARY SERIES
by Dr. Linda Page, N.D., Ph.D.   ISBN - 1884334 -

36-9 **CANCER 96 pages - $8.95**

14-8 **FATIGUE SYNDROMES 46 pages - $3.95**

64-4 **RENEWING FEMALE BALANCE 48 pages - $4.50**

90-3 **MENOPAUSE & OSTEOPOROSIS 64 pages - $5.95**

15-6 **SEXUALITY 96 pages - $8.95**

66-0 **WEIGHT LOSS** & Cellulite Control **96 pages - $8.95**

67-9 **STRESS & ENERGY** Larger Format **96 pages - $9.95**

THE HEALTHY HEALING LIBRARY SERIES
by Dr. Linda Page, N.D., Ph.D.
32 pages, $3.50 each. ISBN - 1884334 -

35-0 **ALLERGY CONTROL & MANAGEMENT**
13-X **REVEALING THE SECRETS OF ANTI-AGING**
27-X **DO YOU WANT TO HAVE A BABY?**
47-4 **COLDS, FLU & YOU** - Building Optimum Immunity
49-0 **DETOXIFICATION & BODY CLEANSING**
34-2 **BOOSTING IMMUNITY WITH POWER PLANTS**
29-6 **FIGHTING INFECTIONS WITH HERBS**
30-X **RENEWING MALE HEALTH & ENERGY**

Continental U.S. shipping info: $4.50 each for books, $1.00 each for Library Series Booklets.

NAME_____ADDRESS_____

CITY_____ STATE_____ZIP_____PHONE_____

☐ Check (Make payable to Healthy Healing)   ☐ Visa   ☐ Mastercard   ☐ American Express   ☐ Discover

CARD #_____EXP. DATE_____SIGNATURE_____

QTY.	BOOK	PRICE	SHIPPING	TOTAL
	CA Residents add 7.25% tax			

Mail to: Healthy Healing Publications, P.O. Box 436, Carmel Valley, CA 93924
Or, fax your order to: 831-659-4044. Or, Call **1-888-447-2939.**
Or order on-line @ www.healthyhealing.com.

TOTAL _____

Code: HH11 - 1.2000

Contents

Practical
Bookkeeping

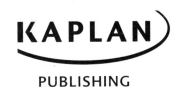

KAPLAN

PUBLISHING

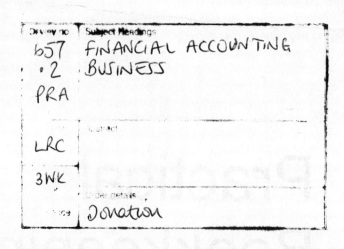
British library cataloguing-in-publication data

A atalgue reord for this bok is available from the British Library.

Published by:
Kaplan Publishing UK
Unit 2 The Business Centre
Molly Millars Lane
Wokingham
Berkshire
RG41 2QZ

ISBN 978-1-84710-714-5

© Kaplan Financial Limited, 2008

Edition 1 published February 2008, amended September 2008

Printed in the UK by CPI William Clowes Beccles NR34 7TL

To help you find your way through the material you will find useful icons throughout each chapter:

Definition	🔍	Key definitions that you will need to learn from the core content.
Key exam points	🔑	Identifies topics that are key to success and are often examined.
Tricky topic	⚠️	When reviewing these areas care should be taken and all illustrations and test your understanding exercises should be completed to ensure that the topic is understood.
Expandable text	📖	Expandable text provides you with additional information about a topic area and may help you gain a better understanding of the core content. Essential text users can access this additional content on-line (read it where you need further guidance or skip over when you are happy with a topic).
Illustration	e.g	Worked examples help you understand the core content better.
Test your understanding	🚀	Exercises for you to complete to ensure that you have understood the topics just learned.

Double entry bookkeeping – introduction

Introduction

This chapter introduces the basic concepts and rules of bookkeeping. In particular, we study:

- the dual effect principle
- the separate entity principle, and
- the accounting equation.

Together these will show how the assets of a business will always equal its liabilities and pave the way for studying double entry bookkeeping in the next chapter.

1 Types of accounting

1.1 Management accounting and financial accounting

Depending on why the accounts are being produced, we can describe them as being either management accounts or financial accounts.

Financial accounts

These are prepared annually, mainly for the benefit of people outside the management of the business, such as the owners of the business, HM Revenue and Customs, banks, customers, suppliers and government.

In this text we focus on financial accounting principles, though most of the ideas would also apply to management accounting.

Management accounts

These are usually prepared on a monthly basis to enable the managers to run the business effectively.

1.2 The two main financial statements

The objective of financial accounting is to provide financial information about a business. This information is given in a set of financial statements (or accounts), which consists of two principal statements.

- The profit and loss account. This is a summary of the business's transactions for a given period.

- The balance sheet. This is a statement of the financial position of the business at a given date (usually the end of the period covered by the profit and loss account).

These financial statements are the final product of the accounting system of a business and it is useful to be aware of where all of the double entry bookkeeping that you will study in this chapter is leading. However, you do not need to know anything about the format or rules governing the preparation of the financial statements.

1.3 Definitions

- An **asset** is something owned by a business, available for use in the business.

- **Fixed asset** – an asset which is to be used for the long term in the business and not resold as part of the trading activities.

- **Current asset** – a short-term asset of the business which is to be used in the business in the near future.

- A **debtor** is an example of a current asset. A debtor is someone who owes the business money.

- A **liability** is an amount owed by the business, i.e. an obligation to pay money at some future date.

- A **creditor** is an example of a liability. A creditor is someone the business owes money to.

- **Capital** is the amount which the owner has invested in the business; this is owed back to the owner and is therefore a special liability of the business.

2 Basic principles of double entry bookkeeping

2.1 Introduction

Double entry bookkeeping is based upon three basic principles:

- the dual effect principle
- the separate entity principle
- the accounting equation.

2.2 The dual effect principle

This states that every transaction has two financial effects.

(a) For example, if you spend £2,000 on a car and pay for it by a cheque, one effect is that you have £2,000 less money in the bank, the second effect is that you have acquired an asset worth £2,000.

(b) Again, if you owe a creditor £100 and send him a cheque for that amount, one effect is that you owe £100 less than before, the second effect is that you have £100 less money in the bank.

2.3 The separate entity principle

This states that the owner of a business is, for accounting purposes, a completely separate entity from the business itself. Therefore the money that the owner pays into the business as initial capital has to be accounted for as an amount that the business owes back to the owner. In just the same way, any money that the owner takes out of the business, known as drawings, is treated as a reduction of the initial capital that is owed back to the owner.

The dual effect principle works here as well. If the owner of the business pays £5,000 into his business, one effect is that the business has £5,000 more cash and the second effect is that the business has a £5,000 liability (called 'capital').

Note that we look at this from the point of view of the business, not from the owner's point of view. This is because when studying bookkeeping we are only interested in the business - we are not considering the owner's personal finances.

2.4 The accounting equation

At its simplest, the accounting equation simply says that:

Assets = Liabilities

If we treat the owner's capital as a special form of liability then the accounting equation is:

Assets = Liabilities + Capital

Or, rearranging:

Assets – Liabilities = Capital

Profit will increase the proprietor's capital and drawings will reduce it, so that we can write the equation as:

Assets – Liabilities = Capital + Profit – Drawings

3 The accounting equation: examples

Illustration 1 – The accounting equation

John starts his business on 1 July and pays £2,000 into his business bank account.

(a) What is the dual effect of this transaction?

(b) What is the accounting equation after this transaction?

Solution

(a) The dual effect

The business bank account has increased by £2,000 (an asset). The business capital has increased by £2,000 (a liability).

(b) The accounting equation
Assets   – Liabilities = Capital
£2,000 – £0   = £2,000

Illustration 2 – The accounting equation

Percy started business on 1 January by paying £20,000 into a business bank account. He then spent £500 on a secondhand van by cheque, £1,000 on purchases of stock for cash, took £500 cash for his own use and bought goods on credit costing £400.

What are the two effects of each of these transactions?

What would the accounting equation look like after each of these transactions?

Solution

(a) Percy pays £20,000 into a business bank account

The bank balance increases from zero to £20,000 (an asset)

and the business now has capital of £20,000 (a liability); capital is the amount that is owed back to the owner of the business, Percy.

Accounting equation:
Assets – Liabilities   =   Capital
£20,000 – £0   =   £20,000

(b) Percy buys a secondhand van for £500 by cheque

The bank balance decreases by £500 (a reduction of assets) but the business has acquired a new £500 asset, the van.

The van is a specific type of asset known as a fixed asset as it is for long-term use in the business rather than an asset that is likely to be sold in the trading activities of the business.

The assets of the business are now:

	£
Van	500
Bank (20,000 – 500)	19,500
	20,000

The liabilities and capital are unchanged.

Accounting equation:
Assets – Liabilities   =   Capital
£20,000 – £0   =   £20,000

(c) Percy spends £1,000 on purchases of goods for cash

The bank balance goes down by £1,000 but the business has another asset, stock of £1,000.

Stock is a short-term asset as it is due to be sold to customers in the near future and is known as a current asset.

The assets of the business are now:

	£
Van	500
Stock	1,000
Bank (19,500 – 1,000)	18,500
	20,000

Accounting equation:
Assets – Liabilities   =   Capital
£20,000 – £0   =   £20,000

(d) Percy took £500 of cash out of the business

The bank balance has decreased by £500 and capital has also decreased as the owner has taken money out of the business – this is known as drawings.

Remember that the owner is a completely separate entity from the business itself and if he takes money out of the business in the form of drawings then this means that the business owes him less.

The assets of the business are now:

	£
Van	500
Stock	1,000
Bank (18,500 – 500)	18,000
	19,500

The capital of the business is now £(20,000 – 500) = £19,500.

Accounting equation:

Assets – Liabilities	=	Capital
£19,500 –– £0		£19,500

(e) Purchased goods on credit for £400

The asset of stock increases by £400 and the business now has a liability of £400, the amount that is owed to the credit supplier. A liability is an amount that is owed by the business.

The assets of the business are now:

	£
Van	500
Stock (1,000 + 400)	1,400
Bank	18,000
	19,900

The liability of the business is £400.

The capital is unchanged.

Accounting equation:

Assets – Liabilities	=	Capital
£19,900 – £400	=	£19,500

General notes

1 Each and every transaction that a business undertakes has two effects. The accounting equation reflects the two effects of each transaction and the accounting equation should always balance.

2 The owner is a completely separate entity from the business, any money the owner puts into the business is known as capital and any amounts taken out by the owner are known as drawings.

Test your understanding 1

State whether each of the following are assets or liabilities:

(i) Money in the business bank account

(ii) A creditor

(iii) Stock of goods for resale

(iv) A computer used in the accounts department

(v) A debtor

(vi) A salesman's car

Test your understanding 2

A worked example

1 Introduce capital

Example 1

You win £10,000 and use it to create a retail business (called TLC) selling hearts and roses. What is the effect?

Answer 1

Dual effect

The business has cash of	£10,000	(asset)
The business owes you	£10,000	(capital)

TLC's position is:

Assets	Capital
£	£

(In this first example, we recorded the dual effect for you just to get you started. In later examples you will need to enter the dual effect yourself, as well as TLC's position after the transaction.)

2 Buy stock with cash

Example 2

TLC buys 500 chocolate hearts. The cost of each heart is £5. What is the effect?

Answer 2

Dual effect

TLC's position is:

Assets	Capital
£	£

3 Buy stock on credit

In reality a business will not always pay for its purchases with cash but is more likely to buy items on credit.

Example 3

TLC buys stock of 200 red roses on credit. Each red rose costs £10. What is the effect?

Answer 3

Dual effect

TLC's position is:

Net assets	Capital
£	£

4 Buy a delivery van

The delivery van is bought for ongoing use within the business rather than for resale. Such assets are known as fixed assets.

Example 4

TLC buys a delivery van for £1,000 cash. What is the effect?

Answer 4

Dual effect

TLC's position is:

Net assets	Capital
£	£

5 Sell stock for profit

Example 5

TLC sells 200 red roses for £15 cash each. What is the effect?

Answer 5

Dual effect

TLC's position is:

Net assets	Capital
£	£

6 Sell stock (on credit) for profit

It is equally likely that a business will sell goods on credit. When goods are sold on credit, an asset of the business called a debtor is generated.

Example 6

TLC sells 400 chocolate hearts to Valentino for £12.50 each on credit. What is the effect?

Answer 6

Dual effect

TLC's position is:

	Net assets £	Capital £

7 Pay expenses

Example 7

In reality, TLC will have been incurring expenses from its commencement. TLC received and paid a gas bill for £500. What is the effect?

Answer 7

Dual effect

TLC's position is:

	Net assets £	Capital £

8 Take out a loan

In order to fund your future expansion plans for TLC, you persuade your Aunt to lend TLC £2,000.

Example 8

TLC is lent £2,000 cash by your Aunt. She expects to be repaid in two years' time. What is the effect?

Answer 8

Dual effect

TLC's position is:

	Net assets	Capital
	£	£

9 **Payment to creditors for purchases**

Example 9

TLC pays cash of £1,500 towards the £2,000 owed to the supplier. What is the effect?

Answer 9

Dual effect

TLC's position is:

	Net assets	Capital
	£	£

10 **Receive cash from debtors**

Example 10

TLC's debtor sends a cheque for £3,000. What is the effect?

Answer 10

Dual effect

TLC's position is:

	Net assets	Capital
	£	£

11 **Drawings**

Example 11

You withdraw £750 from the business. Such a withdrawal

is merely a repayment of the capital you introduced. Your withdrawal is called drawings. What is the effect?

Answer 11

Dual effect

TLC's position is:

	Net assets	Capital
	£	£

Test your understanding 3

1   What is an asset?

2   What is a liability?

3   Why is the owner's capital a liability?

4   Write down the accounting equation when the owner of a business introduces £10,000 capital.

5   Write down the accounting equation for the same business when it buys a van for £1,000.

4   Summary

You must understand the basic definitions covered in this chapter. You must also understand the principles of dual effect and separate entity. The accounting equation underlies the whole of bookkeeping and you should re-work the examples in this chapter if you do not fully understand how it works.

Test your understanding answers

Test your understanding 1

(i) Asset

(ii) Liability

(iii) Asset

(iv) Asset

(v) Asset

(vi) Asset

Test your understanding 2

1

	Assets £		Capital £
Cash	10,000	Capital introduced	10,000

2 Dual effect

Increase stock	£2,500	(↑ asset)
Decrease cash	£2,500	(↓ asset)

	Assets £		Capital £
Stock	2,500	Capital introduced	10,000
Cash	7,500		
	10,000		10,000

3 Dual effect

Increase stock	£2,000	(↑ asset)
Increase creditor	£2,000	(↑ liability)

	Net assets £		Capital £
Stock	4,500	Capital introduced	10,000
Cash	7,500		
	12,000		
Less: Creditors	(2,000)		
	10,000		10,000

4 Dual effect

Increase fixed asset	£1,000	(↑ asset)
Decrease cash	£1,000	(↓ asset)

KAPLAN PUBLISHING

	Net assets £		Capital £
Fixed asset	1,000	Capital introduced	10,000
Stock	4,500		
Cash	6,500		
	12,000		
Less: Creditors	(2,000)		
	10,000		10,000

5   Dual effect

Increase cash	£3,000	(↑ asset)
Decrease stock	£2,000	(↓ asset)
Increase profit	£1,000	(↑profit)

	Net assets £		Capital £
Fixed asset	1,000	Capital introduced	10,000
Stock	2,500	Profit	1,000
Cash	9,500		
	13,000		
Less: Creditors	(2,000)		
	11,000		11,000

6   Dual effect

Increase debtors	£5,000	(↑ asset)
Decrease stock	£2,000	(↓ asset)
Increase profit	£3,000	(↑ profit)

	Net assets £		Capital £
Fixed asset	1,000	Capital introduced	10,000
Stock	500	Profit	4,000
Debtors	5,000		
Cash	9,500		
	16,000		
Less: Creditors	(2,000)		
	14,000		14,000

7   Dual effect

Decrease cash	£500	(↓ asset)
Decrease profit	£500	(↓ profit)

	Net assets £		Capital £
Fixed asset	1,000	Capital introduced	10,000
Stock	500	Profit	3,500
Debtors	5,000		
Cash	9,000		
	15,500		
Less: Creditors	(2,000)		
	13,500		13,500

8 Dual effect

Increase cash	£2,000	(↑ asset)
Increase creditors	£2,000	(↑ liability)

	Net assets £		*Capital* £
Fixed asset	1,000	Capital introduced	10,000
Stock	500	Profit	3,500
Debtors	5,000		
Cash	11,000		
	17,500		
Less: Creditors	(2,000)		
Loan	(2,000)		
	13,500		13,500

The loan will be shown separately from creditors for purchases, which are known as trade creditors.

9 Dual effect

Decrease cash	£1,500	(↓ asset)
Decrease creditors	£1,500	(↓ liability)

	Net assets £		Capital £
Fixed asset	1,000	Capital introduced	10,000
Stock	500	Profit	3,500
Debtors	5,000		
Cash	9,500		
	16,000		
Less: Creditors	(500)		
Loan	(2,000)		
	13,500		13,500

10 Dual effect

Decrease debtors	£3,000	(↓ asset)
Increase cash	£3,000	(↑ asset)

KAPLAN PUBLISHING

	Net assets £	Capital £
Fixed asset	1,000	Capital introduced	10,000
Stock	500	Profit	3,500
Debtors	2,000		
Cash	12,500		
	16,000		
Less: Creditors	(500)		
Loan	(2,000)		
	13,500		13,500

11 Dual effect

Decrease cash	£750	(↓ asset)
Decrease capital	£750	(↓ capital)

	Net assets £	Capital £
Fixed asset	1,000	Capital introduced	10,000
Stock	500	Profit	3,500
Debtors	2,000		
Cash	11,750		
	15,250		13,500
Less: Creditors	(500)	Less: Drawings	(750)
Loan	(2,000)		
	12,750		12,750

We do not simply deduct drawings from profit as we want to show separately the profit or loss for the period before any drawings were made.

Test your understanding 3

1   An asset is something owned by the business.

2   A liability is something owed by the business.

3   The owner's capital is a liability of the business because it represents money/assets that are owed to the owner.

4	Assets		=	Capital	
	Cash	£10,000		Capital	£10,000

5	Assets		=	Capital	
	Van	£1,000		Capital	£10,000
	Cash	£9,000			
		£10,000			£10,000

Ledger accounting

Introduction

Now that we have looked at the basic theory of bookkeeping, it is time to learn and practise how to make the correct double entries for transactions.

We shall start with accounting for cash transactions, and will study a series of the different sorts of things that a business can buy or sell (or pay for or receive) in cash.

We shall then study how to deal with purchases and sales made for credit.

1 Ledger accounts

1.1 Introduction

In practice it would be far too time consuming to write up the accounting equation each time that the business undertook a transaction. Instead the two effects of each transaction are recorded in ledger accounts.

1.2 The ledger account

A typical ledger account is shown below:

Title of account

DEBIT				CREDIT			
Date	Details	Folio	Amount £	Date	Details	Folio	Amount £

It is often called a 'T' account.

The important point to note is that it has two sides. The left hand side is known as the debit side and the right hand side is known as the credit side.

- The date column contains the date of the transaction.

- The details column contains the title of the other account that holds the second part of the dual effect. It may also have a brief description of the nature of the entry (e.g. 'rent 1.1.X3 to 31.3.X3').

- The folio column contains a reference to the source of the information. We shall see some of these sources later on but it could be, for example, 'sales day book p17' or 'payroll month 6'.

- The amount column simply contains the value of the transaction.

- The title of the account is a name that reflects the nature of the transaction ('van account', 'bank account', 'electricity account', etc).

1.3 Simplified account

The ledger account in 1.2 is very detailed and in much of this book we use a simpler form of the account. Part of the reason for this is that it is easier to 'see' the entries being made if there is less detail in the accounts. Thus, we sometimes do without the date or the full description or folio to keep things clear and simple.

For example, we will often use accounts which look like this:

Bank account

	£		£
		Van	500

Van account

	£		£
Bank	500		

It is simple and clearly shows the two sides of the account and the entries that have been made.

1.4 The golden rule for making entries in the ledger accounts

There is a golden rule for making entries in ledger accounts.

Every debit entry must have an equal and opposite credit entry.

This reflects the dual effect of each transaction and causes the accounting equation to always balance.

It is also why we refer to double entry bookkeeping.

1.5 What goes on the debit or credit side?

Step 1

If John pays £2,000 into his business bank account as capital, how do we know on what side of the accounts we should enter the amount. For example, does the payment into the bank go on the debit or credit side of the bank account?

To know this you just have to learn a few simple connected rules.

(a) The bank account

Starting with the bank account, the rule is that:

Money paid into the bank is a debit : Money paid out of the bank is a credit.

All the other rules follow from this.

Thus, if John has paid £2,000 into the bank as capital, this is a debit in the bank account.

(b) The capital account

The other half of the double entry must be a £2,000 credit entry in the capital account.

Bank account

	£		£
Capital	2,000		

Capital account

	£			£
		Bank		2,000

Step 2

If John's business now pays £1,000 out of the bank to buy a van, the double entry will be:

(a) The bank account

Start with the bank account again. Money is paid out so we credit the bank account with £1,000.

(b) The van account

The other half of the transaction must therefore be a debit of £1,000 to the van account.

Bank account

	£		£
Capital	2,000	Van	1,000

Capital account

	£		£
		Bank	2,000

Van account

	£		£
Bank	1,000		

1.6 Which accounts to debit and credit

There are some rules that can help you in finding the correct account to put the debit and credit entries into.

Ledger account

A **debit entry** represents:	A **credit entry** represents:
• money paid into the business bank account	• money paid out of the business bank account
• drawings by the owner	• capital invested by the owner
• an increase in the value of an asset	• a reduction in the value of an asset
• a reduction in the value of a liability, or	• an increase in the value of a liability, or
• an item of expenditure.	• an item of income (revenue).

2 Introducing capital into the business

2.1 Explanation

The owner of a business starts the business by paying money into the business bank account. This is the capital of the business. The business will need this money to 'get going'. It may need to pay rent, buy stock for sale or pay wages to its staff before it has actually sold anything or received any money.

Illustration 1 – Introducing capital into business

Frankie starts a business and pays £5,000 into the business bank account.

What is the double entry for this transaction?

As we have already seen the general rule when dealing with cash transactions is to start with the bank account. Cash paid out of the bank is a credit in the bank account and cash paid into the bank is a debit in the bank account.

Solution

- £5,000 has been paid into the bank account.

  This is therefore a debit in the bank account.

  It represents an asset of the business.

- The business has a liability because it owes Frankie (the owner) £5,000.

  This liability will be a credit in the capital account.

Bank (or cash book)		**Capital**	
Caplital £5,000			Bank £5,000

3 Purchasing goods for resale

3.1 Explanation

A business buys goods for resale to customers – that is how most businesses (eg shops) make their money. These goods are assets which the business owns.

Illustration 2 – Purchasing goods for resale

Frankie buys £300 of chocolate bars for resale. He pays with a cheque to his supplier.

What is the double entry for this transaction?

Solution

- Once again start with the bank account.

  The business has paid £300 out of its bank account.

  Therefore, the £300 will be credited to the bank account.

- The chocolate bars are an asset.

  This asset will be debited to the purchases account.

Purchases		Bank	
Bank £300			Purchases £300

4 Expenditure

4.1 Paying office rent

A business will typically rent office space in order to carry out its operations. It will pay rent to the landlord (owner) of the offices. Rent is an expense of the business.

Illustration 3 – Expenditure

Frankie pays £1,000 per quarter for the rent of his offices. He pays with a cheque to the landlord.

What is the double entry for this transaction?

Solution

- Once again start with the bank account.

  The business has paid £1,000 out of its bank account.

  Therefore, the £1,000 will be credited to the bank account.

- The rent is an expense.

  This expense will be debited to the rent account.

Rent		Bank	
Bank £1,000		Rent £1,000	

4.2 Buying stationery

A business will buy stationery in order to be able to operate. The items of stationery (pens, paper, etc) are not for resale to customers and are used quickly after they are purchased. Stationery is therefore an expense of the business.

Illustration 4 – Expenditure

Frankie pays £200 for items of stationery. He pays with a cheque to the supplier.

What is the double entry for this transaction?

Solution

- Once again start with the bank account.

  The business has paid £200 out of its bank account.

  Therefore, the £200 will be credited to the bank account.

- The stationery is an expense.

  This expense will be debited to the stationery account.

Stationery		Bank	
Bank £200		Stationery £200	

4.3 Buying a computer

A business will buy computers in order to streamline its operations. These computers are not bought with a view to re-sale and are to be used in the business for the long term. They are therefore a fixed asset of the business.

Illustration 5 – Expenditure

Frankie pays £900 to purchase a computer. He pays with a cheque to the supplier.

What is the double entry for this transaction?

Solution

* Once again start with the bank account.

  The business has paid £900 out of its bank account.

  Therefore, the £900 will be credited to the bank account.

* The computer is a fixed asset.

  The £900 will be debited to the fixed asset computer account.

Computer		Bank	
Bank £900			Computer £900

5 Receiving income for services provided

5.1 Receiving income from sales of goods

A business will sell the goods it has purchased for re-sale. This is income for the business and is referred to as 'sales'.

Illustration 6 – Receiving income for services provided

Frankie sells goods for £1,500. The customer pays cash.

What is the double entry for this transaction?

Solution

* Once again start with the bank account.

  The business has received £1,500 into its bank account.

  Therefore, the £1,500 will be debited to the bank account.

* The cash received is income.

  This income will be credited to the sales account.

Sales		Bank	
	Bank £1,500	Sales £1,500	

KAPLAN PUBLISHING

5.2 Receiving income for services provided

A business may provide services to its customers, e.g. it may provide consultancy advice. This is income for the business and will usually be referred to as 'sales'.

Illustration 7 – Receiving income for services provided

Frankie provides consultancy services to a client who pays £2,000 in cash.

What is the double entry for this transaction?

Solution

- Once again start with the bank account.

  The business has received £2,000 into its bank account.

  Therefore, the £2,000 will be debited to the bank account.

- The cash received is income.

  This income will be credited to the sales account.

Sales		Bank	
	Bank £2,000	Sales £2,000	

Illustration 8 – Receiving income for services provided

Percy started business on 1 January and made the following transactions.

1 Paid £20,000 into a business bank account.
2 Spent £500 on a secondhand van.
3 Paid £1,000 on purchases of stock.
4 Took £50 cash for his own use.
5 On 5 January bought goods for cash costing £500.
6 Made sales for cash of £2,000.
7 On 15 January paid £200 of rent.

Task 1

Show how the debit and credit entries for each transaction are determined.

Task 2

Enter the transactions into the relevant ledger accounts.

Solution

Task 1

(1) Capital invested

Percy has paid £20,000 into the bank account – therefore the bank account is debited.

Debit (Dr)   Bank   £20,000

The business now owes the owner £20,000. Capital is the amount owed by the business to its owner – this is a liability, therefore a credit entry in the capital account.

Credit (Cr)   Capital   £20,000

(2) Purchase of van

The business has paid £500 out of the bank account – therefore a credit entry in the cash account.

Cr   Cash   £500

The business now has a van costing £500 – this is an asset therefore a debit entry in the van account. This is a fixed asset of the business.

Dr   Van   £500

(3) Purchase of stock for cash

The business has paid out £1,000 out of the bank account – therefore a credit to the bank account.

Cr   Bank   £1,000

The business has made purchases of stock costing £1,000 – this is an item of expenditure therefore a debit entry in the purchases account. Note that the debit entry is to a purchases account not a stock account. The stock account is a different account altogether and will be considered later in this study text.

Dr   Purchases   £1,000

(4) Drawings

The business has paid £50 out of the bank account – therefore credit the bank account.

Cr   Bank   £50

The proprietor has made drawings of £50 – this is a reduction of capital and therefore a debit entry to the drawings account.

Dr   Drawings   £50

Drawings should not be directly debited to the capital account. A separate drawings account should be used.

(5) Purchase of goods for cash

The business has paid out £500 – therefore credit the bank account.

Cr   Bank   £500

The business has made purchases of stock costing £500 – an expense therefore debit the purchases account.

Dr   Purchases   £500

(6) Sale for cash

The business has paid £2,000 into the bank account – therefore a debit to the bank account.

Dr   Bank   £2,000

The business has made sales of £2,000 – this is income therefore a credit to the sales account.

Cr   Sales   £2,000

(7) Payment of rent

The business now paid £200 out of the bank account – therefore a credit to the bank account.

Cr   Bank   £200

The business has incurred an expense of rent – as an expense item the rent account must be debited.

Dr   Rent   £200

General rule

When dealing with cash transactions think first of all about the cash side.

- Money paid into the business bank account is a debit to the bank account therefore some other account must be credited.
- Money paid out of the business bank account is a credit to the bank account therefore some other account must be debited.

Task 2

Bank

Date			£	Date			£
1 Jan	Capital	(1)	20,000	1 Jan	Van	(2)	500
5 Jan	Sales	(6)	2,000		Purchases	(3)	1,000
					Drawings	(4)	50
				5 Jan	Purchases	(5)	500
				15 Jan	Rent	(7)	200

Capital

Date	£	Date	£
		1 Jan Bank	(1) 20,000

Van

Date	£	Date	£
1 Jan Bank	(2) 500		

Purchases

Date	£	Date	£
1 Jan Bank	(3) 1,000		
5 Jan Bank	(5) 500		

Drawings

Date	£	Date	£
1 Jan Bank	(4) 50		

Sales

Date	£	Date	£
		5 Jan Bank	(6) 2,000

Rent

Date	£	Date	£
15 Jan Bank	(7) 200		

Test your understanding 1

Write up the following cash transactions in the main ledger accounts.

Transaction	Details
1	Set up the business by introducing £150,000 in cash.
2	Purchase property costing £140,000. Pay in cash.
3	Purchase goods costing £5,000. Pay in cash.
4	Sell goods for £7,000. All cash sales.
5	Purchase goods costing £8,000. Pay in cash.
6	Pay a sundry expense of £100, by cheque.
7	Sell goods for £15,000. All cash sales.
8	Pay wages of £2,000 to an employee.
9	Pay postage costs of £100, by cheque.

6   Credit purchases

A **credit purchase** occurs when goods are bought (or a service received) and the customer does not have to pay immediately but can pay after a specified number of days.

Illustration 9 – Credit purchases

We have already seen the double entry for a cash purchase and we shall now contrast this with the double entry for a credit purchase by means of an illustration.

John buys goods from Sam for £2,000.

(a) Record the double entry in John's books if John pays for the goods immediately with a cheque.

(b) Record the double entry in John's books if John buys the goods on credit and pays some time later.

Solution

(a) Cash purchase

The double entry is simply to:

Credit the bank account with £2,000 because £2,000 has been paid out.

Debit the purchases account with £2,000 because goods have been purchased with £2,000.

Bank

	£		£
		Purchases	2,000

Purchases

	£		£
Bank	2,000		

(b) Credit purchase

The double entry will be made at two separate times.

(i)   At the time the purchase is made

At the time the purchase is made we debit £2,000 to the purchases account because a purchase has been made, but we cannot make any entry in the bank account at the time of the purchase because no cash is paid. However, the dual effect principle means that there must be another effect to this transaction, and in this case it is that the business has a creditor (the supplier to whom the £2,000 is owed).

The double entry is:

Debit the purchases account with £2,000 because expenses have increased by £2,000.

Credit creditors account with £2,000 (this is a liability of the business).

Purchases

	£		£
Creditor	2,000		

Creditors

	£		£
		Purchases	2,000

(ii) When John pays the £2,000

The double entry now will be:

Credit the bank account with £2,000 because £2,000 has been paid out.

Debit the creditor account because John has paid and the creditor has been reduced by £2,000.

Creditors

	£		£
Bank	2,000	Purchases	2,000

Purchases

	£		£
Creditor	2,000		

Bank

	£		£
		Creditor	2,000

6.1 Summary

The net effect of the above credit purchase is that the creditor has a nil balance because John has paid, and we are left with a debit in the purchases account and a credit in the cash book. This is exactly as for a cash purchase – we just had to go through the intermediate step of the creditors account to get there.

7 Credit sales

A **credit sale** occurs when goods are sold (or a service provided) and the customer does not have to pay immediately but can pay after a specified number of days.

Illustration 10 – Credit purchases

We have already seen the double entry for a cash sale and we shall now contrast this with the double entry for a credit sale by means of an illustration.

George sells goods to Harry for £1,000.

(a) Record the double entry in George's books if Harry pays for the goods immediately with a cheque.

(b) Record the double entry in George's books if Harry buys the goods on credit and pays some time later.

Solution

(a) Cash sale

The double entry is simply to:

Debit the bank account with £1,000 because £1,000 has been paid in.

Credit the sales account with £1,000 because income has increased by £1,000.

Bank

	£		£
Sales	1,000		

Sales

	£		£
		Bank	1,000

(b) Credit sale

The double entry will be made at two separate times.

(i) At the time the sale is made

At the time the sale is made we credit £1,000 to the sales account because a sale has been made, but we cannot make any entry in the bank account at the time of the sale because no cash is received. However, the dual effect principle means that there must be another effect to this transaction, and in this case it is that the business has acquired a debtor.

The double entry is:

Debit debtors account with £1,000 (this is an asset of the business).

Credit the sales account with £1,000 because income has increased by £1,000.

Debtors

	£		£
Sales	1,000		

Sales

	£		£
		Debtor	1,000

(ii) When Harry pays the £1,000

The double entry now will be:

Debit the bank account with £1,000 because £1,000 has been paid in.

Credit the debtors account because Harry has paid and the debtor has been reduced by £1,000.

Debtors

	£		£
Sales	1,000	Bank	1,000

Sales

	£		£
		Debtor	1,000

Bank

	£		£
Debtor	1,000		

7.1 Summary

The net effect of the above credit sale is that the debtor has a nil balance because Harry has paid and we are left with a credit in the sales account and a debit in the cash book. This is exactly as for a cash sale – we just had to go through the intermediate step of the debtor account to get there.

Test your understanding 2

We shall now revisit our worked example from Chapter 1 and record the transactions with debits and credits to ledger accounts.

Date	Detail
1.1.X5	TLC commenced business with £10,000 introduced by you, the proprietor
2.1.X5	TLC bought stock of 500 chocolate hearts for £2,500 cash
3.1.X5	TLC bought stock of 200 red roses on credit for £2,000
4.1.X5	TLC bought a delivery van for £1,000 cash
5.1.X5	TLC sold all the red roses for £3,000 cash
6.1.X5	TLC sold 400 chocolate hearts for £5,000 on credit
7.1.X5	TLC paid a gas bill for £500 cash
8.1.X5	TLC took out a loan of £2,000
9.1.X5	TLC paid £1,500 to trade creditors
10.1.X5	TLC received £3,000 from debtors
11.1.X5	The proprietor withdrew £750 cash

Record these transactions in the relevant ledger accounts.

Make your entries in the ledger accounts below.

Cash

£	£

Capital

£	£

Purchases

£	£

Creditors

£	£

Delivery van

£	£

Sales

£	£

Debtors

£	£

Gas

£	£

Loan

£	£

Drawings

£	£

Test your understanding 3

1   What is the difference between a cash and a credit transaction?

2   If a business buys goods for cash, is the entry in the bank account a debit or credit?

3   If the business buys a fixed asset for cash, is the entry in the fixed asset account a debit or credit?

4   If the business makes a sale for cash, what is the double entry?

5   If a business provides consultancy services for cash, what will be the entry in the bank account to record this?

6   If cash is paid into the bank account, is this a debit or credit entry in the bank ledger account?

7   Is an asset represented by a debit or credit entry in a ledger account?

8   The owner of a business pays in £1,000 as capital. What is the double entry for this?

9   Is income represented by a debit or credit entry in a ledger account?

8   Summary

In this chapter we have studied cash and credit transactions. It is important to always start with the bank account and remember that cash received is a debit in the bank account and cash paid out is a credit in the bank account. If you get that right then the rest really does fall into place.

You should also be aware of the definitions of assets, expenses and income and the normal entries that you would make in the accounts for these.

Test your understanding answers

Test your understanding 1

The figures in brackets are used here to indicate the transaction number in the activity. They can be used to match the debit entry for the transaction with the corresponding credit entry.

Capital

	£		£
		Cash at bank (1)	150,000

Property

	£		£
Cash at bank (2)	140,000		

Purchases

	£		£
Cash at bank (3)	5,000		
Cash at bank (5)	8,000		

Sales

	£		£
		Cash at bank (4)	7,000
		Cash at bank (7)	15,000

Sundry expenses

	£		£
Cash at bank (6)	100		

Wages payable

	£		£
Cash at bank (8)	2,000		

Postage

	£		£
Cash at bank (9)	100		

KAPLAN PUBLISHING

Cash at bank

	£		£
Capital (1)	150,000	Property (2)	140,000
Sales (4)	7,000	Purchases (3)	5,000
Sales (7)	15,000	Purchases (5)	8,000
		Sundry expenses (6)	100
		Wages payable (8)	2,000
		Postage (9)	100

Test your understanding 2

Cash

Date	Narrative	£	Date	Narrative	£
1.1.X5	Capital	10,000	2.1.X5	Purchases	2,500
5.1.X5	Sales	3,000	4.1.X5	Delivery van	1,000
8.1.X5	Loan	2,000	7.1.X5	Gas	500
10.1.X5	Debtors	3,000	9.1.X5	Creditors	1,500
			11.1.X5	Drawings	750

Capital

Date	Narrative	£	Date	Narrative	£
			1.1.X5	Cash	10,000

Purchases

Date	Narrative	£	Date	Narrative	£
2.1.X5	Cash	2,500			
3.1.X5	Creditors	2,000			

Creditors

Date	Narrative	£	Date	Narrative	£
9.1.X5	Cash	1,500	3.1.X5	Purchases	2,000

Delivery van

Date	Narrative	£	Date	Narrative	£
4.1.X5	Cash	1,000			

Sales

Date	Narrative	£	Date	Narrative	£
			5.1.X5	Cash	3,000
			6.1.X5	Debtors	5,000

Debtors

Date	Narrative	£	Date	Narrative	£
6.1.X5	Sales	5,000	10.1.X5	Cash	3,000

Gas

Date	Narrative	£	Date	Narrative	£
7.1.X5	Cash	500			

Loan

Date	Narrative	£	Date	Narrative	£
			8.1.X5	Cash	2,000

Drawings

Date	Narrative	£	Date	Narrative	£
11.1.X5	Cash	750			

Test your understanding 3

1   A cash transaction is a transaction that is paid for immediately the transaction is made. It is unlikely that an invoice will be raised although a receipt may be provided.

   A credit transaction is one that is paid for at a specified time after the transaction. An invoice will generally be raised.

2   Credit

3   Debit

4   Debit the bank account; credit the sales account

5   Debit

6   Debit

7   Debit

8   Debit bank £1,000; credit capital £1,000

9   Credit

Balancing the ledger accounts

Introduction

At the end of a period of time, for example a month of trading, the owner of the business might wish to know some details about the performance of the business in the period. For example how much sales revenue was earned, how much does the business owe to its creditors, how much money is left in the bank?

These figures can be found by balancing the ledger accounts. So in this chapter we will look at the procedure for balancing a ledger account.

1 Procedure for balancing a ledger account

1.1 Steps to follow

Step 1 Total both the debit and the credit side of the ledger account and make a note of each total.

Step 2 Insert the higher of the two totals as the total on both sides of the ledger account leaving a line beneath the final entry on each side of the account.

Step 3 On the side with the smaller total insert the figure needed to make this column add up to the total. Call this figure the balance carried down (or 'Bal c/d' as an abbreviation).

Step 4 On the opposite side of the ledger account, below the total insert this same figure and call it the balance brought down (or 'Bal b/d' as an abbreviation).

> ### Illustration 1 – Procedure for balancing a ledger account
>
> The bank account of a business has the following entries:
>
> **Bank**
>
> | | £ | | £ |
> |---|---|---|---|
> | Capital | 1,000 | Purchases | 200 |
> | Sales | 300 | Drawings | 100 |
> | Sales | 400 | Rent | 400 |
> | Capital | 500 | Stationery | 300 |
> | Sales | 800 | Purchases | 400 |
>
> **Calculate the balance on the account and bring the balance down as a single amount.**
>
> **Solution**
>
> **Step 1** Total both sides of the account and make a note of the totals. (Note that these totals that are asterisked below would not normally be written into the ledger account itself. They are only shown here to explain the process more clearly.)
>
> **Bank**
>
> | | £ | | £ |
> |---|---|---|---|
> | Capital | 1,000 | Purchases | 200 |
> | Sales | 300 | Drawings | 100 |
> | Sales | 400 | Rent | 400 |
> | Capital | 500 | Stationery | 300 |
> | Sales | 800 | Purchases | 400 |
> | **Sub-total debits*** | **3,000** | **Sub-total credits*** | **1,400** |

Step 2 Insert the higher total as the total of both sides.

Bank

	£		£
Capital	1,000	Purchases	200
Sales	300	Drawings	100
Sales	400	Rent	400
Capital	500	Stationery	300
Sales	800	Purchases	400
Sub-total debits*	**3,000**	**Sub-total credits***	**1,400**
Total	3,000	Total	3,000

Step 3 Insert a balancing figure on the side of the account with the lower sub-total. This is referred to as the 'balance carried down' or 'bal c/d' for short.

Bank

	£		£
Capital	1,000	Purchases	200
Sales	300	Drawings	100
Sales	400	Rent	400
Capital	500	Stationery	300
Sales	800	Purchases	400
Sub-total debits*	**3,000**	**Sub-total credits***	**1,400**
		Bal c/d	1,600
Total	3,000	Total	3,000

Step 4 Insert the balance carried down figure beneath the total on the other side of the account. This is referred to as 'bal b/d' for short.

Bank

	£		£
Capital	1,000	Purchases	200
Sales	300	Drawings	100
Sales	400	Rent	400
Capital	500	Stationery	300
Sales	800	Purchases	400
Sub-total debits*	3,000	Sub-total credits*	1,400
		Bal c/d	1,600
Total	3,000	Total	3,000
Bal b/d	1,600		

The closing balance carried down at the end of the period is also the opening balance brought down at the start of the next period. This opening balance remains in the account as the starting position and any further transactions are then added into the account. In this case the balance brought down is a debit balance as there is money in the bank account making it an asset.

Balancing the ledger accounts

Illustration 2 – Procedure for balancing a ledger account

Consider again the ledger accounts from the example in the previous chapter which are reproduced below and balance them.

Bank

Date			£	Date			£
1 Jan	Capital	(1)	20,000	1 Jan	Van	(2)	500
5 Jan	Sales	(6)	2,000		Purchases	(3)	1,000
					Drawings	(4)	50
				5 Jan	Purchases	(5)	500
				15 Jan	Rent	(7)	200

Capital

Date			£	Date			£
				1 Jan	Bank	(1)	20,000

Van

Date			£	Date		£
1 Jan	Bank	(2)	500			

Purchases

Date			£	Date		£
1 Jan	Bank	(3)	1,000			
5 Jan	Bank	(5)	500			

Drawings

Date			£	Date		£
1 Jan	Bank	(4)	50			

Sales

Date		£	Date			£
			5 Jan	Bank	(6)	2,000

Rent

Date			£	Date		£
15 Jan	Bank	(7)	200			

Solution

(a) The bank account

Bank

Date		£	Date		£
1 Jan	Capital	20,000	1 Jan	Van	500
5 Jan	Sales	2,000		Purchases	1,000
				Drawings	50
			5 Jan	Purchases	500
			15 Jan	Rent	200

Step 1 Total both the debit and the credit side of the ledger account and make a note of each total – debit side £22,000, credit side £2,250.

Step 2 Insert the higher of the two totals, £22,000, as the total on both sides of the ledger account leaving a line beneath the final entry on each side of the account.

Bank

Date		£	Date		£
1 Jan	Capital	20,000	1 Jan	Van	500
5 Jan	Sales	2,000		Purchases	1,000
				Drawings	50
			5 Jan	Purchases	500
			15 Jan	Rent	200
		22,000			22,000

Step 3 On the side with the smaller total insert the figure needed to make this column add up to the total. Call this figure the balance carried down (or Bal c/d as an abbreviation).

Step 4 On the opposite side of the ledger account, below the total insert this same figure and call it the balance brought down (or Bal b/d as an abbreviation).

Bank

Date		£	Date		£
1 Jan	Capital	20,000	1 Jan	Van	500
5 Jan	Sales	2,000		Purchases	1,000
				Drawings	50
			5 Jan	Purchases	500
			15 Jan	Rent	200
			31 Jan	Balance c/d	19,750
		22,000			22,000
1 Feb	Balance b/d	19,750			

This shows that the business has £19,750 left in the bank account

Balancing the ledger accounts

at the end of January and therefore also on the first day of February. As the balance that is brought down to start the next period is on the debit side of the account this is known as a debit balance and indicates that this is an asset – money in the bank account.

(b) Capital

Capital

Date		£	Date		£
			1 Jan	Bank	20,000

As there is only one entry in this account there is no need to balance the account. The entry is on the credit side and is known as a credit balance. A credit balance is a liability of the business and this account shows that the business owes the owner £20,000 of capital.

(c) Van

Van

Date		£	Date		£
1 Jan	Bank	500			

Again, there is no need to balance this account as there is only one entry. This is a debit balance as it is an asset – the fixed asset, the van, which cost £500.

(d) Purchases

Purchases

Date		£	Date		£
1 Jan	Bank	1,000			
5 Jan	Bank	500	31 Jan	Balance c/d	1,500
		1,500			1,500
1 Feb	Balance b/d	1,500			

This now shows that during the month £1,500 of purchases were made. This is a debit balance as purchases are an expense of the business.

(e) Drawings

Drawings

Date		£	Date		£
1 Jan	Bank	50			

This is a debit balance as drawings are a reduction of the capital owed to the owner which is a credit balance.

KAPLAN PUBLISHING

(f) Sales

Sales

Date		£	Date		£
			5 Jan	Bank	2,000

There is no need to balance the account as there is only one entry – a £2,000 credit balance representing income.

(g) Rent

Rent

Date		£	Date		£
15 Jan	Bank	200			

As there is only one entry there is no need to balance the account. This is a debit balance indicating that there has been an expense of £200 of rent incurred during the month.

Test your understanding 1

Given below is a bank ledger account for the month of March. Balance the account.

Bank

Date		£	Date		£
1 Mar	Capital	12,000	3 Mar	Purchases	3,000
7 Mar	Sales	5,000	15 Mar	Fixed asset	2,400
19 Mar	Sales	2,000	20 Mar	Purchases	5,300
22 Mar	Sales	3,000	24 Mar	Rent	1,000
			28 Mar	Drawings	2,000

---

2 Casting and cross-casting

2.1 Introduction

Casting is the way accountants refer to adding a vertical column of figures and cross-casting is the way accountants refer to adding a horizontal row of figures.

It is worth very briefly doing a simple example of this just to show how a valuable check of the accuracy of your additions is provided by these two operations.

Balancing the ledger accounts

Illustration 3 – Casting and cross-casting

The following table of numbers is similar to the contents of accounting records such as the 'sales day book' or the 'analysed cash book' which you will come across in the next few chapters.

This table might represent the sales of products A to E in three geographical areas. We have deliberately chosen some awkward numbers to demonstrate the process.

You should calculate the totals yourself before looking at the solution.

	A	B	C	D	E	Total
UK	221,863	17,327	14,172	189,221	5,863	
USA	17,155	14,327	8,962	27,625	73,127	
Africa	18,627	33,563	62,815	1,003	57,100	
Total						

Solution

	A	B	C	D	E	Total
UK	221,863	17,327	14,172	189,221	5,863	448,446
USA	17,155	14,327	8,962	27,625	73,127	141,196
Africa	18,627	33,563	62,815	1,003	57,100	173,108
Total	257,645	65,217	85,949	217,849	136,090	762,750

If you managed to add the vertical columns and horizontal rows and then produced the overall total of 762,750 correctly for the overall table you have done very well.

This is a very useful technique and provides an excellent check on the accuracy of your addition.

Test your understanding 2

1   In a ledger account, if the total debits are £6,323 and the total credits £5,816, what is the balance on the account and is this balance a debit or a credit?

2   In a ledger account, if the total debits are £4,825 and the total credits are £6,115, what is the balance on the account and is this balance a debit or a credit?

3   In a ledger account if you bring down a debit balance into the new period, were the total debits of the previous period larger or smaller than the total credits?

3   Summary

Balancing an account is a very important technique which you must
be able to master for this Unit. You must understand how to bring the
balance down onto the correct side.

Casting and cross-casting is a simple technique but provides a very
useful check on the accuracy of your calculations.

Test your understanding answers

Test your understanding 1

Bank

Date		£	Date		£
1 Mar	Capital	12,000	3 Mar	Purchases	3,000
7 Mar	Sales	5,000	15 Mar	Fixed asset	2,400
19 Mar	Sales	2,000	20 Mar	Purchases	5,300
22 Mar	Sales	3,000	24 Mar	Rent	1,000
			28 Mar	Drawings	2,000
			31 Mar	Balance c/d	8,300
		22,000			22,000
1 Apr	Balance b/d	8,300			

Test your understanding 2

1 £507 debit

2 £1,290 credit

3 Larger

Credit sales – discounts and VAT

Introduction

In this chapter we will be continuing with our studies of accounting for sales on credit, which were introduced in an earlier chapter, by considering the accounting for VAT and for discounts given to customers.

1 Discounts

1.1 Introduction

There are two main types of discount that a business might offer to its credit customers, a trade discount and a cash (or settlement) discount.

1.2 Trade discounts

A trade discount is a percentage of the list price of the goods being sold that is deducted from the list price for certain customers. This discount may be offered due to the fact that the customer is a frequent and valued customer or because the customer is another business rather than an individual.

A trade discount is deducted from the list price total of the invoice.

1.3 Cash or settlement discounts

A cash or settlement discount is offered to customers if they settle the invoice within a certain time period. It is up to the customer to decide whether or not to pay early and therefore take the settlement discount. The discount is expressed as a percentage of the invoice total but is not deducted from the invoice total as it is not certain when the invoice is sent out whether or not it will be accepted. Instead the details of the settlement discount will be noted at the bottom of the invoice.

A trade discount is a definite amount that is deducted from the list price of the goods. A settlement discount can be offered but it is up to the customer whether or not to take advantage of it.

2 Value added tax

2.1 The operation of VAT

VAT is a tax levied on **consumer** expenditure. However the procedure is that it is collected at each stage in the production and distribution chain. Most businesses (being **taxable persons** as defined later) avoid having to treat VAT as an expense as they may deduct the VAT they have paid on their purchases (**input tax**) from the VAT they charge to customers on their sales (**output tax**) and pay only the difference to HM Revenue and Customs.

2.2 How VAT works

Let us examine a simple illustration. We will assume a standard rate of 17.5%, and follow one article, a wooden table, through the production and distribution chain.

- A private individual cuts down a tree and sells it to a timber mill for £10.

    Tax effect – none. The individual is not a 'taxable person'.

- The timber mill saws the log and sells the timber to a furniture manufacturer for £100 + VAT.

  Tax effect – Being a taxable person, the mill is obliged to charge its customers VAT at 17.5% on the selling price (output tax). There is no input tax available for offset.

  Cash effect – The mill collected £117.50 from the customer (or has a debtor for this sum). Of this, £17.50 has to be remitted to HM Revenue and Customs, and therefore only £100 would be recognised as sales.

- The manufacturer makes a table from the wood, and sells this to a retailer for £400 + VAT.

  Tax effect – The manufacturer is obliged to charge VAT at 17.5% on the selling price (ie £70), but in this instance would be allowed to set off, against this output tax, the input tax of £17.50 charged on the purchase of wood from the mill.

  Cash effect – Tax of £52.50 is remitted to to HM Revenue and Customs (output less input tax = £70 less £17.50). £400 is recognised as sales and £100 as purchases in the accounts.

- The retailer sells the table to a private customer for £851 plus VAT of £149.

  Tax effect – The retailer charges £149 of VAT to the customer but against this output tax may be set off the input tax of £70 charged on the purchase from the manufacturer.

  Cash effect – £79 (£149 – £70) is remitted to to HM Revenue and Customs. Purchases would be shown in the books at £400 and sales at £851.

- **The private customer** – VAT is a tax levied on consumer expenditure and the chain ends here. The customer is not a taxable person, and cannot recover the tax paid.

  You will note that everybody else has passed the VAT on and, though the customer has paid his £149 to the retailer, to HM Revenue and Customs has received its tax by contributions from each link in the chain, as shown below:

	£
Timber mill	17.50
Manufacturer	52.50
Retailer	79.00
	149.00

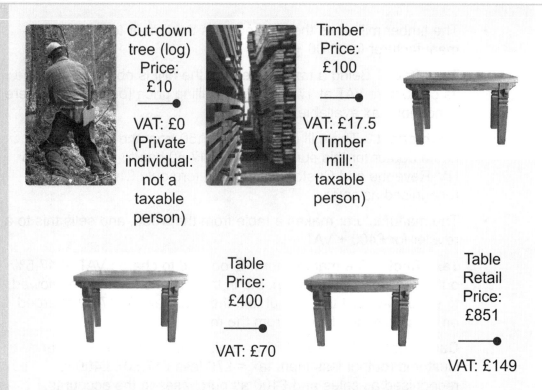

Cut-down tree (log) Price: £10 — VAT: £0 (Private individual: not a taxable person)

Timber Price: £100 — VAT: £17.5 (Timber mill: taxable person)

Table Price: £400 — VAT: £70

Table Retail Price: £851 — VAT: £149

VAT is charged on the **taxable supply of goods and services** in the United Kingdom by a **taxable person** in the course of a business carried on by him.

2.3 Taxable supply of goods and services

Taxable supply is the supply of all items except those which are exempt. Examples of exempt items are as follows:

- certain land and buildings, where sold, leased or hired

- insurance

- Post Office postal services

- betting, gaming and lotteries.

Input tax cannot be reclaimed where the trader's supplies are all exempt.

2.4 Rates of VAT

There are three rates of VAT on taxable supplies. Some items are 'zero-rated' (similar to exempt except that input tax can be reclaimed), there is a special rate of 5% for domestic fuel and power, and all other items are rated at the standard rate of 17.5%. Examples of 'zero-rated' supplies include:

- water and most types of food

- books and newspapers

- drugs and medicines

- children's clothing and footwear.

2.5 Non-deductible VAT

VAT on some items is non-deductible. This means that VAT on any purchases of these items cannot be deducted from the amount of tax payable to HM Revenue and Customs. The business has to bear the VAT as an expense.

Non-deductible items include:

*   motor cars

*   business entertaining.

For the purposes of your studies you will be dealing with taxable supplies at the standard rate of 17.5%.

2.6 Taxable person

A taxable person is any individual, partnership, company, etc who intends to make taxable supplies and is liable to register.

A person is liable to register if the value of his taxable supplies exceeds a specified amount in a 12-month period. Most companies and partnerships and many sole traders are liable to register.

2.7 Calculating the amount of VAT

If you are given the net price of goods, the price excluding VAT, then the amount of VAT is 17.5/100 of this price.

VAT is always rounded down to the nearest penny.

Illustration 1 – Value added tax

A sale is made for £360.48 plus VAT.

What is the amount of VAT to be charged on this sale?

Solution

VAT = £360.48 $\times$ 17.5/100 = £63.08

Remember to round down to the nearest penny.

2.8 VAT inclusive amounts

If a price is given that already includes the VAT then calculating the VAT requires an understanding of the price structure where VAT is concerned.

	%
Selling price including VAT (gross)	117.5
VAT	17.5
Selling price excluding VAT (net)	100.0

Illustration 2 – Value added tax

Goods have a selling price of £2,350 inclusive of VAT.

What is the VAT on the goods and the net price of these goods?

Solution

	£
Net price (£2,350 × 100/117.5)	2,000
VAT (£2,350 × 17.5/117.5)	350
Gross price	2,350

Test your understanding 1

What is the amount of VAT on each of the following transactions?

(i)   £145.37 net of VAT

(ii) £285.47 net of VAT

(iii) £159.80 including VAT

(iv) £575.75 including VAT

3   Cash (or settlement) discount and VAT

3.1   Introduction

When a cash/settlement discount is offered, this makes the VAT calculation slightly more complex.

Invoices should show the VAT payable as 17.5% of the discounted price. The amount paid by the customer is either:

(a) taking discount – discounted amount (excluding VAT) plus discounted VAT, or

(b) not taking discount – full amount (excluding VAT) plus discounted VAT.

The amount of VAT paid is always based on the discounted amount even though when the invoice is being prepared it is not known whether the customer will or will not take advantage of the cash or settlement discount.

Illustration 3 – Cash (or settlement) discount and VAT

A purchase is for 20 items @ £5 each. This totals £100.

A 2% discount is offered for settlement within 30 days.

(a) Calculate the VAT.

(b) Calculate the amount paid if the customer takes the discount.

(c) Calculate the amount paid if the customer does not take the discount.

Solution

(a) The VAT is therefore calculated as:

$(100 \times 98\%) \times 17.5\%$, or
$(100 - (100 \times 2\%)) \times 17.5\% = £17.15$

The amount paid by the customer is either of the following:

(b) Taking discount

	£
Discounted amount	98.00
Discounted VAT	17.15
Total	115.15

(c) Not taking discount

	£
Full amount	100.00
Discounted VAT	17.15
Total	117.15

The invoice looks as follows:

	£
20 items @ £5 each	100.00
VAT @ 17.5%	17.15
Total	117.15

The difference between (b) and (c) is £2, the cash discount on £100.

If no settlement discount were offered the VAT would have been £17.50 and the total of the invoice £117.50.

You may be required to prepare a sales invoice where a cash or settlement discount has been offered and the VAT has to be calculated. You will be required to check invoices that the business has received and to ensure that the VAT has been correctly calculated given any settlement discount offered.

Illustration 4 – Cash (or settlement) discount and VAT

A sales invoice is to be prepared for two adult Fairisle sweaters at a cost of £50.00 each. A settlement discount of 5% for payment within 30 days is offered. What would the sales invoice look like?

Solution

INVOICE
Creative Clothing

3 The Mall, Wanstead, London, E11 3AY, Tel: 0208 491 3200, Fax: 0208 491 3220

Invoice to:	**VAT Registration:**	487 3921 12
Smith & Isaacs	Date/tax point:	14 February 20X0
23 Sloane Street	Invoice number:	149
London	Delivery note no:	41682
SW3	Account no:	SL43

Code	Description	Quantity	VAT rate %	Unit price (£)	Amount exclusive of VAT (£)
FW168	Fairisle Sweater (adult)	2	17.5	50.00	100.00
					100.00
VAT at 17.5%					16.62
Total amount payable					116.62

Terms: Deduct discount of 5% if paid within 30 days

The VAT is calculated as 17.5% × (£100 × 95%) = £16.62.

A customer orders 10 Sansui radios priced at £25 each. The customer is given a 20% trade discount and a 10% cash discount for prompt payment. Calculate the VAT charged on the sale.

4 Accounting for credit sales and VAT

4.1 Accounting entries

We have already seen in this chapter that a business makes no profit out of any VAT charged on its sales. Instead this amount of output tax (less any related input tax) is paid over to HM Revenue and Customs. Therefore when a credit sale is recorded in the sales account it must be at the net of VAT amount.

However, when our customer eventually pays us he will pay the full amount due, i.e. the gross amount including the VAT. Therefore when we record a debtor in the ledger accounts it must be at the full gross amount of the invoice.

The difference between these two amounts, the VAT, is recorded in the VAT account.

4.2 Summary of entries

In summary the accounting entries for a credit sale with VAT are:

Debit   Debtors account with the gross amount

Credit   Sales account with the net amount

Credit   VAT account with the VAT

Illustration 5 – Accounting for credit sales and VAT

A sells goods to X for £500 plus VAT on credit. X pays A in full.

Record these transactions in the accounts.

Solution

Step 1   Calculate the VAT on the sale and enter the transaction in the debtors, sales and VAT accounts.

Calculation of VAT	£
Net value of sale	500.00
VAT at 17.5%	87.50
Gross value of sale	587.50

Debtors

	£		£
Sales and VAT	587.50		

Sales

	£		£
		Debtors	500.00

VAT

	£		£
		Debtors	87.50

Step 2 Enter £587.50 paid by X in the debtors account and the bank account.

Debtors

	£		£
Sales and VAT	587.50	Bank	587.50

Sales

	£		£
		Debtors	500.00

VAT

	£		£
		Debtors	87.50

Bank

	£		£
Debtors	587.50		

Note 1 The VAT that has been credited to the VAT account is a liability of the business. The business has effectively collected this money from X on behalf of HM Revenue and Customs and will have to pay this money to HM Revenue and Customs.

Illustration 6 – Accounting for credit sales and VAT

B sells £1,000 of goods to Y net of VAT on credit. He gives Y a deduction of 20% trade discount from the £1,000 net value. Y pays his account in full.

Enter these amounts in the accounts.

Solution

Step 1 Calculate the value of the sale net of discount and the VAT thereon.

	£
Sales value	1,000
Less: 20% discount	200
Net value	800
VAT at 17.5%	140
Total invoice value	940

KAPLAN PUBLISHING

Step 2 Enter the invoice value in the debtors, sales and VAT accounts.

Debtors

	£		£
Sales and VAT	940		

Sales

	£		£
		Debtors	800

VAT

	£		£
		Debtors	140

Note 1 Note that the trade discount does not feature at all in the accounts. The invoice value is expressed after deduction of the trade discount and it is this invoiced amount that is entered in the accounts.

Step 3 Enter the cash received from Y.

Debtors

	£		£
Sales and VAT	940	Bank	940

Sales

	£		£
		Debtors	800

VAT

	£		£
		Debtors	140

Bank

	£		£
Debtors	940		

Illustration 7 – Accounting for credit sales and VAT

C sells £2,000 of goods net of VAT to Z on credit. He offers Z a 5% settlement discount if Z pays within 30 days. Z does not pay his account within 30 days and so does not take the settlement discount. Z pays after 40 days. Enter these transactions in the accounts.

Solution

Step 1 Calculate the VAT on the sale.

	£
Sales value net of VAT	2,000.00
VAT = 17.5% × (2,000 – (5% × 2,000))	332.50
Invoice value	2,332.50

Note Remember that when a settlement discount is offered, the VAT is calculated on the sales value minus the settlement discount. In this case it turns out that Z does not take the settlement discount but at no stage do we go back to recalculate the VAT.

Step 2 Enter the invoice in the accounts.

Debtors

	£		£
Sales and VAT	2,332.50		

Sales

	£		£
		Debtors	2,000.00

VAT

	£		£
		Debtors	332.50

Step 3 Enter the payment by Z in the accounts.

Debtors

	£		£
Sales and VAT	2,332.50	Bank	2,332.50

Sales

	£		£
		Debtors	2,000.00

VAT

	£		£
		Debtors	332.50

Bank

	£		£
Debtors	2,332.50		

Note As Z does not take the settlement discount, there is no entry for the settlement discount at all in the accounts.

---

e.g **Illustration 8 – Accounting for credit sales and VAT**

Two months later C sells another £2,000 of goods net of VAT to Z on credit. He offers Z a 5% settlement discount if Z pays within 30 days. This time Z does pay his account within 30 days and takes the settlement discount.

Enter these transactions in the accounts.

Solution

Step 1 Calculate the VAT on the sale.

Note This is exactly the same as the previous example because the calculation of VAT with a settlement discount is the same whether the customer takes the settlement discount or not.

	£
Sales value net of VAT	2,000.00
VAT = 17.5% × (2,000 − (5% × 2,000))	332.50
Invoice value	2,332.50

Step 2 Enter the invoice in the accounts.

Note This is exactly the same as the previous example because the value of the invoice is exactly the same as the previous example.

Debtors

	£		£
Sales and VAT	2,332.50		

Sales

	£		£
		Debtors	2,000.00

VAT

	£		£
		Debtors	332.50

Step 3 Calculate the amount paid by Z.

Note The amount paid by Z will be different from the previous example because Z does take the 5% discount.

	£
Sales value net of VAT	2,000.00
Less: settlement discount = 5% x 2,000	(100.00)
VAT (as per the invoice)	332.50
Amount paid by Z	2,232.50

Step 4 Enter this amount in the accounts.

Debtors

	£		£
Sales and VAT	2,332.50	Bank	2,232.50
		Discount allowed	100.00

The amount recorded as a debtor is larger than the amount eventually paid as the settlement discount has been taken by the customer. The difference, the discount allowed, must be credited to the debtors account in order to clear the account and show that nothing more is owed.

Sales

	£		£
		Debtors	2,000.00

VAT

	£		£
		Debtors	332.50

Bank

	£		£
Debtors	2,232.50		

Discount allowed

	£		£
Bank	100.00		

> **Note** Because Z takes the settlement discount, he pays C £100 less than the invoice value. In order to clear the debtors account we have to credit that account with the £100 and debit a discount allowed account with £100. This £100 is an expense of the business as we have allowed our customer to pay less than the invoice value in order to have the benefit of receiving the money earlier.

Test your understanding 3

1 What is a settlement discount?

2 If a customer is given a trade discount, does this discount appear anywhere in the ledger accounts?

3 If a customer takes a settlement discount of £100, what is the double entry to record this settlement discount in the accounts?

4 If goods are sold for £230 including VAT, what is the VAT on the sale?

5 If goods are sold for £230 excluding VAT, what is the VAT on the sale?

5 Summary

We have covered some fairly tricky ideas in this chapter and it is very important that you really do understand them.

The calculations of VAT are fairly straightforward but do make sure that you can calculate the VAT element of a sale when you are given the sales value gross of VAT.

Also quite tricky is the treatment of settlement discounts. You have to be able to do two things.

(a) Calculate the VAT on a sale when a settlement discount is offered. Remember that it is irrelevant whether the customer takes the settlement discount or not.

(b) Calculate the amount paid by the customer if he takes a settlement discount. This will be less than the invoice value and you therefore have to account for the discount allowed.

Test your understanding answers

Test your understanding 1

(i)   £145.37 × 17.5/100   = £25.43

(ii) £285.47 × 17.5/100   = £49.95

(iii) £159.80 × 17.5/117.5 = £23.80

(iv) £575.75 × 17.5/117.5 = £85.75

Test your understanding 2

£31.50

Note: The answer is arrived at as follows:

	£
Sales price (10 × £25)	250.00
Less: Trade discount (250 × 20%)	(50.00)
	200.00
Less: Cash discount (200 × 10%)	(20.00)
	180.00
VAT @ 17.5%	31.50

Test your understanding 3

1   A settlement discount is a percentage reduction from the sales value excluding VAT offered to a customer if he pays within a specified number of days.

2   No

3   Credit Debtors £100; debit discounts allowed £100

4   £34.25

Sales value including VAT	230.00
VAT = 230 ÷ 117.5 × 17.5	34.25

5   £230 × 17.5 = £40.25

The sales day book – main and subsidiary ledgers

Introduction

We have already seen how to calculate the amount of a credit sale, including VAT and any relevant discounts. In this chapter we will deal with the initial recording of credit sales before they are entered into the ledger accounts.

1 Accounting for credit sales

1.1 Introduction

In a typical business there will be a great number of sales transactions to be recorded. We have to record each of these transactions individually but the accounts would be very cluttered if we entered every transaction individually in the main ledger accounts.

In order to simplify the process (and exercise greater control) we divide the recording of the transactions into three parts (we are studying sales invoices here, but similar systems apply to purchases, sales returns, etc as we shall see).

(a) The first part is the books of prime entry. We shall study here the sales day book.

(b) The second part is the main ledger itself where the double entry takes place.

(c) The third part is the subsidiary (sales) ledger which contains the individual debtor accounts.

Sales invoices and cheques are the source documents which will form the basis of accounting entries in all these three parts. Later in this book we study in more detail how invoices and cheques are dealt with.

1.2 Books of prime entry – the sales day book (SDB)

The sales day book is simply a list of the sales invoices that are to be processed for a given period (e.g. a week).

In its simplest form, the sales day book will comprise just the names of the customers and the amount of the invoices issued in the week.

The SDB is not part of the double entry; it is not part of the ledger accounts. It is just a list but we shall use it to perform the double entry. It will look something like this:

Week 1	
Customer	Amount £
X	1,000
Y	2,000
Z	3,000
Total	6,000

1.3 The main ledger

The main ledger is the place where the double entry takes place in the appropriate ledger accounts. The main ledger contains all the accounts you have become familiar with so far, for example:

Capital

Drawings

Van

Rent

Electricity

Purchases

Bank

etc

One of these typical accounts is the debtors account but now we will call this the sales ledger control account.

This account contains (for a given period) the total value of all the invoices issued to customers and the total of all the cash received. It does not contain any detail.

1.4 The subsidiary (sales) ledger

However as well as information about our debtors in total we have to keep track of each individual debtor. How much have we invoiced him with? What has he paid? How much does he owe?

We do this in the subsidiary (sales) ledger. This ledger is not part of the main ledger and it is not part of the double entry.

The subsidiary (sales) ledger contains a separate ledger account for each individual debtor. Every individual invoice and cash receipt is posted to an individual's account in the subsidiary (sales) ledger.

1.5 Fitting it all together

We have now looked at the three elements of a typical accounting system. We must now see how it all fits together.

Consider three credit sales invoices

Customer	Amount
A	£1,500
B	£2,000
C	£2,500

Step 1

Each invoice is recorded in the sales day book and in the personal account of each debtor in the subsidiary sales ledger. The entry required for each invoice is a debit in each debtor account to indicate that this is the amount that each one owes us.

Step 2

At the end of the period the sales day book is totalled and the total is entered into the sales ledger control account (SLCA) (total debtors account) in the main ledger.

The full double entry is as we saw in the previous chapter (ignoring VAT at the moment):

Debit   Sales ledger control account
Credit   Sales

Step 3

Now consider the following cheques being received against these debts.

Customer	Amount
A	£1,000
B	£2,000

Each receipt is recorded in the cash book (see later chapter) and in the personal account of each debtor in the subsidiary sales ledger. The entry for cash received in the individual accounts is a credit entry to indicate that they no longer owe us these amounts.

Step 4

At the end of the period the cash book is totalled and the total is entered into the sales ledger control account (total debtors account) in the main ledger.

The full double entry is:

Debit   Cash account (money in)
Credit   Sales ledger control account

This is illustrated on the next page.

Notes

1   The invoices are entered into the SDB and the cheques are entered into the cash book.

2   The totals from the cash book and SDB are posted to the SLCA.

3   The individual invoices and cash received are posted to the subsidiary (sales) ledger.

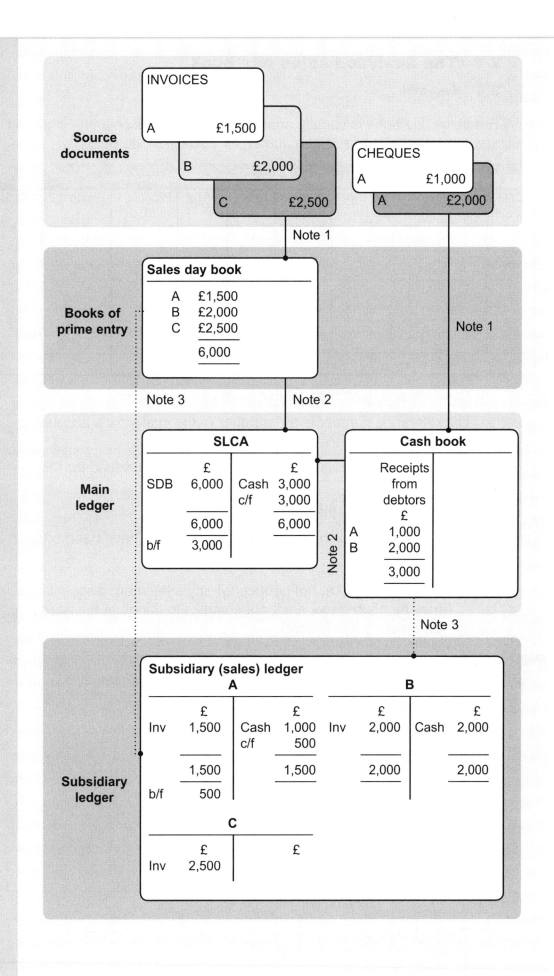

2 The analysed sales day book

2.1 Layout

The sales day book is usually analysed with 'analysis columns' showing how the total value of each customer's invoice is made up.

SALES DAY BOOK

Date	Customer	Reference	Invoice number	Total £	VAT £	Product 1 £	Product 2 £	Product 3 £
		TOTALS						

(a) The date and customer columns are self explanatory.

(b) The reference number is the number of the customer's account in the subsidiary sales ledger.

(c) The invoice number is the number of the invoice issued for this sale.

(d) The total column is the value of the goods sold:

- after deducting any trade discount that may have been offered

- including VAT

- and including (i.e. not deducting) any settlement discount that may be offered (we shall not complicate things at this stage by considering this further).

Illustration 1 – Cash (or settlement) discount and VAT

An invoice to customer A is made up as follows:

	£
Sale of 50 units at £2 per unit	100.00
Less: 20% trade discount	(20.00)
	80.00
VAT @ 17.5% (£80 x17.5%)	14.00
Total invoice value	94.00

The £94 would be entered in the 'total' column.

(e) The VAT column – this column is the value of the VAT on the invoice – in this case £14.00.

(f) Product 1, 2, etc columns – these are columns that analyse the net sales value (i.e. the total value after deducting VAT) into groupings that are of interest to the business.

In this introductory section we shall not complicate things by considering more than one type of product so that there will only be one column for sales.

In this case the entry in the sales column would be £80.

(g) The total boxes – at the end of a period (say a week or a month) the sales day book is totalled and the total values of each column are written in the total boxes.

The sales day book would therefore look as follows for the example above:

SALES DAY BOOK

Date	Customer	Reference	Invoice number	Total £	VAT £	Product 1 £	Product 2 £	Product 3 £
	A			94	14	80		
	TOTALS			94	14	80		

Note: In the pages that follow we shall concentrate on the basic entries in the sales day book using only the customer, total, VAT and one sales column. This will enable us to concentrate on the simple double entry.

Later in this book we shall look at more realistic situations which will involve scenario type material.

Illustration 2 – Cash (or settlement) discount and VAT

Posting the sales day book to the accounts in the ledgers

Consider the following sales transactions made by Roberts Metals.

Customer	Sales value (ex VAT) £	Trade discount %	Net sales value £	VAT £	Total £
A	1,000	10%	900	157.50	1,057.50
B	2,000	20%	1,600	280.00	1,880.00
C	3,000	30%	2,100	367.50	2,467.50

Enter this information in the ledger accounts using the following three steps.

The sales day book – main and subsidiary ledgers

Step 1 Write up the sales day book, and total the columns.

Step 2 Post the totals to the accounts in the main ledger.

Step 3 Post the individual invoices to the subsidiary sales ledger.

Solution

Step 1

SALES DAY BOOK

Date	Customer	Reference	Invoice number	Total £	VAT £	Sales £
	A			1,057.50	157.50	900.00
	B			1,880.00	280.00	1,600.00
	C			2,467.50	367.50	2,100.00
			TOTALS	5,405.00	805.00	4,600.00

Step 2

Main ledger

Sales		VAT		SLCA	
£	£	£	£	£	£
	SDB 4,600.00		SDB 805.00	SDB 5,405.00	

Step 3

Subsidiary (sales) ledger

A		B		C	
£	£	£	£	£	£
SDB 1,057.50		SDB 1,880.00		SDB 2,467.50	

Note to solution

(a) The totals of the SDB are entered in the main ledger.

(b) The individual invoices (total value including VAT) are entered in the individual debtors accounts in the subsidiary ledger. This is the amount that the debtor will pay.

(c) Note that there are no entries for trade discounts either in the SDB or in the ledger accounts.

Test your understanding 1

An analysed sales day book has the following totals for a week.

Date	Invoice no	Customer name	Code	Total	VAT	Europe	Asia	America
				£	£	£	£	£
23/04/X0		Total		63,979	9,529	21,250	15,400	17,800

How would the totals be posted to the main ledger accounts?

3 Sales returns

3.1 Introduction

When customers return goods, the accounting system has to record the fact that goods have been returned. If the goods were returned following a cash sale then cash would be repaid to the customer. If goods were returned following a credit sale then the customer's debtors ledger account will need to be credited with the value of the goods returned.

Illustration 3 – Sales returns

Returns following a cash sale

X sells £500 of goods to A for cash plus £87.50 VAT.

X subsequently agrees that A can return £200 worth of goods (excluding the VAT).

Record these transactions in the ledger accounts.

Solution

Step 1

First of all we need to set up a new account called the 'sales returns account' in the main ledger. This will be used in addition to the sales account and cash book with which you are familiar.

Step 2

Enter the cash sale in the accounts.

Debit bank account for cash received	£587.50
Credit sales with net amount	£500.00
Credit VAT account with VAT	£87.50

Bank account

	£		£
Sales	587.50		

Sales

	£		£
		Cash book	500.00

Sales returns

	£		£

VAT

	£		£
		Cash book	87.50

Step 3

X will repay A £200 plus VAT of (£200 × 17.5%) = £35. We therefore need to enter the sale return, the cash and the VAT in the accounts.

Debit sales returns account	£200.00
Debit VAT account £200 17.5%	£35.00
Credit bank account with cash paid out	£235.00

Bank account

	£		£
Sales	587.50	Sales returns	235.00

Sales

	£		£
		Cash book	500.00

Sales returns

	£		£
Cash book	200.00		

VAT

	£		£
Cash book	35.00	Cash book	87.50

3.2 Sales returns for credit sales

When a credit customer returns goods, he does not receive cash for the return. Instead the seller will issue a credit note to record the fact that goods have been returned. This credit note is sent to the customer and is entered in the seller's books.

Illustration 3 – Sales returns

X sells goods on credit to A for £500. A returns goods worth £200. X sends a credit note for £200 to A. Enter these transactions in the main ledger of X's books. There is no VAT.

Solution

Step 1

Record the invoice issued for the credit sale for £500:

Debit the SLCA in the main ledger with £500.

Credit the sales account in the main ledger with £500.

SLCA

	£		£
Sales	500.00		

Sales

	£		£
		SLCA	500.00

Step 2

Record the credit note for £200. The return is debited to a 'sales returns account' to reflect the reduction in sales. The SLCA is credited to show that the debtor has been reduced.

SLCA

	£		£
Sales	500.00	Sales returns	200.00

Sales

	£		£
		SLCA	500.00

Sales returns

	£		£
SLCA	200.00		

3.3 Sales returns with VAT

When a return is made and we include VAT, the VAT has to be accounted for both on the invoice when the sale is made, and on the credit note when the goods are returned. This VAT has to be entered in the books.

Illustration 4 – Sales returns

X sells goods on credit to B for £1,000 + VAT.

B returns goods worth £400 + VAT.

Enter these transactions in the main ledger of X's books.

Solution

Step 1

Enter the invoice in the usual way, including the VAT.

SLCA

	£		£
Sales	1,175.00		

Sales

	£		£
		SLCA	1,000.00

VAT

	£		£
		SLCA	175.00

Step 2

Enter the credit note. The VAT on the return will be £400 x 17.5% = £70.

SLCA

	£		£
Sales	1,175.00	Sales returns	470.00

Sales

	£		£
		SLCA	1,000.00

VAT

	£		£
SLCA	70.00	SLCA	175.00

Sales returns

	£		£
SLCA	400.00		

The books will reflect the position after the return. The balance on the SLCA is £705. This is made up as:

	£
Sale	1,000
Sale return	400
	600
VAT 600 $\times$ 17.5%	105
	705

4 The sales returns day book

4.1 The sales returns day book

Sales returns are in practice entered in a 'sales returns day book'. This is similar to the sales day book, and the columns are used in the same way. The only difference is that instead of having a column for the invoice number, there is a column for the 'credit note number'. This is because when the goods are received back the business will issue a credit note.

SALES RETURNS DAY BOOK						
Date	Customer	Reference	Credit note number	Total £	VAT £	Sales returns £

Illustration 5 – The sales returns day book

A and B are credit customers of Ellis Electricals. The balances on their accounts in the subsidiary sales ledger are £1,175 and £2,350 because both A and B have made earlier purchases which have not yet been paid.

A returns goods which cost £600 excluding VAT.

B returns goods which cost £400 excluding VAT.

Enter the above returns in the sales returns day book and in the main and subsidiary ledgers of Ellis Electricals.

Solution

Step 1

Enter the original sales invoices in the main ledger.

SLCA

	£		£
SDB	3,525.00		

Sales

	£		£
		SDB	3,000.00

VAT

	£		£
		SDB	525.00

Step 2

Write up the sales returns day book.

SALES RETURNS DAY BOOK						
Date	Customer	Reference	Credit note number	Total £	VAT £	Sales returns £
	A			705.00	105.00	600.00
	B			470.00	70.00	400.00
				1,175.00	175.00	1,000.00

Step 3

Enter the SRDB totals in the main ledger accounts.

SLCA

	£		£
SDB	3,525.00	SRDB	1,175.00

Sales

	£		£
		SDB	3,000.00

VAT

	£		£
SRDB	175.00	SDB	525.00

Sales returns

	£		£
SRDB	1,000.00		

Step 4

Enter the individual amounts in the subsidiary sales ledger.

A

	£		£
SDB	1,175.00	SRDB	705.00

B

	£		£
SDB	2,350.00	SRDB	470.00

4.2 Sales returns in sales day book

In some businesses the level of sales returns are fairly low and therefore it is not justified to keep a separate sales returns day book. In these cases any credit notes that are issued for sales returns are recorded as negative amounts in the sales day book.

Test your understanding 2

Given below are the totals of an analysed sales returns day book for a week.

Date	Customer name	Credit note no	Code	Total £	VAT £	Europe £	Asia £	America £
23/04/X0				3,290	490	1,458	650	692

Post these totals to the main ledger accounts.

1   Does the double entry bookkeeping take place in the main ledger or the subsidiary ledgers?

2   When a credit sale is made, is the debit part of the double entry entered in the sales ledger control account or the individual debtors account?

3   If a supplier gives his customer a trade discount, does this appear in the sales day book?

4   Does the total column of the analysed sales day book include or exclude VAT?

5   Summary

The sales day book, analysed sales day book, and the sales returns day book, are fairly straightforward. Remember that they are simply lists of invoices/credit notes which simplify posting entries to the main ledger.

You should make sure that you are familiar with the material in this chapter and fully understand how the various parts of the accounting system relate to each other. You will often be required to enter invoices and credit notes into the books of prime entry and then to post the entries to the main ledger and subsidiary ledger.

Test your understanding answers

The required double entry is as follows:

Debit	Sales ledger control account	£63,979
Credit	VAT	£9,529
	Europe sales	£21,250
	Asia sales	£15,400
	America sales	£17,800

Note carefully that it is the net amount that is credited to each sales account and the gross amount (including VAT) that is debited to the sales ledger control account. The VAT total is credited to the VAT account.

The ledger entries would appear as follows:

Sales ledger control account

	£		£
SDB	63,979		

VAT

	£		£
		SDB	9,529

Europe sales

	£		£
		SDB	21,250

Asia sales

	£		£
		SDB	15,400

America sales

	£		£
		SDB	17,800

Sales returns – Europe account

	£		£
SRDB	1,458		

Sales returns – Asia account

	£		£
SRDB	650		

Sales returns – America account

	£		£
SRDB	692		

VAT account

	£		£
SRDB	490		

Sales ledger control account

	£		£
		SRDB	3,290

Note carefully that it is the net amount that is debited to each returns account and the gross amount to the sales ledger control account. The difference, the VAT, is debited to the VAT account.

1 Main ledger

2 Sales ledger control account

3 No

4 It includes VAT

The analysed cash receipts book

Introduction

In this chapter we will look in more detail at the recording of cash receipts from customers and in particular from credit customers.

1 The analysed cash receipts book

1.1 Layout

A proforma analysed cash receipts book is shown below.

CASH RECEIPTS BOOK							
Date	Narrative	Reference	Total £	VAT £	Debtors £	Cash sales £	Discount allowed £
		TOTALS					

Notes

(a) The date column contains the date of the transaction.

(b) The narrative column describes the transactions - typically the name of the customer who is paying. It would also contain the subsidiary (sales) ledger code of the debtor.

(c) The reference column contains any other information that may be helpful e.g. 'cash', 'cheque', 'BACS' etc.

(d) The total column contains the total cash received (including any VAT).

(e) The VAT column contains the VAT on the transaction but not if the VAT has already been entered in the sales day book. This is a tricky point and is dealt with later.

(f) The debtors column contains any cash received that has been received from a debtor. The total received including VAT is entered in this column.

(g) The cash sales and discount allowed columns will be dealt with later.

Illustration 1 – Athe analysis cash receipts book

The following is from the example of Roberts Metals in the previous chapter.

Main ledger					
Sales		VAT		SLCA	
£	£	£	£	£	£
	SDB 4,600.00		SDB 805.00	SDB 5,405.00	

Subsidiary (sales) ledger

A		B		C	
£	£	£	£	£	£
SDB 1,057.50		SDB 1,880.00		SDB 2,467.50	

The following transactions took place:

Debtor A pays £1,057.50
Debtor B pays £1,000.00

Enter this information in the cash receipts book and in the ledger accounts given above.

Solution

The following steps are needed.

Step 1 Enter these transactions in the cash book.

Step 2 Total the cash book and post the totals to the main ledger.

Step 3 Post the individual amounts of cash paid by debtors to the subsidiary ledger.

Step 1

CASH RECEIPTS BOOK

Date	Narrative	Reference	Total £	VAT £	Debtors £	Cash sales £	Discount allowed £
	A		1,057.50	See Note 2 of Step 2	1.057.50		
	B		1,000.00		1,000.00		
		TOTALS	2,057.50		2,057.50		

Step 2

We have brought forward the balances from the main ledger in the earlier example and now post the cash received book (CRB) totals to the main ledger.

Main ledger

Sales		VAT		SLCA	
£	£	£	£	£	£
	b/f 4,600.00		b/f 805.00	b/f 5,405.00	CRB 2,057.50

Note 1

We have posted the total of the debtors column of the CRB to the sales ledger control account. This is the same as the total column in this example, but in more complex examples it need not be. The entry to the sales ledger control account is a credit entry as this is reducing the amount owed by our debtors.

Note 2

A common confusion is for people to wonder about the VAT – surely some of the money paid by A and B is actually paying the VAT part of the invoice. Yes it is, but we have already accounted for this VAT element when we entered the invoices themselves into the ledger accounts via the sales day book. Look back at Chapter 5 – the invoices were debited to the debtor accounts **including the VAT** (the VAT and sales entries are the corresponding credits). We therefore now post the total cash including VAT to the sales ledger control account but nothing is posted to the VAT account as this has already been done when dealing with the invoices.

Note 3

This is now the full double entry for the cash received completed.

Debit   Bank account (cash receipts book)
Credit   Sales ledger control account

We have credited the sales ledger control account and the entry in the cash receipts book itself is the related debit entry. So there is no need for any further debit entry.

Step 3

We have brought forward the balance from the subsidiary ledger in the earlier example and now post the cash received to the individual debtor accounts. Again, as with the sales ledger control account, this is a credit entry in each case as the cash received is reducing the amount owed by each debtor.

A			B			C	
	£	£		£	£		£	£
b/f	1,057.50	CRB 1,057.50	b/f	1,880.00	CRB 1,000.00	b/f	2,467.50	

1.2 Balancing the accounts

Below we reproduce the accounts as they have been written up above and we then balance the accounts and bring down the balances.

Main ledger

Sales		VAT		SLCA	
£	£	£	£	£	£
	SDB 4,600.00		SDB 805.00	SDB 5,405.00	CRB 2,057.50
					c/f 3,347.50
				5,405.00	5,405.00
			b/f 3,347.50		

Subsidiary (sales) ledger

A			B			C	
	£	£		£	£		£	£
SDB	1,057.50	CRB 1,057.50	SDB	1,880.00	CRB 1,000.00	SDB	2,467.50	
					c/f 880.00			
	1,057.50	1,057.50		1,880.00	1,880.00			
			b/f	880.00				

Note

The balance on the sales ledger control account in the main ledger (£3,347.50) is the same as the total balances of the individual accounts in the subsidiary sales ledger (£880.00 + £2,467.50 = £3,347.50). We will come back to this important point later in the Study Text.

2 Settlement discounts allowed to customers

2.1 Introduction

Settlement discounts are a small but tricky complication when dealing with the analysed sales day book and cash book.

We shall consider the same example as before with only one change – debtor A is offered an additional 5% settlement discount if he pays his invoice within 30 days.

Illustration 2 – Settlement discounts allowed to customers

The sales day book with settlement discounts

Customer	Sales value (ex VAT) £	Trade discount £	Net sales value £	VAT £	Total £
A	1,000	10%	900	149.62	1,049.62
B	2,000	20%	1,600	280.00	1,880.00
C	3,000	30%	2,100	367.50	2,467.50

Consider again the following sales transactions made by Roberts Metals.

In addition to the trade discount, customer A has been offered an additional 5% discount if he pays his invoice within 30 days.

Enter this information in the sales day book and ledger accounts.

Solution

The following steps are needed.

The analysed cash receipts book

Step 1 Write up the sales day book.

Step 2 Post the totals to the accounts in the main ledger.

Step 3 Post the individual invoices to the subsidiary ledger.

SALES DAY BOOK						
Date	Customer	Reference	Invoice number	Total £	VAT £	Sales £
	A			1,049.62	149.62 (W1)	900.00
	B			1,880.00	280.00	1,600.00
	C			2,467.50	367.50	2,100.00
			TOTALS	5,397.12	797.12	4,600.00

The solution is the same as before except that the VAT for customer A has been recalculated to take account of the settlement discount (W1).

Workings

	£
Sales value	1,000.00
Trade discount	100.00
Net sale value	900.00
VAT £(900 – (900 x 5%)) x 17.5%	149.62
	1,049.62

Step 2

Main ledger

Sales			VAT			SLCA		
£	£		£	£		£		£
	SDB 4,600.00			SDB 797.12		SDB 5,397.12		

Subsidiary (sales) ledger

A			B			C		
£	£		£	£		£		£
SDB 1,049.62			SDB 1,880.00			SDB 2,467.50		

Step 3

As you can see the offering of the settlement discount has had no effect on the entries to the sales day book or the ledgers other than the calculation of the VAT.

KAPLAN PUBLISHING

Illustration 3 – Cash (or settlement) discount and VAT

The analysed cash receipts book with settlement discounts

Now we will look at the cash receipts book.

Debtor A pays his debt within 30 days and therefore takes the 5% discount and debtor B pays £1,000 on account.

Enter these transactions in the cash receipts book and the ledger accounts.

Solution

Notes

The entries in the cash receipts book are different when a debtor takes a settlement discount because a new column is added to the CRB – the 'discount allowed' column. In addition, a new account is opened in the main ledger – the 'discount allowed ledger account'.

The four steps are now:

Step 1 Calculate the cash that A pays after allowing for the discount.

Step 2 Enter the cash received in the CRB (with the additional column for 'discounts allowed'). Total the columns.

Step 3 Enter the totals in the main ledger (including the 'discount allowed account').

Step 4 Enter the individual cash received from debtors A and B in the subsidiary ledger account.

Step 1

Calculate the cash paid by A.

	£
Sale value after trade discount	900.00
VAT (900 – (5% × 900)) × 17.5%	149.62
Invoice value (as entered in SDB)	1,049.62
Less: 5% settlement discount (900 × 5%)	(45.00)
Cash paid by A	1,004.62

Step 2

Enter cash received in the CRB.

CASH RECEIPTS BOOK

Date	Narrative	Total £	VAT £	Debtors £			Discount allowed £
	A	1,004.62		1,004.62			45.00
	B	1,000.00		1,000.00			
		2,004.62		2,004.62			45.00

Note

The CRB does not 'cross-cast', i.e. if you add the totals across (debtors + discounts) this does not equal the total column.

The discount allowed column is known as a 'memorandum column' – it is not really part of the cash book – it is simply there to remind the bookkeeper to make an entry in the main ledger as we shall see below.

Step 3 – posting the CRB totals

The CRB totals are posted as follows to the main ledger.

Sales				VAT			
£		£		£		£	
		SDB 4,600.00				SDB 797.12	

SLCA				Discount allowed			
£		£		£		£	
SDB 5,397.12		CRB 2,004.62		CRB 45.00			
		CRB 45.00					

Note that the discount allowed figure in the CRB is entered in the SLCA (to acknowledge the fact that discount has been taken) and is debited to the discount allowed account.

This debit is an expense of the business – allowing the discount has cost the business £45.

Step 4 – posting to the subsidiary ledger

A				B				C		
£		£		£		£		£		£
SDB 1,049.62		CRB 1,004.62		SDB 1,880.00		CRB 1,000.00		SDB 2,467.50		
		Disk 45.00				c/f 880.00				
1,049.62		1,049.62		1,880.00		1,880.00				
						b/f 880.00				

Note again that the discount is credited to the account of A to show that he has taken the £45 discount which clears his account.

Note also that there is no corresponding debit entry of £45 to a discount account in the subsidiary ledger. The subsidiary sales ledger is simply there to show the detail in the main ledger SLCA. The double entry for the £45 discount only takes place in the main ledger as we have seen between the SLCA and the discounts allowed account.

3 Cash and credit sales contrasted

3.1 Introduction

We studied cash sales at the very start of double entry bookkeeping and saw that the entries were very simple – Debit cash and credit sales. Nothing has happened to change that but it is worth looking at cash and credit sales 'side by side' to appreciate the difference in their treatment, when we consider the sales day book and cash receipts book.

Illustration 4 – Sales returns

Linda's Electricals sells goods to three customers.

Customer A buys an electric fire for £100 cash plus VAT of £17.50.

Customer B buys rolls of electrical wiring on credit for £1,000 plus VAT of £175.00.

Customer C buys 100 switches on credit for £200 plus VAT of £35.00.

Customer B pays his debt in full.

There are no trade or settlement discounts.

Write up the books in the following steps.

Step 1 Enter the cash sale in the analysed cash receipts book in the main ledger.

Step 2 Enter the credit sales in the SDB and cash received in the analysed cash receipts book in the main ledger.

Step 3 Post the totals of the SDB and cash book to the accounts in the main ledger.

Step 4 Post the individual amounts in the SDB and cash book to the subsidiary (sales) ledger.

Solution

Step 1

Enter the cash sale in the cash book.

CASH RECEIPTS BOOK

Date	Narrative	Total £	VAT £	Debtors £	Cash sales £		Discount allowed £
	A	117.50	17.50		100.00		

This is a very simple entry. At the moment of course it is only half of the double entry (the debit side of the entry). We have yet to do the credit entries (see Step 3).

Step 2

Enter the credit sales into the SDB and the cash received into the analysed cash receipts book (which already has the cash received from A per Step 1).

SALES DAY BOOK

Date	Customer	Reference	Invoice number	Total £	VAT £	Net sales value £
	B			1,175.00	175.00	1,000.00
	C			235.00	35.00	200.00
			TOTALS	1,410.00	210.00	1,200.00

CASH RECEIPTS BOOK

Date	Narrative	Total £	VAT £	Debtors £	Cash sales £		Discount allowed £
	A	117.50	17.50		100.00		
	B	1,175.00		1,175.00			
		1,292.50	17.50	1,175.00	100.00		

Note the different treatment of VAT for a cash and credit sale. For the cash sale, the VAT paid by A is entered in the VAT column of the cash book. For the credit sales of B and C, the VAT is entered in the VAT column of the SDB, and because it has already been 'captured' in the books it is not entered again in the cash book when the debt is paid by B.

In Step 3, we will see how the double entry is completed to ensure that all amounts are correctly treated.

Step 3

Post the SDB totals and cash book totals to the main ledger.

Sales				VAT		
£		£		£		£
		SDB 1,200.00				SDB 210.00
		CRB 100.00				CRB 17.50

SLCA		
£		£
SDB 1,410.00		CRB 1,175.00

Note 1

The VAT on the three sales are all now correctly credited to the VAT account, either by way of the SDB for credit sales or the CRB for cash sales.

Note 2

Remember that the CRB is part of the double entry. The total column in the CRB is the debit entry that tells us how much cash has been paid in (£1,292.50), and the entries from the CRB to the other main ledger accounts are the balancing credit entries.

	£
Sales	100.00
VAT	17.50
SLCA	1,175.00
Total credits	1,292.50

Test your understanding 1

Ellis Electricals makes the following credit sales to A and B giving a 20% trade discount plus a 5% settlement discount if customers pay their invoices within 30 days.

	Customer A £	Customer B £
Sales value	1,000	4,000
Trade discount (20%)	200	800
Net sales value	800	3,200
VAT (calculated on the net sales value after allowing for the settlement discount)		
Customer A: $(800 - (800 \times 5\%)) \times 17.5\%$	133	
Customer B: $(3,200 - (3,200 \times 5\%)) \times 17.5\%$		532
Total invoice value	933	3,732

Ellis Electricals also makes a cash sale to C for £300 plus VAT.

Remember that the VAT is calculated as if the settlement discount is taken whether the customer pays within 30 days and takes it or not – there is no going back to recalculate the VAT.

Customer A pays his invoice in full within 30 days and takes the settlement discount. Customer B pays £2,000 on account.

Write up the SDB and the CRB and post the entries to the main and subsidiary ledgers.

Test your understanding 2

1   When a business receives cash from a debtor, is any entry made in the VAT column of the analysed cash book?

2   When a business receives cash from a cash sale, is any entry made in the VAT column of the analysed cash book?

3   When a business raises an invoice offering a settlement discount to the customer, is any entry made to reflect this discount in the analysed sales day book?

4   When a customer pays an invoice having taken a settlement discount, is any entry made in the analysed cash book?

5   What is the double entry in the main ledger to reflect a customer taking a settlement discount?

4   Summary

This has been quite a difficult chapter which has addressed some of the trickier topics. There are two points which typically cause trouble and which you should get to grips with.

(a) Accounting for VAT on cash received from debtors and cash received from cash sales.

(b) Accounting for discounts allowed in the analysed cash book and main ledger accounts.

If you have any doubt at all about the treatment of these you should go back and study these two points in the chapter.

Test your understanding answers

Test your understanding 1

Step 1

Write up the sales day book.

SALES DAY BOOK

Date	Customer	Total £	VAT £	Sales £
	A	933.00	133.00	800.00
	B	3,732.00	532.00	3,200.00
		4,665.00	665.00	4,000.00

Step 2

Write up the cash receipts book.

CASH RECEIPTS BOOK

Date	Narrative	Total £	VAT £	Sales ledger £	Cash sales £		Discount allowed £
	A (W)	893.00		893.00			40.00
	B	2,000.00		2,000.00			
		352.50	52.50		300.00		
		3,245.50	52.50	2,893.00	300.00		40.00

Working

Cash paid by A:

	£
Sale value net of VAT	800
VAT	133
	933
Less: Settlement discount (800 × 5%)	(40)
	893

Step 3

Post the totals to the main ledger.

Sales			VAT		
£		£	£		£
		SDB 4,000.00			SDB 665.00
		CRB 300.00			CRB 52.60

KAPLAN PUBLISHING

	SLCA			Discount allowed	
£		£		£	£
SDB 4,665.00		CRB 2,893.00	CRB 40.00		
		CRB 40.00			

Step 4

Post individual amounts for the SDB and CRB to the subsidiary sales ledger.

	A			B	
£		£		£	£
SDB 933.00		CRB 893.00	SDB 3,732.00		2,000.00
		CRB 40.00			

Test your understanding 2

1 No. Entries relating to the VAT on the sale were initially entered in the sales day book and from there entered in the VAT account in the main ledger.

2 Yes. There are no books of prime entry for a cash sale and therefore no entries regarding VAT will have been made.

   The correct double entry will be: credit VAT account; debit sales ledger control account.

3 No. The sales day book simply lists the value of the invoice which the customer owes and (apart from an adjustment to the calculation of VAT) this is not affected by the settlement discount. If the customer takes the settlement discount and therefore pays less than the books show he owes, this is adjusted for by an entry in the discount allowed account.

4 Yes, the amount of the cash received and the amount of the discount taken.

5 Debit discount allowed account: Credit sales ledger control account.

7

Credit purchases – discounts and VAT

Introduction

In this chapter we move on from considering the accounting entries for sales and look here at the equivalent accounting entries for purchases.

1 Discounts and VAT

1.1 Introduction

We studied discounts and VAT when studying sales. The calculation of VAT and discounts are exactly the same when considering purchases. Remember that it is the seller who offers the discounts and it is the seller who charges the VAT, so the fact that we are now studying purchases does not change how these things are calculated.

The purchaser will receive a 'sales invoice' from the seller. This will have details of discounts and VAT exactly as we saw before when studying sales. The purchaser will call this a 'purchase invoice' and enter it in the books accordingly as we shall see.

We shall not therefore go through all the details of VAT and discounts but will simply revise this with a short example.

Illustration 1 – Discounts and VAT

Carl buys £1,000 of goods from Susan on credit. Susan sends a sales invoice with the goods offering a 5% discount if Carl pays within 30 days. Carl pays within 30 days.

Calculate:

(a) the VAT;

(b) the total value of the invoice; and

(c) the amount that Carl will pay.

Solution

(a) VAT = (£1,000 – (5% × £1,000)) × 17.5% = £166.25

(b) Total value of invoice

	£
Goods	1,000.00
VAT	166.25
Invoice value	1,166.25

(c) Amount Carl will pay

	£
Goods	1,000.00
Less settlement discount	50.00
	950.00
VAT	166.25
	1,116.25

Note: Remember that if Carl does not pay within 30 days the VAT is not recalculated.

2 Credit purchases – double entry

2.1 Basic double entry

The basic double entry for credit purchases with VAT is as follows:

Debit   Purchases account with the net amount
Debit   VAT account with the VAT
Credit   Creditors account with the gross amount

Purchases have been debited with the net amount as the VAT is not a cost to the business. Instead the VAT is an amount that can be set off against the amount of VAT due to HM Revenue and Customs and therefore the VAT is a debit entry in the VAT account. The creditors account is credited with the gross amount as this is the amount that must be paid to the supplier.

As with debtors and the sales ledger control account we will now be calling the creditors account the purchases ledger control account (PLCA).

Work through the following examples to practise the double entry for credit purchases

Illustration 2 – Credit purchases – double entry

B sells goods on credit to Y for £500 plus VAT. Y pays B the full amount due. Record these transactions in the accounts of Y.

Solution

Step 1   Calculate the VAT on the purchase and enter the transaction in the PLCA, purchases and VAT accounts.

Calculation of VAT

	£
Net value of sale	500.00
VAT at 17.5%	87.50
Gross value of purchase	587.50

PLCA

	£		£
		Purchases and VAT	587.50

Purchases

	£		£
PLCA	500.00		

VAT

	£		£
PLCA	87.50		

Step 2 Enter £587.50 paid by Y in the PLCA and the bank account.

PLCA

	£		£
Bank	587.50	Purchases and VAT	587.50

Purchases

	£		£
PLCA	500.00		

VAT

	£		£
PLCA	87.50		

Bank

	£		£
		PLCA	587.50

Illustration 3 – Credit purchases – double entry

B sells £1,000 of goods to Y net of VAT on credit. He gives Y a deduction of 20% trade discount from the £1,000 net value. Y pays his account in full.

Enter these amounts in the accounts of Y.

Solution

Step 1 Calculate the value of the sale net of discount and the VAT thereon.

	£
Sales value	1,000
Less: 20% discount	200
Net value	800
VAT at 17.5%	140
Total invoice value	940

Step 2 Enter the invoice in the PLCA, purchases and VAT accounts.

PLCA

	£		£
		Purchases and VAT	940

Purchases

	£		£
PLCA	800		

VAT

	£		£
PLCA	140		

Note 1

Note that the trade discount does not feature at all in the accounts. The invoice value is expressed after deduction of the trade discount and it is this invoiced amount that is entered in the accounts.

Step 3 Enter the cash paid by Y.

PLCA

	£		£
Bank	940	Purchases and VAT	940

Purchases

	£		£
PLCA	800		

VAT

	£		£
PLCA	140		

Bank

	£		£
		PLCA	940

---

e.g

Illustration 4 – Credit purchases – double entry

C sells £2,000 of goods net of VAT to Z on credit. He offers Z a 5% settlement discount if Z pays within 30 days. Z pays his account within 30 days and takes the settlement discount. Enter these transactions in the accounts of Z.

Solution

Step 1 Calculate the VAT on the purchase.

	£
Invoice value net of VAT	2,000.00
VAT = 17.5% × (2,000 – (5% × 2,000))	332.50
Invoice value	2,332.50

Step 2 Enter the invoice in the accounts of Z.

PLCA

	£		£
		Purchases and VAT	2,332.50

Purchases

	£		£
PLCA	2,000.00		

VAT

	£		£
PLCA	332.50		

Step 3 Calculate the amount paid by Z.

	£
Invoice value net of VAT	2,000.00
Less: settlement discount = 5% x 2,000	(100.00)
VAT (as per the invoice)	332.50
Amount paid by Z	2,232.50

Step 4 Enter this amount in the accounts.

PLCA

	£		£
Bank	2,232.50	Purchases and VAT	2,332.50
Discount received	100.00		

Purchases

	£		£
PLCA	2,000.00		

VAT

	£		£
PLCA	332.50		

Bank

	£		£
		PLCA	2,232.50

Discount received

	£		£
		PLCA	100.00

Note

Because Z takes the settlement discount, he pays C £100 less than the invoice value. In order to clear the creditors account (the PLCA) we have to debit that account with the £100 and credit a discount received account with £100. This £100 is income (reduction of an expense) of the business as the business is paying less than the face value of the invoice.

Test your understanding 1

1   A business purchases goods worth £500 including VAT. What is the VAT on the purchase?

2   A business receives an invoice for goods purchased for £100 plus VAT. The invoice offers the business a 5% settlement discount for payment within 30 days. What is the total value of the invoice including VAT?

3   In the above question the business pays the invoice within 30 days. How much does the business pay the supplier?

4   A business receives £100 settlement discount from a supplier for early payment. What is the double entry in the main ledger?

5   A business receives a trade discount of £200 from a supplier. What is the double entry in the main ledger?

3   Summary

The topics covered in this chapter will have been familiar to you as you have already studied the similar topics for sales.

Make sure you understand the point about VAT when there is a settlement discount offered. You must also understand the double entry for settlement discounts.

Test your understanding answers

Test your understanding 1

1   500 x 17.5 ÷ 117.5 = £74.46

2

	£
Value of goods	100.00
VAT (100 – (100 × 5%)) × 17.5%	16.62
Invoice value	116.62

3

	£
Value of goods	100.00
Less 5% discount	(5.00)
	95.00
VAT (per invoice)	16.62
Total payment	111.62

4   Debit purchase ledger control account £100; credit discounts received £100.

5   There are no entries for trade discounts in the main ledger.

The purchases day book – main and subsidiary ledgers

Introduction

Just as we did for sales on credit we will now consider how purchases on credit are recorded in the books of prime entry and the ledger accounts.

1 Accounting for credit purchases

1.1 Introduction

When we studied accounting for sales in the earlier chapters of this book, we dealt with the three parts of the accounting records as they affected sales.

In the case of purchases, the parts are exactly the same except that instead of a 'sales day book' we have the 'purchases day book', and instead of the 'subsidiary sales ledger' we have the 'subsidiary purchases ledger'. The third part, namely the main ledger, is exactly the same and contains all the main ledger accounts with which you are familiar.

Below we will illustrate how these parts fit together with a diagram.

1.2 Fitting it all together

Consider these three credit purchases invoices

Supplier	Amount
X	£4,000
Y	£5,000
Z	£6,000

Step 1

Each invoice is recorded in the purchases day book by the purchaser.

Step 2

At the end of the period the purchases day book is totalled and the total is entered into the purchases ledger control account in the nominal ledger. The individual entries are recorded in the individual creditor accounts in the subsidiary purchases ledger.

Now consider these cheques being paid to the creditors.

Customer	Amount
X	£2,000
Y	£3,000

Step 1

Each payment is recorded in the cash book.

Step 2

At the end of the period the cash book is totalled and the total is entered into the purchases ledger control account in the nominal ledger. The individual entries are recorded in the individual creditor accounts in the subsidiary purchases ledger.

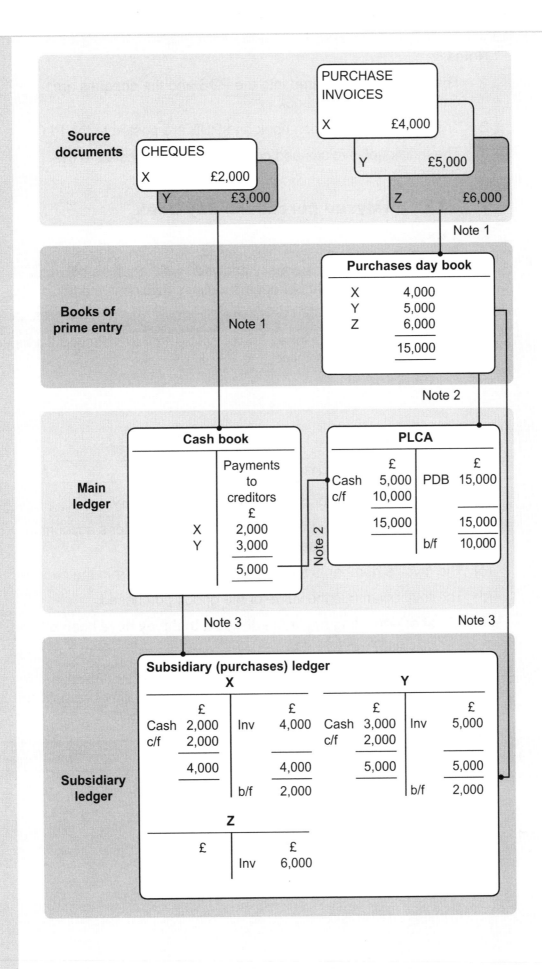

Notes

1 The invoices are entered into the PDB and the cheques are entered into the cash book.

2 The totals from the cash book and PDB are posted to the PLCA.

3 The individual invoices and cash received are posted to the subsidiary (purchases) ledger.

2 The analysed purchases day book

2.1 Layout

The purchases day book is usually analysed with 'analysis columns' showing how the total value of each supplier's invoice is made up.

PURCHASES DAY BOOK								
Date	Supplier	Reference	Invoice number	Total £	VAT £	Product 1 £	Product 2 £	Product 3 £
			TOTALS					

(a) The date and supplier columns are self explanatory.

(b) The reference number is the number of the supplier's account in the subsidiary purchases ledger.

(c) The invoice number is the number of the invoice from the supplier.

(d) The total column is the value of the goods purchased:

  – after deducting any trade discount that may have been offered

  – including VAT

  – and including (i.e. not deducting) any settlement discount that may be offered to the purchaser (we shall not complicate things at this stage by considering this further).

Illustration 1 – The analysed purchases day book

Customer B receives an invoice as follows from supplier X:

	£
50 units at £6 per unit	300
Less: 20% trade discount	60
	240
VAT @ 17.5% (£240 x 17.5%)	42
Total invoice value	282

The £282 would be entered in the 'total' column.

(e) The VAT column – this column is the value of the VAT on the invoice – in this case £42.

(f) Product 1, 2, etc columns – these are columns that analyse the net purchases value (ie the total value after deducting VAT) into groupings that are of interest to the business.

In this introductory section we shall not complicate things by considering more than one type of product so that there will only be one column for purchases.

In this case the entry in the purchases column would be £240.

(g) The total boxes – at the end of a period (say a week or a month) the purchases day book is totalled and the total values of each column are written in the total boxes.

PURCHASES DAY BOOK

Date	Supplier	Reference	Invoice number	Total £	VAT £	Product 1 £	Product 2 £	Product 3 £
	X			282	42	240		
			TOTALS	282	42	240		

The purchases day book would therefore look as follows for the example above:

Note: In the pages that follow we shall concentrate on the basic entries in the purchases day book using only the supplier, total, VAT and one purchases column. This will enable us to concentrate on the simple double entry.

Illustration 2 – The analysed purchases day book

Posting the purchases day book to the accounts in the ledgers

Consider the following purchase invoices received from suppliers by Roberts Metals.

Supplier	Purchases value (ex VAT) £	Trade discount %	Net purchases value £	VAT £	Total £
X	500	10%	450	78.75	528.75
Y	1,750	20%	1,400	245.00	1,645.00
Z	5,000	30%	3,500	612.50	4,112.50

The following three steps are needed to enter this information in the ledger accounts.

Step 1 Write up the purchases day book, and total the columns.

Step 2 Post the totals to the accounts in the main ledger.

Step 3 Post the individual invoices to the subsidiary purchases ledger.

Solution

PURCHASES DAY BOOK

Date	Supplier	Reference	Invoice number	Total £	VAT £	Sales £
	X			528.75	78.75	450.00
	Y			1,645.00	245.00	1,400.00
	Z			4,112.50	612.50	3,500.00
			TOTALS	6,286.25	936.25	5,350.00

Step 1

Main ledger

Purchases		VAT		PLCA	
£	£	£	£	£	£
PDB 5,350.00		PDB 936.25			PDB 6,286.25

Step 2

Subsidiary (purchases) ledger

X		Y		Z	
£	£	£	£	£	£
	PDB 528.75		PDB 1,645.00		PDB 4,112.50

Step 3

Note to solution

(a) The totals of the PDB are entered in the main ledger.

(b) The individual invoices (total value including VAT) are entered in the individual creditor accounts in the subsidiary ledger. This is the amount that will be paid to the creditor.

(c) Note that there are no entries for trade discounts either in the PDB or in the ledger accounts.

Test your understanding 1

An analysed purchases day book has the following totals for a week.

Date	Invoice no	Supplier	Code	Total £	VAT £	Dept 1 £	Dept 2 £	Dept 3 £
		Total		88,125	13,125	20,000	15,000	40,000

How would the totals be posted to the main ledger accounts?

3 Purchases returns – cash customers

3.1 Introduction

When a business buys and then returns goods to a supplier, the accounting system has to record the fact that goods have been returned. If the goods were returned following a cash purchase then cash would be repaid by the supplier to the customer who had bought the goods. If goods were returned following a credit purchase then the supplier's ledger account will need to be debited with the value of the goods returned.

Illustration 2 – Purchases returns – cash customers

Returns following a cash purchase

Y buys £1,000 of goods from B for cash plus £175 VAT.

B subsequently agrees that Y can return £500 worth of goods (excluding VAT).

Record these transactions in the ledger accounts of Y.

Solution

Step 1

First of all we need to set up a new account called the 'purchases returns account' in the main ledger.

Step 2

Enter the cash purchases in the accounts of Y.

Credit cash book for cash paid	£1,175.00
Debit purchases with expense	£1,000.00
Debit VAT account with VAT	£175.00

Cash book

	£		£
		Purchases + VAT	1,175.00

Purchases

	£		£
Cash book	1,000.00		

Purchases returns

	£		£

VAT

	£		£
Cash book	175.00		

Step 3

B will repay Y £500 plus VAT of £87.50. We therefore need to enter the purchase return, the cash and the VAT in the accounts.

Cash book

	£		£
Purchases return + VAT	587.50	Purchases + VAT	1,175.00

Purchases

	£		£
Cash book	1,000.00		

Purchases returns

	£		£
		Cash book	500.00

VAT

	£		£
Cash book	175.00	Cash book	87.50

4 Purchases returns – credit customers

4.1 Introduction

When a credit customer returns goods, he does not receive cash for the return; the seller will issue a credit note to record the fact that goods have been returned. This credit note is sent to the customer and is entered in the customer's books.

4.2 Purchases returns with VAT

When a return is made and we include VAT, the VAT has to be accounted for both on the invoice when the purchase is made, and on the credit note when the goods are returned. This VAT has to be entered in the books.

Illustration 3 – Purchases returns – credit customers

D buys goods from Z for £800 + VAT (= £940).

D returns goods worth £200 + VAT.

Enter these transactions in the main ledger of D's books.

Solution

Step 1

Enter the invoice in the usual way, including the VAT.

PLCA

	£		£
		Purchases	940.00

Purchases

	£		£
PLCA	800.00		

VAT

	£		£
PLCA	140.00		

Step 2

Enter the credit note. The VAT on the return will be £200 × 17.5% = £35. This gives a total credit note of £235.

PLCA

	£		£
Purchases returns	235.00	Purchases	940.00

Purchases

	£		£
PLCA	800.00		

VAT

	£		£
PLCA	140.00	PLCA	35.00

Purchases returns

	£		£
		PLCA	200.00

The books will reflect the position after the return. The balance on the PLCA is £705. This is made up as:

	£
Purchase	800
Purchase return	200
	600
VAT 600 x 17.5%	105
	705

5 The purchases returns day book

5.1 Introduction

Purchases returns are in practice entered in a 'purchases returns day book'. This is similar to the purchases day book, and the columns are used in the same way. The only difference is that instead of having a column for the invoice number, there is a column for the 'credit note number'. This is because when the goods are sent back the business will receive a credit note from the supplier.

PURCHASES RETURNS DAY BOOK						
Date	Supplier	Reference	Credit note number	Total £	VAT £	Purchases returns £

Illustration 4 – The purchase returns day book

John bought goods for £750 + VAT from X and £1,000 + VAT from Y.

John returns goods which cost £200 excluding VAT to X, and goods which cost £400 excluding VAT to Y.

Enter the above purchases and returns in the main and subsidiary ledgers of John, using a purchases returns book.

Solution

Step 1

Enter the original purchases invoices in the main ledger.

PLCA

	£		£
		PDB	2,056.25

Purchases

	£		£
PDB	1,750.00		

VAT

	£		£
PDB	306.25		

Step 2

Write up the purchases returns day book.

PURCHASES RETURNS DAY BOOK

Date	Supplier	Reference	Credit note number	Total £	VAT £	Purchases returns £
	X			235.00	35.00	200.00
	Y			470.00	70.00	400.00
				705.00	105.00	600.00

Step 3

Enter the PRDB totals in the main ledger accounts.

PLCA

	£		£
PRDB	705.00	PDB	2,056.25

Purchases

	£		£
PDB	1,750.00		

VAT

	£		£
PDB	306.25	PRDB	105.00

Purchases returns

	£		£
		PRDB	600.00

Step 4

Enter the individual amounts in the subsidiary purchases ledger. The amounts that will be debited to the individual creditor accounts as the return is reducing the amount that is owed to the creditor.

X

	£		£
PRDB	235.00	PDB (£750 + VAT)	881.25

Y

	£		£
PRDB	470.00	PDB (£1,000 + VAT)	1,175.00

5.2 Purchases returns in purchases day book

In some businesses the level of purchases returns are fairly low and therefore it is not justified to keep a separate purchases returns day book. In these cases any credit notes that are received for purchases returns are recorded as negative amounts in the purchases day book.

Test your understanding 2

Given below are the totals of an analysed purchases returns day book for a week.

Date	Supplier	Credit note no	Code	Total £	VAT £	Dept 1 £	Dept 2 £	Dept 3 £
23/04/X0				9,400	1,400	1,000	2,000	5,000

Post these totals to the main ledger accounts.

chapter 8

Test your understanding 3

1   Does the total column in the analysed purchases day book include or exclude VAT?

2   Why is there no discount received column for settlement discounts in the purchases day book?

3   An analysed purchases day book has the following totals for a week.

Date	Invoice no	Supplier	Code	Total £	VAT £	Dept 1 £	Dept 2 £	Dept 3 £
				19,975	2,975	2,000	5,000	10,000

How would the totals be posted to the main ledger accounts?

4   Given below are the totals of an analysed purchases returns day book for a week.

Date	Supplier	Credit note no	Code	Total £	VAT £	Dept 1 £	Dept 2 £	Dept 3 £
23/04/X0				5,287.50	787.50	500	1,000	3,000

Post these totals to the main ledger accounts.

6   Summary

The purchases day book and the purchases returns day book are simple devices for grouping together purchases invoices for goods purchased and credit notes for goods returned. The topics you need to practise are:

(a) posting the total of these day books to the main ledger accounts, and

(b) posting the individual invoices and credit notes to the creditors accounts in the subsidiary purchases ledger.

It is also useful if you understand how the accounts fit together as shown in the diagram in Section 1.2 of this chapter.

LRS: Somerset College

KAPLAN PUBLISHING

119

The purchases day book – main and subsidiary ledgers

Test your understanding answers

Test your understanding 1

The required double entry is as follows:

Debit		
	VAT	£13,125
	Department 1 purchases	£20,000
	Department 2 purchases	£15,000
	Department 2 purchases	£40,000

Credit	Purchases ledger control account	£88,125

Note carefully that it is the net amount that is debited to each purchases account and the gross amount (including VAT) that is credited to the purchases ledger control account. The VAT total is debited to the VAT account.

The ledger entries would appear as follows:

Purchases ledger control account

	£		£
		PDB	88,125

VAT

	£		£
PDB	13,125		

Department 1 purchases

	£		£
PDB	20,000		

Department 2 purchases

	£		£
PDB	15,000		

Department 3 purchases

	£		£
PDB	40,000		

120

KAPLAN PUBLISHING

Test your understanding 2

Purchases returns – Department 1 account

	£		£
		PRDB	1,000

Purchases returns – Department 2 account

	£		£
		PRDB	2,000

Purchases returns – Department 3 account

	£		£
		PRDB	5,000

VAT account

	£		£
		PRDB	1,400

Purchases ledger control account

	£		£
PRDB	9,400		

Note carefully that it is the net amount that is credited to each returns account and the gross amount to the purchases ledger control account. The difference, the VAT, is credited to the VAT account.

Test your understanding 3

1 Include.

2 There is no discount received column in the purchases day book because for each invoice the amount entered is the total value of the invoice. The value of the invoice which is entered in the day book does not depend on whether the settlement discount is taken or not. Discount received is only accounted for when the payment is made and if the settlement discount is taken it is at this stage that the double entry is put through the main ledger.

3 The required double entry is as follows:

Debit	VAT	£2,975
	Department 1 purchases	£2,000
	Department 2 purchases	£5,000
	Department 2 purchases	£10,00
Credit	Purchases ledger control account	£19,975

Note carefully that it is the net amount that is debited to each purchases account and the gross amount (including VAT) that is credited to the purchases ledger control account. The VAT total is debited to the VAT account.

The ledger entries would appear as follows:

Purchases ledger control account

	£		£
		PDB	19,975

VAT

	£		£
PDB	2,975		

Department 1 purchases

	£		£
PDB	2,000		

Department 2 purchases

	£		£
PDB	5,000		

Department 3 purchases

	£		£
PDB	10,000		

4

Purchases returns – Department 1 account

	£		£
		PRDB	500

Purchases returns – Department 2 account

	£		£
		PRDB	1,000

Purchases returns – Department 3 account

	£		£
		PRDB	3,000

VAT account

	£		£
		PRDB	787.50

Purchases ledger control account

	£		£
PRDB	5,287.50		

The analysed cash payments book

Introduction

In this chapter we will consider how cash payments for cash purchases and to credit suppliers are recorded in the cash payments book and in the ledger accounts.

1 The analysed cash payments book

1.1 Layout

A proforma analysed cash payments book is shown below

CASH PAYMENTS BOOK									
Date	Narrative	Reference	Total £	VAT £	Suppliers/ creditors £	Cash Purchases £	Admin £	Rent and rates £	Discou receive £
		TOTALS							

Notes

(a) The date column contains the date of the transaction.

(b) The narrative column describes the transactions.

(c) The total column contains the total cash paid (including any VAT).

(d) The VAT column contains the VAT on the transaction but not if the VAT has already been entered in the purchases day book. This is a tricky point but is in principle exactly the same as the treatment of VAT that we studied for the cash receipts book.

(e) The suppliers column contains any cash paid that has been paid to a supplier. The total paid including VAT is entered in this column.

(f) The cash purchases column contains cash paid for purchases that are not bought on credit.

(g) We saw with the analysed cash receipts book that nearly all receipts come from debtors or cash sales. In the case of payments, there is a great variety of suppliers who are paid through the cash book; rent and rates, telephone, electricity, marketing, etc. The business will have a separate column for the categories of expense that it wishes to analyse.

1.2 Main ledger payments not entered in the PDB

The PDB is often used only for invoices from suppliers of purchases, i.e. goods for resale. Invoices for rent, electricity, telephone, etc will typically not be entered in the PDB. They will be paid by cheque, and the double entry will be made directly between the cash payments book and the relevant expense account in the main ledger.

One reason for this is that the purchases day book (like the sales day book) is used because the business will typically have a large number of similar transactions (e.g. purchases of goods for resale). To simplify the accounting these are all listed in the PDB and posted in total to the main ledger. Payment of rent or telephone only happens once every three months so there is no need to group these together; they are easily dealt with on an individual basis.

Illustration 1 – The analysed cash payment book

Parma Products buys goods for resale from two suppliers on credit. The business buys £1,000 + VAT of goods from X and £3,000 + VAT of goods from Y. Parma receives an invoice and pays £500 + VAT rent to their landlord. Parma also pays X's invoice in full. Enter these transactions in the accounts of Parma Products. The rent invoice is not entered in the PDB.

Solution

Step 1 Enter the invoices for goods in the PDB

PURCHASES DAY BOOK

Date	Supplier	Reference	Invoice number	Total £	VAT £	Purchases £
	X			1,175	175	1,000
	Y			3,525	525	3,000
				4,700	700	4,000

Step 2 Enter the totals of the PDB in the main ledger.

Purchases

	£		£
PDB	4,000.00		

VAT

	£		£
PDB	700.00		

PLCA

	£		£
		PDB	4,700.00

Step 3 Enter the cash paid in the analysed cash payments book.

CASH PAYMENTS BOOK

Date	Narrative	Reference	Total £	VAT £	Suppliers £	Rent £	Discount received £
	X		1,175.00		1,175.00		
	Rent		587.50	87.50		500.00	
		TOTALS	1,762.50	87.50	1,175.00	500.00	

The analysed cash payments book

Note that the VAT on the payment to the supplier has already been accounted for in the main ledger via the entries in the PDB. However, the rent invoice was not entered in the PDB and so the VAT has to be entered in the VAT column of the cash book from where it will be posted to the VAT account (step 4).

Step 4 Post the cash paid totals from the cash book to the main ledger.

Purchases

	£		£
PDB	4,000.00		

VAT

	£		£
PDB	700.00		
CPB	87.50		

PLCA

	£		£
CPB	1,175.00	PDB	4,700.00

Rent

	£		£
CPB	500.00		

Note 1: All the VAT paid is now debited to the VAT account. You must make sure that you understand how some is posted via the PDB and some via the cash book.

Note 2: All of the entries made from the cash payments book are debit entries. The credit entry is the total of the cash payments (£1,762.50) since the cash payments book is part of the double entry.

Step 5 Enter the amounts in the subsidiary purchases ledger.

X

	£		£
CPB	1,175.00	PDB	1,175.00

Y

	£		£
		PDB	3,525.00

The entries to the subsidiary ledger from the cash payments book are debit entries in the individual creditor accounts as the payment means that less is owed to the creditor.

KAPLAN PUBLISHING

...

2 Settlement discounts received from suppliers

2.1 Introduction

Settlement discounts are a tricky complication when dealing with the analysed purchases day book and cash book.

Illustration 2 – Settlement discounts received from suppliers

Consider a business run by Francis which buys goods costing £2,000 + VAT from Z. Z offers a 5% settlement discount if Francis pays within 30 days. Francis pays within 30 days.

Enter these new transactions in the books of Francis.

Solution

Step 1 Calculate the value of the invoice.

	£
Cost of goods	2,000.00
VAT (2,000 – (5% x 2,000)) x 17.5%	332.50
Total invoice value	2,332.50

Step 2 Enter the invoice from Z in the purchases day book.

PURCHASES DAY BOOK						
Date	Supplier	Reference	Invoice number	Total £	VAT £	Purchases £
	Z			2,332.50	332.50	2,000.00
				2,332.50	332.50	2,000.00

Step 3 Enter the totals of the purchases day book in the main ledger.

Purchases

	£		£
PDB	2,000.00		

VAT

	£		£
PDB	332.50		

PLCA

	£		£
		PDB	2,332.50

Step 4   Calculate the cash paid by Francis.

	£
Cost of goods	2,000.00
5% settlement discount	(100.00)
	1,900.00
VAT (2,000 – (5% × 2,000)) x 17.5%	332.50
Total cash paid	2,232.50

Step 5   Enter the cash paid in the analysed cash payments book.

CASH PAYMENTS BOOK

Date	Narrative	Reference	Total	VAT	Suppliers	Rent	Discount received
			£	£	£	£	£
	Z		2,232.50		2,232.50		100.00
		TOTALS	2,232.50		2,232.50		100.00

Note: Remember that the discount received column is a 'memorandum' account. The cash book only cross-casts if you ignore the discount received column.

Step 6   Post the cash payments book totals to the main ledger.

Purchases

	£		£
PDB	2,000.00		

VAT

	£		£
PDB	332.50		

PLCA

	£		£
CPB	2,232.50	PDB	2,332.50
Discount received	100.00		

Discount received

	£		£
		PLCA	100.00

Test your understanding 1

FFP makes the following payments in respect of various credit invoices and other items:

- Payment of £4,230 on 23/7/X4 to N Hudson for credit purchases. A settlement discount of £130 was taken. This was paid by cheque (cheque number 1003). The purchase ledger reference code is P4153.

- On 24/7/X4, £2,350 to G Farr in respect of an outstanding invoice, by cheque (cheque number 1004). The subsidiary (purchases) ledger reference code is P4778.

- On 28/7/X4, purchase of stock, not on credit, of £940 including VAT of £140 (cheque number 1005).

- On 30/7/X4, payment of a salary by cheque of £2,500, using cheque number 1006. (There is no VAT on wages and salaries.)

Task 1 Enter these transactions in the cash payments book and total the columns.

Task 2 Post the totals to the main ledger.

Task 3 Post the payments to N Hudson and G Farr to the subsidiary (purchases) ledger. The opening balances are N Hudson £10,327.00 and G Farr £8,263.00.

Test your understanding 2

1 Supplier B offers his customer X a 5% settlement discount on an invoice of £1,000 plus VAT if X pays within 30 days. What is the VAT on the invoice?

2 Following on from the question above, if X takes the settlement discount, how much will he pay B?

3 We take a settlement discount of £75 from a supplier when paying an invoice. What is the double entry for this discount?

4 John makes two transactions.

   (a) He pays a rent bill of £150 including VAT which has not been entered in the PDB.

   (b) He pays a supplier £1,175 for an invoice which was entered in the purchases day book.

   Enter these transactions in the cash payments book.

3 Summary

The two main areas covered in this chapter which cause problems are:

(a) the treatment of VAT in the cash payments book; and

(b) the treatment of discount received.

Regarding VAT, remember that if an invoice has been entered in the purchases day book, the VAT will have been captured in the PDB and posted to the VAT account from there. If, however, an invoice is not entered in the purchases day book, the VAT has to be entered in the VAT column of the cash book and posted to the VAT account from there.

Regarding discounts, remember that the discount column in the cash book is simply a memorandum column. The double entry for discount received is entered in the main ledger as: debit PLCA; credit discount received. Remember also that in the subsidiary purchases ledger, the discount received is entered in the suppliers account but there is no corresponding double entry in the discount received account (it has already been posted from the PLCA).

Test your understanding answers

Task 1

ANALYSED CASH PAYMENTS BOOK (CPB)

Date	Cheque number	Payee/ account number	Total £	Creditors £	VAT £	Wages and sala-ries£	Purchases £	Discount received £
23/7/X4	1003	N Hudson, P4153	4,230	4,230				130
24/7/X4	1004	G Farr, P4778	2,350	2,350				
28/7/X4	1005	Purchases	940		140		800	
30/7/X4	1006	Salary	2,500			2,500		
			10,020	6,580	140	2,500	800	130

Task 2

Creditors control account   **2001**

Date	Details	Folio	£	Date	Details	Folio	£
31/7/X4	Bank	CPB	6,580				
31/7/X4	Discounts received	CPB	130				

VAT account   **3215**

Date	Details	Folio	£	Date	Details	Folio	£
31/7/X4	Bank	CPB	140				

Wages and salaries account   **4100**

Date	Details	Folio	£	Date	Details	Folio	£
31/7/X4	Bank	CPB	2,500				

Purchases account   **4200**

Date	Details	Folio	£	Date	Details	Folio	£
31/7/X4	Bank	CPB	800				

Discount received account   **1000**

Date	Details	Folio	£	Date	Details	Folio	£
				31/7/X4	Creditors	CPB	130

N Hudson account   P4153

Date	Details	Folio	£	Date	Details	Folio	£
23/7/X4	Bank	CPB	4,230		b/f		10,327
23/7/X4	Discounts received	CPB	130				

G Farr account   P4778

Date	Details	Folio	£	Date	Details	Folio	£
24/7/X4	Bank	CPB	2,350		b/f		8,263

Test your understanding 2

1    $(£1,000 - (5\% \times £1,000)) \times 17.5\% = £166.25$

2

	£
Cost of goods	1,000.00
Less 5% discount	(50.00)
	950.00
Add VAT	166.25
	1,116.25

3

Purchases ledger control account

	£		£
Discount received	75.00		

Discount received account

	£		£
		PLCA	75.00

4

CASH PAYMENTS BOOK

Date	Narrative	Reference	Total	VAT	Suppliers	Rent	Discount received
			£	£	£	£	£
			150.00	22.34		127.66	
			1,175.00		1,175.00		
			1,325.00	22.34	1,175.00	127.66	

KAPLAN PUBLISHING

10

Credit sales: documents

Introduction

You will be required to deal with many aspects of the sales that a business makes. This will involve the procedure for making the sale and the procedures for receiving the money for the sale.

In this chapter we will take an outline look at the documents required when making a sale.

1 The sales documents

1.1 Introduction

We will now consider the processes involved in making sales to customers. Cash sales are relatively straightforward but credit sales are more involved. The details of all of the aspects covered here will be dealt with in greater depth in later chapters.

1.2 Cash sales

A cash sale will normally be made in a retail environment. A customer will enter the shop, choose the goods they wish to buy then come to the till in order to pay for them. The seller will tell the customer the price of the goods and the customer then offers payment for them.

This may be in the form of notes and coins, in which case it is possible that change will need to be calculated and given to the customer, if they have given more cash than the price of the goods. Most electronic tills calculate the amount of change required and therefore it is a fairly simple task to ensure that the correct amount of change is given.

The customer may alternatively offer to pay for the goods by cheque or by credit or debit card. The detailed procedures for accepting payment by these methods will be considered in later chapters.

Finally, once the customer has paid for the goods, a receipt of some sort will be given to the customer. This may be printed automatically by the till or may be a handwritten receipt in some businesses. The transaction is now complete!

1.3 Credit sales

The procedure for a sale on credit can be rather more involved. The sale process will normally be initiated by the receipt of an order from a customer. This order may be in writing, by fax, over the telephone or by e-mail. When your business receives the order, the first decision that must be made is whether or not to allow the customer credit for this sale.

1.4 Offering credit

Selling goods on credit always involves an element of risk. The goods are being taken away or delivered to the customer now with the promise of payment in the future. Therefore your business must be confident that the payment will be received. The decision process as to whether or not to make the sale on credit will be different depending upon whether this is a sale to an existing credit customer or a new customer.

KAPLAN PUBLISHING

1.5 Existing customers

If an existing credit customer wishes to make a further purchase on credit, it would be normal practice to carry out some basic checks. When the customer was originally taken on as a credit customer, a credit limit will have been set which should not be exceeded. This means that at any time the amount owing from that customer should not exceed the credit limit. Therefore the amount currently owing from the customer should be checked to ensure that the new sale will not take that figure over the credit limit.

It would also be sensible to check that there have been no problems recently with receiving payment from this customer. If the checks are satisfactory then the credit sale can go ahead.

1.6 New customer

If a new customer asks for credit from your business then it would be normal practice to ask the customer to supply some trade references – names of other businesses that they trade with on credit who can vouch for their creditworthiness. Your business may also wish to check the customer's creditworthiness through an agency such as Dun and Bradstreet, or by asking for references from the customer's bank.

If the references and checks are satisfactory then a credit limit will be set for this customer and the sale can go ahead.

2 Summary of a credit sale

The main document flows for a credit sale are illustrated below. The various documents are described in the paragraphs that follow.

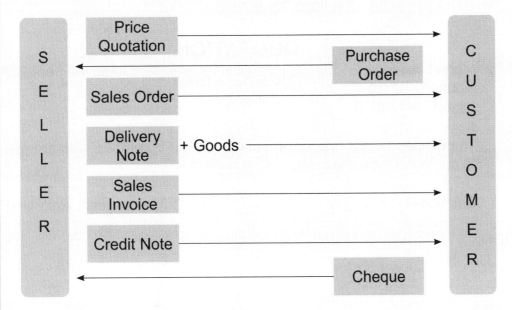

3 Setting up a credit sale

3.1 Price enquiry

The first stage of the process of a credit sale may be the receipt of a price enquiry from a customer.

The price enquiry may be a formal written document or more likely a telephone call. When responding to a price enquiry it is important that you make sure that the price you quote is the correct one as if it is incorrect you may find that you are contracted to sell the goods at that price under contract law (see later chapter in this Study Text).

3.2 Price quotation

In some organisations it is common practice to quote prices to customers over the telephone particularly if there is a catalogue or price list from which there are no deviations in price. However, some businesses will be prepared to offer certain customers goods at different prices. Therefore it is often the case that a price quotation is sent out to a customer showing the price at which the goods that they want can be bought.

A typical price quotation is shown below.

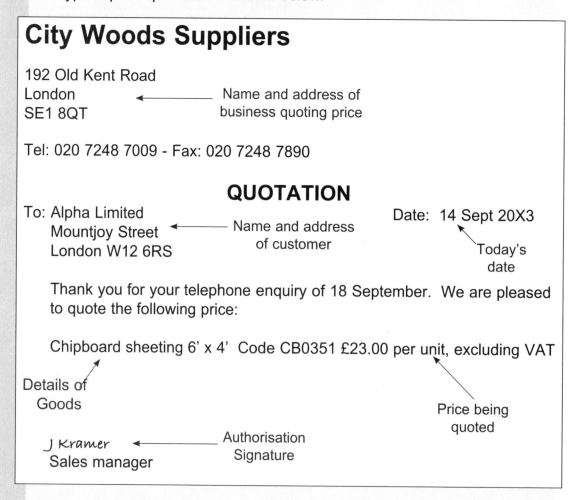

City Woods Suppliers

192 Old Kent Road
London   ←——— Name and address of
SE1 8QT   business quoting price

Tel: 020 7248 7009 - Fax: 020 7248 7890

QUOTATION

To: Alpha Limited   Date: 14 Sept 20X3
    Mountjoy Street ←——— Name and address
    London W12 6RS   of customer   ↖Today's
                                                                    date

Thank you for your telephone enquiry of 18 September. We are pleased to quote the following price:

Chipboard sheeting 6' x 4' Code CB0351 £23.00 per unit, excluding VAT

Details of   ↖
  Goods   Price being
                                                            quoted

  J Kramer ←——— Authorisation
  Sales manager   Signature

The price quotation is an important document as this is the price that your organisation is now contracted to sell the goods at. Therefore it is important that it is authorised by the appropriate person in the organisation.

3.3 The purchase order

If the customer is happy with the price quotation that they have received from your business then they will place a firm order with you. The order may be by telephone or it may be in writing. Whatever method is used for the purchase order, it is important to check all of the details carefully.

- Is the price that which was quoted to the customer?

- Are the delivery terms acceptable?

- Are any discounts

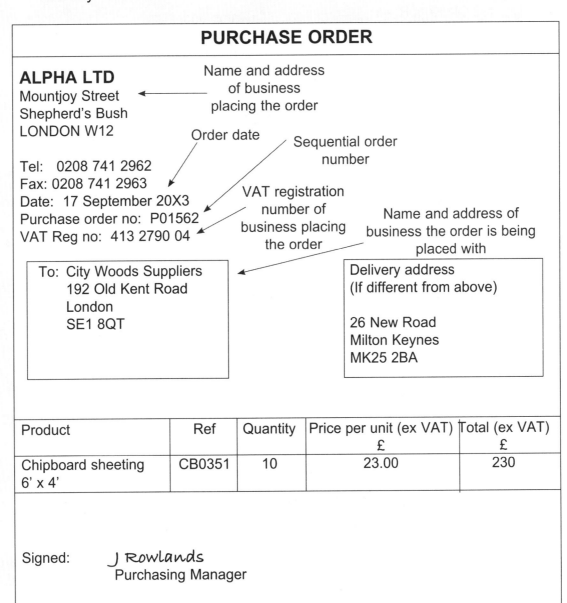

3.4 Confirming sales orders

To avoid misunderstandings, a supplier will normally confirm a customer's order by completing a **sales order**, even if the customer has already sent a written purchase order.

A **sales order** is a document confirming:

*   quantity/type of goods or service

*   date of supply

*   location of supply

*   price and terms.

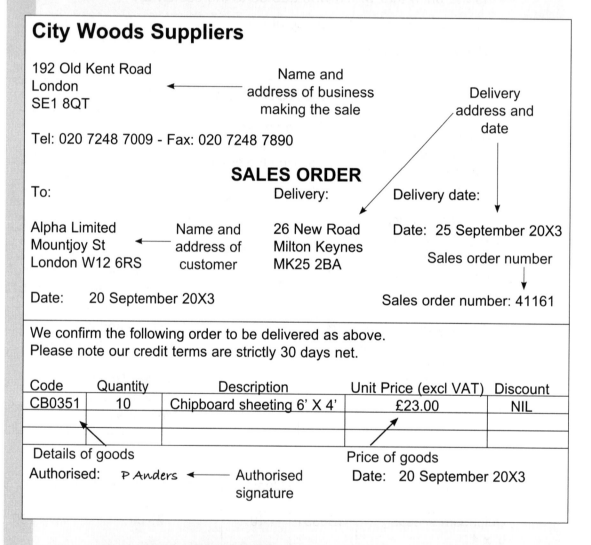

City Woods Suppliers

192 Old Kent Road
London
SE1 8QT

← Name and address of business making the sale

Delivery address and date

Tel: 020 7248 7009 - Fax: 020 7248 7890

SALES ORDER

To: Delivery: Delivery date:

Alpha Limited   Name and   26 New Road   Date: 25 September 20X3
Mountjoy St   ← address of   Milton Keynes
London W12 6RS   customer   MK25 2BA   Sales order number

Date: 20 September 20X3   Sales order number: 41161

We confirm the following order to be delivered as above.
Please note our credit terms are strictly 30 days net.

Code	Quantity	Description	Unit Price (excl VAT)	Discount
CB0351	10	Chipboard sheeting 6' X 4'	£23.00	NIL

Details of goods   Price of goods
Authorised: P Anders ← Authorised   Date: 20 September 20X3
                              signature

4   Supplying the goods

4.1   Introduction

Once all of the negotiations over the price and terms of the credit sale have been completed, then the goods themselves must be delivered.

4.2   Delivery notes

Delivery note – a document accompanying goods despatched to a customer.

Delivery notes should have **sequential numbers** that are either pre-printed for a manual system or computer generated in a computer system, and should be used in order. Spoiled delivery notes should be cancelled and kept.

There will normally be three parts to a delivery note:

Part one   This is kept by the customer in order to compare to the purchase order to ensure that the goods that have been delivered were ordered and then to the sales invoice when they receive it.

Part two   Signed and returned to the supplier of the goods as evidence that they have been received by the customer.

Part three   Signed and kept by the delivery organisation as evidence that they have delivered the goods and that the customer has received them.

City Woods Suppliers

192 Old Kent Road
London
SE1 8QT

Tel: 020 7248 7009 - Fax: 020 7248 7890   DN 005673

DELIVERY NOTE

To: **Delivery:**   **Delivery date:**

Alpha Limited   26 New Road   Date: 25 September 20X3
Mountjoy St   Milton Keynes
London W12 6RS   MK25 2BA

Date: 20 September 20X3   **Sales order number:** 41161

We confirm the following order to be delivered as above.

Product	Code	Quantity
Chipboard 6' x 4'	CB0351	10

Received in good condition: A Patel

4.3 The sales invoice

The next stage is to prepare and send out the sales invoice.

In a manual system, sales invoices must be prepared from the details shown on delivery notes. Delivery notes do not normally show details of prices, discounts or VAT. (This is because the customer might mistake the delivery note for a sales invoice.) Price, discounts and VAT are shown on the sales invoice.

Sales invoices should have **pre-printed sequential numbers** and should be used in order. Spoiled sales invoices should be cancelled and kept.

In a computer system, the sales invoice will generally be produced at the same time as the delivery note and will be identical except that the delivery note may not have details of price, etc.

City Woods Suppliers

192 Old Kent Road
London
SE1 8QT

Tel: 020 7248 7009 - Fax: 020 7248 7890

Invoice no:	I005673
Tax point:	20 September 20X3
VAT reg no:	618 2201 63
Delivery note:	DN005673
Account no:	AL6215

INVOICE

To:

Alpha Limited
Mountjoy St
London W12 6RS

Delivery:

26 New Road
Milton Keynes
MK25 2BA

Delivery date:

Date: 25 September 20X3

Date: 20 September 20X3   **Sales order number:** 41161

We confirm the following order to be delivered as above.

Product	Code	Quantity	Price per unit £	Total £
Chipboard 6' x 4'	CB0351	10	23.00	230.00
			VAT	40.25
				270.25

4.4 Pricing goods and services

Unit prices for goods or services are kept in master files which must be updated regularly. If a price quotation has been sent to a customer then this must be used to find the price to use on the invoice.

Prices will normally be quoted exclusive of value added tax (VAT), as this is the true selling price to the business.

4.5 Customer details

In order to prepare the sales invoice the customer master file must be found. This will show the details of any discounts, etc offered to this customer (see later in this chapter).

4.6 The effect of value added tax

If the selling business is registered for VAT, VAT must be charged on taxable supplies.

Most goods and services are standard-rated (i.e. 17.5% rate of VAT must be charged). This will be considered in more detail later in the chapter.

Test your understanding 1

(AAT CA J92)

List six items of data which you would expect an invoice to contain.

Illustration 1 – Supplying the goods

Preparing a sales invoice

Thelma Goody is the sales invoicing clerk for a clothing wholesaler which trades as a limited company. Thelma prepares the sales invoices to be sent to the customer from the price list and a copy of the delivery note sent up to her by the sales department.

The business is registered for VAT.

Today she has received the following delivery note from the sales department.

Delivery note: 2685

To: Kids Clothes Ltd
       9 Port Street
       MANCHESTER
       M1 5EX

A B Fashions Ltd
3 Park Road
Parkway
Bristol
BR6 6SJ
Tel: 01272 695221
Fax: 01272 695222

Delivery date: 20 August 20X6

Quantity	Code	DESCRIPTION	Colour
90	SSB 330	Shawls (babies)	Assorted
30	CJA 991	Cashmere jumpers (adult)	Cream
30	GGC 442	Gloves (children)	Assorted

Received by: ....

Signature: .... Date: ....

Print name: ....

Code	Description	Colour	Unit price £	VAT rate
SSG 001	Skirt (girls)	Black	13.50	Zero
SSW 002	Skirt (women)	Navy	15.90	Standard
TTW 037	Trousers (women)	Black	21.00	Standard
TTW 038	Trousers (women)	Navy	15.60	Standard
TTW 039	Trousers (women)	Red	15.60	Standard
SSB 330	Shawl (babies)	Assorted	11.50	Zero
SSB 331	Shawl (babies)	White	11.50	Zero
CJA 991	Cashmere jumper (adult)	Cream	65.00	Standard
CJA 992	Cashmere jumper (adult)	Pink	65.00	Standard
CJA 993	Cashmere jumper (adult)	Blue	65.00	Standard
CJA 994	Cashmere jumper (adult)	Camel	65.00	Standard
HHB 665	Hat (babies)	White	3.50	Zero
HHB 666	Hat (babies)	Blue	3.50	Zero
GGC 442	Gloves (children)	Assorted	6.20	Zero
GGC 443	Gloves (children)	White	6.50	Zero
GGC 444	Gloves (children)	Black	6.50	Zero

The customer file shows that Kids Clothes Ltd's account number is KC 0055 and that a trade discount of 10% is offered to this customer.

Thelma must now prepare the sales invoice. Today's date is 22 August 20X6.

Solution

INVOICE

Invoice to:	**AB Fashions Ltd**
	3 Park Road
Kids Clothes Ltd	Parkway
9 Port Street	Bristol BR6 6SJ
Manchester	Tel: 01272 695221
M1 5EX	Fax: 01272 695222

	Invoice no:	95124
Deliver to:	Tax point:	22 August 20X6
	VAT reg no:	488 7922 26
As above	Delivery note no:	2685
	Account no:	KC 0055

Code	Description	Quantity	VAT rate %	Unit price £	Amount excl of VAT £
SSB 330	Shawls (babies) assorted	90	0	11.50	1,035.00
CJA 991	Cashmere Jumper (adult) cream	30	17.5	65.00	1,950.00
GGC 442	Gloves (children) assorted	30	0	6.20	186.00

	3,171.00
Trade discount 10%	(317.10)
VAT at 17.5%	2,853.90
	307.12
Total amount payable	3,161.02

Step 1   Enter today's date on the invoice and the invoice number which should be the next number after the last sales invoice number.

Step 2   Enter the customer details – name, address and account number.

Step 3   Refer now to the delivery note copy and enter the delivery note number and the quantities, codes and descriptions of the goods.

Step 4   Refer to the price list and enter the unit prices of the goods and the rate of VAT (note that the VAT rate for children's clothes is zero).

Step 5   Now for the calculations – firstly multiply the number of each item by the unit price to find the VAT exclusive price – then total these total prices – finally calculate the trade discount as 10% of this total, £3,171 × 10% = £317.10 and deduct it.

Step 6 Calculate the VAT – in this case there is only standard rate VAT on the cashmere jumpers but you must remember to deduct the trade discount (£1,950 – £195) before calculating the VAT amount £1,755 × 17.5% = £307.12 – add the VAT to the invoice total after deducting the trade discount.

Test your understanding 2

A business sells 38 units of a product that is sold for £16.50 per unit and 24 units of a product that is sold for £19.80. The customer is given a 15% trade discount and all of the goods are chargeable to VAT at the standard rate.

Show the figures that would appear on the sales invoice for this sale.

4.7 Other terms found on invoices

You may also find other terms and conditions shown on invoices or other documents. Here are some of the more common:

E & OE – Errors and omissions excepted. The seller is claiming the right to correct any genuine errors on the invoice (e.g. prices) at a later date.

Carriage paid – The invoice value includes delivery of the goods to the customer's premises.

Ex works – Prices quoted do not include delivery to the customer's premises. The customer must organise and pay for the delivery of the goods.

Cash on delivery – The customer is expected to pay for the goods when they are delivered.

Test your understanding 3

A sales order, number 28596, has been received from J Hardy Construction for the following:

    3 Cotswold panels
    5 insulation bricks
    1 red brick roof tile

The file for this customer shows that trade discounts are offered to this customer of 2% and settlement discounts of 3% if payment is within 14 days. The file also includes the customer's address: Poplar Works, Poplar Street, Oldham, OL4 6QB and account number SL07.

An extract from the price list is given.

Description	Code	Unit price £
Insulation bricks	159 SO4	195.50
Red brick roof tiles	874 KL5	56.65
Cotswold panels	950 BB3	300.00

The goods are to be despatched along with despatch note number 68553. The next sales invoice number is 69472. Today's date is 23 August 20X3.

Prepare the sales invoice for this sale on the blank invoice given below.

INVOICE

Invoice to:

A.J. Broom & Company Limited

59 Parkway
Manchester
M2 6EG
Tel: 0161 560 3392
Fax: 0161 560 5322

Deliver to:

Invoice no:
Tax point:
VAT reg no: 625 9911 58
Order no:
Delivery note no:
Account no:

Code	Description	Quantity	VAT rate %	Unit price £	Amount excl of VAT £

Trade discount   %
VAT at 17.5%
Total amount payable
Deduct discount of   % if paid within

5   Issuing credit notes

5.1   Introduction

Credit notes are issued as documentary evidence that goods have been returned and that all or part of a previous sales invoice is cancelled. Therefore a business must keep strict control over the credit notes it issues.

Credit note – Document issued by a supplier to a customer cancelling part or all of a sales invoice.

- business normally issues a credit note:
  - when a customer has returned faulty or damaged goods;
  - when a customer has returned perfect goods by agreement with the supplier; to make a refund for short deliveries; to settle a dispute with a customer.

A credit note is the reversal of a previous invoice or part of the invoice value.

5.2   Return of goods

Returned goods must be inspected, counted and recorded on receipt. They would normally be recorded on a returns inwards note.

5.3   Authorising credit notes

All credit notes must be authorised by a supervisor prior to being issued.

Some credit notes may be issued without a returns inwards note. For example, an error may have been made in pricing on an invoice but the customer is satisfied with the goods and does not need to return them.

These credit notes must be issued only after written authorisation has been received and must be reviewed and approved before being sent to the customer or recorded.

5.4   Preparing credit notes

A credit note is effectively the reverse of an invoice and therefore will tend to include all the details that would normally appear on a sales invoice.

If Alpha Ltd returned two of the chipboard panels, the credit note would be as follows.

KAPLAN PUBLISHING

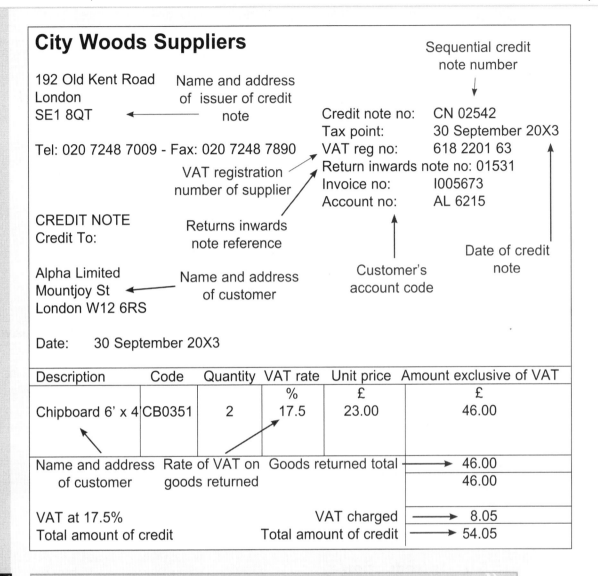

City Woods Suppliers

192 Old Kent Road   Name and address
London   of issuer of credit
SE1 8QT   ←————— note

Tel: 020 7248 7009 - Fax: 020 7248 7890

VAT registration
number of supplier

Sequential credit
note number
↓

Credit note no: CN 02542
Tax point: 30 September 20X3
VAT reg no: 618 2201 63
Return inwards note no: 01531
Invoice no: I005673
Account no: AL 6215

CREDIT NOTE   Returns inwards
Credit To: note reference

Alpha Limited   Name and address
Mountjoy St   ←   of customer
London W12 6RS

Customer's   Date of credit
account code   note

Date: 30 September 20X3

Description	Code	Quantity	VAT rate	Unit price	Amount exclusive of VAT
			%	£	£
Chipboard 6' x 4	CB0351	2	17.5	23.00	46.00

Name and address Rate of VAT on Goods returned total → 46.00
   of customer   goods returned   46.00

VAT at 17.5%   VAT charged → 8.05
Total amount of credit   Total amount of credit → 54.05

Test your understanding 4

You work for A J Broom & Company Limited and have returns inwards note number 01532 in front of you and you have to prepare a credit note to send to K Phipps Builders for one insulation brick, code 159 SO4, that was damaged. The unit price of the insulation brick is £195.50.

The customer file shows that a trade discount of 5% is given to this customer but no settlement discount. The file also shows the customer's address: Hayward House, Manor Estate, Oldham, OL7 4HD, and the customer's account number SL35.

The next credit note number to use is CN 02543 and today's date is 25 August 20X3.

Prepare the credit note on the blank form provided.

CREDIT NOTE

Credit note to:

A.J. Broom & Company Limited
59 Parkway
Manchester
M2 6EG
Tel: 0161 560 3392
Fax: 0161 560 5322

Credit note no:
Tax point:
VAT reg no: 625 9911 58
Returns inwards note no:
Account no:

Code	Description	Quantity	VAT rate %	Unit price £	Amount exclusive of VAT £

Trade discount %	
VAT at 17.5%	
Total amount of credit	

6   Coding sales invoices

6.1   Introduction

Sales invoices should be coded to show:

- product group/type for analysis of sales

- customer account number.

There are several different systems of coding which can be used by a business and the main ones are outlined below.

6.2   Sequence codes

Allocate a number, or a letter, to items in a simple list.

For example:

Code	Name
01	ADAMS, Joan
02	AITKEN, James
03	ALCOCK, Freda
04	BROWN, Joe

6.3 Block codes

These allocate bands of numbers to particular categories.

For example, consider a tobacco manufacturer who produces several types of cigarettes, cigars and pipe tobaccos. He could assign a code to each particular brand as follows:

Product type	Block code
Cigarette	01 – 19
Cigar	20 – 29
Pipe tobacco	30 – 39

6.4 Significant digit codes

These are a particular type of group classification code where individual digits and letters are used to represent features of the coded item. The example given is one used to describe different kinds of vehicle tyres.

Code	Item
TT67015B	Tube Tyre 670 × 15 Blackwall
LT67015W	Tubeless Tyre 670 × 15 Whitewall

6.5 Faceted codes

Faceted codes are another type of group classification code by which the digits of the code are divided into facets of several digits and each facet represents some attribute of the item being coded. These codes are similar to significant digit codes but are purely numerical.

Example: faceted code for types of carpet

Facet 1 = type of weave (1 digit)   1 = cord
2 = twist
3 = short tufted, etc

Facet 2 = material (1 digit)   1 = all wool
2 = 80% wool, 20% nylon
3 = 50% wool, 50% nylon, etc

Facet 3 = pattern (2 digits)   01 = self colour (plain)
02 = self colour (embossed)
03 = fig leaf, etc

Facet 4 = colour (2 digits)   01 = off white
02 = bright yellow
03 = scarlet, etc

A typical code would be 220302 representing a twist carpet in 80% wool, 20% nylon, pattern fig leaf and colour bright yellow.

Note that a two-digit facet allows up to 100 different codings (00 to 99).

6.6 Decimal codes (or hierarchical codes)

These are yet another form of a group classification code. The most obvious example of a decimal code is the Universal Decimal Code (UDC) devised by Dewey and widely used for the classification of books in libraries. UDC divides all human knowledge into more and more detailed categories as shown.

Code	Item
3	Social science
37	Education
372	Elementary
372.2	Kindergarten
372.21	Methods
372.215	Songs and games

Whatever the coding system that is used it is important for further accounting purposes that the invoices and credit notes are coded according to type of sales and the particular customer.

You may be expected to code items included on sales invoices or credit notes according to a coding system that is given to you in an assessment.

Test your understanding 5

Is the cheque number used in a cheque book an example of a sequential code or a hierarchical code?

Test your understanding 6

1   What are the key features that would appear on a sales order?

2   What is a settlement discount?

3   How is a trade discount treated on a sales invoice?

4   Goods have a list price of £268.45 exclusive of VAT. How much VAT at the standard rate should be charged on these goods?

5   Goods have a total VAT inclusive price of £138.65. How much VAT is included in this price?

6   23 items with a list price of £18.60 each have been sent to a customer. A 15% trade discount is allowed to this customer and the goods are all standard rated for VAT purposes. What is the invoice total?

7   14 items at a list price of £23.50 each have been delivered to a customer. The customer is offered a 3% settlement discount and the goods are standard rated for VAT purposes. What is the invoice total?

8   What does the phrase 'E&OE' mean on an invoice?

9   Give three examples of when a credit note might be issued.

10   What are the main items that should be coded on a sales invoice?

7   Summary

In this chapter we have concentrated on the process of actually preparing sales invoices and credit notes. Before preparing an invoice it is necessary to ensure that this is for a valid sale by checking the order and delivery details. When preparing the invoice you need to understand the difference between trade discounts and settlement discounts and their treatment on the invoice and for VAT purposes. You also need to be able to correctly find the price of items from a price list and to correctly transfer this to the invoice together with correct multiplication to arrive at the total. No invoice or credit note should be sent out unless it has been properly authorised and it will also need to be coded to ensure that it is eventually correctly recorded in the accounting records.

Test your understanding answers

Test your understanding 1

Any six from:	Date
	Invoice number
	Customer name and address
	Seller's name and address
	VAT details
	Terms of payment
	Purchase order number
	Number of items that were sold
	Price per item
	Description of goods
	Total amount payable

Test your understanding 2

	£
38 units × £16.50	627.00
24 units × £19.80	475.20
	1,102.20
Less: Trade discount	165.33
	936.87
VAT	163.95
	1,100.82

KAPLAN PUBLISHING

INVOICE

Invoice to:
J Hardy Construction
Poplar Works
Poplar Street
Oldham OL4 6QB

A.J. Broom & Company Limited
59 Parkway
Manchester
M2 6EG
Tel: 0161 560 3392
Fax: 0161 560 5322

Deliver to:
As above

Invoice no:	69472
Tax point:	23 August 20X3
VAT reg no:	625 9911 58
Order no:	28596
Delivery note no:	68553
Account no:	SL07

Code	Description	Quantity	VAT rate %	Unit price £	Amount excl of VAT £
950 BB3	Cotswold Panels	3	17.5	300.00	900.00
159 S04	Insulation Bricks	5	17.5	195.50	977.50
874 KL5	Red Brick Roof Tiles	1	17.5	56.65	56.65
					1,934.15

Trade discount 2%

38.68
1,895.47

VAT at 17.5% *
Total amount payable
Deduct discount of 3% if paid within 14 days

321.75
2,217.22

* VAT is calculated as 17.5% × (£1,895.47 × 0.97), i.e. assuming that the settlement discount is taken.

Note that the trade discount is deducted on the face of the invoice whereas the only effect of the settlement discount is in the calculation of the VAT.

CREDIT NOTE

Credit note to:
K Phipps Builders
Hayward House
Manor Estate
Oldham
OL7 4HD

A.J. Broom & Company Limited
59 Parkway
Manchester
M2 6EG
Tel: 0161 560 3392
Fax: 0161 560 5322

Credit note no:	CN02543
Tax point:	25 August 20X3
VAT reg no:	625 9911 58
Returns inwards note no:	01532
Account no:	SL35

Code	Description	Quantity	VAT rate %	Unit price £	Amount exclusive of VAT £
159 S04	Insulation Brick	1	17.5	195.50	195.50

	195.50
Trade discount 5%	9.77
	185.73
VAT at 17.5%	32.50
Total amount of credit	218.23

Test your understanding 5

A sequential code (the numbers run in sequential order).

KAPLAN PUBLISHING

Test your understanding 6

1 – Quantity and type of goods

  – Date of supply

  – Location of supply

  – Price and terms

  – Delivery address

  – Name and address of seller

  – Name and address of buyer

  – Sales order number

  – Authorisation

2 A settlement discount is a discount that is offered to a customer for payment of the invoice within a certain time period.

3 A trade discount is deducted from the list price of the goods on a sales invoice.

4 £268.45 × 17.5/100   = £46.97 (remember to round down)

5 £138.65 × 17.5/117.5 = £20.65

6

	£
23 × £18.60	427.80
Trade discount@ 15%	(64.17)
	363.63
VAT @ 17.5%	63.63
Invoice total	427.26

7

	£
14 × £23.50	329.00
VAT (17.5% × (£329 × 97%)	55.84
Invoice total	384.84

8 Errors and omissions excepted.

9 – When a customer has returned faulty or damaged goods

  – As a refund for short delivery

  – To settle a dispute with a customer

10 – Type of product

  – Type of sale

  – Customer account number

Debtors' statements

Introduction

In this chapter we consider communication with our debtors. If we are to receive the money owed to us on time it is important to ensure that the customers are fully aware of the amount they owe us and our credit terms.

1 Accounting for credit sales and receipts from customers

1.1 Introduction

Before we consider the preparation of debtors' statements, we will firstly bring together all of the accounting that has taken place for credit sales and receipts from credit customers in one example so that you can see how it all fits together. It is important that you understand how the amount owed by customers is calculated and recorded.

Illustration 1 – Acounting for credit sales and receipts from customers

Given below is the sales day book, sales returns day book and cash receipts book for the first month of trading by Nick Brookes.

Sales day book

Date	Invoice No	Customer name	Code	Total	VAT	Net
20X2				£	£	£
03/04	001	Mayer Ltd	SL1	185.65	27.65	158.00
04/04	002	Elizabeth & Co	SL2	257.34	37.34	220.00
07/04	003	Hofen Partners	SL3	129.25	19.25	110.00
10/04	004	Penken Bros	SL4	157.91	22.91	135.00
14/04	005	Mayer Ltd	SL1	206.80	30.80	176.00
18/04	006	Hofen Partners	SL3	122.20	18.20	104.00
21/04	007	Mayer Ltd	SL1	253.80	37.80	216.00
24/04	008	Penken Bros	SL4	167.27	24.27	143.00
26/04	009	Mayer Ltd	SL1	192.70	28.70	164.00
28/04	010	Elizabeth & Co	SL2	233.95	33.95	200.00
28/04	011	Penken Bros	SL4	138.03	20.03	118.00
				2,044.90	300.90	1,744.00

Sales returns day book

Date	CN No	Customer name	Code	Total	VAT	Net
20X2				£	£	£
10/04	CN001	Mayer Ltd	SL1	49.35	7.35	42.00
17/04	CN002	Penken Bros	SL4	39.77	5.77	34.00
				89.12	13.12	76.00

Cash receipts book						
Date	Narrative	Total	VAT	Debtors	Cash sales	Discount
			£	£	£	£
20X2						
07/04	Cash sales	374.23	55.73		318.50	
15/04	Elizabeth & Co	250.74		250.74		6.60
18/04	Mayer Ltd	136.30		136.30		
21/04	Cash sales	566.93	84.43		482.50	
21/04	Penken Bros	115.11		115.11		3.03
28/04	Hofen Partners	129.25		129.25		
		1,572.56	140.16	631.40	801.00	9.63

Solution

First we must post the totals from each of the books of prime entry to the main ledger accounts. As this is the first month of trading there will of course be no opening balances on any of the ledger accounts.

Sales ledger control account

		£			£
30/04	SDB	2,044.90	30/04	SRDB	89.12
			30/04	CRB	631.40
			30/04	CRB – discount	9.63

VAT account

		£			£
30/04	SRDB	13.12	30/04	SDB	300.90
			30/04	CRB	140.16

Sales account

		£			£
			30/04	SDB	1,744.00
			30/04	CRB	801.00

Sales returns account

		£		£
30/04	SRDB	76.00		

Discounts allowed account

		£		£
30/04	CRB	9.63		

Once the entries have been made in total to the main ledger accounts then each individual invoice, credit note, cash receipt and discount must be entered into the individual debtor accounts in the subsidiary ledger.

Mayer Ltd

		£			£
03/04	001	185.65	10/04	CN001	49.35
14/04	005	206.80	18/04	CRB	136.30
21/04	007	253.80			
26/04	009	192.70			

Elizabeth & Co

		£			£
04/04	002	257.34	15/04	CRB	250.74
28/04	010	233.95	15/04	CRB – discount	6.60

Hofen Partners

		£			£
07/04	003	129.25	28/04	CRB	129.25
18/04	006	122.20			

Penken Bros

		£			£
10/04	004	157.91	17/04	CN002	39.77
24/04	008	167.27	21/04	CRB	115.11
28/04	011	138.03	21/04	CRB – discount	3.03

From this you can see how the full accounting system for credit sales works and the information that is accumulated in each of the individual debtor accounts in the subsidiary ledger.

2   Debtors' statements

2.1   Introduction

The sales ledger clerk prepares monthly statements to send to debtors:

- to remind them that certain invoices are due for payment;
- to reconfirm amounts outstanding where credit notes have been issued.

A **statement** is a document issued (normally monthly) by a supplier to a customer showing unpaid sales invoices and the amount due in total.

2.2   Layout of statement

Statements can be prepared in a number of different ways. Some also have remittance advices attached to them in order to encourage early payment.

A remittance advice is a blank document that the customer fills out when making a payment to the supplier. It shows the total payment being made and which invoices (less credit notes) the payment is paying off.

2.3 Preparing a debtors' statement

A debtors' statement will normally be prepared from the information in the debtors' individual account in the subsidiary ledger. Different businesses will use different formats but the basics that must be shown are all invoices, credit notes, payments received and discounts for the period together with usually a running total of the balance.

2.4 Procedure for preparing a debtors' statement

When preparing a statement for a credit customer, it is important that all details are correct therefore a logical and accurate approach is required.

Step 1 Find the customer's account in the filing system for the subsidiary ledger.

Step 2 Work through the account by date order listing each transaction in turn on the statement – invoices as a debit and credit notes, payments and discounts as credits.

Step 3 Return to the start of the statement and calculate the balance at each transaction date to appear in the balance column.

Illustration 2 – Debtors' statements

Given below are the subsidiary ledger accounts for two of Nick Brookes' customers. We will start by balancing each account to show the total amount due by each customer.

Mayer Ltd   SL01

		£			£
03/04	001	185.65	10/04	CN001	49.35
14/04	005	206.80	18/04	CRB	136.30
21/04	007	253.80			
26/04	008	192.70		Balance c/d	653.30
		838.95			838.95
Balance b/d		653.30			

Penken Bros   SL04

		£			£
10/04	004	157.91	17/04	CN002	39.77
24/04	008	167.27	21/04	CRB	115.11
28/04	011	138.03	21/04	CRB – discount	3.03
				Balance b/d	305.30
		463.21			463.21
Balance c/d		305.30			

We can now use this information to prepare statements for these two customers as at the end of April 20X2.

Solution

		NICK BROOKES
To:	Mayer Ltd	225 School Lane
		Weymouth
		Dorset WE36 5NR
		Tel: 0149 29381
		Fax: 0149 29382
		Date: 30/04/X2

	STATEMENT			
Date	**Transaction**	**Debit** £	**Credit** £	**Balance** £
03/04	INV001	185.65		185.65
10/04	CN001		49.35	136.30
14/04	INV005	206.80		343.10
18/04	Payment		136.30	206.80
21/04	INV007	253.80		460.60
26/04	INV008	192.70		653.30

May we remind you that our credit terms are 30 days
With 3% discount for payment within 14 day

		NICK BROOKES
To:	Penken Bros	225 School Lane
		Weymouth
		Dorset WE36 5NR
		Tel: 0149 29381
		Fax: 0149 29382
		Date: 30/04/X2

	STATEMENT			
Date	**Transaction**	**Debit** £	**Credit** £	**Balance** £
10/04	INV004	157.91		157.91
17/04	CN002		39.77	118.14
21/04	Payment		115.11	
21/04	Discount		3.03	0.00
24/04	INV008	167.27		167.27
28/04	INV011	138.03		305.30

May we remind you that our credit terms are 30 days
With 3% discount for payment within 14 days

These are documents that are being sent to customers, therefore it is extremely important that it is completely accurate. Always check your figures and additions.

You are to prepare a statement to be sent out to one customer, Jack Johnson, for the month of May 20X6. At the start of May this customer did not owe your business, Thames Traders, any money. The subsidiary ledger account for Jack for the month of May is given below.

Jack Johnson

Date		£	Date		£
03 May	Invoice 1848	38.79	08 May	Credit note 446	12.40
07 May	Invoice 1863	50.70	15 May	Cash receipt	77.09
10 May	Invoice 1870	80.52	24 May	Credit note 458	16.50
18 May	Invoice 1881	42.40			
23 May	Invoice 1892	61.20			
30 May	Invoice 1904	27.65			

You are required to prepare a statement for Jack on the blank statement given below.

Thames Traders

To: Date:

STATEMENT

Date	Transaction £	Debit £	Credit £	Balance £

May we remind you that our credit terms are 30 day

3 Communication with customers

If there is a problem with a customer's balance then it will be normal practice to write a polite letter to the customer requesting payment and enquiring if there is any problem with the amounts shown in the statement. If there are no problems or disputed invoices but payment is still not received within a reasonable time then this initial letter should be followed by a letter with a firmer tone requesting payment. This may include a statement that the matter will be put into the hands of your business's solicitors if payment if not received. However, this will be a matter of policy within each business.

Illustration 3 – Communication with customers

You are the credit controller for GoGo Limited, a wholesaler of discount children's clothing. You have been reviewing the aged debtors' listing. The following customer is causing you concern:

	Total £	Current £	30+ days £	60+ days £
Candy Limited	556.78	0	0	556.78

You must write a letter to this customer to ask for payment.

Solution

GoGo Limited
225 Western Road
Anytown
Anyshire AN1 2RN

Creditors' Ledger Clerk   23 August 20X4
Candy Limited
53 High Street
Anytown
Anyshire AN1 6BN

Dear Sir

Outstanding balance

According to our records your company has an outstanding balance of £556.78.

Our normal credit terms are 30 days. As this debt is now over 60 days old we would be very grateful if you could send us your payment immediately.

If you have any queries please do not hesitate to contact me.

Yours faithfully

AN Smith

Credit Controller

Do not be tempted to write a letter that sounds angry or threatening. Polite efficiency is what is required.

KAPLAN PUBLISHING

Test your understanding 2

The following is an extract from an aged debt analysis report prepared on 1 June.

Name	Balance £	Up to 1 month £	Up to 3 months £	Over 3 months £
West & Co	4,860	3,400	1,460	0
Star Limited	2,719	0	0	2,719
Norwood Limited	3,116	1,200	1,900	16
Just Electric	1,391	1,320	0	71

(a) **With which one of the four accounts might you be most concerned?**

(b) **Explain briefly the reason for your answer.**

Test your understanding 3

1   **What is the procedure for preparing a debtor's statement?**

2   **What is a debtor's statement?**

4   Summary

In this chapter all of the accounting entries for sales invoices, credit notes and receipts from debtors were brought together. We also saw how to produce a statement to be sent to a customer from the customer's account in the subsidiary ledger.

We have also introduced an aged debt analysis. You do not need to be able to produce one but you do need to be able to use it to determine any customers who appear to be causing problems with debt collection. It is important when communicating with customers that you deal effectively but politely at all times.

Test your understanding answers

Test your understanding 1

Thames Traders

To: Jack Johnson

Date: 31 May 20X6

STATEMENT

Date	Transaction	Debit £	Credit £	Balance £
03 May	Inv 1848	38.79		38.79
07 May	Inv 1863	50.70		89.49
08 May	CN 446		12.40	77.09
10 May	Inv 1870	80.52		157.61
15 May	Payment		77.09	80.52
18 May	Inv 1881	42.40		122.92
23 May	Inv 1892	61.20		184.12
24 May	CN 458		16.50	167.62
30 May	Inv 1904	27.65		195.27

May we remind you that our credit terms are 30 days

Test your understanding 2

(a) Star Limited

(b) The balance has been outstanding for over three months with no sales since.

Test your understanding 3

1 – Find the customer's account in the subsidiary ledger.

  – List each transaction in turn on the statement.

  – Calculate the balance after each transaction.

2 A debtor's statement is a document sent to a customer detailing unpaid invoices and the total amount due.

12

Accounting for sales – summary

Introduction

We have studied the double entry bookkeeping for sales and receipts in detail at the start of this book.

At that time we concentrated on the basic entries so that the double entry would be clear. It is now time to 'put some flesh on the bones' and study these transactions again using more realistic material.

1   The sales day book

Illustration 1 – The sales day book

Given below are three invoices that have been sent out by your organisation today. You are required to record them in the sales day book

---

INVOICE

Invoice to:	**A.J. Broom & Company Limited**
T J Builder	59 Parkway Manchester
142/148 Broadway	M2 6EG
Oldham	Tel: 0161 560 3392
OD7 6LZ	Fax: 0161 560 5322

Deliver to:		
As above	Invoice no:	69489
	Tax point:	28 August 20X3
	VAT reg no:	625 9911 58
	Delivery note no:	68612
	Account no:	SL21

Code	Description	Quantity	VAT rate %	Unit price £	Amount exclusive of VAT £
874 KL7	Brown Brick Roof Tiles	40	17.5	43.95	1,758.00

	1,758.00
Trade discount 5%	87.90
	1,670.10
VAT at 17.5%	283.49
Total amount payable	1,953.59

Deduct discount of 3% if paid within 21 days

INVOICE

Invoice to:	**A.J. Broom & Company Limited**
McCarthy & Sons	59 Parkway Manchester M2 6EG
Shepherds Moat	Tel: 0161 560 3392
Manchester M6 9LF	Fax: 0161 560 5322

Deliver to:		
	Invoice no:	69490
	Tax point:	28 August 20X3
As above	VAT reg no:	625 9911 58
	Delivery note no:	68610
	Account no:	SL08

Code	Description	Quantity	VAT rate %	Unit price £	Amount exclusive of VAT £
617 BB8	Red Wall Bricks	400	17.5	2.10	840.00
294 KT6	Insulation Brick	3	17.5	149.90	449.70

	1,289.70
Trade discount 4%	51.58
	1,238.12
VAT at 17.5%	216.67
Total amount payable	1,454.79

INVOICE

Invoice to:	A.J. Broom & Company Limited
Trevor Partner	59 Parkway Manchester
Anderson House	M2 6EG
Bank Street	Tel: 0161 560 3392
Manchester M1 9FP	Fax: 0161 560 5322

Deliver to:	Invoice no:	69491
As above	Tax point:	28 August 20X3
	VAT reg no:	625 9911 58
	Delivery note no:	68613
	Account no:	SL10

Code	Description	Quantity	VAT rate %	Unit price £	Amount exclusive of VAT £
611 TB4	Bathroom Tiles	160	17.5	5.65	904.00
					904.00
Trade discount 2%					18.08
					885.92
VAT at 17.5%					151.93
Total amount payable					1,037.85

Deduct discount of 2% if paid within 21 days

Solution

Sales day book						
Date	Invoice No	Customer name	Code	Total £	VAT £	Net £
28/08/X3	69489	T J Builder	SL21	1,953.59	283.49	1,670.10
28/08/X3	69490	McCarthy & Sons	SL08	1,454.79	216.67	1,238.12
28/08/X3	69491	Trevor Partner	SL10	1,037.85	151.93	885.92

2 The analysed sales day book

2.1 Introduction

Many organisations analyse their sales into different groups. This may be analysis by different products or by the geographical area in which the sale is made. If the sales are eventually to be analysed in this manner in the accounting records then they must be analysed in the original book of prime entry, the sales day book.

Illustration 2 – The analysesd sales day book

You work for an organisation that makes sales to five different geographical regions. You are in charge of writing up the sales day book and you have listed out the details of the invoices sent out yesterday, 15 August 20X1. They are given below and must be entered into the sales day book and the totals of each column calculated.

The invoice details are as follows:

	£
Invoice number 167 – France	
Worldwide News – (Code W5)	
Net total	2,500.00
VAT	437.50
Gross	2,937.50
Invoice number 168 – Spain	
Local News – (Code L1)	
Net total	200.00
VAT	35.00
Gross	235.00
Invoice number 169 – Germany	
The Press Today – (Code P2)	
Net total	300.00
VAT	52.50
Gross	352.50
Invoice number 170 – Spain	
Home Call – (Code H1)	
Net total	200.00
VAT	35.00
Gross	235.00
Invoice number 171 – France	
Tomorrow – (Code T1)	
Net total	100.00
VAT	17.50
Gross	117.50
Invoice number 172 – Russia	
Worldwide News – (Code W5)	
Net total	3,000.00
VAT	525.00
Gross	3,525.00

Solution

Sales day book										
Date	Invoice No	Customer name	Code	Total	VAT	Russia	Poland	Spain	Germany	France
15/08/X1	167	Worldwide	W5	2,937.50	437.50					2,500.00
	168	Local News	L1	235.00	35.00			200.00		
	169	The Press Today	P2	352.50	52.50				300.00	
	170	Home Call	H1	235.00	35.00			200.00		
	171	Tomorrow	T1	117.50	17.50					100.00
	172	Worldwide News	W5	3,525.00	525.00	3,000.00				
				7,402.50	1,102.50	3,000.00	–	400.00	300.00	2,600.00

When you have totalled the columns you can check your additions by 'cross-casting'. If you add together the totals of all of the analysis columns and the VAT column, they should total the figure in the 'Total' column.

Test your understanding 1

Sweepings Ltd is a wall covering manufacturer. It produces four qualities of wallpaper:

01	–	Anaglypta
02	–	Supaglypta
03	–	Lincrusta
04	–	Blown Vinyl

Francis is a sales ledger clerk and he is required to write up the sales day book each week from the batch of sales invoices he receives from the sales department.

He has just received this batch of sales invoices which show the following details. All sales are standard-rated for VAT.

Invoice no	Date	Customer	Description	Amount (inc VAT) £
1700	06.09.X1	Gates Stores	Anaglypta, 188 rolls	470.00
1701	06.09.X1	Texas	Blown Vinyl, 235 rolls	1,762.50
1702	07.09.X1	Dickens	Blown Vinyl, 188 rolls	1,410.00
1703	07.09.X1	Hintons DIY	Supaglypta, 470 rolls	1,880.00
1704	08.09.X1	Co-op Stores	Anaglypta, 94 rolls	235.00
1705	08.09.X1	B & Q Stores	Lincrusta, 125 rolls	1,175.00
1706	09.09.X1	Ferris Décor	Supaglypta, 235 rolls	940.00
1707	09.09.X1	Ferris Décor	Blown Vinyl, 94 rolls	705.00
1708	10.09.X1	Homestyle	Lincrusta, 25 rolls	235.00
1709	10.09.X1	Quick Style	Anaglypta, 47 rolls	117.50

Show how this information would appear in the sales day book given below, including the totals of the relevant columns.

Sales day book

Date	Invoice	Customer	Code	Total	VAT	Group 01	Group 02	Group 03	Group 04
				£	£	£	£	£	£

Test your understanding 2

Given below are the totals from the analysed sales day book for an organisation for a week.

Sales day book

	Gross £	VAT £	Sales Type 1 £	Sales Type 2 £
Totals	8,471.75	1,261.75	4,320.00	2,890.00

You are required to post these totals to the main ledger accounts given below:

SLCA account

£		£

Sales – Type 1 account

£		£

Sales – Type 2 account

£		£

VAT account

£		£

3   The sales returns day book

3.1   Introduction

When goods are returned by customers and credit notes sent out then these credit notes are also recorded in their own book of prime entry, the sales returns day book.

3.2   Sales returns day book

The sales returns day book is effectively the reverse of the sales day book but will have the same entries, the total of the credit note, including VAT, the VAT element and the net amount, excluding the VAT.

Accounting for sales – summary

Illustration 3 – The sale return day book

Given below are the totals from three credit notes that your organisation has sent out this week, the week ending 21 January 20X4. They are to be recorded in the sales returns day book.

Credit note no:	03556	To: J Slater & Co	Code: SL67

	£
Goods total	126.45
VAT	22.12
Credit note total	148.57

Credit note no:	03557	To: Paulsons	Code: SL14

	£
Goods total	58.40
VAT	10.22
Credit note total	68.62

Credit note no:	03558	To: Hudson & Co	Code: SL27

	£
Goods total	104.57
VAT	18.29
Credit note total	122.86

Solution

Sales returns day book

Date	Credit note no	Customer name	Code	Total £	VAT £	Net £
21/01/X4	03556	J Slater & Co	SL67	148.57	22.12	126.45
21/01/X4	03557	Paulsons	SL14	68.62	10.22	58.40
21/01/X4	03558	Hudson & Co	SL27	122.86	18.29	104.57

3.3 Analysed sales returns day book

If the business keeps an analysed sales day book then it will also analyse its sales returns day book in exactly the same manner.

Illustration 4 – The sale return day book

In an earlier example we considered the sales day book for an organisation that makes sales to five different geographical regions. The sales returns day book would also be analysed into these geographical regions. The details of two credit notes issued this week are given and are to be written up in the sales returns day book. Today's date is 21 October 20X6.

Credit note no: 0246 - Poland	To: Russell & Sons	Code: R3
	£	
Goods total	85.60	
VAT	14.98	
	100.58	

Credit note no: 0247 - Germany	To: Cleansafe	Code: C7
	£	
Goods total	126.35	
VAT	22.11	
	148.46	

Solution

Sales returns day book										
Date	Credit	Customer	Code	Total	VAT	Russia	Poland	Spain	Germany	France
21/10/X6	0246	Russell & Sons	R03	100.58	14.98		85.60			
21/10/X6	0247	Cleansafe	C07	148.46	22.11				126.35	

Test your understanding 3

A business analyses its sales into Product 1 sales and Product 2 sales. During the week ending 14 March 20X4 the following credit notes were sent out to customers.

CN3066
£120.00 plus VAT – Product 2, Customer K Lilt, Code L04
CN3067
£16.00 plus VAT – Product 1, Customer J Davis, Code D07
CN3068
£38.00 plus VAT – Product 1, Customer I Oliver, Code O11
CN3069
£80.00 plus VAT – Product 2, Customer D Sharp, Code S02

Enter the credit notes in the analysed sales returns day book given below and total the day book for the week.

Sales returns day book

Date	Credit Note No	Customer Name	Code	Total £	VAT £	Product 1 £	Product 2 £

Test your understanding 4

Given below are the totals from the analysed sales returns day book for an organisation for a week:

Date	Customer Name	Credit note no	Code	Total £	VAT £	Sales Type 1 £	Sales Type 2 £
25/09/X2				589.26	87.76	327.00	174.50

Post these totals to the main ledger accounts.

3.4 Posting to the subsidiary ledger accounts

As well as posting the totals from the books of prime entry to the main ledger accounts each individual invoice and credit note must also be posted to the individual customer's account in the subsidiary sales ledger.

Illustration 5 – The analysesd sales day book

Here is an account from the subsidiary sales ledger of Frosty Limited, a glass manufacturer which specialises in glassware for the catering trade.

Account name: **Account code:**

	£		£

You have taken over writing up the subsidiary ledger because the ledger clerk has been ill for several months.

You have gathered together the following information about sales. The customer is a new customer whose name is Arthur Pickering.

The account code will be SP05.

Sales invoices

Date	Invoice Number	Gross £	VAT £	Net £
02/05/X1	325	585.60	87.21	498.39
03/06/X1	468	238.90	35.58	203.32
15/06/X1	503	113.43	16.89	96.54
16/06/X1	510	48.70	7.25	41.45
24/06/X1	CN048	27.73	4.13	23.60
17/07/X1	604	441.12	65.69	375.43

Solution

Account name: Arthur Pickering   **Account code:** SP05

		£			£
02/05/X1	Inv 325	585.60	24/06/X1	CN048	27.73
03/06/X1	Inv 468	238.90			
15/06/X1	Inv 503	113.43			
16/06/X1	Inv 510	48.70			
17/07/X1	Inv 604	441.12			

Remember that sales invoices are always entered on the debit side of the customer's account and credit notes on the credit side of the account.

4 The analysed cash book

4.1 Introduction

In order to revise the layout of the cash receipts book consider the following example.

Cash receipts book for the week commencing 15 September 20X4

Date	Narrative	Total £	VAT £	Debtors £	Cash/cheque Sales £	Discount allowed £
15 Sept	Paying-in slip 584	653.90		653.90		
16 Sept	Paying-in slip 585	864.60		864.60		
17 Sept	Paying-in slip 586	953.58	9.84	887.54	56.20	
18 Sept	Paying-in slip 587	559.57		559.57		
19 Sept	Paying-in slip 588	234.23	27.74	48.00	158.49	
		3,265.88	37.58	3,013.61	214.69	

The bankings are a mixture of cash sales and cheques from debtors. The VAT is just the VAT on the cash/cheque sales. There are no discounts.

Check that the three analysis column totals add back to the total column total.

Illustration 6 – The analysesd cash book

Returning to the cash receipts book, post the totals to the main ledger accounts.

Cash receipts book

Date	Narrative	Total £	VAT £	Debtors £	Cash/cheque Sales £	Discount allowed £
15 Sept	Paying-in slip 584	653.90		653.90		
16 Sept	Paying-in slip 585	864.60		864.60		
17 Sept	Paying-in slip 586	953.58	9.84	887.54	56.20	
18 Sept	Paying-in slip 587	559.57		559.57		
19 Sept	Paying-in slip 588	234.23	27.74	48.00	158.49	
		3,265.88	37.58	3,013.61	214.69	

Solution

The double entry for posting the cash receipts book totals is:

		£	£
DR	Bank account	3,265.88	
CR	VAT account		37.58
	Sales ledger control account		3,013.61
	Sales account		214.69

Bank account

	£		£
Cash receipts book (CRB)	3,265.88		

VAT account

	£		£
		CRB	37.58

Sales ledger control account

	£		£
		CRB	3,013.61

Sales account

	£		£
		CRB	214.69

Note that the description of each transaction is the primary record that it came from, the cash receipts book, shortened to CRB.

Test your understanding 5

The cheques received from customers of Passiflora Products Ltd, a small company which produces herbal remedies and cosmetics and supplies them to shops and beauty parlours, for a week are given below:

Cheques received

	Paying-in slip/customer	Amount £	Discount allowed £
01/5/X6	Paying-in slip 609		
	Natural Beauty	11,797.05	176.95
	Grapeseed	417.30	6.26
	New Age Remedies	6,379.65	95.69
	The Aromatherapy Shop	9,130.65	136.96
03/5/X6	Paying-in slip 610		
	Comfrey Group	5,689.20	85.34
	Natural Elegance	2,056.89	30.85
08/5/X6	Paying-in slip 611		
	The Herbalist	8,663.45	129.95
12/5/X6	Paying-in slip 612		
	Edwards Pharmacy	106.42	
	Healthworks	17,213.94	258.21
19/5/X6	Paying-in slip 613		
	The Beauty Box	11,195.85	167.94
	Crystals	54.19	
25/5/X6	Paying-in slip 614		
	The Village Chemist	7,662.55	114.94
29/5/X6	Paying-in slip 615		
	Brewer Brothers	2,504.61	37.57
30/5/X6	Paying-in slip 616		
	Lapis Lazuli	112.58	
31/5/X6	Paying-in slip 617		
	Lorelei	5,618.40	84.27
	Spain & Co, Chemists	197.93	

(a) **Enter the totals for each paying-in slip (including discounts) into the cash receipts book given below.**

(b) **Total the cash receipts book and post the totals for the month to the main ledger accounts given.**

Check that the three analysis column totals add back to the total column total.

(a) **Cash receipts book**

Date	Narrative	Total £	VAT £	Debtors £	Other £	Discount £

(b) **Main ledger**

Sales ledger control account

£		£

Discount allowed account

£		£

Test your understanding 6

Given below are the details of paying-in slip 609 from the previous activity, Passiflora Products Ltd.

You are required to enter the details in the subsidiary ledger accounts given.

Paying-in slip 609

	Amount £	Discount allowed £
Natural Beauty	11,797.05	176.95
Grapeseed	417.30	6.26
New Age Remedies	6,379.65	95.69
The Aromatherapy Shop	9,130.65	136.96

Natural Beauty

	£		£
Opening balance	17,335.24		

The Aromatherapy Shop

	£		£
Opening balance	12,663.42		

New Age Remedies

	£		£
Opening balance	6,475.34		

Grapeseed

	£		£
Opening balance	423.56		

Test your understanding 7

1   Why is there no discount allowed column in the analysed sales day book?

2   Calculate the VAT on a credit sale for £1,000 where a 5% settlement discount is offered to the customer.

3   A customer takes a settlement discount of £57 when paying his invoice. What is the double entry for this £57 in the books of the seller?

4   A customer returns goods which were invoiced to him for £400 plus VAT and which have been paid for. What is the double entry in the main ledger of the books of the seller to record the original sale and payment and the raising of the credit note?

5   When customer X pays £500 including VAT for a sale made on credit to the seller Y, what entries does Y make in his analysed cash received book?

Date	Narrative	Total £	VAT £	Debtors £	Cash/ cheque Sales £	Discount allowed £

6   When customer Z pays £500 including VAT to the seller Y for a cash sale, what entries does Y make in his analysed cash received book?

Date	Narrative	Total £	VAT £	Debtors £	Cash/ cheque Sales £	Discount allowed £

5   Summary

In this chapter we have pulled together into one place all the main documents and double entry for the sales cycle. If you have had any trouble with any of these points, you should refer again to the earlier chapters of the textbook where the double entry is explained in basic terms.

Test your understanding answers

Date	Invoice	Customer	Code	Total	VAT	Group 01	Group 02	Group 03	Group 04
				£	£	£	£	£	£
06/09/X1	1700	Gates Stores		470.00	70.00	400.00			
06/09/X1	1701	Texas		1,762.50	262.50				1,500.00
07/09/X1	1702	Dickens		1,410.00	210.00				1,200.00
07/09/X1	1703	Hintons DIY		1,880.00	280.00		1,600.00		
08/09/X1	1704	Co-op Stores		235.00	35.00	200.00			
08/09/X1	1705	B & Q Stores		1,175.00	175.00			1,000.00	
09/09/X1	1706	Ferris Décor		940.00	140.00		800.00		
09/09/X1	1707	Ferris Décor		705.00	105.00				600.00
10/09/X1	1708	Homestyle		235.00	35.00			200.00	
10/09/X1	1709	Quick Style		117.50	17.50	100.00			
				8,930.00	1,330.00	700.00	2,400.00	1,200.00	3,300.00

Sales day book

SLCA

	£		£
SDB	8,471.75		

Sales – Type 1 account

	£		£
		SDB	4,320.00

Sales – Type 2 account

	£		£
		SDB	2,890.00

VAT account

	£		£
		SDB	1,261.75

183

Test your understanding 3

Sales returns day book

Date	Credit Note No	Customer Name	Code	Total £	VAT £	Product 1 £	Product 2 £
14/3	3066	K Lilt	L04	141.00	21.00		120.00
14/3	3067	J Davis	D07	18.80	2.80	16.00	
14/3	3068	I Oliver	O11	44.65	6.65	38.00	
14/3	3069	D Sharp	S02	94.00	14.00		80.00
				298.45	44.45	54.00	200.00

Test your understanding 4

Sales ledger control account

	£		£
		SRDB	589.26

Sales returns – Type 1

	£		£
SRDB	327.00		

Sales returns – Type 2

	£		£
SRDB	174.50		

VAT account

	£		£
SRDB	87.76		

KAPLAN PUBLISHING

Test your understanding 5

(a) Cash receipts book

Date	Narrative	Total £	VAT £	Debtors £	Others £	Discount £
01/05/X6	Cheques – 609	27,724.65		27,724.65		415.86
03/05/X6	Cheques – 610	7,746.09		7,746.09		116.19
08/05/X6	Cheques – 611	8,663.45		8,663.45		129.95
12/05/X6	Cheques – 612	17,320.36		17,320.36		258.21
19/05/X6	Cheques – 613	11,250.04		11,250.04		167.94
25/05/X6	Cheques – 614	7,662.55		7,662.55		114.94
29/05/X6	Cheques – 615	2,504.61		2,504.61		37.57
30/05/X6	Cheques – 616	112.58		112.58		
31/05/X6	Cheques – 617	5,816.33		5,816.33		84.27
		88,800.66	–	88,800.66	–	1,324.93

(b) Main ledger

Sales ledger control account

	£		£
		CRB	88,800.66
		CRB – discount allowed	1,324.93

Discount allowed account

	£		£
CRB	1,324.93		

Test your understanding 6

Natural Beauty

	£		£
Opening balance	17,335.24	CRB	11,797.05
		CRB – discount	176.95

The Aromatherapy Shop

	£		£
Opening balance	12,663.42	CRB	9,130.65
		CRB – discount	136.96

New Age Remedies

	£		£
Opening balance	6,475.34	CRB	6,379.65
		CRB – discount	95.69

Grapeseed

	£		£
Opening balance	423.56	CRB	417.30
		CRB – discount	6.26

Test your understanding 7

1   There is no discount allowed column because the value of an invoice entered in the sales day book is always the amount before the discount as you do not know whether or not the customer will take the discount.

2   $(£1,000 - (5\% \times £1,000)) \times 17.5\% = £166.25$

3   Debit discount allowed £57; credit SLCA £57

    (Note that £57 will also be entered on the credit side of the individual debtors account in the subsidiary sales ledger.)

4

Sales

	£			£
		SLCA	(1)	400

Sales returns

		£		£
SLCA	(3)	400		

VAT

		£			£
SLCA	(3)	70	SLCA	(1)	70

SLCA

		£			£
Sales plus VAT	(1)	470	Bank	(2)	470
			Sales returns plus VAT	(3)	470

Bank

		£		£
SLCA	(2)	470		

5

Date	Narrative	Total £	VAT £	Debtors £	Cash/ cheque Sales £	Discount allowed £
	X	500		500		

6

Date	Narrative	Total £	VAT £	Debtors £	Cash/ cheque Sales £	Discount allowed £
	Z	500	74.46		425.54	

13

Credit purchases: documents

Introduction

You will be required to deal with many aspects of the purchases that a business makes. This will involve the procedure for making the purchase and the procedures for paying for the purchase.

In this chapter we will study the documents required when making a purchase.

1   Summary of a credit purchase

The main document flows for a credit purchase are illustrated below. The various documents are described in the paragraphs that follow.

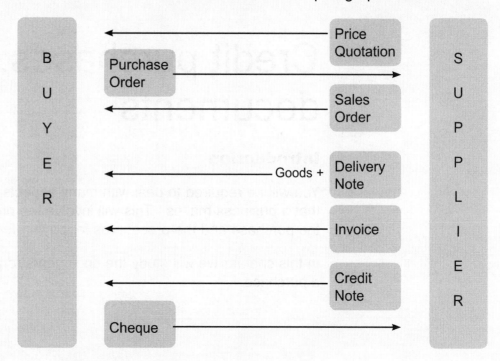

2   Ordering goods and services

2.1   Introduction

There are a variety of different methods of placing an order with a supplier.

(a) **Telephone**

If an order is made by telephone then it is important that the details are confirmed with the supplier in writing. This may be by the supplier sending your organisation an order confirmation or alternatively by you following up the telephone order with a written confirmation of the details.

(b) **In writing**

If an order is to be made in writing then again you would expect an order confirmation to be sent back to you by the supplier confirming all of the details of the order, for example, price, discounts and delivery details.

(c) **Fax**

An order could be made with a supplier by sending a fax. This is similar to sending an order in writing, only that it is received sooner by the supplier. However again you would expect to receive an order confirmation from the supplier.

(d) **Internet**

These days it is also possible to order many goods over the internet as there are many websites that allow you to purchase goods directly online. This should only be considered if it is a procedure that is allowed by your organisation's policy manual and this course of action should be authorised by the appropriate person before any order is placed. It is advisable to only order goods from reputable, well-known organisations but if the organisation is unknown then try to find one that at least has a telephone number that will allow you to verify their authenticity. A copy of the order placed over the internet should be printed out to act as a purchase order and be filed accordingly.

In all instances of ordering, a copy of the order or order confirmation should be filed so that it can be compared with the actual goods when they arrive and eventually with the purchase invoice.

2.2 **An internal purchasing system**

When a department needs goods and services from outside suppliers it may make an internal request using a purchase requisition.

A purchase requisition is an internal document by which a department requests purchases from an outside supplier.

When the purchasing department of a business receives a purchase requisition then it will start the procedures of the purchasing system.

This will normally start with price enquiries being made of a number of different suppliers in order to identify the supplier who will provide the goods at the best price and with the best terms. The suppliers will then send a price quotation in order for the purchasing department to be able to compare prices and terms.

A typical quotation is shown below. Note that this is exactly the same as the quotation received in the examples in Chapter 10 where we studied the sales order systems. The purchasing system is the 'mirror image' of the sales system and the documents are the same. We are simply looking at these systems from the point of view of the customer rather than the supplier.

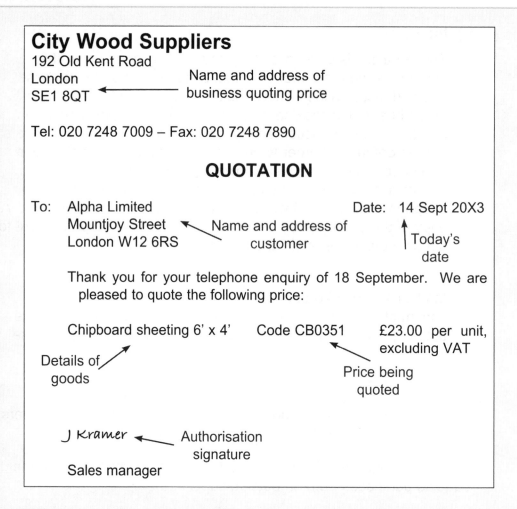

City Wood Suppliers
192 Old Kent Road
London   Name and address of
SE1 8QT ◄─────── business quoting price

Tel: 020 7248 7009 – Fax: 020 7248 7890

QUOTATION

To: Alpha Limited   Date: 14 Sept 20X3
     Mountjoy Street ◄──── Name and address of
     London W12 6RS   customer   Today's
                                                    date

Thank you for your telephone enquiry of 18 September. We are
pleased to quote the following price:

Chipboard sheeting 6' x 4'   Code CB0351   £23.00 per unit,
                                                excluding VAT
Details of
goods   Price being
                                            quoted

J Kramer ◄──── Authorisation
                signature
Sales manager

When the supplier has been chosen then a purchase order will be sent
out to that supplier.

2.3   Purchase order

A purchase order is a document sent to a supplier confirming an order
for goods or services.

Each purchase order must be authorised by the relevant department
head or supervisor before being sent to the supplier. Each department
head has an authorisation limit. Orders above that value must be
authorised by a director, eg managing director.

Only approved suppliers (shown on an official list) should be used.

Purchase orders should be sequentially numbered and carefully
controlled and filed in numerical order for later use.

An example purchase order is shown overleaf:

Illustration 1 – Ordering goods and services

PURCHASE ORDER

Alpha Ltd   Name and address
Mountjoy Street ←——— of business
Shepherd's Bush   placing the order
LONDON W12
                    Order date
Tel: 0208 741 2962   Sequential order
Fax: 0208 741 2963   number
Date: 17 September 20X3 ↙ VAT registration
Purchase order no: P01562   number of   Name and address
VAT Reg no: 413 2790 04   business placing   of business the order
                              ←——— the order   is being placed with

To:	City Wood Suppliers	**Delivery address**
	192 Old Kent Road	(If different from above)
	London	26 New Road
	SE1 8QT	Milton Keynes
		MK25 2BA

Product	Ref	Quantity	Price per unit (ex VAT) £	Total (ex VAT) £
Chipboard sheeting 6' x 4'	CB0351	10	23.00	230

Signed: *J Rowlands*

              Purchasing Manager

2.4 Confirming sales orders

To avoid misunderstandings, a supplier will normally confirm a customer's order by completing a sales order, even if the customer has already sent a written purchase order.

A sales order is a document confirming:

- quantity/type of goods or service
- date of supply
- location of supply
- price and terms.

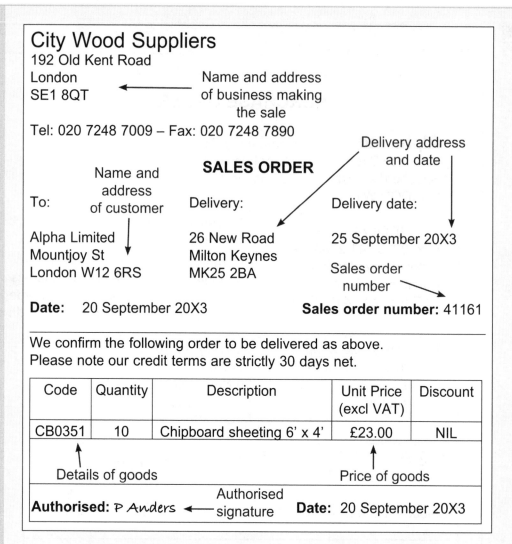

City Wood Suppliers
192 Old Kent Road
London
SE1 8QT

Name and address of business making the sale

Tel: 020 7248 7009 – Fax: 020 7248 7890

SALES ORDER

Delivery address and date

Name and address of customer

To:

Delivery:

Delivery date:

Alpha Limited
Mountjoy St
London W12 6RS

26 New Road
Milton Keynes
MK25 2BA

25 September 20X3

Sales order number

Date: 20 September 20X3

Sales order number: 41161

We confirm the following order to be delivered as above.
Please note our credit terms are strictly 30 days net.

Code	Quantity	Description	Unit Price (excl VAT)	Discount
CB0351	10	Chipboard sheeting 6' x 4'	£23.00	NIL

Details of goods

Price of goods

Authorised: P Anders ← *Authorised signature* **Date:** 20 September 20X3

3 Receipt of the goods

3.1 Introduction

Once the order has been placed with the supplier then the next stage will be for the goods to be received.

3.2 Delivery note

When the supplier sends the goods they will normally be accompanied by a delivery note.

A delivery note is a document that accompanies the goods when they are delivered by the supplier.

The delivery note details the goods that have been delivered to your organisation. When the goods are received by the business they must be checked by the stores or warehouse to ensure that the goods that are detailed on the delivery note are indeed the goods that have been delivered. The goods must also be checked to ensure that they are in good condition. The person in your organisation who has checked the goods will then sign the delivery note.

KAPLAN PUBLISHING

There will normally be three parts to a delivery note:

Part one – This is kept by your organisation in order to compare to the purchase order to ensure that the goods that have been delivered were ordered and then to the purchase invoice when it is received.

Part two – Returned to the supplier as evidence that you have received the goods detailed on the delivery note.

Part three – Kept by the delivery organisation as evidence that they have delivered the goods and that your organisation has received them.

City Wood Suppliers

192 Old Kent Road
London
SE1 8QT
Tel: 020 7248 7009 – Fax: 020 7248 7890

DN 005673

DELIVERY NOTE

To: **Delivery:**   **Delivery date:**

Alpha Limited   26 New Road   25 September 20X3
Mountjoy St   Milton Keynes
London W12 6RS   MK25 2BA

Date: 21 September 20X3   Sales order number: 41161

We confirm the following order to be delivered as above.

Product	Code	Quantity
Chipboard 6' x 4'	CB0351	10

Received in good condition: *A Patel*

---

4 The purchase invoice

4.1 Introduction

The final stage in the purchasing system will normally be the receipt of the purchase invoice from the supplier detailing the cost of the goods purchased and the payment terms.

A typical invoice is shown below.

City Wood Suppliers

192 Old Kent Road
London
SE1 8QT
Tel: 020 7248 7009
Fax: 020 7248 7890

Invoice no: I005673
Tax point: 21 September 20X3
VAT reg no: 618 2201 63
Delivery note: DN005673
Account no: AL6215

INVOICE

To: **Delivery:**   **Delivery date:**

Alpha Limited   26 New Road   25 September 20X3
Mountjoy St   Milton Keynes
London W12 6RS   MK25 2BA

Date: 21 September 20X3   **Sales order number:** 41161

Product	Code	Quantity	Price per unit £	Total £
Chipboard 6' x 4'	CB0351	10	23.00	230.00
			VAT	40.25
				270.25

4.2   Checks on purchase invoices

Once the purchase invoice arrives then a number of checks need to be made on it before it can be passed for payment.

4.3   Order and receipt of goods

Firstly the purchase invoice must be checked to the purchase order and to the delivery note. This is to ensure that not only is this an invoice for goods that were ordered but also for goods that were received. In particular check the description and the quantity of the goods.

For example suppose that the purchase order for goods shows that 100 packs were ordered and the delivery note shows that 100 packs were received. If when the invoice arrives it is for 120 packs then the supplier should be politely informed of the error and a credit note requested.

4.4 Calculations

All of the calculations on the invoice should also be checked to ensure that they are correct. This will include the following:

- all pricing calculations

- any trade discount or bulk discount calculations

- the VAT calculations remembering any cash discounts that may be offered

- the total addition of the invoice.

4.5 Trade discounts

Remember that trade discounts are a definite amount that is deducted from the list price of the goods for the supplies to some customers. As well as checking the actual calculation of the trade discount on the face of the invoice, the supplier's file or the price quotation should be checked to ensure that the correct percentage of trade discount has been deducted.

Even if no trade discount appears on the purchase invoice, the supplier's file or price quotation must still be checked as it may be that a trade discount should have been deducted but has been inadvertently forgotten by the supplier.

4.6 Bulk discounts

A bulk discount is similar to a trade discount in that it is deducted from the list price on the invoice. However, a bulk discount is given by a supplier for orders above a certain size. As with a trade discount the calculation of any bulk discount must be checked to the supplier's file to ensure that the correct discount has been given.

4.7 Settlement or cash discounts

Settlement or cash discounts are offered to customers in order to encourage early payment of invoices. The details of the settlement discount will normally be shown at the bottom of the purchase invoice and it is up to the customer to decide whether to pay the invoice early enough to benefit from the settlement discount or whether to delay payment and ignore the settlement discount.

Again the supplier's file should be checked to ensure that the correct percentage of settlement discount according to the correct terms has been offered.

If there is no settlement discount offered the supplier's details must still be checked to ensure that the settlement discount has not been forgotten by the supplier.

A trade discount or a bulk discount is a definite reduction in price from the list price whereas a cash or settlement discount is only a reduction in price if the organisation decides to take advantage of it by paying earlier.

4.8 VAT calculations and cash discounts

You will remember from an earlier chapter that when a cash or settlement discount is offered then the VAT calculation is based upon the assumption that the customer will take the settlement discount and pay the discounted price for the goods.

Illustration 1 – The purchase invoice

An invoice has a list price of goods of £400.00 with a trade discount of 10% then deducted. A settlement discount of 5% is also offered for payment within 10 days. The goods are charged to VAT at a rate of 17.5%.

How much should the VAT charge on the invoice be and what would be the invoice total?

Solution

	£
List price	400.00
Less: Trade discount 10%	40.00
	360.00
VAT (17.5% × (360 × 95%))	59.85
Invoice total	419.85

Test your understanding 1

A business receives an invoice for £2,400 (exclusive of VAT) from a supplier offering a 5% cash discount.

What should be the total of the invoice inclusive of VAT at 17.5%?

KAPLAN PUBLISHING

Illustration 2 – The purchase invoice

Given below are two invoices; they must be thoroughly checked to ensure that they are correct.

Invoice 7761B

Barrett & Company
Ewe House, Parkside, Oldham.

J Hardy Construction,
Poplar Works,
Poplar Street,
Oldham OL4 6QB

Tel: 0161 338 4444
Fax: 0161 338 5555
Tax Point: 28 August 20X3
VAT Reg No: 268 9104 07

Code	Supply	Description	Quantity	VAT rate	Unit price £	Amount (£) exclusive of VAT
734 226	Sale	Insular Bricks	40	17.50%	16.25	650.00
874 KL5	Sale	Brick Tiles	15	17.50%	43.12	664.80
Total						1,296.80
VAT at 17.5%						226.94
Total amount payable						1,523.74

A settlement discount of 5% is offered for payment within 20 days of the invoice date.

Invoice 68553

A.J. Broom & Company Limited.
59 Parkway, Manchester M2 6EG

J Hardy Construction,
Poplar Works,
Poplar Street,
Oldham OL4 6QB

Tel: 0161 560 3392
Fax: 0161 560 5322
Tax Point: 23 August 20X3
VAT Reg No: 417 1066 22

Code	Supply	Description	Quantity	VAT rate	Unit price £	Amount (£) exclusive of VAT
950 BB3	Sale	Cotswold Bricks	3	17.50%	300.00	900.00
159 504	Sale	Roof Tiles – Red	5	17.50%	195.50	977.50
874 KL5	Sale	Brick Tiles	1	17.50%	56.65	56.65
Total						1,934.15
Less: trade discount 2%						28.68
						1,905.47
VAT at 17.5%						333.46
Total amount payable						2,238.93

Solution

Invoice from Barrett & Co

- the calculation of the brick tiles total is incorrect - it should be 15 x £43.12 = £646.80;

- the VAT has been incorrectly calculated as it has been taken on the invoice total instead of on the figure that would be due if the cash discount were taken. The VAT should be 95% x 17.5% x £1,296.80 = £215.59.

Invoice from A J Broom & Co

- the trade discount of 2% has been incorrectly calculated and this means that the VAT is also incorrect. The supplier should be notified of these errors and a credit note requested.

In assessments you should thoroughly check every figure and every calculation on a purchase invoice just as you would in practice.

Test your understanding 2

(AAT CA D92)

When passing a purchase invoice for payment, what two aspects need to be checked, other than calculations?

4.9 Invoices for services

Invoices or bills can also be received for services such as rent, electricity, cleaning, etc. There will be no delivery note, however the accuracy of the invoice can be checked and it should be sent to the appropriate person to be authorised. This person should be able to assess whether the service has in fact been received and was required.

5 Credit notes

5.1 Introduction

A credit note is simply the reverse of an invoice. It is sent by a supplier to a customer either to correct an error on a previous invoice or because the customer has returned some goods that do not therefore need to be paid for. Exactly the same checks should be made on credit notes as on invoices. The reason for the credit note and the amount that has been credited should be checked, so should all of the calculations and the VAT.

If Alpha Ltd retained two panels of wood, the credit note would be as follows.

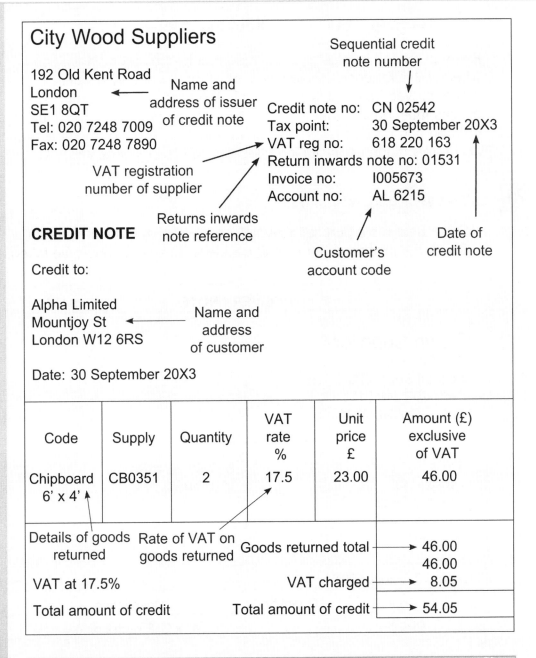

City Wood Suppliers

192 Old Kent Road
London
SE1 8QT
Tel: 020 7248 7009
Fax: 020 7248 7890

Name and address of issuer of credit note

Sequential credit note number

Credit note no: CN 02542
Tax point: 30 September 20X3
VAT reg no: 618 220 163
Return inwards note no: 01531
Invoice no: I005673
Account no: AL 6215

VAT registration number of supplier

Returns inwards note reference

CREDIT NOTE

Customer's account code

Date of credit note

Credit to:

Alpha Limited
Mountjoy St
London W12 6RS

Name and address of customer

Date: 30 September 20X3

Code	Supply	Quantity	VAT rate %	Unit price £	Amount (£) exclusive of VAT
Chipboard 6' x 4'	CB0351	2	17.5	23.00	46.00

Details of goods returned   Rate of VAT on goods returned

Goods returned total → 46.00
                                     46.00

VAT at 17.5%   VAT charged → 8.05

Total amount of credit   Total amount of credit → 54.05

Test your understanding 3

(AAT CA D92)

State the document appropriate to each of the following stages for purchasing and paying for goods.

(a) Notification to purchasing manager of need to order.

(b) Request to supplier to supply goods.

(c) Form accompanying goods sent by supplier.

5.2 The importance of checking documents

Every purchase invoice or credit note received by an organisation, whether it is for goods or services, must be thoroughly checked and approved before it is entered into the accounting records. The checks must ensure that the invoice is for goods or services actually ordered and received, and also ensure that the invoice or credit note is accurately made up, including checks on all calculations and VAT.

Test your understanding 4

Given below is a purchase invoice and associated documentation. Check the invoice carefully and decide what action should be taken.

DELIVERY NOTE		**94511**

Town Suppliers
111 City Road
London SE21 2TG
Tel: 020 7248 7123
Fax: 020 7248 7234

To:
Omega Ltd
27 Holly Road
Birmingham
B27 4XL

Delivery address:
(if different):

Date: 19 October 20X1

Code	Quantity	Description
PP0292	90	4" x 2" Piranha pine 6'

Received by: . . . . Date: . . . . . .

PURCHASE ORDER	263

Omega Ltd
27 Holly Road
Birmingham
B27 4XL

To: Town Suppliers
       111 City Road
       London SE21 2TG

Date: 6 October 20X1

PLEASE SUPPLY TO THE ABOVE ADDRESS

Code	Quantity	Description	Unit price (exclusive of VAT) £
PP0292	100	6' Piranha pine (4" x 2")	3.50

INVOICE	94511

Town Suppliers
111 City Road
London SE21 2TG
Tel: 020 7248 7123
Fax: 020 7248 7234

To:
Omega Ltd
27 Holly Road
Birmingham
B27 4XL

Tax point: 19 October 20X1

VAT Reg No: 234 4610 23

Code	Quantity	Amount exclusive of VAT £	VAT rate %	VAT net £
PP0292	100	350.00	17.5	61.25
	Total	350.00		
	VAT	61.25		
		411.25		

Test your understanding 5

1   When your business wishes to purchase goods from a supplier what document will normally be sent to the supplier?

2   When goods are received from a supplier what document will normally accompany the goods?

3   If goods are returned to a supplier what document would you expect to receive from the supplier?

4   What are the main checks that should be made when a purchase invoice is received?

5   If a bulk discount has been agreed with a supplier how should this be treated on the purchase invoice?

6   A purchase invoice is received for goods with a list price of £1,000 net of VAT. The supplier has agreed a trade discount of 10% and a settlement discount of 2% has been offered. What is the amount of VAT that should be charged on the invoice?

6   Summary

In this chapter the documentation that is used in the purchases system is firstly considered. The different methods of ordering goods and services are covered, as well as the documents that are required when goods are received: the delivery note, the purchase invoice and possibly any credit notes. The most important aspect of the chapter, however, are the thorough and accurate checks that must be made on all purchase invoices and credit notes received from suppliers. The invoices and credit notes must be checked to supporting documentation such as the delivery note, purchase order, returns note, etc. All of the calculations on the invoice or credit note should be checked as well as the percentage of trade, bulk and settlement discounts that have been stated on the invoice or credit note.

Test your understanding answers

Test your understanding 1

£2,799

Note: This answer is arrived at as follows:

	£
Goods/services	2,400
VAT @ 17.5% × 2,400 x 95%	399
	2,799

Test your understanding 2

(i) That the goods or services invoiced are as ordered.

(ii) That the goods or services invoiced have been received in good condition or carried out properly.

Test your understanding 3

(a) Purchase requisition

(b) Purchase order

(c) Delivery note

Test your understanding 4

The delivery note shows that only 90 units were delivered, not the 100 units that were ordered and invoiced.

You should write to the supplier requesting a credit note for the 10 missing units. Once the supplier has agreed the situation, the invoice can then be passed for payment.

Test your understanding 5

1 Purchase order.

2 Delivery note.

3 Credit note.

4   –   Check to the purchase order and delivery note

      –   Check all prices and price extensions

      –   Check calculations of trade/bulk discounts and that the correct

      –   percentage has been used

      –   Check VAT calculations

      –   Check total addition of the invoice

5 A bulk discount should be deducted from the list price.

6 £1,000 – 100 = £900

    VAT = £900 $\times$ 98% $\times$ 17.5% = £154.35

KAPLAN PUBLISHING

Accounting for purchases – summary

Introduction

We have studied the double entry bookkeeping for purchases and payments in detail at the start of this book.

At that time we concentrated on the basic entries so that the double entry would be clear. It is now time to 'put some flesh on the bones' and study these transactions again using more realistic material.

1 Coding of purchase invoices

1.1 Introduction

As we have seen in the purchases day book the purchase invoices are normally given an internal invoice number and are also recorded under the supplier's purchase ledger code and possibly the type of purchase.

1.2 Authorisation stamp

This is often done by stamping an authorisation stamp or grid stamp onto the invoice once it has been thoroughly checked and the relevant details entered onto the authorisation stamp. A typical example of an authorisation stamp is shown below:

	Purchase order no	04618	
	Invoice no	04821	
	Cheque no		
	Account code	PL06	
	Checked	L Finn	
	Date	23/02/X2	
	ML account	07	

1.3 Entries on the authorisation stamp

At this stage of entering the invoice in the purchases day book it has been checked to the purchase order and the delivery note, therefore the purchase order number is entered onto the authorisation stamp.

The purchase invoice will then be allocated an internal code number which will be sequential and therefore the next number after the last invoice entered into the purchases day book.

At this stage the invoice will not necessarily have been authorised for payment (see earlier chapter), therefore the cheque number will not yet be entered onto the authorisation stamp.

The purchase invoice details such as trade and settlement discounts should have been checked to the supplier's file to ensure that the correct percentages have been used and at this point the supplier's subsidiary ledger code can be entered onto the authorisation stamp.

The person checking the invoice should then sign and date the authorisation stamp to show that all details have been checked.

Finally, the main ledger account code should be entered. We have seen that in some businesses a simple three column purchases day book will be used with a total, VAT and net column. In such cases all of the invoices will be classified as 'purchases' and will have the main ledger code for the purchases account.

However, if an analysed purchases day book is used then each analysis column will be for a different type of expense and will have a different main ledger code.

If your organisation does have an authorisation stamp procedure then it is extremely important that the authorisation is correctly filled out when the invoice has been checked. Not only is this evidence that the invoice is correct and is for goods or services that have been received, it also provides vital information for the accurate accounting for this invoice.

Illustration 1 – Coding of purchase invoices

Given below are three purchase invoices received and the authorisation stamp for each one. They are to be entered into the purchases day book. Today's date is 25 April 20X1.

INVOICE

Invoice to:
Keller Bros
Field House
Winstead
M16 4PT

Deliver to:
above address

Anderson Wholesale
Westlife Park
Gripton
M7 1ZK
Tel: 0161 439 2020
Fax: 0161 439 2121
Invoice no: 06447
Tax point: 20 April 20X1
VAT reg no: 432 1679 28
Account no: SL14

Code	Description	Quantity	VAT rate	Unit price	Amount exclusive of VAT £
PT417	Grade A Compost	7 tonnes	17.5	15.80	110.60

	110.60
Trade discount 5%	5.53
	105.07
VAT at 17.5%	18.38
Total amount payable	123.45

Purchase order no	34611	
Invoice no	37240	
Cheque no		
Account code	PL14	
Checked	C Long	
Date	25/04/X1	
ML account	020	

INVOICE

Invoice to:
Keller Bros
Field House
Winstead
M16 4PT

Deliver to:
above address

Better Gardens Ltd
Broom Nursery
West Lane
Farforth   M23 4LL
Tel: 0161 380 4444
Fax: 0161 380 6128

Invoice no: 46114
Tax point: 21 April 20X1
VAT reg no: 611 4947 26
Account no: K03

Code	Description	Quantity	VAT rate	Unit price	Amount exclusive of VAT £
B4188	Tulip bulbs	28 dozen	17.5	1.38	38.64
B3682	Daffodil bulbs	50 dozen	17.5	1.26	63.00
					101.64
VAT at 17.5%					17.25
Total amount payable					118.89

Deduct discount of 3% if paid within 14 days

Purchase order no	34608	
Invoice no	37241	
Cheque no		
Account code	PL06	
Checked	C Long	
Date	25/04/X1	
ML account	020	

INVOICE

Invoice to:
Keller Bros
Field House
Winstead
M16 4PT

Winterton Partners
28/32 Coleman Road
Forest Dene
M17 3AT
Tel: 0161 224 6760
Fax: 0161 224 6761

Deliver to:
above address

Invoice no:	I21167
Tax point:	22 April 20X1
VAT reg no:	980 3012 74
Account no:	SL44

Code	Description	Quantity	VAT rate	Unit price	Amount exclusive of VAT £
A47BT	Seedlings	120	17.5	0.76	91.20
					91.20

Trade discount 7%

	6.38
	84.82

VAT at 17.5%

	14.55

Total amount payable

	99.37

Deduct discount of 2% if paid within 14 days

	Purchase order no	34615	
	Invoice no	37242	
	Cheque no		
	Account code	PL23	
	Checked	C Long	
	Date	25/04/X1	
	ML account	020	

Solution

Purchases day book

Date	Invoice no	Code	Supplier	Total £	VAT £	Net £
25/04/X1	37240	PL14	Anderson Wholesale	123.45	18.38	105.07
25/04/X1	37241	PL06	Better Gardens Ltd	118.89	17.25	101.64
25/04/X1	37242	PL23	Winterton Partners	99.37	14.55	84.82

Note that the net total is the invoice amount after deducting any trade discount as the trade discount is a definite reduction in the list price of the goods. At this stage any settlement discount is ignored as it will not necessarily have been decided whether or not to take advantage of the settlement discount.

Test your understanding 1

You are a purchases clerk for Robins, a soft drink manufacturer. Here is part of the layout of the purchases day book.

Purchases day book

Date	Invoice no	Code	Supplier	Total £	VAT £	01 £	02 £	03 £	04 £

01 represents purchases of parts or raw materials for manufacture

02 represents advertising expenditure

03 represents entertaining expenditure

04 represents purchases of fixed assets

Here are five documents that are to be written up in the purchases day book on 10.11.X2 as necessary.

Document 1

No: 511 X

SALES INVOICE   **Drip Farm**
Lover's Lane
To: Robins Ltd   **Norwich NO56 2EZ**
      Softdrink House
      Wembley   **Tax point: 7.11.X2**
      London   **VAT Reg No: 566 0122 10**
      NW16 7SJ

Quantity	Description	VAT rate	Price/unit	Total
50 litre drum	Apple juice (inferior)	17.5%	£2/litre	100.00
			VAT	17.50
				117.50

Grid stamp on reverse of invoice.

Invoice no	4221	
Account code	DF2	
Checked	R Robins	
Date	9.11.X2	
ML account	01	

Document 2

Sales Invoice   Inv No: 5177

DAILY NEWS PLC
Europe Way, Southampton, SO3 3BZ

Tax point 5.11.X2
VAT Reg No: 177 0255 01

To: Robins Ltd
      Softdrink House Wembley LONDON NW16 7SJ

Sale details:
4 line advertisement   £
3 weeks   04.10.X2 @ £100/week
               11.10.X2   Net price   300.00
               18.10.X2   VAT 17.5%   52.50
                                                352.50

Grid stamp on reverse of invoice.

Invoice no	4222	
Account code	DN1	
Checked	R Robins	
Date	9.11.X2	
ML account	02	

Document 3

RECEIPT

9/11/X2

Yellow River Restaurant

Received with thanks the sum of £17.50

T W Wang

Document 4

SALES ORDER 562

Robins Ltd
Softdrink House
Wembley
BTEB Stores   LONDON
Gateshead   NW16 7SJ

Quantity	Description	Price
20 cases	0.75 bottles of Norfolk apple juice	£2/bottle

Document 5

SALES INVOICE P261

To: Robins Ltd
     Softdrink House
     Wembley
     LONDON
     NW16 7SJ

STANDARD MACHINES
Starlight Boulevard, Milton Keynes
MK51 7LY

Tax point: 6.11.X2
VAT Reg No: 127 0356 02

Quantity	Description	VAT	Price (£)/unit
1	Bottling machine	17.5%	2,000
		VAT	350
			2,350

Grid stamp on reverse of invoice.

Invoice no.	4223	
Account code	SM4	
Checked	R Robins	
Date	9.11.X2	
ML account	04	

2 Returns of goods

2.1 Introduction

Returns may be made for various reasons, e.g.

- faulty goods

- excess goods delivered by supplier

- unauthorised goods delivered.

All returned goods must be recorded on a returns outwards note.

2.2 Credit notes

The return should not be recorded until the business receives a credit note from the supplier. This confirms that there is no longer a liability for these goods. A credit note from a supplier is sometimes requested by the organisation issuing a debit note.

The credit note should be checked for accuracy against the returns outwards note. The calculations and extensions on the credit note should also be checked in just the same way as with an invoice.

2.3 Purchases returns day book

When credit notes are received from suppliers they are normally recorded in their own primary record, the purchases returns day book. This has a similar layout to a purchases day book. If the purchases day book is analysed into the different types of purchase that the organisation makes then the purchases returns day book will also be analysed in the same manner.

2.4 Coding of credit notes

In just the same way as with purchase invoices, credit notes must also be thoroughly checked for accuracy and then coded on an authorisation stamp or grid stamp. This will then provide all of the details that are necessary in order to enter the credit note into the purchases returns day book.

Illustration 2 – Ruturns of goods

Today, 5 February 20X5, three credit notes have been passed as being checked. The details of each credit note and the authorisation stamp are given below. The credit note details are to be entered into the purchases returns day book.

From Calderwood & Co	£
Goods total	16.80
VAT	2.94
Credit note total	19.74

Purchase order no	41120
Credit note	C461
Cheque no	–
Account code	053
Checked	J Garry
Date	05/02/X5
ML account	02

From Mellor & Cross	£
Goods total	104.50
Less: Trade discount 10%	10.45
	94.05
VAT	16.45
Credit note total	110.50

Purchase order no	41096
Credit note	C462
Cheque no	–
Account code	259
Checked	J Garry
Date	05/02/X5
ML account	02

From Thompson Bros Ltd	£
Goods total	37.60
Less: Trade discount 5%	1.88
	35.72
VAT	6.25
Credit note total	41.97

Purchase order no	41103
Credit note	C463
Cheque no	–
Account code	360
Checked	J Garry
Date	05/02/X5
ML account	01

KAPLAN PUBLISHING

> ## Solution
>
> | Date | Credit note no | Code | Supplier | Total £ | VAT £ | 01 £ | 02 £ | 03 £ | 04 £ |
> |------|------|------|----------|---------|-------|------|------|------|------|
> | 05/02/X5 | C461 | 053 | Calderwood & Co | 19.74 | 2.94 | | 16.80 | | |
> | 05/02/X5 | C462 | 259 | Mellor & Cross | 110.50 | 16.45 | | 94.05 | | |
> | 05/02/X5 | C463 | 360 | Thompson Bros Ltd | 41.97 | 6.25 | 35.72 | | | |
>
> Note that it is the credit note total which is entered into the total column and the VAT amount into the VAT column. The amount entered into the analysis columns is the goods total less the trade discount. The analysis column is taken from the main ledger code on the authorisation stamp.

> ## Test your understanding 2
>
> A newsagents shop has received the following invoices. Write them up in the purchases day book using the format provided. The last internal invoice number to be allocated to purchase invoices was 114.
>
> | | | |
> |---|---|---|
> | 1.1.X1 | Northern Electric – invoice | £235 including VAT at 17.5% |
> | | Northern Gas – invoice | £235.00 (no VAT) |
> | 2.1.X1 | Post Office Counters – invoice | £117.50 (no VAT) |
> | | Northern Country – invoice | £58.75 including VAT at 17.5% |
> | 3.1.X1 | South Gazette – invoice | £352.50 including VAT at 17.5% |
>
> The supplier codes are as follows:
>
> | | |
> |---|---|
> | Northern Country (a newspaper) | N1 |
> | Northern Electric | N2 |
> | Northern Gas | N3 |
> | Post Office Counters | P1 |
> | South Gazette (a newspaper) | S1 |
>
> ### Purchases day book
>
> | Date | Invoice no | Code | Supplier | Total £ | VAT £ | Goods for resale £ | Heat and light £ | Postage and stationery £ |
> |------|-----------|------|----------|---------|-------|--------------------|------------------|--------------------------|
> | | | | | | | | | |
> | | | | | | | | | |
> | | | | | | | | | |

3 Accounting entries in the main ledger

3.1 Introduction

In an earlier chapter we have already come across the main ledger which is the collection of ledger accounts for all of the assets, liabilities, income and expenses of the business. The accounting entries that are to be made in the main ledger are the same as those that have been considered in previous chapters and are made from the totals of the columns in the purchases day book and purchases returns day book.

3.2 Analysed purchases day book

If an analysed purchases day book is being used then there will be a debit entry in an individual purchases or expense account for each of the analysis column totals.

Remember that these totals are the net of VAT purchases/expenses totals.

Illustration 3 – Accounting entries in the main ledger

Reproduced below is a purchases day book for the first week of February 20X5. Each column has been totalled and it must be checked that the totals of the analysis columns agree to the 'Total' column. Therefore you should check the following sum:

	£
01	744.37
02	661.23
03	250.45
04	153.72
VAT	296.15
	2,105.92

Purchases day book

Date	Invoice no	Code	Supplier	Total £	VAT £	01 £	02 £	03 £	04 £
20X5									
1 Feb	3569	265	Norweb	148.29	22.09	126.20			
2 Feb	3570	053	Calderwood & Co	98.60			98.60		
3 Feb	3571	259	Mellor & Cross	661.09	98.46		562.63		
4 Feb	3572	360	Thompson Bros Ltd	260.18	38.75	221.43			
5 Feb	3573	023	Cooplin Associates	18.90				18.90	
	3574	056	Heywood Suppliers	272.07	40.52			231.55	
	3575	395	William Leggett	45.37	6.76				38.61
	3576	271	Melville Products	366.49	54.58	311.91			
	3577	301	Quick-Bake	99.68	14.85	84.83			
	3578	311	Roger & Roebuck	135.25	20.14				115.11
				2,105.92	296.15	744.37	661.23	250.45	153.72

The totals of the purchases day book will now be posted to the main ledger accounts.

Solution

Purchase ledger control account

	£		£
		PDB	2,105.92

VAT account

	£		£
PDB	296.15		

Purchases – 01 account

	£		£
PDB	744.37		

Purchases – 02 account

	£		£
PDB	661.23		

Purchases – 03 account

	£		£
PDB	250.45		

Purchases – 04 account

	£		£
PDB	153.72		

3.3 Purchases returns day book

The purchases returns day book is kept in order to record credit notes received by the business. The totals of this must also be posted to the main ledger.

Illustration 4 – Accounting entries in the main ledger

Given below is a purchases returns day book for the week. The totals are to be posted to the main ledger accounts.

Purchases returns day book

Date	Credit note no	Code	Supplier	Total £	VAT £	01 £	02 £	03 £	04 £
20X3									
4 May	CN 152	PL21	Julian R Partners	129.25	19.25		110.00		
6 May	CN 153	PL07	S T Trader	79.90	11.90			68.00	
8 May	CN 154	PL10	Ed Associates	68.85	10.25		58.60		
8 May	CN 155	PL03	Warren & Co	105.28	15.68	89.60			
				383.28	57.08	89.60	168.60	68.00	–

Solution

First, check that each of the column totals add back to the total column total:

	£
VAT	57.08
01	89.60
02	168.60
03	68.00
04	–
	383.28

Then post the totals to the main ledger accounts:

Purchases ledger control account

	£		£
Purchases return day book (PRDB)	383.28		

VAT account

	£		£
		PRDB	57.08

Purchases returns – 01

	£		£
		PRDB	89.60

Purchases returns – 02

	£		£
		PRDB	168.60

Purchases returns – 03

	£		£
		PRDB	68.00

If the purchases returns day book is analysed then there will be an account in the main ledger for each different category of purchases returns.

Test your understanding 3

Given below is the purchases day book. You are required to check the total of each analysis column and that the total of each analysis column agrees to the total column, and then to enter the totals in the correct main ledger accounts.

Purchases day book

Date	Invoice no	Code	Supplier	Total £	VAT £	01 £	02 £	03 £	04 £
01.01.X1	115	N2	Northern Electric	235.00	35.00		200.00		
	116	N3	Northern Gas	235.00			235.00		
02.01.X1	117	P1	Post Office	117.50				117.50	
	118	N1	Northern Country	58.75	8.75	50.00			
03.01.X1	119	S1	South Gazette	352.50	52.50	300.00			
				998.75	96.25	350.00	435.00	117.50	

4   Accounting entries in the subsidiary (purchases) ledger

4.1   Subsidiary ledger

So that a business knows how much it owes to each credit supplier, it maintains a subsidiary ledger which consists of records of amounts owed to each supplier (or creditor). Each supplier has their own page or card (or account) in the ledger.

4.2   Typical supplier's account

Purchase invoices are recorded on the right hand side (credit side) just as they are in the purchases ledger control account in the main ledger. Individual transactions are transferred from the purchases day book.

Note that the amount recorded for each purchase invoice is the total including VAT, as this is what is owed to each supplier.

Account name: Robert Jones   **Code: J53**

Date	Transaction	£	Date	Transaction	£
			01.8.X3	Invoice 0992	236.93
			03.8.X3	Invoice 0996	92.58
			10.8.X3	Invoice 1032	69.53

Illustration 5 – Accounting entries in the subsidiary (purchases) ledger

Here is an account from the subsidiary (purchases) ledger of Frosty Limited.

Account name: **Code:**

Date	Transaction	£	Date	Transaction	£

We will write up the account for Jones Brothers, account number PJ06. This is a new supplier.

Frosty Limited has only been trading for a short time and is not yet registered for VAT.

Purchase invoices and credit notes

02.5.X1	9268	£638.26
06.6.X1	9369	£594.27
15.6.X1	9402	£368.24
17.6.X1	C Note 413	£58.62
19.6.X1	9568	£268.54

Solution

Account name: Jones Brothers   **Account number: PJ06**

Date	Transaction	£	Date	Transaction	£
17.6.X1	Credit note 413	58.62	02.5.X1	Invoice 9268	638.26
			06.6.X1	Invoice 9369	594.27
			15.6.X1	Invoice 9402	368.24
			19.6.X1	Invoice 9568	268.54

Each purchase invoice from the Purchases Day Book must be entered on the credit side of that individual suppliers account in the subsidiary ledger. Any credit notes recorded in the Purchases Returns Day Book must be recorded on the debit side of the supplier's account. Where there is VAT involved the amount to be recorded for an invoice or credit note is the gross amount or VAT inclusive amount.

5 The impact of value added tax

5.1 Introduction

Having looked at the accounting for purchase invoices and credit notes, we will now move on to consider the accounting for payments to suppliers. First we will consider the impact of VAT in this area.

When writing up the payments side of the cash book VAT must be considered.

Any payments to suppliers or creditors included in the Purchases ledger column need have no analysis for VAT as the VAT on the purchase was recorded in the purchases day book when the invoice was initially received.

However any other payments on which there is VAT must show the gross amount in the Total column, the VAT in the VAT column and the net amount in the relevant expense column.

Illustration 6 – The impact of value added tax

Peter Craddock is the cashier for a business which manufactures paper from recycled paper. The payments that were made for one week in September are as follows:

15 September	Cheque no 1151 to K Humphrey (credit supplier)	£1,034.67
	Cheque no 1152 to Y Ellis (credit supplier)	£736.45
	Cheque no 1153 to R Phipps (credit supplier)	£354.45
	Standing order for rent	£168.15
	Direct debit to the electricity company (including VAT of £22.92)	£130.98
16 September	Cheque no 1154 to L Silton (credit supplier)	£1,092.75
	Cheque no 1155 to the insurance company	£103.18
17 September	Cheque no 1156 to F Grange (credit supplier)	£742.60
	Cheque no 1157 to Hettler Ltd for cash purchases	£420.00 plus VAT
18 September	Cheque no 1158 to J Kettle (credit supplier)	£131.89
	BACS payment of wages	£4,150.09
19 September	Cheque no 1159 to Krane Associates for cash purchases	£186.00 plus VAT

Enter these transactions into the cash payments book, total the columns and post the totals to the main ledger.

Solution

Date	Details	Cheque no	Total £	VAT £	Purchases ledger £	Cash purchases £	Rent £	Elec-tricity £	Wages £	Insurance £
15/9	K Humphrey	1151	1,034.67		1,034.67					
	Y Ellis	1152	736.45		736.45					
	R Phipps	1153	354.45		354.45					
	Rent	SO	168.15				168.15			
	Electricity	DD	130.98	22.92				108.06		
16/9	L Silton	1154	1,092.75		1,092.75					
	Insurance	1155	103.18							103.18
17/9	F Grange	1156	742.60		742.60					
	Hettler Ltd	1157	493.50	73.50		420.00				
18/9	J Kettle	1158	131.89		131.89					
	Wages	BACS	4,150.09						4,150.09	
19/9	Krane Ass	1159	218.55	32.55		186.00				
			9,357.26	128.97	4,092.81	606.00	168.15	108.06	4,150.09	103.18

The analysis column totals should add back to the Total column – this must always be done to check the accuracy of your totalling.

	£
VAT	128.97
Purchases ledger	4,092.81
Cash purchases	606.00
Rent	168.15
Electricity	108.06
Wages	4,150.09
Insurance	103.18
	9,357.26

Purchase ledger control account

		£		£
19/9	CPB	4,092.81		

VAT account

		£		£
19/9	CPB	128.97		

Purchases account

		£		£
19/9	CPB	606.00		

Electricity account

		£		£
19/9	CPB	108.06		

Salaries account

		£		£
19/9	CPB	4,150.09		

Rent account

		£		£
19/9	CPB	168.15		

Insurance account

		£		£
19/9	CPB	103.18		

All of the entries in the main ledger accounts are debit entries. The credit entry is the total column of the cash payments book and these individual debit entries form the double entry.

6 Cash (settlement) discounts

6.1 Introduction

If a business takes advantage of cash discounts on items purchased, the discount is treated as income as it is a benefit to the business i.e. although the invoice is paid earlier, the amount paid is less than the invoice net amount due to the discount.

Cash or settlement discounts are recorded in a memorandum column in the cash book. The memorandum column does not form part of the double entry. It requires an entire piece of double entry itself (see below).

The business must record these settlement discounts. Trade discounts are not recorded in the cash book.

An extra column is included in the analysed cash payments book. This should be the final right hand column.

Illustration 7 – Cash (settlement) discounts

The following four payments have been made today, 12 June 20X6:

Cheque number 22711 B Caro
     Purchases ledger code CL13
     £342.80 after taking a settlement discount of £14.20
Cheque number 22712 S Wills
     Cash purchases of £235.00 inclusive of VAT
Cheque number 22713 P P & Co
     Purchases ledger code CL22   £116.40
Cheque number 22714 W Potts
     Purchases ledger code CL18   £162.84

The relevant subsidiary (purchases) ledger accounts are shown over the page.

B Caro (CL 13)

	£		£
		PDB Invoice	357.00

W Potts (CL 18)

	£		£
PRDB Credit note	10.00	PDB Invoice	172.84

P P & Co (CL 22)

	£		£
		PDB Invoice	116.40
		PDB Invoice	121.27

In this example we will:

- write up the cash payments book for the day;

- total the columns to check that they add back to the total of the Total column;

- enter the totals in the main ledger;

- write up each individual entry in the subsidiary ledger.

Solution

Date	Details	Cheque	Code	Total £	VAT £	Purchases ledger £	Cash purchases £	Other £	Discounts £
12 Jun	B Caro	22711	CL13	342.80		342.80			14.20
	S Wills	22712		235.00	35.00		200.00		
	PP&Co	22713	CL22	116.40		116.40			
	W Potts	22714	CL18	162.84		162.84			
				857.04	35.00	622.04	200.00	–	14.20

Total Check

	£
Purchases ledger	622.04
Cash purchases	200.00
VAT	35.00
	857.04

Note that the discount received column is not included in the total check as this is simply a memorandum column.

Main ledger

Purchase ledger control account

	£		£
CPB	622.04		
CPB – discount	14.20		

Purchases account

	£		£
CPB	200.00		

VAT account

	£		£
CPB	35.00		

Discounts received account

	£		£
		CPB	14.20

When posting the cash payments book to the main ledger there are two distinct processes. Firstly enter the totals of each of the analysis columns as debits in their relevant accounts in the main ledger. Then do the double entry for the discounts received –

debit the purchase ledger control account and credit the discounts received account.

Subsidiary ledger

B Caro (CL 13)

		£			£
CPB	Payment	342.80	PDB	Invoice	357.00
CPB	Discount	14.20			

Note that the discount is entered here as well as the cash payment.

W Potts (CL 18)

		£			£
PRDB	Credit note	10.00	PDB	Invoice	172.84
CPB	Payment	162.84			

P P & Co (CL 22)

		£			£
CPB	Payment	116.40	PDB	Invoice	116.40
			PDB	Invoice	121.27

Test your understanding 4

Given below is a completed cash payments book.

You are required to:

(a) Total each of the columns and check that the totals add across to the total column.

(b) Post the totals to the main ledger accounts given.

(c) Post the individual creditor entries to the creditors' accounts in the subsidiary ledger, also given.

Date	Details	Cheque no	Code	Total £	VAT £	Purchases ledger £	Cash purchases £	Wages £
1/7	G Hobbs	34	PL14	325.46		325.46		
1/7	Purchases	35	ML03	66.98	9.98		57.00	
2/7	Purchases	36	ML03	49.53	7.37		42.16	
3/7	P Taylor	37	PL21	157.83		157.83		
3/7	S Dent	38	PL06	163.58		163.58		
4/7	K Smith	39	ML07	24.56				24.56

Test your understanding 5

1 Why is there no discount received column in the purchases day book?

2 When cross-casting the analysed cash payments book, do you include the discount received column in your calculations?

3 What is the double entry for a settlement discount received of £100?

4 In the subsidiary purchases ledger, would a settlement discount received of £75 be entered on the debit or credit side of the individual creditor account?

5 In the subsidiary purchases ledger, why is there no corresponding double entry in a discount received account corresponding to the entry in the individual creditor account?

7 Summary

In this chapter we have pulled together into one place all the main documents and double entry for the purchases cycle. If you have had any trouble with any of these points, you should refer again to the earlier chapters of the textbook where the double entry is explained.

Test your understanding answers

Test your understanding 1

Purchases day book

Date	Invoice no	Code	Supplier	Total £	VAT £	01 £	02 £	03 £	04 £
10/11X2	4221	DF2	Drip Farm	117.50	17.50	100.00			
10/11X2	4222	DN1	Daily News plc	352.50	52.50		300.00		
10/11X2	4223	SM4	Standard Machines	2,350.00	350.00				2,000.00
				2,820.00	420.00	100.00	300.00	–	2,000.00

Document 3 receipt is not a purchase invoice, it is a receipt for cash paid.

Document 4 is a sales order to supply 20 cases of bottled juice. It is not a purchase invoice so would not appear in the purchases day book.

Test your understanding 2

Date	Invoice no	Code	Supplier	Total £	VAT £	Goods for resale £	Heat and light £	Postage and stationery £
01.01.X1	115	N2	Northern Electric	235.00	35.00		200.00	
	116	N3	Northern Gas	235.00	–		235.00	
02.01.X1	117	P1	Post Office Counters	117.50	–			117.50
	118	N1	Northern Country	58.75	8.75	50.00		
03.01.X1	119	S1	South Gazette	352.50	52.50	300.00		
				998.75	96.25	350.00	435.00	117.50

Test your understanding 3

	£
Goods for resale	350.00
Heat and light	435.00
Postage and stationery	117.50
VAT	96.25
Total	998.75

Purchases (goods for resale)

	£		£
PDB	350.00		

Heat and light

	£		£
PDB	435.00		

Postage and stationery

	£		£
PDB	117.50		

VAT

	£		£
PDB	96.25		

Creditors control/Purchase ledger control accounts/PLCA

	£		£
		PDB	998.75

Test your understanding 4

Date	Details	Cheque no	Code	Total £	VAT £	Purchases ledger £	Cash purchases £	Wages £
1/7	G Hobbs	34	PL14	325.46		325.46		
1/7	Purchases	35	ML03	66.98	9.98		57.00	
2/7	Purchases	36	ML03	49.53	7.37		42.16	
3/7	P Taylor	37	PL21	157.83		157.83		
3/7	S Dent	38	PL06	163.58		163.58		
4/7	K Smith	39	ML07	24.56				24.56
				787.94	17.35	646.87	99.16	24.56

Check that totals add across:

	£
VAT	17.35
Purchases ledger	646.87
Cash purchases	99.16
Wages	24.56
	787.94

(b) Main ledger accounts

Purchases ledger control account

	£		£
CPB	646.87		

Cash purchases account

	£		£
CPB	99.16		

Wages account

	£		£
CPB	24.56		

VAT account

	£		£
CPB	17.35		

(c) Subsidiary ledger

G Hobbs   PL14

	£		£
CPB	325.46		

P Taylor   PL21

	£		£
CPB	157.83		

S Dent   PL06

	£		£
CPB	163.58		

Test your understanding 5

1   The purchases day book lists the value of the invoice sent by the supplier. This value is not affected by the settlement discount and so there is no column for the discount.

2   No. The discount received column is a memorandum column to remind the bookkeeper to make the double entry in the main ledger.

3   Debit purchases ledger control account £100; credit discount received account £100.

4   The £75 would be entered on the debit side of the individual creditor account. The discount received represents a reduction in the creditor – hence a debit entry.

5   The purpose of the subsidiary (purchases) ledger is to provide the detailed entries in each individual creditor account that goes to make up the total entries in the PLCA. The discounts received are therefore entered as debits in the individual creditor accounts but there is no need to make the corresponding entries in a discount received account. The subsidiary (purchases) ledger account contains just memorandum accounts which are effectively single entry.

Petty cash systems

Introduction

As well as making payments from the business bank account by cheque or other methods considered in the previous chapter, most businesses will also carry a certain amount of cash on the premises known as petty cash. The purpose of this cash is in order to make small business payments for which writing a cheque would not be appropriate, such as payment in the local shop for tea, coffee and milk for the staff kitchen. In this chapter we will consider how a petty cash system will work, the documentation required and how petty cash payments are accounted for.

1 Petty cash systems

1.1 Introduction

We have seen in the previous chapters how most business payments are made out of the business bank account by cheque, standing order, direct debit or other automated payment mechanisms. However, most businesses will require small amounts of cash for payment for items such as stamps, coffee, tea, taxi fares, train fares, etc. The cash that is held is known as petty cash.

Petty cash is the small amount of cash that most businesses will hold in order to make small cash payments.

1.2 Petty cash box

Cash being held on business premises is obviously a security risk. Therefore it is important that the petty cash is secure. It will normally be kept in a locked petty cash box and usually this itself will be held in the safe. Only the person responsible for the petty cash should have access to the petty cash box.

1.3 Payment of petty cash

Petty cash will usually be paid out to employees who have already incurred a small cash expense on behalf of the business, such as buying coffee and milk in the local shop or paying for a train fare that the business is to reimburse. It is obviously important that payments are only made out of the petty cash box for valid business expenses that have been incurred. For this reason petty cash should only ever be given to an employee on receipt by the petty cashier of an authorised petty cash voucher and, where appropriate, VAT receipt.

A petty cash voucher is an internal document that details the business expenditure that an employee has incurred out of his own money.

This voucher must be authorised before any amounts can be paid to that employee out of the petty cash box.

A typical petty cash voucher is shown below:

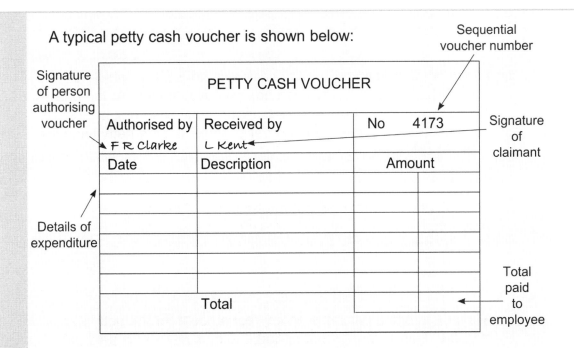

Sequential
voucher number

Signature
of person
authorising
voucher

PETTY CASH VOUCHER

Authorised by	Received by	No	4173
F R Clarke	L Kent		
Date	Description	Amount	
	Total		

Signature
of
claimant

Details of
expenditure

Total
paid
to
employee

Test your understanding 1

Give two ways in which the company might attempt to maintain security over the petty cash.

1.4 The imprest system

Many businesses use the imprest system for petty cash. Using an imprest system makes petty cash easier to control and therefore reduces the possibility of error and fraud.

The business decides on a fixed amount of petty cash (the imprest) which is just large enough to cover normal petty cash requirements for a period (usually a week). This amount of petty cash is withdrawn from the bank.

Claims are paid out of petty cash by a voucher being completed for each amount of petty cash paid out. The vouchers are kept in the petty cash box so that the amount of cash held decreases and is replaced by vouchers.

At any given time, the total contents of the box (i.e. petty cash plus amounts withdrawn represented by vouchers) should equal the amount of the imprest.

At the end of the period, a cheque is drawn for the total of the vouchers which restores the petty cash float to the amount of the imprest. The vouchers are removed from the petty cash box and filed.

Illustration 1 – Petty cash systems

The imprest amount for a petty cash system is £150, which is the amount paid into the petty cash box on 1 November. At the end of the week the total of the vouchers in the petty cash box is £125.05. How much cash is required in order to replenish the petty cash box to the imprest amount?

Solution

£125.05, the amount paid out on the basis of the petty cash vouchers.

Test your understanding 2

Allsports Limited maintains an imprest amount for the petty cash of £250. During the current period, the sum of £180 is paid out, supported by petty cash vouchers.

At the end of the period, what amount should be drawn out of the bank?

1.5   Non-imprest petty cash system

An imprest petty cash system as in the previous example is the most common method of dealing with and controlling petty cash. However some businesses may use a non-imprest system. This might be where a set amount of cash is withdrawn each week and paid into the petty cash box no matter what the level of expenditure in that week.

For example it may be an organisation's policy to cash a cheque for £50 each Monday morning for use as petty cash for the week. The danger here is either that petty cash requirements are more than £50 in the week in which case the petty cash box will run out of money. Alternatively week after week expenditure is significantly less than £50 each week, leading to a large amount of cash building up in the petty cash box.

Test your understanding 3

You receive the following memorandum:

HAIRDRESSING SUPPLIES LIMITED

M E M O R A N D U M

To: Chris   Date: 29 March 20X2
From: Phyllis Cranborne
Subject: Petty cash

Marjorie Thistlethwaite mentioned to me yesterday that she wanted me to take responsibility for petty cash commencing on 1 June.

Could you please let me have a brief summary of how the petty cash imprest system works?

Thanks.

Phyllis

Draft a suitable reply.

2   Petty cash vouchers

2.1   Introduction

We have already seen the importance of petty cash vouchers as any payment of petty cash should not be made unless supported by a properly completed petty cash voucher which has been authorised.

2.2   Completing a petty cash voucher

If an employee wishes to be reimbursed for a business expense that he has incurred himself then he must complete a petty cash voucher. Different businesses will have different policies regarding amounts that can be paid out as petty cash but most organisations will require that petty cash vouchers are supported by documentation to show that the expenditure has occurred.

Most businesses will require petty cash vouchers to be supported by a receipt or other evidence of the payment such as a train ticket for a train fare.

Petty cash systems

Illustration 2 – Ruturns of goods

The petty cashier for your organisation is on holiday and you have been asked to act as petty cashier in her absence. You have been given the policy documents relating to petty cash and have discovered the following:

- a petty cash imprest system is operated with an imprest amount of £300 per week;

- no single petty cash voucher for more than £30 can be paid out of petty cash; any claims for amounts greater than £30 must be made using a cheque requisition;

- all petty cash claims other than taxi fares (see below) must include a valid receipt or evidence of payment;

- taxi fares of less than £5 can be paid without a receipt; all others must be supported by a receipt from the taxi;

- other transport expenses such as rail or underground fares exceeding £3 must be supported by a ticket showing the price of the fare or evidence of payment of the fare;

- other transport expenses of less than £3 do not need evidence of payment;

- no single employee can make claims of more than £30 on any one day.

On your first day of acting as petty cashier you have to deal with the following petty cash vouchers.

PETTY CASH VOUCHER				
Authorised by	Received by P Mallins		No	3562
Date	Description		Amount	
12 June X6	Tea and biscuits for office		12	73
	Total		12	73

Receipt attached

PETTY CASH VOUCHER			
Authorised by	Received by N Nixon	No	3563
Date	Description		Amount
12 June X6	Taxi	3	80
	Total	3	80

PETTY CASH VOUCHER			
Authorised by	Received by J KARL	No	3564
Date	Description		Amount
12 June X6	Bus fare	2	50
	Total	2	50

PETTY CASH VOUCHER			
Authorised by	Received by G Hull	No	3565
Date	Description		Amount
12 June X6	Taxi	6	00
	Total	6	00

PETTY CASH VOUCHER			
Authorised by	Received by F Trent	No	3566
Date	Description		Amount
12 June X6	Train fare	12	80
	Total	12	80

Ticket attached

PETTY CASH VOUCHER

Authorised by	Received by P Phillips		No	3567
Date	Description			Amount
12 June X6	Entertaining		35	00
	Total		35	00

PETTY CASH VOUCHER

Authorised by	Received by V Close		No	3568
Date	Description			Amount
12 June X6	Underground ticket		3	60
	Total		3	60

PETTY CASH VOUCHER

Authorised by	Received by P Mallins		No	3569
Date	Description			Amount
12 June X6	Entertaining		20	00
	Total		20	00

Restaurant bill attached

For each voucher explain whether you would be able to authorise it for payment from petty cash.

You must check each petty cash voucher carefully, together with any supporting documentation, to ensure that a valid payment can be made.

Solution

Voucher 3562 – Amount is less than £30 and supported by receipt – authorise for payment.

Voucher 3563 – Taxi fare of less than £5 therefore no receipt required – authorise for payment.

Voucher 3564 – Bus fare of less than £3 therefore no receipt required – authorise for payment.

Voucher 3565 – Taxi fare of more than £5 but no receipt – cannot authorise for payment.

Voucher 3566 – Train fare with ticket attached – authorise for payment.

Voucher 3567 – Claim for more than £30 – cannot authorise for payment – cheque requisition required.

Voucher 3568 – Underground ticket for more than £3 but no evidence of payment – cannot authorise for payment.

Voucher 3569 – Claim made by P Mallins who has already claimed £12.73 today (voucher no 3562) making a total of £32.73 – cannot authorise for payment.

2.3 VAT and petty cash vouchers

If an expense includes an amount of VAT, then the amounts recorded on the petty cash vouchers should be the net amount, the amount of VAT and the total payment.

Test your understanding 4

You are the petty cashier for your organisation. During your lunch break five receipts have appeared on your desk from employees making petty cash claims.

The receipts are as follows:

£2.99   Chocolate biscuits
£5.58   Stationery (includes VAT)
£20.00 Computer disks (includes VAT)
£8.90   Train fare
£3.95   Coffee and milk

The last petty cash voucher to be used was number 158. You are required to fill out and authorise petty cash vouchers for each of these receipts ready for payment of the petty cash to the employees concerned. Use the blank petty cash vouchers given.

Today's date is 7 September 20X1.

PETTY CASH VOUCHER

Authorised by	Received by	No
Date	Description	Amount
	Total	

PETTY CASH VOUCHER

Authorised by	Received by	No
Date	Description	Amount
	Total	

PETTY CASH VOUCHER

Authorised by	Received by	No
Date	Description	Amount
	Total	

PETTY CASH VOUCHER		
Authorised by	Received by	No
Date	Description	Amount
	Total	

PETTY CASH VOUCHER		
Authorised by	Received by	No
Date	Description	Amount
	Total	

3   Maintaining petty cash records

3.1   Introduction

The petty cash vouchers are recorded in their own book of prime entry which is known as the petty cash book. The petty cash book, similar to the cash receipts book and the cash payments book, is not only a primary record but is normally also kept as part of the main ledger double entry system.

The petty cash book is a primary record and is also part of the main ledger.

3.2   Layout of the petty cash book

The petty cash book is normally set out as a large ledger account with a small receipts side and a larger analysed payments side. A typical petty cash book is set out below.

Receipts			Payments								
Date	Narrative	Total	Date	Narrative	Voucher no	Total £	Postage £	Cleaning £	Tea & coffee £	Sundry £	VAT £
1 Nov	Bal b/f	35.50									
1 Nov	Cheque 394	114.50	1 Nov	ASDA	58	23.50			23.50		
			2 Nov	Post Office Ltd	59	29.50	29.50				
			2 Nov	Cleaning materials	60	14.76		12.56			2.20
			3 Nov	Postage	61	16.19	16.19				
			3 Nov	ASDA	62	10.35		8.81			1.54
			4 Nov	Newspapers	63	18.90				18.90	
			5 Nov	ASDA	64	11.85				10.09	1.76

3.3 Receipts side of the petty cash book

The receipts side of the petty cash book only requires one column, as the only receipt into the petty cash box is the regular payment into the petty cash box of cash drawn out of the bank account.

The only receipt into the petty cash box is the cash regularly paid into the petty cash box from the bank account.

3.4 Payments side of the petty cash book

Payments out of the petty cash box will be for a variety of different types of expense and an analysis column is required for each type of expense in the same way as the cash payments book is analysed. Note that a column is also required for VAT, as if a petty cash expense includes VAT this must also be analysed out. Remember that any VAT included in a petty cash expense must be shown separately on the petty cash voucher.

Any VAT shown on the petty cash voucher must be analysed out into the VAT column and the net amount shown in the expense analysis column.

3.5 Writing up the petty cash book

When cash is originally paid into the petty cash book then this will be recorded on the receipts side (debit side) of the petty cash book.

Each petty cash voucher will then in turn be written up in the petty cash book on the payments side.

Petty cash vouchers are pre-numbered to ensure that none are mislaid and they will be written into the petty cash book in number order with each item of expenditure being recorded in the correct analysis column.

Illustration 4 – Maintaining petty cash records

A business has just started to run an imprest petty cash system with an imprest amount of £100. £100 is withdrawn from the bank account and paid into the petty cash box on 3 April 20X1.

During the first week the following authorised petty cash vouchers were paid.

These transactions will now be recorded in the petty cash book.

PETTY CASH VOUCHER

Authorised by T Smedley	Received by P Lannall	No	0001	
Date	Description		Amount	
3 April 20X1	Tea/coffee/milk	4	73	
	Total	4	73	

PETTY CASH VOUCHER

Authorised by T Smedley	Received by R Sellers	No	0002	
Date	Description		Amount	
3 April 20X1	Train fare	14	90	
	Total	14	90	

PETTY CASH VOUCHER

Authorised by T Smedley	Received by F Dorne	No	0003	
Date	Description		Amount	
4 April 20X1	Stationery	4	00	
	VAT	0	70	
	Total	4	70	

PETTY CASH VOUCHER

Authorised by	Received by	No	0004
T Smedley	P Dent		
Date	Description		Amount
5 April 20X1	Postage costs	16	35
	Total	16	35

PETTY CASH VOUCHER

Authorised by	Received by	No	0005
T Smedley	H Polly		
Date	Description		Amount
7 April 20X1	Train fare	15	30
	Total	15	30

PETTY CASH VOUCHER

Authorised by	Received by	No	0006
T Smedley	P Lannall		
Date	Description		Amount
8 April 20X1	Milk/biscuits	3	85
	Total	3	85

> ### Solution
>
> | Receipts | | | Payments | | | | | | | | |
> |---|---|---|---|---|---|---|---|---|---|---|---|
> | Date | Narrative | Total | Date | Narrative | Voucher no | Total £ | Postage £ | Travel £ | Tea & coffee £ | Sundry £ | VAT £ |
> | 20X1 03/04 | Cash | 100.00 | 20X1 03/04 | Tea/coffee | 0001 | 4.73 | | | 4.73 | | |
> | | | | 03/04 | Train fare | 0002 | 14.90 | | 14.90 | | | |
> | | | | 04/04 | Stationery | 0003 | 4.70 | | | | 4.00 | 0.70 |
> | | | | 05/04 | Postage | 0004 | 16.35 | 16.35 | | | | |
> | | | | 07/04 | Train fare | 0005 | 15.30 | | 15.30 | | | |
> | | | | 08/04 | Milk/biscuits | 0006 | 3.85 | | | 3.85 | | |

4 Posting the petty cash book

4.1 Introduction

Now that we have seen how the petty cash book is written up we must next post the totals of the petty cash book to the main ledger accounts.

Remember that the petty cash book is part of the main ledger double entry system. Therefore the receipt of cash is the debit entry in the petty cash account and only the related credit entry is the cash coming out of the bank account and therefore recorded in the cash payments book .

The total of the payments is effectively the credit entry in the petty cash account and therefore the only postings that are required are the related debit entries to the relevant expense accounts.

4.2 Posting the petty cash receipt

The receipt into the petty cash box has come from cash being withdrawn from the bank account. This will have been done by writing out a cheque for cash and withdrawing this from the bank. Therefore the cheque should be recorded in the cash payments book as a payment when the cash payments book is written up.

The receipt of the cash into the petty cash box is recorded in the receipts side of the petty cash book, debit side.

As both the petty cash book and the cash payments book are normally part of the main ledger double entry system, the double entry has been completed. The debit is the entry into the petty cash book and the credit entry is the entry in the cash payments book.

4.3 Posting the petty cash payments

The petty cash book is part of the main ledger double entry system so the total column in the petty cash payments side is the credit entry to the petty cash account.

All that is required is therefore the debit entries to match this. These debit entries are taken from the totals of each of the analysis columns.

The total from each analysis column is debited to the relevant main ledger account.

Illustration 5 – Posting the petty cash book

The petty cash book written up in an earlier example is given again below. This is to be posted to the main ledger accounts.

Petty cash book

Receipts			Payments								
Date	Narrative	Total	Date	Narrative	Voucher no	Total £	Postage £	Travel £	Tea & coffee £	Sundry £	VAT £
20X1 03/04	Cash	100.00	20X1 03/04	Tea/coffee	0001	4.73			4.73		
			03/04	Train fare	0002	14.90		14.90			
			04/04	Stationery	0003	4.70				4.00	0.70
			05/04	Postage	0004	16.35	16.35				
			07/04	Train fare	0005	15.30		15.30			
			08/04	Milk/biscuits	0006	3.85			3.85		

Solution

Step 1 Each of the columns in the petty cash payments side must be totalled.

The accuracy of your totalling should be checked by ensuring that all of the analysis column totals add back to the total of the 'total' column in the petty cash book payments side.

Petty cash book

Receipts			Payments								
Date	Narrative	Total	Date	Narrative	Voucher no	Total £	Postage £	Travel £	Tea & coffee £	Sundry £	VAT £
20X1 03/04	Cash	100.00	20X1 03/04	Tea/coffee	0001	4.73			4.73		
			03/04	Train fare	0002	14.90		14.90			
			04/04	Stationery	0003	4.70				4.00	0.70
			05/04	Postage	0004	16.35	16.35				
			07/04	Train fare	0005	15.30		15.30			
			08/04	Milk/biscuits	0006	3.85			3.85		
						59.83	16.35	30.20	8.58	4.00	0.70

Check the totals:

	£
Postage	16.35
Travel	30.20
Tea and coffee	8.58
Sundry	4.00
VAT	0.70
	59.83

Step 2 Each of the analysis column totals must now be entered into the main ledger accounts as debit entries.

VAT account

	£		£
Petty cash book (PCB)	0.70		

The entry has come from the petty cash book and this is the reference – this is now shortened to PCB.

Postage account

	£		£
PCB	16.35		

Travel account

	£		£
PCB	30.20		

Tea and coffee account

	£		£
PCB	8.58		

Sundry expenses account

	£		£
PCB	4.00		

Test your understanding 5

Summary of petty cash vouchers in hand at 31 October 20X7

Date	Description	Total £	VAT included £
1/10	Envelopes (Administration)	19.72	2.93
4/10	Cleaner (Administration)	8.75	
6/10	Food for staff lunch (Marketing)	17.13	
6/10	Taxi fares (Marketing)	16.23	
6/10	Rail fares (Marketing)	43.75	
10/10	Postage (Administration)	4.60	
15/10	Tea and coffee (Production)	4.39	
17/10	Light bulbs and refuse sacks (Distribution)	8.47	1.26
20/10	Flowers for reception (Administration)	21.23	
26/10	Cleaner (Administration)	8.75	

(a) Write up the payments side of the petty cash book for October 20X7 from the information given.

You should allocate a sequential voucher number to each entry in the petty cash book. The last voucher number to be allocated in September was 6578.

Use the blank petty cash book provided.

(b) Total each of the columns in the petty cash book and cross-cast them.

(c) Post the totals to the main ledger accounts given.

PETTY CASH BOOK – PAYMENTS

Date	Voucher no	Total £	Production £	Distribution £	Marketing £	Administration £	VAT £

Production expenses account

£		£

Distribution expenses account

£		£

Marketing expenses account

£		£

Administration expenses account

£		£

VAT account

£		£

5 Petty cash control account

5.1 Introduction

In most cases the petty cash book is not only a book of prime entry but also part of the main ledger. However in other businesses the petty cash book will be simply a book of prime entry and a petty cash control account will be maintained in the main ledger.

5.2 Petty cash control account

The petty cash control account summarises the information in the petty cash book and is posted from the petty cash book. When cash is put into the petty cash box the petty cash control account will be debited and the total of the petty cash payments for the period will be credited to the petty cash control account.

Illustration 6 – Petty cash control account

A business runs a petty cash imprest system with an imprest amount of £100. At 1 May there was £32.56 remaining in the petty cash box and £67.44 of cash was withdrawn from the bank and put into the petty cash box to restore the imprest amount. During the month of May the total payments from the petty cash book were £82.16.

Write up the petty cash control account.

Solution

Petty cash control account

	£		£
Balance b/f	32.56	Payments	82.16
Receipt	67.44	Balance b/f	17.84
	100.00		100.00

5.3 Reconciliation of the petty cash with the petty cash control account

The balance on the petty cash control account at the end of each period should be equal to the amount of cash remaining in the petty cash box. If there is a difference then this must be investigated.

5.4 Possible causes of difference

If there is more cash in the petty cash box than the balance on the petty cash control account this could be due to an error in writing up the petty cash book as more has been recorded in payments than has actually been paid out. In this case the entries in the petty cash book should be checked to the underlying petty cash vouchers to discover the error.

If there is less cash in the petty cash box than the balance on the petty cash control account this could also be due to an error in writing up the petty cash book as this time less payments have been recorded in the petty cash control account than were actually made. This may be due to a petty cash voucher having been omitted from the petty cash book and therefore again the underlying petty cash vouchers should all be checked to their entries in the petty cash book.

If no accounting errors or posting errors can be found then the cause is likely to be one of the following:

- an error has been made in paying a petty cash voucher and more money was handed out than was recorded on the voucher;

- cash has been paid out of the petty cash box without a supporting voucher

- cash could have been stolen from the petty cash box.

In such cases the matter should be investigated and security of the petty cash and petty cash procedures improved.

Illustration 7 – Petty cash control account

The petty cash control account from the previous example is reproduced.

Petty cash control account

	£		£
Balance b/f	32.56	Payments	82.16
Receipt	67.44	Balance b/f	17.84
	100.00		100.00
Balance b/f	17.84		

What action should be taken if when the petty cash was counted at 31 May the amount held in the box was:

(a) £27.84

(b) £7.84

Solution

(a) If the amount of cash in the box was £27.84 then this is £10 more than expected.   The following checks should be made:

  – Has the balance on the petty cash control account been correctly calculated?

  – Have the receipt and payments totals been correctly posted to the petty cash control account?

  – Have the payments in the petty cash book been correctly totalled?

  – Has each individual petty cash voucher been correctly recorded in the petty cash book?

(b) If the amount of cash in the box is only £7.84 then this is £10 less than expected. All of the above checks should be carried out and if no accounting errors can be found then it will have to be assumed that either £10 too much has been paid out on a petty cash voucher, £10 has been paid out of the petty cash box without a supporting voucher or that £10 has been stolen from the petty cash box.

6 Reconciling the petty cash

6.1 Introduction

We saw earlier in the chapter that when an imprest system is being used for petty cash then at any point in time the amount of cash in the petty cash box plus the total of the vouchers in the petty cash box should equal the imprest amount.

At regular intervals, usually at the end of each week, this check will be carried out.

6.2 Procedure for reconciling the petty cash box

The total amount of cash in the petty cash box will be counted. The vouchers that have been paid during the week are also in the petty cash box and they must also be totalled.

When the amount of cash is added to the total of the vouchers in the box they should equal the imprest amount.

The petty cash vouchers for the week will then be removed from the box and filed.

Illustration 8 – Reconciling the petty cash

The amount of cash remaining in a petty cash box at the end of a week is as follows:

Notes/coins	Quantity
£10	1
£5	2
£2	3
£1	7
50p	9
20p	11
10p	15
5p	7
2p	16
1p	23

The imprest amount is £100 and the vouchers in the petty cash box at the end of the week are as follows:

PETTY CASH VOUCHER			
Authorised by C Alexi	*Received by* P Trant	*No* 0467	
Date	*Description*	*Amount*	
4 May 20X3	Window cleaner	15	00
	Total	15	00

PETTY CASH VOUCHER			
Authorised by C Alexi	*Received by* F Saint	*No* 0468	
Date	*Description*	*Amount*	
5 May 20X3	Train fare	9	80
	Total	9	80

PETTY CASH VOUCHER			
Authorised by C Alexi	Received by A Paul	No 0469	
Date	Description	Amount	
5 May 20X3	Stationery	8	00
	VAT	1	40
	Total	9	40

PETTY CASH VOUCHER			
Authorised by C Alexi	Received by P Peters	No 0470	
Date	Description	Amount	
7 May 20X3	Postage	6	80
	Total	6	80

PETTY CASH VOUCHER

Authorised by C Alexi	Received by C Ralph	No	0471	
Date	Description		Amount	
5 May 20X3	Train fare	16	90	
	Total	16	90	

The cash and vouchers in the petty cash box at the end of the week are to be reconciled.

Solution

The petty cash must be totalled:

Notes/coins	Quantity	Amount £
£10	1	10.00
£5	2	10.00
£2	3	6.00
£1	7	7.00
50p	9	4.50
20p	11	2.20
10p	15	1.50
5p	7	0.35
2p	16	0.32
1p	23	0.23
		42.10

Now the vouchers must be totalled.

	£
0467	15.00
0468	9.80
0469	9.40
0470	6.80
0471	16.90
	57.90

Finally, total the cash and the vouchers to ensure that they add back to the imprest amount.

	£
Cash	42.10
Vouchers	57.90
	100.00

Test your understanding 6

Your business runs a petty cash box based upon an imprest amount of £60.

This morning you have emptied the petty cash box and found the following notes, coins and vouchers.

Notes
£5 × 2

Coins
£1 × 3
50p × 5
20p × 4
10p × 6
5p × 7
2p × 10
1p × 8

Vouchers	£
2143	10.56
2144	3.30
2145	9.80
2146	8.44
2147	2.62
2148	6.31
2149	1.44

You are required to reconcile the cash and the vouchers in the petty cash box.

Test your understanding 7

1   Explain how an imprest petty cash system works.

2   What are the important features of a properly completed petty cash voucher?

3   A petty cash imprest system is run with an imprest amount of £120. During a week the total of the petty cash vouchers that have been reimbursed was £83. How much should be withdrawn from the bank to reimburse the petty cash box?

4   A cheque for cash is drawn and £58.00 in cash taken from the bank for petty cash. How should this be recorded in the petty cash book?

5   If the petty cash book is part of the main ledger then how are

the totals of the analysis columns of the payment side of the petty cash book entered into the ledger accounts?

6   A business has a petty cash box run on an imprest system with an imprest amount of £80. The actual cash in the box at the end of the week totalled £36.44. How much should the petty cash vouchers for the week total?

7   Summary

In this chapter we have considered the entire petty cash system. Cash is paid into the petty cash box in order to meet the requirements for actual cash in a business's life. This will normally be in the form of reimbursing employees for business expenses that they have incurred on their own behalf. In order to be reimbursed for the expense, the employee must fill out a petty cash voucher which will normally be accompanied by a receipt for the expense and must then be authorised. At this point the employee can be paid the cash out of the petty cash box.

All petty cash is recorded in the petty cash book which is normally both a book of prime entry and part of the main ledger. The cash paid into the petty cash box is recorded as a receipt in the petty cash book and as a payment in the cash payments book, an amount of cash being taken out of the bank account. The payments of petty cash vouchers are recorded as payments in the petty cash book and are analysed as to the type of payment. These payments are then recorded as debit entries in the appropriate expense account.

At the end of a period, a week or a month possibly, the cash in the petty cash box will be counted and reconciled to the vouchers in the box. In an imprest system the total of the vouchers in the box plus the total of the cash in the box should equal the imprest amount.

KAPLAN PUBLISHING

Test your understanding answers

Test your understanding 1

Any two from the following:

(i)   Should be kept securely in a locked box or safe, etc.

(ii) All payments should be properly authorised.

(iii) Should be the responsibility of one person.

(iv) The amount of any one payment should be restricted.

Test your understanding 2

£180

Test your understanding 3

HAIRDRESSING SUPPLIES LIMITED

MEMORANDUM

To: Phyllis Cranborne   Date: 29 March 20X2
From: Chris

Subject: Petty cash system

Marjorie has already notified me that she would like you to take charge of petty cash from 1 June next.

The main features of our present system are as follows:

(1) The petty cash imprest system is one in which a fixed amount of money is advanced to the cashier, sufficient to meet normal petty cash disbursements over an agreed period (in our case one month).

(2) Payments are made out of petty cash only if evidenced by properly authorised petty cash vouchers, supported by invoices or receipts.

(3) At the end of each period, the petty cashier presents a return to the cashier giving details of the total amount spent, which is repaid to the petty cashier. The amount then held is the originally agreed fixed sum.

(4) Periodically, Marjorie checks that the amount held agrees with the fixed amount, less expenditure since the last reimbursement date.

Please let me know if you have any further queries regarding the petty cash system.

Chris

Test your understanding 4

PETTY CASH VOUCHER				
Authorised by A Student	Received by		No	159
Date	Description		Amount	
07/09/X1	Chocolate biscuits		2	99
		Total	2	99

PETTY CASH VOUCHER				
Authorised by A Student	Received by		No	160
Date	Description		Amount	
07/09/X1	Stationery		4	75
	VAT		0	83
		Total	5	58

PETTY CASH VOUCHER				
Authorised by A Student	Received by		No	161
Date	Description		Amount	
07/09/X1	Computer disks		17	03
	VAT		2	97
		Total	20	00

PETTY CASH VOUCHER

Authorised by A Student	Received by	No	162	
Date	Description	Amount		
07/09/X1	Train fare	8	90	
	Total	8	90	

PETTY CASH VOUCHER

Authorised by A Student	Received by	No	163	
Date	Description	Amount		
07/09/X1	Coffee and milk	3	95	
	Total	3	95	

If any petty cash expenses include VAT then the VAT must be shown on the petty cash voucher so that it can eventually be correctly posted to the petty cash book and expense accounts.

Test your understanding 5

(a), (b)

PETTY CASH BOOK – PAYMENTS

Date	Voucher no	Total £		Production £		Distribution £		Marketing £		Administration £		VAT £	
01/10/X7	6579	19	72							16	79	2	93
04/10/X7	6580	8	75							8	75		
06/10/X7	6581	17	13					17	13				
06/10/X7	6582	16	23					16	23				
06/10/X7	6583	43	75					43	75				
10/10/X7	6584	4	60							4	60		
15/10/X7	6585	4	39	4	39								
17/10/X7	6586	8	47			7	21					1	26
20/10/X7	6587	21	23							21	23		
26/10/X7	6588	8	75							8	75		
		153	02	4	39	7	21	77	11	60	12	4	19

Production expenses account

	£		£
PCB	4.39		

Distribution expenses account

	£		£
PCB	7.21		

Marketing expenses account

	£		£
PCB	77.11		

Administration expenses account

	£		£
PCB	60.12		

VAT account

	£		£
PCB	4.19		

Test your understanding 6

Notes and coins

	£	£
£5 × 2	10.00	
£1 × 3	3.00	
50p × 5	2.50	
20p × 4	0.80	
10p × 6	0.60	
5p × 7	0.35	
2p × 10	0.20	
1p × 8	0.08	
		17.53

Vouchers

	£	
2143	10.56	
2144	3.30	
2145	9.80	
2146	8.44	
2147	2.62	
2148	6.31	
2149	1.44	
		42.47
Imprest amount		60.00

Test your understanding 7

1   An imprest amount is initially set and paid into the petty cash box. At any point in time the amount of cash in the box plus the value of the vouchers should total to the imprest amount. At the end of each period the amount of cash to be withdrawn to reimburse the petty cash box to the imprest amount is the total of the vouchers that have been paid during the period.

2   – Sequential number

    – Details of the expenditure

    – Name of the claimant

    – Authorisation signature

    – Date of claim

3   £83

4   As a receipt on the receipts side of the petty cash book.

5   The totals of the analysis columns are debited to the appropriate expense accounts.

6   £80 – £36.44 = £43.56

Bank reconciliations

Introduction

You may be required to prepare the cash book, compare the entries in the cash book to details on the bank statement and then finally to prepare a bank reconciliation statement.

1 Writing up the cash book

1.1 Introduction

Earlier in this text you learnt how to write up the cash receipts book and the cash payments book. This will be practised again here.

Most businesses will have a separate cash receipts book and a cash payments book which are part of the double entry system. If this form of record is used, the cash balance must be calculated from the opening balance at the beginning of the period, plus the receipts shown in the cash receipts book and minus the payments shown in the cash payments book.

1.2 Balancing the cash book

You will need to be able to find the balance on the cash book. This is done using the following brief calculation:

	£
Opening balance on the cash book	X
Add: Receipts in the period	X
Less: Payments in the period	(X)
Closing balance on the cash book	X

Illustration 1 – Writing up the cash book

Suppose that the opening balance on the cash book is £358.72 on 1 June. During June the Cash Payments Book shows that there were total payments made of £7,326.04 during the month of June and the Cash Receipts Book shows receipts for the month of £8,132.76.

What is the closing balance on the cash book at the end of June?

Solution

	£
Opening balance at 1 June	358.72
Add: Receipts for June	8,132.76
Less: Payments for June	(7,326.04)
Balance at 30 June	1,165.44

Take care if the opening balance on the cash book is an overdraft balance. Any receipts in the period will reduce the overdraft and any payments will increase the overdraft.

Test your understanding 1

The opening balance at 1 January in a business cash book was £673.42 overdrawn. During January payments totalled £6,419.37 and receipts totalled £6,488.20.

What is the closing balance on the cash book?

Illustration 2 – Writing up the cash book

The following transactions are to be written up in the cash book of Jupiter Limited and the balance at the end of the week calculated. The opening balance on the bank account on 1 July 20X1 was £560.61.

2 July   Received a cheque for £45.90 from Hill and French Limited (no settlement discount allowed) – paying in slip 40012.

2 July   Corrected a salary error by paying a cheque for £56.89 – cheque number 100107.

3 July   Paid £96.65 by cheque to Preston Brothers after deducting a settlement discount of £1.65 – cheque number 100108.

3 July   Banked £30 of cash held – paying in slip 40013.

4 July   Received a cheque from Green and Holland for £245.89. They were allowed a settlement discount of £3.68 – paying in slip 40014.

5 July   Reimbursed the petty cash account with £34.89 of cash drawn on cheque number 100109.

The cash receipts and payments books are to be written up and the closing balance calculated.

Solution

Step 1   Enter all of the transactions into the receipts and payments cash books.

Step 2   Total the cash book columns.

Cash receipts book

Date	Narrative		Total £	VAT £	Sales ledger £	Other £	Discount £
20X1							
2 July	Hill and French	40012	45.90		45.90		
3 July	Cash	40013	30.00			30.00	
4 July	Green and Holland	40014	245.89		245.89		3.68
			321.79	–	291.79	30.00	3.68

Cash payments book

Date	Details	Cheque	Code no	Total £	VAT £	Purchases ledger £	Cash purchases £	Other £	Discounts received £
20X1									
2 July	Salary error	100107		56.89				56.89	
3 July	Preston Bros	100108		96.65		96.65			1.65
5 July	Petty cash	100109		34.89				34.89	
				188.43	–	96.65	–	91.78	1.65

Step 3 Find the balance on the cash book at the end of the week.

	£
Opening balance at 1 July	560.61
Add: Receipts total	321.79
Less: Payments total	(188.43)
Balance at the end of the week	693.97

When totalling the cash book columns always check your additions carefully as it is easy to make mistakes when totalling columns of numbers on a calculator. Check that the totals of each analysis column (excluding the discounts columns) add back to the total of the total column.

2 Preparing the bank reconciliation statement

2.1 Introduction

At regular intervals (normally at least once a month) the cashier must check that the cash book is correct by comparing the cash book with the bank statement.

2.2 Differences between the cash book and bank statement

At any date the balance shown on the bank statement is unlikely to agree with the balance in the cash book for two main reasons.

(a) Items in the cash book not on the bank statement

Certain items will have been entered in the cash book but will not appear on the bank statement at the time of the reconciliation. Examples are as follows.

– Cheques received by the business and paid into the bank which have not yet appeared on the bank statement, due to the time lag of the clearing system. These are known as outstanding lodgements.

– Cheques written by the business but which have not yet

appeared on the bank statement, because the recipients have not yet paid them in, or the cheques are in the clearing system. These are known as unpresented cheques.

- Errors in the cash book (e.g. transposition of numbers, addition errors).

(b) Items on the bank statement not in the cash book

At the time of the bank reconciliation certain items will appear on the bank statement that have not yet been entered in the cash book. These occur because frequently the cashier will not know of the existence of these items until he receives the bank statements. Examples are:

- direct debit or standing order payments that are in the bank statement but have not yet been entered in the cash payments book

- BACS or other receipts paid directly into the bank account by a customer

- bank charges or bank interest that are unknown until the bank statement has been received and therefore will not be in the cash book

- errors in the cash book that may only come to light when the cash book entries are compared to the bank statement

- returned cheques i.e. cheques paid in from a customer who does not have sufficient funds in his bank to pay the cheque (see later in this chapter).

2.3 The bank reconciliation

A bank reconciliation is simply a statement that explains the differences between the balance in the cash book and the balance on the bank statement at a particular date.

A bank reconciliation is produced by following a standard set of steps.

Step 1: Compare the cash book and the bank statement for the relevant period and identify any differences between them.

This is usually done by ticking in the cash book and bank statement items that appear in both the cash book and the bank statement. Any items left unticked therefore only appear in one place, either the cash book or the bank statement. We saw in 2.2 above the reasons why this might occur.

Step 2: Enter in the cash book items that appear on the bank statement which do not yet appear in the cash book.

Tick these items in both the cash book and the bank statement once they are entered in the cash book.

At this stage there will be no unticked items on the bank statement.

(You clearly cannot enter on the bank statement items in the cash book that do not appear on the bank statement – the bank prepares the bank statement, not you. These items will either be unpresented cheques or outstanding lodgements – see 2.2 above.)

Step 3: Bring down the new cash book balance following the adjustments in step 2 above.

Step 4: Prepare the bank reconciliation statement.

This will typically have the following proforma.

Bank reconciliation as at 31.0X.200X

	£
Balance as per bank statement	X
Less unpresented cheques	(X)
Add outstanding lodgements	X
Balance as per cash book	X

Think for a moment to ensure you understand this proforma.

We deduct the unpresented cheques (cheques already entered in the cash book but not yet on the bank statement) from the bank balance, because when they are presented this bank balance will be reduced.

We add outstanding lodgements (cash received and already entered in the cash book) because when they appear on the bank statement they will increase the bank balance.

2.4 Debits and credits in bank statements

When comparing the cash book to the bank statement it is easy to get confused with debits and credits.

- When we pay money into the bank, we debit our cash book but the bank credits our account.

- This is because a debit in our cash book represents the increase in our asset 'cash'. For the bank, the situation is different: they will debit their cash book and credit our account because they now owe us more money; we are a creditor.

- When our account is overdrawn, we owe the bank money and consequently our cash book will show a credit balance. For the bank an overdraft is a debit balance.

On the bank statement a credit is an amount of money paid into the account and a debit represents a payment.

Illustration 3 – Preparing a bank reconcilliation statement

Given below are the completed cash books for Jupiter Limited from the previous example.

Cash receipts book

Date	Narrative		Total £	VAT £	Sales ledger £	Other £	Discount received £
20X1							
2 July	Hill and French	40012	45.90		45.90		
3 July	Cash	40013	30.00			30.00	
4 July	Green and Holland	40014	245.89		245.89		3.68
			321.79	–	291.79	30.00	3.68

Cash payments book

Date	Details	Cheque	Code no	Total £	VAT £	Purchases ledger £	Cash purchases £	Other £	Discounts received £
20X1									
2 July	Salary error	100107		56.89				56.89	
3 July	Preston Bros	100108		96.65		96.65			1.65
5 July	Petty cash	100109		34.89				34.89	
				188.43	–	96.65	–	91.78	1.65

You have now received the bank statement for the week commencing 1 July 20X1 which is also shown below.

FIRST NATIONAL BANK
Cheque Account
SHEET NUMBER 012
ACCOUNT NUMBER 38 41 57 33794363

			Paid in £	Paid out £	Balance £
28 June	Balance brought forward				560.61
1 July	CT	A/C 38562959	123.90		684.51
4 July	CHQ	100107		56.89	
4 July	CR	40013	30.00		657.62
5 July	CR	40012	45.90		
5 July	DR	Bank charges		5.23	
5 July	DD	English Telecom		94.00	
5 July	CHQ	100109		34.89	569.40

CHQ	Cheque	CT	Credit transfer	CR	Payment in
DR	Payment out	DD	Direct debit		

You are required to compare the cash book and the bank statement and determine any differences. Tick the items in the bank statement and in the cash book above, then prepare the bank reconciliation statement at 5 July 20X1.

The balance on the cash book at 28 June was £560.61.

Solution

Step 1   The cash book, duly ticked, appears below.

Cash receipts book

Date	Narrative		Total £	VAT £	Sales ledger £	Other £	Discount allowed £
20X1							
2 July	Hill and French	40012	45.90 ✓		45.90		
3 July	Cash	40013	30.00 ✓			30.00	
4 July	Green and Holland	40014	245.89		245.89		3.68
			321.79	–	291.79	30.00	3.68

Cash payments book

Date	Details	Cheque	Code no	Total £	VAT £	Purchases ledger £	Cash purchases £	Other £	Discounts received £
20X1									
2 July	Salary error	100107		56.89 ✓				56.89	
3 July	Preston Bros	100108		96.65		96.65			1.65
5 July	Petty cash	100109		34.89 ✓				34.89	
				188.43	–	96.65	–	91.78	1.65

The bank statement should have been ticked as shown below.

```
FIRST NATIONAL BANK
Cheque Account
SHEET NUMBER 012
ACCOUNT NUMBER 38 41 57 33794363
                                    Paid in    Paid out    Balance
                                       £           £           £
     28 June  Balance brought forward                        560.61
     1 July   CT    A/C 38562959     123.90                  684.51
     4 July   CHQ   100107                       56.89 ✓
     4 July   CR    40013            30.00 ✓                 657.62
     5 July   CR    40012            45.90 ✓
     5 July   DR    Bank charges                  5.23
     5 July   DD    English Telecom             94.00
     5 July   CHQ   100109                       34.89 ✓     569.40

CHQ  Cheque          CT    Credit transfer    CR    Payment in
DR   Payment out     DD    Direct debit
```

Step 2 A comparison of the items in the cash book with those in the bank statement reveals unticked items in both.

(a) We will first consider the items that are unticked on the bank statement;

  – there is a credit transfer on 1 July of £123.90 – this must be checked to the related documentation and then entered into the cash receipts book;

  – the bank charges of £5.23 must be entered into the cash payments book;

  – the direct debit of £94.00 should be checked and then entered into the cash payments book.

(b) We will now consider the items that are unticked in the cash book. Remember that no adjustment is needed to these but we have to decide where they will appear in the bank reconciliation statement.

  – the cheque paid in on 4 July has not yet appeared on the bank statement due to the time it takes for cheques to clear through the clearing system – an outstanding lodgement;

  – cheque number 100108 has not yet cleared through the banking system – an unpresented cheque.

The cash receipts and cash payments book will now appear as follows after the adjustments in (a) above.

Bank reconciliations

Date	Narrative		Total £	VAT £	Sales ledger £	Other £	Discount allowed £
20X1							
2 July	Hill and French	40012	45.90	✓	45.90		
3 July	Cash	40013	30.00	✓		30.00	
4 July	Green and Holland	40014	245.89		245.89		3.68
1 July	Credit transfer		123.90	✓	123.90		
			445.69	–	415.69	30.00	3.68

Cash payment book

Date	Details	Cheque	Code no	Total £	VAT £	Purchases ledger £	Cash purchases £	Other £	Discounts received £
20X1									
2 July	Salary error	100107		56.89	✓			56.89	
3 July	Preston Bros	100108		96.65		96.65			1.65
5 July	Petty cash	100109		34.89	✓			34.89	
5 July	Bank charges			5.23	✓			5.23	
5 July	English Telcom	DD		94.00	✓	94.00			
				287.66	–	190.65	–	97.01	1.65

Note that the items we have entered in the cash book from the bank statement are ticked in both. There are no unticked items on the bank statement (not shown) and two unticked items in the cash book.

Step 3 Find the amended cash book balance.

	£
Balance at 28 June	560.61
Cash receipts in first week of July	445.69
Cash payments in first week of July	(287.66)
Balance at 5 July	718.64

Step 4 Reconcile the amended cash book balance to the bank statement balance.

Bank reconciliation as at 5 July 20X1

	£
Balance per bank statement	569.40
Less: unpresented cheque	(96.65)
Add: outstanding lodgement	245.89
Balance per cash book	718.64

This is the completed bank reconciliation.

KAPLAN PUBLISHING

The following are summaries of the cash receipts book, cash payments book and bank statement for the first two weeks of trading of Gambank, a firm specialising in selling cricket bats.

Cash receipts book

Date	Narrative	Total £	VAT £	Sales ledger £	Other £	Discount £
20X0						
01 Jan	Capital	2,000			2,000	
05 Jan	A Hunter	1,000		1,000		
09 Jan	Cancel chque no 0009	90				90
10 Jan	IM Dunn	4,800		4,800		

Cash payments book

Date	Details	Cheque	Code no	Total £	VAT £	Purchases ledger £	Cash purchases £	Other £	Discounts received £
20X0									
01 Jan	Wages	0001		50				50	
02 Jan	Fine	0002		12				12	
03 Jan	Dodgy Dealers	0003		1,500		1,500			
04 Jan	E L Pubo	0004		45		45			
05 Jan	Drawings	0005		200				200	
07 Jan	EL Wino	0007		30		30			
08 Jan	Toby	0008		1,400		1,400			
09 Jan	EL Pubo	0009		70		70			
10 Jan	Marion's Emp	0010		200		200			
11 Jan	Speeding	0011		99				99	

FINANCIAL BANK plc   CONFIDENTIAL

10 Yorkshire Street   **Account** CURRENT Sheet No.   1
Headingley   GAMBANK
Leeds LS1 1QT
Telephone: 0113 633061

Statement date 14 Jan 20X0   **Account Number** 40023986

Date	Details	Withdrawals (£)	Deposits (£)	Balance (£)
01 Jan	CR		2,000	2,000
02 Jan	0001	50		1,950
04 Jan	0003	1,500		450
05 Jan	0005	200		250
07 Jan	CR		1,000	
	0002	12		
	0004	45		
	0006	70		1,123
08 Jan	0007	30		1,093
10 Jan	0009	70		
	0009		70	
	0010	200		893
11 Jan	0012	20		
	Charges	53		820

SO Standing order	DD Direct debit	CRCredit
AC Automated cash	OD Overdrawn	TRTransfer

Prepare a bank reconciliation statement at 14 January 20X0.

2.5   Opening balances disagree

Usually the balances on the bank statement and in the cash book do not agree at the start of the period for the same reasons that they do not agree at the end, e.g. items in the cash book that were not on the bank statement. When producing the reconciliation statement it is important to take this opening difference into account.

Illustration 4 – Preparing a bank reconcilliation statement

The bank statement and cash book of Jones for the month of December 20X8 start as follows.

Bank statement

		Debit £	Credit £	Balance £
1 Dec 20X8	Balance b/d (favourable)			8,570
2 Dec 20X8	0073	125		
2 Dec 20X8	0074	130		
3 Dec 20X8	Sundries		105	

Cash book

	£			£
1 Dec 20X8 b/d	8,420	Cheque 0076	Wages	200
Sales	320	Cheque 0077	Rent	500
	X			X
	X			X

Explain the difference between the opening balances.

Solution

The difference in the opening balance is as follows.

£8,570 – £8,420 = £150

This difference is due to the following.

	£
Cheque 0073	125
Cheque 0074	130
	255
Lodgement (sundries)	(105)
	150

These cheques and lodgements were in the cash book in November, but only appear on the bank statement in December. They will therefore be matched and ticked against the entries in the November cash book. The December reconciliation will then proceed as normal.

3 Returned cheques

A customer C may send a cheque in payment of an invoice without having sufficient funds in his account with Bank A.

The seller S who receives the cheque will pay it into his account with Bank B and it will go into the clearing system. Bank B will credit S's account with the funds in anticipation of the cheque being honoured.

Bank A however will not pay funds into the S's account with Bank B and Bank B will then remove the funds from S's account.

The net effect of this is that on S's bank statement, the cheque will appear as having been paid in (a credit on the bank statement), and then later will appear as having been paid out (a debit on the bank statement).

The original credit on the bank statement will be in S's cash book as a debit in the normal way. But the debit on the bank statement (the dishonour of the cheque) will not be in S's cash book. This will have to be credited into the cash book as money paid out.

These cheques are technically referred to as 'returned cheques', but they are also called 'dishonoured cheques' or 'bounced cheques'.

Illustration 5 – Preparing a bank reconcilliation statement

C sends a cheque to S in payment of an invoice for £300.

(a) S will enter this cheque into his accounts as follows:

Cash book

	£		£
SLCA	300		

SLCA

	£		£
		Cash book	300

The cheque will appear on S's bank statement as a credit entry.

(b) When the cheque is dishonoured S will enter this cheque into his accounts as follows:

Cash book

	£		£
		SLCA	300

SLCA

	£		£
Cash book	300		

The journal entry will be

Dr	SLCA	300	
Cr	Cash book		300

This reinstates the debtor

The dishonoured cheque will appear on the bank statement as a debit entry.

Test your understanding 3

1   The opening balance on a business cash book was an overdraft of £200. During the period there were cash receipts totalling £2,500 and cash payments totalling £1,800. What was the closing balance on the cash book?

2   What differences might be discovered by comparing the cash receipts and payments books to the bank statement?

3   If a standing order payment appears on the bank statement but not in the cash book what action, if any, is required?

4   A cash receipt of £500 has been entered into the cash receipts book but is not in the bank statement. What would the receipt be known as and what action, if any, is required?

5   The bank statement for a business at the end of June shows a debit balance of £320. Does this mean that the business has money in the bank or an overdraft?

6   The bank statement for a business at the end of March shows a credit balance of £440. There are items totalling £600 in the cash receipts book which do not appear in the bank statement and items totalling £800 in the cash payments book which do not appear in the bank statement. Assuming that the cash books are correct what is the balance on the cash book at the end of March?

4   Summary

In this chapter you have had to write up the cash receipts and cash payments books and then total and balance the cash book. However, most importantly a comparison has to be made between the cash book and the bank statement and a bank reconciliation prepared. Do note that when comparing the bank statement to the cash book, figures appearing on the bank statement may be from the cash book some time ago due to the nature of the clearing system and the general timing of cheques being sent out and then presented to a bank.

Test your understanding answers

Test your understanding 1

	£
Opening balance	(673.42)
Payments	(6,419.37)
Receipts	6,488.20
Closing balance	(604.59)

The closing balance is £604.59 overdrawn.

Test your understanding 2

Step 1 Tick the cash books and bank statement to indicate the matched items.

Date	Narrative	Total £	VAT £	Sales ledger £	Other £	Discount £
20X1						
01 Jan	Capital	2,000 ✓			2,000	
05 Jan	A Hunter	1,000 ✓		1,000		
09 Jan	Cancel chque no 0009	90			90	
10 Jan	I M Dunn	4,800		4,800		
		7,890	–	5,800	2,090	–

Cash payments book

Date	Details	Cheque	Code no	Total £	VAT £	Purchases ledger £	Cash purchases £	Other £	Discounts received £
20X0									
01 Jan	Wages	0001		50 ✓				50	
02 Jan	Fine	0002		12 ✓				12	
03 Jan	Dodgy Dealers	0003		1,500 ✓		1,500			
04 Jan	E L Pubo	0004		45 ✓		45			
05 Jan	Drawings	0005		200 ✓				200	
07 Jan	EL Wino	0007		30 ✓		30			
08 Jan	Toby	0008		1,400		1,400			
09 Jan	EL Pubo	0009		70 ✓		70			
10 Jan	Marion's Emp	0010		200 ✓		200			
11 Jan	Speeding Fine	0011		99				99	
				3,606	–	3,245	–	361	

FINANCIAL BANK plc   CONFIDENTIAL

Account CURRENT Sheet No.   1

10 Yorkshire Street
Headingley   GAMBANK
Leeds LS1 1QT
Telephone: 0113 633061

Statement date 14 Jan 20X0   **Account Number** 40023986

Date	Details	Withdrawals (£)	Deposits (£)	Balance (£)
01 Jan	CR		2,000✓	2,000
02 Jan	0001	50 ✓		1,950
04 Jan	0003	1,500 ✓		450
05 Jan	0005	200 ✓		250
07 Jan	CR		1,000✓	
	0002	12✓		
	0004	45✓		
	0006	70		1,123
08 Jan	0007	30✓		1,093
10 Jan	0009	70✓		
	0009		70	
	0010	200✓		893
11 Jan	0012	20		
	Charges	53		820

SO Standing order	DD Direct debit	CRCredit
AC Automated cash	OD Overdrawn	TRTransfer

Step 2 Deal with each of the unticked items.

Cash receipts book

- cheque number 0009 does appear to have been cancelled as it has appeared as a debit and a credit entry in the bank statement – however the bank statement shows that the cheque was for £70 and not the £90 entered into the cash receipts book – this must be amended in the cash book.

- the receipt from I M Dunn has not yet cleared through the banking system and is therefore not on the bank statement – it is an outstanding lodgement.

Cash payments book

- cheque number 0008 to Toby and cheque number 0011 have not yet cleared through the clearing system – they are unpresented cheques.

Bank statement

- cheque number 0006 has not been entered into the cash

payments book but it has cleared the bank account – the cash book must be amended to show this payment.

- cheque number 0012 has not been entered into the cash payments book but it has cleared the bank account – the cash book must be amended to show this payment.

- the bank charges of £53 must be entered into the cash payments book.

Step 3 Amend the cash books and total them.

Cash receipts book

Date	Narrative	Total £	VAT £	Sales ledger £	Other £	Discount £
20X1						
01 Jan	Capital	2,000	✓		2,000	
05 Jan	A Hunter	1,000	✓	1,000		
09 Jan	Cancel chque no 0009	90	✓		90	
10 Jan	I M Dunn	4,800		4,800		
10 Jan	Cancelled cheque adjustment 0009	(20)	✓		(20)	
		7,890	–	5,800	2,070	–

Cash payments book

Date	Details	Cheque	Code no	Total £	VAT £	Purchases ledger £	Cash purchases £	Other £	Discounts received £
20X0									
01 Jan	Wages	0001		50	✓			50	
02 Jan	Fine	0002		12	✓			12	
03 Jan	Dodgy Dealers	0003		1,500	✓	1,500			
04 Jan	E L Pubo	0004		45	✓	45			
05 Jan	Drawings	0005		200	✓			200	
07 Jan	EL Wino	0007		30	✓	30			
08 Jan	Toby	0008		1,400		1,400			
09 Jan	EL Pubo	0009		70	✓	70			
10 Jan	Marion's Emp	0010		200	✓	200			
11 Jan	Speeding Fine	0011		99				99	
10 Jan		0006		70	✓	70			
10 Jan		0012		20	✓	20			
11 Jan	Bank charges			53	✓			53	
				3,749	–	3,335	–	414	

Step 4 Determine the amended cash book balance

	£
Opening balance	–
Cash receipts	7,870
Cash payments	(3,749)
Amended cash book balance	4,121

Step 5 Reconcile the amended cash book balance to the bank statement balance

		£	£
Balance per bank statement			820
Add: outstanding lodgement			4,800
Less: unpresented cheques	0008	1,400	
	0011	99	
			(1,499)
Amended cash book balance			4,121

Test your understanding 3

1

	£
Opening balance	(200)
Receipts	2,500
Payments	(1,800)
	500 in credit

2 – errors in the cash book

– direct debits/standing orders omitted from the cash book

– direct bank giro credits omitted from the cash book

– bank charges/interest not entered into the cash book

– unpresented cheques/outstanding lodgements

3 The cash payments book should be amended to reflect the payment.

4 Outstanding lodgement. No alteration is required although this will be a reconciling item in the bank reconciliation statement.

5 A debit balance on the bank statement is an overdraft.

6

	£
Balance per bank statement	440
Add: Outstanding lodgements	600
Less: Unpresented cheques	(800)
Balance per cash book	240

17

Ledger balances and control accounts

Introduction

In this chapter we will be finding the correct ledger account balances by revising balancing off ledger accounts (covered in an earlier chapter) as the basis for drafting an initial trial balance. In particular we will be looking at ways of ensuring the accuracy of the balances for debtors (sales ledger control account) and creditors (purchases ledger control account).

1 Balancing ledger accounts

1.1 Introduction

The purpose of maintaining double entry ledger accounts is to provide information about the transactions and financial position of a business. Each type of transaction is gathered together and recorded in the appropriate ledger account, for example all sales are recorded in the sales account. Then at intervals it will be necessary to find the total of each of these types of transactions.

This is done by balancing each ledger account. This has been covered earlier in this text but is worth revising here, by attempting the following activity.

Test your understanding 1

You are required to balance off the following ledger accounts:

Sales ledger control account

	£		£
SDB – invoices	5,426.23	CRB	3,226.56
		Discounts allowed	315.47

VAT account

	£		£
PDB	846.72	SDB	1,036.54

Sales account

	£		£
		SDB	2,667.45
		SDB	1,853.92

2   Opening balances

2.1   Introduction

If an account has a balance on it at the end of a period then it will have the same balance at the start of the next period. This is known as an opening balance.

2.2   Debit or credit?

The key to determining whether an opening balance on a ledger account is a debit or a credit is to understand the general rules for debit and credit balances.

2.3   Debit and credit balance rules

Asset account   –   debit balance
Liability account   –   credit balance
Expense account   –   debit balance
Income account   –   credit balance

It may be difficult to see why assets and expenses are both debit balances. The reason is that both are the result of an outflow of cash to acquire the asset or to pay the expense. Similarly, the incurring of a liability and the receipt of income are both the result of an inflow of cash.

Illustration 1 – Opening balance

You are told that the opening balance on the sales ledger control account is £33,600, the opening balance on the purchases account is £115,200 and the opening balance on the purchases ledger control account is £12,700.

You are required to enter these into the relevant ledger accounts.

Solution

Sales ledger control account

	£		£
Balance brought forward	33,600		

Purchases account

	£		£
Balance brought forward	115,200		

Purchases ledger control account

£		£
	Balance brought forward	12,700

Assets and expenses normally have opening debit balances.

Liabilities and income normally have opening credit balances.

Test your understanding 2

Would the balances on the following accounts be debit or credit balances?

(a) Sales account

(b) Discounts allowed account

(c) Discounts received account

(d) Wages expense account

Test your understanding 3

The following transactions all occurred on 1 December 20X1 and have been entered into the relevant books of prime entry (given below). However, no entries have yet been made into the ledger system. VAT has been calculated at a rate of 17.5%.

Purchases day book

Date	Details	Invoice no	Total £	VAT £	Purchases £	Stationery £
20X1						
1 Dec	Bailey Limited	T151	235	35	200	
1 Dec	Byng & Company	10965	940	140	800	
1 Dec	Office Supplies Ltd	34565	329	49		280
1 Dec	O'Connell Frames	FL013	4,935	735	4,200	
	Totals		6,439	959	5,200	280

Purchases returns day book

Date	Details	Invoice no	Total £	VAT £	Purchases £	Stationery £
20X1						
1 Dec	O'Connell Frames	C011	2,115	315	1,800	40
1 Dec	Office Supplies Ltd	CR192	47	7		
	Totals		2,162	322	1,800	40

Sales day book

Date	Details	Invoice no	Total £	VAT £	Sales £
20X1					
1 Dec	Bentley Brothers	H621	1,645	245	1,400
1 Dec	J & H Limited	H622	4,230	630	3,600
1 Dec	Furniture Galore	H623	4,700	700	4,000
1 Dec	The Sofa Shop	H624	2,585	385	2,200
	Totals		13,160	1,960	11,200

Balances

The following are some of the balances in the accounting records and are all relevant to you at the start of the day on 1 December 20X1:

	£
Credit Suppliers	
Bailey Limited	11,750
Byng & Company	1,269
Office Supplies Limited	4,230
O'Connell Frames	423
Creditors' control	82,006
Debtors' control	180,312
Purchases	90,563
Sales	301,492
Purchases returns	306
Stationery	642
Discounts received	50
VAT (credit balance)	17,800

Receipts on 1 December 20X1

	Total £
Lili Chang (cash sale including VAT)	517
Bentley Brothers (credit customer)	5,875

Cheque issued

	Total £
Bailey Limited (in full settlement of debt of £819)	799

Task 1

Enter the opening balances listed above into the following accounts, blanks of which are provided on the following pages:

Bailey Limited
Byng & Company
Office Supplies Limited
O'Connell Frames
Creditors' control
Debtors' control

Purchases
Sales
Purchases returns
Stationery
Discounts received
VAT

Task 2

Using the data shown above, enter all the relevant transactions into the accounts in the subsidiary (purchases) ledger and main ledger. Entries to the subsidiary (sales) ledger for debtors are not required.

Task 3

Enter the receipts and payments shown above into the cash book given on the following pages.

Task 4

Transfer any relevant sums from the cash book into the subsidiary ledger for creditors and main ledger.

Task 5

Balance off all of the accounts and the cash book, showing clearly the balances carried down. The opening cash balance was £3,006. Find the closing balance on the cash book.

Tasks 1, 2, 4 and 5

Subsidiary (purchases) ledger

Bailey Limited

£	£

Byng & Company

£	£

Office Supplies Limited

£	£

O'Connell Frames

£		£

Main ledger

Creditors' control

£		£

Debtors' control

£		£

Purchases

£		£

Sales

£		£

Purchases returns

£		£

Stationery

£		£

Discounts received

£		£

VAT

£	£

Tasks 3, 4 and 5

Cash receipts book

Date	Narrative £	Total £	VAT £	Sales ledger £	Other £	Discounts allowed

Cash payments book

Date	Details	Cheque no	Code	Total £	VAT £	Purchases ledger £	Cash purchases £	Other £	Discounts received £

3   Accounting for debtors

3.1   Sales ledger control account

Within the main ledger the total amount outstanding from debtors is shown in the sales ledger control account or debtors' control account.

The totals of credit sales (from the sales day book), returns from customers (from the sales returns day book) and cash received and discounts (from the analysed cash book) are posted to this account.

This account therefore shows the total debtors outstanding. It does not give details about individual customers' balances. This is available in the subsidiary ledger for debtors.

However, as both records are compiled from the same sources, the total balances on the customers' individual accounts should equal the outstanding balance on the control account at any time.

3.2 Double entry system

The double entry system operates as follows.

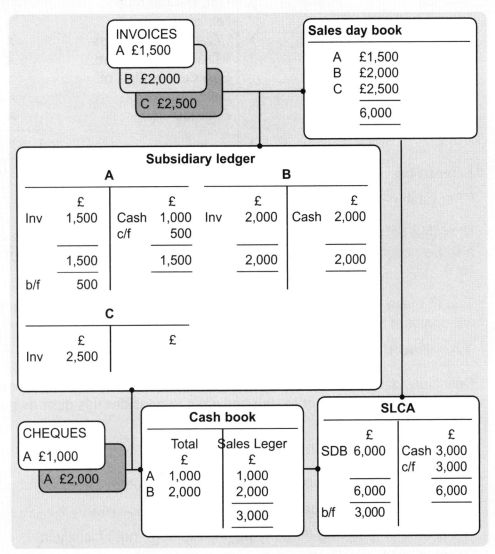

Notice that the remaining balance on the control account (£3,000) is equal to the sum of the remaining balances on the individual debtors' accounts (A £500 + C £2,500).

If all of the accounting entries have been made correctly then the balance on the sales ledger control account should equal the total of the balances on each of the individual debtors' accounts in the subsidiary (sales) ledger.

3.3 Proforma sales ledger control account

A sales ledger control account normally appears like this.

Sales ledger control account

	£		£
Balance b/f	X	Returns per sales returns day book	X
Sales per sales day book	X	* Cash from debtors	X
		* Discounts allowed	X
		Bad debt written off	X
		Contra entry	X
		Balance c/f	X
	X		X
Balance b/f	X		

* Per cash receipts book

Note that balances brought forward (b/f) and carried forward (c/f) can also be described as balances brought down (b/d) and carried down (c/d).

Two of these entries, bad debts and contra entry, are new to you so we will consider them now.

3.4 Bad debts

Definition: A bad debt is a debt which is highly unlikely to be received; it is therefore not prudent for the business to consider this debt as an asset.

3.5 Reasons for bad debts

A business may decide that a debt is bad for a number of reasons:

- customer is in liquidation – no cash will be received

- customer is having difficulty paying although not officially in liquidation

- customer disputes the debt and refuses to pay all or part of it.

3.6 Accounting for bad debts

The business must make an adjustment to write off the bad debt from the customer's account in the subsidiary ledger and to write it off in the main ledger. The double entry in the main ledger is:

DR Bad debt expense

    CR Sales ledger control account

Notice that the bad debt becomes an expense of the business. Writing off bad debts decreases the profits made by a business. (Note that the bad debt is not deducted from sales.) The sale was made in the anticipation of receiving the money but, if the debt is not to be received, this does not negate the sale it is just an added expense of the business.

The bad debt must also be written off in the individual debtor's account in the subsidiary ledger by crediting the customer's account as this amount is not going to be received.

To write off a bad debt, it is necessary to debit the bad debt expense account in the main ledger and credit the sales ledger control account. In the subsidiary (sales) ledger the customer's account must be credited with the amount of the bad debt.

3.7 Contra entries

A further type of adjustment that may be required to sales ledger and purchases ledger control accounts is a contra entry.

3.8 Why a contra entry is required

In some instances a business will be both a debtor and a creditor of another business as it both buys from the business and sells to it. If this is the case then there will be money owed to the business and money owing from it. This can be simplified by making an adjustment known as a contra entry.

Illustration 2 – Accounting for debtors

James Associates has a customer, X Brothers. X Brothers also sells goods to James Associates. Therefore X Brothers is both a debtor and a creditor of James Associates. The subsidiary ledger accounts of James Associates show the following position:

Subsidiary ledger – debtors

X Brothers

	£		£
Balance b/f	250		

Subsidiary ledger – creditors

X Brothers

	£		£
		Balance b/f	100

The problem here is that X Brothers owes James Associates £250 and is owed £100 by James Associates. If both parties are in agreement it makes more sense to net these two amounts off and to say that X Brothers owes James Associates just £150. This is achieved in accounting terms by a contra entry.

Solution

Step 1 Take the smaller of the two amounts and debit the subsidiary ledger account for the creditor and credit the subsidiary ledger account for the debtor with this amount.

Subsidiary ledger – debtors

X Brothers

	£		£
Balance b/f	250	Contra	100

Subsidiary ledger – creditors

X Brothers

	£		£
Contra	100	Balance b/f	100

Step 2 Balance off the accounts in the subsidiary ledgers.

Subsidiary ledger – debtors

X Brothers

	£		£
Balance b/f	250	Contra	100
		Balance c/f	150
	250		250
Balance b/f	150		

Subsidiary ledger – creditors

X Brothers

	£		£
Contra	100	Balance b/f	100

This now shows that X Brothers owes £150 to James Associates and is owed nothing by James Associates.

Step 3 The double entry must also be carried out in the main ledger accounts. This is:

DR Purchases ledger control account

    CR Sales ledger control account

When a contra entry is made you must remember not just to deal with the entries in the subsidiary ledgers but also to put through the double entry in the main ledger accounts, the sales ledger and purchases ledger control accounts.

3.9   Main ledger and subsidiary ledger

We will now return to the relationship between the sales ledger control account in the main ledger and the individual accounts for debtors in the subsidiary ledger.

Illustration 3 – Accounting for debtors

James has been trading for two months. He has four credit customers. James is not registered for VAT. Here is the day book for the first two months:

Sales day book (SDB)

Date	Customer	Invoice	£
02.2.X4	Peter Brown	01	50.20
05.2.X4	Ian Smith	02	80.91
07.2.X4	Sid Parsons	03	73.86
23.2.X4	Eva Lane	04	42.30
	Total		247.27
09.3.X4	Ian Smith	05	23.96
15.3.X4	Sid Parsons	06	34.72
20.3.X4	Peter Brown	07	12.60
24.3.X4	Sid Parsons	08	93.25
31.3.X4	Total		164.53

Here is the receipts side of the analysed cash book for March 20X4 (no cash was received from debtors in February).

Cash receipts book (CRB)

Date	Narrative	Total £	Cash sales £	Sales ledger £	Rent £
01.3.X4	Peter Brown	50.20		50.20	
03.3.X4	Clare Jones	63.80	63.80		
04.3.X4	Molly Dell	110.00			110.00
12.3.X4	Sid Parsons	50.00		50.00	
13.3.X4	Emily Boyd	89.33	89.33		
20.3.X4	Frank Field	92.68	92.68		
25.3.X4	Eva Lane	42.30		42.30	
31.3.X4	Total	498.31	245.81	142.50	110.00

We will write up the subsidiary ledger and the sales ledger control account and compare the balances.

Solution

Subsidiary ledger – debtors

Peter Brown

		£			£
02.2.X4	01	50.20	28.2.X4	c/f	50.20
		50.20			50.20
01.3.X4	b/f	50.20	01.3.X4	Cash	50.20
20.3.X4	07	12.60	31.3.X4	c/f	12.60
		62.80			62.80
01.4.X4	b/f	12.60			

Eva Lane

		£			£
23.2.X4	04	42.30	28.2.X4	c/f	42.30
		42.30			42.30
01.3.X4	b/f	42.30	25.3.X4	Cash	42.30

Sid Parsons

		£			£
07.2.X4	03	73.86	28.2.X4	c/f	73.86
		73.86			73.86
01.3.X4	b/f	73.86	12.3.X4	Cash	50.00
15.3.X4	06	34.72	31.3.X4	c/f	151.83
24.3.X4	08	93.25			
		201.83			201.83
01.4.X4	b/f	151.83			

Ian Smith

		£			£
05.2.X4	02	80.91	28.2.X4	c/f	80.91
		80.91			80.91
01.3.X4	b/f	80.91	31.3.X4	c/f	104.87
09.3.X4	05	23.96			
		104.87			104.87
01.4.X4	b/f	104.87			

Sales ledger control account

		£			£
28.2.X4	SDB	247.27	28.2.X4	c/f	247.27
		247.27			247.27
01.3.X4	b/f	247.27	31.3.X4	CRB	142.50
31.3.X4	SDB	164.53	31.3.X4	c/f	269.30
		411.80			411.80
01.4.X4	b/f	269.30			

Let us compare balances at 31 March 20X4.

Subsidiary ledger – debtors

	£
Peter Brown	12.60
Eva Lane	–
Sid Parsons	151.83
Ian Smith	104.87
	269.30
Sales ledger control account	269.30

As the double entry has been correctly carried out, the total of the balances on the individual debtors' accounts in the subsidiary ledger is equal to the balance on the sales ledger control account.

4   Sales ledger control account reconciliation

4.1   Introduction

Comparing the control account balance with the total of the subsidiary ledger accounts is a form of internal control. The reconciliation should be performed on a regular basis by the sales ledger clerk and reviewed and approved by an independent person.

If the total of the balances on the subsidiary (sales) ledger do not equal the balance on the sales ledger control account then an error or errors have been made in either the main ledger or subsidiary ledger, and these must be discovered and corrected.

4.2   Journal entries

Any corrections or adjustments made to the sales ledger control account must be documented as a journal entry.

A journal entry is a written instruction to the bookkeeper to enter a double entry into the main ledger accounts.

This will be a double entry that has not been recorded in the primary records as these are posted automatically to the main ledger when the primary records are posted. Therefore journal entries are used for unusual items that do not appear in the primary records or for the correction of errors or making of adjustments to ledger accounts.

A typical journal entry to write off a bad debt is shown below:

Authorisation

Description of why double entry is necessary

Double entry

Sequential journal number

JOURNAL ENTRY		No: 06671		
Prepared by:	P Freer			
Authorised by:	P Simms			
Date:	3 October 20X2			
Narrative:				
To write off bad debt from L C Hamper				
Account	Code	Debit	Credit	
Bad debts expense	ML28	102.00		
Debtors' control	ML06		102.00	
TOTALS		102.00	102.00	

Equal totals as journal must balance

Illustration 4 – Sales ledger control reconcilliation

The total sales for the month was posted from the sales day book as £4,657.98 instead of £4,677.98. This must be corrected using a journal entry.

Solution

The journal entry to correct this error will be as follows:

JOURNAL ENTRY		No: 97	
Prepared by:	A Grimm		
Authorised by:	L R Ridinghood		
Date:	23.7.X3		
Narrative:			
To correct error in posting to debtors'			
control account			
Account	Code	Debit	Credit
Sales ledger control	ML11	20	
Sales	ML56		20
TOTALS		20	20

The adjustment required is to increase debtors and sales by £20 therefore a debit to sales ledger control and a credit to sales is needed.

4.3 Adjustments in the subsidiary ledger

Adjustments in the subsidiary ledger do not need to be shown in a journal entry. Journal entries are only required for adjustments to the main ledger.

These adjustments should be recorded in memorandum form, with proper authorisation.

4.4 Procedure for a sales ledger control account reconciliation

(1) The balances on the subsidiary ledger accounts for debtors are extracted, listed and totalled.

(2) The sales ledger control account is balanced.

(3) If the two figures differ, then the reasons for the difference must be investigated.

Reasons may include the following:

- An error in the casting of the day book. (The total is posted to the control account whereas the individual invoices are posted to the individual accounts and, therefore, if the total is incorrect, a difference will arise.)

- A transposition error which could be made in posting either:

  (a) to the control account (the total figure), or

  (b) to the individual accounts (the individual transactions).

- A casting error in the cash book column relating to the control account. (The total is posted.)

- A balance omitted from the list of individual accounts.

- A credit balance on an individual account in the subsidiary ledger for debtors which has automatically and wrongly been assumed to be a debit balance.

(4) Differences which are errors in the control account should be corrected in the control account.

(5) Differences which are errors in the individual accounts should be corrected by adjusting the list of balances and, of course, the account concerned.

Test your understanding 4

Would the following errors cause a difference to occur between the balance of the debtors' control account and the total of the balances in the subsidiary (sales) ledger?

(a) The total column of the sales day book was overcast by £100.

(b) In error H Lambert's account in the sales ledger was debited with £175 instead of M Lambert's account.

(c) An invoice for £76 was recorded in the sales day book as £67.

Illustration 5 – Sales ledger control reconcilliation

The balance on the sales ledger control account for a business at 31 March 20X3 is £14,378.37. The total of the list of subsidiary ledger balances for debtors is £13,935.37.

The difference has been investigated and the following errors have been identified:

- the sales day book was overcast by £1,000

- a credit note for £150 was entered into the individual debtors' account as an invoice

- discounts allowed of £143 were correctly accounted for in the subsidiary ledger but were not entered into the main ledger accounts

- a credit balance on one debtor's account of £200 was mistakenly listed as a debit balance when totalling the individual debtor accounts in the subsidiary ledger.

Prepare the reconciliation between the balance on the sales ledger control account and the total of the individual balances on the subsidiary ledger accounts.

Solution

Step 1 Amend the sales ledger control account for any errors that have been made

Sales ledger control account

	£		£
Balance b/f	14,378.37	SDB overcast	1,000.00
		Discounts allowed	143.00
		Balance c/f	13,235.37
	14,378.37		14,378.37
Balance b/f	13,235.37		

Step 2 Correct the total of the list of balances in the subsidiary (sales) ledger.

		£
Original total		13,935.37
Less:	Credit note entered as invoice (2 × 150)	(300.00)
	Credit balance entered as debit balance (2 × 200)	(400.00)
		13,235.37

Test your understanding 5

The balance on Diana's sales ledger control account at 31 December 20X6 was £15,450. The balances on the individual accounts in the subsidiary ledger have been extracted and total £15,705. On investigation the following errors are discovered:

(a) a debit balance of £65 has been omitted from the list of balances

(b) discounts totalling £70 have been recorded in the individual accounts but not in the control account

(c) the sales day book was 'overcast' by £200

(d) a contra entry for £40 has not been entered into the control account, and

(e) an invoice for £180 was recorded correctly in the sales day book but was posted to the debtors' individual account as £810.

Prepare the sales ledger control account reconciliation.

5 Accounting for creditors

5.1 Introduction

As we have seen in earlier chapters, the total amount payable to creditors is recorded in the main ledger in the purchases ledger control account. The total of credit purchases from the purchases day book, returns to suppliers from the purchases returns day book and the total payments to creditors and discounts received taken from the cash payments book are all posted to this account.

The purchases ledger control account shows the total amount that is payable to creditors but it does not show the amount owed to individual suppliers. This information is provided by the subsidiary ledger which contains an account for each individual creditor.

Each individual invoice from the purchases day book and each individual credit note from the purchases returns day book is posted to the relevant creditor's account in the subsidiary ledger. Similarly each individual payment to creditors and discounts received are posted from the cash payments book to the individual creditors' accounts in the subsidiary ledger.

5.2 Relationship between the purchases ledger control account and the balances in the subsidiary ledger

The information that is being posted to the purchases ledger control account in total and to the individual accounts in the subsidiary ledger as individual entries are from the same sources and should in total be the same figures.

Therefore, just as with the sales ledger control account, if the double entry and entries to the subsidiary ledger have been correctly carried out then the balance on the purchases ledger control account should be equal to the total of the list of balances on the individual creditors' accounts in the subsidiary ledger.

5.3 Proforma purchases ledger control account

A purchases ledger control account normally appears like this.

Purchases ledger control account

	£		£
Payments to suppliers per analysed cash book		Balance b/f	X
		Purchases per purchases	
Cash	X	day book	X
Discount received	X		
Returns per purchases			
returns day book	X		
Contra entry	X		
Balance c/f	X		
	X		X
	Balance b/f	X

If all of the accounting entries have been correctly made then the balance on this purchases ledger control account should equal the total of the balances on the individual supplier accounts in the subsidiary ledger.

6 Purchases ledger control account reconciliation

6.1 Introduction

At each month end the purchases ledger clerk must reconcile the purchases ledger control account and the subsidiary ledger, just as the sales ledger clerk performed the sales ledger control account reconciliation.

Remember that as well as investigating and discovering the differences, the control account and the individual accounts in the subsidiary ledger must also be amended for any errors.

6.2 Adjustments to the purchases ledger control account

Any corrections or adjustments made to the purchases ledger control account can be documented as a journal entry.

Illustration 6 – Purchase ledger control account reconcilliation

The total purchases for the month were posted from the purchases day book as £2,547.98 instead of £2,457.98. Prepare a journal to correct this error.

Solution

The journal entry to correct this error will be as follows:

JOURNAL ENTRY	No: 253		
Prepared by: P Charming			
Authorised by: U Sister			
Date: 29.8.X5			
Narrative:			
To correct error in posting to debtors' control account			
Account	Code	Debit	Credit
Purchases ledger control	ML56	90	
Purchases	ML34		90
TOTALS		90	90

In this case both creditors and purchases need to be reduced by £90. Therefore a debit to the purchases ledger control and a credit to purchases are required.

6.3 Adjustments in the subsidiary ledger

Adjustments in the subsidiary ledger do not need to be documented in a journal entry. Journal entries are only required for adjustments to the main ledger.

Illustration 7 – Purchase ledger control account reconcilliation

The balance on the purchases ledger control account for a business at 30 June was £12,159. The total of the balances on the individual creditors' accounts in the subsidiary ledger was £19,200.

The following errors were also found:

*   the cash payments book had been undercast by £20;

*   an invoice from Thomas Ltd, a credit supplier, for £2,350 was correctly entered in the subsidiary ledger but had been missed out of the addition of the total in the purchases day book;

*   an invoice from Fred Singleton for £2,000 plus VAT was included in his individual account in the subsidiary ledger at the net amount;

*   an invoice from Horace Shades for £6,000 was entered into the individual account in the subsidiary ledger twice;

*   the same invoice is for £6,000 plus VAT but the VAT had not been included in the subsidiary ledger;

*   returns to Horace Shades of £111 had been omitted from the subsidiary ledger.

You are required to reconcile the purchases ledger control account with the balances on the subsidiary ledger accounts at 30 June.

Solution

Step 1   Amend the purchases ledger control account to show the correct balance.

Purchases ledger control account

	£		£
Undercast of CPB	20	Balance b/f	12,159
Balance c/f	14,489	Invoice omitted from PDB	2,350
	14,509		14,509
		Amended balance b/f	14,489

Step 2   Correct the total of the list of subsidiary ledger balances.

		£
Original total		19,200
Add:	Fred Singleton VAT	350
Less:	Horace Shades invoice included twice	(6,000)
Add:	Horace Shades VAT	1,050
Less:	Horace Shades returns	(111)
Amended control account balance		14,489

Remember that invoices from suppliers should be included in the individual suppliers' accounts in the subsidiary ledger at the gross amount, including VAT.

Test your understanding 6

How would each of the following be dealt with in the purchases ledger control account reconciliation?

(a) A purchase invoice for £36 from P Swift was credited to P Short's account in the subsidiary ledger.

(b) A purchase invoice for £96 not entered in the purchases day book.

(c) An undercast of £20 in the total column of the purchases day book.

(d) A purchase invoice from Short & Long for £42 entered as £24 in the purchases day book.

The examiner will sometimes ask you to say what has caused the difference between the control account and the list of balances. If you are asked to do this, the difference will usually be caused by just one error.

An example will illustrate this.

Illustration 8 – Purchase ledger control account reconcilliation

XYZ Ltd has made the following entries in the sales ledger control account

	£
Opening balance 1 April 20X7	49,139
Credit sales posted from the sales day book	35,000
Discounts allowed	328
Bad debt written off	127
Cash received from debtors	52,359

The list of balances from the subsidiary (sales) ledger totals £31,679.

(a) Calculate the closing balance on the SLCA at 31 April 2007.

(b) State one reason for the difference between the SLCA balance and the total of the list of balances.

Solution

(a) The SLCA

Sales ledger control account

	£		£
Balance b/d	49,139	Discount allowed	328
SDB – sales	35,000	Bad debt	127
		Cash received	52,359
		Balance c/d	31,325
	84,139		84,139

(b) Total of subsidiary (sales) ledger balances — 31,679
    Balance of SLCA at 30 April 20X7 — 31,325

    Difference — 354

One cause of the difference may have been that the bad debt written off was entered on the debit side of the relevant account in the subsidiary (sales) ledger.

Tutorial note

You have to look for the fairly obvious clues and also make some assumptions

(i) It's reasonable to assume that the control account is correct – it may not, so be careful.

(ii) Calculate the difference and determine whether the list total is larger than the SLCA balance or vice versa.

(iii) See if one of the figures given in the question is the same as the difference or double the difference.

If a figure given is the same as the difference then it is likely that a number has been left out of an account.

If a figure given is double the difference then it is likely that a number has been entered on the wrong side of an account, or possibly entered twice.

– In the above question, the difference is £354.

– The total of the list of ledger balances is bigger than the SLCA balance.

– £354 is not a figure given in the question but the amount £127 is given and the difference is twice this figure.

One possible reason for this is that the bad debt write off (£127) was entered on the debit side of a ledger account in the subsidiary (sales) ledger – that would have made the total of the list £354 larger. Of course there are a million possible reasons – perhaps there was an invoice for £354 and it was entered twice in a ledger account – that would have caused the difference, but the examiner is looking for something obvious in the figures he's given you – not some speculative reason.

8 Batch control

8.1 Introduction

Throughout this book we have been dealing with control accounts in the main ledger and individual debtors and creditors accounts in the subsidiary ledgers. We have noted that there will sometimes be a discrepancy between the balance on the control account in the main ledger and the total of the balances in the subsidiary ledgers. Sometimes this difference is caused by correctly entered items that can be reconciled. However, sometimes the difference is caused by an error in the entering of the data. These latter errors can be eliminated or minimised by the use of batch control.

8.2 How a lack of batch control causes problems

Consider the situation where a small business has received 40 cheques from debtors and is going to post these into the accounts for the week. A typical system might be as follows.

(a) John writes the cheques into the debtors column of the analysed cash received book. John then totals the cash received book for the week and posts the total of the debtors column to the sales ledger control account. He then writes out the bank paying-in slip and pays the cheques into the bank.

(b) George writes up the individual accounts in the subsidiary (sales) ledger from the entries in the main cash book.

The above is a fairly typical system and of course all sorts of things can go wrong.

(a) A cheque could go missing and not be paid into the bank, causing a discrepancy between the entries in the cash book and the bank statement.

(b) John could write the values of one or more of the cheques incorrectly in the cash book, causing the cash book total and the sales ledger control account entry to be incorrect.

(c) George could also write the values of the cheques incorrectly in the subsidiary (sales) ledger.

8.3 How batch control helps reduce errors

To improve the system the company employs a system of batch control.

(a) Before the cheques are entered in the cash book, a person unconnected with entering the cheques in the books (Jemima) will total the cheques using a computer spreadsheet such as Excel or an adlisting calculating machine (i.e. a machine which will print out the value of the amounts entered). She will not disclose the total of the cheques.

(b) John will now write the cheques into the cash book and total the cash book as before. He will then compare his total with Jemima's total. If the totals are different, Jemima and John will both check their work until they can agree on a total. This clearly minimises any errors that are likely to be made when entering the cheques in the books of account.

(c) George will write up the subsidiary (sales) ledger as before. As a further check, the subsidiary (sales) ledger could be passed to another person who would total the entries that George has just made and then compare that total with Jemima's total.

As you can see, by batching the cheques together and producing a total of their value before any entries are made in the books, the company has an excellent check on the accuracy of the entries that are made.

Of course nothing is foolproof. The accountants could enter incorrect amounts in the ledger which compensate for each other thereby still giving the correct total. Alternatively, a cheque might be lost thereby giving an incorrect banking total. But at least the possibility of human error is reduced.

Test your understanding 7

1   Would the year end balance on the sales returns account be a debit balance or a credit balance?

2   What is the double entry for writing off a bad debt?

3   What is the double entry for a contra?

4   The sales day book has been undercast by £100. What is the double entry to correct this?

5   A credit note from a supplier for £50 was omitted from the purchases returns day book. What is the double entry to correct this?

6   The total of the sales returns day book of £360 was posted as £630. What is the double entry to correct this?

7   When carrying out the sales ledger control account reconciliation it was discovered that an invoice to a customer for

£200 has been omitted from the sales day book. How would this be treated in the reconciliation?

8 When carrying out the sales ledger control account reconciliation it was discovered that a credit balance for a customer of £100 had been included in the list of balances as a debit balance. How would this be treated in the reconciliation?

9 When carrying out the purchases ledger control account reconciliation it was discovered that the purchases day book total of £4,750 had been posted as £4,570. How would this be treated in the reconciliation?

10 When carrying out the purchases ledger control account reconciliation it was discovered that a discount taken from a supplier of £20 had not been recorded in the cash payments book. How would this be treated in the reconciliation?

10 Summary

We started this chapter with a revision of balancing accounts and extended this to entering opening balances in the ledger accounts in preparation for posting transactions for a period which is a favourite assessment topic. Then the chapter moved on to aspects of control and the use of control accounts and control account reconciliations in order to determine the accuracy of the figures in the ledger accounts.

Test your understanding answers

Test your understanding 1

Sales ledger control account

	£		£
SDB – invoices	5,426.23	CRB	3,226.56
		Discounts allowed	315.47
		Balance c/f	1,884.20
	5,426.23		5,426.23
Balance b/f	1,884.20		

VAT account

	£		£
PDB	846.72	SDB	1,036.54
Balance c/f	189.82		
	1,036.54		1,036.54
		Balance b/f	189.82

Sales account

	£		£
		SDB	2,667.45
Balance c/f	4,521.37	SDB	1,853.92
	4,521.37		4,521.37
		Balance b/f	4,521.37

Test your understanding 2

(a) Credit balance

(b) Debit balance

(c) Credit balance

(d) Debit balance

KAPLAN PUBLISHING

Test your understanding 3

Subsidiary (purchases) ledger

Bailey Limited

		£			£
01 Dec	Bank	799	01 Dec	Balance b/f	11,750
01 Dec	Discount received	20	01 Dec	Purchases	235
01 Dec	Balance c/f	11,166			
		11,985			11,985
			02 Dec	Balance b/f	11,166

Byng & Company

		£			£
			01 Dec	Balance b/f	1,269
01 Dec	Balance c/f	2,209	01 Dec	Purchases	940
		2,209			2,209
			02 Dec	Balance b/f	2,209

Office Supplies Limited

		£			£
01 Dec	Purchases returns	47	01 Dec	Balance b/f	4,230
01 Dec	Balance c/f	4,512	01 Dec	Purchases	329
		4,559			4,559
			02 Dec	Balance b/f	4,512

O'Connell Frames

		£			£
01 Dec	Purchases returns	2,115	01 Dec	Balance b/f	423
01 Dec	Balance c/f	3,243	01 Dec	Purchases	4,935
		5,358			5,358
			02 Dec	Balance b/f	3,243

Main ledger

Creditors' control

		£			£
01 Dec	Purchases returns	2,162	01 Dec	Balance b/f	82,006
01 Dec	Bank	799	01 Dec	Purchases	6,439
01 Dec	Discounts received	20			
01 Dec	Balance c/f	85,464			
		88,445			88,445
			02 Dec	Balance b/f	85,464

Debtors' control

		£			£
01 Dec	Balance b/f	180,312	01 Dec	Bank	5,875
01 Dec	Sales	13,160	01 Dec	Balance c/f	187,597
01 Dec					
		193,472			193,472
02 Dec	Balance b/f	187,597			

Purchases

		£			£
01 Dec	Balance b/f	90,563			
01 Dec	Creditors	5,200	01 Dec	Balance c/f	95,763
		95,763			95,763
02 Dec	Balance b/f	95,763			

Sales

		£			£
			01 Dec	Balance b/f	301,492
			01 Dec	Debtors	11,200
01 Dec	Balance c/f	313,132	01 Dec	Cash sale	440
		313,132			313,132
			02 Dec	Balance b/f	313,132

Purchases returns

		£			£
			01 Dec	Balance b/f	306
01 Dec	Balance c/f	2,106	01 Dec	Creditors	1,800
		2,106			2,106
			02 Dec	Balance b/f	2,106

Stationery

		£			£
01 Dec	Balance b/f	642	01 Dec	Purchases returns	40
01 Dec	Creditors	280	01 Dec	Balance c/f	882
		922			922
02 Dec	Balance b/f	882			

Discounts received

		£			£
			01 Dec	Balance b/f	50
01 Dec	Balance c/f	70	01 Dec	Creditors	20
		70			70
			02 Dec	Balance b/f	70

VAT

		£			£
01 Dec	Purchases	959	01 Dec	Balance b/f	17,800
			01 Dec	Purchases returns	322
			01 Dec	Sales	1,960
01 Dec	Balance c/f	19,200	01 Dec	Cash sale	77
		20,159			20,159
			02 Dec	Balance b/f	19,200

Cash receipts book

Date 20X1	Narrative £	Total £	VAT £	Sales ledger £	Other £	Discounts allowed
01 Dec	Lili Chang	517	77		440	
01 Dec	Bentley Brothers	5,875		5,875		
		6,392	77	5,875	440	–

Cash payments book

Date 20X1	Details	Cheque no	Code	Total £	VAT £	Purchases ledger £	Cash purchases £	Other £	Discounts received £
01 Dec	Bailey Ltd			799	–	799	–	–	20

	£
Opening balance	3,006
Add: Receipts	6,392
Less: Payments	(799)
Closing balance	8,599

Test your understanding 4

(a) Yes, because the detailed entries in the sales day book are posted to the sales ledger accounts and the incorrect total used in the control account.

(b) No, because the arithmetical balance is correct even though the wrong account is used.

(c) No, because the double entry will be for £67 and the entry in the subsidiary ledger will also be for £67.

Test your understanding 5

- We must first look for those errors which will mean that the sales ledger control account is incorrectly stated. The control account is then adjusted as follows:

Sales ledger control account

	£		£
Balance b/f	15,450	Discounts allowed	70
		Overcast of sales day book	200
		Contra with creditors' control account	40
		Adjusted balance c/f	15,140
	15,450		15,450
Balance b/f	15,140		

- We must then look for errors in the total of the individual balances per the debtors' ledger. The extracted list of balances must be adjusted as follows:

	£
Original total of list of balances	15,705
Debit balance omitted	65
Transposition error (810 – 180)	(630)
	15,140

- As can be seen, the adjusted total of the list of balances now agrees with the balance per the control account.

Test your understanding 6

(a) A correction would simply be made in the subsidiary ledger.

(b) This must be adjusted for in the purchase ledger control account and in the subsidiary ledger.

(c) This is just an adjustment to the purchase ledger control account.

(d) This will require alteration in both the control account and the subsidiary ledger.

Test your understanding 7

1	Debit balance			
2	Debit	Bad debts expense		
	Credit	Sales ledger control		
3	Debit	Purchase ledger control		
	Credit	Sales ledger control		
4	Debit	Sales ledger control	£100	
	Credit	Sales	£100	
5	Debit	Purchase ledger control	£50	
	Credit	Purchase returns	£50	
6	Debit	Sales ledger control	£270	
	Credit	Sales returns	£270	
7	Debit	Sales ledger control	£200	
	and			
	Increase list of debtor balances total by		£200	
8	Decrease list of debtor balances total by		£200	(2 x £100)
9	Credit	Purchase ledger control account	£180	
10	Debit	Purchase ledger control account	£20	
	and			
	Decrease list of creditor balances total by		£20	

319

Drafting an initial trial balance

Introduction

This chapter covers the is the preparation of an initial trial balance. We will consider the trial balance and its purpose and look at how to deal with discrepancies on the trial balance and particularly the correction of errors using a suspense account and journal entries.

1 Main ledger accounts

1.1 Introduction

As you have seen earlier in your studies, as each transaction is made by a business it is recorded in a primary record and then in the main ledger accounts. Therefore at any point in time the main ledger accounts should include all the transactions of the business to date.

1.2 Checking the accounting

You have also seen that it is relatively easy for errors to be made when entering the transactions into the accounting records. Therefore it is important that on a regular basis the business checks that the ledger accounts have been correctly written up.

1.3 Balancing the main ledger accounts

This process of checking the overall accounting is done at regular intervals by balancing each of the main ledger accounts and then listing each of the balances in what is known as a trial balance.

We have already come across ways of checking bank, cash, debtor and creditor balances and the trial balance is a further final check on these and the other balances.

2 The trial balance

2.1 List of balances

The trial balance is a list showing the balance on each ledger account. An example of a simple trial balance is given below:

	Debit £	Credit £
Sales		5,000
Opening stock	100	
Purchases	3,000	
Rent	200	
Car	3,000	
Debtors	100	
Creditors		1,400
	6,400	6,400

Note that the trial balance contains a figure for opening stock not closing stock. This will always be the case but you do not need to worry about the reasons why.

The trial balance is produced immediately after the double entry has been completed and balances extracted on the accounts. If the double entry has been done correctly, the total of the debits will equal the total of the credits.

2.2 Reasons for extracting a trial balance

- To ensure that the double entry has been completed. Note however, that there are some types of error that will not be picked up merely by extracting a trial balance (see below).

- As a first stage in the preparation of the financial statements.

2.3 Errors identified by extracting a trial balance

- **Single entry**

  The debit entry may have been made correctly but the associated credit entry has been overlooked. The result will be that the total of the debits will exceed the total of the credits. Equally if a credit entry has been made but no corresponding debit the credits will exceed the debits.

- **Casting error**

  An account itself or the trial balance in total may have been added up incorrectly. In this case the trial balance will not balance.

- **Transposition error**

  For example, an amount of £7,532 may have been incorrectly written as £7,352. If one such error has occurred, the difference on the trial balance will be divisible by nine (this is often a useful tip if you find an account or trial balance does not balance when you expect it to).

- **Extraction error**

  An account may be correct in the ledger but has been copied out incorrectly (or not at all) onto the trial balance. Or indeed the account balance may have been entered as the correct amount, but on the wrong side of the trial balance, e.g. as a credit rather than a debit.

2.4 Errors not identified by extracting a trial balance

- **Errors of original (prime) entry**

  Where the original figure is incorrectly entered in both parts of the double entry then the trial balance will still balance.

- **Compensating errors**

  Quite simply where one error is compensated exactly by another in the opposite direction. Again, the trial balance will still balance.

- **Errors of omission**

  Here, an entry is left out altogether on both sides of the double entry. There will be no effect on the trial balance.

- **Errors of commission**

  Here the double entry is completed but between the wrong accounts, for example where a payment of £50 for rates is debited to the wages account.

- **Errors of principle**

  Similar to errors of commission but these items are treated in fundamentally the wrong type of account, ie treating a fixed asset as an expense (meaning capital expenditure being treated as revenue expenditure).

A trial balance will pick up some types of errors but there are others that will not be found by producing a trial balance.

2.5 Computerised accounting systems

The same basic principles apply to all accounting systems, whether manual or computerised. Most computer systems, however, automatically post both sides of the double entry, meaning that the trial balance will always balance.

Where the accounting system is computerised, certain errors cannot occur:

- single entries (the computer will not accept them)
- casting errors (the computer will total accounts automatically)
- transposition errors (the computer posts the double entry automatically)
- extraction errors (the computer posts the double entry automatically).

But human errors can still occur:

- errors of original entry
- errors of commission
- errors of principle.

Illustration 1 – The trial balance

The following are the balances on the accounts of Ernest at 31 December 20X8.

	£
Sales	47,140
Purchases	26,500
Debtors	7,640
Creditors	4,320
General expenses	9,430
Loan	5,000
Plant and machinery at cost	7,300
Motor van at cost	2,650
Drawings	7,500
Rent and rates	6,450
Insurance	1,560
Bank overdraft	2,570
Capital	10,000

Prepare Ernest's trial balance as at 31 December 20X8.

Solution

Step 1 Set up a blank trial balance

TRIAL BALANCE AT 31 DECEMBER 20X8

	£	£
Sales		
Purchases		
Debtors		
Creditors		
General expenses		
Loan		
Plant and machinery at cost		
Motor van at cost		
Drawings		
Rent and rates		
Insurance		
Bank overdraft		
Capital		

Step 2 Work down the list of balances one by one using what you have learned so far about debits and credits. Assets and expenses are debit balances and liabilities and income are credit balances.

TRIAL BALANCE AT 31 DECEMBER 20X8

	£	£
Sales		47,140
Purchases	26,500	
Debtors	7,640	
Creditors		4,320
General expenses	9,430	
Loan		5,000
Plant and machinery at cost	7,300	
Motor van at cost	2,650	
Drawings	7,500	
Rent and rates	6,450	
Insurance	1,560	
Bank overdraft		2,570
Capital		10,000
	69,030	69,030

Take care with drawings. These are a reduction of the capital owed back to the owner therefore as a reduction of a liability they must be a debit balance.

The bank overdraft is an amount owed to the bank therefore it must be a credit balance.

Test your understanding 1

The following balances have been extracted from the books of Fitzroy at 31 December 20X2:

	£
Capital on 1 January 20X2	106,149
Freehold factory at cost	360,000
Motor vehicles at cost	126,000
Stocks at 1 January 20X2	37,500
Debtors	15,600
Cash in hand	225
Bank overdraft	82,386
Creditors	78,900
Sales	318,000
Purchases	165,000
Rent and rates	35,400
Discounts allowed	6,600
Insurance	2,850
Sales returns	10,500
Purchases returns	6,300
Loan from bank	240,000
Sundry expenses	45,960
Drawings	26,100

Prepare a trial balance at 31 December 20X2.

The main problem is usually in determining whether each balance is a debit balance or a credit balance. Remember that assets and expenses are debit balances, and liabilities and income are credit balances. So think carefully about the nature of each of the accounts listed.

Some balances could be either a debit or a credit (e.g. VAT). The question would have to indicate which balance it was.

3 Discrepancies on the trial balance

3.1 Introduction

As we saw earlier in this chapter the trial balance should balance, ie the total of debit balances should equal the total of credit balances. However we also saw how various different types of error might mean that the trial balance will not balance. If a discrepancy is discovered on the trial balance then it must be investigated.

3.2 Checks on the trial balance

However, before investigating any discrepancies some basic checks should be carried out.

Firstly check that the debit and credit columns have been correctly added up.

When totalling a long list of figures it is very easy to make an error.

If the column totals are correct then go back to the ledger accounts and check that each of those has been correctly balanced and that the correct balance has been extracted and entered onto the trial balance.

If the discrepancy still exists then it will need to be investigated.

Test your understanding 2

Enter the following details of transactions for the month of May into the appropriate ledger accounts.

You should also extract a trial balance as at 30 May 20X6. Transactions with debtors and creditors are to be recorded in the control accounts for debtors and creditors in the main ledger. You can ignore VAT.

20X6

1 May	Started in business with £6,800 in the bank
3 May	Bought goods on credit from the following: J Johnson £400, D Nixon £300 and J Agnew £250
5 May	Cash sales £300 paid into the bank account
6 May	Paid rates by cheque £100
8 May	Paid wages £50 by cheque.
9 May	Sold goods on credit: K Homes £300, J Homes £300 and B Hood £100
10 May	Bought goods on credit: J Johnson £800, D Nixon £700
11 May	Return goods to J Johnson £150
15 May	Bought office fixtures £600 by cheque
18 May	Bought a motor vehicle £3,500 by cheque
22 May	Goods returned by J Homes £100
25 May	Paid J Johnson £1,000, D Nixon £500, both by cheque
26 May	Paid wages £150 by cheque

4 The suspense account

4.1 Introduction

A suspense account is used in two circumstances.

- When the destination of a posting is uncertain the amount may be entered in a suspense account until further information is available regarding the nature of the item.

- When the trial balance totals disagree the difference may be temporarily recorded in a suspense account. This will enable final accounts to be prepared and in the course of this work some or all of the errors giving rise to the balance on the suspense account may be discovered and the balance on the account reduced or eliminated.

Illustration 2 – The suspense account

A cheque for £200 is received through the post with no indication of what it is for. The drawer of the cheque is the local government authority. It is posted to the suspense account. Investigation reveals that it is a rates rebate.

Show these entries in the ledger accounts.

Solution

Step 1

The amount is entered as a debit entry in the cash book (cash receipt) and as a credit in the suspense account as it is not yet known what this receipt is for.

Suspense

	£		£
		Cash	200

Step 2

Transfer this amount to the rates account.

Suspense

	£		£
Rates	200	Cash	200
	200		200

Rates			
	£		£
		Suspense	200

4.2 When the trial balance totals disagree

We have so far assumed that the trial balance can be easily made to balance. However, it is often the case that any misbalance is due to a large number of items and hence the reasons may not be immediately pinpointed. The difference is recorded in a suspense account temporarily until the errors are discovered and can be corrected.

We have already come across errors which are likely to cause a difference on the trial balance and these include the following:

*   Transposition, e.g. a debit of £67 and a credit of £76 for the same transaction. As mentioned already, this kind of error leads to an imbalance that is divisible by 9.

*   One-side omission, e.g. a cheque for rent of £150 entered in the cash account but not in the rent account.

*   Two entries on one side and none on the other, e.g. purchases of goods debited to purchases account and also debited to purchases ledger control account.

*   An account entered on the wrong side of the trial balance or omitted from the trial balance.

Only those errors which cause a difference on the trial balance need to be adjusted by means of an entry in the suspense account. For example, if an item has been posted to the wrong account, this will not cause a difference on the trial balance, although the error must be adjusted by means of a journal entry.

Illustration 3 – The suspense account

The trial balance is found to be £90 out, the total credits being £25,190 and the total debits being £25,100. In order to make the trial balance totals agree, £90 is debited to the suspense account. It is subsequently discovered that cash paid for stationery was credited in the cash book as £211 (the correct amount) and debited in the stationery account as £121 by mistake.

(a) Enter the amount in the suspense account.

(b) Show that this makes the trial balance balance.

(c) Correct the error using a journal.

Solution

Step 1 Enter the amount in the suspense account.

Suspense

	£		£
Difference in trial balance	90		

Step 2 The trial balance now balances.

	Debit £	Credit £
Original totals	25,100	25,190
Suspense account	90	
	25,190	25,190

Step 3 Correct the error.

Identify the actual entry made and establish what the correct entry should have been.

	Actual entry		Correct entry	
	Dr £	Cr £	Dr £	Cr £
Stationery	121		211	
Cash		211		211

The stationery account is understated by £90. Prepare a journal to correct the error.

	£	£
Debit Stationery account	90	
Credit Suspense account		90

Being incorrect posting of cash paid for stationery.

The ledger accounts will now look as follows:

Suspense

	£		£
Balance b/d	90	Stationery	90
	90		90

Stationery

	£		£
Balance b/d	121		
Suspense	90	Balance c/d	211
	211		211
Balance b/d	211		

We now have the correct figure in the stationery account, the suspense account has been cleared and the trial balance balances.

5   Journals

5.1   Introduction

Journal entries have been considered briefly in earlier sections but will now be looked at in more detail.

The journal is a formal, written instruction to the bookkeeper to put an item of double entry through the main ledger.

Whenever an error has to be corrected or an adjustment made to the ledgers then it is important that this is correct and that it is properly authorised. This can only be done with a formal system such as the journal.

5.2   Use of the journal

The journal consists of a debit and credit entry and the ledger accounts that these entries are to be made to. However there are also other important details for journals.

*   The journal must be dated.

*   They must be consecutively numbered so that it can be checked that all journals have been entered into the ledgers.

*   There must be adequate description of the journal so that the person authorising it knows exactly what it is for.

Illustration 4 – Journals

A business wishes to write off a debt from N Jones for £200 that it now considers to be bad. Today's date is 30 June and the last journal entry was numbered 336.

We will draft the journal entry for this adjustment.

Solution

JOURNAL ENTRY		No: 337	
Prepared by:			
Authorised by:			
Date: 30 June			
Narrative: To write off bad debt from N Jones			
Account	Code	Debit	Credit
Bad debts expense	ML	200	
Sales ledger control	ML		200
TOTALS		200	200

In examination, you are often asked to prepare journal entries. However, many examination do not require the narrative so read the instructions carefully.

5.3 Correction of errors where the suspense account is not affected

We have seen that not all errors that are found in the ledgers affect the balancing of the trial balance. However even if the trial balance still balances but errors are discovered they must still be corrected using a journal entry.

Illustration 5 – Use of journal and suspense account

When performing the sales ledger control account reconciliation the following errors were discovered:

- the sales day book was overcast by £1,000;

- the discounts allowed total in the cash receipts book of £140 was not posted at all;

- a receipt from H Fisher of £870 was entered into H Fisher's individual account in the subsidiary ledger as £780.

We will write up the journal entries to correct these errors starting with journal number 1658.

Solution

JOURNAL ENTRY	No: 1658		
Prepared by:			
Authorised by:			
Date:			
Narrative: To correct overcast of sales day book			
Account	Code	Debit	Credit
Sales	ML	1,000	
Sales ledger control	ML		1,000
TOTALS		1,000	1,000

JOURNAL ENTRY		No: 1659		
Prepared by:				
Authorised by:				
Date:				
Narrative: To post discounts allowed omitted				
Account	Code	Debit	Credit	
Discounts allowed	ML	140		
Sales ledger control	ML		140	
TOTALS		140	140	

The error in H Fisher's individual account in the subsidiary ledger needs to be corrected but this will not be done with a journal entry as no double entry is required.

When correcting errors with journal entries, firstly work out what has been done in the accounts and then determine the double entry necessary to put it right.

Test your understanding 3

Discounts received of £50 have not been posted to the main ledger at all.

Draft a journal entry to correct this. The last journal number was 152. Today's date is 12 September 20X1.

Test your understanding 4

John

On 31 December 20X8 the trial balance of John, a small manufacturer, failed to agree and the difference was entered in a suspense account. After the final accounts had been prepared the following errors were discovered and the difference was eliminated.

- The purchase day book was undercast by £200.

- Machinery purchased for £150 had been debited to the purchases account.

- Discounts received of £130 had been posted to the debit of the discounts received account.

- Rates of £46 paid by cheque had been posted to the debit of the rates account as £64.

- Cash drawings by the owner of £45 had been entered in the cash account correctly but not posted to the drawings account.

- The balance on the stock account representing the opening stock of £1,200 had been omitted from the trial balance.

(a) **Show the journal entries necessary to correct the above errors.**

(b) **Show the entries in the suspense account to eliminate the differences.**

6 Use of journal and suspense account

Very often, some of the errors made will affect the suspense account and some will not. In the exam you need to be clear when sorting out a difference which are which.

Illustration 6 – Use of journal and suspense account

The following summary trial balance has been extracted from the ledger accounts.

	£	£
Capital		150,000
Profit and loss		75,000
Freehold property	560,000	
Motor vehicles	30,000	
Depreciation on motor vehicles		2,500
Stock	40,000	
Sales ledger control account	25,000	
Bank (overdrawn)	2,600	
Purchases ledger control account		20,000
Sales		585,000
Purchases	175,000	
Electricity	2,300	
Rent and rates	900	
Discount allowed		670
Discount received	820	
Stationery	600	
Travel expenses	800	
	838,020	833,170

Task 1

(a) Certain items that have been entered on the wrong side of the trial balance. Rewrite the Trial Balance with these amounts corrected, and with a suspense account for any residual difference.

(b) On inspection of the books the following mistakes are

discovered.

(i) An electricity invoice for £200 was entered in the rent account.

(ii) An invoice for stationery for £300 was entered as a credit note in the purchases day book

(iii) A cash purchase for a train ticket costing £280 was credited to the travel account.

(iv) An invoice for a cash purchase of stationery for £320 was entered in the stationery account as a debit of £230.

Produce journal entries to correct these errors.

(c) Enter the journals in part (b) in the suspense account if they are relevant to that account.

Solution

(a)

	£	£
Capital		150,000
Profit and loss		75,000
Freehold property	560,000	
Motor vehicles	30,000	
Depreciation on motor vehicles		2,500
Stock	40,000	
Sales ledger control account	25,000	
Bank (overdrawn)		2,600
Purchases ledger control account		20,000
Sales		585,000
Purchases	175,000	
Electricity	2,300	
Rent and rates	900	
Discount allowed	670	
Discount received		820
Stationery	600	
Travel expenses	800	
Suspense	650	
	835,920	835,920

Tutorial note

(i) The bank is overdrawn – this has to be a credit balance

(ii) Discount allowed is what the business has allowed other people – money given away – an expense – a debit balance

(iii) Discount received is what the business has received – a type of income – a credit balance

Learn these entries – don't be one of the people who always get them wrong.

chapter **18**

(b)

			£	£
(i)	Dr	Electricity	200	
	Cr	Rent		200
(ii)	Dr	Purchases	600	
	Cr	PLCA		600
(iii)	Dr	Travel expenses	560	
	Cr	Suspense account		560
(iv)	Dr	Stationery	90	
	Cr	Suspense account		90

(c)

Suspense account

	£		£
Balance b/d	650	Travel expenses	560
		Stationery	90
	650		650

Test your understanding 5

Whilst preparing the purchases ledger control account the following errors were discovered:

(a) the purchases day book was undercast by £100;

(b) the discounts received total in the cash payments book of £390 had not been posted at all.

The last journal number used was 153. Draft the journal entries required to correct these errors.

Test your understanding 6

1 What are the two reasons for extracting a trial balance?

2 What types of error will affect the balancing of the trial balance?

3 What is an error of commission?

4 Are drawings a debit or a credit balance on the trial balance?

5 A cheque payment has been made but the bookkeeper does not immediately know what the payment is for. How would this be treated in the ledger accounts whilst the nature of the payment was investigated?

6 A trial balance has a total of debit balances of £36,540 and credit balances of £34,700. If a suspense account is set up how much would it be for and would it be a debit or credit balance?

7 Discounts allowed have been entered correctly as £1,540 in the sales ledger control account but have been entered as £1,450 in the discounts account. What double entry is required to correct this?

8 The electricity account balance of £866 has been omitted from the trial balance. What is the journal entry required to correct this?

9 A £200 telephone bill has been incorrectly posted to the rent account. What is the double entry required to correct this?

10 The purchases returns day book was undercast by £100. What is the double entry required to correct this?

7 Summary

In this chapter we have covered the preparation of the trial balance, the identification of any discrepancies and the rectification of errors and omissions to ensure that the trial balance does in fact balance. Once the trial balance has been initially drawn up if it does not balance it is worthwhile carrying out basic checks to ensure that all balances have been correctly transferred and that the debits and credits have been correctly totalled. Then you will need to set up a suspense account and finally to try to clear the suspense account by putting through the correcting double entry. Remember that not all errors affect the balancing of the trial balance and therefore not all adjustments will affect the suspense account.

Test your understanding answers

Test your understanding 1

Trial balance at 31 December 20X2

	Dr £	Cr £
Capital on 1 January 20X2		106,149
Freehold factory at cost	360,000	
Motor vehicles at cost	126,000	
Stocks at 1 January 20X2	37,500	
Debtors	15,600	
Cash in hand	225	
Bank overdraft		82,386
Creditors		78,900
Sales		318,000
Purchases	165,000	
Rent and rates	35,400	
Discounts allowed	6,600	
Insurance	2,850	
Sales returns	10,500	
Purchases returns		6,300
Loan from bank		240,000
Sundry expenses	45,960	
Drawings	26,100	
	831,735	831,735

Test your understanding 2

Bank account

		£			£
01 May	Capital	6,800	06 May	Rates	100
05 May	Cash sales	300	08 May	Wages	50
			15 May	Office fixtures	600
			18 May	Motor vehicle	3,500
			25 May	Creditors	
				(1,000 + 500)	1,500
			26 May	Wages	150
			31 May	Balance c/f	1,200
		7,100			7,100
1 June	Balance b/f	1,200			

Purchase ledger control account

		£			£
11 May	Purchases returns	150	03 May	Purchases (400 + 300 + 250)	950
25 May	Bank	1,500	10 May	Purchases (800 + 700)	1,500
31 May	Balance c/f	800			
		2,450			2,450
			1 June	Balance b/f	800

Sales ledger control account

		£			£
9 May	Sales (300 + 300 + 100)	700	22 May	Sales returns	100
			31 May	Balance c/f	600
		700			700
1 June	Balance b/f	600			

Capital account

		£			£
31 May	Balance c/f	6,800	1 May	Bank	6,800
			1 June	Balance b/f	6,800

Purchases account

		£			£
03 May	J Johnson	400			
	D Nixon	300			
	J Agnew	250			
10 May	J Johnson	800			
	D Nixon	700			
			31 May	Balance c/f	2,450
		2,450			2,450
1 June	Balance b/f	2,450			

Sales account

		£			£
			05 May	Cash	300
			09 May	K Homes	300
				J Homes	300
31 May	Balance c/f	1,000		B Hood	100
		1,000			1,000
			1 June	Balance b/f	1,000

Rates account

		£			£
06 May	Bank	100	31 May	Balance c/f	100
1 June	Balance b/f	100			

Wages account

		£			£
08 May	Bank	50			
26 May	Bank	150	31 May	Balance c/f	200
		200			200
1 June	Balance b/f	200			

Purchases returns account

		£			£
31 May	Balance c/f	150	11 May	Johnson	150
			1 June	Balance b/f	150

Office fixtures account

		£			£
15 May	Bank	600	31 May	Balance c/f	600
1 June	Balance b/f	600			

Motor vehicle account

		£			£
18 May	Bank	3,500	31 May	Balance c/f	3,500
1 June	Balance b/f	3,500			

Sales returns account

		£			£
22 May	J Homes	100	31 May	Balance c/f	100
1 June	Balance b/f	100			

Tutorial note

Balances have been brought forward on all accounts. As noted earlier in this text, it is not customary to bring forward balances on accounts with only a single item on them.

Trial balance as at 30 May 20X6

	Dr £	Cr £
Bank	1,200	
Purchase ledger control		800
Sales ledger control	600	
Capital		6,800
Purchases	2,450	
Sales		1,000
Rates	100	
Wages	200	
Purchase returns		150
Office fixtures	600	
Motor vehicles	3,500	
Sales returns	100	
	8,750	8,750

Test your understanding 3

JOURNAL ENTRY		No: 153		
Prepared by:				
Authorised by:				
Date: 12 September 20X1				
Narrative: To enter discounts received omitted				
Account		Code	Debit £	Credit £
Purchases ledger control		ML	50	
Discounts received		ML		50
TOTALS			50	50

Test your understanding 4

(a) Journal Entries

		Debit £	Credit £
1	**Purchases**	200	
	Purchases ledger control account		200
	Being correction of undercast of purchases day book. (No effect on suspense account as control account is the double entry. However, the error should have been found during the reconciliation of the control account).		
2	**Machinery (fixed assets)**	150	
	Purchases		150
	Being adjustment for wrong entry for machinery purchased (no effect on suspense account).		
3	**Suspense account**	260	
	Discount received		260
	Being correction of discounts received entered on wrong side of account		
4	**Suspense account**	18	
	Rates		18
	Being correction of transposition error to rates account		
5	**Drawings**	45	
	Suspense account		45
	Being completion of double entry for drawings		
6	**Stock per trial balance**	1,200	
	Suspense account		1,200
	Being inclusion of opening stock. There is no double		

(b)

Suspense account

	£		£
Difference in TB (balancing figure)	967	Drawings	45
Discounts received	260	Stock per trial balance	1,200
Rates	18		
	1,245		1,245

Test your understanding 5

JOURNAL ENTRY	No: 154		
Prepared by:			
Authorised by:			
Date:			
Narrative: To correct undercast of the purchases day book			
Account	Code	Debit	Credit
		£	£
Purchases	ML	100	
Purchases ledger control	ML		100
TOTALS		100	100

JOURNAL ENTRY	No: 155		
Prepared by:			
Authorised by:			
Date:			
Narrative: To correct omission of discounts received			
Account	Code	Debit	Credit
		£	£
Purchases ledger control	ML	390	
Discounts received	ML		390
TOTALS		390	390

KAPLAN PUBLISHING

chapter **18**

Test your understanding 7

1 – As a check on the double entry

– As a starting point for the preparation of final accounts

2 – Single entry

– Casting error

– Transposition error

– Extraction error

– Balance on the wrong side of the trial balance

– Balance omitted from the trial balance

3 An error of commission is where the double entry has been completed but between the wrong accounts.

4 Debit balance.

5 Debit   Suspense account
Credit   Cash payments book.

6 £1,840 credit balance.

7 Debit   Discounts allowed account   £90
Credit   Suspense account   £90

8 Debit   Electricity account in trial balance   £866
Credit   Suspense   £866

Being omission of electricity account balance from the trial balance.

9 Debit   Telephone account   £200
Credit   Rent account   £200

10 Debit   Purchases ledger control   £100
Credit   Purchases returns   £100

Final accounts and accounting concepts

Introduction

Financial statements are prepared under a number of well-established and generally accepted accounting concepts or principles.

1 Financial statements

1.1 Introduction

Periodically all organisations will produce financial statements in order to show how the business has performed and what assets and liabilities it has. The two main financial statements are the profit and loss account and the balance sheet.

1.2 Profit and loss account

The profit and loss account summarises the transactions of a business over a period and determines whether the business has made a profit or a loss for the period.

A typical profit and loss account is shown below.

Trading and profit and loss account of Stanley for the year ended 31 December 20X2

		£	£
Sales			X
Less: Cost of sales			
Stock, at cost on 1 January (opening stock)		X	
Add: Purchases of goods		X	
		X	
Less: Stock, at cost on 31 December (closing stock)		(X)	
			(X)
Gross profit			X
Sundry income:			
Discounts received		X	
Commission received		X	
Rent received		X	
			X
			X
Less:	Expenses:		
	Rent	X	
	Rates	X	
	Lighting and heating	X	
	Telephone	X	
	Postage	X	
	Insurance	X	
	Stationery	X	
	Office salaries	X	
	Depreciation	X	
	Accountancy and audit fees	X	
	Bank charges and interest	X	
	Bad and doubtful debts	X	
	Delivery costs	X	
	Van running expenses	X	
	Advertising	X	
	Discounts allowed	X	
			(X)
Net profit			X

Technically the first part of the profit and loss account, from sales down to gross profit, is known as the trading account. The profit and loss account itself is the bottom part of the statement starting with gross profit, then showing any sundry income and expenses and finally leading to a figure for net profit.

However, in practice, the whole trading and profit and loss account combined is often referred to as the profit and loss account.

The trading account section is the comparison of sales to the cost of the goods sold. This gives the gross profit. Note how the cost of goods sold is made up of:

Opening stock	X
Purchases	X
	X
Less: closing stock	(X)
Cost of sales	X

The profit and loss account shows any other sundry income and then a list of all of the expenses of the business. After all of the expenses have been deducted the final figure is the net profit or loss for the period.

1.3 Balance sheet

 The balance sheet is a list of all of the assets and liabilities of the business on the last day of the accounting period.

An example of a typical sole trader's balance sheet is given below:

Balance sheet of Stanley at 31 December 20X2

	Cost	Depreciation	
	£	£	£
Fixed assets			
Freehold factory	X	X	X
Machinery	X	X	X
Motor vehicles	X	X	X
	X	X	X
Current assets			
Stocks		X	
Debtors	X		
Less: provision for doubtful debts	(X)		
		X	
Prepayments		X	
Cash at bank		X	
Cash in hand		X	
		X	
Current liabilities			
Trade creditors	X		
Accrued charges	X		
		(X)	
Net current assets			X
Total assets less current liabilities			X
Long-term liabilities			
12% loan			(X)
Net assets			X
Capital at 1 January			X
Net profit for the year			X
			X
Less: drawings			(X)
Proprietor's funds			X

Note that the balance sheet is split into two sections.

(a) The top part of the balance sheet lists all of the assets and liabilities of the organisation. This is then totalled by adding together all of the asset values and deducting the liabilities.

The assets are split into fixed assets and current assets.

 Fixed assets are assets for long-term use within the business.

 Current assets are assets that are either currently cash or will soon be converted into cash.

The current assets are always listed in the reverse order of liquidity. Therefore stock is always shown first as this has to be sold to a customer, become a debtor and then be converted into cash. Next shown are debtors who will become cash when the customer pays and prepayments (these will be considered in a later chapter). Finally the most liquid of all assets are listed, the bank balance and any cash in hand.

Current liabilities are the short term creditors of the business. This generally means creditors who are due to be paid within twelve months of the balance sheet date.

Long-term liabilities are creditors who will be paid after more than 12 months. These are deducted to give the net assets.

(b) The bottom part of the balance sheet shows how all of these assets less liabilities have been funded. For a sole trader this is made up of the capital at the start of the year plus the net profit for the year less any drawings that the owner made during the year. This part of the balance sheet is also totalled and it should have the same total as the top part of the balance sheet.

Test your understanding 1

How is cost of sales calculated in the profit and loss account?

2 FRS 18 Accounting Policies

2.1 Introduction

When a sole trader or a partnership is preparing their final accounts and dealing with accounting transactions on a day to day basis they will find that there are many choices about the accounting treatment of transactions and events. The way in which the accountant deals with these choices is dependent on a number of well known and well understood accounting concepts and also according to the organisation's own accounting policies. There are also rules from the Companies Act. Although sole traders are not required to follow these they may wish to as these are best accounting practice, as are rules from accounting standards as to how to treat items in the final accounts.

The choices that an organisation makes when preparing final accounts are known as their accounting policies. The choice of accounting policies that an organisation makes is fundamental to the picture shown by the final accounts and therefore an accounting standard has been issued on this area – FRS 18 Accounting Policies.

FRS 18 sets out the principles that organisations should follow when selecting their accounting policies. The basic principle is that an organisation should select the accounting policies that are judged to be the most appropriate to its particular circumstances so guidance is given in the form of accounting concepts, objectives and constraints in order to help organisations choose the most appropriate accounting policies.

2.2 Accounting concepts

Over the years a number of accounting concepts have been judged to be fundamental to the preparation of final accounts. Some of these have their origins in the Companies Act whereas others have come about through best accounting practice. FRS 18 identifies two of these concepts as playing a pervasive role in the preparation of final accounts and therefore also in the selection of accounting policies - the going concern concept and the accruals concept.

2.3 Going concern concept

FRS 18 requires that final accounts should be prepared on the going concern basis unless the directors believe that the organisation is not a going concern. The going concern basis is that the final accounts are prepared with the underlying assumption that the business will continue for the foreseeable future. This concept or basis affects the valuation of assets shown in the balance sheet in particular. If the business is a going concern then assets will continue to be shown in the balance sheet at the amount that they cost. However, if the business were not a going concern and was due to close down in the near future then assets such as specialised premises or machinery may have a very low value, much lower than their original cost, as they would not easily be sold when the business closed.

2.4 Accruals concept

FRS 18 also requires final accounts to be prepared on the accruals basis of accounting. The accruals basis of accounting requires that transactions should be reflected in the final accounts for the period in which they occur and not simply in the period in which any cash involved is received or paid.

This means that the amount of any income or expense that appears in the final accounts should be the amount that was earned or incurred during the accounting period rather than the amount of cash that was received or paid.

For example, consider credit sales and credit purchases. When a sale is made on credit the sales account is credited immediately even though it may be a considerable time before the cash is actually received from the debtor. In just the same way when goods are purchased on credit from a supplier, the purchases account is debited immediately although it will be some time before the creditor is paid. We will come across further examples of applying the accruals basis of accounting when we deal with accruals and prepayments.

2.5   Objectives in selecting accounting policies

As well as the two underlying accounting concepts of going concern and accruals accounting, FRS 18 sets out four objectives against which an organisation should judge the appropriateness of accounting policies to its own particular circumstances. These objectives are relevance, reliability, comparability and understandability.

2.6   Relevance

Financial information is said to be relevant if it has the ability to influence the economic decisions of the users of that information and is provided in time to influence those decisions. Where an organisation faces a choice of accounting policies they should choose the one that is most relevant in the context of the final accounts as a whole.

2.7   Reliability

As you will start to see in this text there are many estimates and management decisions which have to be made when determining the figures that will appear in the final accounts. It may not be possible to judge whether such estimates are absolutely correct or not but the accounting policies chosen by an organisation must ensure that the figures that appear in the final accounts are reliable.

There are a number of aspects to providing reliable information in the final accounts.

- The figures should represent the substance of the transactions or events.

- The figures should be free from bias or neutral.

- The figures should be free of material errors.

- Where there is uncertainty, a degree of caution should be applied in making the judgements.

The last factor, the degree of caution, is also known as prudence. The prudence concept was initially one of the fundamental accounting concepts stated by the Companies Act and SSAP 2 (now withdrawn and replaced by FRS 18). However, FRS 18 now views prudence as part of the objective of reliability. Prudence is only relevant in conditions of uncertainty and in such conditions it requires more evidence of the existence of an asset or gain than for the existence of a liability or loss. When the value of the asset, liability, gain or loss is uncertain then prudence requires a greater reliability of measurement for assets and gains than for liabilities and losses.

2.8   Comparability

Information in final accounts is used by many different people and organisations such as the employees, investors, potential investors, creditors and the organisation's bank. The information provided in the final accounts is much more useful to these users if it is comparable over time and also with similar information about other organisations. The selection of appropriate accounting policies and their consistent use should provide such comparability.

2.9 Understandability

If the final accounts of an organisation are to be useful then they must be understandable. Accounting policies should be chosen to ensure ease of understanding for users of the final accounts who have a reasonable knowledge of business and economic activities and accounting and a willingness to studythe information diligently.

2.10 Constraints in selecting accounting policies

As well as requiring an organisation's accounting policies to meet these four objectives of relevance, reliability, comparability and ease of understanding, FRS 18 also sets out two constraints on the choice of accounting policies:

* the need to balance the four objectives - particularly where there might be a conflict between relevance and reliability

* the need to balance the cost of providing information with the likely benefit of that information to the users of the final accounts.

2.11 Materiality

An item is deemed to be material if its omission or misstatement will influence the economic decisions of the users of the accounts taken on the basis of the financial statements.

One further important accounting concept is that of materiality.

Accounting standards do not apply to immaterial items and judgement is required when determining whether or not an item is material.

An example might be the purchase of a stapler for use in the office. Technically this should be treated as a fixed asset as it is presumably for fairly long term use in the business. However rather than including it on the balance sheet and then depreciating it (see later chapter), it is more likely that on the basis of it being an immaterial item it would be written off as an expense in the profit and loss account.

Test your understanding 2

What affect does the concept of materiality have on the preparation of final accounts?

Test your understanding 3

1   What is the final figure calculated in the trading account known as?

2   What elements make up the cost of sales?

3   What is the distinction between fixed assets and current assets?

4   What is the rule regarding the order in which current assets are listed in the balance sheet?

5   What are current liabilities?

6   What is meant by the going concern concept?

7   What is meant by the accruals concept?

8   What are the four objectives against which an organisation should judge the appropriateness of its accounting policies?

9   What are the two constraints from FRS 18 regarding the choice of accounting policies?

10 What is materiality?

3   Summary

At this stage you need to be familiar with the proforma for a profit and loss account and a balance sheet. You also need to appreciate that accounting is not an exact science and that when dealing with transactions and events the accountant is faced with many choices regarding accounting treatment. The accounting methods chosen are known as the organisation's accounting policies and, according to FRS 18, these should be chosen on the basis of the four objectives of relevance, reliability, comparability and understandability.

For the ICB level II syllabus, you will need to be able to draw up a balance sheet and profit and loss account from a trial balance. It is therefore very important that you understand the layouts of these financial statements. If you are doing an ICB distance learning course, there will be practice questions on this area in your revision material.

Test your understanding answers

Test your understanding 1

Opening stock	X
Purchases	X
	X
Less: closing stock	(X)
Cost of sales	X

Test your understanding 2

The effect of materiality on the preparation of final accounts is that only material items are subject to the accounting conventions and policies of the business.

Test your understanding 3

1   Gross profit.

2   Opening stock + purchases – closing stock

3   Fixed assets are for long-term use in the business, whereas current assets are due to be used up in the trading process and converted into cash.

4   They are listed from the least liquid first, stock, to the most liquid last, cash in hand.

5   Amounts that are due to be paid within 12 months of the balance sheet date.

6   The going concern concept is that the final accounts are prepared on the basis that the business will continue for the foreseeable future.

7   The accruals concept is that transactions are accounted for in the period in which they take place rather than the period in which the cash is received or paid.

8   Relevance, reliability, comparability and understandability.

9   –   The need to balance the four objectives.

    –   The need to balance cost and benefit.

10 Materiality is an underlying concept which states that accounting policies and standards need only apply to material items. A material item is one which has the ability to influence the economic decisions of users of the final accounts.

Capital expenditure and revenue expenditure

Introduction

This chapter covers all areas of accounting for fixed assets, acquisition, disposal and depreciation. In this chapter we will start to look at the details of authorisation and accounting for capital expenditure.

1 Capital and revenue expenditure

1.1 Introduction

In an earlier chapter it was noted that in the balance sheet assets are split between fixed assets and current assets.

1.2 Fixed assets

The fixed assets of a business are the assets that were purchased with the intention of being for long term-use within the business.

Examples of fixed assets include buildings, machinery, motor vehicles, office fixtures and fittings and computer equipment.

1.3 Capital expenditure

Capital expenditure is expenditure on the purchase of fixed assets.

The purchase of fixed assets is known as capital expenditure as it is capitalised. This means that the cost of the fixed asset is initially taken to the balance sheet rather than the profit and loss account. We will see in a later chapter how this cost is then charged to the profit and loss account over the life of the fixed asset by the process of depreciation.

1.4 Revenue expenditure

Revenue expenditure is all other expenditure incurred by the business other than capital expenditure.

Revenue expenditure is charged to the profit and loss account in the period that it is incurred.

Capital expenditure is shown as a fixed asset in the balance sheet. Revenue expenditure is shown as an expense in the profit and loss account.

1.5 Authorising capital expenditure

Many types of fixed asset are relatively expensive. Most fixed assets will be used to generate income for the business for several years into the future. Therefore they are important purchases. Timing may also be critical. It may be necessary to arrange a bank overdraft or a loan, or alternatively capital expenditure may have to be delayed in order to avoid a bank overdraft.

For these reasons, most organisations have procedures whereby capital expenditure must be authorised by a responsible person. In small organisations, most fixed asset purchases are likely to be authorised by the owner of the business. In large organisations, there is normally a system whereby several people have the authority to approve capital expenditure up to a certain limit which depends on the person's level of seniority.

KAPLAN PUBLISHING

The method of recording the authorisation is also likely to vary according to the nature and size of the organisation and according to the type of fixed asset expenditure it normally undertakes. In a small business, there may be no formal record other than a signature on a cheque.

In a large company, the directors may record their approval of significant expenditure in the minutes of the board meeting. Other possibilities include the use of requisition forms or memos and signing of the invoice.

In most organisations, disposals of fixed assets must also be authorised in writing.

Where standard forms are used, these will vary from organisation to organisation, but the details for acquisition of an asset are likely to include:

* date
* description of asset
* reason for purchase
* supplier
* cost/quotation
* details of quotation (if applicable)

* details of lease agreement (if applicable)
* authorisation (number of signatures required will vary according to the organisation's procedures)
* method of financing.

2 Recording the purchase of fixed assets

2.1 Introduction

We have seen that the cost of a fixed asset will appear in the balance sheet as capitalised expenditure. Therefore it is important that the correct figure for cost is included in the correct ledger account.

2.2 Cost

The cost figure that will be used to record the fixed asset is the full purchase price of the asset. Care should be taken when considering the cost of some assets, in particular motor cars, as the invoice may show that the total amount paid includes some revenue expenditure for example petrol and road fund licences. These elements of revenue expenditure must be written off to the profit and loss account and only the capital expenditure included as the cost of the fixed asset.

Cost should also include the cost of getting the asset to its current location and into working condition. Therefore this may include freight costs, installation costs and test runs.

2.3 Ledger accounts

If a fixed asset is paid for by cheque then the double entry is:

DR   Fixed asset account
CR   Bank account

If the fixed asset was bought on credit the double entry is:

DR   Fixed asset account
CR   Creditors account

In practice most organisations will have different fixed asset accounts for the different types of fixed assets, for example:

* land and buildings account

* plant and machinery account

* motor vehicles account

* office fixtures and fittings account

* computer equipment account.

2.4 Purchase of fixed assets and VAT

When most fixed assets are purchased VAT will be added to the purchase price and this can normally be recovered from HM Revenue and Customs as input VAT. Therefore the cost of the fixed asset is the amount net of VAT.

2.5 Purchase of cars and VAT

When new cars are purchased the business is not allowed to reclaim the VAT. Therefore the cost to be capitalised for the car must include the VAT.

Illustration 1 – Recording the purchase of fixed assets

Your business has just purchased a new car by cheque and an extract from the invoice shows the following:

	£
Cost of car	18,000
Road fund licence	155
Petrol	20
	18,175
VAT on cost of car	3,150
Total cost	21,325

Record this cost in the ledger accounts of the business.

Motor Cars Account

	£		£
Bank (18,000 + 3,150)	21,150		

Motor Expenses Account

	£		£
Bank (155 + 20)	175		

Bank Account

	£		£
		Motor vehicle + expenses	21,325

Note that only the motor cars account balance would appear in the balance sheet, ie be capitalised, while the motor expenses account balance would appear in the profit and loss account as an expense for the period.

Test your understanding 1

A piece of machinery has been purchased on credit from a supplier for £4,200 plus VAT at 17.5%.

Record this purchase in the ledger accounts.

2.6   Transfer journal

Fixed asset acquisitions do not normally take place frequently in organisations and many organisations will tend to record the acquisition in the transfer journal.

The transfer journal is a primary record which is used for transactions that do not appear in the other primary records of the business.

The transfer journal will tend to take the form of an instruction to the bookkeeper as to which accounts to debit and credit and what this transaction is for.

An example of a transfer journal for the purchase of a fixed asset is given below.

Journal entry		No: 02714		
Date	20 May 20X1			
Prepared by	C Jones			
Authorised by	F Peters			
Account		Code	Debit £	Credit £
Computers: Cost		0120	5,000	
VAT		0138	875	
Cash at Bank		0163		5,875
Totals			5,875	5,875

A transfer journal is used for entries to the ledger accounts that do not come from any other primary records.

Illustration 2 – Recording the purchase of fixed assets

Produce a journal entry for the example on the previous page, reproduced below

	£
Cost of car	18,000
Road fund licence	155
Petrol	20
	18,175
VAT (18,000 x 0.175)	3,150
	21,325

Solution

Ref		Dr (3)	Cr (£)
	Motor car a/c (18,000 + 3,150)	21,150	
	Motor expenses a/c (155 + 20)	175	
	Bank a/c	.	21,325

2.7 Fixed assets produced internally

In some instances a business may make its own fixed assets. For example a construction company may construct a new Head Office for the organisation.

Where fixed assets are produced internally then the amount that should be capitalised as the cost is the production cost of the asset.

Production cost is the direct cost of production (materials, labour

and expenses) plus an appropriate amount of the normal production overheads relating to production of this asset.

2.8 Capitalising subsequent expenditure

It is frequently the case that there will be further expenditure on a fixed asset during its life in the business. In most cases this will be classed as revenue expenditure and will therefore be charged to the profit and loss account. However in some cases the expenditure may be so major that it should also be capitalised as an addition to the cost of the fixed asset.

FRS 15 Tangible Fixed Assets, states that subsequent expenditure should only be capitalised in three circumstances:

*   where it enhances the value of the asset

*   where a major component of the asset is replaced or restored

*   where it is a major inspection or overhaul of the asset.

Illustration 3 – Recording the purchase of fixed assets

A four-colour printing press is purchased in 20X1 for £150,000. Annual maintenance expenditure is £15,000 in 20X1 and 20X2, £20,000 in 20X3 and £30,000 in 20X4. In 20X5, £30,000 is spent on the machine to improve its running and add a facility for it to print in five colours. Annual maintenance expenditure in 20X5 is cut to £10,000. What accounting entries would be made from 20X1 to 20X5 in respect of this machine? Ignore VAT.

Solution

		£	£
20X1			
Dr	Fixed assets	150,000	
	Maintenance	15,000	
	Cr Creditors/cash		165,000
20X2			
Dr	Maintenance	15,000	
	Cr Creditors/cash		15,000
20X3			
Dr	Maintenance	20,000	
	Cr Creditors/cash		20,000
20X4			
Dr	Maintenance	30,000	
	Cr Creditors/cash		30,000
20X5			
Dr	Fixed assets	30,000	
	Maintenance	10,000	
	Cr Creditors/cash		40,000

2.9 Financing fixed asset acquisitions

Fixed assets generally cost a lot of money and are purchased with the intention that they be used over a period of years. For most businesses the full purchase cost cannot be funded from cash available in the business, and so other financing methods must be found, including the following.

Borrowing – a bank or other lender lends the business cash to pay for the asset, at a negotiated interest rate. Often the loan will be secured on the asset, so that it can be sold directly for the benefit of the bank or lender in the event of non-payment or liquidation.

Hire purchase – the business makes regular payments to the finance company (comprising capital amounts plus interest) but the asset remains the finance company's property until the last regular payment is made, when the business can elect to take over the asset's full ownership.

Leasing – the business makes regular payments to the finance company and makes full use of the asset, but never actually becomes the asset's owner.

Part exchange – part of the purchase price of the asset is satisfied by transferring ownership of another asset to the seller. This is frequently seen in the case of motor vehicles, and represents a disposal and a purchase at the same time.

3 SSAP 21: Accounting for Leases and Hire Purchase Contracts

3.1 Definitions

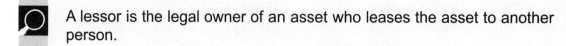

A lessor is the legal owner of an asset who leases the asset to another person.

A lessee is the person to whom the asset is leased - they are not the legal owner.

SSAP 21 deals with definitions of leases and the accounting treatment of leases and hire purchase contracts.

According to SSAP 21 there are two types of leases – finance leases and operating leases.

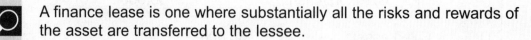

A finance lease is one where substantially all the risks and rewards of the asset are transferred to the lessee.

An operating lease is any lease other than a finance lease.

KAPLAN PUBLISHING

3.2 Explanation

A finance lease is a financial arrangement between the owner of the asset (the lessor) and the lessee whereby the lessee substantially (although not legally) becomes the owner of the asset. The lessee assumes all the costs and risks associated with ownership, eg maintenance, insurance, etc. The lessee in these circumstances normally leases the asset for the whole of its useful life. You can therefore think of a finance lease as being a long-term lease (the lease term is similar to the asset's useful life), while an operating lease is often a short-term lease.

3.3 Accounting for finance leases and hire purchase contracts

The only difference between a finance lease asset and one purchased under a hire purchase contract is that when the final payment is made on hire purchase the purchaser becomes the legal owner. The lessee under a finance lease never becomes the legal owner of the asset.

In essence the lessee's accounting treatment of assets purchased under finance leases and under hire purchase contracts is the same.

Step 1 The asset must be treated as a fixed asset in the lessee's balance sheet at its fair value or cash cost (exactly as if they had actually bought the asset outright).

Step 2 A creditor is also set up in the balance sheet for the same amount. For a finance lease this creditor is known as 'obligations under finance leases' and for a hire purchase contract as a 'hire purchase creditor'.

Step 3 The fixed asset is then treated as any other fixed asset and is depreciated over its useful life (see later chapter).

Step 4 When each lease or hire purchase payment is made the payment must be split between the amount that is paying off the capital cost of the asset and the amount that is the finance charge for the period. The element of capital cost is debited to the creditor account whilst the finance charge is charged to the profit and loss account as an expense.

You will not be asked to perform this bookkeeping for finance leases in detail.

3.4 Accounting for operating leases

The accounting for operating leases is very simple. The asset is not included in the lessee's balance sheet, instead each lease payment is charged in full to the profit and loss account as an expense.

A finance lease asset is capitalised and included in the lessee's balance sheet as a fixed asset whereas an operating lease asset is not treated as a fixed asset by the lessee.

Test your understanding 2

When a company purchases data disks for the new word-processor, the amount of the purchase is debited to fittings and equipment (cost) account.

(a) Is this treatment correct?

(b) If so, why; if not, why not?

4 Types of fixed assets

4.1 Introduction

We have seen how the fixed assets of a business will be classified between the various types, e.g. buildings, plant and machinery, etc. However there is a further distinction in the classification of fixed assets that must be considered. This is the distinction between tangible fixed assets and intangible fixed assets.

4.2 Tangible fixed assets

Tangible fixed assets are assets which have a tangible, physical form.

Tangible fixed assets therefore are all of the types of assets that we have been considering so far such as machinery, cars, computers, etc.

4.3 Intangible fixed assets

Intangible fixed assets are assets for long-term use in the business that have no physical form.

4.4 Goodwill

Many businesses will have a particular intangible fixed asset known as goodwill. Goodwill is the asset arising from the fact that a going concern business is worth more in total than the value of its tangible net assets in total. The reasons for this additional asset are many and varied but include factors such as good reputation, good location, quality products and quality after sales service.

4.5 Accounting treatment of goodwill

Although it is recognised that goodwill exists in many businesses, it is generally not included as a fixed asset on the balance sheet. This is for a number of reasons including the difficulty in valuation of goodwill and also its innate volatility. Consider a restaurant with an excellent reputation which suddenly causes a bout of food poisoning. The asset, goodwill, could literally be wiped out overnight.

Even though goodwill will not generally be included in the balance sheet, you need to be aware of its existence.

5 Fixed asset register

5.1 Introduction

Obviously the fixed assets of a business will tend to be expensive items that the organisation will wish to have good control over. In particular the organisation will wish to keep control over which assets are kept where and check on a regular basis that they are still there.

Therefore most organisations that own a significant number of fixed assets will tend to maintain a fixed asset register as well as the ledger accounts that record the purchase of the fixed assets.

5.2 Layout of a fixed asset register

The purpose of a fixed asset register is to record all relevant details of all of the fixed assets of the organisation. The format of the register will depend on the organisation, but the information to be recorded for each fixed asset of the business will probably include the following:

- asset description
- asset identification code
- asset location
- date of purchase
- purchase price
- supplier name and address
- invoice number
- any additional enhancement expenditure
- depreciation method
- estimated useful life
- estimated residual value
- accumulated depreciation to date
- net book value
- disposal details.

A typical format for a fixed asset register is shown overleaf.

5.3 Example of a fixed asset register

Date of purchase	Invoice number	Serial number	Item	Cost £	Accum'd depreciation b/f at 1.1.X8 £	Date of disposal	Depreciation charge in 20X8 £	Accumulated depreciation c/f £	Disposal proceeds £	Loss/gain on disposal £
3.2.X5	345	3488	Chair	340						
6.4.X6	466	–	Bookcase	258						
10.7.X7	587	278	Chair	160						
				758						

There may also be a further column or detail which shows exactly where the particular asset is located within the business. This will facilitate checks that should be regularly carried out to ensure that all of the assets the business owns are still on the premises.

Test your understanding 3

1   What is capital expenditure?

2   What is revenue expenditure?

3   What is the double entry for recording a fixed asset purchased on credit?

4   What is included in the cost of a fixed asset that is capitalised?

5   What are the three occasions where subsequent expenditure on a fixed asset can be capitalised according to FRS 15?

6   What is a finance lease?

7   How is a finance lease accounted for by the lessee?

8   What is the essential difference between a finance lease asset and a hire purchase contract asset?

9   How is an operating lease accounted for by the lessee?

10 Should goodwill always be included as a fixed asset in a business's balance sheet?

6 Summary

In this chapter we have considered the acquisition of fixed assets. The acquisition of a fixed asset must be properly authorised and the most appropriate method of funding the purchase used. The correct cost figure must be used when capitalising the fixed asset and care should be taken with VAT and exclusion of any revenue expenditure in the total cost. The details of the acquisition of the asset should also be included in the fixed asset register.

Test your understanding answers

Machinery account

	£		£
Creditors	4,200		

VAT account

	£		£
Creditors	735		

Purchases ledger control account

	£		£
		Machinery and VAT	4,935

(a) No.

(b) Although, by definition, they are probably fixed assets, their treatment would come within the remit of the concept of materiality and would probably be treated as office expenses – revenue expenditure.

1   Expenditure on the purchase of fixed assets.

2   All other expenditure other than capital expenditure.

3   Debit   Fixed asset account

     Credit   Purchases ledger control account

4   The full purchase price of the asset plus the cost of getting the asset to its location and into working condition.

5   –   Where the expenditure enhances the economic benefits of the asset.

     –   Where the expenditure is on a major component which is being replaced or restored.

     –   Where the expenditure is on a major inspection or overhaul of the asset.

6   A lease agreement where the lessee enjoys substantially all of the rewards of an asset and bears the risks of the asset.

7   The fair value is capitalised as a fixed asset and a matching creditor is set up in the balance sheet. When each payment is made, the creditor is reduced by the capital element of the payment and the finance charge is an expense to the profit and loss account.

8   The asset becomes legally owned by the purchaser under a hire purchase contract upon payment of the final instalment. However, under a finance lease the asset never becomes legally owned by the lessee.

9   The operating lease rentals are charged to the profit and loss account as an expense and the asset does not appear on the balance sheet.

10 No. Its value is too uncertain to be recognised as an asset.

Depreciation

Introduction

You need to be able to understand the purpose of depreciation, calculate the annual depreciation charge using one of two standard methods, account correctly for the annual depreciation charge and to treat the depreciation accounts in the trial balance correctly in a set of final accounts. All of this will be covered in this chapter.

1 The purpose of depreciation

1.1 Introduction

We have already seen that fixed assets are capitalised in the accounting records which means that they are treated as capital expenditure and their cost is initially recorded in the balance sheet and not charged to the profit and loss account. However this is not the end of the story and this cost figure must eventually go through the profit and loss account by means of the annual depreciation charge.

1.2 Accruals concept

The accruals concept states that the costs incurred in a period should be matched with the income produced in the same period. When a fixed asset is used it is contributing to the production of the income of the business. Therefore in accordance with the accruals concept some of the cost of the fixed asset should be charged to the profit and loss account each year that the asset is used.

1.3 What is depreciation?

Depreciation is the measure of the cost of the economic benefits of the tangible fixed assets that have been consumed during the period. Consumption includes the wearing out, using up or other reduction in the useful economic life of a tangible fixed asset whether arising from use, effluxion of time or obsolescence through either changes in technology or demand for the goods and services produced by the asset. (Taken from FRS 15 Tangible Fixed Assets.)

This makes it quite clear that the purpose of depreciation is to charge the profit and loss account with the amount of the cost of the fixed asset that has been used up during the accounting period.

1.4 How does depreciation work?

The basic principle of depreciation is that a proportion of the cost of the fixed asset is charged to the profit and loss account each period and deducted from the cost of the fixed asset in the balance sheet. Therefore as the fixed asset gets older its value in the balance sheet reduces and each year the profit and loss account is charged with this proportion of the initial cost.

Net book value is the cost of the fixed asset less the accumulated depreciation to date.

	£
Cost	X
Less: Accumulated depreciation	(X)
Net book value (NBV)	X

The aim of depreciation of fixed assets is to show the cost of the asset that has been consumed during the year. It is not to show the true or market value of the asset. So this net book value will probably have little relation to the actual market value of the asset at each balance sheet date. The important aspect of depreciation is that it is a charge to the profit and loss account of the amount of the fixed asset consumed during the year.

2 Calculating depreciation

2.1 Introduction

The calculation of depreciation can be done by a variety of methods (see later in the chapter) but the principles behind each method remain the same.

2.2 Factors affecting depreciation

There are three factors that affect the depreciation of a fixed asset:

*   the cost of the asset (dealt with in the previous chapter);
*   the length of the useful economic life of the asset;
*   the estimated residual value of the asset.

2.3 Useful economic life

The useful economic life of an asset is the estimated life of the asset for the current owner.

This is the estimated number of years that the business will be using this asset and therefore the number of years over which the cost of the asset must be spread via the depreciation charge.

One particular point to note here is that land is viewed as having an infinite life and therefore no depreciation charge is required for land. However, any buildings on the land should be depreciated.

2.4 Estimated residual value

Many assets will be sold for a form of scrap value at the end of their useful economic lives.

The estimated residual value of a fixed asset is the amount that it is estimated the asset will be sold for when it is no longer of use to the business.

The aim of depreciation is to write off the cost of the fixed asset less the estimated residual value over the useful economic life of the asset.

2.5 The straight line method of depreciation

The straight line method of depreciation is a method of charging depreciation so that the profit and loss account is charged with the same amount of depreciation each year.

The method of calculating depreciation under this method is:

Annual depreciation charge $= \dfrac{\text{Cost} - \text{estimate residual value}}{\text{Useful economic life}}$

Illustration 1 – Calculating depreciation

An asset has been purchased by an organisation for £400,000 and is expected to be used in the organisation for 6 years. At the end of the six-year period it is currently estimated that the asset will be sold for £40,000.

What is the annual depreciation charge on the straight line basis?

Solution

Annual depreciation charge $= \dfrac{400,000 - 40,000}{6}$

$= £60,000$

Test your understanding 1

An asset was purchased on 1 January 20X0 for £85,000. It is expected to have an expected useful life of five years at the end of which it is estimated that the asset would be scrapped for £5,000.

What is the annual depreciation charge for this asset using the straight line method?

2.6 The reducing balance method

The reducing balance method of depreciation allows a higher amount of depreciation to be charged in the early years of an asset's life compared to the later years.

The depreciation is calculated using this method by multiplying the net book value of the asset at the start of the year by a fixed percentage.

Illustration 2 – Calculating depreciation

A fixed asset has a cost of £100,000 and is to be depreciated using the reducing balance method at 30% over its useful economic life of four years after which it will have an estimated residual value of approximately £24,000.

Show the amount of depreciation charged for each of the four years of the asset's life.

Solution

	£
Cost	100,000
Year 1 depreciation 30% × 100,000	(30,000)
Net book value at the end of year 1	70,000
Year 2 depreciation 30% × 70,000	(21,000)
Net book value at the end of year 2	49,000
Year 3 depreciation 30% × 49,000	(14,700)
Net book value at the end of year 3	34,300
Year 4 depreciation 30% × 34,300	(10,290)
Net book value at the end of year 4	24,010

Test your understanding 2

A business buys a machine for £20,000 and depreciates it at 10% per annum by the reducing balance method.

What is the depreciation charge for the second year of the machine's use and the asset's net book value at the end of that year?

2.7 Choice of method

Whether a business chooses the straight line method of depreciation or the reducing balance method (or indeed any of the other methods which are outside the scope of this syllabus) is the choice of the management.

The straight line method is the simplest method to use. Often however the reducing balance method is chosen for assets which do in fact reduce in value more in the early years of their life than the later years. This is often the case with cars and computers and the reducing balance method is often used for these assets.

Once the method of depreciation has been chosen for a particular class of fixed assets then this same method should be used each year in order to satisfy the accounting objective of comparability. The management of a business can change the method of depreciation used for a class of fixed assets but this should only be done if the new method shows a truer picture of the consumption of the cost of the asset than the previous method.

Give one reason why a business might choose reducing balance as the method for depreciating its delivery vans.

3 Accounting for depreciation

3.1 Introduction

Now we have seen how to calculate depreciation we must next learn how to account for it in the ledger accounts of the business.

3.2 Dual effect of depreciation

The two effects of the charge for depreciation each year are:

*   there is an expense to the profit and loss account – therefore there is a debit entry to a depreciation expense account;

*   there is a reduction in the value of the fixed asset in the balance sheet – therefore we create a provision for accumulated depreciation account and there is a credit entry to this account.

The provision for accumulated depreciation account is used to reduce the value of the fixed asset in the balance sheet.

Illustration 3 – Accounting for depreciation

An asset has been purchased by an organisation for £400,000 and is expected to be used in the organisation for six years. At the end of the six-year period it is currently estimated that the asset will be sold for £40,000. The asset is to be depreciated on the straight line basis.

Show the entries in the ledger accounts for the first two years of the asset's life and how this asset would appear in the balance sheet at the end of each of the first two years.

Solution

Step 1 Record the purchase of the asset in the fixed asset account.

Fixed Asset Account

	£		£
Year 1 Bank	400,000		

Step 2 Record the depreciation expense for Year 1.

Depreciation charge $= \dfrac{£400,000 - £40,000}{6}$

$= £60,000$ per year

DR   Depreciation expense account
CR   Provision for accumulated depreciation account

Depreciation Expense Account			
	£		£
Year 1 Provision account	60,000		

Provision for Accumulated Depreciation Account			
	£		£
		Expense account	60,000

Step 3 Show the fixed asset in the balance sheet at the end of year 1

Balance Sheet			
	Cost	Accumulated depreciation	Net book value
	£	£	£
Fixed asset	400,000	60,000	340,000

Note the layout of the balance sheet – the cost of the asset is shown and the accumulated depreciation is then deducted to arrive at the net book value of the asset.

Depreciation Expense Account			
	£		£
Year 2 Provision account	60,000		

Provision for Accumulated Depreciation Account			
	£		£
		Balance b/d	60,000
		Expense account	60,000

Step 4 Show the entries for the year 2 depreciation charge

Note that the expense account has no opening balance as this was cleared to the profit and loss account at the end of year 1. However the provision account being a balance sheet account is a continuing account and does have an opening balance being the depreciation charged so far on this asset.

Step 5 Balance off the provision account and show how the fixed asset would appear in the balance sheet at the end of year 2.

Provision for accumulated depreciation account

	£		£
		Balance b/d	60,000
Balance c/d	120,000	Expense account	60,000
	120,000		120,000
		Balance b/d	120,000

Balance Sheet

	Cost	Accumulated depreciation	Net book value
	£	£	£
Fixed asset	400,000	120,000	280,000

3.3 Net book value

As you have seen from the balance sheet extract the fixed assets are shown at their net book value. The net book value is made up of the cost of the asset less the accumulated depreciation on that asset or class of assets.

The net book value is purely an accounting value for the fixed asset. It is not an attempt to place a market value or current value on the asset and it in fact often bears little relation to the actual value of the asset.

Test your understanding 4

At 31 March 20X3, a business owned a motor vehicle which had a cost of £12,100 and accumulated depreciation of £9,075.

(a) **What is the net book value of the motor vehicle? What does this figure represent?**

(b) **What would the net book value of the motor vehicle have been if the company had depreciated motor vehicles at 50% per annum on a reducing-balance basis and the vehicle had been purchased on 1 April 20X0?**

3.4 Ledger entries with reducing balance depreciation

No matter what method of depreciation is used the ledger entries are always the same. So here is another example to work through.

Illustration 4 – Accounting for depreciation

On 1 April 20X2 a machine was purchased for £12,000 with an estimated useful life of 4 years and estimated scrap value of £4,920. The machine is to be depreciated at 20% reducing balance. The ledger accounts for the years ended 31 March 20X3, 31 March 20X4 and 31 March 20X5 are to be written up. Show how the fixed asset would appear in the balance sheet at each of these dates.

Solution

Step 1 Calculate the depreciation charge.

	£
Cost	12,000
Year-end March 20X3 – depreciation 12,000 × 20% =	2,400
	9,600
Year-end March 20X4 – depreciation 9,600 × 20% =	1,920
	7,680
Year-end March 20X5 – depreciation 7,680 × 20% =	1,536
	6,144

Step 2 Enter each year's figures in the ledger accounts bringing down a balance on the machinery account and provision account but clearing out the entry in the expense account to the profit and loss account.

Machinery Account

		£			£
April 20X2	Bank	12,000	Mar 20X3	Balance c/d	12,000
April 20X3	Balance b/d	12,000	Mar 20X4	Balance c/d	12,000
April 20X4	Balance b/d	12,000	Mar 20X5	Balance c/d	12,000
April 20X5	Balance b/d	12,000			

Depreciation Expense Account

		£			£
Mar 20X3	Provision for dep'n a/c	2,400	Mar 20X3	P&L a/c	2,400
Mar 20X4	Provision for dep'n a/c	1,920	Mar 20X4	P&L a/c	1,920
Mar 20X5	Provision for dep'n a/c	1,536	Mar 20X5	P&L a/c	1,536

Depreciation

Machinery: Provision for Accumulated Depreciation Account		£			£
Mar 20X3	Balance c/d	2,400	Mar 20X3	Depreciation expense	2,400
			April 20X3	Balance b/d	2,400
Mar 20X4	Balance c/d	4,320	Mar 20X4	Depreciation expense	1,920
		4,320			4,320
			April 20X4	Balance b/d	4,320
Mar 20X5	Balance c/d	5,856	Mar 20X5	Depreciation expense	1,536
		5,856			5,856
			April 20X5	Balance b/d	5,856

Step 3 Prepare the balance sheet entries.

Make sure that you remember to carry down the provision at the end of each period as the opening balance at the start of the next period.

Balance Sheet				
Fixed assets		Cost	Accumulated depreciation	Net book value
		£	£	£
At 31 Mar 20X3	Machinery	12,000	2,400	9,600
At 31 Mar 20X4	Machinery	12,000	4,320	7,680
At 31 Mar 20X5	Machinery	12,000	5,856	6,144

Test your understanding 5

ABC Co owns the following assets as at 31 December 20X6:

	£
Plant and machinery	5,000
Office furniture	800

Depreciation is to be provided as follows:

(a) plant and machinery, 20% reducing-balance method;

(b) office furniture, 25% on cost per year, straight-line method.

The plant and machinery was purchased on 1 January 20X4 and the office furniture on 1 January 20X5.

Show the ledger accounts for the year ended 31 December 20X6 necessary to record the transactions.

380

KAPLAN PUBLISHING

4 Assets acquired during an accounting period

4.1 Introduction

So far in our calculations of the depreciation charge for the year we have ignored precisely when in the year the fixed asset was purchased. This can sometimes be relevant to the calculations depending upon the policy that you are given in the exam or simulation for calculating depreciation. There are two main methods of expressing the depreciation policy and both of these will now be considered.

4.2 Calculations on a monthly basis

The policy may be stated that depreciation is to be charged on a monthly basis. This means that the annual charge will be calculated using the depreciation method given and then pro-rated for the number of months in the year that the asset has been owned.

> ### Illustration 5 – Assets acquired during an accounting period
>
> A piece of machinery is purchased on 1 June 20X1 for £20,000. It has a useful life of 5 years and zero scrap value. The organisation's accounting year ends on 31 December.
>
> **What is the depreciation charge for 20X1? Depreciation is charged on a monthly basis using the straight line method.**
>
> **Solution**
>
> Annual charge $= \dfrac{£20,000}{5} = £4,000$
>
> Charge for 20X1: £4,000 × 7/12 (i.e. June to Dec) = £2,333

> ### Test your understanding 6
>
> A business buys a machine for £40,000 on 1 January 20X3 and another one on 1 July 20X3 for £48,000. Depreciation is charged at 10% per annum on cost, and calculated on a monthly basis.
>
> **What is the total depreciation charge for the two machines for the year ended 31 December 20X3?**

4.3 Acquisition and disposal policy

The second method of dealing with depreciation in the year of acquisition is to have a depreciation policy as follows:

'A full year's depreciation is charged in the year of acquisition and none in the year of disposal.'

Ensure that you read the instructions in any question carefully.

A business purchased a motor van on 7 August 20X3 at a cost of £12,640. It is depreciated on a straight-line basis using an expected useful economic life of five years and estimated residual value of zero. Depreciation is charged with a full year's depreciation in the year of purchase and none in the year of sale. The business has a year end of 30 November.

What is the net book value of the motor van at 30 November 20X4? What does this amount represent?

5 Depreciation in the fixed asset register

5.1 Introduction

In the previous chapter we considered how the cost of fixed assets and their acquisition details should be recorded in the fixed asset register.

5.2 Recording depreciation in the fixed asset register

Let us now look at recording depreciation in the fixed asset register.

Illustration 6 – Depreciation in the fixed asset register

Date of purchase	Invoice number	Serial number	Item	Cost £	Accum'd depreciation b/f at 1.1.X8 £	Date of disposal	Depreciation charge in 20X8 £	Accumulated depreciation c/f £	Disposal proceeds £	Loss/ gain on disposal £
3.2.X5	345	3488	Chair	340						
6.4.X6	466	–	Bookcase	258						
10.7.X7	587	278	Chair	160						
				758						

Using the example from the previous chapter, reproduced above, we have now decided that fixtures and fittings (including office furniture) should be depreciated at 10% per annum using the straight-line method.

A full year's depreciation is charged in the year of purchase and none in the year of disposal.

The current year is the year to 31 December 20X8.

The chair acquired on 10.7.X7 was sold on 12.7.X8. A new table was purchased for £86 on 30.8.X8.

Do not worry at this stage about the disposal proceeds. We will look at disposals in the next chapter.

Solution

Date of purchase	Invoice number	Serial number	Item	Cost £	Accum'd deprecia-tion b/f at 1.1.X8 £	Date of disposal	Depreciation charge in 20X8 £	Accumulated depreciation c/f £	Disposal proceeds £	Loss/ gain on disposal £
3.2.X5	345	3488	Chair	340	102 (W1)		34	136		
6.4.X6	466	–	Bookcase	258	52 (W2)		26	78		
10.7.X7	587	278	Chair	160	16 (W3)	12.7.X8	–	–		
30.8.X8	634	1228	Table	86			9 (W4)	9		
				844	170		69	223		

W1 3 years' depreciation – £340 x 10% × 3 = £102
W2 2 years' depreciation – £258 x 10% × 2 = £52
W3 1 year's depreciation – £160 x 10%   = £16
W4 No depreciation in year of sale

Note how the depreciation charge is calculated for each asset except the one disposed of in the year as the accounting policy is to charge no depreciation in the year of sale. If the policy was to charge depreciation even in the year of disposal, then the charge would be calculated and included in the total.

The total accumulated depreciation should agree with the balance carried forward on the accumulated depreciation ledger account in the main ledger.

6   Summary

This chapter considered the manner in which the cost of fixed assets is charged to the profit and loss account over the life of the fixed assets, known as depreciation. There are a variety of different methods of depreciation though only the straight-line method and reducing balance method are required. Whatever the method of depreciation, the ledger entries are the same. The profit and loss account is charged with the depreciation expense and the provision for depreciation account shows the accumulated depreciation over the life of the asset to date. The provision balance is netted off against the cost of the fixed asset in the balance sheet in order to show the fixed asset at its net book value. Finally the depreciation must also be entered into the fixed asset register each year

Test your understanding answers

Test your understanding 1

Annual depreciation charge $= \dfrac{£85,000 - 5,000}{5} = £16,000$

Test your understanding 2

		£
Cost		20,000
Depreciation year 1	10% × £20,000	(2,000)
NBV at end of year 1		18,000
Depreciation year 2	10% × £18,000	(1,800)
NBV at end of year 2		16,200

Test your understanding 3

The reducing balance method is used to equalise the combined costs of depreciation and maintenance over the vehicle's life (i.e. in early years, depreciation is high, maintenance low; in later years, depreciation is low, maintenance is high). The reducing balance method is also used for fixed assets that are likely to lose more value in their early years than their later years such as cars or vans.

Test your understanding 4

(a) NBV = £3,025. The NBV is the amount of the original cost of the motor vehicle which remains to be written off over the rest of its useful life.

(b)

		£
Original cost	1 April 20X0	12,100
50%		6,050
Net book value	31 March 20X1	6,050
50%		3,025
Net book value	31 March 20X2	3,025
50%		1,512
Net book value	31 March 20X3	1,513

Test your understanding 5

Plant and machinery account

Date		£	Date		£
1.1.X6	Balance b/d	5,000	31.12.X6	Balance c/d	5,000
1.1.X7	Balance b/d	5,000			

Office furniture account

Date		£	Date		£
1.1.X6	Balance b/d	800	31.12.X6	Balance c/d	800
1.1.X7	Balance b/d	800			

Depreciation expense account

Date		£	Date		£
31.12.X6	Provision for dep'n a/c – plant and machinery	640	31.12.X6	Trading and profit and loss account	840
31.12.X6	Provision for dep'n a/c – office furniture	200			
		840			840

Provision for depreciation account – Plant and machinery

Date		£	Date		£
31.12.X6	Balance c/d	2,440	1.1.X6	Balance b/d	1,800
			31.12.X6	Dep'n expense	640
		2,440			2,440
			1.1.X7	Balance b/d	2,440

Provision for depreciation account – Office furniture

Date		£	Date		£
31.12.X6	Balance c/d	400	1.1.X6	Balance b/d	200
			31.12.X6	Dep'n expense	200
		400			400
			1.1.X7	Balance b/d	400

The opening balance on the provision for depreciation account is calculated as follows:

		Plant and machinery £	Office furniture £
20X4	20% × £5,000	1,000	–
20X5	20% × £(5,000 – 1,000)	800	
	25% × £800		200
Opening balance 1.1.X6		1,800	200

The depreciation charge for the year 20X6 is calculated as follows:

	Plant and machinery £	Office furniture £	Total £
20% × £(5,000 – 1,800)	640		
25% × £800		200	840

Test your understanding 6

		£
Machine 1	£40,000 × 10%	4,000
Machine 2	£48,000 × 10% × 6/12	2,400
		6,400

Test your understanding 7

Annual depreciation $= \dfrac{£12,640}{5} = £2,528$

NBV $= £12,640 - (2 × £2,528) = £7,584$

This is the cost of the van less the provision for depreciation to date. It is the amount remaining to be depreciated in the future. It is not a market value.

22

Accruals and prepayments

Introduction

In this chapter we will look at how income and expenditure will be recognised in the accounts

1 Recording income and expenditure

1.1 Introduction

We saw in an earlier chapter that one of the fundamental accounting concepts is the accruals concept. This states that the income and expenses recognised in the accounting period should be that which has been earned or incurred during the period rather than the amounts received or paid in cash in the period.

1.2 Recording sales and purchases on credit

Sales on credit are recorded in the ledger accounts from the sales day book. The double entry is to credit sales and debit the sales ledger control account (debtors account). Therefore all sales made in the period are accounted for in the period whether the money has yet been received by the seller or not.

Purchases on credit are recorded in ledger accounts from the purchases day book and debited to purchases and credited to the purchases ledger control account (creditors account). Again this means that the purchases are already recorded whether or not the creditor has yet been paid.

1.3 Recording expenses of the business

Most of the expenses of the business such as rent, rates, telephone, power costs etc will tend to be entered into the ledger accounts from the cash payments book. This means that the amount recorded in the ledger accounts is only the cash payment. In order to accord with the accruals concept the amount of the expense to be recognised in the profit and loss account may be different to this cash payment made in the period.

Expenses should be charged to the profit and loss account as the amount that has been incurred in the accounting period rather than the amount of cash that has been paid during the period.

2 Accruals

2.1 Introduction

If an expense is to be adjusted then the adjustment may be an accrual or a prepayment.

An accrual is an expense that has been incurred during the period but has not been paid for by the period end and has therefore not been entered in the ledger accounts.

Illustration 1 – Accruals

A business has a year end of 31 December. During the year 20X1 the following electricity bills were paid:
It is estimated that the average monthly electricity bill is £100.

What is the total charge for the year 20X1 for electricity?

		£
15 May	4 months to 30 April	400
18 July	2 months to 30 June	180
14 Sept	2 months to 30 August	150
15 Nov	2 months to 31 October	210

Solution

	£
Jan to April	400
May to June	180
July to August	150
Sept to Oct	210
Accrual for Nov/Dec (2 3 £100)	200
Total charge	1,140

Test your understanding 1

Neil commenced business on 1 May 20X0 and is charged rent at the rate of £6,000 per annum. During the period to 31 December 20X0, he actually paid £3,400.

What should his charge in the profit and loss account for the period to 31 December 20X0 be in respect of rent?

2.2 Accounting for accruals

The method of accounting for an accrual is to:

(a) debit the expense account to increase the expense to reflect the fact that an expense has been incurred, and

(b) credit an accruals account (or the same expense account) to reflect the fact that there is a creditor for the expense.

Note that the credit entry can be made in one of two ways:

(a) credit a separate accruals account, or

(b) carry down a credit balance on the expense account.

Illustration 2 – Accruals

Using the electricity example from above, the accounting entries will now be made in the ledger accounts.

Solution

Method 1 – separate accruals account

Electricity Account

		£		£
15 May	CPB	400		
18 July	CPB	180		
14 Sept	CPB	150		
15 Nov	CPB	210		
31 Dec	Accrual	200	P&L Account	1,140
		1,140		1,140

Accruals Account

	£		£
		Electricity account	200

Using this method the profit and loss account is charged with the full amount of electricity used in the period and there is an accrual or creditor to be shown in the balance sheet of £200 in the accruals account. Any other accruals such as telephone, rent, etc would also appear in the accruals account as a credit balance. The total of the accruals would appear in the balance sheet as a creditor.

Electricity Account

		£		£
15 May	CPB	400		
18 July	CPB	180		
14 Sept	CPB	150		
15 Nov	CPB	210		
31 Dec	Balance c/d	200	P&L Account	1,140
		1,140		1,140
			Balance b/d	200

Method 2 – using the expense account

Again with this method the profit and loss account charge is the amount of electricity used in the period and the credit balance on the expense account is shown as an accrual or creditor in the balance sheet.

You will normally use a separate accruals account.

Test your understanding 2

Neil commenced business on 1 May 20X0 and is charged rent at the rate of £6,000 per annum. During the period to 31 December 20X0, he actually paid £3,400.

Write up the ledger account for rent for the period to 31 December 20X0.

2.3 Opening and closing balances

When the accrual is accounted for in the expense account then care has to be taken to ensure that the accrual brought down is included as the opening balance on the expense account at the start of the following year.

Illustration 3 – Accruals

Continuing with our earlier electricity expense example the closing accrual at the end of 20X0 was £200. During 20X1 £950 of electricity bills were paid and a further accrual of £220 was estimated at the end of 20X1.

Write up the ledger account for electricity for 20X1 clearly showing the charge to the profit and loss account and any accrual balance.

Solution

Electricity Account

	£		£
Cash paid during the year	950	Balance b/d – opening accrual	200
Balance c/d – closing accrual	220	P&L account	970
	1,170		1,170
		Balance b/d	220

Test your understanding 3

The rates account of a business has an opening accrual of £340. During the year rates payments of £3,700 were made and it has been calculated that there is a closing accrual of £400.

Write up the ledger account for rates for the year showing clearly the charge to the profit and loss account and the closing accrual.

3 Prepayments

3.1 Introduction

The other type of adjustment that might need to be made to an expense account is to adjust for a prepayment.

A prepayment is a payment made during the period (and therefore debited to the expense account) for an expense that relates to a period after the year end.

> ### Illustration 4 – Prepayments
>
> The rent of a business is £3,000 per quarter payable in advance. During 20X0 the rent ledger account shows that £15,000 of rent has been paid during the year.
>
> **What is the correct charge to the profit and loss account for the year and what is the amount of any prepayment at 31 December 20X0?**
>
> **Solution**
>
> The profit and loss account charge should be £12,000 for the year, four quarterly charges of £3,000 each. The prepayment is £3,000 (£15,000 – £12,000), rent paid in advance for next year.

> ### Test your understanding 4
>
> Graham paid £1,300 insurance during the year to 31 March 20X6. The charge in the profit and loss account for the year to 31 March 20X6 is £1,200.
>
> **What is the amount of the prepayment at 31 March 20X6?**

3.2 Accounting for prepayments

The accounting for prepayments is the mirror image of accounting for accruals.

There is:

(a) a credit entry to the ledger account to reduce the expense by the amount of the prepayment; and

(b) a debit in the books to show that the business has an asset (the prepayment) at the period end.

The debit entry can appear in one of two places:

- a debit to a separate prepayments account, or

• a debit balance carried down on the expense account.

Illustration 5 – Prepayments

The rent of a business is £3,000 per quarter payable in advance. During 20X0 the rent ledger account shows that £15,000 of rent has been paid during the year.

Show how these entries would be made in the ledger accounts.

Solution

Method one – separate prepayments account

Rent Account

	£		£
Cash payments	15,000	Prepayments account	3,000
		P&L account	12,000
	15,000		15,000

Prepayments Account

	£		£
Rent account	3,000		

The charge to the profit and loss account is now the correct figure of £12,000 and there is a debit balance on the prepayments account.

This balance on the prepayments account will appear as a debtor or prepayment in the balance sheet.

Method two – balance shown on the expense account.

Rent Account

	£		£
Cash payments	15,000	P&L account	12,000
		Balance c/d	
		– prepayment	3,000
	15,000		15,000
Balance b/d			
– prepayment	3,000		

The expense to the profit and loss account is again £12,000 and the debit balance on the account would appear as the prepayment on the balance sheet.

You will normally use a separate prepayments account.

3.3 Opening and closing balances

Again as with accounting for accruals, care must be taken with opening prepayment balances on the expense account. If there is a closing prepayment balance on an expense account then this must be included as an opening balance at the start of the following year.

Illustration 6 – Prepayments

Continuing with the previous rent example the prepayment at the end of 20X0 was £3,000. The payments for rent during the following year were £15,000 and the charge for the year was £14,000.

Write up the ledger account for rent clearly showing the charge to the profit and loss account and the closing prepayment at 31 December 20X1.

Rent Account

	£		£
Balance b/d – opening prepayment	3,000	P&L account charge	14,000
Cash payments	15,000	Balance c/d – prepayment (bal fig)	4,000
	18,000		18,000
Balance b/d – prepayment	4,000		

Solution

Note that you were given the charge for the year in the question and therefore the prepayment figure is the balancing amount.

Test your understanding 5

The following information relates to a company's rent and rates account:

	Opening balance	Closing balance
	£	£
Rates prepayment	20	30
Rent accrual	100	120

Cash payments of £840 were made in respect of rent and rates during the year.

What is the charge to the profit and loss account for the year?

3.4 Approach to accruals and prepayments

There are two approaches to writing up expenses accounts with accruals or prepayments. This will depend upon whether the charge to the profit and loss account is the balancing figure or whether the accrual or prepayment is the balancing figure.

Approach 1 – enter any opening accrual /prepayment

  – enter the cash paid during the period

  – enter the closing accrual/prepayment that has been given or calculated

  – enter the charge to the profit and loss account as a balancing figure.

Approach 2 – enter any opening accrual/prepayment

  – enter the cash paid during the period

  – enter the profit and loss account charge for the period

  – enter the closing accrual/prepayment as the balancing figure.

4 Income accounts

4.1 Introduction

As well as having expenses some businesses will also have sundry forms of income. The cash received from this income may not always be the same as the income earned in the period and therefore similar adjustments to those for accruals and prepayments in the expense accounts will be required.

4.2 Accruals of income

If the amount of income received in cash is less than the income earned for the period then this additional income must be accrued for. This is done by:

- a credit entry in the income account;

- a debit entry/debtor in the balance sheet for the amount of cash due.

4.3 Income prepaid

If the amount of cash received is greater than the income earned in the period then this income has been prepaid by the payer. The accounting entries required here are:

- a debit entry to the income account;

- a credit entry/creditor shown in the balance sheet for the amount of income that has been prepaid.

  Write up separate rent accounts for properties A and B showing the income credited to the profit and loss account and any closing balances on the income accounts. Explain what each balance means.

Illustration 7 – Income statement

A business has two properties, A and B, that are rented out to other parties. The rental on property A for the year is £12,000 but only £10,000 has been received. The rental on property B is £15,000 and the client has paid £16,000 this year.

Solution

Rent Account – A

	£		£
P&L account	12,000	Cash received	10,000
		Balance c/d	
		– income accrued	2,000
	12,000		12,000
– income accrued	2,000		

This would be a debtor balance in the balance sheet showing that £2,000 is owed for rent on this property.

Rent Account – B

	£		£
P&L account	15,000	Cash received	16,000
Balance c/d			
– income prepaid	1,000		
	16,000		16,000
		Balance b/d	
		– income prepaid	1,000

This would be a creditor balance in the balance sheet indicating that too much cash has been received for this rental.

Test your understanding 6

An acquaintance wishes to use your shop to display and sell framed photographs. She will pay £40 per month for this service.

(a) How would you account for this transaction each month?

(b) If, at the end of the year, the acquaintance owed one month's rental, how would this be treated in the accounts?

5 Journal entries

5.1 Introduction

As with the depreciation expense, the accruals and prepayments are adjustments to the accounts which do not appear in the accounting records from the primary records. Therefore the adjustments for accruals and prepayments must be entered into the accounting records by means of a journal entry.

Illustration 8 – Journal entries

An accrual for electricity is to be made at the year end of £200. Show the journal entry required for this adjustment.

Solution

Journal entry			No:
Date			
Prepared by			
Authorised by			
Account	Code	Debit £	Credit £
Electricity account	0442	200	
Accruals	1155		200
Totals		200	200

Test your understanding 7

1   What is an accrued expense?

2   What is the double entry for an accrual of £400 for telephone charges if a separate accruals account is used?

3   What is a prepaid expense?

4   What is the double entry for a prepayment of £650 of rent if a separate prepayments account is used?

5   A sole trader has a year end of 30 September. In the year to 30 September 20X2 he has paid insurance of £2,400 for the year ending 30 April 20X3. What is the journal entry required for the year end adjustment?

6   A sole trader rents out some surplus office space to another business. At the sole trader's year end he is owed £200 in outstanding rent. What is the journal entry required for the year end adjustment?

6   Summary

In order for the final accounts of an organisation to accord with the accruals concept, the cash receipts and payments for income and expenses must be adjusted to ensure that they include all of the income earned during the year and expenses incurred during the year. The sales and purchases are automatically dealt with through the sales ledger and purchases ledger control account. However the expenses and sundry income of the business are recorded in the ledger accounts on a cash paid and received basis and therefore adjustments for accruals and prepayments must be made by journal entries.

Test your understanding answers

Test your understanding 1

$$\frac{8}{12} \times £6{,}000 = £4{,}000$$

Test your understanding 2

Rent account

	£		£
Cash payments	3,400	Profit and loss account $(6{,}000 \times \frac{8}{12})$	4,000
Balance c/d – accrual	600		
	4,000		4,000
		Balance b/d – accrual	600

Test your understanding 3

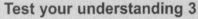

Rent account

	£		£
Cash payments	3,700	Balance b/d – opening accrual	340
Balance c/d –closing accrual	400	P & L account charge (bal fig)	3,760
	4,100		4,100
		Balance b/d – accrual	400

Test your understanding 4

The prepayment is £1,300 – 1,200 = £100.

Test your understanding 5

Rent and rates expense

	£		£
Balance b/d	20	Balance b/d	100
Cash	840		
Balance c/d	120	Profit and loss account	
		(bal fig)	850
		Balance c/d	30
	980		980
Balance b/d	30	Balance b/d	120

Test your understanding 6

(a) DR Debtor account
   CR Sundry Income a/c (or any other sensible account name)

   On payment:
   DR Bank
   CR Debtor account

(b) A sundry debtor

   – revenue in the Profit and Loss a/c

   – current asset in the Balance Sheet

Test your understanding 7

1 An expense that has been incurred in the accounting period but which will not be paid for until after the end of the accounting period.

2 Debit Telephone charges account £400
   Credit Accruals account £400

3 An item of expense which has been paid for during the accounting period but which will not be incurred until after the end of the accounting period.

4 Debit Prepayments account £650
   Credit Rent account £650

5 Debit Prepayments account (2,400 × 7/12) £1,400
   Credit Insurance account £1,400

6 Debit Rent due account (debtor account) £200
   Credit Rental income account £200

23

VAT – registration and administration

Introduction

This is the first of three chapters covering VAT, and in this chapter we are going to be looking at the registration and administration of VAT.

VAT (Value Added Tax) is a European tax which applies throughout the European Community (EC). We are going to look at VAT within the United Kingdom only (this includes England, Wales, Northern Ireland and Scotland, and excludes the Channel Islands).

As well as being able to complete a VAT return you also need to understand how the VAT system works and how VAT is administered – we shall be covering all of these things in this chapter.

1 Value added tax (VAT) – how it works

1.1 How does VAT work?

VAT is a tax paid by consumers but it is collected by businesses on behalf of HM Revenue and Customs.

- Businesses who make taxable supplies collect the tax from their customers. (The definition of taxable supplies is wider than just sales. It includes goods taken from the business for personal use.)

The VAT charged on sales or taxable supplies is known as output VAT.

- Those businesses (taxable persons) have to assess the amount of tax payable on goods and services provided (output tax). They pay it over on a regular basis to HM Revenue and Customs.

- When a business makes purchases or pays expenses it will also be paying the VAT on those purchases/expenses.

VAT on purchases or expenses is known as input VAT.

- As the businesses themselves are not being taxed, they are allowed to reclaim tax on their own expenditure (input VAT).

- The input VAT is deducted from the output VAT and the net amount is paid each quarter to HM Revenue and Customs, or recovered from them.

Illustration 1 – Value added tax (VAT – how it works

A business makes sales of £10,000 plus £1,750 of VAT. Its expenditure totals £7,000 plus £1,225 of VAT. How much VAT is due to Revenue and Customs?

Solution

	£
Output VAT	1,750
Less: Input VAT	1,225
	525

1.2 VAT place of supply

A supply must take place within the United Kingdom to be a taxable supply under United Kingdom VAT law.

Generally, if a business makes a supply of goods from stocks held in the United Kingdom, then the supply takes place in the United Kingdom. If the business must install the goods at the customer's premises, then the supply takes place at those premises.

When supplying services, the place of supply is the place where the supplier belongs, e.g. where a supplier has fixed business premises.

1.3 Time of supply

Most businesses account for input and output VAT according to the dates that they issue and receive invoices. The time of supply is known as the tax point and this is covered in more detail in the next chapter.

1.4 VAT Guide

HM Revenue and Customs issue a booklet called the VAT Guide which is a guide to the main VAT rules and procedures. If you are dealing with accounting for VAT and VAT returns in practice then you should become familiar with the contents of the VAT Guide in order to be able to refer to it when necessary.

2 Registration for VAT

2.1 Compulsory registration for VAT

Anyone in business whose taxable supplies exceed a certain annual limit must register. This includes sole traders, partnerships and limited companies. Penalties for failing to register can be severe.

A business must register if:

- at the end of any month the value of taxable supplies in the past year has exceeded the annual limit of £60,000, or

- at any time there are reasonable grounds for believing that the value of taxable supplies to be made in the next 30 days will exceed the annual limit of £60,000, or

- their acquisitions from other EC member states are more than £60,000 in the calendar year.

2.2 Voluntary registration for VAT

A business may volunteer to register for VAT. HM Revenue and Customs may refuse registration if the applicant is unable to show that supplies are being made in the course of business. The reason why someone might wish to voluntarily register for VAT will be considered later in the chapter.

2.3 More than one business

It is the person not the business which is required to register. So, if a person is carrying on several businesses, only a single registration is required and the turnovers of all businesses carried on by that person must be considered together when considering registration limits.

Illustration 2 – Value added tax (VAT – how it works

Robert Parker is a sole trader with three businesses: a hairdressing business (taxable turnover £29,000 per annum), a printing business (taxable turnover £15,000 per annum) and he also deals in second-hand cars (taxable turnover £17,000 per annum). Does he have to register for VAT?

Solution

The VAT registration limit applies to the total taxable turnover of all the business interests of a taxable person. In this case each business venture is below the limit, but in total they exceed the limit. Robert Parker would have to register for VAT.

Let us now assume that the hairdressing business is a partnership with Peter Green. The partnership would be treated as a different taxable person from Robert Parker trading alone. Both taxable persons (Robert Parker and the partnership) would avoid registration.

2.4 Deregistration for VAT

A taxable person may deregister if the value of his taxable supplies (net of VAT) is expected to be less than £60,000 in the following 12 months. If the taxable person changes – for example, when a sole trader incorporates – then the registration of the sole trader will be cancelled.

If a person reaches the registration limit for VAT then they must register immediately. If not it is entirely possible that they will have to pay the VAT that should have been charged out of their own pockets.

3 Types of supply

3.1 Rates of VAT

There are three types of supply: standard-rated (with a reduced rate for domestic fuel and power), zero-rated and exempt. These are examples of zero-rated and exempt items.

Zero-rated	Exempt
• Water and most types of food	• Land (including rent on property)
• Books and newspapers	• Insurance
• Drugs and medicines	• Postal services
• Public transport	• Betting, gaming and lorries
• Children's clothing and footwear	• Finance (e.g. making loans)
• Sewerage + water services	• Non profit-making education
• New house building	• Health services provided by doctors and dentists

All supplies that are not zero-rated or exempt are standard-rated at 17.5%. The exception is the supply of domestic fuel and power which is at a rate of 5%.

The turnover limits for registration mentioned above include both zero-rated and standard-rated supplies. They do not include exempt supplies.

3.2 Zero-rated and exempt supplies

The distinction between zero-rated supplies and exempt supplies is important. If a person makes zero-rated supplies then input VAT can be reclaimed from HM Revenue and Customs. However if a person makes exempt supplies he cannot register for VAT and therefore cannot reclaim any input tax from HM Revenue and Customs.

3.3 Voluntary registration for VAT

The reason a person may voluntarily register for VAT is if they have zero-rated supplies and wish to register in order to reclaim their input tax.

3.4 Partial exemption for VAT

A taxable person who makes both taxable supplies (standard and zero–rated) and exempt supplies is referred to as 'partially exempt'. For this purpose, zero-rated supplies are treated as taxable. The problem which arises from partial exemption is that taxable supplies entitle the supplier to a credit for input tax, whereas exempt supplies do not. It is therefore necessary to apportion input tax between taxable and exempt supplies, using a method set out by HM Revenue and Customs.

VAT can only be reclaimed if it is incurred in making taxable supplies.

3.5 Non-reclaimable input tax

There are some items of expense upon which VAT is charged but the VAT cannot be reclaimed from HM Revenue and Customs. These include:

- business entertainment expenses

- purchase of a car for use within the business

- goods and services purchased but not used within the business i.e. used by the owner instead.

Test your understanding 1

In the most recent quarter a business has made standard-rated supplies of £22,400 (net of VAT) and zero-rated supplies of £5,500. The total of purchases and expenses on which VAT has been charged for the quarter are £16,300 (net of VAT).

How much VAT is due to or from HM Revenue and Customs?

4 Administration of VAT

4.1 Introduction

The main source of law on VAT is the VAT Act 1994, the annual Finance Acts and other regulations issued by the government.

HM Revenue and Customs is the government department that is responsible for administering VAT in the United Kingdom. VAT offices across the country are responsible for the local administration of VAT within a particular geographical area.

Officers from the local VAT office deal with registration, visit taxpayers to check returns and deal with routine enquiries. They are also responsible for enforcing the tax.

Taxpayers send their returns and payments to the VAT Central Unit at Southend-on-Sea that keeps central records.

4.2 HM Revenue and Customs power

HM Revenue and Customs has certain powers that helps it administer the tax. It has the power to examine records, inspect premises, make assessments for underpaid tax and raise penalties for breaches of VAT law. Penalties may be made for (amongst other things) failing to register for VAT, failing to make returns or failing to make payments on time. They also decide whether or not supplies are liable to VAT.

The decisions of HM Revenue and Customs are not legally binding.

There are inevitably disputes between the taxpayer and HM Revenue and Customs. HM Revenue and Customs has its own administrative procedures to deal with disputes. In certain cases the taxpayer may appeal to a VAT tribunal. The taxpayer may appeal against the decision of a VAT tribunal to the High Court (on a point of law only). Beyond that appeals may go to the Court of Appeal and then to the House of Lords. The ultimate legal authority on VAT is the European Court of Justice.

4.3 VAT records

The form of records must allow HM Revenue and Customs to check VAT returns adequately. Generally, the business must keep records of:

*   all taxable and exempt supplies made in the course of business

*   all taxable supplies received in the course of business

*   a summary of the total output tax and input tax for each tax period – the VAT account (see later chapter).

4.4 Details to be kept

The business must keep records to prove the figures shown on the VAT returns for the previous six years. These records might include the following:

*   orders and delivery notes

*   relevant business correspondence

*   appointment and job books

*   purchases and sales books

*   cash books and other account books

*   bank statements, paying-in slips and cheque stubs

*   purchase invoices and copy sales invoices

*   recordings of daily takings, including till rolls

*   annual accounts

*   import and export documents

*   VAT accounts

*   any credit notes issued or received.

Registered businesses may be visited by a VAT officer on occasion to ensure that their records are being correctly maintained.

A business can keep its records on microfilm. The business must tell HM Revenue and Customs. It must be possible to inspect the records.

Any business that maintains its records on computer must tell HM Revenue and Customs. The system must comply with VAT regulations.

Some businesses send or receive invoices by electronic means. Again they must tell HM Revenue and Customs and check that they are complying with regulations.

You must be able to list the records that must be kept for VAT purposes.

4.5 Special schemes

Normally a VAT return is completed by a registered person every three months and any amounts of VAT due paid over to HM Revenue and Customs with the return or a claim made for VAT to be reimbursed.

However, there are some special schemes that are different – the two that you are required to be aware of are the annual accounting scheme and the cash accounting scheme. We also include brief details of the flat rate accounting scheme.

4.6 VAT: Annual accounting scheme

Under this scheme a VAT return is only made once a year rather than quarterly.

In order to qualify for this scheme the registered person must have annual taxable supplies of no more than £660,000 and have been VAT registered for 12 months. An estimate is made of the likely annual VAT due, this agreed figure is divided by ten, and nine equal monthly payments are made by direct debit, starting four months into the year. Businesses with a taxable turnover of £150,000 need not wait for 12 months.

The balance is then due with the annual VAT return within two months after the end of the VAT year.

The benefit of this scheme to a sole trader is that he does not have to spend valuable time every quarter completing a VAT return. However it does mean that his VAT records must be kept accurately as the VAT return is only completed once a year.

4.7 VAT: cash accounting scheme

Normally VAT is due from the date invoices are sent out and can be reclaimed from the date a supplier's invoice is received (details in the next chapter). However under the cash accounting scheme a business accounts for VAT due on the basis of the time when the payment is actually received from customers or made to suppliers.

In order to qualify for this scheme the registered person must have expected annual taxable supplies of £660,000 or less and have a clean VAT record. The trader must leave the scheme if turnover exceeds £850,000.

If registered under this scheme invoices will still be sent out to customers and received from suppliers but the key record that must be kept is a cash book summarising all payments made and received and their date with a separate column for VAT.

The benefit of this scheme is in terms of cash flow for a trader who must pay his suppliers promptly but has to wait a considerable time before being paid by his customers. It also means that there is automatic relief for VAT on bad debts because, if the customer does not pay, then the VAT is not due (bad debt relief in normal circumstances is considered in a later chapter).

4.8 VAT: flat rate accounting scheme

This is intended to simplify the way small businesses account for VAT. Under this scheme, businesses with a taxable turnover up to £150,000 do not have to keep records of the VAT charged on each individual purchase and sales invoice.

Instead, their net VAT liability is calculated by applying a flat rate percentage to the business's total turnover. The actual percentage used depends upon the particular industry sector in which the business operates.

This cuts down on the paperwork involved in accounting for VAT, thereby offering administrative cost savings. However, VAT invoices will still need to be issued to VAT registered customers for their own VAT requirements.

Test your understanding 2
1   Who ultimately (i) bears the cost of; (ii) gains benefit from VAT?
2   Why might a business voluntarily register for VAT even if not required to?
3   Give two examples each of (i) zero-rated and (ii) exempt supplies.
4   What records must a business keep for VAT purposes and for how long?
5   How do the special VAT schemes help the small business?

5 Summary

This chapter has served as an introduction to the VAT system. You should now understand how VAT is collected by businesses but is a tax paid by the final consumer.

You must know when a person should register for VAT and deregister if relevant. You should also be clear as to the different types of supply and the difference to a trader between making zero-rated supplies and exempt supplies.

We also considered how VAT is administered by local VAT officers and the documents and records that must be kept for six years in order to ensure that the correct amount of VAT has been paid.

Finally we considered two special schemes for VAT payment – the annual accounting scheme and the cash accounting scheme.

Test your understanding answers

Test your understanding 1

	£
Output VAT	
Standard-rated (22,400 × 17.5%)	3,920.00
Zero-rated	–
	3,920.00
Less: input VAT (16,300 × 17.5%)	2,852.50
VAT due to HMRC	1,067.50

Test your understanding 2

1 (i) The final consumer (customer) who buys goods/services from a VAT registered supplier.

   (ii) The government – businesses simply act as collection agencies between the two.

2 Registering for VAT means that the business will have to add VAT onto its sales invoices (unless they are exempt supplies), but they can also reclaim VAT on their purchases and expenses. Provided it is felt that the addition to VAT on sales prices will not result in a significant loss of demand (e.g. if their customers are mainly registered themselves to whom VAT is not a cost) the benefits may well outweigh the costs – particularly if the business makes largely exempt supplies.

3 (i) Zero-rated: water/most types of food; books/newspapers; drugs; public transport; children's clothes; sewerage and water services; new house building.

   (ii) Exempt: land; insurance; postal services; education; health services; finance; betting.

4 The records must be sufficient to show details of all taxable and exempt supplies made and all supplies received in the course of business (invoices, cash books, day books, etc), along with a summary of total input and output tax for each period (in a VAT account). They must be kept for six years.

5 The annual accounting scheme, cash accounting scheme and flat rate scheme are all designed to 'ease the impact of VAT on small businesses' – the annual accounting scheme by removing the need for a VAT return to be prepared each quarter, the cash accounting scheme by helping cash flow in that VAT is only paid/recovered once the cash from the related transactions has actually been received/paid, and the flat rate and purchase.

KAPLAN PUBLISHING

VAT – invoices and tax points

Introduction

In this second chapter covering the preparation of VAT returns we are going to look at how VAT is collected via a VAT invoice and all of the details that are required to be shown on such an invoice. We will also be looking at the rules regarding tax points (i.e. the time period in which VAT is to be accounted for) and therefore the figures that will eventually appear on the VAT return. There are lots of important rules concerning VAT covered in this chapter and it is important that you remember them when performing VAT calculations.

1 VAT invoices

1.1 Introduction

All businesses that are registered for VAT must collect tax on taxable supplies. In order to do this the supplier must give or send to the purchaser a VAT invoice within 30 days of the supply.

1.2 Form of a VAT invoice

There is no standard format for invoices. The exact design is the choice of the business, but it must show the following details (unless the invoice is a less detailed tax invoice that you will see later):

- identifying number
- date of supply (or tax point – see below) and the date of issue of the invoice
- supplier's name and address and registration number
- name and address of customer, i.e. the person to whom the goods or services are supplied
- type of supply
  - sale
  - hire purchase, credit sale, conditional sale or similar transaction
  - loan
  - exchange
  - hire, lease or rental
  - process (making goods using the customer's own materials)
  - sale on commission (e.g. by an estate agent)
  - supply on sale or return
- description of the goods or services
- quantity of goods or extent of services.
- rate of tax and amount payable (in sterling) excluding VAT for each separate description
- total amount payable (excluding VAT) in sterling
- rate of any cash discount offered (these are also called settlement discounts)
- separate rate and amount of VAT charged for each rate of VAT
- total amount of VAT chargeable.

A VAT invoice is not strictly required where the purchaser is not registered for VAT, however as the seller will not know whether a purchaser is registered, one will be sent.

1.3 VAT and discounts

If a trade discount is given then this is deducted before the VAT is calculated. If a settlement discount is offered then the VAT is always calculated on the lowest amount that the customer may pay. You must assume that the customer will take the discount.

1.4 What a VAT invoice looks like

Here is an example of a tax invoice.

<table>
<tr><td colspan="5" align="center">MICRO TRAINING GROUP LTD
Unit 34
Castlewell Trading Estate
Manchester
M12 5RHF</td></tr>
<tr><td colspan="2">To: JF Jenkins & Co
      65 Green Street
      Manchester
      M12 4ED</td><td colspan="3">Sales invoice nummber: 35
VAT registered number: 234 5566 87

Tax point: 12 September 20X2</td></tr>
<tr><td colspan="5">Sales:</td></tr>
<tr><td>Quantity</td><td>Description and price</td><td>Amount ex VAT</td><td>VAT rate</td><td>VAT</td></tr>
<tr><td align="center">6</td><td>Programmable calculators</td><td></td><td></td><td></td></tr>
<tr><td></td><td>FR34 at £24.76</td><td>148.56</td><td>17.5%</td><td></td></tr>
<tr><td align="center">12</td><td>Programmable calculators</td><td></td><td></td><td></td></tr>
<tr><td></td><td>GT60 at £36.80</td><td>441.60</td><td>17.5%</td><td></td></tr>
<tr><td></td><td></td><td>590.16</td><td></td><td>101.21</td></tr>
<tr><td></td><td>Delivery</td><td>23.45</td><td>17.5%</td><td>4.02</td></tr>
<tr><td colspan="2">**Terms: Cash discount of 2% if paid within 10 days**</td><td>613.61</td><td></td><td>105.23</td></tr>
<tr><td colspan="2">**VAT**</td><td>105.23</td><td></td><td></td></tr>
<tr><td colspan="2">**TOTAL**</td><td>718.84</td><td></td><td></td></tr>
</table>

Test your understanding 1

An invoice is issued for standard-rated goods with a list price of £380.00 (excluding VAT). A 10% trade discount is given and a 4% settlement or cash discount is offered.

How much VAT should be included on the invoice?

1.5 Rounding VAT

Usually, the amount of VAT calculated will not be a whole number of pounds and pence. You will therefore need a rounding adjustment. The rules governing this adjustment are quite tricky, and permit more than one method. For simplicity, the following approach is recommended.

- On an invoice containing several lines, where the VAT is shown separately for each line, calculate the amount of VAT for each line by rounding to the nearest 1p. For example, 87.7p would be rounded up to 88p. Then simply add up the VAT for each line to arrive at the total VAT.

- On an invoice containing just one (total) figure for VAT, calculate the amount of VAT by rounding down to the nearest 1p. For example £20.877 would be rounded down to £20.87.

Test your understanding 2

(a) Given below is an extract from a VAT invoice:

Quantity	Description and price	Net of VAT	VAT rate	**VAT**
16	6 metre hosepipes @ £3.23	51.68	17.5%	
24	12 metres hosepipes @ £5.78	138.72	17.5%	

   Calculate the VAT for each line of the invoice and the total VAT charged.

(b) An invoice includes a net total for goods of £1,084.50.

   How much VAT should be charged for these goods?

1.6 Less detailed VAT invoices

Retailers do not have to issue a detailed VAT invoice every time they make a sale. This would make trading impossible. If the total amount of the supply (including VAT) by the retailer does not exceed £100.00, a retailer may issue a **less detailed tax invoice**. However, if requested by a customer a full VAT invoice must be issued. The supplier only needs to show the following details on the invoice:

- supplier's name and address
- supplier's VAT registration number
- date of supply
- description sufficient to identify the goods or services
- amount payable (including VAT) for each rate (standard and zero)
- each rate of VAT.

The main differences here are that the customer's name and address can be omitted, and the total on the invoice includes the VAT without the VAT itself being shown separately.

Although this invoice shows less detail, it is still a valid tax invoice.

All retailers must keep a record of their daily gross takings so that VAT can be calculated on the total of cash takings, not individual invoices. This means that the retailer will need to keep a careful note of any money taken for own use.

1.7 Calculating the VAT

When a less detailed VAT invoice is issued or received it will be necessary to calculate the amount of the VAT that is included in the invoice total in order to record the sale or purchase in the accounting records.

The VAT element is calculated by multiplying the invoice total (for standard-rated goods) by the fraction 17.5/117.5 or 7/47.

Illustration 1 – VAT invoices

If the VAT inclusive amount is £48.66 what is the VAT element?

Solution

$$VAT = 48.66 \times \frac{17.5}{117.5} = £7.24$$

or

$$VAT = 48.66 \times \frac{7}{47} = £7.24$$

Remember that the VAT is rounded down to the nearest penny.

Test your understanding 2

The total of a less detailed invoice for standard-rated goods is £68.90.

How much VAT is included in this amount?

1.8 Modified invoices

For a sale of any amount, if the buyer agrees, then a modified invoice can be issued. This shows the VAT inclusive amount for each item sold and then at the bottom of the invoice the following amounts must be shown:

- the overall VAT inclusive total

- the total amount of VAT included in the total

- the total value of the supplies net of VAT

- the total value of any zero-rated and exempt supplies.

1.9   Proforma invoices

When a business issues a sales invoice that includes VAT, the VAT becomes payable to HM Revenue and Customs next time the business submits a return. This can cause cashflow problems if the customer has not yet paid the invoice, because the business then has to pay the VAT before collecting it from the customer.

To avoid this, a business may issue a **proforma invoice**, which essentially is a demand for payment. Once payment is received, the business will then issue a 'live' invoice to replace the proforma.

Because a proforma invoice **does not rank as a VAT invoice** the supplier is not required to pay VAT to HM Revenue and Customs until the 'live' invoice is issued. By the same token, the customer cannot reclaim the VAT on a proforma invoice, but must instead wait until the valid tax invoice is received.

Pro-forma invoices should be clearly marked 'THIS IS NOT A VAT INVOICE'.

1.10   Credit notes and VAT

A credit note involving a taxable supply must show:

*   the identifying number and date of issue
*   the supplier's name, address and registration number
*   the customer's name and address
*   the reason for the credit (e.g. goods returned)
*   a description of the goods or services for which the credit is being allowed
*   the quantity and amount credited for each description
*   the total amount credited, excluding VAT
*   the rate and amount of VAT credited.

The number and date of the original tax invoice should also appear on the credit note.

If the supplier issues the credit note without making a VAT adjustment the credit note must say: **'This is not a credit note for VAT'**.

A supplier is **not allowed to issue a credit note to recover VAT on bad debts**.

2   Tax points

2.1   Introduction

The **tax point** is the date on which the liability for output tax arises – it is the date on which it is recorded as taking place for the purposes of the tax return.

Most taxable persons make a VAT return each quarter. The return must include all supplies whose tax points fall within that quarter.

2.2   The basic tax point

The 'basic tax point' is the date of delivery of goods or the date the customer takes the goods away or the date of completion/performance of services.

2.3   Actual tax point

Where an invoice is issued or payment received before the basic tax point, this earlier date becomes the 'actual tax point'.

If a supplier issues an invoice within 14 days after the basic tax point, the invoice date becomes the actual tax point and is used as the tax point for the tax return, unless payment has been received earlier, in which case the payment date is the actual tax point.

Provided that written approval is received from the local VAT office the 14-day rule can be varied, for example to accommodate a supplier who issues all of his invoices each month on the last day of the month.

2.4   Deposits received in advance

Any deposits received in advance create a basic tax point. The business must account for the VAT element. The VAT included in the deposit must be calculated and entered in the accounting records.

Illustration 2 – Tax points

A £50.00 deposit is received in advance of the goods being delivered. What is the VAT on this amount?

Solution

The amount of VAT included in the deposit = £50.00 $\times \dfrac{7}{47}$ = £7.44.

Test your understanding 4

In each of the following cases state the date of the tax point and whether it is a basic tax point or actual tax point:

(i) Goods delivered to a customer on 10 July, invoice sent out on 15 July and payment received on 30 July.

(ii) Invoice sent out to a customer on 12 August, goods delivered to the customer on 16 August, payment received 20 September.

(iii) Payment received from customer on 4 September, goods sent to customer on 5 September together with the invoice.

(iv) Goods delivered to a customer on 13 September, invoice sent out on 30 September and payment received on 31 October.

Test your understanding 5

1   How are trade/settlement discounts dealt with when computing VAT on an invoice?

2   What is the advantage of issuing a proforma invoice?

3   In what circumstances will a business become liable for output tax prior to goods being delivered to the customer?

3   Summary

This chapter has covered two important areas for VAT – invoicing and tax points. VAT invoices must include certain details and in normal circumstances must be given or sent to a VAT registered purchaser. In practice this means that all purchasers will be provided with a VAT invoice whether they are registered or not. However, retailers are allowed to issue less detailed or modified invoices if the customer is happy with this, showing only the total amount due without any breakdown of the VAT included. Any credit notes sent out by a business must include the same details as the invoices.

The tax point for a supply of goods is important as this determines the date on which the VAT becomes accountable therefore determining which VAT return the VAT for that supply of goods appears on. You must know the rules for the basic tax point and for actual tax points.

Test your understanding answers

Test your understanding 1

	£
List price	380.00
Less: trade discount 10%	38.00
	342.00

VAT $= £342.00 \times 96\% \times 17.5\%$

$\quad\;\; = £57.45$

Test your understanding 2

Part (a)

Quantity	Description and price	Net of VAT	VAT rate	VAT
16	6 metre hosepipes @ £3.23	51.68	17.5%	9.04
24	12 metre hosepipes @ £5.78	138.72	17.5%	24.28

Part (a)

VAT $= £1{,}084.50 \times 17.5\%$

$\quad\;\; = £189.78$

Test your understanding 3

VAT $= £68.90 \times 17.5/117.5$

$\quad\;\; = £10.26$

Test your understanding 4

(i)   15 July actual tax point

(ii) 12 August actual tax point

(iii) 4 September actual tax point

(iv) 13 September basic tax point

25

VAT returns

Introduction

In the final chapter of this study text we are going to conclude our VAT studies by looking at how to complete a VAT return correctly and on time. Businesses must complete a VAT return (a VAT 100 form) at the end of each quarter. The purpose of a VAT return is to summarise the transactions of a business for a period. In an assessment you are likely to be required to complete an organisation's VAT return so that it is ready for authorisation and despatch.

We shall also be looking at situations that may give rise to VAT penalties and how to avoid them.

1   The VAT return

1.1   Introduction

The tax period for VAT is three months, or one month for taxpayers who choose to make monthly returns (normally taxpayers who receive regular refunds).

The taxpayer must complete a VAT return (a VAT 100 form) at the end of each quarter. The return summarises all the transactions for the period.

1.2   Timing of the VAT return

The taxpayer must make the return within one month of the end of the tax period. The taxable person must send the amount due at the same time (i.e. output tax collected less input tax deducted). Payment may be by cheque (made payable to 'HM Revenue and Customs only') or by credit transfer.

If VAT is due from HM Revenue and Customs the VAT return must still be completed and submitted within one month of the end of the quarter in order to be able to reclaim the amount due.

1.3   What a VAT return looks like

Given below is an example of a VAT return:

Value Added Tax Return

For the period

to

Your VAT Office telephone number 0123-4567

For Official Use

Registration number   Period

You could be liable to a financial penalty if your completed return and all the VAT payableare not received by the due date.

Due date:

For Official Use

Before you fill in this form please read the notes on the back and the VAT Leaflet 'Filling in your VAT return'. Fill in all boxes clearly in ink and write 'none' where necessary. Don't put a dash or leave any box blank. If there are no pence write '00' in the pence column. Do not enter more than one amount in any box.

For official use		
VAT due in this period on sales and other outputs	1	
VAT due in this period on acquisitions from other EC Member states	2	
Total VAT due (the sum of boxes 1 and 2)	3	
VAT reclaimed in this period on purchases and other inputs (including acquisitions from the EC)	4	
Net VAT to be paid to Customs or reclaimed by you (Difference between boxes 3 and 4)	5	
Total value of sales and all other outputs excluding any VAT. Include your box 8 figure.	6	
Total value of purchases and all other inputs excluding any VAT. Include your box 9 figure.	7	
Total value of all supplies of goods and related services excluding any VAT to other EC Member States.	8	
Total value of all acquisitions of goods and related services excluding any VAT, from other EC Member States.	9	

If you are enclosing a payment please tick this box.

DECLARATION: You, or someone on your behalf, must sign below.
I .... declare that the information given
(Full name of signatory in BLOCK LETTERS)
above is true and complete.
Signature .... Date   20
A false declaration can result in prosecution.

VAT 100 (full)   PT1 (April 2004)

As you will see there are nine boxes to complete with the relevant figures. Boxes 2, 8 and 9 are to do with supplies of goods and services to other European Community (EC) Member States and acquisitions from EC Member States. Therefore we will now consider how VAT is affected by exports and imports.

1.4   VAT: Exports and imports to or from non-EC members

(a)   Generally, goods exported from the United Kingdom to a non-EC country are normally zero-rated (i.e. there is no tax charged on them, even if there normally would be) provided there is documentary evidence of the export.

(b) Goods that are imported from outside the EC have to have customs duty paid on them when they enter the country (these are outside the scope of this syllabus and we will not consider them further). However, goods that would be taxed at the standard rate of VAT if supplied in the United Kingdom are also subject to VAT. The amount payable is based on their value including customs duty. This applies to all goods whether or not they are for business use. The aim of the charge is to treat foreign goods in the same way as home-produced goods. The VAT is paid at the port of entry and the goods will typically not be released until it is paid.

If the imported goods are for business use and the business uses them to make taxable supplies, it can reclaim the VAT paid in the usual way as input tax on the VAT return (Box 4).

1.5 Exports and imports to and from countries within the EC

When both the exporting and importing country are EC members the situation is rather complicated and we shall look at it carefully.

Movements of goods between EC Member States are no longer known as imports and exports but as acquisitions.

In what follows we refer to HM Revenue and Customs as the collecting authority, even though in different countries it will have a different name.

(a) Sale to a VAT registered business

When an EC member sells goods to a VAT registered business in another EC country, it is the buyer who pays over the VAT to HM Revenue and Customs (or the equivalent in the buyer's country). Provided the seller has the buyer's VAT number, the seller sells the goods zero-rated to the buyer. The buyer will then pay VAT to HM Revenue and Customs at the appropriate rate. The buyer can also reclaim the VAT from HM Revenue and Customs.

We can summarise this as follows:

The seller

The seller will supply the goods zero-rated.

The seller makes no entries in Boxes 1 to 4 of the VAT return.

The seller will enter the value of the sale in Box 8.

The buyer

The VAT registered buyer will pay the seller the sale price of the goods (excluding any VAT) .

The buyer will enter the VAT output tax in Box 2 of the return and the VAT input tax in Box 4 of the return. Thus, the net amount of

VAT the buyer pays to HM Revenue and Customs is nil.

The buyer will also enter the VAT exclusive price of the goods in Box 9.

(b) Sale to a non-VAT registered buyer

When a sale is made to a non-VAT registered buyer, the seller has to charge VAT at the standard rate. The buyer will pay the VAT inclusive price to the seller.

We can summarise this as follows:

The seller

The seller supplies the goods and charges VAT.

The seller enters the VAT in Box 2.

The seller enters the VAT exclusive price in Box 8.

The buyer

The non-VAT registered buyer pays the VAT inclusive price to the seller and of course makes no entries in a VAT return because he is not registered.

2   Completing the VAT return

2.1   The VAT account

The main source of information for the VAT return is the VAT account which must be maintained to show the amount that is due to or from HM Revenue and Customs at the end of each quarter.

2.2 How the VAT account should look

Given below is a pro-forma of a VAT account as suggested by the VAT Guide.

1 April 20X5 to 30 June 20X5

VAT deductible - input tax		VAT payable - output tax	
VAT on purchases		VAT on sales	
April	X	April	X
May	X	May	X
June	X	June	X
VAT on imports	X		
VAT on acquisition from EC	X	VAT on acquisiton from EC	X

Adjustments of previous errors (if £2,000 or less)			
Net underclaim	X	Net overclaim	X
Bad debt relief	X		
Less: Credit notes received	(X)	Less: Credit notes issued	(X)
Total tax deductible	X	Total tax payable	X
		Less: total tax deductible	(X)
		Payable to HM Revenue and Customs	X

You will note that the VAT shown is not strictly a double entry account as the VAT on credit notes received is deducted from input tax and the VAT on credit notes issued is deducted from output tax instead of being credited and debited respectively.

2.3 Information required for the VAT return

Boxes 1 to 4 of the VAT return can be fairly easily completed from the information in the VAT account. However, Boxes 6 and 7 require figures for total sales and purchases excluding VAT. This information will need to be extracted from the totals of the accounting records such as sales day book and purchases day book totals.

Boxes 8 and 9 require figures, excluding VAT, for the value of supplies to other EC Member States and acquisitions from other EC Member States. Therefore the accounting records should be designed in such a way that these figures can also be easily identified.

Test your understanding 1

Panther

You are preparing the VAT return for Panther Alarms Ltd and you must first identify the sources of information for the VAT account.

Suggest the best sources of information for the following figures:

(a) sales

(b) credit notes issued

(c) purchases

(d) credit notes received

(e) capital goods sold

(f) capital goods purchased

(g) goods taken from business for own use

(h) bad debt relief.

Illustration 1 – Completing the VAT return

Given below is a VAT account for Thompson Brothers for the second VAT quarter of 20X5.

Thompson Brothers Ltd

1April 20X5 to 30 June 20X5

VAT deductible - input taxVAT payable - output tax

VAT on purchases	£	VAT on sales	£
April	525.00	April	875.00
May	350.00	May	1,750.00
June	350.00	June	700.00
	1,225.00		3,325.00
EC acquisitions	210.00		210.00

Other adjustments

Less: Credit notes received (17.50)	Less: Credit notes issued (105.00)
Total tax deductible 1,417.50	Total tax payable 3,430.00
	Less: total tax deductible (1,417.50)
	Payable to HM Revenue and Customs 2,012.50

You are also given the summarised totals from the day books for the three-month period:

Sales Day Book

	Net £	VAT £	Total £
Standard-rate	19,000.00	3,325.00	22,325.00
Zero-rated	800.00	–	800.00
EC Member States	1,500.00	–	1,500.00

Sales Returns Day Book

	Net £	VAT £	Total £
Standard-rate	600.00	105.00	705.00
Zero-rated	40.00	–	40.00
EC Member States	–	–	–

Purchase Day Book

	Net £	VAT £	Total £
Standard-rate	7,000.00	1,225.00	8,225.00
Zero-rated	2,000.00	-	2,000.00
EC Member States	1,200.00	210.00	1,410.00

Purchases Returns Day Book

	Net £	VAT £	Total £
Standard-rate	100.00	17.50	117.50
Zero-rated	–	–	–
EC Member States	–	–	–

We also need the address and VAT registration number of the business:

Thompson Brothers Ltd
Arnold House
Parkway
Keele
KE4 8US

VAT registration number 165 4385 32.

We are now in a position to complete the VAT return.

Solution

Step 1

Fill in the VAT registration number, VAT period, name and address of the business and the due date of the return which is one month after the end of the quarter.

Step 2

Fill in Box 1 with the VAT on sales less the VAT on credit notes issued - this can be taken either from the VAT account or from the day book summaries: £3,325 - £105 = £3,220.00.

Note that the instructions at the top of VAT return require '00' to be shown if there are no pence in the total.

Step 3

Fill in Box 2 with the VAT payable on acquisitions from other EC Member States - this figure of £210.00 can be taken either from the VAT account or from the Purchases Day Book.

Note that this figure will be included here on the VAT return as output tax payable to HM Revenue and Customs and also in Box 4 as input tax reclaimable.

Step 4

Complete Box 3 with the total of Boxes 1 and 2.

Step 5

Fill in Box 4 with the total of VAT on all purchases (including acquisitions from EC Member States) less the total VAT on any credit notes received. These figures can either be taken from the VAT account or from the day book totals: £1,225.00 + £210.00 - £17.50 = £1,417.50.

Step 6

Complete Box 5 by deducting the figure in Box 4 from the total in Box 3. This is the amount due to HM Revenue and Customs and should equal the balance on the VAT account.

If the Box 4 figure is larger than the Box 3 total then there is more input tax reclaimable than output tax to pay - this means that this is the amount being reclaimed from HM Revenue and Customs.

Step 7

Fill in Box 6 with the VAT exclusive figure of all sales less credit notes issued - this information will come from the day books - this figure includes sales to EC Member States: £19,000 + £800.00 + £1,500.00 - £600.00 - £40.00 = £20,660.

Note that this figure includes zero-rated supplies and any exempt supplies that are made.

Step 8

Fill in Box 7 with the VAT exclusive total of all purchases less credit notes received - again this will be taken from the day books: £7,000

+ £2,000 + £1,200.00 - £100.00 = £10,100.00.

Step 9

Fill in Box 8 with the VAT exclusive total of all supplies made to EC Member States (less any credit notes) - this figure is taken from the Sales Day Book: £1,500.00.

Step 10

Fill in Box 9 with the VAT exclusive total of all acquisitions from other EC Member States (less any credit notes) - this figure is taken from the Purchases Day Book: £1,200.00.

Note that no pence are required for the final four boxes. Also note the instruction that if there is no entry for any box then 'none' should be written in the box.

Step 11

Write in the name of the person within the organisation (senior management or owner) who will be authorising the VAT return with their signature.

Step 12

If VAT is due to HM Revenue and Customs a cheque must be sent with the VAT return and the box at the bottom of the return must be ticked.

Value Added Tax Return
For the period
1/4/X5 to 30/6/X5

For Official Use

Thompson Brother Ltd
Arnold House
Parkway
Keele
KE4 8US

Your VAT Office telephone number 0123-4567

Registration number	Period
165 4385 32	20X5

You could be liable to a financial penalty if your completed return and all the VAT payable are not received by the due date.

Due date: **31 July 20X5**

For Official Use	

Before you fill in this form please read the notes on the back and the VAT Leaflet 'Filling in your VAT return'. Fill in all boxes clearly in ink and write 'none' where necessary. Don't put a dash or leave any box blank. If there are no pence write '00' in the pence column. Do not enter more than one amount in any box.

For official use				
	VAT due in this period on sales and other outputs	1	3,220	00
	VAT due in this period on acquisitions from other EC Member States	2	210	00
	Total VAT due (the sum of boxes 1 and 2)	3	3,430	00
	VAT reclaimed in this period on purchases and other inputs (including acquisitions from the EC)	4	1,417	50
	Net VAT to be paid to Customs or reclaimed by you (Difference between boxes 3 and 4)	5	2,012	50
	Total value of sales and all other outputs excluding any VAT. Include your box 8 figure.	6	20,660	00
	Total value of purchases and all other inputs excluding any VAT. Include your box 9 figure.	7	10,100	00
	Total value of all supplies of goods and related services excluding any VAT to other EC Member States.	8	1,500	00
	Total value of all acquisitions of goods and related services excluding any VAT, from other EC Member States.	9	1,200	00

If you are enclosing a payment please tick this box.

☑

DECLARATION: You, or someone on your behalf, must sign below.
I ....A Thompson........................... declare that the information given
(Full name of signatory in BLOCK LETTERS)
above is true and complete.
Signature .... Date   20

A false declaration can result in prosecution.

VAT 100 (full)   PT1 (April 2004)

If the business makes sales or purchases for cash then the relevant net and VAT figures from the cash receipts and payments books should also be included on the VAT return.

Test your understanding 2

Given below is a summary of the day books of a business for the three months ended 31 March 20X1. The business is called Long Supplies Ltd and trades from Vale House, Lilly Road, Trent, TR5 2KL. The VAT registration number of the business is 285 3745 12.

Sales Day Book

	Net £	VAT £	Total £
Standard-rate	15,485.60	2,709.98	18,195.58
Zero-rated	1,497.56	–	1,497.56

Sales Returns Day Book

	Net £	VAT £	Total £
Standard-rate	1,625.77	284.50	1,910.27
Zero-rated	106.59	–	106.59

Purchase Day Book

	Net £	VAT £	Total £
Standard-rate	8,127.45	1,422.30	9,549.75
Zero-rated	980.57	–	980.57
EC Member States	669.04	117.08	786.12

Purchases Returns Day Book

	Net £	VAT £	Total £
Standard-rate	935.47	163.70	1,099.17
Zero-rated	80.40	–	80.40
EC Member States	–	–	–

(a) **Write up the VAT account to reflect these figures.**

(b) **Complete the VAT return given.**

KAPLAN PUBLISHING

Value Added Tax Return

For the period

to

⌐   ⌐

∟   ⌐

Your VAT Office telephone number 0123-4567

■▬ ▮ ▬■ ▮ ▮

For Official Use

Registration number	Period

You could be liable to a financial penalty if your completed return and all the VAT payable are not received by the due date.

Due date:

For Official Use	

Before you fill in this form please read the notes on the back and the VAT Leaflet 'Filling in your VAT return'. Fill in all boxes clearly in ink and write 'none' where necessary. Don't put a dash or leave any box blank. If there are no pence write '00' in the pence column. Do not enter more than one amount in any box.

For official use			
	VAT due in this period on sales and other outputs	1	
	VAT due in this period on acquisitions from other EC Member States	2	
	Total VAT due (the sum of boxes 1 and 2)	3	
	VAT reclaimed in this period on purchases and other inputs (including acquisitions from the EC)	4	
	Net VAT to be paid to Customs or reclaimed by you (Difference between boxes 3 and 4)	5	
	Total value of sales and all other outputs excluding any VAT. Include your box 8 figure.	6	
	Total value of purchases and all other inputs excluding any VAT. Include your box 9 figure.	7	
	Total value of all supplies of goods and related services excluding any VAT to other EC Member States.	8	
	Total value of all acquisitions of goods and related services excluding any VAT, from other EC Member States.	9	

If you are enclosing a payment please tick this box.	DECLARATION: You, or someone on your behalf, must sign below. I .... declare that the information given (Full name of signatory in BLOCK LETTERS) above is true and complete. Signature .... Date 20 A false declaration can result in prosecution.

VAT 100 (full)   PT1 (April 2004)

2.4   VAT: Adjustment of previous errors

You will notice in the pro-forma VAT account that there are entries for net underclaims and net overclaims. Net errors made in previous VAT returns of £2,000 or less can be adjusted for on the VAT return through the VAT account.

Net error means the difference between any earlier errors in output tax and any earlier errors in input tax.

The one single figure for net errors will then be entered as additional input tax if there has been an earlier net underclaim of VAT and as additional output tax if the net error was a net overclaim in a previous return.

2.5   Errors of more than £2,000

If the net error from a previous return totals more than £2,000 then the VAT office should be informed immediately either by a letter or on Form VAT 652. This is known as voluntary disclosure. The information provided to the VAT office should be:

*   the amount of the error

*   the VAT period in which it occurred

*   whether the error was involving input or output tax

*   whether the error is in favour of the business or HM Revenue and Customs.

2.6   VAT: Bad debt relief

You will notice that there is an entry in the pro-forma VAT account for bad debt relief as additional input tax.

When a supplier invoices a customer for an amount including VAT, the supplier must pay the VAT to HM Revenue and Customs. If the customer then fails to pay the debt, the supplier's position is that he has paid output VAT which he has never collected. This is obviously unfair, and the system allows him to recover such amounts.

We saw earlier that **suppliers cannot issue credit notes to recover VAT on bad debts.**

Instead, the business must make an **adjustment through the VAT return.**

The business can reclaim VAT already paid over if:

*   output tax was paid on the original supply

*   six months have elapsed between the date of supply and the date of the VAT return, and

- the debt has been written off as a bad debt in the accounting records.

If the business receives a **repayment of the debt later**, it must make an adjustment to the VAT relief claimed.

The bad debt relief is entered in box 4 of the return along with the VAT on purchases.

Be very careful when computing the VAT on the bad debt. The amount of the bad debt will be VAT inclusive because the amount the debtor owes is the amount that includes VAT. To calculate the VAT you have to multiply the bad debt by 17.5/117.5.

Be careful also that the examiner may try and confuse you by giving you a purchases figure (which also goes into box 4) that is net of VAT – and you calculate the VAT on that by simply multiplying by 17.5/% ie 0.175.

Illustration 1 – Completing the VAT return

A business has made purchases of £237,000 (net of VAT) in the VAT quarter and has written off a bad debt of £750. Calculate the figure that will be entered on the VAT return for the quarter in Box 4.

Solution

	£	£
Purchases (net of VAT)	237,000	
VAT thereon (237,000 × 0.175)		41,475.00
Bad debt	750	
VAT thereon (750 × 17.5/117.5)		111.70
Total VAT for Box 4		41,586.70

3 VAT penalties

3.1 Late notification

If a trader **trades** in **excess of the registration limits** without informing HM Revenue and Customs, a penalty is levied for failing to register by the proper date.

This penalty is a **proportion of the net tax due** from the date registration should have taken place. The proportion percentage varies as follows:

Period of failure to register	Percentage of tax
9 months or less	5%
Over 9 months, but not over 18 months	10%
Over 18 months	15%

A **minimum penalty** of £50 exists. If the trader can show a reasonable excuse for not registering, the penalty may be mitigated.

3.2 Default surcharge

A **default** occurs when a trader submits his VAT return late or submits the return on time but pays the VAT late. On default, HM Revenue and Customs serve a **default liability notice** on the taxpayer which identifies a surcharge period which runs from the date of the notice until the anniversary of the end of the period for which the taxpayer is in default.

If a **second default** occurs in the surcharge period it is further extended until the anniversary of the end of the period to which the new default relates.

If **VAT is paid late in a surcharge period**, a surcharge is payable as follows:

Default involving late payment of VAT in the surcharge period	Surcharge, % of outstanding VAT
1st	2%
2nd	5%
3rd	10%
4th and above	15%

(The minimum charge is £30.)

3.3 Misdeclaration penalties

Making returns which understate the trader's VAT liability incurs a penalty of 15% of the lost tax. Errors of up to £2,000 can be rectified on the usual quarter-end VAT 100 return.

3.4 Default interest

Interest is charged on VAT due on an assessment from HM Revenue and Customs. Interest runs from the date the VAT should have been paid (up to a maximum of three years).

Test your understanding 3

1   Company X is based in an EC Member State, in which the VAT rate is 8%, and sells goods worth £100 to Company Y, a VAT-registered company in the UK. How much VAT, if any, is payable and from whom is it collected?

2   Box 6 on the VAT return is for 'total value of sales and all other outputs excluding any VAT'. Does this include (i) zero-rated and/or (ii) exempt supplies?

3   Under what three conditions can bad debt relief be claimed?

5   Summary

In this final chapter the actual completion of the VAT return was considered. A business should keep a VAT account which summarises all of the VAT from the accounting records and this can be used to complete the first five boxes on the VAT return. The figure for VAT due to or from HM Revenue and Customs on the VAT return should equal the balance on the VAT account.

In order to complete the remaining boxes on the VAT return information will be required from the accounting records of the business, normally in the form of the day books.

Test your understanding answers

Test your understanding 1

Panther

The two basic records needed are the sales day book and purchase day book for the **sales** and **purchases.**

For **cash sales** and **purchases** the cash book should be analysed.

Information about **credit notes received and issued** should be in the purchase returns and sales returns day books.

The **capital goods purchased and sold** will probably be in a separate assets account under plant and machinery unless the company maintains analysed purchase and sales day books which include asset purchases and disposals.

The goods taken for own use should be recorded in the sales day book and the drawings account.

The **bad debt relief** is generally found in the bad and doubtful debts account.

Test your understanding 2

Part (a)

Long Supplies Ltd
VAT account 1 January to 31 March 20X1

	£		£
VAT on purchases	1,422.30	VAT on sales	2,709.98
EC acquisitions	117.08	EC acquisitions	117.08
	1,539.38		2,827.06
Less: credit notes received	163.70	Less: credit notes issued	284.50
Total tax deductible	1,375.68	Total tax payable	2,542.56
		Less: total tax deductible	1,375.68
		Payable to HM Revenue and Customs	1,166.88

KAPLAN PUBLISHING

Part (b)

**Value Added Tax
Return**

For the period
1/1/X1 to 31/3/X1

Long Supplies Ltd
Vale House
Lily Road
Trent
TR5 2KL

Your VAT Office telephone number 0123-4567

For Official Use

Registration number	Period
285 3745 12	01X1

You could be liable to a financial penalty
if your completed return and all the VAT
payable are not received by the due date.

Due date: 30 April 20X1

For Official Use	

Before you fill in this form please read the notes on the back and the VAT Leaflet 'Filling in your VAT return'. Fill in all boxes clearly in ink and write 'none' where necessary. Don't put a dash or leave any box blank. If there are no pence write '00' in the pence column. Do not enter more than one amount in any box.

For official use				
	VAT due in this period on sales and other outputs	1	2,425	48
	VAT due in this period on acquisitions from other EC Member States	2	117	08
	Total VAT due (the sum of boxes 1 and 2)	3	2,542	56
	VAT reclaimed in this period on purchases and other inputs (including acquisitions from the EC)	4	1,375	68
	Net VAT to be paid to Customs or reclaimed by you (Difference between boxes 3 and 4)	5	1,166	88
	Total value of sales and all other outputs excluding any VAT. Include your box 8 figure.	6	15,251	00
	Total value of purchases and all other inputs excluding any VAT. Include your box 9 figure.	7	8,761	00
	Total value of all supplies of goods and related services excluding any VAT to other EC Member States.	8	None	
	Total value of all acquisitions of goods and related services excluding any VAT, from other EC Member States.	9	669	00

If you are enclosing a payment please tick this box.

✓

DECLARATION: You, or someone on your behalf, must sign below.
I .... declare that the information given
(Full name of signatory in BLOCK LETTERS)
above is true and complete.
Signature .... Date   20

A false declaration can result in prosecution.

VAT 100 (full)   PT1 (April 2004)

Workings

Box 1	£
VAT on sales	2,709.98
Less: VAT on credit notes	(284.50)
	2,425.48

Box 4	£
VAT on purchases	1,422.30
EC Member States acquisitions	117.08
	1,539.38
Less: VAT on credit notes	(163.70)
	1,375.68

Box 6	£
Standard-rated sales	15,485.60
Zero-rated sales	1,497.56
	16,983.16
Less: credit notes	
Standard-rated	(1,625.77)
Zero-rated	(106.59)
	15,250.80

Box 7	£
Standard-rated purchases	8,127.45
Zero-rated purchases	980.57
EC acquisitions	669.04
	9,777.06
Less: credit notes	
Standard-rated	(935.47)
Zero-rated	(80.40)
	8,761.19

Test your understanding 3

1   The VAT on transfers between EC Member States is payable at the rate prevalent in the buyer's country and is collected from the buyer. Thus, £17.50 will be payable by Company Y (via Box 2 on the VAT Return) and can be reclaimed (via Box 4).

2   It includes both zero-rated and exempt supplies.

3   Output tax was paid on original supply. There has been at least six months between the supply date and the VAT return date. The debt has been written off as a bad debt in the books.

Legal background

Introduction

You need a basic knowledge of the law surrounding business transactions. In this final chapter we cover the areas of legal knowledge that you require for this syllabus.

1 Nature of a contract

1.1 Introduction

When a business agrees to buy goods or services from a supplier or to sell goods to a customer, then the business is entering into a contract.

A contract is a legally binding agreement. The law of contract is the branch of the civil law which determines whether or not a particular agreement is legally binding, that is enforceable by a court of law.

When you are dealing with customers and suppliers you will be entering into legally binding contracts, therefore it is important that you understand contract law in outline.

1.2 The essential characteristics of a contract

The main requirements if a contract is to be valid are:

*   offer and acceptance, that is, an agreement

*   the intention to create legal relations, that is, the parties must be willing to accept the authority of the law, and to be bound by their contracts

*   consideration, in that both parties must do, or promise to do, something as their side of the contract

*   written formalities must be observed in some situations

A brief outline understanding is required of each of these characteristics so each one will be considered in turn.

2 Offer and acceptance

2.1 Agreement

The first essential of a contract is that there must be an agreement between the parties.

Agreement is usually expressed in the terms of offer and acceptance. It must be shown that an offer was made by one party (the offeror) and accepted by the other party (the offeree) and that legal relations were intended. Therefore:

OFFER + ACCEPTANCE = AGREEMENT

2.2 The offer

An offer is an expression of willingness to contract on certain terms, made with the intention that it shall become binding as soon as it is accepted by the person to whom it is addressed.

(a) An offer may be made to a specific person, to a group of people, or to the world at large.

Example of an offer to the world at large:

- offering coupons on the packets of products to exchange for gifts.

(b) The offer may be conditional, but it must be certain.

Examples of conditions:

- collecting coupons

- while stocks last.

(c) The offer may be express or implied.

Implied offer: boarding a bus is an implied offer to buy a ticket.

(d) The offer must be communicated to the offeree: a person who returns property without knowing that a reward has been offered would not be entitled to the reward.

2.3 Invitation to treat

An offer must be distinguished from an invitation to another party to make an offer himself (referred to as an invitation to treat).

In the case of an offer, the agreement is complete when the offeree agrees unconditionally to the terms of the offer. However, with an invitation to treat it is the person to whom the invitation is directed who may make the offer, which the party issuing the invitation (now the offeree) is free to accept if he wishes to do so.

No agreement (and hence no contract) arises until acceptance is made by the party originating the invitation.

Examples of invitations to treat include:

- notices in shop windows

- advertisements for goods for sale

- mail order 'bargain offers', and

- the display of goods in supermarkets.

Take care that you understand the distinction between an offer and an invitation to treat as this is highly significant in determining whether or not a contract exists.

Due to a printer's error, one of the items in Hairdressing Supplies' equipment catalogue was under-priced. Subsequently a letter was received from a customer ordering one of these items.

(a) Are Hairdressing Supplies obliged to supply the goods at this price? Yes/No

(b) Explain briefly why.

2.4 The acceptance

Acceptance is a final expression of assent to the terms of an offer. Offer and acceptance constitute agreement.

In order to be effective, the acceptance must be:

- made while the offer is still in force, ie before it has been revoked or before it has lapsed

- absolute and unqualified: if the terms of the offer are altered, then there has been a counter-offer

- communicated to the offeror in cases where notification of acceptance is specifically or tacitly required.

Generally, silence does not constitute acceptance.

3 Intention to create legal relations

3.1 Introduction

Even if an accepted offer creates an agreement, it does not automatically make the agreement a contract. If one of the parties wishes the help of the law in enforcing the terms of the agreement against the other party, he must show, amongst other things, that there had been an intention by both parties that the agreement was to create legal relations.

3.2 Social or domestic agreements

There is a presumption in social or domestic agreements that legal relations are not intended.

Agreements between spouses living together are usually assumed to be of a domestic nature only.

3.3 Commercial agreements

In commercial agreements there is a presumption that legal relations are intended, although this can be changed by an 'honourable pledge' clause which expressly states that the agreement is not to be legally binding: if this is the case, the agreement will not be legally enforceable.

As you will be dealing with commercial agreements there will therefore normally be an intention to create legal relations.

4 Consideration

4.1 Introduction

The essence of a contract is that it is an agreed bargain between two parties. We have considered the agreement side of a contract, now we must consider the bargain element.

4.2 What is consideration?

Consideration is quite a complex legal concept but in essence it is the fact that there is value given by both parties to the contract. When your business agrees to sell goods to a customer then your business is promising to deliver the goods and the seller is providing consideration by promising to pay for the goods.

Illustration 1 – Consideration

A sells goods on credit to B and a third party C promises to pay for the goods. If A did not deliver the goods then could B sue A?

Solution

B could not sue A for breach of contract as B has provided no consideration. The promise to pay for the goods came from C.

4.3 Amount of consideration

The legal rule is that consideration must be sufficient but need not be adequate. This means that the consideration must have some value but it need not necessarily be what the goods are worth.

4.4 Past consideration

A further aspect of consideration is that it must not be past. In practical terms this means that if you help a friend for a morning in her shop with no thoughts of payment and a few days later she thanks you and promises to pay you £20 for your time, you cannot sue your friend for the £20 if she then does not pay you. The consideration, the work in the shop, preceded the promise of payment.

5 Formality

5.1 The requirement of formality

The general rule of English law is that contracts can be made quite informally, even verbally in numerous situations, and the form in which a contract is made does not matter and will have no effect upon the validity of the contract.

There are, however, certain exceptions, especially:

- contracts which must be made by deed, and
- contracts which must be in writing.

Where the required formality is not observed, the contract is generally unenforceable or void.

5.2 Contracts made by deed

A contract under deed is a written document which is signed and often sealed. Such contracts are described as 'speciality contracts', all others being simple contracts.

The types of contract which must be made by deed are as follows.

- Contracts where one of the parties provides no consideration (for example a contract to establish a covenant to a charity for a number of years whereby the charity claims the amount paid plus the related income tax). Such contracts are often referred to as 'deeds of gift'.
- Contracts for the transfer of a British registered ship or aeroplane.
- Documentation for the legal conveyance of land or leases of land (for more than three years); therefore for house purchases or sales, the completion documents must be made by deed.

5.3 Contracts which must be in writing

The following simple contracts are required to be wholly in writing otherwise they are invalid and of no legal effect.

- Contracts for the future sale of interests in land:
  - such contracts must be signed; and
  - all terms which the parties have expressly agreed must be included in the document (or be identifiable by reference to some other document).
- Contracts of marine insurance.
- Regulated agreements under the Consumer Credit Act 1974, for example hire purchase contracts.
- Transfers of company shares.

- Bills of exchange, whereby one party (A) instructs another party (B) to pay money to a third party (C) to settle a debt due from A to C (e.g. cheques).

6 Sale of Goods Act

6.1 Introduction

Customers may sometimes return goods and ask for a refund. The customer has certain rights under the Sale of Goods Act.

6.2 Right to a refund

The customer has a legal right to receive a refund only in the following cases:

- The items bought are faulty (e.g. electrical goods which do not work).

- The items bought are not as described (e.g. a tin marked 'peaches' actually contains sardines).

- The items bought are not of satisfactory quality. This means they are not fit for their usual purpose. This may only become obvious once the items have been used for that purpose (e.g. underwear which still contains chemicals used in the manufacturing process and which make the underwear unwearable).

- The items bought are not fit for the particular purpose. This means that the customer must have told the retailer of the specific purpose, or made it clear through his actions (eg the customer wishes to use a particular type of paint to paint the outside of his house).

- The retailer agrees, at the time of the sale, that the goods can be returned, even if they are perfect (this is the policy of Marks and Spencer and certain other retailers).

Note that contracts of sale are between the buyer and the seller, not the buyer and the manufacturer. The customer is entitled to a refund if any of the above conditions apply, regardless of whether a fault (for example) is the responsibility of the manufacturer.

The customer does not, by law, have to produce his receipt to get a refund in the above cases. A retailer cannot insist on a receipt as a proof of purchase. A receipt makes the refund more straightforward and many retailers therefore encourage their customers to keep their receipts. Otherwise the retailer must accept the customer's word that he paid for the goods.

In some cses the customer may change his or her mind about the goods, but the retailer has not agreed a refund in advance. The retailer can choose whether or not to accept the goods and make a refund. Some shops allow their customers to return goods but will only issue a credit note for the value of the goods which the customer can then use to buy something else in the same shop or another branch of the same chain.

This legal knowledge is important background information for Unit 30 which you need to understand in outline although no great detail is required.

Test your understanding 2

1   What are the main requirements for a valid contract?

2   Is an advertisement for goods for sale an offer or an invitation to treat?

3   What is consideration?

---

7   Summary

When dealing with the buying and selling of goods within the business that you work for, you need to be aware that you are taking part in the formation of a legally binding contract. For practical purposes probably the most important area to understand is the concept of offer and acceptance. An offer is made by the offeror to the offeree and it is the responsibility of the offeree to accept within a reasonable time. The acceptance must be unconditional, as if additional terms are introduced then this is deemed to be a counter-offer which rejects the original offer. Care should also be taken to distinguish between an offer and an invitation to treat. If an offer is made then acceptance or rejection is required. If an invitation to treat is made then an offer is required, followed by acceptance or rejection. The other areas of contract law are less important but an outline knowledge is required.

If you are working in a retail environment then it is important to understand the rules from the Sale of Goods Act for the granting of refunds for sales.

Test your understanding answers

Test your understanding 1

(a) No

(b) Offer and acceptance are essential elements of a valid contract.

Goods advertised in catalogues are invitations to treat (i.e. inviting offers). The customer's letter is therefore an offer, which Hairdressing Supplies are not obliged to accept.

Test your understanding 2

1 – Offer and acceptance

   – Intention to create legal relations

   – Consideration

   – Written formalities (in some contracts)

2 Invitation to treat.

3 Consideration is where value is given by both parties to a contract.

Index

Index

KAPLAN PUBLISHING